Pediatric Orthopaedics: Core Knowledge in Orthopaedics

PEDIATRIC ORTHOPAEDICS: CORE KNOWLEDGE IN ORTHOPAEDICS

JOHN P. DORMANS, MD

Chief of Orthopaedic Surgery
The Children's Hospital of Philadelphia
Philadelphia, PA;
Professor of Orthopaedic Surgery
University of Pennsylvania School of Medicine
Philadelphia, PA

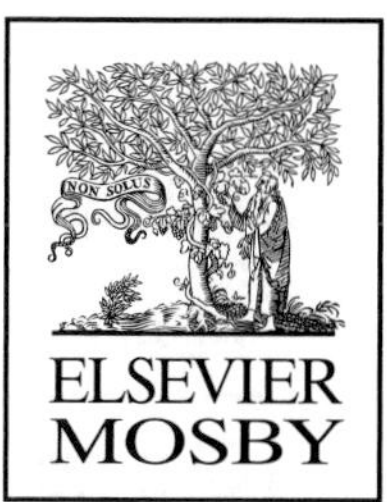

ELSEVIER
MOSBY

ELSEVIER
MOSBY

The Curtis Center
170 S Independence Mall W 300 E
Philadelphia, Pennsylvania 19106

 ISBN 0-323-02590-0

Notice

Orthopaedics is an ever-changing field. Standard safety precautions must be followed, but as new research and clinical experience broaden our knowledge, changes in treatment and drug therapy may become necessary or appropriate. Readers are advised to check the most current product information provided by the manufacturer of each drug to be administered to verify the recommended dose, the method and duration of administration, and contraindications. It is the responsibility of the treating physician, relying on experience and knowledge of the patient, to determine dosages and the best treatment for each individual patient. Neither the Publisher nor the editor assumes any liability for any injury and/or damage to persons or property arising from this publication.

The Publisher

Library of Congress Cataloging-in-Publication Data

Pediatric orthopaedics: core knowledge in orthopaedics/[edited by] John P. Dormans.– 1 st ed.
p. ; cm.
ISBN 0-323-02590-0
1. Pediatric orthopedics. I Dormans, John P.
[DNLM: 1. Musculoskeletal Diseases–Child 2. Orthopedics–methods. 3. Pediatrics–methods. 4. Wounds and Injuries–Child. WS 270 P3711 2005]
RD732.3.C48P4315 2005
618.92'7–dc22

2004057887

Publishing Director: Kim Murphy
Senior Developmental Editor: Anne Snyder
Publishing Services Manager: Joan Sinclair
Production Manager: Mary Stermel
Marketing Manager: Robert Kolton

Printed in the United States of America

Last digit is the print number: 9 8 7 6 5 4 3 2 1

Contributors

Allan C. Beebe,
MD, Orthopaedic Faculty, Department of Orthopaedic Surgery, Children's Hospital, Columbus, OH; Assistant Program Director, Department of Orthopaedic Surgery, Mount Carmel Medical Center, Columbus, OH

Benjamin Chang,
MD, FACS, Plastic Surgeon, The Children's Hospital of Philadelphia; Assistant Professor of Surgery, Division of Plastic Surgery, University of Pennsylvania Medical School, Philadelphia, PA

Lawson A.B. Copley,
MD, Assistant Professor of Orthopaedic Surgery, University of Texas Southwestern, Dallas, TX; Staff Orthopaedic Surgeon, Texas Scottish Rite Hospital for Children, Children's Medical Center of Dallas, Dallas, TX

Randy Q. Cron,
MD, PhD, Attending Physician, Division of Rheumatology, The Children's Hospital of Philadelphia, Philadelphia, PA; Assistant Professor of Pediatrics, University of Pennsylvania, Philadelphia, PA

Richard S. Davidson,
MD, Orthopaedic Surgeon, The Children's Hospital of Philadelphia and Shriners Hospital, Philadelphia, PA; Associate Professor, University of Pennsylvania School of Medicine, Philadelphia, PA

John P. Dormans,
MD, Chief of Orthopaedic Surgery, The Children's Hospital of Philadelphia, Philadelphia, PA; Professor of Orthopaedic Surgery, University of Pennsylvania School of Medicine, Philadelphia, PA

Denis S. Drummond,
MD, Professor Emeritus, University of Pennsylvania School of Medicine, Philadelphia, PA; Chief Emeritus, Orthopaedic Surgery, The Children's Hospital of Philadelphia, Philadelphia, PA

Bülent Erol,
MD, Attending Surgeon, Department of Orthopaedic Surgery, The Hospital of University of Marmara, Marmara University School of Medicine, Istanbul, Turkey

Richard S. Finkel,
MD, Pediatric Neurologist, Director, Neuromuscular Program, Division of Neurology and Neurology Research, The Children's Hospital of Philadelphia, Philadelphia, PA

John M. Flynn,
MD, Attending Surgeon, Division of Orthopaedic Surgery, The Children's Hospital of Philadelphia, Philadelphia, PA; Associate Professor, Department of Orthopaedics, University of Pennsylvania, Philadelphia, PA

Steven L. Frick,
MD, Residency Program Director, Pediatric Orthopaedic Surgery, Carolinas Medical Center, Department of Orthopaedic Surgery, Charlotte, NC

Theodore J. Ganley,
MD, Orthopaedic Surgeon, Division of Orthopaedic Surgery; and Orthopaedic Director, Sports Medicine and Performance Center, The Children's Hospital of Philadelphia, Philadelphia, PA; Assistant Professor of Orthopaedic Surgery, University of Pennsylvania School of Medicine, Philadelphia, PA

†**John R. Gregg,**
MD, Orthopaedic Surgeon, Division of Orthopaedic Surgery, The Children's Hospital of Philadelphia, Philadelphia, PA

Harish S. Hosalkar,
MD, Resident, Orthopaedic Surgery, University of Pennsylvania, Philadelphia, PA

James M. Kerpsack,
MD, The Center for Orthopaedic Surgery and Sports Medicine, Indianapolis, IN

Emily A. Kolze,
Clinical Research Coordinator, Division of Orthopaedic Surgery, The Children's Hospital of Philadelphia, Philadelphia, PA

Scott H. Kozin,
MD, Hand Surgeon, Shriners Hospital for Children, Philadelphia, PA; Associate Professor, Department of Orthopaedic Surgery, Temple University, Philadelphia, PA

James J. McCarthy,
MD, Assistant Professor, Temple University, Philadelphia, PA; Assistant Chief of Staff, Shriners Hospital for Children, Philadelphia, PA

Jennifer E. Millman,
BA, Clinical Research Coordinator, Division of Orthopaedic Surgery, The Children's Hospital of Philadelphia, Philadelphia, PA

Leslie A. Moroz,
BA, Clinical Research Coordinator, Division of Orthopaedic Surgery, The Children's Hospital of Philadelphia, Philadelphia, PA

Kristan A. Pierz,
MD, Surgeon, Department of Orthopaedics, Connecticut Children's Medical Center, Hartford, CT; Assistant Professor of Orthopaedics, University of Connecticut School of Medicine, Hartford, CT

Benjamin D. Roye,
MD, MPH, Attending Surgeon, Division of Pediatric Orthopaedics, Department of Orthopaedic Surgery, Beth Israel Medical Center, New York, NY

Lee S. Segal,
MD, Associate Professor of Orthopaedics and Pediatrics, Chief, Division of Pediatric Orthopaedics, Department of Orthopaedics and Rehabilitation, Milton S. Hershey Medical Center, Pennsylvania State University College of Medicine, Hershey, PA

David A. Spiegel,
MD, Associate Professor of Orthopaedic Surgery, University of Pennsylvania, Philadelphia, PA; Staff Surgeon, The Children's Hospital of Philadelphia, Philadelphia, PA

Paul D. Sponseller,
MD, MBA, Professor of Orthopaedic Surgery, Johns Hopkins University, Baltimore, MD; Chief, Division of Pediatric Orthopaedics, Johns Hopkins Medical Institutions, Baltimore, MD

David M. Wallach,
MD, Orthopaedic Surgeon, the Milton S. Hershey Medical Center, Hershey, PA; Assistant Professor, Orthopaedics and Rehabilitation, Pennsylvania State University

Lawrence Wells,
MD, Assistant Professor of Orthopaedic Surgery, University of Pennsylvania School of Medicine, Philadelphia, PA; Attending Physician, The Children's Hospital of Philadelphia, Philadelphia, PA

†Deceased

Contents

1. **Normal Growth and Development in Pediatric Orthopaedics** 1
Steven L. Frick

2. **Pediatric Musculoskeletal Examination** 15
Allan C. Beebe and James M. Kerpsack

3. **Introduction to Trauma** 36
Paul D. Sponseller

4. **Upper Extremity Injuries** 47
John M. Flynn and Emily A. Kolze

5. **Trauma Related to the Lower Extremity** 85
Lawrence Wells and Jennifer E. Millman

6. **Spine and Pelvis Trauma** 116
Lee S. Segal

7. **Pediatric Sports Medicine** 138
Theodore J. Ganley, Emily A. Kolze, and John R. Gregg

8. **Upper Extremity Disorders** 159
Benjamin Chang and Scott H. Kozin

9. **Pediatric Lower Limb Disorders** 197
David M. Wallach and Richard S. Davidson

10. **Hip Disorders** 224
Bülent Erol and John P. Dormans

11. Spinal Disorders 265
Kristan A. Pierz and John P. Dormans

12. Musculoskeletal Tumors in Children 290
Bülent Erol and John P. Dormans

13. Musculoskeletal Infections 337
Lawson A.B. Copley and John P. Dormans

14. Skeletal Dysplasias 353
Bülent Erol, Leslie A. Moroz, and John P. Dormans

15. Metabolic Disorders of Bone 386
Bülent Erol and John P. Dormans

16. Synovial Disorders 403
Randy Q. Cron and James J. McCarthy

17. Neuromuscular Disorders: Cerebral Palsy 418
David A. Spiegel and John P. Dormans

18. Neuromuscular Disorders of Infancy and Childhood and Arthrogryposis 454
Harish S. Hosalkar, Leslie A. Moroz, Denis S. Drummond, and Richard S. Finkel

19. Neuromuscular Disorders: Myelomeningocele 483
Benjamin D. Roye

Index 505

Acknowledgments

A lot of people must be acknowledged whenever you embark on as grandiose a project as creating a new book. Many people deserve credit for this book. These special people can be grouped into four categories: chapter authors, reviewers, *Core Knowledge in Orthopaedics (CKO)*/Elsevier staff, and colleagues.

Chapter Authors: I am indebted to the many friends and colleagues who took time away from their busy lives to contribute to this book. I know this project took valuable time away from other projects and your families; I appreciate the time and effort. Many of the chapter authors are past fellows or trainees at The Children's Hospital of Philadelphia (CHOP) or the University of Pennsylvania. It is very rewarding to see you doing so well in your academic careers.

Reviewers: Leslie Moroz has been a valuable organizer and helper with this project, and has kept my research, academic affairs, and the papers moving forward while I was preoccupied with the book. Additional thanks go to Bea Chestnut, Catherine O'Shea, and Jennifer Millman in CHOP Orthopaedics.

CKO/Elsevier staff: To Anne Snyder, Senior Developmental Editor; Mary Stermel, Production Manager; Anne Williams, Production Editor; and the many others at Elsevier, thank you. You have been a terrific team to work with.

Colleagues: My colleagues in pediatric orthopaedic surgery at CHOP and the University of Pennsylvania also deserve credit. These colleagues who put up with my preoccupation with "The Book" and other projects—Denis Drummond, Richard Davidson, Bong Lee, Malcolm Ecker, Jack Flynn, Ted Ganley, David Horn, Larry Wells, Angela Smith, Ben Chang, and Roger Cornwall—are in my opinion, the greatest group of pediatric orthopaedic surgeons assembled in one Division. I would like to acknowledge the lifetime of contributions to our hospital and our specialty by John Gregg, who passed away this past year—John will be missed and remembered by each of us. And finally, thanks to all of my current and past fellows, who have provided me with endless educational experiences and who have created the vitality necessary for learning. *You* make *us* better surgeons. Each of you is very special to me. I am biased, but I believe that there is no better place to practice the art and science of pediatric orthopaedic surgery.

John P. Dormans, M.D.
Chief of Orthopaedic Surgery
The Children's Hospital of Philadelphia
Professor of Orthopaedic Surgery
University of Pennsylvania
School of Medicine

Preface

The overall *Core Knowledge in Orthopaedics (CKO)* series is an attempt to concisely summarize a "core knowledge" of orthopaedics for a broad group of medical and surgical specialists. *CKO* is an up-to-date text for understanding the common pediatric orthopaedic conditions faced by providers of musculoskeletal care. We have attempted to assemble the essential fund of pediatric orthopaedic knowledge and choose topics that could be considered a "curriculum" or "refresher course" for students, nurse practitioners, resident physicians, primary care providers, and other specialists. We have included the most common pediatric orthopaedic conditions that physicians and surgeons caring for infants, children, and adolescents need to know and understand. The book includes practical information and illustrations demonstrating the technique of appropriate and proper physical examination, major points for each condition, imaging pearls, and up-to-date treatment recommendations.

We intended to have fun writing this book and to make it fun to read. At the same time, we strove to cover the material well enough that this would be the only book you'd need to read to get a thorough introduction to pediatric orthopaedic surgery—the "core knowledge." We believe that if you have the perseverance to read this book from cover to cover, you'll have the foundation for being better able to care for these children when they present to you for evaluation and care. Try to stick with it, and you will find the material rewarding in your practice, be it primary care, pediatrics, radiology, surgery, orthopaedic surgery, pediatric orthopaedic surgery, and so on. We hope you enjoy and benefit from *Pediatric Orthopaedics: Core Knowledge in Orthopaedics.*

John P. Dormans, M.D.
Chief of Orthopaedic Surgery
The Children's Hospital of Philadelphia
Professor of Orthopaedic Surgery
University of Pennsylvania
School of Medicine

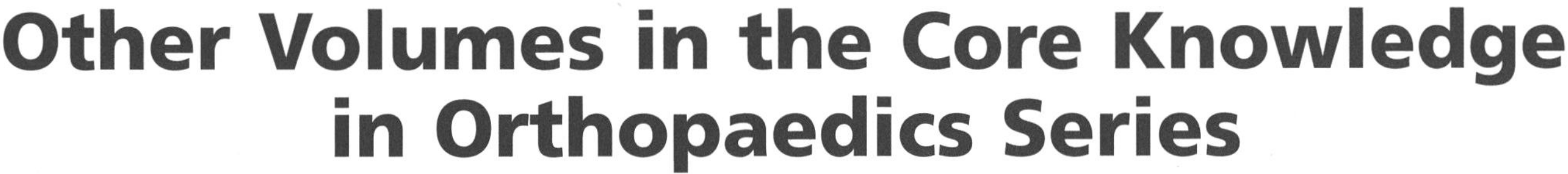

Other Volumes in the Core Knowledge in Orthopaedics Series

Spine

Hand and Upper Extremity

Sports Medicine

Trauma

Adult Reconstruction and Arthroplasty

Foot and Ankle

Normal Growth and Development in Pediatric Orthopaedics

Steven L. Frick

MD, Residency Program Director, Pediatric Orthopaedic Surgery, Carolinas Medical Center, Department of Orthopaedic Surgery, Charlotte, NC

Introduction

Defining normal in pediatric orthopaedics has many potential ramifications. Parents may desire their children to be not "just normal" but supranormal or exceptional. In statistical terms, defining normal is straight-forward—it is the 95% of a population that falls within two standard deviations of the mean from any given measurement. Mercer Rang has pointed out, however, that statistically normal is not the same as ideal or desirable[1] (Figure 1–1). It has also been noted that by statistical definition 1 of 33 children would be declared abnormal.[2]

The challenge for the orthopaedic surgeon caring for children is to understand which deviations from normal are likely to result in impairment of function, progressive deformity, or premature degeneration and pain. The pediatric orthopaedic surgeon may also be asked to alter conditions that are primarily cosmetic, and in these situations a careful risk–benefit analysis, and an honest and complete discussion with the parents, is essential. Many of these deviations or conditions, although not desirable in the eyes of parents, will resolve with time or will have no adverse effect on function.

Most studies of normal growth, and of the natural history of many orthopaedic disorders, have been done on small and often homogenous populations and then generalized to larger, diverse groups. The information available to help orthopaedic surgeons make decisions is thus flawed and incomplete and is likely always to be so. The art of medicine involves making decisions in the face of such uncertainties. Physicians need to recognize the limitations of the knowledge base and, given the potential for individual variations from "normal" patterns, to understand that it is often most helpful to follow each patient at regular intervals and to document the patient's own growth pattern (Box 1–1).

Terminology to Describe Deviations from Normal

- *Congenital*—An anomaly that is apparent at birth
- *Developmental*—A deviation that occurs over time; one that may not be present or apparent at birth
- *Malformation*—A structure that is wrongly built; failure of embryologic development or differentiation resulting in abnormal or missing structures
- *Dysplasia*—A tissue that is abnormal or wrongly constructed; abnormal development resulting in abnormal anatomy
- *Disruption*—A structure undergoing normal development that stops developing or is destroyed or removed
- *Deformation*—A normally formed structure that is pushed out of shape by mechanical forces
- *Deformity*—A body part altered in shape from normal, outside the normal range

When considering birth defects or congenital anomalies, it is convenient to group them into two categories:

1. *Packaging problems*—Deformations caused by mechanical factors, usually from the effects of intrauterine molding. These will usually grow straight and resolve with time.
2. *Production problems*—Abnormalities caused by malformation, dysplasia, or disruption. These will not spontaneously resolve.

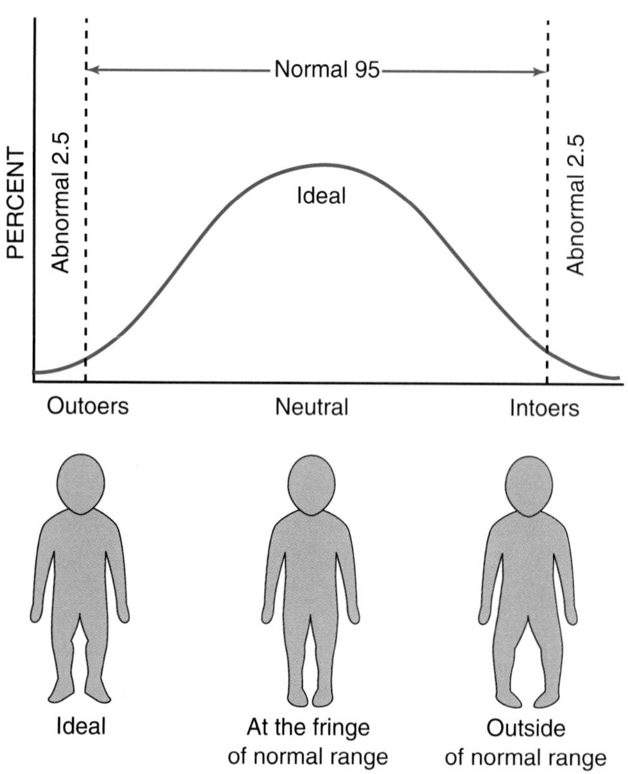

Figure 1–1: Being statistically normal is not the same as being desirable or ideal, and parents may seek treatment for conditions within the range of normal. **From Wenger DR, Rang M (1993) The Art and Practice of Children's Orthopaedics. New York: Raven Press, Figure 1–2.**

Growth problems can be characterized as follows:

- Congenital
- Acquired
- Excessive—Too much
- Recessive—Too little
- Generalized—Symmetric
- Localized—Asymmetric

Introduction to Concepts

- Understanding normal and abnormal growth, particularly as they relate to specific anatomical regions, is critically important for the orthopaedic surgeon caring for children. Consideration of growth and development is what differentiates pediatric from adult orthopaedics.
- When confronted with orthopaedic problems in children, the physician must always consider how growth will be affected and whether growth is likely to improve or worsen the clinical problem. Surgical and nonsurgical treatment strategies should be designed to preserve or restore normal growth potential.

Box 1–1 Origin of the Profession

In 1741, Nicholas Andry, a Parisian pediatrician, wrote the book founding orthopaedics. He was 83 years old at the time. The title of the book was formed from two Greek words.

1. *Orthos,* meaning straight or free from deformity
2. *Paedis,* meaning child

The subtitle was *The Art of Correcting and Preventing Deformities.* This is still a good description of what pediatric orthopaedic surgeons strive to do today.[1]

The symbol of orthopaedics was taken from Andry's book and is a crooked tree bound to an upright stake. Deformed children, like this crooked tree, can be helped to grow straight by the application of appropriate forces.[23]

Orthopaedics has grown into the specialty of medicine that diagnoses and treats musculoskeletal disorders in children and adults. This involves injuries, diseases, malformations, and disorders of the body's bones, joints, ligaments, muscles, and tendons. Consideration of growth is the main factor differentiating pediatric from adult orthopaedics.

- Growth potential and time are related and must be considered together. Time can be an ally or an enemy depending on whether normal growth potential is present. If it is, then growth will frequently improve deformity (e.g., remodeling of an angular deformity after a fracture). If normal growth potential is not present, however, deformity will often increase with further growth (e.g., physeal bar or scoliosis).
- Growth is not constant (Figure 1–2) and is subject to many variables (e.g., genetics, nutrition, overall health, endocrine status, mechanical forces [Box 1–2], and physiological age). The velocity of growth is most rapid in the first few years; thus, there is greater opportunity to alter bone growth patterns in younger children.
- Growth is known to vary by anatomical region and even between two bones in the same region (e.g., tibia and fibula in the leg).
- It is preferable, given individual variations in the rate and timing of growth, to follow patients at regular intervals and make measurements to develop a trend of progression or resolution of discrepancies or deformities.

Embryology[3]

- Two periods of embryogenesis:
  1. Embryonic—Fertilization to 8 weeks of gestation
  2. Fetal—8 weeks to birth
- Growth does not start at birth but in the first trimester.
- By 8 weeks of gestation, the organism's shape is fully formed, and tissue and organ differentiation is complete. The remainder of embryogenesis involves growth and maturation.

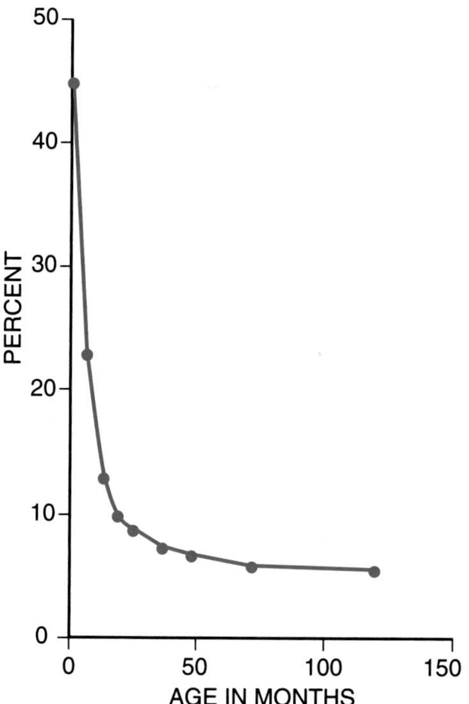

Figure 1–2: Growth velocity decelerates significantly early in childhood and then levels off by 50 months. **From Wenger DR, Rang M (1993) The Art and Practice of Children's Orthopaedics. New York: Raven Press, Figure 2–16.**

Clinical Significance of Embryology

- Birth defects occur in 6% of all births.
- Among newborns, 3% have significant structural abnormalities.
- Of infant deaths, 20% are related to congenital anomalies.
- Limb deficiencies occur in 3-8 per 1000 births; 50% are associated with other malformations.

Box 1–2 Mechanical Influences on Growth

The application of forces to the growing skeleton can improve or worsen deformities in children.

Wolff's Law

The direct translation of Wolff's law of bone remodeling is difficult to understand.[1] It can be paraphrased in different ways:

1. Bone alters its shape in response to the stresses placed on it.
2. Bone is laid where it is needed.
3. Bone is added to the compression side (concavity) and subtracted from the tension side (convexity) of long bones.
4. Bone responds to the stresses placed upon it in mathematically predictable ways, changing internal architecture and external form.

Hueter-Volkmann's Law

Excessive compression inhibits physeal growth (e.g., medial proximal tibia in infantile tibia vara), and tension or distraction across the physis accelerates growth.[1]

- Defective vertebral formation or segmentation can lead to scoliosis, kyphosis, or both.
- Failure of neural tube closure is believed to cause myelomeningocele. Folate supplementation appears to decrease the risk of neural tube defects (mechanism unknown).
- Rests of notochordal cells in cervical and sacral regions can result in the development of chordomas later in life.
- Many types of skeletal dysplasias exist—the primary abnormality may be in the epiphysis, physis, metaphysis, diaphysis, or spine. Studying these abnormalities improves our understanding of normal development, and in many types of skeletal dysplasias specific genetic abnormalities have been identified.

Control of Development

In this active area of research, studies have revealed a remarkable conservation across species of genes and gene products that regulate development, including the following:

- Homeobox (Hox) genes convey body plan or position information.
- Sonic hedgehog proteins (Shh) and genes are involved in limb development.
- Retinoic acid regulates cells that produce shh; the Hox gene is an intermediate.
- Shh and Hox genes are involved regulating the expression of bone morphogenetic proteins.

Axial Skeleton

- The axial skeleton is composed of the skull, vertebrae, ribs, and sternum.
- It is derived from sclerotome of somites.
- The notochord is the organizing structure of the axial skeleton.
  - Appears at 15 days of gestation
  - A rod of cells stretching along the cranial–caudal axis of embryo
- Somites (paired mesodermal condensations) appear on either side of notochord between 19 and 32 days of gestation.
- The neural tube closes in a cranial-to-caudal direction.
- Normally by 28 days, the neural tube is closed, all somites are present, and the anlage of the vertebrae and intervertebral disks are present.

Appendicular Skeleton

- The appendicular skeleton is composed of the pectoral and pelvic girdles and the long and short bones of limbs.
- Limb bud appears at 4 weeks.
- Soon after forming, the surface ectoderm thickens to form the apical ectodermal ridge that guides subsequent limb development.
- By the eighth week of gestation, tissue differentiation is largely complete.

Apical Ectodermal Ridge

- The apical ectodermal ridge is needed for sustained outgrowth of the limb bud.
- It is responsible for proximal-to-distal positional information.
- Hox genes seem to control mass and subsequent local growth of condensing mesenchyme.
- Local growth factors may also be signaling molecules to direct a pattern along the dorsoventral axis.

Limb Rotational Alignment

- Embryonic period—All four limbs have parallel axes.
- Preaxial borders (thumb and hallux) are cephalad, and postaxial borders are caudad.
- The radius–tibia and ulna–fibula are homologous.
- During the fetal period, limb rotation occurs around the axes of the long finger and the second toe.
- The upper limb rotates 90 degrees externally, and the lower limb rotates 90 degrees internally.

Articular Joint Development

- Begins in the sixth week
- A three-step process:
  1. Segmentation of the chondrogenic core
  2. Cavitation by apoptosis
  3. Development of intra-articular structures

Bone Formation or Ossification

Endochondral

- Mesenchymal cells condense, undergo chondrogenesis, and form cartilage.
- Cartilage matures and hypertrophies.
- Cartilage calcifies or is mineralized.
- Vascular invasion occurs and calcified cartilage is replaced by bone.
- Most bones of the appendicular and axial skeleton are formed this way.

Intramembraneous

- Direct differentiation of mesenchymal cells into osteoblasts
- No cartilage precursor or model; no intermediate stage
- Flat bones of the skull and clavicle are formed this way

Origin of the Growth Plate

- Apparent by light microscopy at the end of the embryonic and the beginning of the fetal period
- Chondrocytes in the midshaft of long bone anlagen hypertrophy and elicit vascular invasion
- Form primary centers of ossification in the middle of the bone
- Growth from primary ossification centers lengthens bones

Secondary Centers of Ossification

- Secondary centers appear in chondroepiphysis.
- A few form prenatally, but most appear postnatally (Box 1–3).
- Physis becomes plate-like between the bone of the secondary ossification center (the epiphysis) and the metaphysic.
- Physeal cartilage directs the formation of bone throughout growth.

Anatomy of the Growing Skeletal System[4-7]

Skeleton

- The skeleton is composed of two tissues—cartilage and bone.
- Three basic cell types are involved in skeletal construction and remodeling:
  1. Chondrocytes
  2. Osteoblasts
  3. Osteoclasts

Skeletal Functions

- Controls rate and extent of longitudinal growth
- Provides lever arms and insertion sites for muscles to move joints

Box 1–3 Timing of the Appearance of Ossification Centers: Pearls

The following ossification centers are typically present at birth:

- Distal femur
- Proximal tibia (within 2 months)
- Calcaneus
- Talus

The proximal femoral epiphysis usually begins to ossify between 4 and 6 months after birth.

The ossification centers about the elbow ossify according to the eponym CRITOE:

- C—Capitellum
- R—Radial head
- I—Internal or medial epicondyle
- T—Trochlea
- O—Olecranon
- E—External or lateral epicondyle

If you estimate that the capitellum ossifies around 1 year and then add 2 years for each successive ossification center, the order is reasonably accurate.

The medial clavicular ossification center is the last to (appear around 17 years) and is the last to fuse (around 25 years).

From Gross R. The Pediatric Orthopaedic Society of North America Core Curriculum, http://www.posna.org.

- Protects vital organs
- Maintains bone mass and mineral homeostasis

Anatomy of Long Bones

- Physis—The growth plate, one located on each end of the bone
- Diaphysis—The shaft, central part of long bones
- Metaphysis—The bone adjacent to the physis on the side away from the joint
- Epiphysis—The secondary ossification center; the bone with physis on one side and articular cartilage of one end of a long bone (joint) on the other

The growth plate, or epiphyseal plate or physis, is the growth organ of the skeleton. Physeal anatomy, potential for growth, and biomechanical behavior or responsiveness varies by location in the skeleton.

Physis

- Basic mechanism of endochondral ossification
- Usually perpendicular to the long axis of bone
- Responsible for the enlargement of all components of the axial and appendicular skeleton
- Cellular zones well defined at birth—growth, cartilage formation, and cartilage transformation (Figure 1–3)

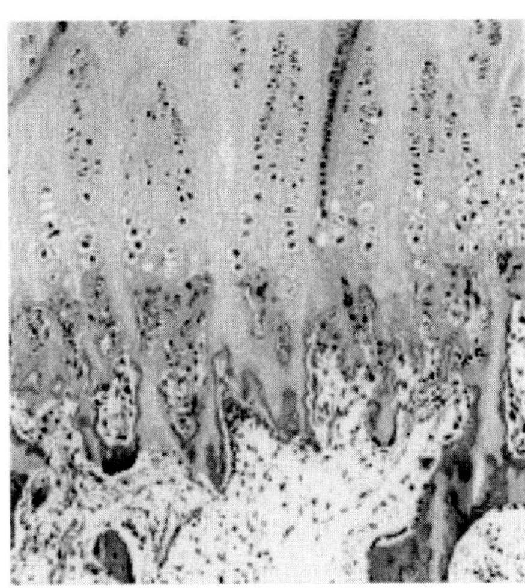

Figure 1–3: The zones of the growth plate have been well described and consist of layers of chondrocytes that proliferate and then hypertrophy before undergoing apoptosis, mineralization, and ossification. **From Ballock RT, O'Keefe RJ. (2003) The biology of the growth plate. J Bone Joint Surg 85A: Figure 1,** ***A*****.**

Growth Zone

- Cellular addition and mitosis
- Resting cells intimately associated with epiphyseal blood vessels
- Active cell division (primarily longitudinal)
- Cell column formation

Cartilage Formation Zone

- Increasing extracellular matrix formation
- Chondrocytes hypertrophy
- Calcification of matrix

Cartilage Transformation Zone

- Vascular invasion of calcified cartilage by metaphyseal blood vessels
- Provides cellular components (osteoblasts or osteoclasts) for initial bone formation on the calcified cartilage precursor

Zone of Ranvier

- Groove bordered by outer fibrous periosteum, metaphyseal cortex, and inner epiphyseal and physeal cartilage
- Responsible for transverse growth of physis

Perichondral Fibrous Ring of LaCroix

- Band of fibrous tissue that merges with periosteum
- Provides mechanical support in response to loads on the physis

Lappet Formation

- Zone of Ranvier turns from planar orientation toward metaphysis
- Lappet—A fold or flap
- Resulting circumferential overlap of the zone of Ranvier with physis–metaphysis
- Provides stability to physeal–metaphyseal interface
- Overlap amount may vary considerably by anatomical region and individual (some believe abnormal lappets may predispose patients to slipped capital femoral epiphysis)

Apophysis

- Simplistically a physis that is primarily exposed to tensile (rather than compressive) forces by tendon insertions
- Histologically different
- Fibrocartilage in the zone of hypertrophy
- Ongoing membranous and endochondral ossification
- Examples—Tibial tubercle and olecranon; not greater trochanter (compression by vastus lateralis or external rotators)

Bipolar Physes

- Example—Triradiate cartilage
- Unique confluence of three primary ossification centers expanding toward each other
- Allows acetabulum to grow spherically with an enlarging femoral head

Spherical Physes

- Located in carpal and tarsal bones
- Progressive centrifugal expansion

- Secondary physes in long bones, but they do not contribute to longitudinal growth
- Gradually grow to assume the shape of epiphysis, carpal bone, or tarsal bone

Periosteum

- Tissue covering the outside of the long bones
- Thicker in children and more osteogenic than in adults
- Contributes to growth in the width of bones
- Considered a tether connecting the two physes of long bones—disruption of the periosteal tether by injury or surgery can lead to localized increased growth (e.g., progressive valgus overgrowth of the proximal tibia after nondisplaced fractures)
- Useful in the reduction of displaced children's fractures because the periosteum on the concavity is typically intact and can be used as a hinge for reduction

How Do Bones Grow?[4-7]

The physis or growth plate is the organ of bone growth, primarily in length but also contributing to growth in diameter or width.

- Paired human limbs reach the same adult length through tight regulation of longitudinal growth of the skeleton
- Regulated by the interaction of systemic hormones and locally produced peptide growth factors, resulting in altered gene expression in growth plate chondrocytes
- Leads to changes in chondrocyte size, the production of extracellular matrix, secreted enzymes and growth factors, and the expression of cell surface receptors
- Results in the calcification of matrix, chondrocyte apoptosis, vascular invasion, and endochondral bone formation

Vascular Invasion

- Pivotal event in endochondral ossification
- Controlled by vascular endothelial growth factor
- Physis is essentially avascular—oxygen and nutrients reach it by diffusion
- Metaphyseal vessels—longitudinal ascending and descending capillaries

Life Cycle of Growth Plate Chondrocytes

- Proliferation
- Maturation
- Hypertrophy
- Mineralization
- Ossification

Growth Plate Zones

The following growth plate zones are shown in Figure 1–3:

- Resting zone
- Proliferative zone
- Zone of hypertrophy
- Zone of provisional calcification

Growth of Long Bones

- Long bones grow in length only from the physes at their ends.
- The rate of growth and the extent of contribution to eventual overall length of proximal and distal physes are different.
- Growth occurs by two mechanisms—cell division and cell hypertrophy.

Parameters Influencing Rate of Growth

1. Growth fraction (percentage of proliferating cells)
2. Cell cycling time
3. Degree of hypertrophy

Unanswered Questions about Growth

- How is growth regulated so that different growth plates grow at different rates at the same time?
- How does the growth rate of a specific physis increase and decrease from birth to skeletal maturity?

Growth Plate Regulation

- Programmed cartilage development or growth, endocrine or local factors, and physical forces
- Autocrine or paracrine regulation—physeal cells self-regulate and regulate neighboring cells
- The size of the proliferation zone and variations in cell cycles control proliferation activity of individual growth plates

Parathyroid Hormone-Related Peptide

- Regulates the conversion of chondrocytes in physis from a small cell to a hypertrophic cell phenotype
- Controls the transition between chondrocyte proliferation and differentiation
- The primary regulator of cell proliferation in the growth plate is the parathyroid hormone-related peptide (PTH-rP) → the Indian hedgehog (Ihh) and transforming growth factor beta (TGF-β) feedback loop; insulin-like growth factor 1 and fibroblast growth factor also are involved

Cell Proliferation

- Estimated eight new cells per day; varies with age
- Regulated by PTH-rP (also by Ihh and TGF-β)
- Controls the rate at which growth plate cells leave the proliferative zone and irreversibly commit to becoming terminally differentiated hypertrophic cells

Chondrocyte Hypertrophy

- Chondrocyte hypertrophy is essential for longitudinal growth.

- There is a five- to tenfold increase in intracellular volume, with an increase in the number of intracellular organelles—not just passive swelling.
- Chondrocyte height increases—44 to 59% of long bone growth (the remainder is from proliferation and matrix synthesis).
- Different rates of growth in different bones appear to be related to differences in the amount of chondrocyte hypertrophy (size, not number), such as femur versus radius.
- Hypertrophic chondrocytes prepare the extracellular matrix for calcification (high levels of alkaline phosphatase and type X collagen).
- Bone morphogenetic proteins and their receptors appear to be responsible for the maturation of chondrocytes.
- Autocrine signaling loops in the growth plate mediate hypertrophy.

Collagens in the Growth Plate

- Primarily type II
- Type IX—Covalently linked to type II; may mediate interactions between type II and the extracellular matrix
- Type X—In hypertrophic zone only; thought to have a role in matrix mineralization

Skeletal Maturity

- Such maturity is reached when growth ceases as the physes in the body undergo physiological epiphysiodesis and fusion occurs from the epiphysis to the metaphysic.
- This process appears to be related to and possibly controlled by estrogen levels in both males and females.

Physiological Epiphysiodesis

- Occurs in females earlier than in males
- Begins with ossified bridge formation from the epiphyseal ossification center to metaphysis
- Cartilaginous physis replaced by trabecular bone
- Often leaves a residual plate of bone (physeal ghost or scar)

Physeal Closure

- Decreased rate of longitudinal growth
- Decreased proliferation of chondrocytes
- Structural changes in physis—Decreased width and length of the proliferative and hypertrophic zones; decreased cell size in the hypertrophic zone
- Growth plate resorbed or replaced → fusion of epiphysis to metaphysis

Growth Slowdown Lines

- May also be called *Harris* or *Park lines* (Figure 1–4)
- Reflect alterations in the rate of longitudinal growth from physis
- Transversely oriented trabecular bands of increased radiodensity within metaphysis
- Thickened, transversely connected trabecular networks with typical, longitudinally oriented trabecular bone on either side
- Appear after a temporary slowdown of rapid longitudinal bone formation
- Parallels contours of physis after the resumption of normal growth
- If not parallel to physis, indicates the persistent growth slowdown of part of physis or growth acceleration
- Helpful after physeal injury to identify localized area of physeal damage (the line will "point" to the bar, see Figure 1–4)

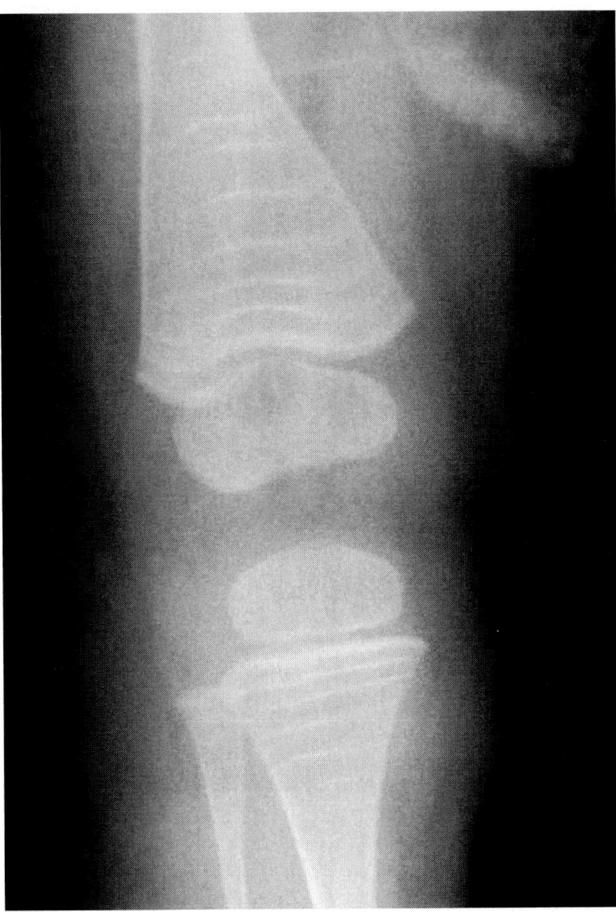

A

Figure 1–4: Growth slowdown lines appear after trauma or other stresses to the body and signal a temporary slowing of growth followed by resumption of growth. When normal growth resumes, the line of increased radiodensity will parallel the physis (A, an example of parallel lines after each pamidronate treatment in a child with osteogenesis imperfecta), but in situations with abnormal growth, the slowdown line will not parallel the growth plate. This can be helpful in identifying physeal bars after trauma because the slowdown line will be angled and will "point" to the bar (B).

Continued

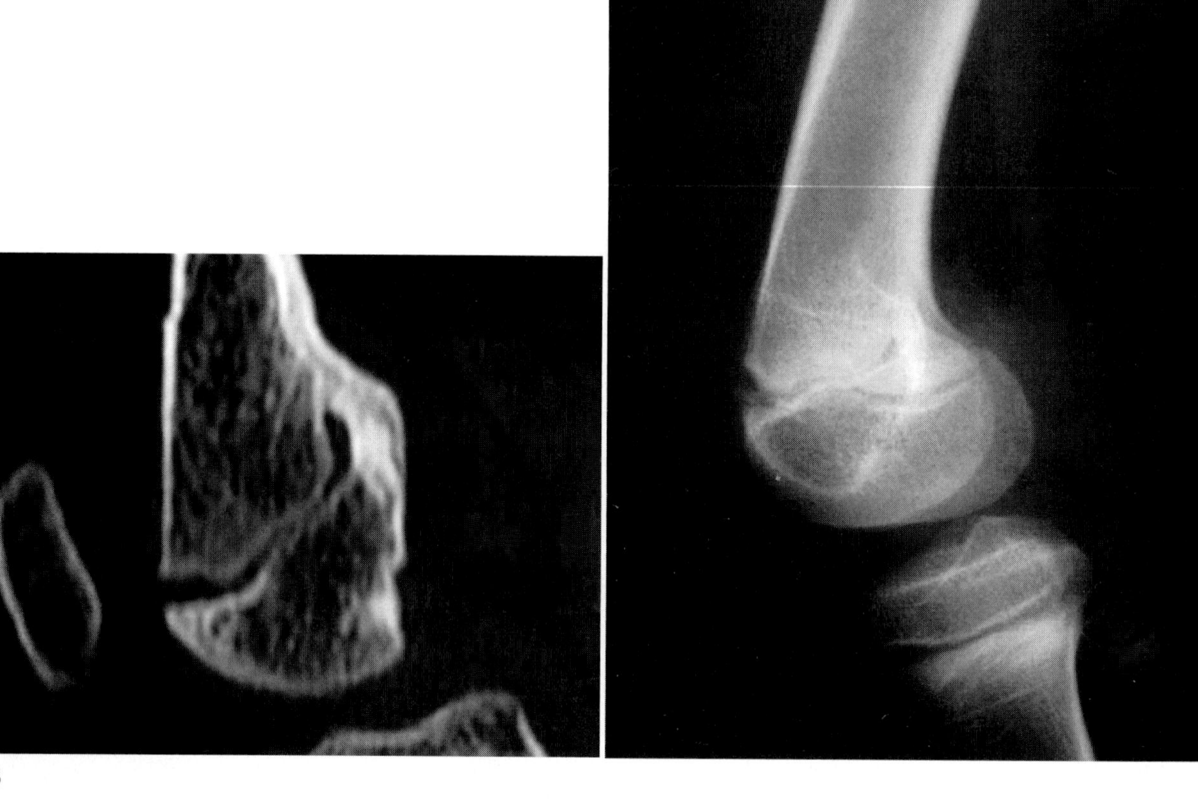

B

Figure 1–4, cont'd.

Basic Terminology and Concepts Important to Skeletal Growth

- *Chondrogenesis*—Growth and development of chondrocytes and cartilage tissue
- *Growth plate chondrocytes*
  - Cartilage cells that produce a highly specialized extracellular matrix
  - Extracellular matrix function promotes the calcification of cartilage
  - Serves as a template for bone formation by osteoblasts
- *Matrix vesicles*
  - Produced by the budding of chondrocyte plasma membranes
  - Serve as nidus for calcification, typically between columns of hypertrophic chondrocytes
  - Contain alkaline phosphatase and matrix metalloproteases
  - The initial site of mineralization in the hypertrophic zone
  - Critical for the calcification of the extracellular matrix
  - Calcification occurs between and not within chondrocyte columns
- *Matrix metalloproteases*
  - Involved in the catabolism and turnover of the cartilage matrix
  - Cleave type II collagen
  - Activate TGF-β
  - Critical for angiogenesis
  - Necessary for normal calcification and bone formation
- *Alkaline phosphatase*
  - Increases the concentration of phosphate ions necessary for calcification
  - Involved in pyrophosphate hydrolysis, which stimulates the mineralization of matrix
  - Deficient in hypophosphatasia, leading to poorly mineralized bone and widened physes
- *Apoptosis*
  - Programmed cell death (physiologic) necessary for homeostasis and normal development
  - Terminally differentiated chondrocytes in physes undergo apoptosis
  - Cell death → active and regulated, not a passive process

- Induced by capsases (enzymes)
- Radiation and glucocorticoids—Increased rate apoptosis
- Phosphate levels may trigger fully differentiated cells to begin apoptosis
- Morphology—Condensed nuclear chromatin, cell shrinkage, and plasma membrane blebbing

- *Vascular endothelial growth factor*
  - Targets vascular endothelial cells
  - Stimulates their proliferation and the formation of blood vessels
  - Expressed by hypertrophic chondrocytes
  - Vascularity brings chondroclasts and osteoclasts to calcified cartilage
- *Aggrecan*
  - Principal proteoglycan molecule in the cartilage matrix
  - Provides osmotic properties necessary to withstand compressive loads
- *Integrins*
  - Cell surface receptors
  - Transduce extracellular forces leading to changes in the cytoskeleton

Basic Growth Considerations[8]

- Standing height equals sitting height (trunk) plus subischial height (lower limbs).
- Abnormal stature may be assessed as proportionate or disproportionate by comparing the ratio of sitting height (pelvis/trunk/head) with subischial limb length.
- Arm span is normally almost equal to standing height.
- Body proportions change significantly during growth. The head is disproportionately large at birth, with a ratio of head height to total height of 1:4. At skeletal maturity, the ratio is 1:7.5 (Figure 1–5).
- Lower limbs account for about 15% of height at birth and 30% at skeletal maturity.
- At birth, the average child is about 50 to 54 cm long (30% of final height); by skeletal maturity, the child will have grown to about 175 cm, more than three times the length of a baby.
- The rate of height and growth increase is not constant, with an initially high rate of growth (0-2 years), a slowing of the rate for a few years, and a quiescent period before the adolescent growth spurt. Standardized charts are available to plot normal growth in height and weight.
- The average 2-year-old has reached about half of his or her adult height.
- By age 5, birth height has doubled and the child is at 60% of final height.
- From age 5 to 10—with the deceleration of growth—height increases about 5.5 cm per year. The child is 80% of final height at 9 years.
- Puberty—The beginning is best characterized by the acceleration in the velocity of growth: age 11 for girls and age 13 for boys. There are four main characteristics of puberty
  1. A dramatic increase in stature
  2. Change in the proportions of the upper and lower body segments
  3. Change in overall morphology (e.g., shoulder and pelvic width and fat distribution)
  4. Development of sexual characteristics
- During puberty, standing height increases by approximately 1 cm per month. The increase in height is derived more from growth of the trunk than growth of the lower limbs.
- Puberty in girls—Menarche occurs about 2 years after breast budding, and final height usually achieved 2.5-3

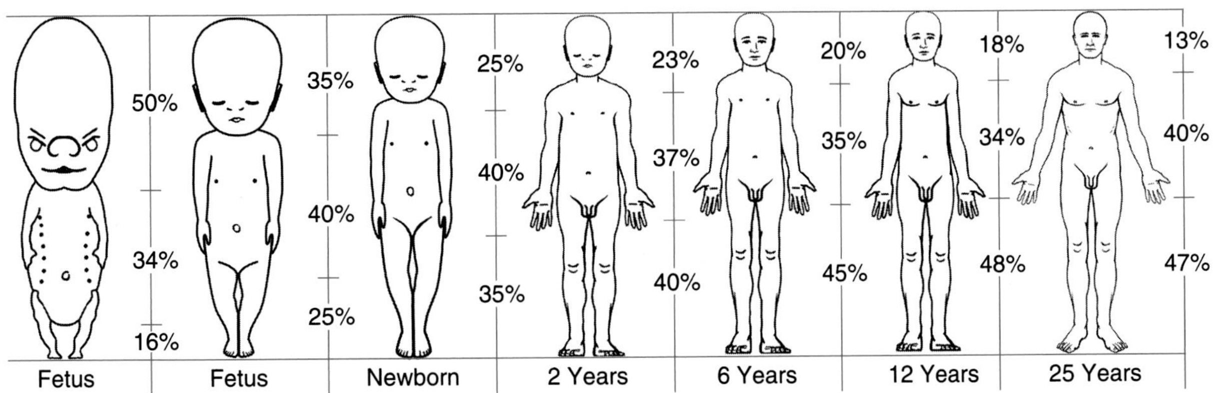

Figure 1–5: Body proportions change significantly with growth; in particular, note that the head is proportionately large in early childhood. **From Dimeglio A (2001) Growth in pediatric orthopaedics. In: Lovell & Winter's Pediatric Orthopaedics, 5th edition (Morrissy R, Weinstein S, eds). Philadelphia: Lippincott-William & Wilkins Publishers, Figure 2–4.**

years after menarche. After menarche, girls typically will gain 3-5 cm.
- Weight gain also is not constant—the average boy weighs 10 kg at age 1, 20 kg at age 5, 30 kg at age 10, and 60 kg at age 17. These estimates are from studies decades ago, and newer studies may show that children now are heavier.
- Weight doubles between 10 and 17 years.
- Body mass index = weight (kg)/height (m^2): 20-25 is normal, 25-30 shows moderate obesity, 30-40 indicates major obesity, and more than 40 is morbid obesity
- Bone age or physiological age is more important than chronological age in determining future growth. Unfortunately, accurate determination of bone age can be difficult. Commonly employed methods include using wrist or hand radiographs and the Greulich and Pyle atlas and staging secondary sexual development using the Tanner and Whitehouse method.

Pearls about Growth by Anatomical Region

Spine Growth[1,8-10]

- Sitting height equals 60% spine, 20% pelvis, and 20% head.
- Spinal height triples from birth to adulthood.
- Space available for the spinal cord reaches adult volume by age 5.
- Curve progression in idiopathic scoliosis is related to growth. Maximal curve progression is associated with the adolescent growth peak, with a marked reduction in progression after growth has stopped. Chronological age, Risser sign, and menarcheal age are historical markers used to assess growth potential. Peak height velocity has been recently noted to be helpful.
- Menarche is typically preceded by a growth spurt, and on average, growth continues for 2-3 years after menarche.
- The Risser sign (the degree of ossification of the iliac apophysis) is commonly used in scoliosis to measure skeletal maturation and is loosely correlated with menstrual age. A general rule of thumb is as follows:
  - Risser 0—premenarchal
  - Risser 1—6 months postmenarche
  - Risser 2—1 year postmenarche
  - Risser 3—18 months postmenarche
  - Risser 4—2 years postmenarche
- There is significant individual variation in the timing of the adolescent growth spurt and the timing of cessation of growth.
- Two-thirds of girls have ceased growing at Risser stage 4, but to be 90% certain of cessation of spinal growth clinicians must wait on average another 19 months until Risser stage 5 is achieved.
- Boys may continue to grow and have curve progression in late adolescence; one study noted that only 61% of boys who were Risser 5 had ceased growing.
- Measurement of peak height velocity is helpful in predicting the cessation of growth (height velocity less than 2 cm per year) and the risk of curve progression. It has been reported to be more accurate than Risser sign, menarcheal status, or chronological age for predicting the length of time of remaining growth and the risk of curve progression. If a patient's height velocity is increasing, the risk of curve progression is high.
- By the time they are Risser 1, 85% of girls are past their growth peak.
- Crankshaft phenomenon—Solid posterior fusion with continued anterior spinal growth produces spine rotation and curve progression. Patients who have not reached peak height velocity, who are Tanner I, or who have open triradiate cartilage are reported to be at the greatest risk for crankshaft.

Hip Growth[11-14]

- Normal growth and development of the hip is under the influence of genetic, endocrine, environmental, morphological, and mechanical stimuli over a prolonged period.
- The acetabulum forms at the convergence of three primary ossification centers—the ischium, the pubis, and the ilium (triradiate cartilage).
- Growth in the triradiate cartilage occurs primarily before 8 years, with later secondary ossification centers within the arms of the triradiate cartilage developing and contributing to final growth of the acetabulum in adolescence.
- The depth of the acetabulum and its cup-like shape are determined by the presence of a spherical femoral head within the socket during growth.
- The proximal femoral epiphysis is entirely cartilaginous at birth, with a confluence of the proximal femoral physis and the greater trochanteric physis in the first few years of life.
- The ossification center of the proximal femoral epiphysis appears usually between 4 and 6 months.
- Understanding the normal blood supply to the proximal femur and how it changes with growth is important in pediatric orthopaedics. The proximal femoral physis is a barrier to blood flow between the epiphysis and the metaphysis. The predominant blood supply to the proximal femoral epiphysis is from the ascending cervical arteries of the medial femoral circumflex artery.[15,16]
- Developmental hip dysplasia seems to be primarily a deformation rather than a malformation, and restoration of an appropriate, stable articulation between the proximal femur and the acetabulum can remodel the deformity and normalize the morphology of the hip (the concept of developmental plasticity).

- Normal growth and development of the hip is often radiographically determined.

Lower Limb Growth[17-20]

Key point—Most of the lower extremity longitudinal growth occurs around the knee, in the distal femoral and the proximal tibial physes.

Femur

- Contribution of individual physis to longitudinal growth—proximal 30%, distal 70%
- Doubles in length from birth to 4 years
- Roughly 1cm per year for the distal femur

Tibia—Fibula

- Contribution of individual physis to longitudinal growth—60% proximal tibia, 40% distal tibia
- Tibia and fibula are interdependent and have harmonious growth
- If not harmonious, the growth can lead to genu varum and ankle valgus

Predicting Growth Remaining to Equalize Limb Lengths

Westh and Menelaus Method

- Distal femur grows 10 mm per year
- Proximal tibia grows 6 mm per year
- Boys grow until 16 years; girls grow until 14 years
- Bone age should be within 1 year of chronological age to be accurate
- Limb length discrepancy—predicting at maturity and predicting the effect of epiphysiodeses[20]

Straight-Line Graph Method

1. Assess past growth
2. Predict future growth
3. Predict effects of surgical epiphysiodesis

Alignment

Tibiofemoral Angle Changes with Growth[19]

Figure 1–6 shows the natural history of angular deformities in children.

- From birth to 1 year, the tibiofemoral angle is in marked varus.
- Between 1.5 and 2 years, the knees straighten to neutral tibiofemoral alignment.
- Between 2 and 3 years, the angle changes to valgus, with maximum valgus achieved between 3 and 3.5 years.
- The valgus corrects until 6 to 7 years, when the angle stabilizes at a mean of 5 to 6 degrees valgus.

If alignment of the lower extremities remains varus at 2 years, then infantile tibia vara may be present.

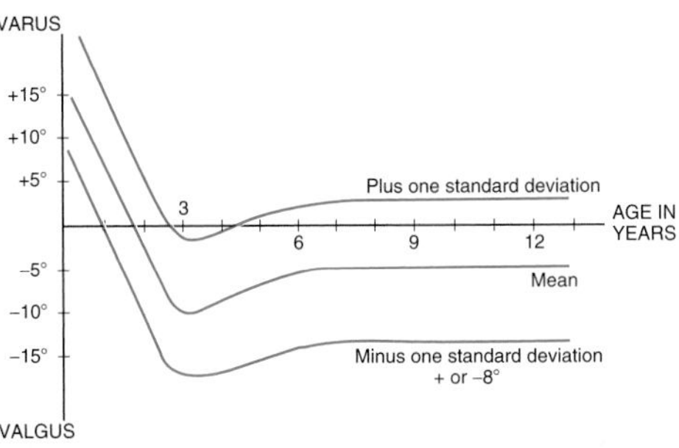

Figure 1–6: Classic study by Salenius and Vankka demonstrated the normal pattern of varus to neutral to valgus alignment of the lower extremities in the first few years of life. **From Wenger DR, Rang M (1993) The Art and Practice of Children's Orthopaedics. New York: Raven Press, Figure 7–2.**

Normal Values for Rotational Alignment in Children[18]

- Foot-progression angle—The angular difference between the long axis of the foot and the line of forward progression. It is used to quantify in-toeing or out-toeing gait. The angle is variable within a great range in infancy but stabilizes in childhood with a mean of 10 degrees outward and a normal range of 3 degrees inward to 20 degrees outward.
- Thigh–foot angle and transmalleolar axis—These are methods to measure the transverse plane or rotational alignment of the tibia and fibula. The thigh–foot axis from middle childhood averages 10 degrees with a normal range of −5 to 30 degrees. The transmalleolar angle average from middle childhood is 20 degrees, with a range of normal from 0 to 45 degrees.
- Hip rotation—Medial and lateral rotation is measured prone with the knees flexed 90 degrees to indirectly assess the amount of femoral anteversion. Medial hip rotation increases in the first few years of life, peaks around age 7 or 8, and then decreases with age. From middle childhood on, the mean for males is 50 degrees, with a normal range from 25 to 65 degrees. For females, the mean is 40 degrees, with a normal range of 15 to 60 degrees. Lateral hip rotation is greatest in infancy and declines throughout childhood. From middle childhood on, the average is 45 degrees, with a normal range of 25 to 65 degrees.
- Recommendations for treatment of torsional deformities—Generally, these resolve spontaneously with growth and no treatment is needed. Staheli has recommended age 8 as a cutoff beyond which further spontaneous correction is less likely. Corrective osteotomies may be indicated for medial tibial torsion greater than 15 degrees, lateral tibial torsion greater than 30 degrees, and severe femoral anteversion greater than 50 degrees, with medial hip rotation exceeding 85 degrees and lateral hip rotation less than 10 degrees.

Foot Growth

Postnatal Foot Growth

- At birth, the foot is about 40% of its final length.
- It grows to half of the adult foot length by age 1 (girl) or age 1½ (boy).
- There is a sharply decreasing rate of growth from birth to age 5.
- Average yearly growth is 0.9 cm after 5 years until 12 years (girl) or 14 years (boy).
- At age 10, a girl's foot is 90% of its final length and a boy's foot is 85% of its final length.

The foot is the first musculoskeletal structure to have a growth spurt in puberty and the first structure to stop growing.

The foot contributes 10-15% to standing height and should be considered in limb length inequality cases.

Upper Extremity Growth8

Key point—The upper extremity grows longitudinally primarily from physes far from the elbow, with the proximal humeral physis and the distal radial and ulnar physes contributing a greater amount than the physes close to the elbow (opposite of the lower extremity growth pattern in which most growth occurs about the knee) (Figure 1–7).

- Fractures are more common in the upper extremities of children and are most frequently treated nonoperatively.
- Fractures near rapidly growing physes in the upper extremity (distal radius or proximal humerus) have great potential for remodeling with growth. Residual deformity after fracture healing in these areas is typically observed for 6 to 12 months to see whether significant improvement occurs with growth.
- The general pattern of growth is similar in the upper and lower extremities, with accelerated growth in the first 5 years of life, a plateau from 5 until puberty, and then a growth spurt at puberty.

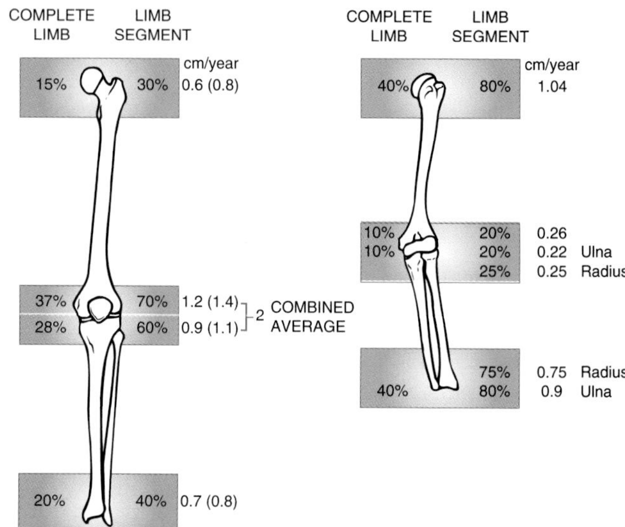

Figure 1–7: Physes around the knee contribute the greatest amount to the length of the lower extremity, but in the upper extremity, the physes furthest from the elbow contribute the greatest amount to longitudinal growth. **Panels show the contribution (%) of each physis to the overall length of the extremities, either of the complete limb or the limb segment. Panel A—lower extremity, Panel B—upper extremity. From Dimeglio A (2001) Growth in pediatric orthopaedics. In: Lovell & Winter's Pediatric Orthopaedics, 5th edition (Morrissy R, Weinstein S, eds). Philadelphia: Lippincott-William & Wilkins Publishers, Figures 2–18 and 2–21.**

Neurodevelopmental "Norms"2

The orthopaedic surgeon will frequently be consulted for delays in the achievement of motor developmental milestones, although often children with motor developmental delay will also have delayed development in other areas. Table 1–1 provides the ages at which more than 75% of children should have attained the listed motor milestone.

Developmental Red Flags

The following red flags should prompt referral or evaluation:

- Not rolling over by 6 months
- Not sitting by 8 months
- Handedness before 12 months
- Not walking by 18 months
- No words by 14 months

Parents will frequently ask whether a nonambulatory child with motor developmental delay will ever walk. Some poor prognostic signs for future ambulation include the following:

- Persistent head lag when pulled to sit at 9 months
- Not sitting independently by 2 years
- Not cruising by 4 years

It may be helpful to know that adults with neuromuscular disorders do not rank independent ambulation highest on

Table 1–1: Motor Milestones

AGE	MILESTONE
4 months	No head lag when pulling to a sitting position
5 months	Rolls over
6-7 months	Sits without support
9-11 months	Pulls to stand
12 months	Cruises; walks with support (hands held)
14 months	Walks alone
18 months	Runs
19 months	Walks up steps
36 months	Walks up stairs, alternating feet
48 months	Hops on one foot

their priority list of desired capabilities; it falls after communication skills, independence with activities of daily living, and general mobility.

Maturation of Gait[22]

Learning and maturation of the central nervous system contribute to the development of mature gait.

Gait Terminology

- *Gait cycle*—From foot strike to foot strike
- Phases of the gait cycle—*Stance phase* (60%) and *swing phase* (40%)
- *Velocity*—Average horizontal speed of the body along the plane of progression
- *Cadence*—Number of steps per unit of time
- *Step length*—Distance from one foot to the other foot in stance phase
- *Stride length*—Distance from the initial contact of one foot to the following initial contact on the same foot

Instrumented gait analysis by Sutherland has characterized the *stages of maturation* of gait (309 normal children, 1-7 years).

Beginning Ambulation

- Wide base gait
- Hyperflexion of hips and knees
- Arms abducted and elbows extended
- No reciprocal arm swing
- Initial contact with toes
- Circumduction to clear foot

By 2 Years

- Width of base diminishes
- Smoother movements
- Reciprocal arm swing for most children
- Initial contact with heel
- Increased step length and walking velocity

By 3 Years

- Adult kinematic patterns
- Higher cadence and diminished stride length compared with adults

By 7 Years

- Time–distance parameters that reach adult values (cadence, velocity, and step length)

Five Parameters of Gait Maturity

1. Single limb stance duration increases with age and maturity.
2. Walking velocity increases with age and limb length.
3. Cadence decreases with age and limb length.
4. Step length increases with age and limb length.
5. Ratio of interankle distance to pelvic width decreases with age and maturation.

References

1. Wenger DR, Rang M (1993) The Art and Practice of Children's Orthopaedics. New York: Raven Press.
   Pediatric orthopaedic textbook that covers topics by anatomical region, diagnoses, or both and that contains the wisdom of two experienced practitioners. It also provides informative historical vignettes and minibiographies of influential people in orthopaedics. Highly recommended.

2. Gross R. The Pediatric Orthopaedic Society of North America Core Curriculum, http://www.posna.org.
   This curriculum was developed to enhance pediatric orthopaedic education in residency programs and contains sections on growth and development with listed objectives and discussion points. It also provides brief discussion sections for each topic and a list of pertinent references.

3. Dietz FR, Morcuende JA (2001) Embryology and development of the musculoskeletal system. In: Lovell & Winter's Pediatric Orthopaedics, 5th edition (Morrissy R, Weinstein S, eds). Philadelphia: Lippincott-William & Wilkins Publishers, pp 1-31.
   An excellent overview and introduction to the embryology of the musculoskeletal system.

4. Uhthoff H, Wiley JJ, eds (1988) Behavior of the Growth Plate. New York: Raven Press.
   A textbook devoted to defining normal parameters for the growth plate. There are chapters on growth plate injuries, mechanisms of altering bone length, management of osseous bridges, infections and the physis, and the physeal response to developmental disorders.

5. Buckwalter JA, Ehrlich MG, Sandell LJ, Trippel SB, eds (1998) Skeletal Growth and Development. Rosemont, IL: American Academy of Orthopaedic Surgeons.
   An update on basic science and clinical applications with sections on the formation of the bony skeleton, synovial joints, and growth plate; function and regulation; disturbances in skeletal morphogenesis and growth; and therapeutic interventions for these disturbances.

6. Ogden J (2000) Anatomy and physiology of skeletal development. In: Skeletal Injury in the Children, 3rd edition. New York: Springer-Verlag, pp 1-37.
   Detailed descriptions of the development of the skeleton by the foremost authority on the anatomy of the growing skeleton, with numerous clinical and histological photographs.

7. Ballock RT, O'Keefe RJ. (2003) The biology of the growth plate. J Bone Joint Surg 85A: 715-726.
   An excellent review of the basic science of the physis, particularly of the mechanisms thought to regulate physeal growth and mineralization.

8. Dimeglio A (2001) Growth in pediatric orthopaedics. In: Lovell & Winter's Pediatric Orthopaedics, 5th edition (Morrissy R, Weinstein S, eds). Philadelphia: Lippincott-William & Wilkins Publishers, pp 33-62.
   An experienced clinician and researcher of growth provides valuable insight into patterns of growth in the pediatric musculoskeletal system.

9. Song KM, Little DG (2000) Peak height velocity as a maturity indicator for males with idiopathic scoliosis. J Pediatr Orthop 20(3): 286-288.

10. Little DG, Song KM, Katz D, Herring JA (2000) Relationship of peak height velocity to other maturity indicators in idiopathic scoliosis in girls. J Bone Joint Surg 82A(5): 685-693.
    The two preceding articles provide data relating that peak height velocity may be the most sensitive marker of the risk of scoliosis curve progression in growing adolescents. They also describe other methods of evaluating growth potential and the risk of curve progression.

11. Ponseti IV (1978) Growth and development of the acetabulum in the normal child. J Bone Joint Surg 60A: 575-585.
    Morphologic, radiographic, and histological study of the hip in infants and children, detailing the triradiate cartilage and its three secondary ossification centers.

12. Lindstrom J, Ponseti I, Wenger D (1979) Acetabular development after reduction in congenital dislocation of the hip. J Bone Joint Surg 61A: 112-118.

13. Scoles PV, Boyd A, Jones PK (1987) Roentgenographic parameters of the normal infant hip. J Pediatr Orthop 7(6): 656-663.

14. Kahle WK, Coleman SS. The value of the teardrop figure in assessing pediatric hip disorders. J Pediatr Orthop 12: 586-591, 1992.
    These articles are among many that describe the normal and abnormal radiographic development of the hip. Many children with hip dysplasia are asymptomatic during childhood and adolescence and have a normal physical examination; thus, radiographic evaluation is used to follow the development of the hip.

15. Chung SM (1976) The arterial supply of the developing proximal end of the human femur. J Bone Joint Surg Am 58(7): 961-970.

16. Gautier E, Ganz K, Krügel N, Gill T, Ganz R (2000) Anatomy of the medial femoral circumflex artery and its surgical implications. J Bone Joint Surg 82B(5): 679-683.
    These articles describe the anatomy of the blood supply to the proximal femur, its changes with age, and surgical approaches that preserve it. Pediatric orthopaedic surgeons need to be knowledgeable about the proximal femoral blood supply to avoid osteonecrosis when treating pediatric hip disorders.

17. Staheli LT, Corbett M, Wyss C, King H (1985) Lower-extremity rotational problems in children. J Bone Joint Surg 67A(1): 39-47.
    This article documents the normal values for rotational alignment of the lower limbs in children of varying ages through the study of 1000 normal lower extremities. Most rotational variations fall within the broad range of normal and do not require treatment.

18. Staheli LT (1989) Torsion—Treatment indications. Clin Orthop Rel Res 247: 61-66.
    The author defines torsional deformities—that is, those rotational problems that fall outside the range of normal—and offers guidelines for the treatment of the few deformities that do not improve with growth.

19. Salenius P, Vankka E (1975) The development of the tibiofemoral angle in children. J Bone Joint Surg 57A(2): 259-261.
    Classic article about normal children studied radiographically with measurements of the tibiofemoral angle, and the progression from varus in infancy, to neutral by 1.5-2 years, to maximum valgus by 3-3.5 years, and then to physiological valgus by 6-7 years.

20. Moseley CF (1977) A straight-line graph for leg-length discrepancies. J Bone Joint Surg Am 59(2): 174-179.
    Classic article based on growth charts to plot predicted limb length discrepancy at skeletal maturity and determine the effects of surgical epiphysiodesis on equalizing limb lengths.

21. Westh RN, Menelaus MB (1981) A simple calculation for the timing of the epiphyseal arrest. J Bone Joint Surg 63B(1): 117-119.
    The arithmetic method of calculating the effects of epiphysiodesis by estimating that the distal femoral physis contributes about ⅜ inch per year to length and the proximal tibia contributes about ¼ inch per year.

22. Davids JR (2001) Normal gait and assessment of gait disorders. In: Lovell & Winter's Pediatric Orthopaedics, 5th edition (Morrissy R, Weinstein S, eds). Philadelphia: Lippincott-William & Wilkins Publishers, pp 131-156.
    This chapter expertly summarizes normal gait and how it develops. It also introduces concepts of gait analysis and how common gait deviations are analyzed.

23. Salter R (1984) Textbook of Disorders and Injuries of the Musculoskeletal System, 2nd edition. Baltimore: Williams & Wilkins.
    This textbook is an excellent introductory text for a student of the musculoskeletal system. The first part of the textbook covers normal structure and function, principles of diagnosis, and treatment of disorders and injuries.

CHAPTER 2

Pediatric Musculoskeletal Examination

Allan C. Beebe* and James M. Kerpsack†

*MD, Orthopaedic Faculty, Department of Orthopaedic Surgery, Children's Hospital, Columbus, OH; Assistant Program Director, Department of Orthopaedic Surgery, Mount Carmel Medical Center, Columbus, OH
†MD, The Center for Orthopaedic Surgery and Sports Medicine, Indianapolis, IN

Introduction

- History and physical examination are the basis for all decision making in medicine.
- Pediatric orthopaedic surgery is unique in that there are usually many participants in the concern and evaluation of the child (e.g., parents, grandparents, siblings, aunts, uncles, and teachers).
- The pediatric orthopaedic surgeon must be artful in negotiating the various complaints, concerns, anxieties, and findings in the infant or child.
- The orthopaedic surgeon is often the first consultant to evaluate deformities or developmental abnormalities in children.
- The surgeon must be familiar with the "norms" of development and function.
- The orthopaedic examination must be performed expeditiously to maintain the cooperation of an understandably anxious or uncooperative patient.
- The examiner must keep in mind that the family is anticipating a thorough examination of a problem they perceive as important.
- Depending on the severity of the problem, the examination may vary from focused to comprehensive.

Chief Complaint

- Discover the reason for the visit.
- Determine whether there are true complaints from the child or the evaluation is desired because of the concerns of family, friends, or referring physicians.
- Establish a clear and concise timeline of the child's or family's complaints.
- Decide whether the child's problem is diffuse or generalized.
- Determine whether pain or swelling interferes with the child's function or there are concerns of stiffness, weakness, limp, or deformity.
- Discover whether the child will continue to participate in chosen activities or the complaints interfere with play or sleep. (Pain at night is unusual in the pediatric population and can indicate a reason for further investigative efforts.)

Orthopaedic History

- Orthopaedic history is a vital part of the examination in pediatric patients.
- A comprehensive history should include questions about the mother's prenatal health (Box 2–1).
- Perinatal history can also be important in the evaluation of the developing child. Delays in development can be related to difficulties around the time of birth (Box 2–2).
- Developmental milestones can reveal the child's neurological development (Table 2–1).

Box 2–1 Mother's Prenatal Questionnaire

Smoking
Prenatal vitamins
Illicit drug or narcotic use
Alcohol history
Diabetes
Rubella
Sexually transmitted diseases

- A family history of illness may play a role in expectations for the child's future development (e.g., clubfoot, scoliosis, developmental dysplasia of the hip, or skeletal dysplasias).
- Do any siblings or immediate relatives have conditions similar to those of the child?
- Social history should include questions about child's educational standing in school, emotional development, daily behavior, and regular activities or sports.
- The past medical and surgical history should include any previous procedures and significant medical conditions (e.g., sickle cell, diabetes, malignancies, connective tissue disorders, or dysplasias).
- The child's history of growth and development should be noted, as should allergies, present medications, and immunizations.
- Orthopaedic-specific questions should focus on extremity, joint, muscular, or axial skeleton complaints (Box 2–3).

Orthopaedic Physical Examination

- Examination of the orthopaedic patient includes a thorough evaluation of the musculoskeletal system and a comprehensive neurological examination.
- The dividing line between a neurological evaluation and an orthopaedic evaluation is often blurred.

Box 2–2 Child's Perinatal Questionnaire

Length of the pregnancy
Prematurity
Length of labor
Labor induced or spontaneous
Infant position at delivery (breech versus vertex)
Infant distress at delivery
Requirements for oxygen following delivery
Birth length and weight
Apgar score
Muscle tone at birth
Feeding history
Discharged status from hospital (with mother or after a prolonged hospitalization)

Table 2–1: Motor Developmental Milestones

AGE	MILESTONE
2 months	Maintains head position when prone
3 months	Lifts head above body when prone
4 months	Lifts head and chest when prone leaning on forearms
6 months	Lifts head and chest when prone with weight on hands, sits with support
8 months	Sits without support, reaches for objects
10 months	Crawls, pulls to sitting position, stands with assistance (by holding on)
12 months	Walks with no or minimal assistance
14 months	Walks without assistance, stoops and recovers balance
18 months	Ascends stairs with support, handedness becoming evident
24 months	Ascends stairs without support one step at a time, jumps, kicks a ball
36 months	Ascends stairs one foot at a time, stands on one foot momentarily
48 months	Hops on one foot, throws a ball overhand
60 months	Skips, hops without support

- A basic neurological examination including sensation, motor function, and reflex evaluation appropriate for the age of the child should be performed in most

Box 2–3 Orthopaedic-Specific History

Joint Complaints

- Character—Stiffness or limitation of motion, swelling or erythema and warmth, single or multiple joint involvement, constant or activity-related pain, deformity
- Associated factors—Activity, injuries (recent or remote), time of day
- Temporal factors—Slow versus fast onset, sequence of pain during day (better or worse)
- Previous treatments—Rest, exercise, nonsteroidal anti-inflammatory drugs (NSAIDs)

Muscular Complaints

- Character—Limitation of movement, weakness, fatigue, falling, pain
- Precipitating factors—Injury, new onset activity, strenuous activity
- Previous treatments—Ice, immobilization, NSAIDs

Skeletal Complaints

- Character—Limp or gait abnormality, pain with movement, deformity
- Associated factors—Recent injury, recent fracture, frequent repetitive activity, present at birth or acquired
- Previous treatments—Rest, immobilization, NSAIDs

Injury

- Mechanism—Fall, overuse, crush, motor vehicle accident
- Pain—Location, gradual or immediate onset, most comfortable position
- Swelling—Location, gradual or immediate onset

orthopaedic evaluations ranging from birth to adolescence.
- The examination will often include observation, palpation, and evaluation of motion and stability.
- The orthopaedic physical examination requires basic knowledge of anatomy, "norms" as far as joint range of motion and alignment, and a glossary of basic terminology to standardize communication regarding the patient's findings.
- It is necessary to define deformity, contractures, spasticity (increased muscle tone), range of motion, and neurological function in an effort to identify the problem of the patient.

Deformity

- The examining physician must identify the site of the deformity.
- The area can usually be localized by the complaint of the patient or family (Box 2–4).
- Once the site of deformity has been identified, the magnitude of the deformity must be determined.
- Deformity is usually measured with a goniometer and stated in degrees.
- Deformity can occur in both the sagittal (lateral) and the coronal (frontal) planes.
- Deviations in the coronal plane are termed *varus,* angulation toward the midline of the distal segment, or *valgus,* angulation away from the midline of the distal segment (e.g., cubitus varus, genu valgus, or coxa valgus).
- There can be developmental changes in the normal amount of varus or valgus of various joints depending on age (Box 2–5).[1]
- Angulation is usually stated in degrees with a direction as a modifier (e.g., 30 degrees apex anterior angulation).
- Deformities of the spine are termed *scoliosis* in the coronal plane and *kyphosis* or *lordosis* in the sagittal plane.

Contractures

- Contractures are a loss of mobility of a joint from either a congenital or acquired etiology.
- They can form from fibrosis of the soft tissues immediately surrounding a joint or from loss of elasticity of the muscles crossing a joint.

Box 2–4 Anatomical Area of Complaint

Cervical spine
Shoulder
Thoracic or lumbar spine
Cubitus—Elbow
Coxa—Hip
Genu—Knee
Pes—Foot

Box 2–5 Normal Knee Alignment by Age

Neonates—10-15 degrees of varus
14-22 months—Neutral
36-45 months—Maximum valgus of 10-15 degrees
6-8 years—Gradual return to normal of 5-7 degrees

- Contractures can be acquired following bony or muscle trauma, inflammatory arthritis, or a congenital origin such as in arthrogryposis.
- Numerous authors have documented that newborns will normally have flexion contractures of the upper and lower extremities that will resolve with growth and maturation.

Spasticity

- Spasticity is the abnormal increase in tone that can come from a variety of causes.
- Cerebral palsy (static encephalopathy) is the most common cause of increased muscle tone in the pediatric population.
- Other upper motor neuron lesions such as head injury or spinal cord injury can increase muscle tone.
- It is important to isolate the individual muscle groups when examining the limb of a child with spasticity. (e.g., What is the range of ankle dorsiflexion of a child with the knee both flexed and extended? Is there gastrocnemius tightness?)
- Remember that several muscle–tendon units cross two joints and that the excursion of one joint can be affected by the position of the other (Box 2–6).

Range of Motion

- Motion can be evaluated actively (the patient moves the joint) or passively (the examiner moves the joint).
- Both active and passive motions should be recorded in the evaluation of the joint.
- Passive motion evaluates the mobility of the joint.
- Active motion evaluates both the mobility of the joint and the neuromuscular function crossing the joint.
- Pain from injury or illness can affect both active and passive motions.
- Joint motion should always be compared with the opposite side because joint motion is normally the same on the right and left sides.

Box 2–6 Muscle–Tendon Units Crossing Two Joints

Hamstrings, rectus femoris, gracilis, and sartorius—Hip and knee
Gastrocnemius—Knee and ankle
Biceps—Shoulder and elbow
Wrist flexors and extensors—Elbow and wrist

- Joint motion, like contracture, is measured in degrees with a goniometer.
- To allow conformity, the zero starting position is determined to be the fully extended position of the joint to be evaluated.
- The American Academy of Orthopaedic Surgeons has published standards of joint motion.[2]
- Joints are capable of many planes of motion, and directions are used to define their motion (Box 2–7).

Cervical Spine

- Motions available to the cervical spine are flexion, extension, lateral bending, and rotation.
- The cervical spine is the most flexible portion of the spine.
- C1-C2 provides 50% of the rotation of the cervical spine.
- The remaining levels share fairly evenly the rest of the rotation available.
- Occiput-C1 provides 50% of the flexion and extension of the cervical spine with the remaining motion shared among C1-C7.[3]
- A goniometer is the most accurate way to evaluate motion of the cervical spine.
- Clinical measurement is a more common method of conveying motion (Figure 2–1).
- Limitations of motion suggest abnormalities such as torticollis, congenital vertebral abnormalities, instability, infection, tumor, or trauma.

Box 2–7 Direction of Joint Motion

Flexion—Bending a joint from the starting position
Extension—Bending a joint toward the starting position
Abduction—Movement from the midline
Adduction—Movement toward the midline
Supination—With the elbow flexed 90 degrees, rotating the palm upward
Pronation—With the elbow flexed 90 degrees, rotating the palm downward
Inversion—Rotating inward, usually referring to the subtalar joint
Eversion—Rotating outward, usually referring to the subtalar joint
Internal Rotation—Turning inward toward the body
External Rotation—Turning outward from the body

- The evaluation of the brachial plexus and the neurological examination of the lower extremity are important in the face of a suspected cervical spine injury.

Thoracolumbar Spine

- Motions of flexion, extension, lateral bending, and rotation are coupled motions in the thoracic and lumbar spine.
- Flexion and extension are greatest in the lower lumbar spine, where rotation is limited.
- Motion at individual levels can often be difficult to quantify.

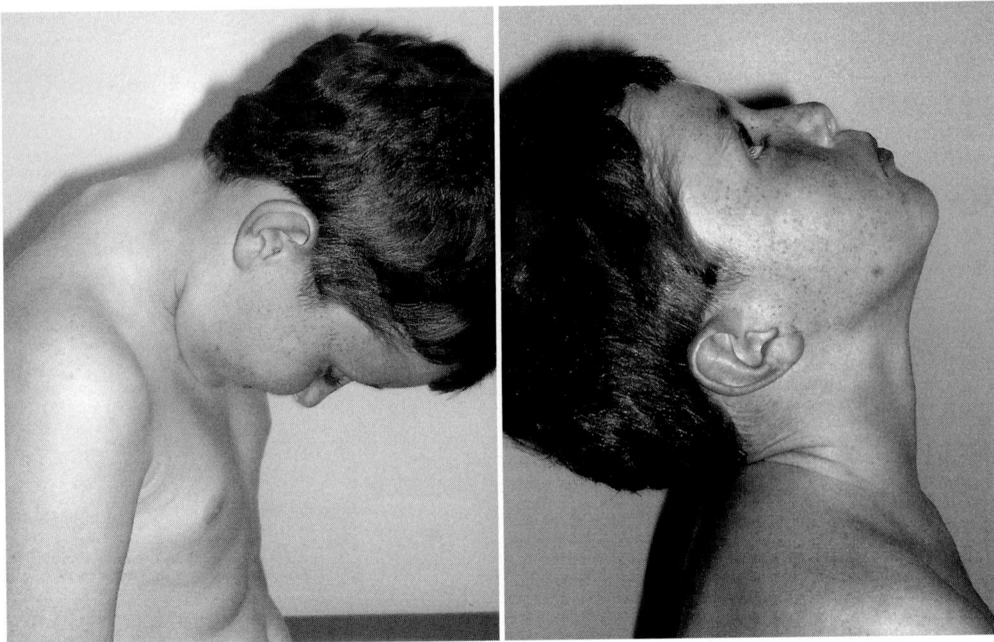

Figure 2–1: Clinical evaluation of the cervical spine motion is most common. **Note the position of the chin on flexion and extension, the position of the ear in relation to the shoulder on lateral tilt, and the position of the nose in relation to the shoulder on rotation.**

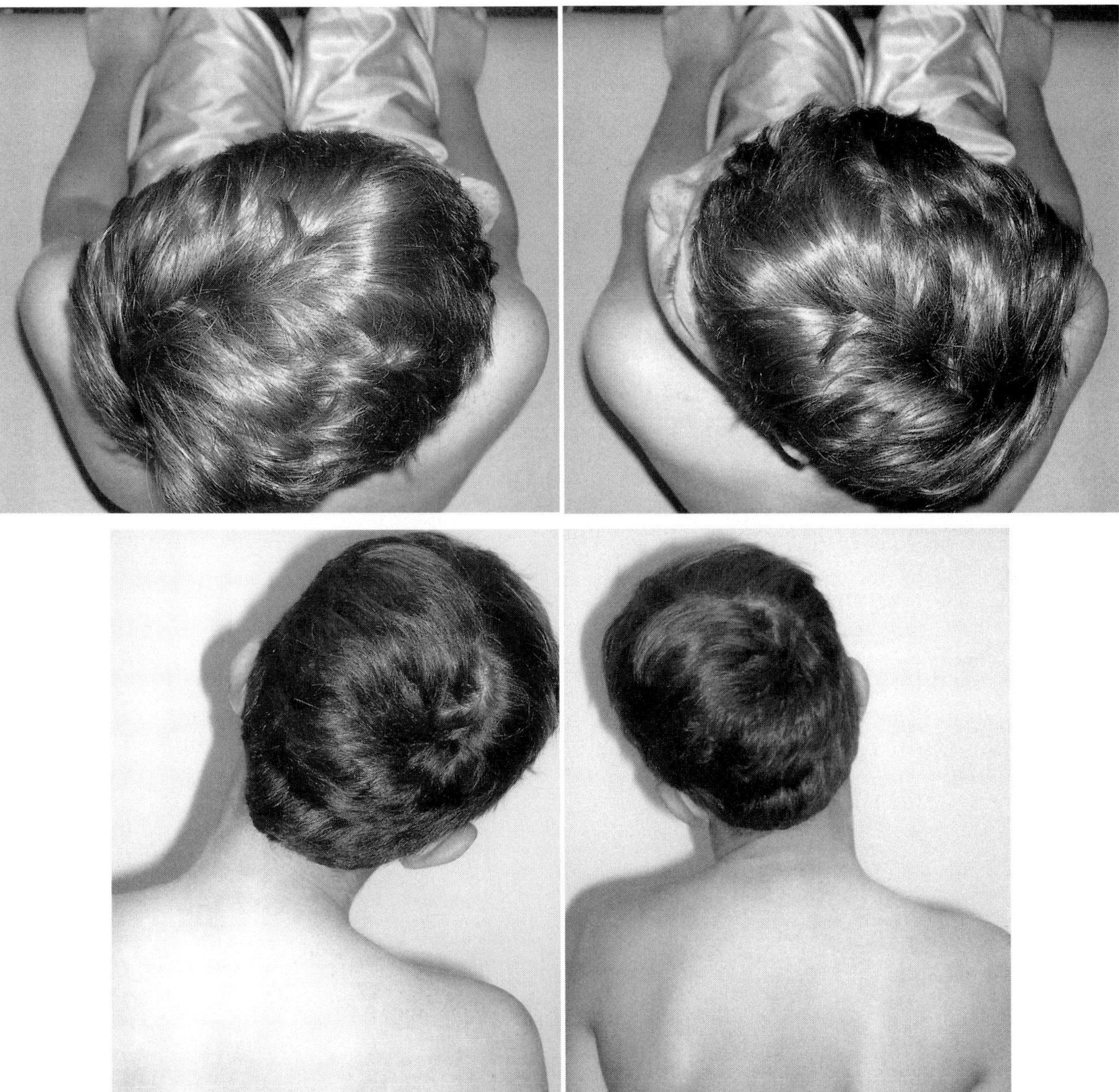

Figure 2–1, cont'd.

- Motion, alignment, and rotational changes are all evaluated in examining the thoracic and lumbar spine.
- Goniometers, visual estimation, and inclinometers or scoliometers are ways commonly used to attempt to quantify motion and rotation in the thoracic and lumbar spine (Figures 2–2 through 2–4).
- Simple clinical evaluation is sometimes the easiest way to have the child cooperate with the examination of the thoracolumbar spine.

Shoulder

- Inspection of symmetry is an important first step in the examination of the shoulder. (Are the shoulder heights symmetrical and the muscular contours normal?)
- The level of the clavicles, acromium, and scapula should be visualized.
- The range of motion of the shoulder is the greatest of any joint in the body.

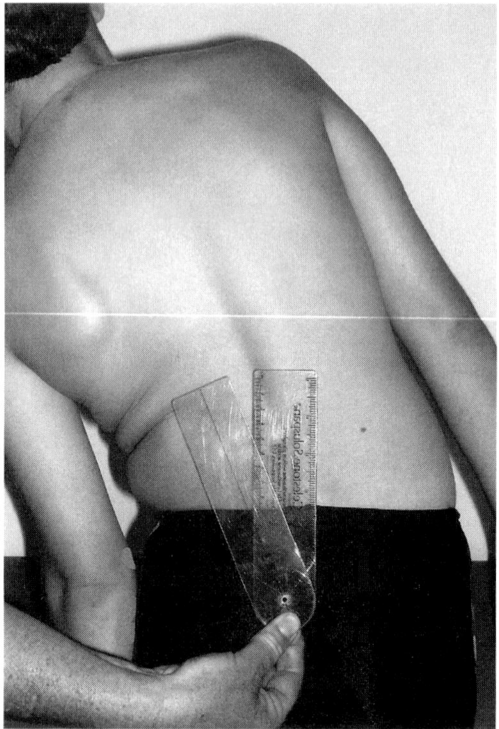

A

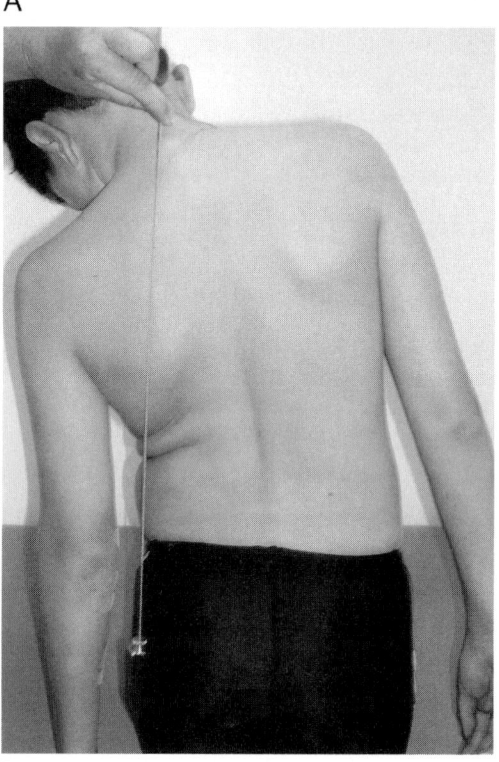

B

Figure 2–2: Lateral bending can be evaluated by marking T1-T2 and measuring with a goniometer the angular displacement in relation to the midline (A) or by dropping a plumb line from the spinous process of C7 and determining the lateral displacement from the midline (B).

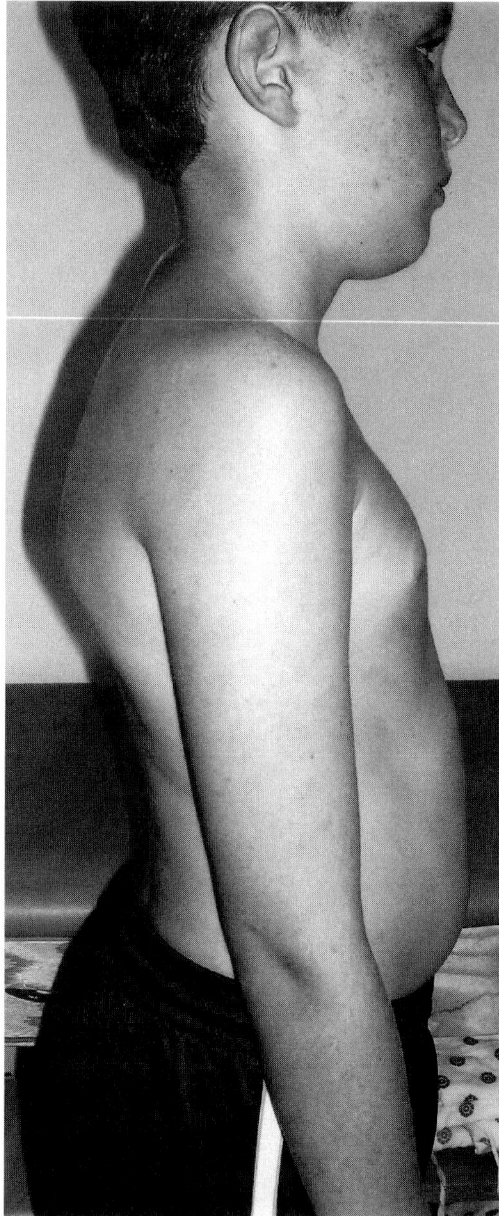

Figure 2–3: Sagittal alignment is evaluated from the side of the patient, and the appearance of the normal kyphosis and lordosis is appreciated.

- Forward flexion, abduction, adduction, internal and external rotation, and extension make up the six planes of motion of the shoulder (Figure 2–5 through 2–7).
- Maximal abduction is accomplished by a combination of abduction and external rotation as the articulating surface of the humeral head is increased with external rotation.
- Shoulder stability can be evaluated in an older child by the apprehension test, performed by abducting the shoulder 90 degrees, externally rotating the arm, and attempting to translate the humeral head anterior.

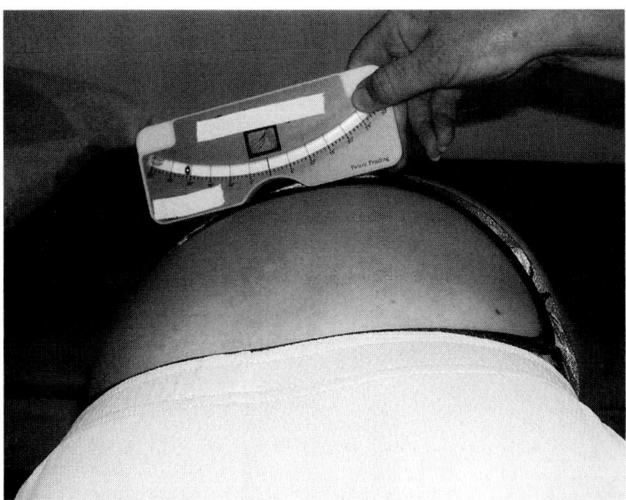

Figure 2–4: Deformity of the spine often results in rotational deformities that can be evaluated with a scoliometer. The patient is asked to bend forward, and the prominence of the right or left hemithorax or lumbar paraspinal musculature is evaluated from behind.

A patient with instability will become uncomfortable or begin to guard the shoulder.

- Anterior, inferior, or posterior translation can also be performed by stabilizing the scapula and stressing the proximal humerus.
- Abnormal laxity can be present in younger children or adolescents (e.g., habitual or voluntary dislocation or subluxation, or congenital laxity such as Marfan or Ehlers-Danlos syndromes).

Elbow

- The elbow is a hinge (ginglymus) joint composed of three articulations: radial–capitellar, radial–ulnar, and humeral–ulnar.
- The carrying angle of the elbow is the natural valgus angle of the humerus in relation to the forearm with the elbow extended (Figure 2–8).
- The patient should be able to easily touch a shoulder with a hand in maximal flexion (Figure 2–9).
- Individuals with congenital laxities will often be able to hyperextend an elbow beyond 0 degrees of extension (Ehlers-Danlos or Marfan syndromes).
- The elbow is more superficial than the shoulder; therefore, it is easier to identify areas of tenderness.
- The bony landmarks of the medial and lateral epicondyles, olecranon, and radial head are easily palpated.
- Displacement of the radial head can be detected by palpation while rotating the forearm.
- Extension or flexion supracondylar injuries to the elbow can result in malunions that will produce an altered arc of motion.

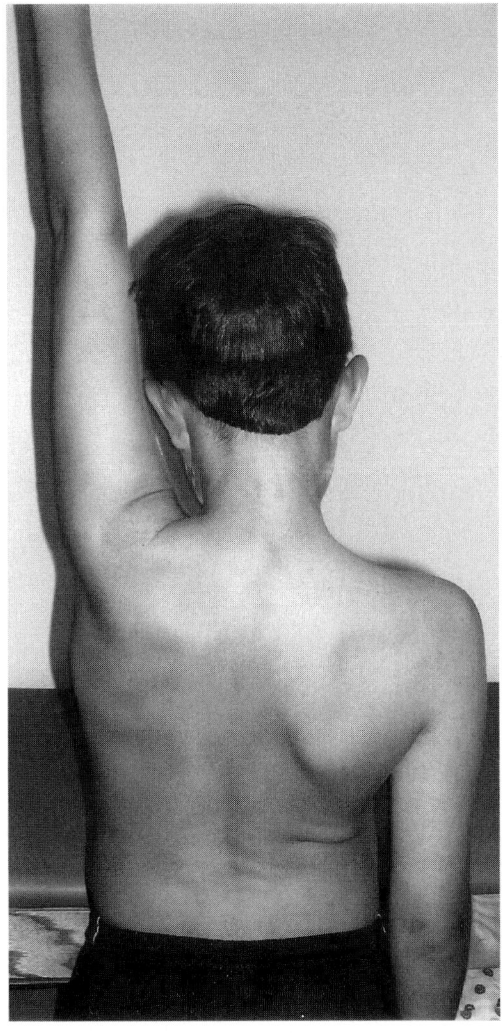

Figure 2–5: Abduction of the shoulder is a combination of glenohumeral motion (2/3) and scapulothoracic motion (1/3); it encompasses 180 degrees of motion.

Forearm, Wrist, and Hand

- Pronation (palm down) and supination (palm up) should be evaluated with the arm at the side and the elbow flexed 90 degrees (Figure 2–10).
- Wrist dorsiflexion and palmar flexion are measured from the neutral starting position with the hand parallel to the forearm (Figure 2–11).
- Young children are often not interested in voluntarily participating in an extensive hand examination.
- Observation of children using their hands to grasp and interact with parents or siblings is an excellent initial evaluation of hand function.
- All children should be able to fully flex their fingers into their palm and extend them fully.
- Inspection for abnormal palmar creases can suggest underlying genetic abnormalities such as Down's syndrome.

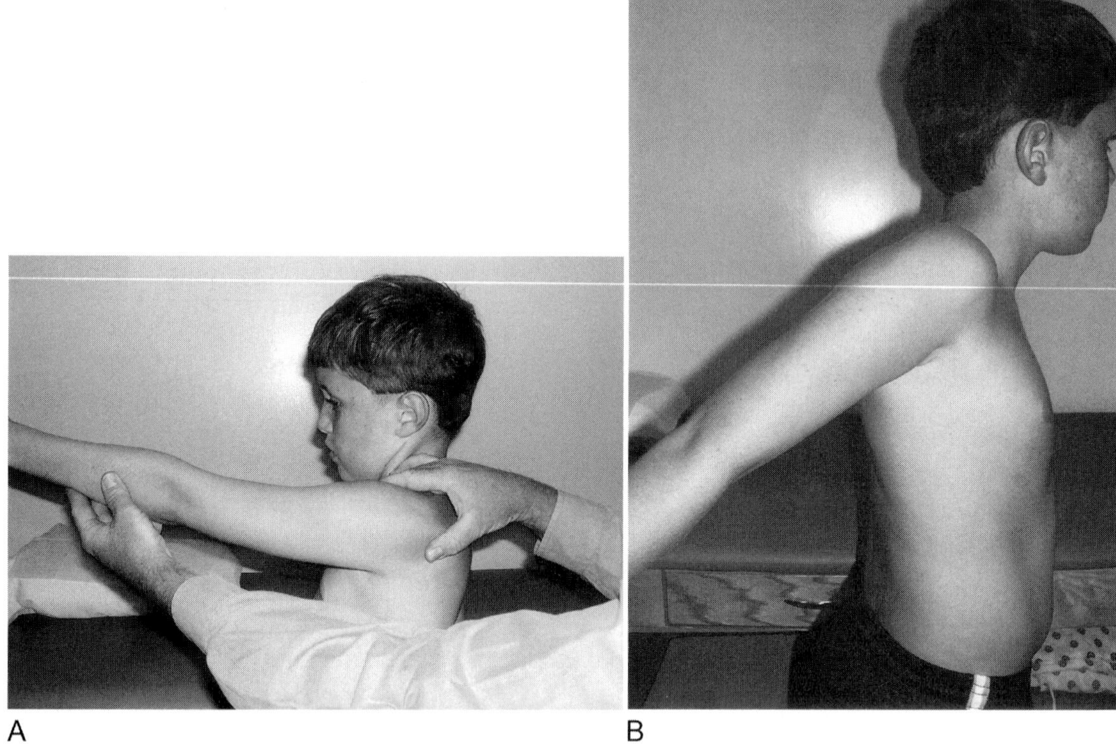

Figure 2–6: The examiner must stabilize the scapula and acromium to evaluate flexion and extension of the shoulder. Forward flexion is possible to 90 degrees (A) and extension is possible to 45 degrees in the normal shoulder (B).

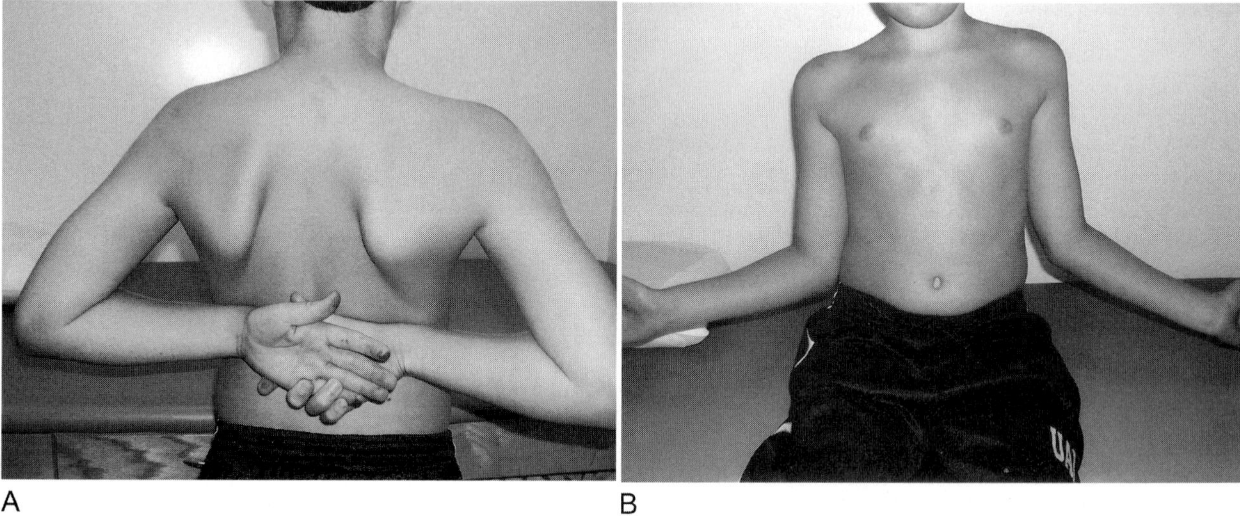

Figure 2–7: Internal and external rotation can be evaluated by placing the patient's arm at his or her side with the elbow flexed 90 degrees and assessing the rotation possible (A). The neutral starting point is with the hand and forearm directed forward (B).

- Clinodactyly (angular deformity of any finger in the coronal plane) and camptodactyly (flexion deformity of the fifth finger proximal interphalangeal joint) are two common angular deformities of the fingers that have a genetic link.[4]
- Polydactaly and syndactaly are usually obvious and are the most common types of genetic hand abnormalities.

Hip

- The hip is a ball and socket joint capable of a large range of motion in all planes.
- The limits of motion are dictated by the depth of the acetabulum.

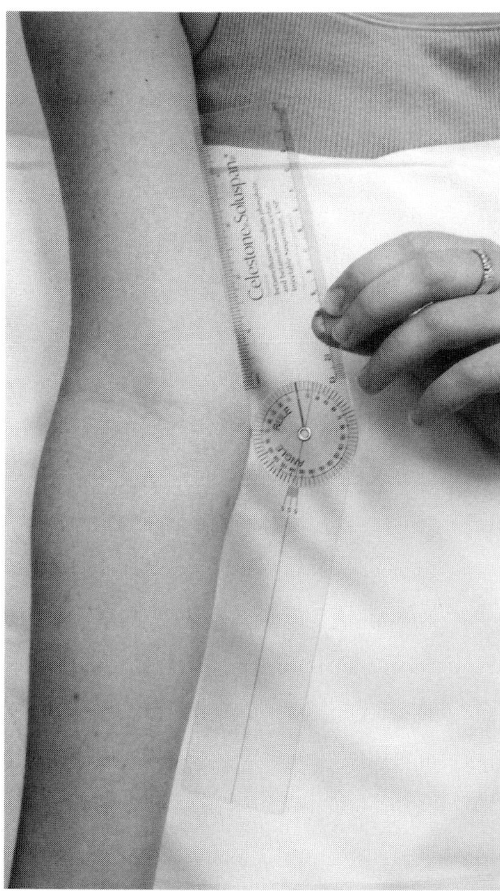

Figure 2–8: The normal carrying angle of the elbow is between 5 and 15 degrees.

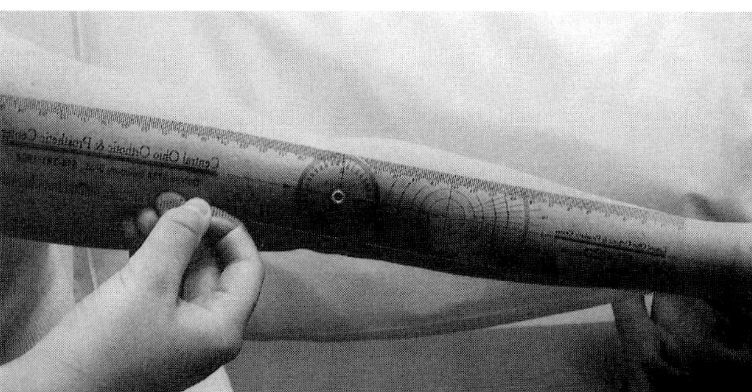

A

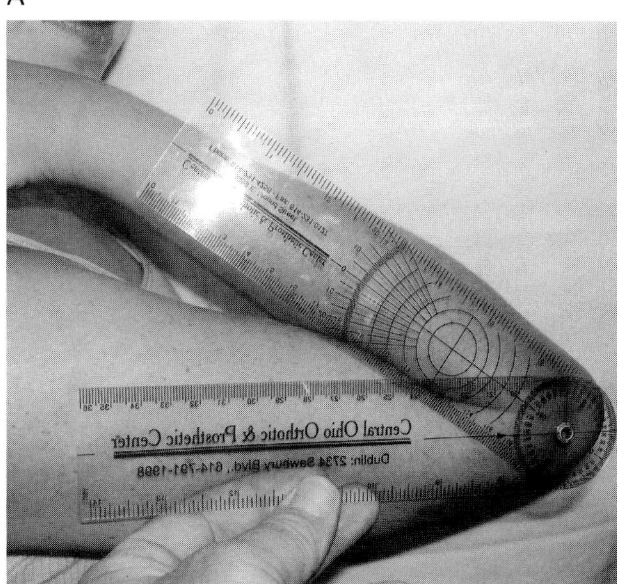

B

Figure 2–9: Flexion and extension of the elbow should be possible from full extension (0 degrees, A) to between 135 and 150 degrees of flexion (B).

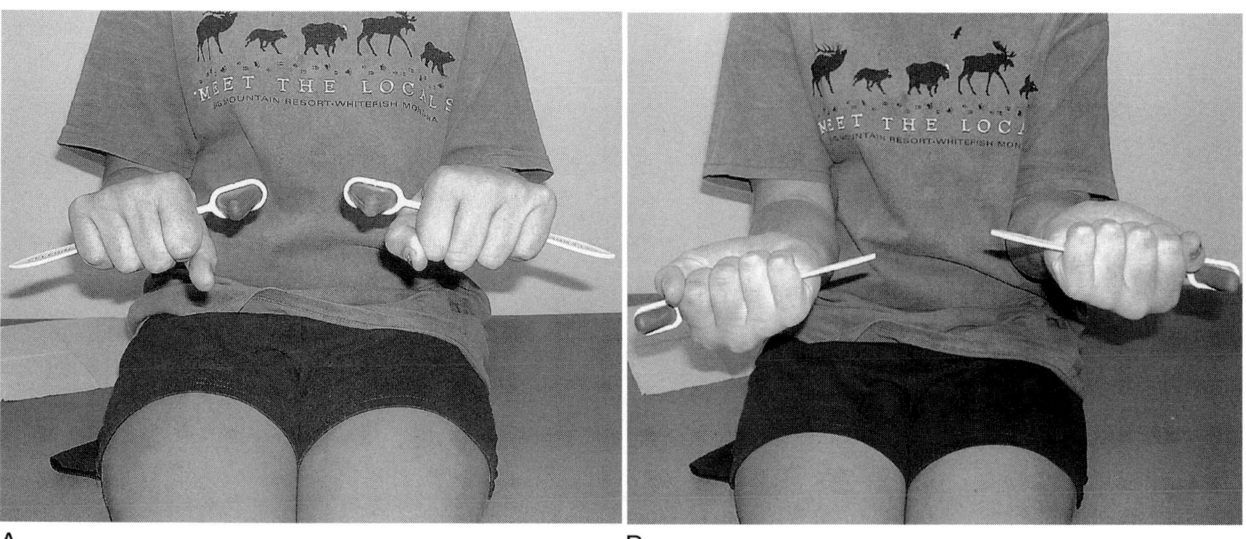

A B

Figure 2–10: A pencil, reflex hammer, or ruler in a clasped hand can help to measure pronation and supination of the forearm. Normal pronation (A) and supination (B) should be from 0 degrees to between 80 and 90 degrees each.

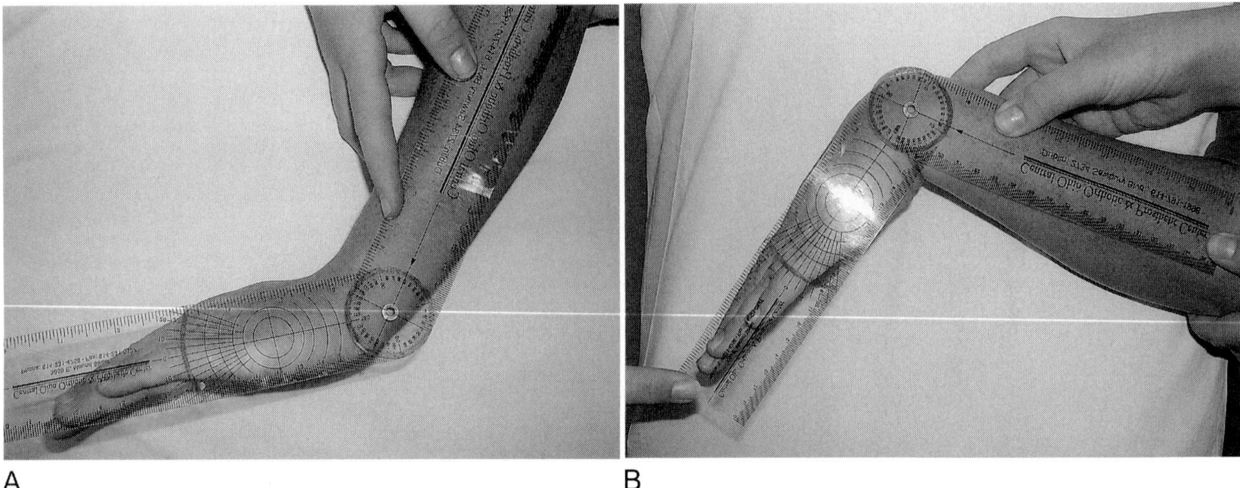

Figure 2–11: Wrist motion should be from 0-70 degrees of extension (dorsiflexion, A) to 0-80 degrees of flexion (palmar flexion, B).

- Normal newborns have an approximately 30-degree flexion contracture that usually resolves itself by 1 year (Figure 2–12).
- Staheli has described a prone test for determining hip flexion deformities[5] (Figure 2–13).
- Children with a significant hip flexion contracture will compensate during gait with an increased lumbar lordosis or, if severe, will ambulate with a flexed knee and only touch the ground with their toes, falsely suggesting leg length inequality.
- Abduction and adduction needs to be evaluated with the pelvis stable and the hip in both the flexed and extended positions (Figure 2–14).
- The infant is sometimes easier to evaluate for adduction and abduction in the lateral position.
- Internal and external rotation of the hips should be evaluated in the flexed and extended positions (Figure 2–15).
- Younger children may become anxious in the prone position (Figure 2–16). This may be overcome by allowing them to be held prone on their parent's lap or to evaluate the rotation available in the supine position using the patella as the indicator of hip rotation (Figure 2–17).

Thigh and Knee

- Inspection is an important first step in the examination of the knee.
- Is there redness, swelling, bruising, or skin changes?
- In evaluating the knee, the examiner should *always* be thinking about the possibility of hip pathology.

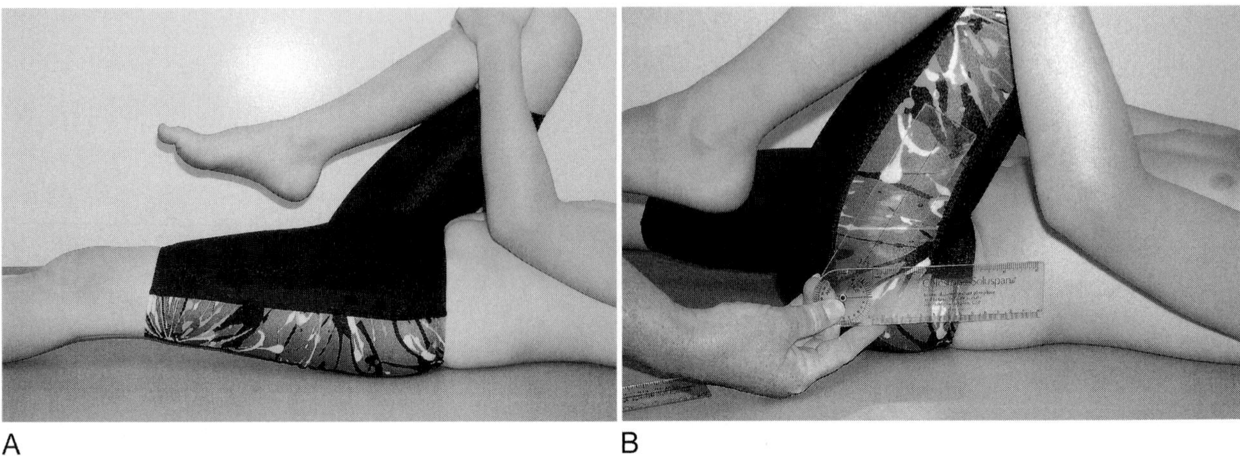

Figure 2–12: Normal range of motion of the hip is from 20 degrees of extension (A) to between 0 and 120 degrees of flexion (B). Maximally flexing the opposite hip can help to evaluate the presence of a hip flexion contracture on the examined side.

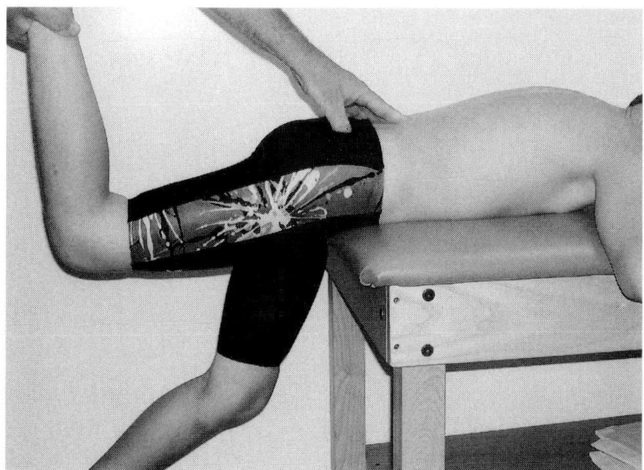

Figure 2–13: Place the child prone with his or her legs over the edge of the table, allow the opposite hip to flex, and evaluate the amount of extension, or lack of full extension, while stabilizing the pelvis.

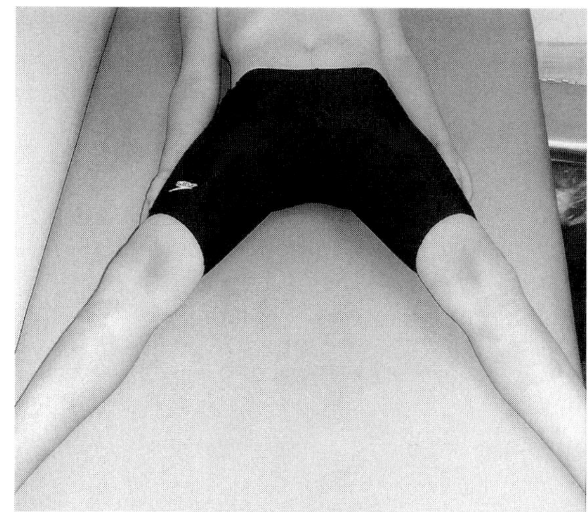

Figure 2–14: Normal range of abduction of the hip in the extended position is 0-45 degrees.

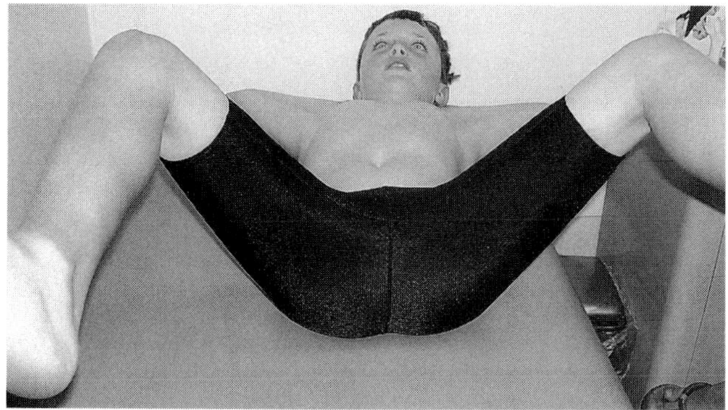

Figure 2–15: Hip abduction can be evaluated in the flexed position by grasping the patient's heels, flexing the knees, and evaluating the amount of angular displacement from the midline as the hips abduct.

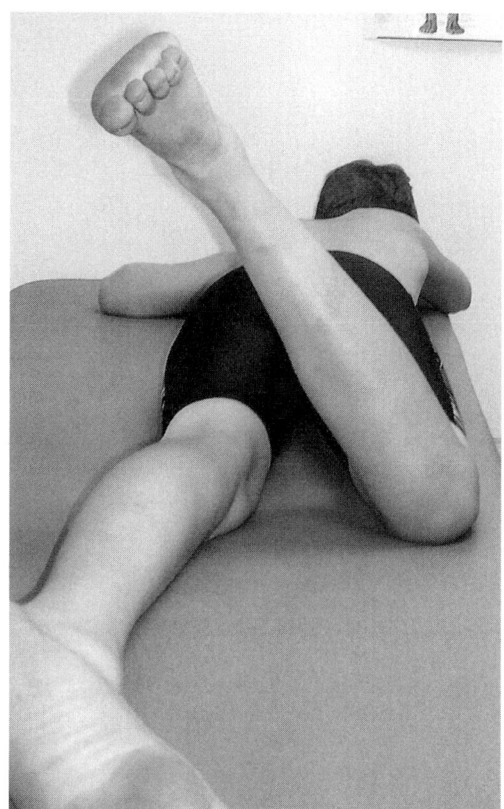

A

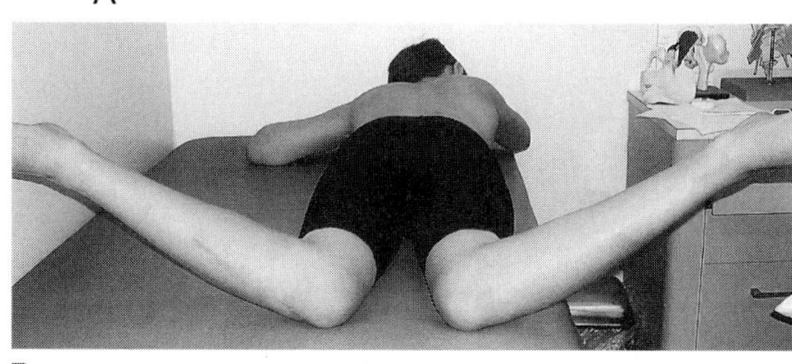

B

Figure 2–16: The prone position allows the knees to be flexed and the lower leg to be used as a goniometer to assess the amount of internal (A) and external (B) rotation at the hip in the extended position.

- The hip is innervated by both the obturator and the femoral nerves, which also supply sensation to the anterior and medial thigh and knee. Referred pain to the knee from the hip is not an uncommon presentation for slipped capital femoral epiphysis.
- Thigh circumference asymmetry can sometimes indicate occult hip pathology such as Perthes disease.
- The examiner should document both the active and the passive ranges of motion of the knee (Figure 2–18).
- Where are the areas of maximal tenderness?
- Popliteal cysts when present can usually be felt quite easily in the posterior aspect of the knee.
- With the patient supine, evaluate the presence or absence of an effusion. Is there a ballottable patella?

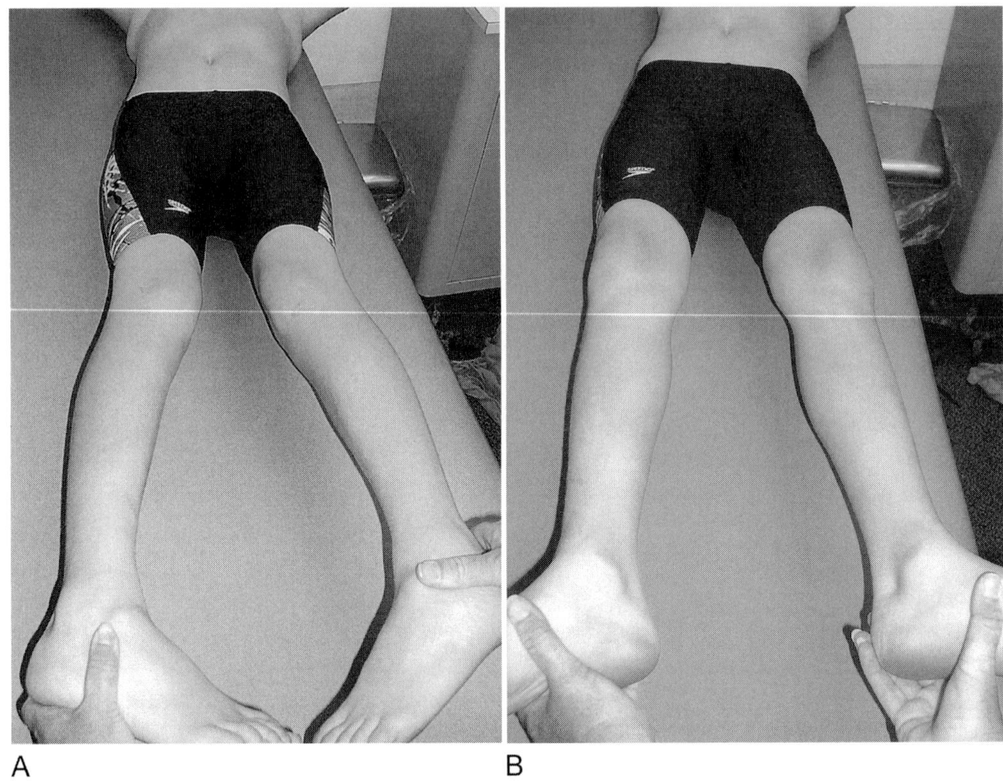

Figure 2–17: Hip rotation in the extended position is evaluated with the patient supine by using the patella as the indicator of maximal internal (A) and external (B) rotation.

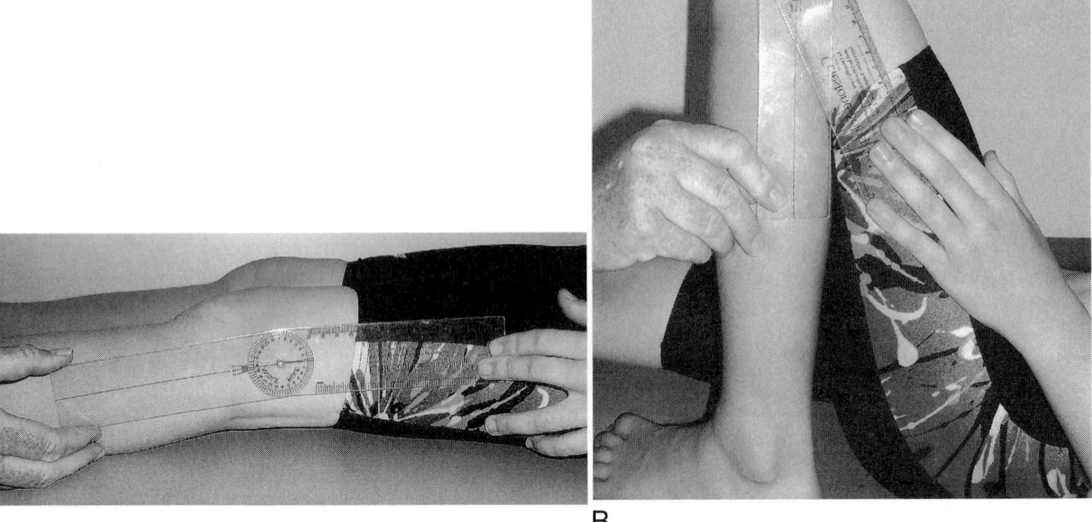

Figure 2–18: The knee should range from full extension (0 degrees, A) to 135 degrees of flexion (B).

- Evaluate the position of the patella and whether there is any tenderness at the superior or inferior pole of the patella (Sinding-Larsen-Johansson condition versus quadriceps tendonitis).
- Attempt to translate the patella in the medial and lateral directions and watch for any discomfort (positive apprehension sign).
- Palpate directly the tibial tubercle for any sign of tenderness (Osgood-Schlatter syndrome).
- Palpate the medial and lateral joint lines to evaluate any potential tenderness and the possibility of meniscal injuries (Box 2–8).
- Perform the Lachman and anterior drawer tests and compare the results with the stability of the opposite extremity[6] (Figure 2–19).
- Abnormal anterior laxity in the face of trauma can represent a tibial spine avulsion, an anterior cruciate ligament injury, or an epiphyseal plate injury in the skeletally immature child.
- Gentle varus and valgus stress can be applied in the face of trauma to evaluate the integrity of the medial and lateral collateral ligaments. Caution should be exercised in the immature child because an epiphyseal plate fracture can simulate an injury to the medial and lateral collateral ligaments in an adult.

Ankle and Foot

- Ankle range of motion is determined using the tibia as a reference with the neutral position defined as the lateral border of the foot perpendicular to the axis of the tibia.
- Ankle motion should be evaluated both actively and passively with the knee both flexed and extended.
- Supination of the foot can lock the hindfoot and allow isolated evaluation of passive ankle dorsiflexion.
- Flexibility of the midfoot can sometimes mislead an examiner into believing there is more dorsiflexion at the ankle than is truly there.
- Inversion and eversion of the hindfoot occurs primarily through the subtalar joint[7] (Figure 2–20).

Neurological Examination

- The neurological examination is an important part of any orthopaedic evaluation regardless of whether the child is a newborn or adolescent.

Box 2–8 Pathological Knee Diagnosis Based on Tenderness

Tibial tubercle—Osgood-Schlatter disease
Inferior pole patella—Patellar tendonitis (Sinding-Larsen-Johansson)
Superior pole patella—Quadriceps tendonitis
Medial or lateral joint line—Possible meniscal injury

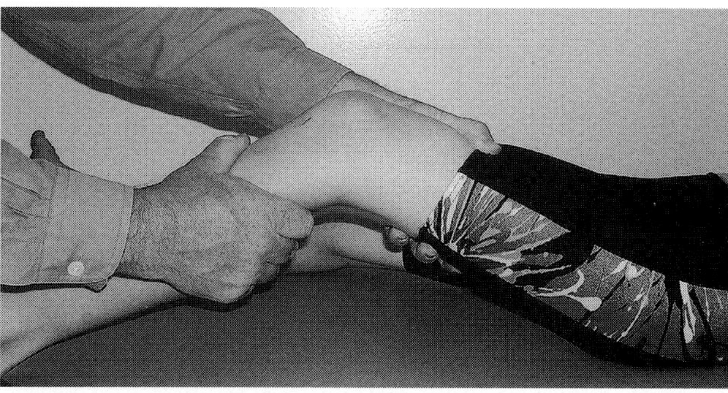

A

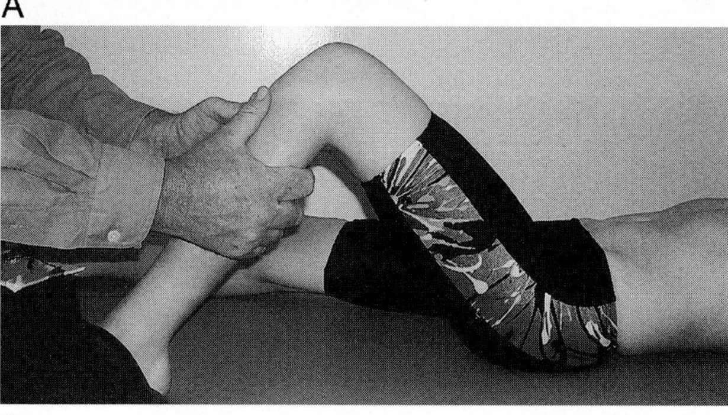

B

Figure 2–19: **The Lachman test is performed with the knee flexed 25-30 degrees, and the tibia is translated anteriorly (A). The anterior drawer test is performed with the knee flexed 90 degrees; again, the tibia is translated anteriorly in relation to the femoral condyles (B).**

- In the face of trauma, the neurological examination helps to determine the extent of the soft tissue component of the injury and the function of the neurological elements distal to the level of the injury.
- For developmental abnormalities, assessment of neurological function helps to better determine the appropriate level of function for a child of a particular age.
- Neurological assessment should include the evaluation of muscle strength, reflexes, muscle tone, sensation, and—in the infant—developmental milestones[8] (Box 2–9).
- The examiner must determine whether the weakness is diffuse or localized.
- Localized weakness may involve a single muscle group or a group of muscles similarly innervated (isolated nerve or spinal cord level).
- Diffuse weakness can involve an entire limb (monoplegia), lower limbs (diplegia), the right or left half of the body (hemiplegia), or all four extremities (quadriplegia).
- Absence of motor function in the lower limbs is usually termed *paraplegia*.
- Motor innervation is determined by the cerebral cortex, the corticospinal tracts of the spinal cord, individual segmental nerve roots, and the peripheral nerves.

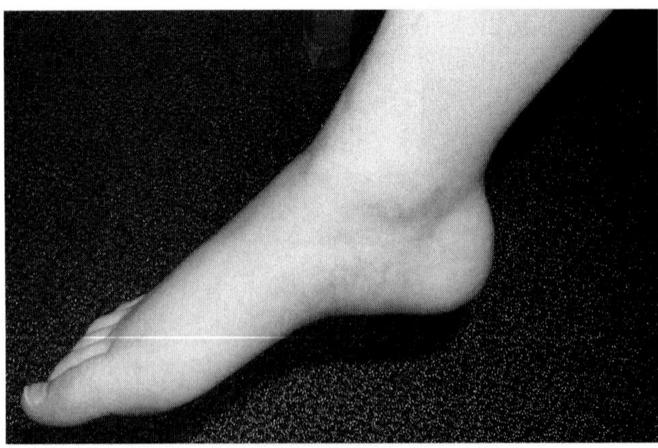

A

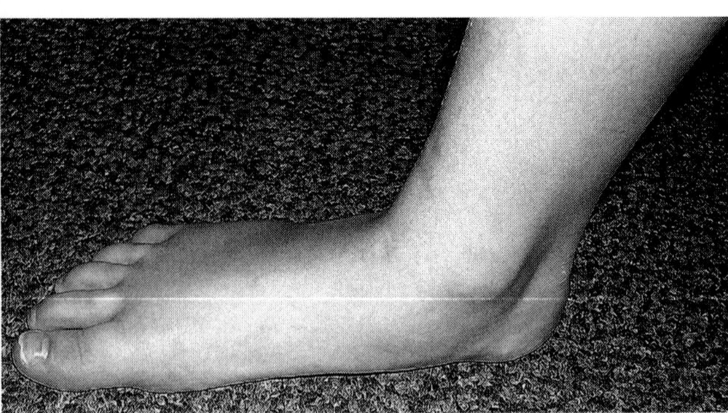

B

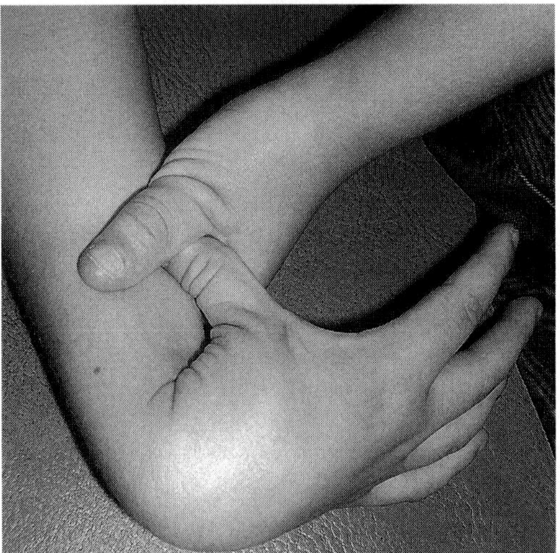

C

Figure 2–20: The appearance of the foot should be evaluated in the weight-bearing and non–weight-bearing modes. **Young children will often have a normal-appearing arch in the non–weight-bearing position (A) and develop a flat foot appearance when weight bearing (B). The examiner can also ask the child to stand on tiptoe and can observe the appearance of the arch that will develop in a flexible foot. These children will often demonstrate other evidence of ligamentous laxity (C).**

- Physical examination can help to determine the level of abnormality regardless of whether it is peripheral or central (Table 2–2).

Deep Tendon Reflexes

- Deep tendon reflexes in the infant can be variable.
- Depending on the development of the corticospinal tracts, they can be present or absent.
- The most commonly performed examinations include the biceps, triceps, patellar tendon, and Achilles reflexes.

Box 2–9 Clinical Muscle Grading

0—No active contraction
1—Trace contraction
2—Active motion without gravity
3—Active motion against gravity
4—Active motion against gravity and resistance
5—Normal strength against resistance

According to Lovett RW, Martin EG (1916) Certain aspects of infantile paralysis, with a description of a method of muscle testing. JAMA 66: 729.

- Ankle clonus (alternating contraction and relaxation of the gastroc–soleus) can also be tested by quickly dorsiflexing the infant's ankle with the hip and knee flexed. Sustained clonus is often a sign of neurological abnormality requiring further testing.

Developmental Reflexes

- Developmental reflexes in the newborn can be normal.
- As neurological maturation occurs, the developing cortex will often inhibit the rudimentary reflexes present at birth.
- Absence or persistence of these reflexes can sometimes indicate an underlying neurological abnormality.

Palmar Grasp Reflex

- Palmar grasp is normally present in infants up to 4 months.
- Palmar grasp can be elicited by stimulation of the palmar aspect of the hand on the ulnar side and will result in flexion of the fingers around the object grasped (Figure 2–21).
- There will also be synergistic flexion of the other muscles in the upper extremity.

Table 2–2: Motor Innervation

MUSCLE	NERVE	SPINAL CORD LEVEL
UPPER EXTREMITY		
Deltoid	Axillary	C5
Coracobrachialis	Musculocutaneous	C5, C6
Teres major	Lower subscapular	C5, C6
Supraspinatus	Suprascapular	C5, C6
Pectoralis major	Medial or lateral anterior thoracic	C5, C6, C7, C8, T1
Latissimus dorsi	Thoracodorsal	C6, C7, C8
Infraspinatus	Suprascapular	C5, C6
Teres minor	Axillary	C5
Trapezius	Spinal accessory	Cranial 11
Rhomboid major or minor	Dorsal scapular	C5
Serratus anterior	Long thoracic	C5, C6, C7
Brachialis	Musculocutaneous	C5, C6
Biceps	Musculocutaneous	C5, C6
Triceps	Radial	C7
Extensor carpi radialis or ulnaris	Radial	C6, C7
Flexor carpi radialis	Median	C7
Flexor carpi ulnaris	Ulnar	C8-T1
Finger extensors	Radial	C7
Flexor digitorum profundus (radial 2)	Anterior interosseous branch–median	C6, C7, T1
Flexor digitorum profundus (ulnar 2)	Ulnar	C8, T1
Lumbricals (radial 2)	Median	C7
Lumbricals (ulnar 2)	Ulnar	C8
Dorsal interosseous	Ulnar	C8, T1
Abductor digiti minimi	Ulnar	C8, T1
Palmar interosseous	Ulnar	C8, T1
Extensor pollicis brevis	Radial	C7
Extensor pollicis longus	Radial	C7
Flexor pollicis brevis (medial)	Ulnar	C8
Flexor pollicis brevis (lateral)	Median	C6, C7
Flexor pollicis longus	Anterior interosseous branch–median	C8, T1
Abductor pollicis longus	Radial	C7
Abductor pollicis brevis	Median	C6, C7
Adductor pollicis	Ulnar	C8
Opponens pollicis	Median	C6, C7
Opponens digiti minimi	Ulnar	C8
LOWER EXTREMITY		
MUSCLE	**NERVE**	**SPINAL CORD LEVEL**
Iliopsoas	Femoral	L1, L2, L3
Gluteus maximus	Inferior gluteal	S1
Gluteus medius	Superior gluteal	L5
Adductor longus	Obturator	L2, L3, L4
Quadriceps	Femoral	L2, L3, L4
Semimembranosus	Tibial portion sciatic	L5
Semitendinosus	Tibial portion sciatic	L5
Biceps femoris	Tibial portion sciatic	S1
Tibialis anterior	Deep peroneal	L4
Extensor hallucis	Deep peroneal	L5
Extensor digitorum longus	Deep peroneal	L5
Gastrocnemius–soleus	Tibial	S1, S2
Flexor hallucis longus	Tibial	L5
Flexor digitorum longus	Tibial	L5
Tibialis posterior	Tibial	L5

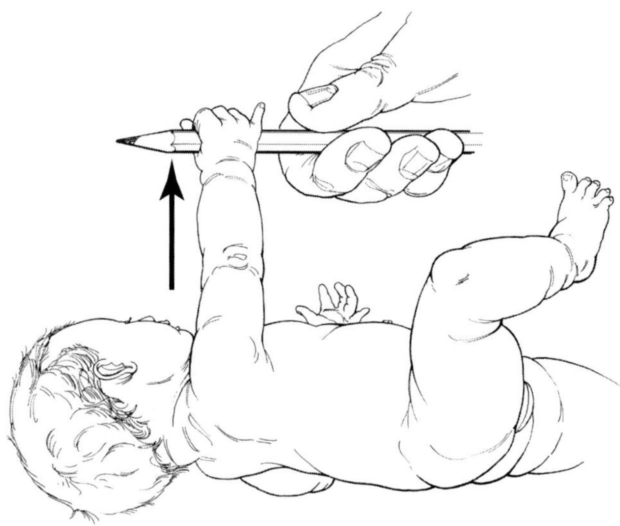

Figure 2–21: Palmar grasp reflex in an infant.

- Asymmetry of this reflex may indicate hypertonicity, such as in spastic hemiplegia. Absence of this reflex may indicate flaccid paralysis, such as in brachial plexus palsy. Continued presence of the palmar grasp reflex in infants beyond 4 months may indicate hypertonicity, possibly associated with cerebral palsy.

Startle Reflex

- The startle reflex is elicited with a loud noise or percussion on the infant's sternum.
- Stimulation causes a flexion of the infant's knees and of the elbow with a clenched fist.
- The startle reflex appears at birth and remains throughout life. Absence of the startle reflex suggests the possibility of significant weakness; asymmetry may suggest brachial plexus paralysis.

Stepping Reflex

- The stepping reflex is normally present in children at birth and usually disappears by 2 months.
- The reflex is elicited by suspending the infant beneath the arms, allowing the feet to gently touch the examination table, and leaning the child forward.
- The child will initiate an alternating flexion and extension of the lower limbs, which appears to be a walking behavior (Figure 2–22).
- Continued presence of this stepping reflex beyond 4 months suggests the possibility of neurological impairment.

Parachute Reaction

- The parachute reaction usually becomes present by 6 months and continues throughout life.
- The parachute reaction is initiated by supporting the patient at the waist in the prone position. The child is then moved toward the floor, simulating a drop. A positive

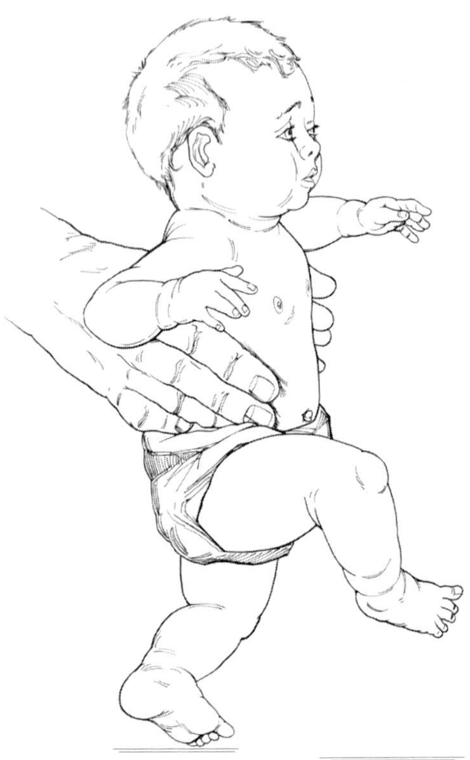

Figure 2–22: Stepping reflex.

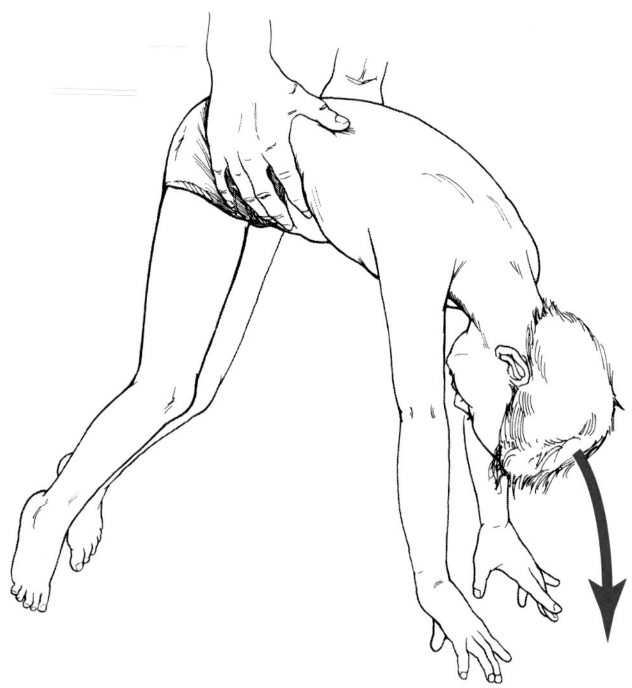

Figure 2–23: Parachute reaction.

response has the arms extended in a protected position (Figure 2–23).

- A parachute reaction does not depend on vision and can be elicited in children who are blind or who are blindfolded.
- Failure to develop this reflex suggests severe neurological impairment.

Symmetrical Tonic Neck Reflex

- The symmetrical tonic neck reflex is performed with the child prone and supported by the torso.
- The child's head is then extended. The upper extremities will extend and the lower extremities will flex. When the head is flexed, the upper limbs will flex and the lower limbs will extend (Figure 2–24).
- The symmetrical tonic neck reflex usually appears by 8 months. Failure to demonstrate this reflex suggests that the child will be unable to kneel or crawl.
- This reflex often diminishes by 14 months, and persistence of this reflex can make it difficult to develop the alternating limb motion needed for crawling.

Asymmetrical Tonic Neck Reflex

- The asymmetrical tonic neck reflex is usually present at birth and disappears by 6 months.
- The reflex is elicited by rotating the head, holding the rotated position of the head for 5-10 seconds, then rotating it to the opposite side (Figure 2–25).

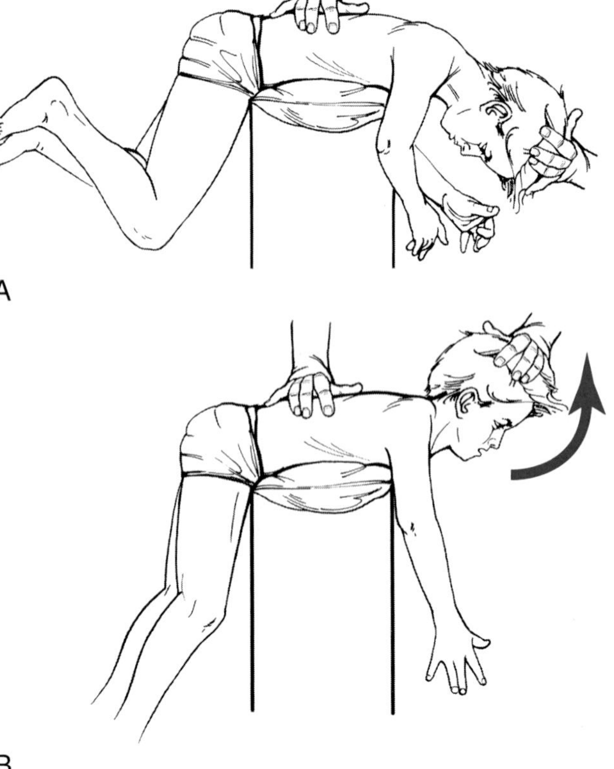

Figure 2–24: Symmetrical tonic neck reflex.

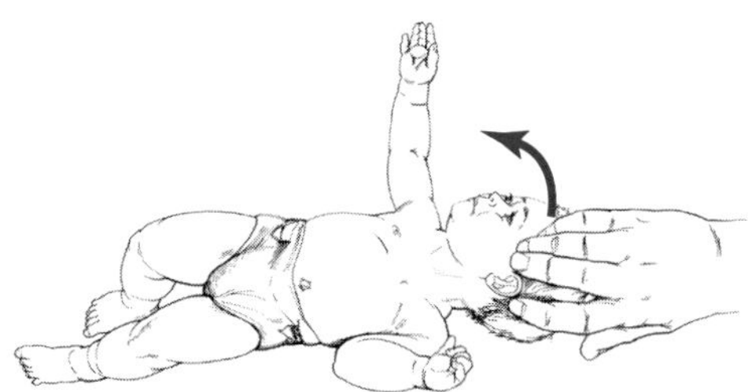

Figure 2–25: Asymmetrical tonic neck reflex.

- A positive response is one in which the infant's arm extends on the side to which the chin is turned, with knee flexion on the same side. Occasionally, the arm on the opposite side will go into flexion, simulating a fencer's position.
- The reflex may persist or become more severe in individuals with cerebral palsy.

Babinski Reflex

- A normal Babinski reflex is elicited by stimulating the plantar lateral aspect of the foot. A normal response is one in which the ankle dorsiflexes in a withdrawal maneuver but the toes flex (Figure 2–26).
- An abnormal response is one in which the great toe withdraws in a slow, hyperextended position.
- Persistence of the Babinski reflex may persist in infants, sometimes up to 2 years.
- A positive Babinski sign in an older child suggests an upper motor neuron abnormality.

Abdominal Reflexes

- Abdominal reflexes are normal in the older child and are elicited by gently stroking the abdomen from lateral to medial toward the umbilicus.
- An abnormal response is usually asymmetrical and may suggest an intraspinal abnormality, such as syringomyelia.
- Abdominal reflexes should be evaluated in all children being seen for scoliosis regardless of whether they are infantile, juvenile, or adolescent.

Sensation

- Sensation in the infant can sometimes be difficult to evaluate.

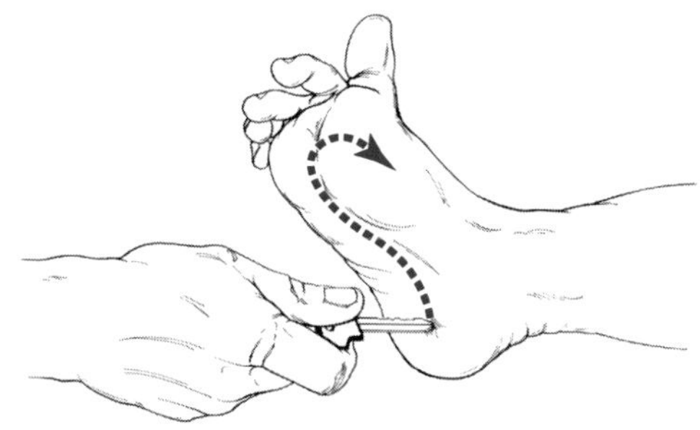

Figure 2–26: Positive (abnormal) Babinski reflex.

- Withdrawal in an infant from a noxious stimulus will help to establish pain and temperature pathways in the lateral spinothalamic tracts and to establish an intact motor response.
- As the child matures and is able to cooperate with an examination, sensation to light touch and symmetry of examination becomes easier to accomplish.
- Sensation follows predictable dermatomal patterns.

Gait and Gait Analysis

Introduction

- The fundamental goal of normal gait is to move safely and efficiently from one point to another.
- Instrumented gait analysis has become the gold standard for the evaluation of any abnormalities in gait patterns so that an effective treatment plan can be formulated and the appropriate surgery is performed.[9]
- Children typically begin walking between 12 and 16 months.[10]
- Children do not develop sufficient abductor strength until 30 to 36 months to maintain single leg stance for long periods.[10]
- A short stride length, a fast cadence with a slow velocity, and a wide base stance characterize early ambulation.
- A mature gait develops by 7 years.
  - Velocity is normally 114 cm/sec with 143 steps/min at this age.[9]
- Walking speed is usually the speed at which the energy cost per unit of distance is minimized.
- Regardless of the abnormality of gait, the energy expenditure per minute remains the same. A decrease in the speed of ambulation is the most common method of maintaining constant energy expenditure. The result is a shorter distance in which the body is propelled in the same period compared with a normal gait.[11]

Gait Cycle

- The *gait cycle* is a single sequence of functions by one limb (Figure 2–27).
- Definitions[12]
  - *Cadence*—Number of steps per minute
  - *Step period*—Time measured from an event in one foot to the same event in the opposite foot
  - *Step length*—Distance covered during one step (typically heel strike to opposite foot heel strike)
  - *Stride period*—Time from heel strike of one foot to the next heel strike of the same foot and composed of two sequential steps
  - *Stride length*—Distance covered during one stride (typically heel strike to same-foot heel strike); thus, each stride length comprises one right and one left step length

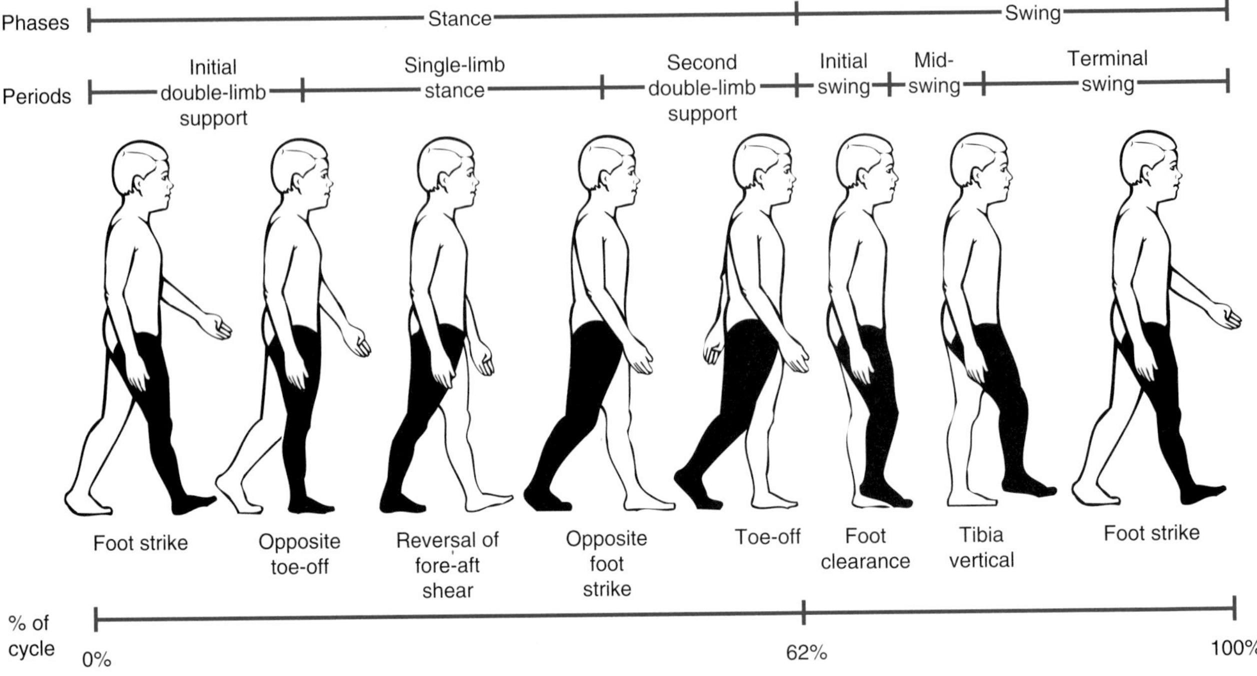

Figure 2–27: Normal gait cycle of an adult and all of its components.

- Each gait cycle has two components[12]:
  - Stance phase—Duration of foot contact with the ground
  - *Swing phase*—Time during which the foot is in the air for limb advancement
- The stance phase comprises 60% of the gait cycle and is divided into three periods. It begins with a heel strike and ends with the toe off of the same limb.
  1. Initial double limb support or initial contact
  2. Single limb stance
  3. Second double limb support or preswing
- The swing phase comprises 40% of the gait cycle and is divided into three periods. It begins with the toe off and ends with a heel strike of the same limb.
  1. Initial swing
  2. Midswing
  3. Terminal swing
- As speed increases and the patient begins to run, a double float phase is added to the cycle and the total stance and swing times decrease.
- To maintain a normal gait, the central cerebral control and the end muscles must all work correctly and in a coordinated fashion. Any central or muscular aberration can lead to a pathological gait.
- Hip abductors control tilt in the swing phase. Thus, when the right leg is in the swing phase, the left abductors must function correctly to keep the pelvis level while the right side is unsupported.
- The low point of the center of gravity is during double limb support, and the high point occurs at midstance.
- The average total displacement of the center of gravity during a stride is less than 5 cm in both the horizontal and the vertical planes. This combined vertical and horizontal motion describes a double sinusoidal curve. Impaired gait patterns increase excursion and decrease energy efficiency.
- Leg clearance requires coordinated events and can be altered significantly in the disabled child because of muscle imbalances.
- Lifting the foot for clearance requires knee flexion during the preswing phase, hip and knee flexion during midswing, and ankle dorsiflexion in late swing phase. This shortens the swing leg to allow adequate clearance.
- The stance leg also ensures limb clearance of the swing leg by elevating the center of gravity with midstance ankle dorsiflexion and knee extension and with terminal stance ankle plantar flexion.

Prerequisites for Normal Gait

- Described by Perry[13]
  - Stability of the weight-bearing foot throughout the stance phase
  - Clearance of the non–weight-bearing foot during the swing phase
  - Appropriate prepositioning during the terminal swing of the foot for the next gait cycle
  - Adequate step length
  - Energy conservation (added by Gage[14])

Motion Analysis Laboratory

- Simple observation is helpful and should always be the first step.
- It is often necessary to ask the child and parents to walk down the hallway.
- The physician should observe the child's gait pattern and document a rotational profile (Table 2–3).
- The rotational profile includes the foot-progression angle, the internal rotation of the hips, the external rotation of the hips, the thigh–foot angle, and any foot deformities.
- The *foot-progression angle* is a comparison of an imaginary line drawn on the floor with the axis of the foot. The foot axis is a straight line that connects the center of the second metatarsal head with the center of the heel. This angle measures the degree of intoeing or outtoeing compared with an imaginary straight line drawn on the floor[15] (Figure 2–28).
- The normal foot-progression angle in children from 1 to 4 years varies between 40 degrees of internal rotation to 40 degrees of external rotation.
- Hip rotation measures the internal or the external femoral *version* or any torsional deformity of the femur.
- The thigh–foot angle compares the axis of the foot with the axis of the thigh and is measured with the knee bent 90 degrees (Figure 2–29). This angle determines any degree of tibial version or torsional deformity.[16]
- An examination of the foot determines any deformities of the foot such as metatarsus adductus that may be contributing to intoeing or outtoeing.[16]
- The speed and complexity of gait combined with the many deviations and possible compensations limit the quantitative information that can be obtained through simple observation.
- The gait laboratory is used to measure kinetics and muscular activity to define the source of abnormalities so that a treatment plan can be formulated.
- There are three components of the quantitative gait analysis:
  - Electromyogram (EMG)—Analysis of muscle activity and identification of the period and relative intensity of muscle function[10]
  - Kinetics—Analysis of forces or loads that cause motion[9]
  - Kinematics—Temporal stride measures and motion analysis[9]

Table 2–3: Recording Basic Elements of Observational Analysis

	RIGHT	LEFT
Foot-progression angle		
Hip medial rotation		
Hip lateral rotation		
Thigh–foot angle		
Foot		

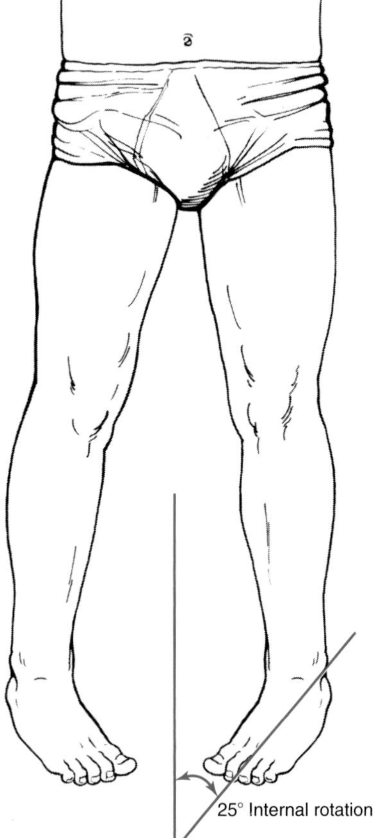

Figure 2–28: Measuring the foot-progression angle of a child.

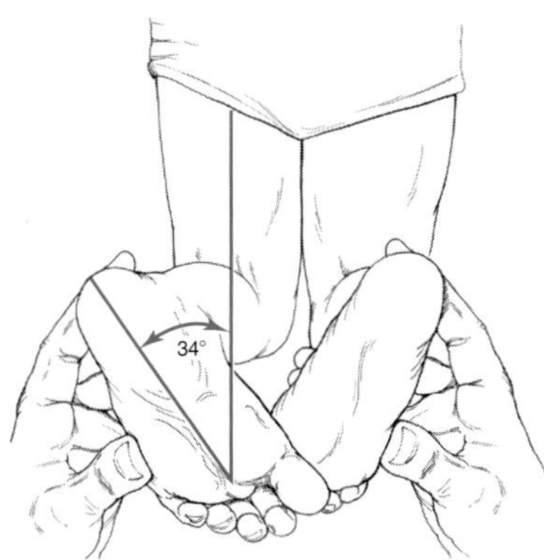

Figure 2–29: Thigh–foot angle in a child.

- EMG provides information about the timing, duration, and relative strength of muscle activation. This information is used to identify a muscle causing an aberrant movement.
- Surface electrodes can be taped to the skin for superficial muscles such as the adductors or gastrocnemius–soleus complex. Indwelling fine-wire electrodes are inserted through a hypodermic needle for deep muscles such as the tibialis posterior or flexor digitorum profundus.

- Kinetics is studied with the use of foot plates to determine the ground reaction forces. Foot plates measure a vector force of all the components acting at a focal point.
- Foot plates measure vertical and shear forces in the anterior–posterior and medial–lateral planes. *Vertical force* is similar to body weight measured on a scale. Anterior–posterior *shear* is the push against the floor that allows propulsion. There are similar shear forces in the medial–lateral plane.
- The three forces comprise the *total force*.
- Two foot plates are arranged adjacent to each other so that both legs can be recorded. Ultrathin Mylar pressure sensors can also be placed in the shoes so that the patient does not have to step on prearranged foot plates.
- The reaction forces are plotted as a function of time and reported as a percentage of body mass. This is compared with standard values.

Box 2–10 Common Deviations of Gait

Equinus Gait, Toe Walking

- Excessive ankle plantar flexion
  - Cerebral palsy (Gastroc–soleus spasticity)
  - Clubfoot
  - Idiopathic tight Achilles tendon
  - Muscle diseases (e.g., Duchenne muscular dystrophy)
  - Post-traumatic (e.g., compartment syndrome)
  - Limb-length inequality

Calcaneus Foot

- Excessive ankle dorsiflexion
  - Low lumbar myelodysplasia
  - Overlengthening of the heel cord in cerebral palsy
  - Compensation for forefoot pain

Steppage Gait

- Increased knee flexion to facilitate limb clearance
  - Cerebral palsy (hamstring spasticity)
  - Myelodysplasia (Gastroc–soleus weakness)
  - Charcot-Marie-Tooth disease (weak tibialis anterior)
  - Friedreich ataxia

Circumduction or Vaulting Gait

- Excessive abduction of the hip with increased pelvic rotation and upward pelvic obliquity
- Limb-length discrepancy to clear long limb
- Cerebral palsy (abductor spasticity)
- Scoliosis with pelvic obliquity
- Any cause of ankle or knee stiffness

Trendelenburg Gait

- Contralateral pelvic drop during stance phase
  - Cerebral palsy (adductor spasticity)
  - Legg-Calve'-Perthes disease
  - Developmental dysplasia of the hip
  - Slipped capital femoral epiphysis
  - Muscle disease

- The information in the report is used to evaluate the dynamic basis for an observed gait deviation. It can be used to select surgical intervention, guide a gait retraining program, select an appropriate brace treatment or assistive device, or choose a combination of these actions (Box 2–10).
- Repeat analysis should always be performed to assess the effectiveness of intervention and to guide the postoperative rehabilitation.[17]

References

1. Wenger DR, Rang M (1993) The Principles and Practice of Children's Orthopaedics. New York: Raven Press.

2. Greene WB, Heckman JD (1994) The Clinical Measurement of Joint. Rosemont, IL: American Academy of Orthopaedic Surgeons.

3. Hoppenfeld S (1976) Physical Examination of the Spine and Extremities. New York: Appleton-Century-Crofts.

4. Green DP, Hotchkiss RN, Pederson WC (1999) Green's Operative Hand Surgery. New York: Churchill Livingstone.

5. Staheli LT (1977) The prone hip extension test: A method of measuring hip flexion deformity. Clin Orthop Rel Res 123: 12-15.

   This is a description of an alternative method of evaluating the amount of hip flexion contracture in children.

6. Fu FH, Harner CD, Vince KG (1994) Knee Surgery. Baltimore: William and Wilkins.

7. Mann RA (1992) Principles of Examination of the Foot and Ankle. St. Louis: CV Mosby.

8. Lovett RW, Martin EG (1916) Certain aspects of infantile paralysis, with a description of a method of muscle testing. JAMA 66: 729.

   This classic article describes a now well-accepted way of grading muscle strength.

9. Sutherland DH, Olshen R, Cooper L, Woo SLY (1980) The development of mature gait. J Bone Joint Surg Am 62: 336-353.

   This observational paper determined the changes that occur in the gait cycle and the milestones achieved as the child grows.

10. Chambers HG, Sutherland DH (2002). A practical guide to gait analysis. JAAOS 10: 222-231.

    This article gives an overview of the components of the gait cycle and a detailed description of gait analysis, including the motion analysis laboratory.

11. Cotes J, Meade F (1960) The energy expenditure and mechanical energy demand in walking. Ergonomics 3: 97-119.

    Energy expenditure during normal and abnormal walking was determined by measuring the oxygen and carbon dioxide exhaled in a kinesiology laboratory.

12. Inman VT, Ralston HJ, Todd F (1981) Human Walking. Baltimore: Williams & Wilkins.

This textbook is an overview of all aspects of the human gait and defined many of the terms used to describe the gait cycle. It also describes the use of EMG to record multiple muscle group activity during ambulation.

13. Perry J, ed (1992) Gait Analysis: Normal and Pathological Function. Thorofare, NJ: SLACK.
    This textbook summarizes the process of gait analysis and defined the four prerequisites of normal human gait.
14. Gage JR, DeLuca PA, Renshaw TS (1995) Gait analysis: Principles and applications with emphasis on its use in cerebral palsy. J Bone Joint Surg Am 77: 1607-1623.
    This instructional course lecture gives an overview of kinetics and kinematics and their measurement in the gait analysis laboratory. The information is specifically applied to children with cerebral palsy.
15. Yngve D (1990) Foot-progression angle in clubfeet. J Pediatr Orthop 10: 467.
    A case-control study of 52 clubfeet treated by surgical release compared with 43 age-matched controls showed 13 degrees of inturning from the normal mean of 8 degrees.
16. Staheli LT, Corbett M, Wyss C, King H (1985) Lower-extremity rotational problems in children: Normal values to guide management. J Bone Joint Surg Am 67: 39.
    For this study, 1000 normal lower extremities of children and adults were examined to establish the normal values of the rotational profile of the lower extremity.
17. Kay RM, Dennis S, Rethlefsen S, Reynolds RA, Skaggs DL, Tolo VT (2000) The effect of preoperative gait analysis on orthopaedic decision making. Clin Orthop 20: 210-216.
    The average number of surgical procedures performed was reduced by 1.5 per patient as a result of preoperative gait analysis. Of 70 patients who had preoperative treatment plans, 62 plans were changed as a result of the preoperative gait analysis.

Bibliography

Gage JR (1990) An overview of normal walking. In: Instructional Course Lectures XXXIX (Greene WB, ed). Park Ridge, IL: American Academy of Orthopaedic Surgeons, pp 291-303.

Herring JA, ed (2002) Tachdjian's Pediatric Orthopaedics, 3rd edition. Philadelphia: WB Saunders Company.

Iida H, Yamamuro T (1987) Kinetic analysis of the center of gravity of the human body in normal and pathological gaits. J Biomech 20: 987-995.

Inman VT, Ralston HJ, Todd F, eds (1981) Human Walking. Baltimore: Williams & Wilkins.

Lamoreux LW (1971) Kinematic measurements in the study of human walking. Bull Prosthet Res 10: 3-84.

Morrisey RT, Weinstein SL (1996) Lovell and Winter's Pediatric Orthopaedics, 4th edition. Philadelphia: Lippincott-Raven.

Murray MP, Drought AB, Kory RC (1964) Walking patterns of normal men. J Bone Joint Surg Am 46A(2): 335-360.

Perry J (1993) Determinants of muscle function in the spastic lower extremity. Clin Orthop 288: 10-26.

Saunders JB, Inman VT, Eberhart HD (1953) The major determinants in normal and pathological gait. J Bone Joint Surg Am 35: 543-558.

Staheli LT (1992) Fundamentals of Pediatric Orthopedics. New York: Raven Press.

Sutherland DH, ed (1984) Gait Disorders in Childhood and Adolescence. Baltimore: Williams & Wilkins.

Sutherland DH, Kaufman KR, Moitoza JR (1994) Kinematics of normal human walking. In: Human Walking, 2nd edition (Rose J, Gamble JG, eds). Baltimore, MD: Williams & Wilkins, pp 23-44.

Wenger DR, Rang M (1993) The Principles and Practice of Children's Orthopaedics. New York: Raven Press.

Introduction to Trauma

Paul D. Sponseller

MD, MBA, Professor of Orthopaedic Surgery, Johns Hopkins University, Baltimore, MD;
Chief, Division of Pediatric Orthopaedics, Johns Hopkins Medical Institutions, Baltimore, MD

Trauma in children is distinguished from that in adults by differences in the following:

- Mechanisms of injury—The ones more common in children include the following:
  - Pedestrian struck by vehicle
  - Falls from low heights
  - Nonaccidental injury in infants or toddlers
  - Power-implement injuries in preschool ages
  - Vehicle operators and falls from heights in teens
- Fracture patterns (greenstick, buckle, and physeal injuries)
- Multiple acceptable treatment options in some cases
  - Femur fractures do well after traction, spica, external fixator, flexible nails, and plates
  - Forearm fractures do well with cast, plates, and intramedullary rods
  - Age-based guidelines for some injuries (e.g., femoral shaft fractures)
- Associated system injuries (described later)
- Mortality in pediatric polytrauma—Less than 3% overall
- Residual morbidity—Mainly related to head injury or growth disturbance

This chapter will expand upon those themes and provide examples. Further chapters will describe specific fracture management.

Principles of Pediatric Fractures

Altered Fracture Patterns

- Physeal or metaphyseal bone is the most likely site of failure.
- Ligaments and other factors protect some physes.
  - The proximal tibial physis is protected by collateral ligaments and fibula; it is rarely injured.
  - The distal femoral physis is four times more likely than the proximal tibial physis to fracture.
- Ligamentous disruption is less likely than in adults.
  - Anterior cruciate ligament, medial collateral ligament, and elbow dislocations rare but occasionally occur
  - Shoulder dislocations rare under age 14
  - Knee dislocations virtually never before physeal closure
  - Vertical shear pelvis fractures rare before teens
- Bone is less brittle; it absorbs more energy before a fracture.

In Compression

- The torus (buckle) fracture is unique to children (Figure 3–1).
- Fracture does not propagate through the entire bone.
- Bone is stable to limited use; diagnosis may be delayed.
- Comminution is less extensive than in mature patients for a given injury.

In Tension or Torsion

- Plastic deformation sometimes occurs without visible fracture (Figure 3–2).
- *Greenstick* pattern provides an intact cortex and periosteal sleeve.
- Closed reduction is more feasible because of these factors.
- Undisplaced fractures are more common (Figure 3–3).

Transitional Fracture Patterns

- As physis is partially closing, changes pattern of failure
  - Tillaux fracture of distal tibia

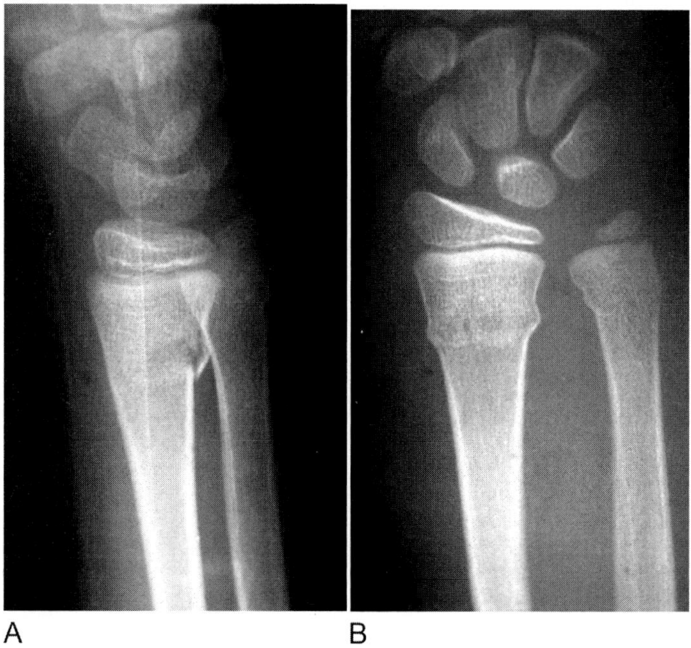

Figure 3–1: Buckle fracture is a partial failure in compression. A, Lateral view. B, Anteroposterior view.

- Anteromedial physis closes first
- Triplane fracture (Figure 3–4)
- Type III tibial tubercle avulsion

Soft Tissue Factors

- Stiffness less of a problem
  - OK to immobilize joints in casts 6 weeks, if needed
  - Less need for physical therapy
- Coverage by granulation rapid
  - Less need for flap coverage
- Slightly lower infection rate after open fractures

Remodeling

- Much more pronounced than in adults (Figure 3–5)
  - Approximately 10 degrees per year in the average metaphysis
- Proportional to growth in a region
  - Example—Slow in the supracondylar region of the humerus
- Least in the torsional plane
- Angulation most evident in the midportion of a limb (knee or elbow)

Physeal Fractures

- Occur primarily through the zone of hypertrophy, but some variation exists
- Growth disturbance because of the following:
  - Damage to cells in the proliferative layer (may be invisible)[1]

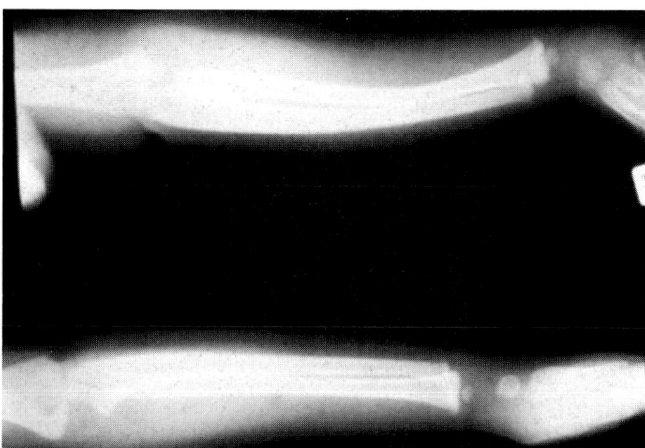

Figure 3–2: Plastic deformation is a microfailure in tension without a visible fracture line.

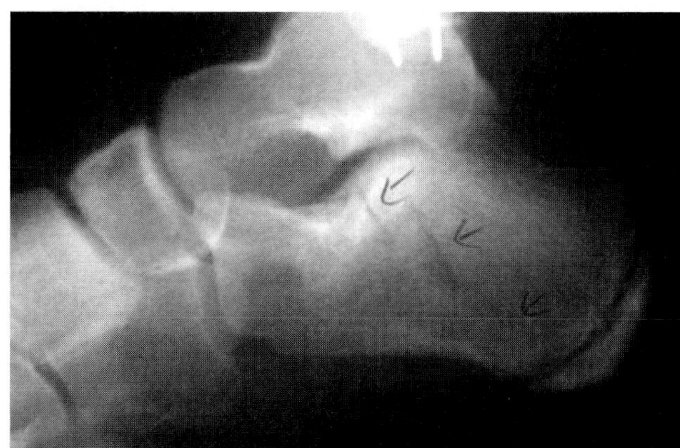

Figure 3–3: Undisplaced fractures are more common in children because of metaphyseal and periosteal properties.

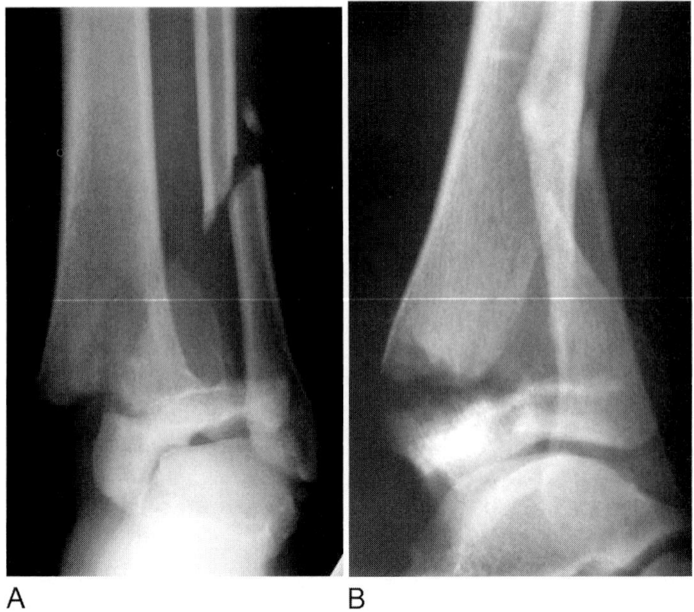

Figure 3–4: The triplane fracture is a transitional fracture, changing directions to propagate into the metaphysis where the physis has closed.

- Malalignment causing bar formation
  a. Gap
  b. Longitudinal offset

Areas Aided by Classification

- Prognosis for the following:
  - Growth disturbance
  - Articular incongruity
- Communication
- Decision making
  - Relative stability of fracture (II > III > IV)
  - Location of bone for fixation

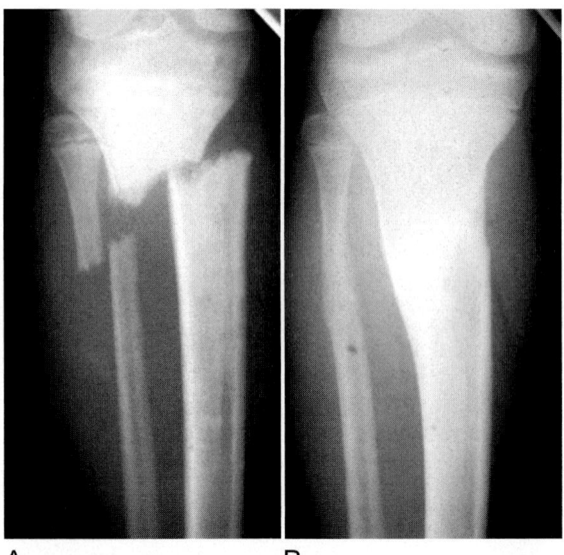

Figure 3–5: Remodeling in children is often extensive, such as in this proximal tibial fracture (A) seen 1 year later (B).

  - Operative versus nonoperative treatment (based on the preceding results)

Salter-Harris Classification

More details on the Salter-Harris classification are shown in Figure 3–6, *A*.

I. Through and parallel to the physis
II. Includes the metaphyseal triangle
   A. May be useful for fixation
   B. Junction is the common site for growth disturbance
III. Right angle through the physis and joint
   A. Semistable
IV. Vertical fracture perpendicular to the physis
   A. Low risk of bar if anatomically reduced
V. Crush of the physis
   A. Rarely seen

Peterson Classification[2]

- Shown in Figure 3–6, *B*
- Adds categories for the following:
  - Missing physis—Peripherally or centrally
  - Metaphyseal comminution reaching the physis
- Less commonly used than Salter-Harris

Accuracy of Classification in Predicting Growth Disturbance

- Varies with joint because of the unique anatomy of each physis and its stabilizers[1]
- Varies with degree of trauma
- Most predictive in the ankle
- Least predictive in the knee, even after anatomical reduction[1]

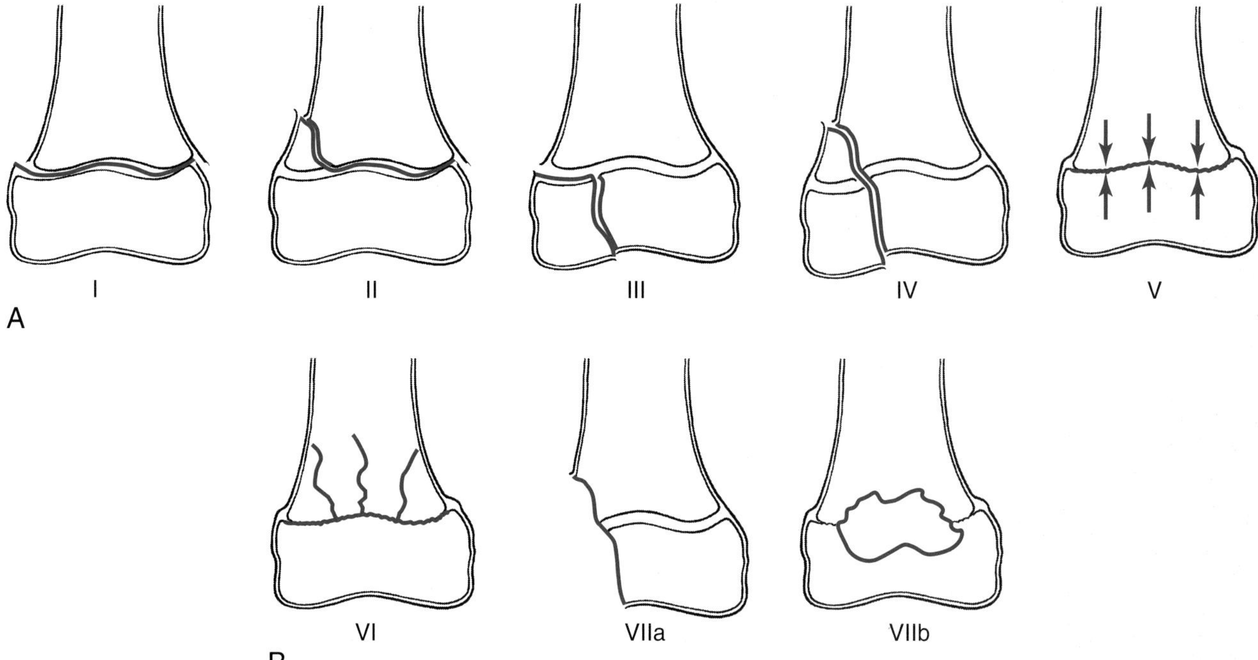

Figure 3–6: Classification of physeal fractures. A, Salter-Harris classification of physeal fractures, types I-V. B, Two additional types added by Peterson: Metaphyseal fractures extending to the physis and complete physeal absence, central or peripheral.

- Risk after Salter-Harris II greater than after Salter-Harris IV
- Because of crushing or unseen damage to the physis

Physeal Growth Disturbances

- Major "negative" in pediatric fractures
- First noted usually 6-9 months after injury[12]
  - Park–Harris lines (Figure 3–7)
- Follow-up rationale explained to parents
  - Most physeal fractures require a 6-month follow-up

Overgrowth after Fracture

- Occurs primarily in long bones, 2-10 years
  - 1-1.5 cm in femur over 18 months after the fracture; not related to the method of treatment
- Approximately 7 mm after a tibia fracture or a humerus fracture
- Compensates for shortening in the cast after the fracture

Epidemiology of Pediatric Trauma

Fracture rate varies with high-risk behaviors and environment.[3]

Behavioral or Individual Risk Factors

- Lower socioeconomic status
- Increased population density
- Single-parent families
- Maternal smoking
- Attention-deficit hyperactivity disorder
- Peak ages for fracture—6-9 years old
- Males > females

Environmental Risk Factors[4]

- Traffic[3]
- Crime (gunshot wounds in adults and children)

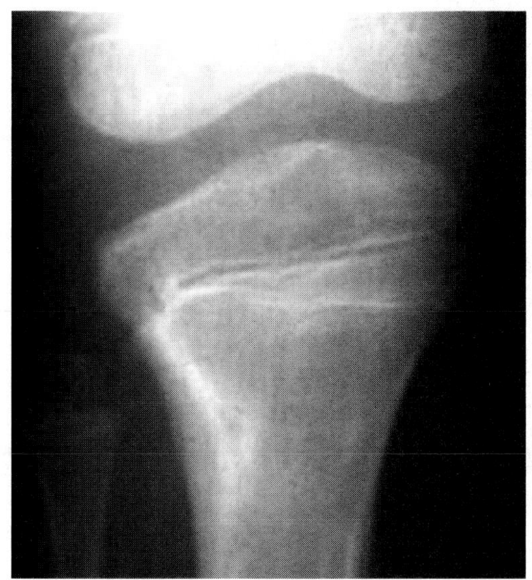

Figure 3–7: Growth arrest line at the knee.

- Poorly built playgrounds[5]
- Improper pediatric seating in a vehicle
- Specialized activities
  - Farming implements
  - Lawnmower

Activities Not Recommended by the American Academy of Pediatrics

- Trampoline use
  - Especially with more than one child at a time
- All-terrain vehicles or equivalents
  - Should not be used under 14-16 years
- Power implements or tools
  - Children should not be out of the yard under age 5
  - Should not operate under age 12

Principles of Polytrauma Management in Children

Physiological Factors

- Increased metabolic rate (twice that of an adult per unit of weight)
- Greater surface area-to-mass ratio—More risk of hypothermia
- Decreased blood volume—Critical traumatic blood loss not as apparent
- Inability to alter stroke volume as much—Risk of sudden arrest
- Tongue relatively larger—Risk of airway obstruction
- Short trachea—Increased risk of mainstem intubation

Determinants of Morbidity

- Head injury
- Intrathoracic injury
- Increased injury severity score (over 25)

Examination of Polytrauma Patient

- Primary survey—Remember your "ABCDEs"[6]
  - Airway (assure patency)
  - Breathing (chest wall movement and breath sounds)
  - Circulation (pulse, pressure, and capillary refill)
  - Disability
  - Exposure (take temperature and prevent hypothermia)
- Secondary survey
  - Detailed reexamination of all systems to detect non–life-threatening injury
  - Careful palpation of all regions; active range of motion of joints if able
  - Order appropriate diagnostic tests
  - Obtunded patient (order x-rays of the entire spine, chest, abdomen, and pelvis)
  - Skull films if large laceration, hematoma, or tenderness
  - Abdominal computerized tomography (CT) scan if blunt trauma
- Repeat physical examination as patient recovers to rule out missed skeletal injury

Head Injury

- Primary determinant of morbidity after pediatric trauma[7]
- Cerebral perfusion pressure
  - Mean arterial pressure minus intracranial pressure
  - Should be greater than 60 mm Hg
- Factors that increase intracranial pressure
  - Inhalational anesthetics
  - Ketamine
- Factors that decrease intracranial pressure
  - Hyperventilation
  - Mannitol
  - Barbiturates
- Glasgow coma score (GCS, Table 3–1) rates severity
  - Scores for eye opening, best motor response, and best verbal response
  - Slight scoring differences for children under 5 (Table 3–1)
  - Moderate injury—GCS 9-12
  - Severe injury—GCS <8
- Indications for hospital admission after head injury
  - Loss of consciousness greater than 5 minutes
  - Seizure after trauma
  - Neurological change
  - Question of nonaccidental injury
- Indications for CT scan after head injury
  - Altered consciousness
  - Depressed skull fracture
- Indications for intracranial pressure measurement
  - GCS less than 8
  - CT scan that suggests intracranial swelling
- Timing of orthopaedic surgery in patients with head injury
  - No evidence that acute fracture stabilization helps intracranial pressure
  - Pressures are stable and cleared by an anesthesiologist and neurosurgeon
- Orthopaedic treatment for a child surviving trauma
  - Should assume good outcome
  - Should optimize function
- Criteria for brain death
  - No cerebral or brainstem function
  - No hypothermia or pharmacotherapy
  - Two separate determinations

Thoracic Injury

- Second most significant cause of morbidity (after head injury)
- Child's chest more compliant than an adult's
  - Risk of pulmonary contusion without rib fracture
  - Treatment—Positive pressure ventilation and fluid restriction
- Pneumothorax—Treat with a chest tube or tubes, emergently if needed

Table 3–1: Pediatric Glasgow Coma Scale

SCORE	OLDER THAN 5 YEARS	1 TO 5 YEARS	YOUNGER THAN 1 YEAR
Best Motor Response	**(of 6)**	**(of 6)**	**(of 5)**
6	Obeys commands	Obeys commands	
5	Localizes pain	Localizes pain	Localizes pain
4	Withdrawal	Withdrawal	Abnormal withdrawal
3	Flexion to pain	Abnormal flexion	Abnormal flexion
2	Extensor rigidity	Extensor rigidity	Abnormal extension
1	None	None	None
Best Verbal Response			
5	Oriented	Appropriate words	Smiles or cries appropriately
4	Confused	Inappropriate words	Cries
3	Inappropriate words	Cries/screams	Cries inappropriately
2	Incomprehensible	Grunts	Grunts
1	None	None	None
Eye Opening			
4	Spontaneous	Spontaneous	Spontaneous
3	To speech	To speech	To shout
2	To pain	To pain	To pain
1	None	None	None

- Hemothorax
  - Thoracentesis if mild
  - Thoracotomy if ongoing or severe bleeding
- Posterior rib fractures may be a sign of nonaccidental injury

Abdominal Injury

Unique Factors

- Rib cage more pliable
- Abdominal muscles less well developed
- Pelvis relatively smaller
- Solid organs relatively larger
- Increased relative risk of abdominal organ injury

Physical Examination Findings

- Ecchymosis
- Abdominal guarding
- Lap belt marks

Imaging

- CT with contrast
- Worrisome findings
  - Pneumoperitoneum
  - Fluid in the abdomen without solid organ injury

Treatment: Laparotomy

Splenic Laceration

- Usually nonoperative treatment
- 3-4 days of rest in hospital
- 3 months of quiet activity in home
- Decreased incidence of late immune problems
- Indications for splenectomy
  - Estimated blood loss of more than 50% of blood volume
  - Vital signs (VS) unstable

Liver Laceration

- Longer period of bed rest
- Similar indications for surgery

Intestinal Injury: Observation versus Segmental Resection

- Diaphragmatic hernia
  - Respiratory distress
  - Bowel in chest
  - Emergent repair
- Renal laceration
  - Follow up for hydronephrosis and hypertension

Genitourinary

- Beware urethral injury with the following:
  - Anterior pelvic fractures (2% incidence)
  - Blood at the meatus

Management

- Pediatric polytrauma survival best in a pediatric center or in a general center with pediatric consultants available

Nutrition

- Initial resuscitation may use intraosseous infusion if needed
- Enteral nutrition preferred if possible

- Parenteral nutrition if gastrointestinal (GI) injuries
- Consider total parenteral nutrition if no GI function expected within 5 days

Timing of Orthopaedic Surgery

- No evidence that emergent fracture fixation improves outcomes in children unless there is ongoing bleeding or a severe open injury
- When most appropriate for patient and team

Classification of Open Fractures

- Grade I—Clean laceration <2 cm
- Grade II—Laceration 2-10 cm
- Grade III—Laceration >10 cm or significant crush
  - A—Adequate soft tissue coverage
  - B—Incomplete coverage
  - C—Neurovascular injury
- Mangled extremity score—Similar to adults[8]

Imaging of Pediatric Fractures

Fracture Definition

Plain Films

- Coned anteroposterior (AP) lateral and obliques if needed
  - Specify area of symptoms for detail
  - Include joint above and below in most cases
- Comparison films
  - Not on a routine basis if experienced
  - Skeletally immature elbows if needed

Computerized Tomography

- CT with multiplanar reconstruction may be helpful in complex fractures
  - Triplane angle (optional, not obligatory)
  - Salter-Harris IV fractures of the distal femur
  - Acetabular fractures
  - Hip dislocations after reduction to rule out entrapment
  - Some spine fractures poorly seen on plain films
  - Sternoclavicular injuries before and after reduction

Magnetic Resonance Imaging for Acute Fractures

- Distinguishing Salter-Harris II versus IV in pediatric elbow
- Spinal injury with neurological deficit
  - Spinal cord injury without radiographic abnormality

Arthrogram

- Elbow fractures–dislocations (Figure 3–8)
- Usually performed in the operating room
- Inject from the lateral side—the radiocapitellar joint

Bone Scan

- Advocated for unresponsive patients
- Rules out occult injuries (10% positive—Heinrich)

Growth Plate Injury

- Plain films first begin to show problem about 3 months after injury.
  - Park–Harris lines should be parallel to the physis and should move from it (Figures 3–9 and 3–10).

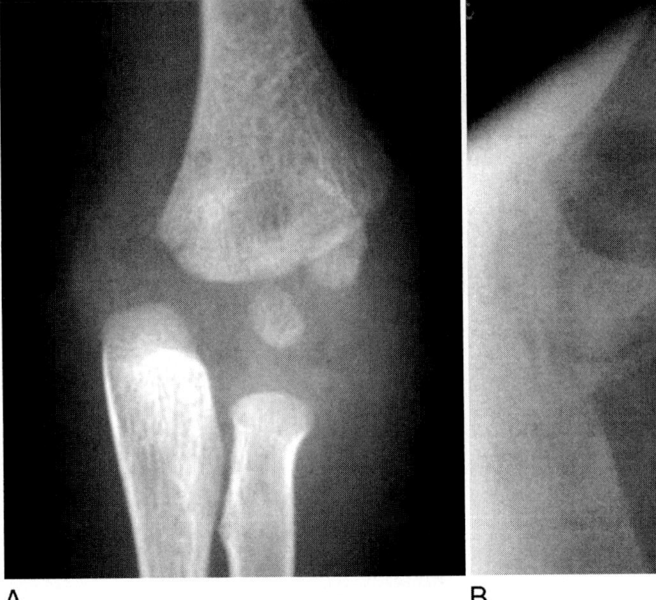

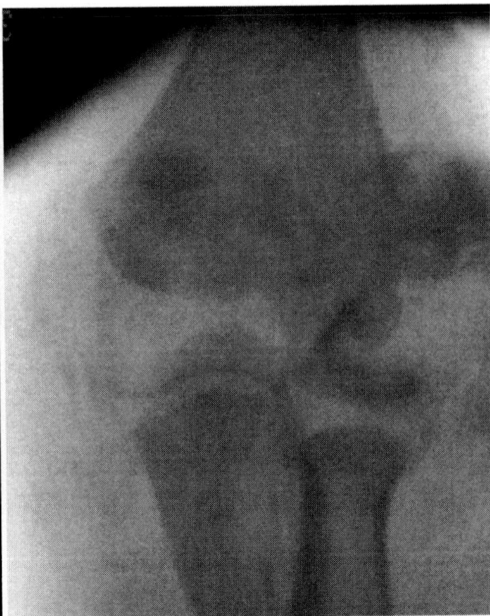

Figure 3–8: This elbow arthrogram may be useful for illustrating articular fracture lines in a fracture (A, before the arthrogram; B, after the arthrogram).

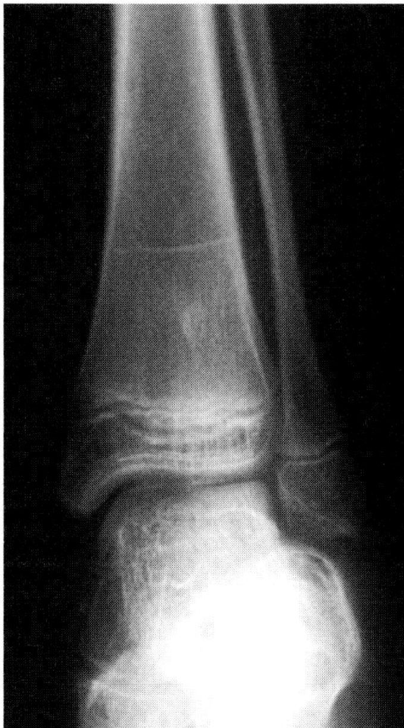

Figure 3–9: Park–Harris growth lines are seen in the metaphysis (in which they run parallel to the physis), in the epiphysis of the tibia, and in the talus (in which they are parallel to the articular surface), indicating normal growth.

- CT scanograms are helpful for measuring length and angulation; they are also reliable in the presence of joint contracture.
- Magnetic resonance imaging (MRI)—Specify imaging of the physis rather than of the joint or bone.
  - Order gradient echo sequence; "rule out physeal bar" (Figure 3–11).

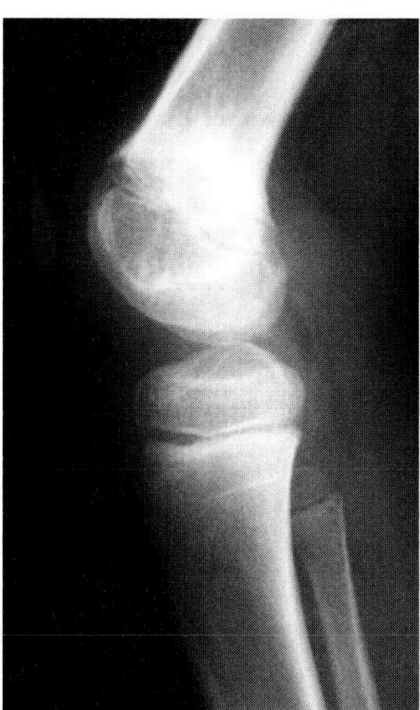

Figure 3–10: Park–Harris lines are seen moving normally from the proximal tibial physis but are not seen at the distal femur, signaling a bar.

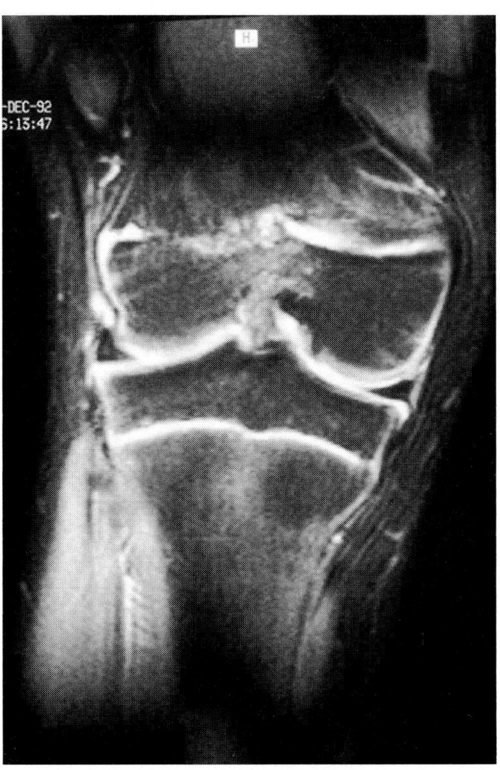

Figure 3–11: MRI with a gradient echo sequence, clearly illustrating the distal femoral physeal bar.

  - CT with multiplanar reconstruction may be helpful in defining bony versus fibrous tissue.
- Bone age and a growth chart may be helpful in defining the growth remaining.
- Indications for physeal bar resection:
  - Bar less than about 40% of the physeal width
  - At least 2 years of growth remaining

Nonaccidental Injury

Epidemiology

- Approximately 1% of all children are victims of abuse.[9]
  - Of these, 35% will be reinjured.
  - Approximately 1-5% will die if returned to the original environment.
- Most are under 1 year; some are up to 3 years.
  - Some experts allege that up to 30% of all fractures under age 3 are nonaccidental.
  - Others allege that this occurs mainly under age 1.[10]

Presentation

Have an index of suspicion in young children.

Risk Factors

- Families "in crisis"
  - Parental substance abuse

- Children
  - Age < 3
  - Premature infants; stepchildren
  - Disability

Evaluation

History

- What was mechanism? Is it plausible? Who witnessed it?
- Time from injury until treatment
- Interview each caregiver separately if necessary
- Who has access to the child?
- Work history
- Supervision patterns
- Interview siblings
- Interview child if possible

Physical Examination

- Look for bruises. Photograph if found.
  - Bruises on the buttocks, perineum, or backs of the legs are the most suspicious.
- Perform an ophthalmological examination for hemorrhages.
- Use a head CT scan for hematoma if there are unexplained neurological findings.
- Examine siblings if relevant.

Orthopaedic Injuries

- Orthopaedic injuries are seen in 30-50% of nonaccidental injuries.
- Fractures highly specific for nonaccidental injury include the following:
  - Corner or bucket-handle fractures
  - Scapular fractures
  - Posterior rib fractures
  - Old fractures
  - Multiple fractures of different ages
  - Spinous process fractures
- Spiral fractures are not pathognomonic for abuse.
- Many fractures resulting from abuse resemble those in accidental trauma.
- Include spine radiographs in suspicious cases.

Imaging for Abuse

- Perform a skeletal survey if suspicious.
  - AP or lateral skull
  - Lateral cervical, thoracic, and lumbar spine
  - AP pelvis and extremities
  - AP chest
- Repeat films in 2 weeks *if needed* to rule out other injuries and determine the date.
- Use a CT head scan if the fracture or neurological finding is questionable.
- Bone scan is an *option* to document all subtle fractures.

Estimating Fracture Age

- Bone scan positive less than 1 day
- Fracture edges become indistinct at 7 days
- Periosteal new bone appears around 7 days
- Abundant callus around 14 days
- Well-defined periosteal sleeve at 3 weeks
- Remodeling 2-3 months

Differential Diagnosis

- Caffey disease—Infantile cortical hyperostosis (Figure 3–12)
- Osteogenesis imperfecta
  - Usually bones gracile, thin or thick, and bowed
  - Use DNA testing as needed
- Rickets
- Syphilis—Multiple lytic lesions and periosteal reaction; positive serological test
- Scurvy
- Osteopetrosis
- Congenital insensitivity to pain—Check sensory examination

Management

- Treat orthopaedic injuries appropriately.
  - Parents can still consent.
- Reporting is an obligation for *all suspected cases.*
  - Can happen at all socioeconomic levels; explain your requirement to the parents.
  - There is greater liability for not reporting than for reporting; *legal* immunity is granted to all reporting physicians.
  - Contact the child protective services team.
- Make detailed documentation with the expectation that it will be used in court.
- Avoid dogmatic statements about mechanism unless they are well supported.
- The child should be protected against reinjury.
  - At home if deemed safe by social services
  - In a relative's custody
  - Hospitalization and foster care

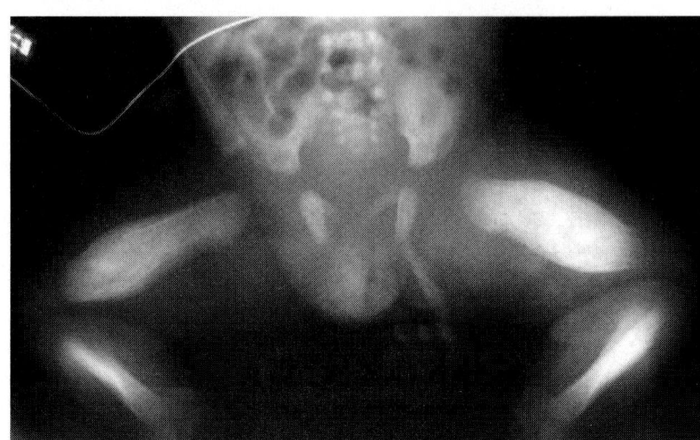

Figure 3–12: Caffey disease (infantile cortical hyperostosis).

- Perform further evaluations over time if needed to diagnose and document injuries.

Complications of Trauma

Compartment Syndrome

- Impaired muscle perfusion because of compartmental pressure
  - Clinical findings—Pain on passive stretch and unexplained sensory or motor deficit
  - Pressure measurement—More than 40 mm Hg and within 30 mm Hg of diastolic blood pressure
- Harder to detect in children because of communication differences
- Results better even after late detection
- Greatest in the following:
  - Open tibia
  - Ipsilateral open femur fracture (10% risk)

Osteomyelitis

- Risks lower than adult
- Vary with grade of fracture

Deep vein thrombosis

- Reports rare under 16 years

Fat Embolism

- Mainly occurs in older teens or young adults
- Altered sensorium, oxygenation, and petechiae

Stiffness

- Much less common than in adult injuries
- Risk factors
  - Intra-articular fractures (Figure 3–13)
  - Muscle or capsular damage
  - Nerve injury
  - Compartment syndrome

Growth Disturbance

- Risk factors
  - Major physeal displacement
  - High energy
  - Unreduced Salter-Harris III or IV

Residual Disability

- Related to head injury and skeletal damage

Trauma Prevention

Trauma can be treated by a "disease model" and frequency can be decreased[11]

- Most effective if there are structural, legal, or permanent interventions
  - Traffic "calming"[3]
  - Operator licensing
  - Playground codes
  - Handgun legislation
  - Smoke detector regulations
- Behavioral changes are the hardest and the least permanent
  - Trauma education in schools, including traffic rules
  - "Safe seating" practices for children in vehicles
  - Bike helmets can decrease the severity of head injury 85%

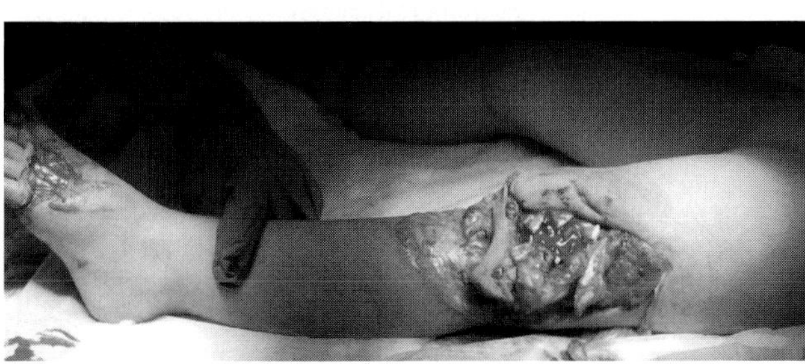

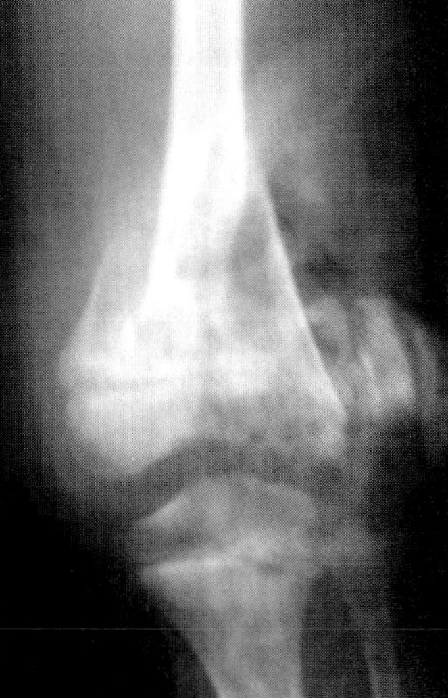

A

Figure 3–13: Lawnmower injury, a grade IIIB injury resulting in residual disability because of articular stiffness and growth disturbance. A, Before treatment.

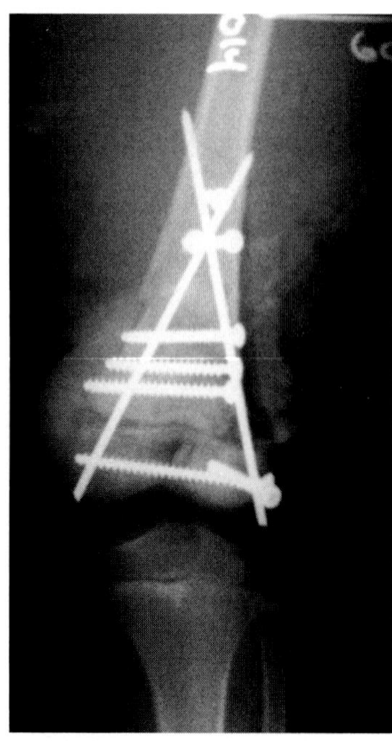

B

Figure 3–13, cont'd **B, After treatment.**

- Seating guidelines for children in vehicles
  - Prevent airbag injuries, chance fractures, and seat belt injuries
  - Do not allow in the front seat until the child is 12 and weighs more than 100 lbs
  - Rear-facing car seats for infants
  - Booster seats for children until age 8 and 60-80 lbs
  - Allow shoulder harnesses to fit more anatomically

References

1. Riseborough E, Barrett I, Shapiro F (1983) Growth disturbances following distal femoral physeal fracture–separations. J Bone Joint Surg Am 65: 885-892.
   Growth disturbances followed more than half of these injuries, although not all were severe.

2. Peterson HA (1994) Physeal fractures: Classification. J Pediatr Orthop 14: 439-448.
   Peterson provides an alternate, more comprehensive classification than that of Salter-Harris.

3. Merrell GA, Driscoll JC, Degutis LC, Renshaw TS (2002) Prevention of childhood pedestrian trauma: A study of interventions over 6 years. J Bone Joint Surg 84A: 863-869.
   Some interventions were more effective than others.

4. Kelm J, Ahlhelm F, Pape D, Pitxch W, Engel C (2001) School sports accidents: Analysis of causes, modes, and frequencies. J Pediatr Orthop 21: 165-168.
   This article is an excellent reference for those interested in prevention.

5. Sheehan E, Mulhall KJ, Kearns S, O'Connor P, McManus F, Stephens M, McCormack D (2003) Impact of dedicated skate parks on severity and incidence of skateboard and rollerblade related pediatric fractures. J Pediatric Orthop 23(4): 440-442.
   Skate parks can decrease the incidence and severity of injury.

6. Sanchez JI, Paidas CN (1999) Childhood trauma: Now and in the new millennium. Surg Clin N Am 79: 1503-1535.
   Excellent overview of trauma.

7. Ziv I, Rang M (1983) Treatment of femoral fracture in the child with head injury. J Bone Joint Surg Br 65: 276-278.
   Femur fractures in the head-injured patient are more prone to shortening and angulation as the patients recover and become spastic. Definitive fixation is preferred.

8. Fagelman MF, Epps HR (2002) Mangled extremity severity score in children. J Pediatr Orthop 22: 182-184.
   This article describes a way to quantitate severe injury.

9. Akbarnia B, Campbell R (2001) The role of the orthopaedic surgeon in child abuse. In: Lovell and Winter's Pediatric Orthopaedics, 5th edition (Morrissy RT, Weinstein SL, eds). Philadelphia: Lippincott-Williams and Wilkins, pp 1423-1443.
   Excellent overview of nonaccidental injury.

10. Schwend R, Werth C, Johnston A (2000) Femur fractures in toddlers and young children: Rarely from abuse. J Pediatr Orthop 20: 475-481.
    After age 1, the number of these fractures that are nonaccidental drops sharply.

11. Rivara FP, Grossman DC (1996) Prevention of traumatic deaths to children in the United States: How far have we come? Pediatrics 97: 791-797.
    Details progress in the prevention of serious trauma.

12. Wattenbarger JM (2002) Physeal fractures: Part I—Histologic features, Part II—Fate of interposed periosteum. J Pediatr Orthop 22(6): 701-716.
    Histological analysis of physeal fractures.

CHAPTER 4

Upper Extremity Injuries

John M. Flynn* and Emily A. Kolze†

*MD, Attending Surgeon, Division of Orthopaedic Surgery, The Children's Hospital of Philadelphia, Philadelphia, PA; Associate Professor, Department of Orthopaedics, University of Pennsylvania, Philadelphia, PA
†Clinical Research Coordinator, Division of Orthopaedic Surgery, The Children's Hospital of Philadelphia, Philadelphia, PA

Introduction

- Injuries to the hand, forearm, arm, and shoulder are the most common musculoskeletal injuries sustained by children.[1]
- Most injuries can be successfully treated and heal uneventfully; however, careful attention to principles of diagnosis and management are crucial to a consistently good outcome.[2]
- Many skeletal injuries in children involve the growth plate. These injuries are commonly classified into five types: Salter-Harris I, II, III, IV, and V (Figure 4–1).

Injuries to the Hand

General Principles

- The pediatric hand is a common site for injury.
- The incidence of hand fractures increases sharply after age 8, and the peak in boys is at age 13, when they are often participating in contact sports.
- Physeal injuries represent between 10 and 40% of hand fractures.[3]
  - The most common physeal fracture is the Salter-Harris II variant.
  - The thumb and the little finger are the most commonly injured fingers.
- The anatomy of the immature hand includes epiphyses at both the proximal and the distal ends of all tubular bones.
  - Secondary ossification centers develop in the proximal end of only the thumb metacarpal and in the distal ends of the other four metacarpals.
  - As children reach skeletal maturity, the irregularity of the physeal zones increases.[4] Salter-Harris I and II fractures occur more often in younger patients, and Salter-Harris III and IV fractures are seen more commonly as children approach skeletal maturity.[5]
- The ligaments of a child are stronger than the physeal and epiphyseal bone.
  - Tendon and ligamentous injuries are uncommon.
  - Extensor tendons insert into the epiphysis of the terminal phalange.
  - The flexor digitorum profundus inserts into the distal phalanx, and the flexor digitorum superficialis inserts into the middle phalanx.
  - All interphalangeal joints have collateral ligaments that insert into the metaphysis and epiphysis of the respective bones. The ligaments also insert into the volar plate. The volar plate is a soft tissue structure that functions to stabilize the joint from hyperextension forces.
- Nail bed injuries are common in children.
  - An awareness and understanding of nail bed anatomy is essential for treating these injuries.
  - Figure 4–2 diagrams the anatomy of the distal phalanx in a child.
  - The nail bed is composed of a germinal matrix and a sterile matrix.

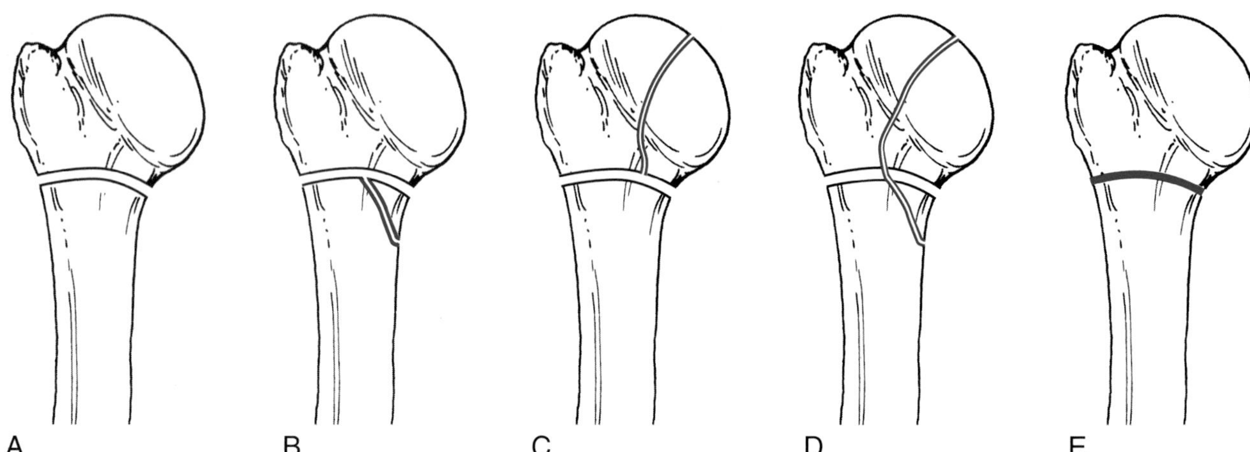

Figure 4–1: This schematic depicts the five Salter-Harris fracture types as they might occur in the proximal humerus. A, Salter-Harris I fracture involving only the physis. B, Salter-Harris II fracture with a metaphyseal fragment. C, Salter-Harris III fracture in which the fracture line breaks into the epiphysis. D, Salter-Harris IV fracture in which the fracture breaks into both the epiphysis and the metaphysis. E, Salter-Harris V fracture involving a crushing type injury to the physis. Redrawn from Flynn JM, Nagda S (2004) Upper extremity injuries. In: Requisites in Pediatrics: Pediatric Orthopaedics and Sports Medicine (Dormans J, ed). Philadelphia, Mosby.

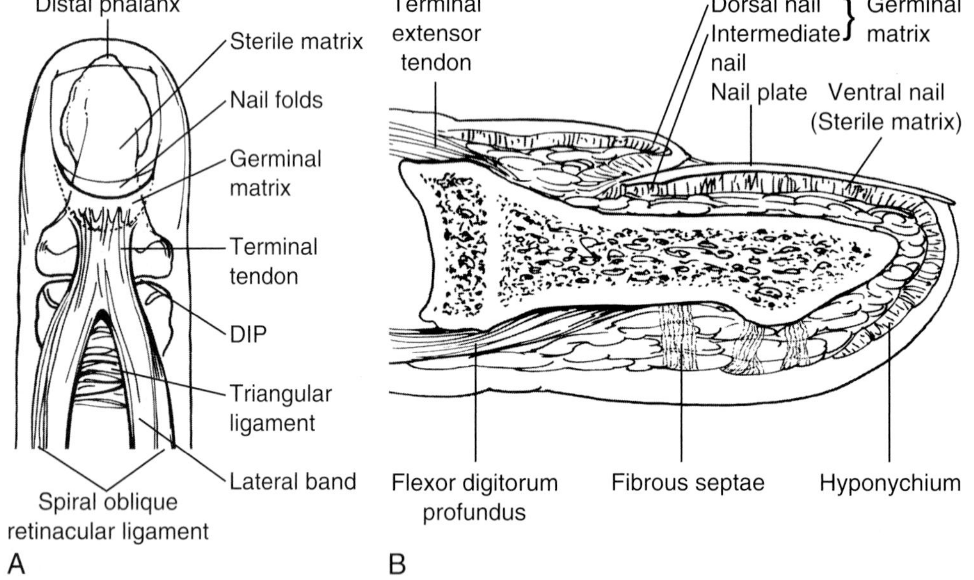

Figure 4–2: The anatomy of the nail bed. Redrawn from Rockwood C, Wilkins K, Beaty J (1996) Fractures in Children, 4th edition. Philadelphia, Lippincott-Raven.

- The germinal matrix produces the cells that make up the overlying nail.

- Evaluation of the pediatric hand can be a difficult task.
  - Injured children are usually apprehensive about allowing anyone to come near them.
  - Calming both parents and children is critical before any examination.
  - Examining uninvolved areas first can give the child some comfort and allow you to ease into the examination.
  - The first thing to assess is whether there is an open injury.
  - Palpation of the hand provides an indication of injured areas, although bony landmarks are often difficult to feel.
  - Tenderness at the insertion site of a ligament or tendon can provide clues to soft tissue injuries.
  - Range of motion, both passive and active, should be measured at every joint, and stability of all joints to varus and valgus forces should be checked.
  - Assessment of volar plate integrity by gentle hyperextension testing should be done.
  - Neurological examination can be difficult in children.
  - One clue to possible nerve injury can be excessive bleeding from a wound around the area of the digital

nerve, because laceration of the digital artery is often associated with a digital nerve injury.
  - One helpful examination to assess nerve injury is the "wrinkle test."
    1. Immerse the digit in warm water for 5 minutes.
    2. Denervated digits will not have any wrinkling of the volar skin.
- X-ray evaluation includes anteroposterior (AP), lateral, and oblique views. Oblique views are helpful for assessing intra-articular injuries.
- Treatment of any hand injury begins with proper pain control.
  - Conscious sedation is used when manipulation of a fracture is required.
  - Digital blocks are effective for phalangeal and nail bed injuries.
  - Lidocaine is effective, but epinephrine should never be used.
    1. You should inject lidocaine from the dorsal surface of the hand on both sides of the metacarpophalangeal (MCP) joint.
    2. Inject almost to the volar surface and retract as the anesthetic is injected.
  - Never inject in a circular wheel around the digit; it can compromise the circulation to the digit.
- Manipulation of a fracture will require further examination and treatment.
- Repeated attempts to reduce physeal fractures will increase the chances of premature growth arrest.
- Early reduction before swelling occurs will make the reduction easier and can help to prevent increased swelling.
- The hand should be immobilized immediately after the reduction.

Phalangeal Fractures

- Fractures of the distal phalanx are common (Figure 4–3). They can range from closed avulsion fractures to high-energy crush injuries.
- Further examination and treatment may be necessary for crush injuries of the distal phalanx. Patients can have severe comminution of the underlying bone, disruption of the nail bed, and significant soft tissue injury.
- Care must be taken to preserve all possible tissue during evaluation and treatment.
- The nail is removed if it is not already off.
- The nail bed injury often appears as a stellate laceration.
- The wound is irrigated because this is an open fracture.
- Antibiotics and tetanus prophylaxis are given.
- The nail bed should be loosely approximated with a 6.0 or smaller absorbable suture.
- The healing potential in children is excellent, and loose approximation will allow this.
- Treatment of the nail bed injury will often act as a splint to bring the underlying fracture together.
- After repair of the nail bed, the nail is replaced onto the bed with the end of it inserted under the nail fold. It should also be sutured in place.
- A nail substitute can be fashioned from the sterile suture packaging.
  - Using the contralateral nail as a guide, you can cut a piece off the wrapping and use it in place of a destroyed or missing nail.

Mallet Finger Deformities

- A mallet finger deformity is a common distal phalanx injury (Figure 4–4).

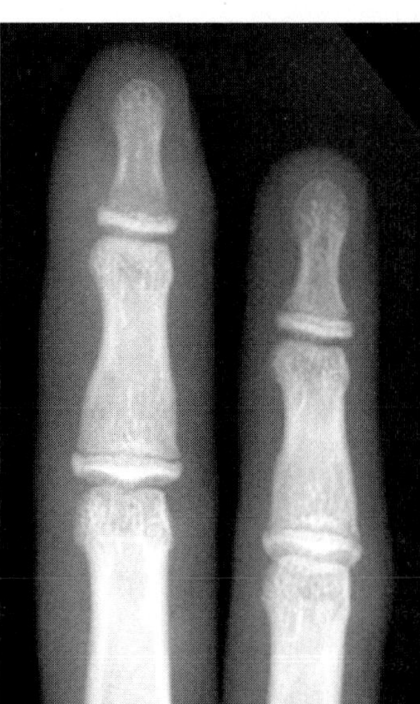

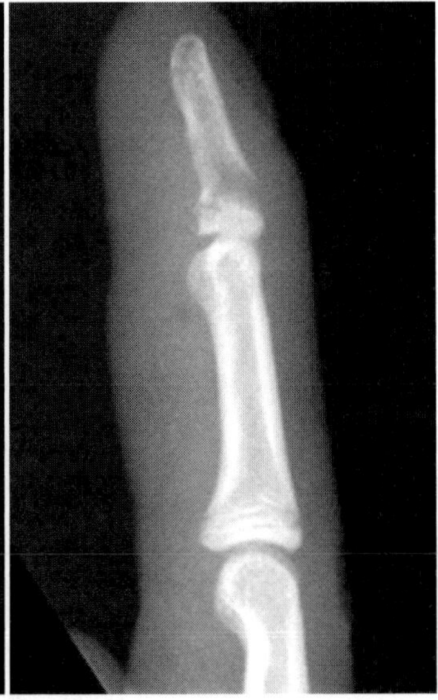

Figure 4–3: An open fracture of the distal phalanx. **A,** This AP radiograph of the injured finger and adjacent digits shows radiolucency in the area of the physis of the distal phalanx. **B,** The lateral radiograph shows the relationship between the base of the nail bed and the location of the fracture. A common mistake is to miss the fact that a nail bed injury can be associated with this fracture; thus, it is an open fracture.

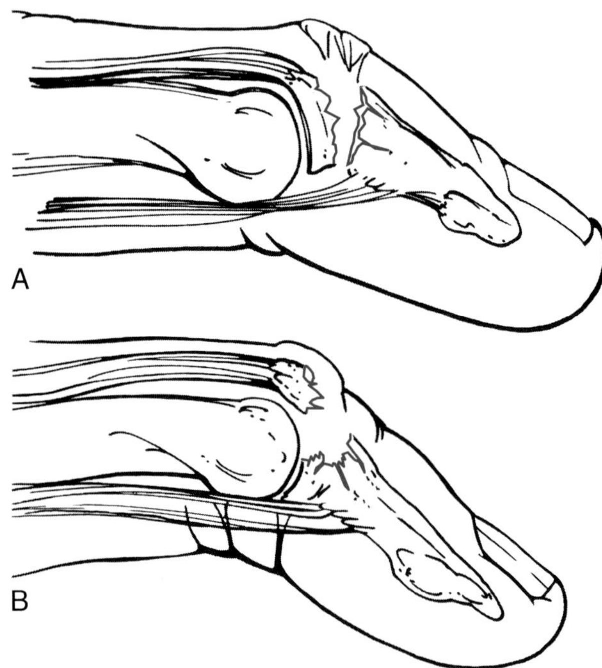

Figure 4–4: This schematic shows two types of a mallet finger, one involving the entire epiphysis (A) and the other involving the dorsal surface of the epiphysis (Salter-Harris III fracture) (B). **Redrawn from Morrissy RT, Weinstein SL (eds) (2001) Lovell & Winter's Pediatric Orthopaedics, 5th edition. Philadelphia, Lippincott-Raven.**

- The child will complain of pain and inability to extend the distal portion of the digit after a hyperextension injury.
- This is similar to the mallet finger injury in adults; however, the underlying pathology is different.
  - Unlike in adults, where a disruption of the tendon is the cause, children will usually have avulsion fractures.
  - Children younger than 5 years will have a Salter-Harris I or II injury with the flexor tendon still attached to the distal piece, pulling it in a volar direction.
  - Children closer to adolescence will usually have a Salter-Harris III injury.
- Plain radiographs should be obtained regardless of the obvious nature of the diagnosis assess the displacement of the fracture.
- The patient should be splinted with the digit in extension for 3-4 weeks.
- Some patients closer to skeletal maturity may require operative fixation for severely displaced fractures.
- Another easily overlooked injury is the "jersey finger" injury.
  - This injury is the opposite of the mallet finger and usually occurs in adolescents near skeletal maturity.
  - It is most often the result of a true flexor tendon avulsion and is classically seen in football players who get their fingers caught in an opposing player's jersey.
  - The patient will have a history of a forced extension of a flexed digit and will be unable to flex the digit at the distal interphalangeal (DIP) joint.
  - AP or lateral and oblique radiographs should be obtained.
  - Surgical intervention is usually required to reattach the tendon and should be performed within 7-10 days of the injury.
- Fractures of the proximal and middle phalanx can be classified into one of four groups: physeal, shaft, neck (Figure 4–5), or intra-articular (condylar) (Figure 4–6).
  - Careful examination with observation, palpation, and range of motion testing should reveal any associated soft tissue injuries or rotational deformities.
  - It is essential to assess the level of rotational deformity.
  - There can often be a significant deformity with only a subtle finding on initial examination.
- Plain radiographs are essential in the diagnosis and in pretreatment planning.
  - Oblique views may show intra-articular extension better than AP or lateral views.
  - Lateral views will detail any sagittal plane deformity.
  - Surgical treatment should be considered for any displaced or intra-articular fractures.
  - A pencil may be used as a fulcrum over which angulation can be reduced.
- Salter-Harris II fractures (Figure 4–7) are common and can be managed with immobilization alone if there is no significant displacement.
- Overall, most proximal and middle phalangeal fractures can be treated with nonoperative management using closed reduction and casting for 3-4 weeks.
- Outcomes are usually excellent because healing and remodeling in children is significant.

Fingertip Amputations

- Distal fingertip amputations and avulsions can be gruesome injuries presented by hysterical patients and parents.

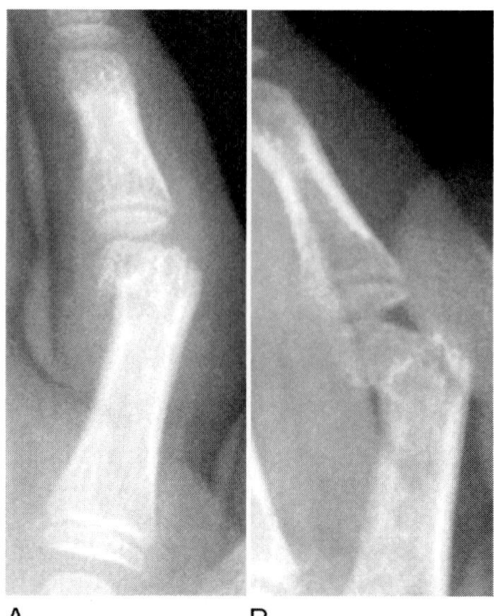

Figure 4–5: An AP radiograph (A) and a lateral radiograph (B) show a neck fracture of the proximal phalanx.

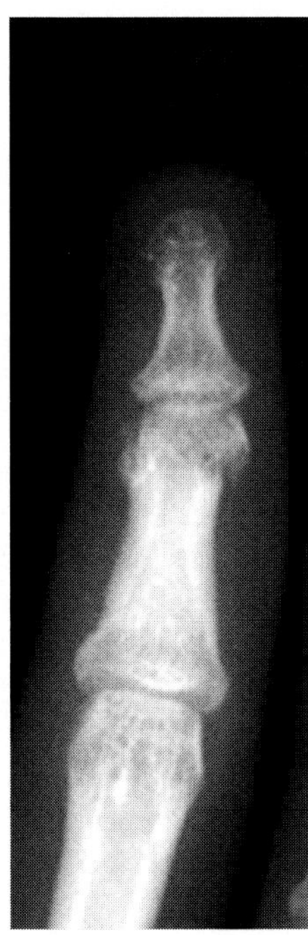

Figure 4–6: This AP radiograph shows a fracture of the middle phalanx that extends into the DIP joint.

- The history is often similar to that of a crush injury, but the force causes an avulsion rather than a true crush.
- An evaluation of the extent of tissue deficit, the amount of visible bone, and the presence of vessel or nerve injury must be completed.
- The avulsed part may be missing or too damaged to salvage.
- If the parents bring in the part, it is important to assess its quality.
- Even if the tissue is not viable, it may serve as a short-term biological dressing to cover any visible bone.
- It should be irrigated and placed in damp saline-soaked gauze until after the finger has been cleaned.
- A motor and sensory examination should be made on the proximal portion before any digital block is performed.
- Excessive bleeding signals a digital vessel injury, and direct pressure should be applied until bleeding stops.
- Antibiotic and tetanus prophylaxis should be administered.
- The wound should be irrigated after a good digital nerve block has been obtained. You can reassess the wound after irrigating and debride any nonviable tissue.
- Significant tissue deficit should be evaluated and managed by an experienced hand surgeon.
- If the distal piece is intact, it can be placed on the proximal piece and approximated with 5.0 or 6.0 absorbable sutures.
- If the amputation traverses through the nail bed, a meticulous repair should be performed and the nail fold should be splinted using the technique mentioned in the preceding section on crush injuries. Once the repair is complete, the wound should be dressed with sterile gauze and copious amounts of padding.
- Close follow-up is essential to monitor any signs of infection or necrosis of the distal piece.
- Outcomes are variable and are usually better for extremely young children.

Nail Bed Injuries

- Nail bed injuries (Figure 4–8) are common injuries in children and can easily be missed.

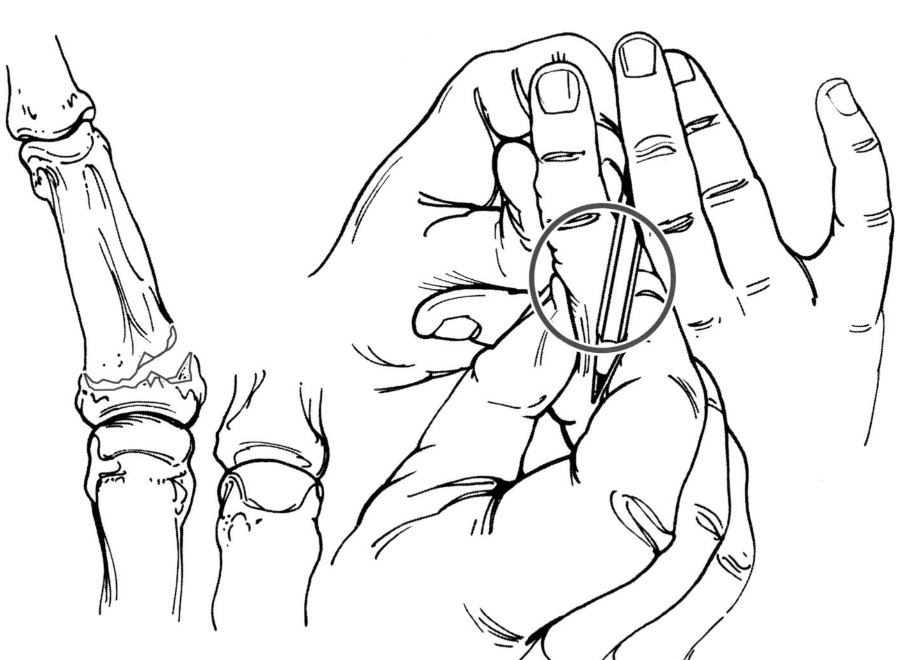

Figure 4–7: This schematic shows a displaced, angulated Salter-Harris II fracture of the proximal phalanx and a reduction maneuver in which a pencil is placed between the index and the long fingers and the index finger is pushed ulnar ward to reduce the fracture. **Redrawn from Morrissy RT, Weinstein SL (eds) (2001) Lovell & Winter's Pediatric Orthopaedics, 5th edition. Philadelphia, Lippincott-Raven.**

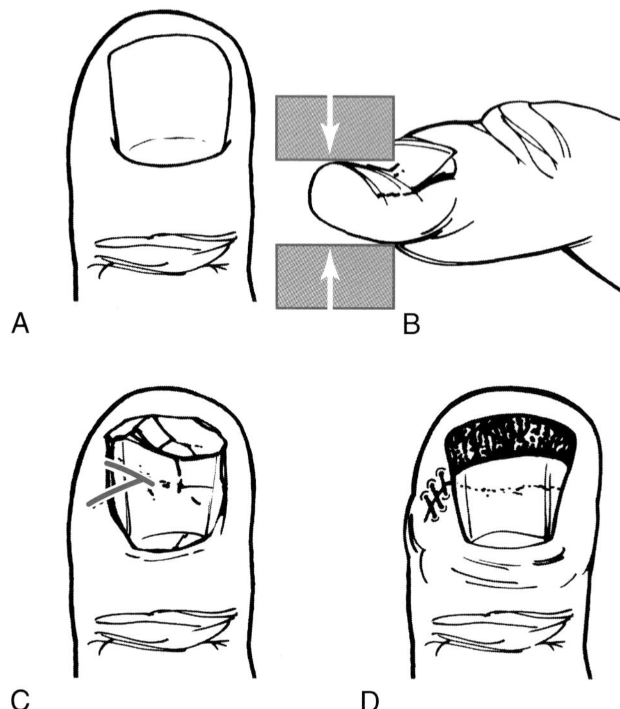

Figure 4–8: This schematic depicts an injury to the nail bed. **A, The normal finger. B, A crush injury of the distal phalanx involving the nail. C, The injured finger with a crushed nail and a stellate laceration. D, The injured digit after repair. Redrawn from Morrissy RT, Weinstein SL (eds) (2001) Lovell & Winter's Pediatric Orthopaedics, 5th edition. Philadelphia, Lippincott-Raven.**

- Often the only clue during physical examination may be a subungual hematoma. A hematoma greater than 25% of the nail bed should raise suspicion and prompt a direct visual evaluation of the nail bed.
- Plain radiographs should be obtained to assess for a concomitant fracture.
- A digital block is established by injecting 1% plain lidocaine around the radial and ulnar digital nerve at the proximal end of the digit to be treated. After this has been performed, the nail should be elevated with a blunt instrument such as a freer elevator.
- If a laceration is identified, it should be repaired meticulously. A 6.0 chromic suture can be used to approximate the edges.
- The nail should be used as a splint.
  - This repair can be performed in an emergency department setting.
  - The patient should have close hand surgery follow-up.
- Outcomes are good overall.
- Meticulous repair of the laceration will improve the chances of a good outcome.

Metacarpal Fractures

- The relative mobility of the metacarpals varies; the second and third metacarpals have less mobility.
- Fractures can occur at the head, neck, shaft, or base.
- The neck is the most common site for fracture.
- Fracture patterns of the shaft are similar to those of the phalangeal shaft.
- Fractures of the second and third metacarpals tend to have less displacement because of the surrounding soft tissue.
- The injury can occur from a direct blow, a rotational force, or an axial load.
- Fractures of the metacarpal head are seen most commonly as Salter-Harris II fractures of the fifth digit in adolescent patients.
- Physeal injuries of the other metacarpals are rarely seen.[6]
- X-ray evaluation of the hand will usually show the fracture.
  - This is taken with the dorsum of the hand against the cassette with the MCP joint flexed 65 degrees.
  - The beam is angled 15 degrees to the ulnar side of the hand.
- There is a risk of avascular necrosis of the metacarpal head. It is postulated that the risk is increased from hematoma collection at the fracture site.[7] Therefore, some authors advocate aspiration of the hematoma.
- Most of these fractures can be treated with closed reduction and splinting in the safe position.
- Fractures that are reduced but remain unstable will require pin fixation.
- Displaced fractures of the metacarpal head will often require open reduction and internal fixation.
- Fractures of the metacarpal neck are the most common metacarpal fractures in children.[8] These fractures are analogous to the boxer's fracture in adults.
- Examination of the hand will show significant swelling over the area. An obvious bump may be visible over the fracture site.
- Routine radiographs will show the fracture.
  - X-ray evaluation of the degree of angulation of the fracture can often be difficult because of superimposed digits on the lateral view.
  - Oblique views can often aid delineation of the digits.
- Neck fractures are usually treated with closed methods.
  - The Jahss reduction maneuver is performed by flexing the MCP joint 90 degrees.
  - This is followed by the application of pressure on the dorsal aspect of the metacarpal proximal to the fracture.
  - Pressure on the volar side of the distal fragment can aid the reduction.
  - The hand should then be placed in the safe position with the wrist extended 10-15 degrees, the MCP joint flexed, and the proximal interphalangeal (PIP) joint extended.
  - Postreduction radiographs should always be obtained.
  - Some patients near skeletal maturity with unstable fractures may require closed reduction and pin fixation.
- Fractures of the metacarpal shaft can be transverse, oblique, or spiral.
- These fractures must be evaluated for rotational deformity.

- This can be done by asking the patient to make a fist (Figure 4–9).
- All fingers should point to the scaphoid, and all the nail beds should be parallel.

- Angular and rotational deformity must be corrected before splinting or casting.
  - After reduction is obtained, the patient should be splinted in the safe position.
  - Unstable fractures with residual rotational malalignment may require pin fixation.
  - A rotational deformity of even 10 degrees can be enough to cause overlapping of the fingers.
- Fractures of the base of the metacarpal (Figure 4–10) are infrequent in children.
  - They are usually the result of high-energy trauma.
    1. They can occur because of an axial load resulting in a stable compression fracture.
    2. High-energy trauma will usually result in a fracture–dislocation at the carpometacarpal level.
  - Radiographic evaluation should include a 30-degree pronated or supinated oblique view. This aids the assessment of joint dislocation or subluxation.
  - Significant fracture–dislocations should alert you to search for associated soft tissue injury.
  - Reduction of the dislocation or fracture should be followed by a thorough examination to assess stability of the joint. Splinting in the safe position is an option. However, some authors will leave the PIP joint free to move.
- Fractures of the head and shaft of the thumb metacarpal are treated just as in the other digits.
- Fractures of the base of the thumb metacarpal can present as simple transverse fractures or intra-articular fractures (Figure 4–11).
  - Salter-Harris III and IV fractures of the base most closely resemble the adult Bennett's fracture.
  - Examination of the thumb will show swelling similar to other metacarpal fractures.
  - Malrotation can be assessed by using the perpendicular relationship of the thumb's nail plate with the other nail plates.
- Fractures of the base of the thumb without intra-articular extension can be treated with closed reduction and immobilization. Angulation of up to 20 degrees can be accepted.
- Unstable fractures should be stabilized with reduction and pin fixation in the operating room.
- Displaced intra-articular fractures will also require operative intervention.

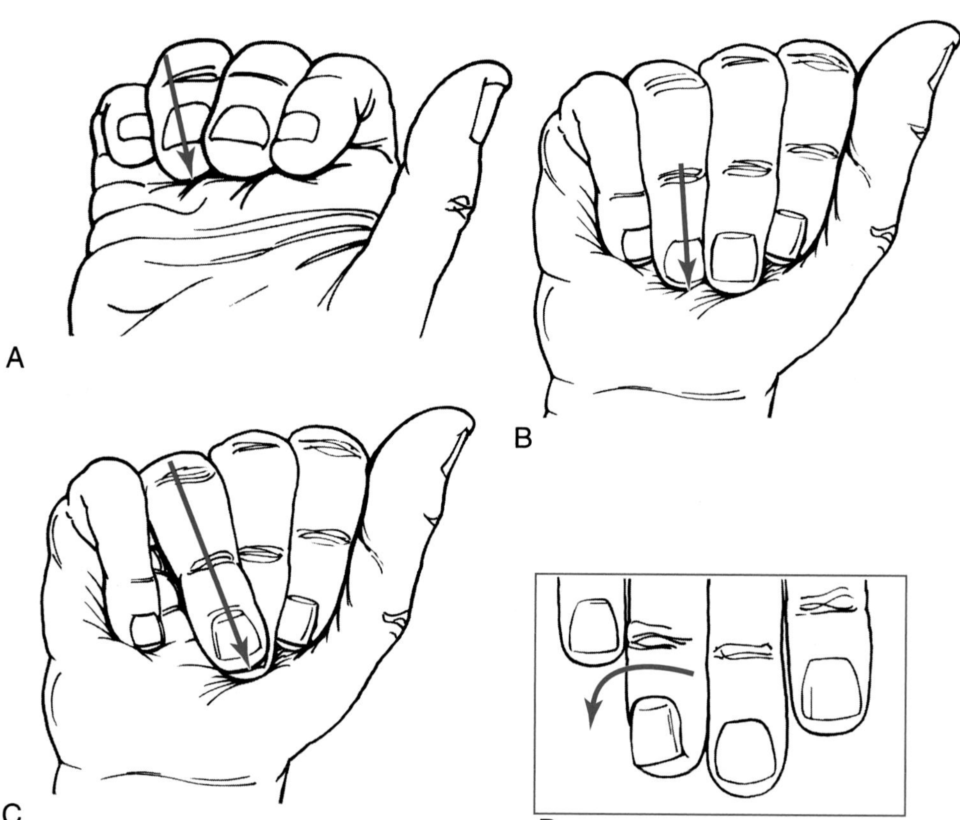

Figure 4–9: This schematic depicts an important physical examination test to note possible rotational malalignment after a hand fracture. **Redrawn from Morrissy RT, Weinstein SL (eds) (2001) Lovell & Winter's Pediatric Orthopaedics, 5th edition. Philadelphia, Lippincott-Raven.**

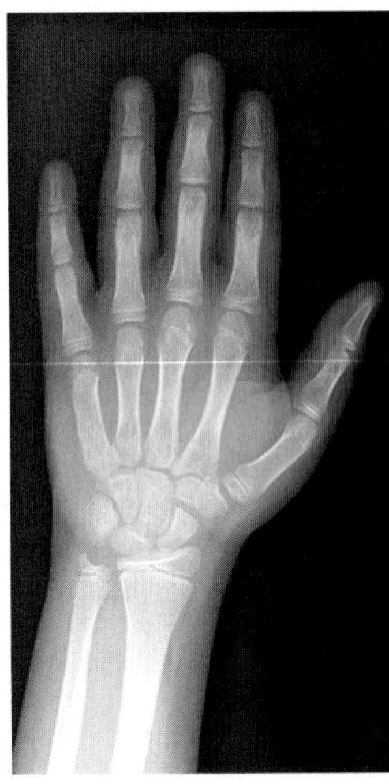

Figure 4–10: This AP radiograph of the hand shows a fracture at the base of the fifth metacarpal with minimal displacement.

 - The outcomes are usually good.
 - The immobilization period is usually 4-6 weeks.
- Ulnar collateral ligament (UCL) injuries of the thumb (also known as Gamekeeper's thumb) are usually encountered in adolescent patients, not in young children.
 - Usually the result of an abduction force applied to the thumb, the injury can range from a sprain of the UCL to an avulsion fracture from the proximal phalanx.
 - The patient will have pain over the ulnar side of the thumb.
 - Examination should include stressing the MCP joint of the thumb in extension and flexion.
 - Lack of a distinct endpoint or a joint that opens greater than 45 degrees more than the contralateral side is indicative of a tear in the UCL.
 - Routine radiographs will differentiate between an avulsion fracture and a tear.
 - Stress x-rays may be required to appreciate the fracture.
 - Immobilization in a cast for 3-4 weeks is usually all that is needed for fractures and incomplete tears.
 - A complete tear will require operative repair.
- Immobilization of metacarpal fractures is usually 3-4 weeks. This should be followed by an examination to assess tenderness at the fracture site. The correlation between tenderness at the fracture site and radiographic evidence of a nonunion should prompt you to consider immobilization for longer than 4 weeks.
- Outcomes for metacarpal fractures are excellent if you address any rotational malalignment or angular deformity during primary treatment.

Carpal Bone Fractures

- Fractures of the carpal bones in young children are exceedingly rare.
 - Most occur in the adolescent patient from a fall on an outstretched hand.
 - The patient will complain of pain over the dorsum of the hand.
 - The physical examination will be consistent with pain over the affected bone.

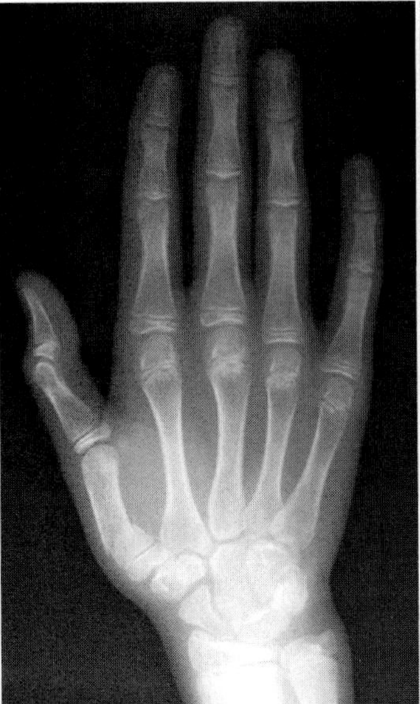

A

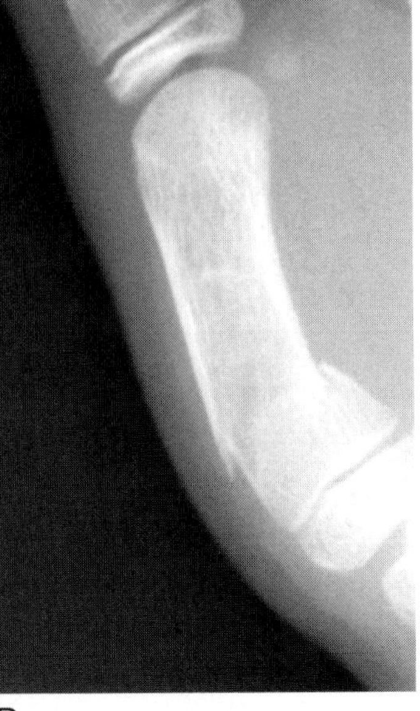

B

Figure 4–11: A fracture of the base of the thumb metacarpal. A, This AP radiograph of the hand shows a fracture at the base of the metacarpal. B, This close-up of the fracture shows minimal displacement and angulation.

- The most commonly fractured carpal bone is the scaphoid.
  - Pain will typically be in the anatomical snuff box.
  - Good quality radiographs (AP, lateral, and scaphoid views) should be obtained.
  - Scaphoid fractures will have a false, negative x-ray about 10% of the time.
- It is essential that this fracture be diagnosed because most complications result from late presentations or missed diagnosis.
- Any patient with pain in the snuff box should be treated using a thumb spica cast for 10-14 days even if radiographs are negative.
  - The patient should be reexamined after this time with repeat x-rays.
  - Continued pain with negative x-rays should prompt a bone scan or magnetic resonance image.
  - Treatment for nondisplaced fractures is with a thumb spica cast for 4-6 weeks.
  - Reduction and internal fixation is necessary for displaced fractures.
  - Outcomes are usually good; nonunion and avascular necroses are the main complications.

Hand Dislocations

- Dislocations of the hand in children are uncommon.
- The collateral ligaments and volar plate are stronger than the physeal bone.
- Any force strong enough to produce a dislocation will usually produce a fracture.
- Occasionally a patient will have an acute dislocation.
  - Physical examination will usually show an obvious deformity and inability to move a certain joint.
  - An inspection to evaluate for the presence of an open dislocation is important. A prereduction neurovascular examination is also important.
  - The blood supply distally can be compromised and the nerve can be placed into excessive traction.
  - Radiographs are equally important to assess for any fractures.
  - Reduction can be attempted after a digital block or under conscious sedation. Slight traction followed by the reduction of the joint is usually all that is required.
- Occasionally, you will encounter an irreducible joint dislocation.
  - It is likely that an interposed ligament or volar plate is hindering the reduction.
  - Operative reduction may be necessary.
- Also, postreduction stressing of the joint is important to evaluate for ligamentous and volar plate injury. Immobilization of the joint with buddy taping for a few weeks is usually all that is required.
- A "jammed finger" is a common injury, but it is not a dislocation.
  - Patients usually complain of tenderness at a joint and have a history of a longitudinal force applied to the finger.
  - Physical examination will reveal tenderness and swelling over a joint.
  - Motion will be painful.
  - The diagnosis is one of exclusion.
  - All bony and soft tissue injury should be ruled out.
- The etiology of this common entity is unknown. However it may be caused by a sprain of one of the collateral ligaments.
- Patients and parents should be warned that discomfort may last up to 9 months after the injury.
  - Swelling about the joint may remain as a residual thickening about the joint.
  - Treatment is symptomatic with warm compresses and buddy taping during activities.

Fractures of the Wrist and Forearm

Fractures of the Distal Radius and Ulna

General Principles

- Fractures of the wrist and forearm are common in children, accounting for nearly half of all fractures seen in the skeletally immature.
- The most common mechanism of injury is a fall on the outstretched hand.
- About 80% of forearm fractures are injuries to the distal third of the radius and ulna, 15% involve the middle third, and the rest are the rare fractures to the proximal third of the radius or ulnar shaft.
- Most fractures, especially in younger children, are greenstick or buckle fractures.
- Several important anatomical features should be considered in managing these injuries.
  - The ulna is a straight, triangular-shaped bone.
  - The radius is rectangular distally, triangular in the middle third, and cylindrical in the proximal third.
  - The radius has a gentle bow throughout the extent of its shaft, which is critical in allowing its rotation around the ulna during pronation and supination (Figure 4–12).
  - The interosseous membrane attaches along the lateral border of the ulna and along the medial border of the radius.
  - The radius has a tuberosity just below its proximal neck that is the site of insertion of the biceps tendon.
  - This tuberosity is located opposite the radial styloid. Understanding this relationship can be valuable in determining rotational alignment after fracture reduction.
- Fracture management is greatly aided by an understanding of the connection (Figure 4–13) between the radius and the ulna. With an articulation proximally

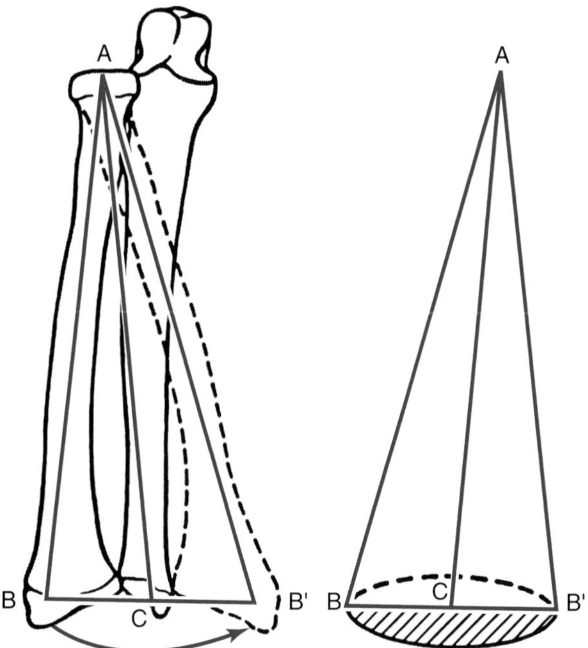

Figure 4–12: This schematic demonstrates the mechanism by which the radius rotates around the ulna during forearm supination and pronation. Redrawn from Green NE (1998) Skeletal Trauma in Children, 2nd edition. Philadelphia, WB Saunders.

and distally and an interosseous membrane in the middle, the radius and the ulna act as a two-bone complex.

- Managing these injuries requires an understanding of this relationship, because a significantly displaced injury to one bone usually is associated with an injury to the other.
- Detecting this second subtle injury (e.g., a radial head dislocation with a greenstick ulnar fracture) is based on an understanding of the radioulnar relationship.
  - The interosseous membrane is stretched to its full length when the forearm is in a neutral to a 30-degree supination.[9]
  - As the forearm is pronated, the radius rotates around the ulna and the interosseous membrane relaxes.
  - Distally, the triangular fibrocartilage complex (TFCC) includes an articular disk and several fibers that connect the ulna to the carpus and to the distal radius.
  - The ulnar styloid, sometimes fractured in wrist injuries, is a key source of attachment of these ligaments. Fortunately, unlike adults, young children rarely sustain injuries to the TFCC that require treatment.
  - Proximally, the radius articulates with the capitulum and is connected to the ulna by a complex of tissues that includes the angular ligament.
- Important developmental features include the following:
  - The distal radial physis, a common location of injury, closes late in development. Typical closure is about age 17 in girls and age 18 in boys.
  - The distal ulnar physis closes about 1 year earlier.

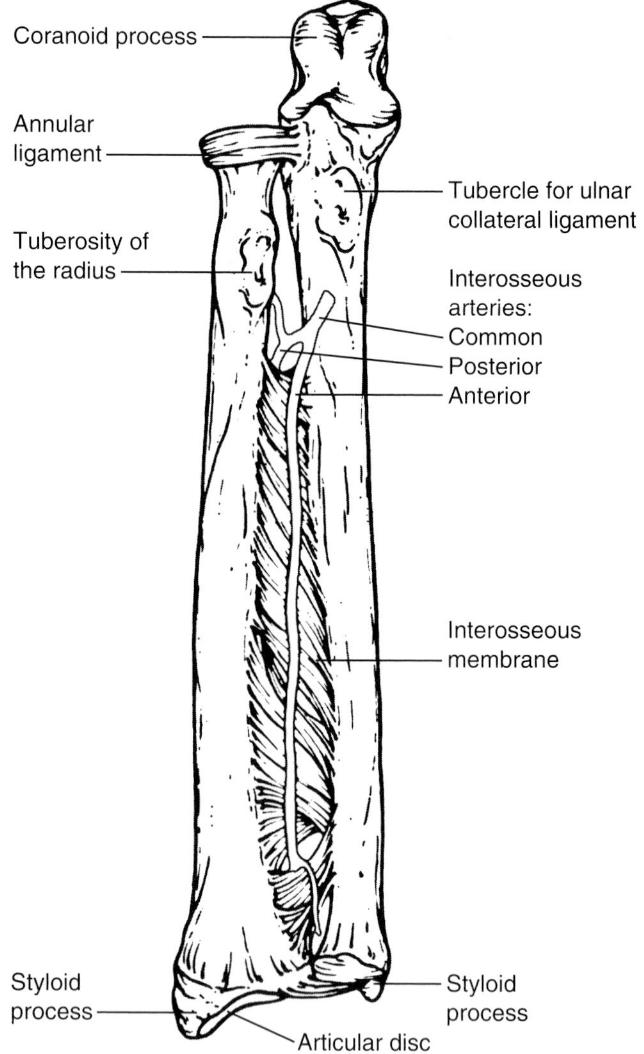

Figure 4–13: This schematic depicts the important connections between the radius and the ulna. Redrawn from Green NE (1998) Skeletal Trauma in Children, 2nd edition. Philadelphia, WB Saunders.

  - A separate ossification center at the radial styloid can be mistaken for a fracture in children between 1 and 2 years.
  - At the elbow, the proximal ulnar ossification center appears around age 10. This can have a bipartite ossification center commonly mistaken for an avulsion fracture.
- The orthopaedic surgeon must understand the muscles attached to the radius and ulna and the forces they exert to understand typical patterns of fracture displacement and the deforming forces on the bones after reduction (Figure 4–14).
  - Distally, the pronator quadratus, some extensors and adductors, and wrist extensors tend to pronate and extend a distal radius fracture fragment.
  - The stronger force, however, is the brachioradialis, which inserts laterally above the radial styloid.
  - More proximally, the pronator quadratus inserts into the middle third of the radius and will pronate the shaft in all fractures proximal to its insertion.

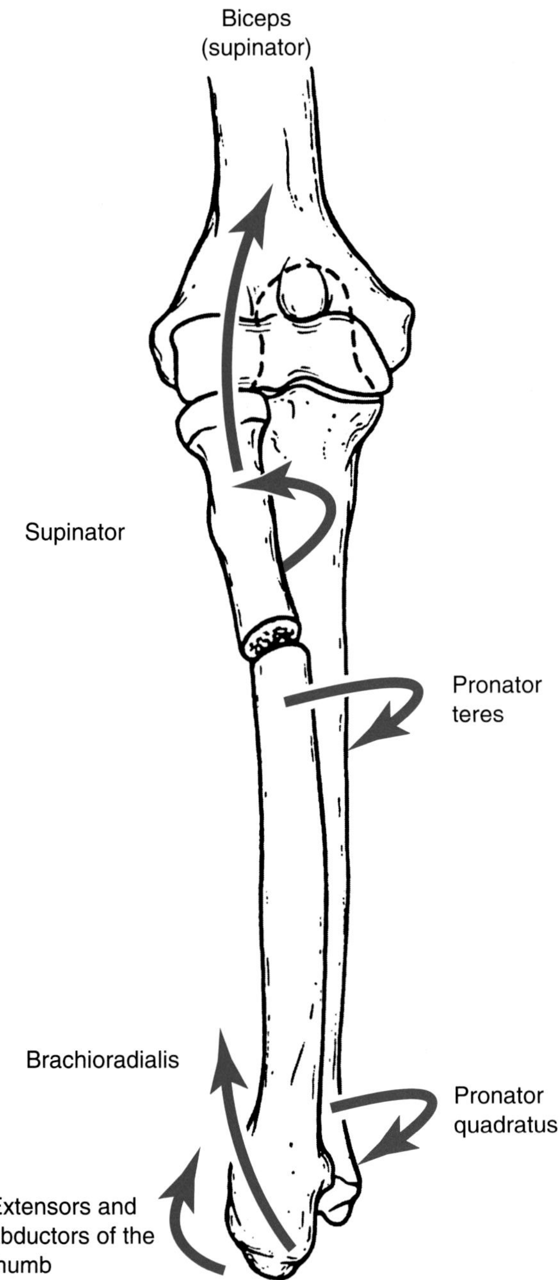

Figure 4–14: This schematic demonstrates the muscular forces acting on the radius that can lead to displacement after a fracture. **Understanding these forces is critical to obtaining and maintaining a reduction of a diaphyseal forearm fracture. Redrawn from Green NE (1998) Skeletal Trauma in Children, 2nd edition. Philadelphia, WB Saunders.**

- In the proximal third of the radius, there is a strong supination force from the supinator and the biceps. The biceps also flex a proximal radius fragment.
- Understanding these forces, most surgeons will treat proximal fractures with forearm supination and middle or distal third fractures with a neutral forearm or slight forearm pronation.

- In addition to understanding the mechanism of injury, anatomy, development, and forearm mechanics, the orthopaedic surgeon must understand the tremendous remodeling potential of the forearm in children.
- This remodeling potential is the most important reason that most forearm fractures in children can be treated with cast immobilization but many similar fractures in adults require operative reduction and internal fixation.[10]
- Remodeling is greatest in young children, in fractures near a rapidly growing physis, in fractures in the plane of motion of the adjacent joint, and in fractures with a greater angulation.
- Thus, the typical apex–volar angulation of the distal radius fracture in a 5-year-old has tremendous remodeling potential—adjacent to the distal radius physis, it is in the plane motion of the wrist joint, and the child has nearly 12 years of physeal growth to drive the remodeling.
- Typically, angulation of about 10 degrees per year is corrected with remodeling.
- Radialward angulation of the distal radius, cause by the pull of the brachioradialis, corrects more slowly.
- Bayonet apposition remodels reliably in younger children (Figure 4–15).
- Rotational malalignment will not remodel, although shoulder abduction can functionally compensate for loss of pronation.

Physeal Distal Radius and Ulna Injuries

- Distal radial physeal fractures are the most common growth plate injury in children.
  - Most occur after age 10 (younger children are more likely to sustain a metaphyseal buckle fracture).
  - Most distal radial physeal fractures are of the Salter-Harris II type.
  - Type I fractures are less common. Although many fractures are called type I, careful inspection of radiographs will often reveal a small Thurston-Holland metaphyseal fragment.
  - Most distal radial and ulnar physeal fractures occur from a fall on an outstretched hand.
  - Many of these injuries in teenagers are high energy, sustained during rollerblading, skateboarding, or sports.
- On physical examination, displaced fractures will show deformity, tenderness, and swelling at the fracture site.
- Because the fracture usually displaces dorsally, the volar periosteum is often disrupted.
- It is critical that the initial evaluation includes a careful inspection of the skin around the forearm, because subtle pinpoint openings in the skin represent an open fracture caused by the sharp volar metaphyseal fragment.
- Careful neurological examination is also important. Higher-energy injuries may cause a neuropraxia of the median nerve or an acute carpal tunnel syndrome.
- Physical examination should include palpation of the hand below and the elbow above in a search for associated injuries.
- In fractures without significant swelling and deformity, diagnosis of a nondisplaced distal radius fracture is

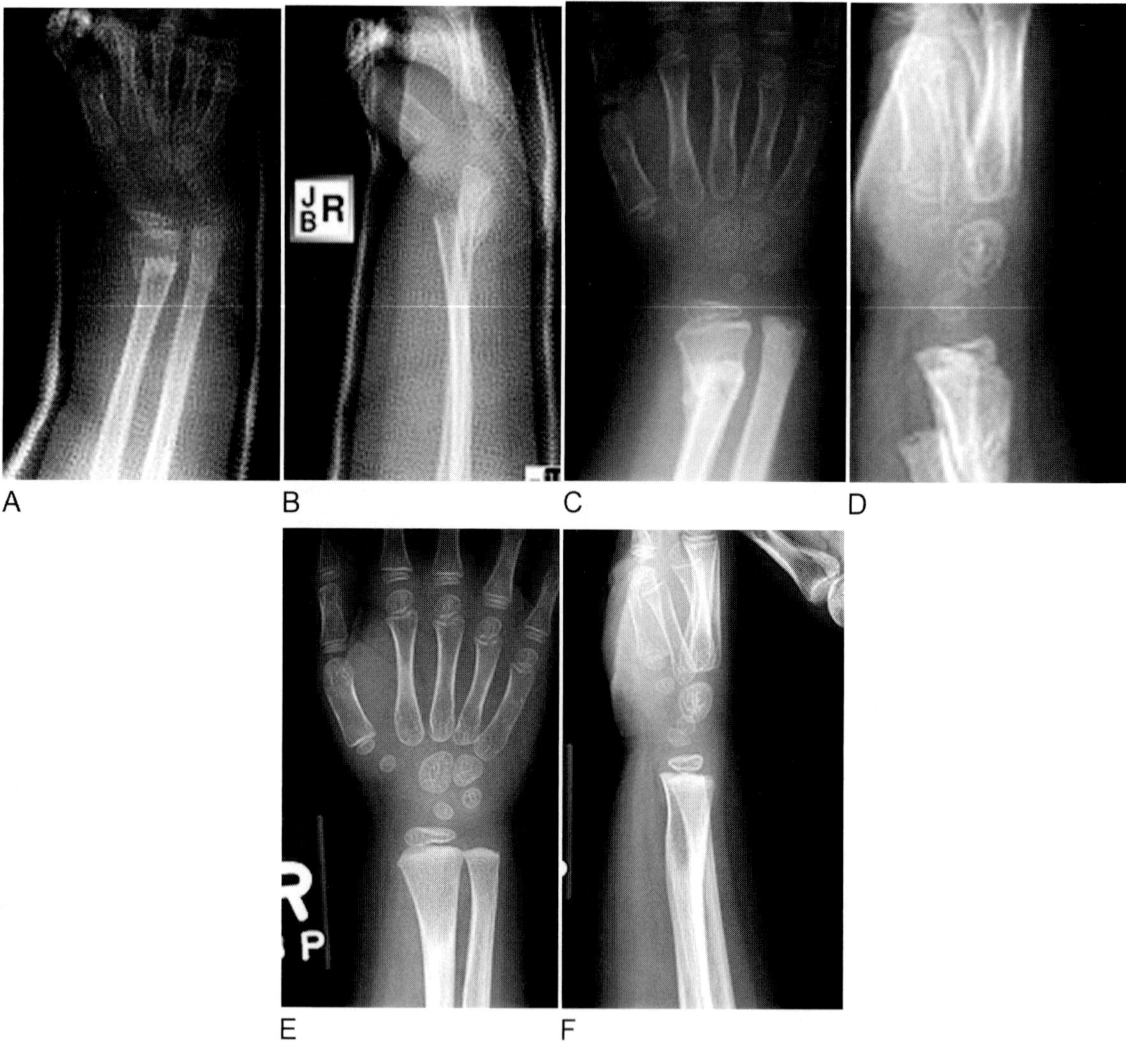

Figure 4–15: Typical dramatic remodeling that can be expected after distal radius fracture in a young child. The child in this case is 3 years old. AP (A) and lateral (B) radiographs were taken after attempted closed reduction of a complete distal radial metaphyseal fracture. Note that there is no three-point mold on the cast and that the wrist is in radial deviation after reduction. An AP radiograph (C) and a lateral radiograph (D) were taken after the fracture healed in malangulation, 3 weeks after reduction. Finally, an AP radiograph (E) and a lateral radiograph (F) of the wrist show dramatic remodeling of the distal radius and ulna 7 months after reduction.

confirmed by specific tenderness over the distal radial physis.

- Radiographs should include good quality AP and lateral views centered at the wrist. In addition, radiographs of the whole forearm, including the elbow, are valuable to rule out associated injuries.
- In occult or nondisplaced fractures, the pronator fat pad sign may alert the physician to the presence of an injury.
- Nondisplaced Salter-Harris I fractures at the distal radius or ulna can be splinted, with an evaluation and management appointment scheduled within a few days. If there is minimal swelling, a short arm cast can be applied in the emergency department.
  - A simple, well-padded volar splint from the metacarpal heads to the proximal forearm safely gives sufficient comfort to the injured child.
  - If an elastic ace wrap is used, wrap with no tension to avoid the finger swelling commonly seen a few days later if the ace wrap is stretched during splint application.
- Displaced fractures should be reduced under conscious sedation or general anesthesia.
  - Most fractures are dorsally displaced with disruption of the volar periosteum (Figure 4–16).
  - The reduction maneuver involves volarward pressure on the distal fragments with slight traction. Too much traction tightens the periosteum, making reduction more difficult.
- A long arm splint or cast is used to hold reduction.
  - A three-point mold, with volarward pressure at the fracture, works with the intact periosteum to maintain reduction during the 4 weeks in a cast.
  - In children with more than 1-2 years of growth remaining, up to 50% displacement is acceptable.

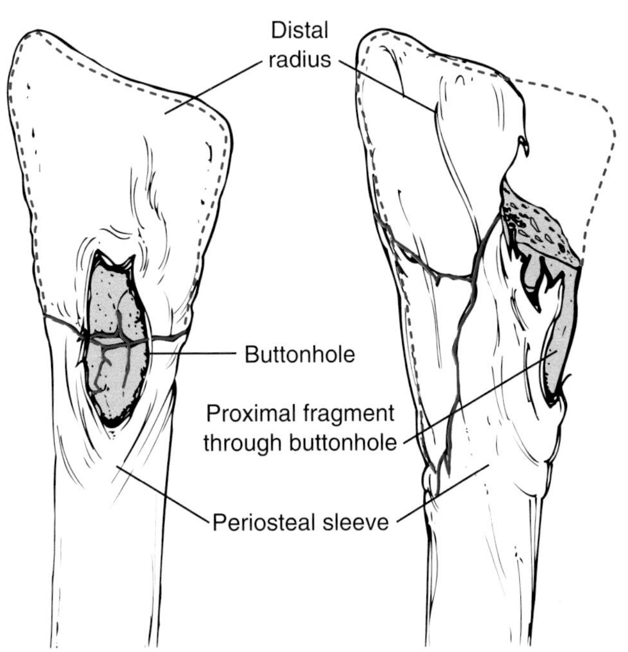

Figure 4–16: This schematic demonstrates the location of the periosteal injury in a completely dorsally displaced distal radius metaphyseal fracture. **Understanding the anatomy of the periosteal sleeve is essential to obtaining a safe and satisfactory reduction.**

  - Repeat reductions more than 3 days after injury are thought to risk physeal arrest.
  - Irreducible fractures may result from interposed tissue, especially on the volar side. The tissue may include the median nerve or radial artery, so careful examination is important.
  - Open or closed reduction with Kirschner wire (K-wire) fixation is used rarely—only for irreducible fractures, for fractures associated with acute carpal tunnel syndrome, and after irrigation and debridement of open fractures. During pinning, care should be taken to avoid the radial sensory nerve and extensor tendons.
- The long-term outcome after distal radius and ulnar physeal fractures is usually excellent.
- Up to 30-40 degrees of dorsal angulation will remodel satisfactorily in a child who has more than 3 years of growth remaining.
- Physeal arrest after distal radius fractures is rare, occurring in less than 10% of these common injuries.
- Follow a displaced distal radial physeal fracture for up to 1 year to be certain that there is not growth arrest.

Metaphyseal Distal Radius and Ulnar Fractures

- Metaphyseal fractures to the arm occur during early childhood and during the adolescent growth spurt, when the trabecular bone of the metaphysis is thought to weaken temporarily during rapid growth.
- Most are caused by a fall on an outstretched hand, usually with some pronation to the wrist.
- Most displace dorsally.
- Nondisplaced buckle fractures can be splinted or casted at the time of injury.
- A short arm cast worn for 3-4 weeks allows healing of most buckle fractures.
- In children younger than 3, it may be necessary to take the cast above the elbow because the toddler can often wiggle out of a short arm cast and return for recasting.
- Greenstick fractures, which involve a break on the tension (usually volar) cortex, are treated similarly with slightly longer protection.
- After 4 weeks in a short or long arm cast, most fractures will be healed and the child will have no tenderness at the fracture site.
  - The orthopedist can place a short arm cast then test pronation and supination in the cast.
  - If the child is comfortable, there is no need to take the cast above the elbow.
- Complete fractures require closed reduction.
  - Once adequate conscious sedation is obtained, the fracture is reduced by re-creation of the deformity (extreme volar angulation) and reduction with a volarward pressure. Unlike in the comminuted adult Colles, traction will make reduction more difficult.
  - A carefully prepared cast, with three-point molding (Figure 4–17), is applied.

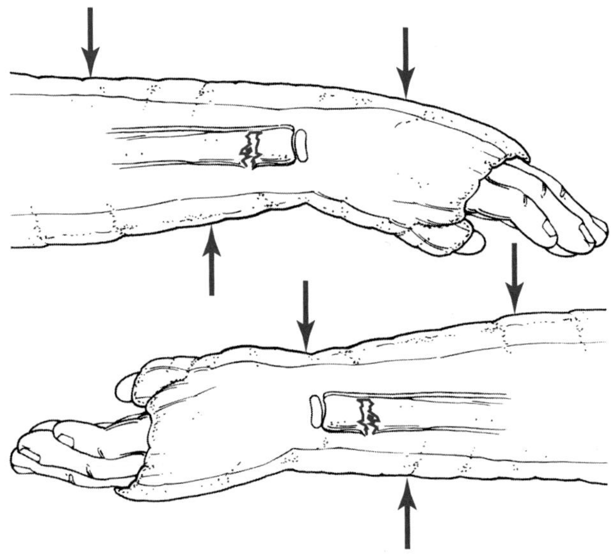

Figure 4–17: This schematic demonstrates the location of a three-point mold for a distal radial metaphyseal fracture and how this mold is influenced by the location of the periosteal disruption. Redrawn from Rockwood C, Wilkins K, Beaty J (1996) Fractures in Children, 4th edition. Philadelphia, Lippincott-Raven.

- Neutral or slight pronation of the forearm is preferred.
- A long arm cast is used for completely displaced fractures.
- An initial follow-up with x-rays occurs between 5 and 10 days.
- If the angulation is unacceptable at this time, a repeat reduction can be performed.
- In children younger than 10 years, up to 30 degrees of dorsal angulation or 20 degrees of radial angulation will yield a good result.
- After age 10, less than half of this displacement should be accepted.
- Pinning is used in rare circumstances (Figure 4–18).

Galeazzi Fractures

- A Galeazzi fracture is a distal radius fracture with disruption (or its equivalent) of the TFCC (Figure 4–19).
- A Galeazzi fracture is a relatively rare injury in children.

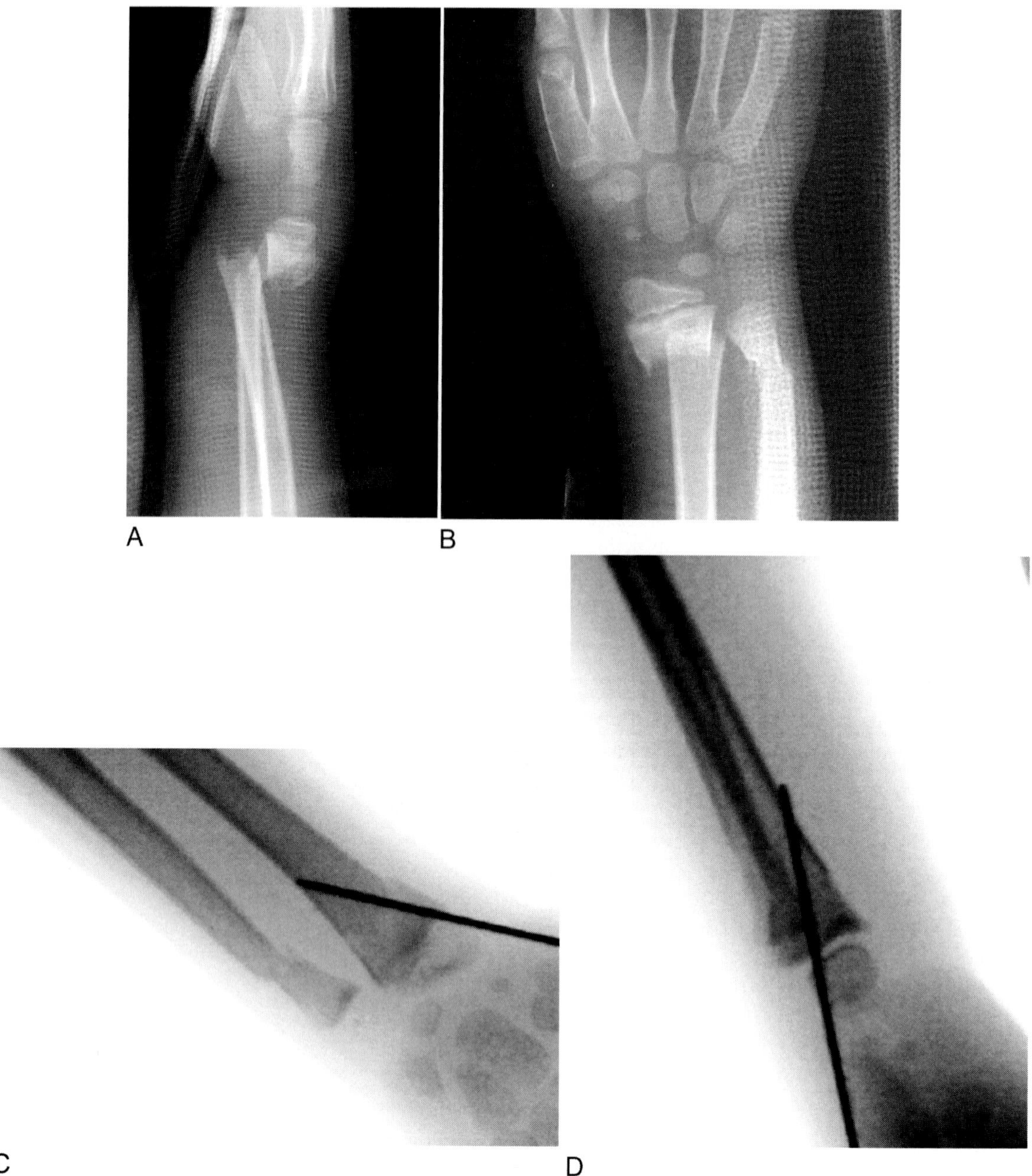

Figure 4–18: Intramedually pinning of a distal radius fracture. A lateral radiograph (A) and an AP radiograph (B) demonstrated a completely displaced distal radius and ulnar fracture in a child who also had a supracondylar fracture. An AP radiograph (C) and a lateral radiograph (D) after closed reduction and pinning.

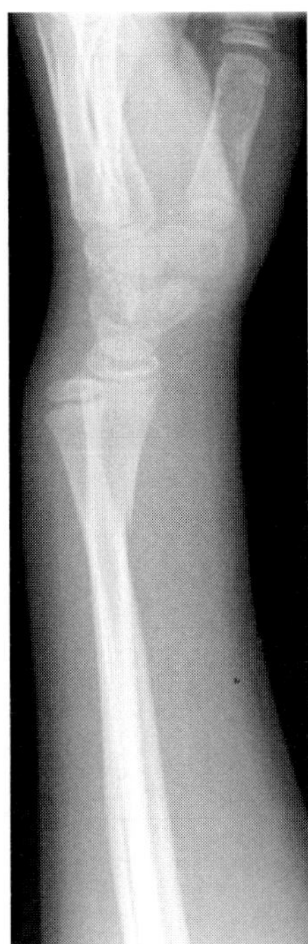

Figure 4–19: A Galeazzi fracture involving the distal–radial metaphyseal–diaphyseal junction and the distal–radial ulnar joint.

- In adults, a Galeazzi fracture is more common than a Monteggia lesion. This incidence is reversed in children.
- Galeazzi fractures are thought to occur by a fall on the outstretched hand with extreme hand or wrist pronation.
- The equivalent fractures in children include a radius fracture with a distal ulnar physeal injury.
- Generally, these fractures can be successfully treated by closed reduction and a long arm cast for 6 weeks. The forearm should be casted in slight pronation.
- Open reduction or pinning is rarely necessary in children.

Injuries to the Shafts of the Radius and Ulna

Radius and Ulna Diaphyseal Fractures

- Radial and ulnar diaphyseal fractures can be more difficult to treat because the limits of acceptable reduction are more stringent than those for distal radial fractures.
- A significant malunion of a forearm diaphyseal fracture can lead to a permanent loss of pronation and supination and sometimes an unsightly curvature or prominence in the forearm.
- Fortunately, diaphyseal fractures are four times less common than distal radius fractures and are seen more frequently in younger children, where remodeling potential is better.
- Like most other fractures in the upper extremity, these injuries are typically caused by a fall on an outstretched arm, usually with a significant rotational component.
- Understanding this rotational component is valuable in performing the reduction, especially in greenstick fractures.
- The examiner should note the rotation of the arm, the neurovascular status, the location of the deformity, and the status of the compartment pressures.
- Although upper extremity compartment syndrome is rare, the most common cause is a severe radial and ulnar diaphyseal fracture.
- Radiographs should include two views at right angles to one another that include the entire extent of the forearm on the same film.
  - The wrist and the elbow should be clearly visualized.
  - The fracture location and pattern should be noted.
- In fractures with the dorsal angulation, the distal fragment is pronated; in fractures with a volar angulation, the distal fragment is supinated. The key to reduction of these greenstick fractures (Figure 4–20) is reversal of this rotation (Figure 4–21).
- In complete fractures, the widths of the diaphyseal fragments at the fracture site should be studied. A significant discrepancy in the width of the bone ends adjacent to the fracture suggests a rotational deformity. In addition, the relationship of the bicipital tuberosity to the radial styloid should be noticed—in anatomical alignment, the bicipital tuberosity should be opposite the radial styloid.
- In all angulated or displaced radius and ulna diaphyseal fractures, a manipulative closed reduction under conscious sedation or general anesthesia should be performed.
  - Once the child is comfortably sedated, the fracture can be reduced by rotating the palm toward the angulation (e.g., supinate the hand to correct the pronation deformity of a dorsally angulated fracture).
  - Acceptable reduction is 10-20 degrees of angulation in children younger than 10 years but no more than 10 degrees of angulation in older children and adolescents.
  - Bayonet apposition is acceptable at union, but correction to near-anatomical alignment should be sought at the time of injury.
- Because diaphyseal fractures heal more slowly than distal metaphyseal fractures, clinical and radiograph evaluation should be performed about 1 and 2 weeks after injury.
  - Loss of reduction is common.
  - If loss of reduction causes an unacceptable alignment, repeat manipulation or limited internal fixation with wires or plates can be used even several weeks after injury.
  - Cast immobilization should be continued for at least 6 weeks. Sometimes, in high-energy fractures, open fractures, or fractures in adolescents, up to 8 weeks of cast immobilization may be required.
  - Immobilization should be in a well-molded long arm cast with a flat ulnar border and a good interosseous mold (Figure 4–22).

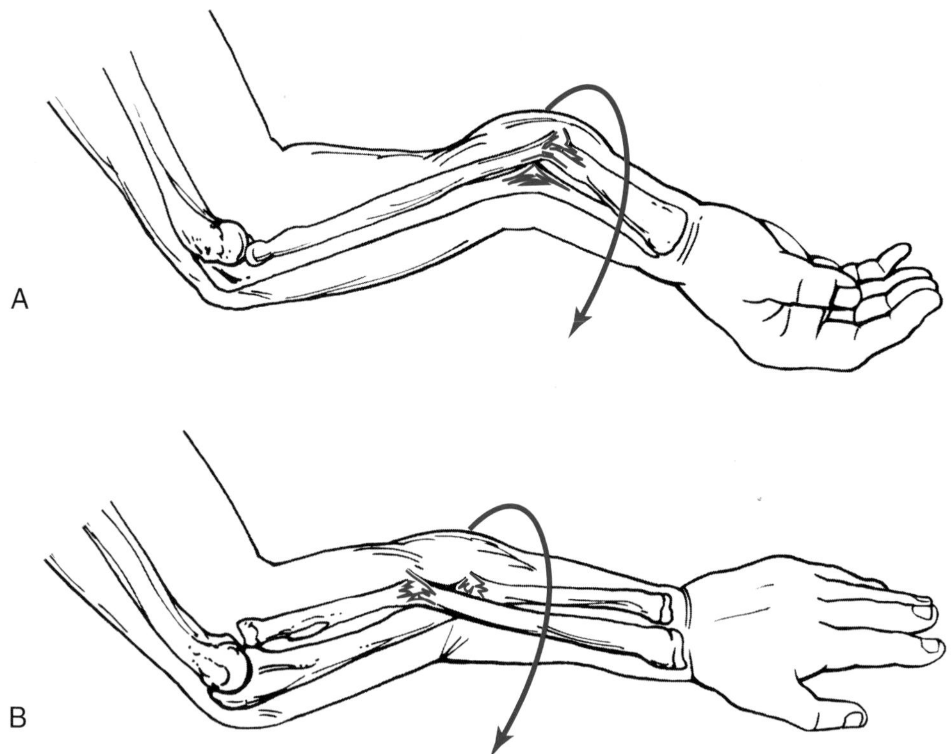

Figure 4–20: This schematic shows the importance of rotation to the understanding a greenstick fracture of the diaphysis of the radius and ulna. Redrawn from Rockwood C, Wilkins K, Beaty J (1996) Fractures in Children, 4th edition. Philadelphia, Lippincott-Raven.

  - Some prefer to include the thumb, though this is not the author's practice.
- The major causes of failed treatment of these fractures are a lack of understanding of the rotational component of the fracture and poor technical skills in making the cast.
- If reduction is inadequate or there is loss of reduction, operative intervention is warranted.[10]
- Intramedullary K-wires or titanium nails have been used with success to stabilize one or both bones.
- Preferred entry is proximally for the ulna and, if necessary, distally for the radius (through Lister's tubercle, or radially, with caution to avoid the radial nerve).
- Single-bone fixation, with supplemental casting, often is adequate for many pediatric diaphyseal forearm fractures[11] (Figure 4–23).
- As children approach maturity, adult-style plating, allowing rapid mobilization, is preferred (Figure 4–24).

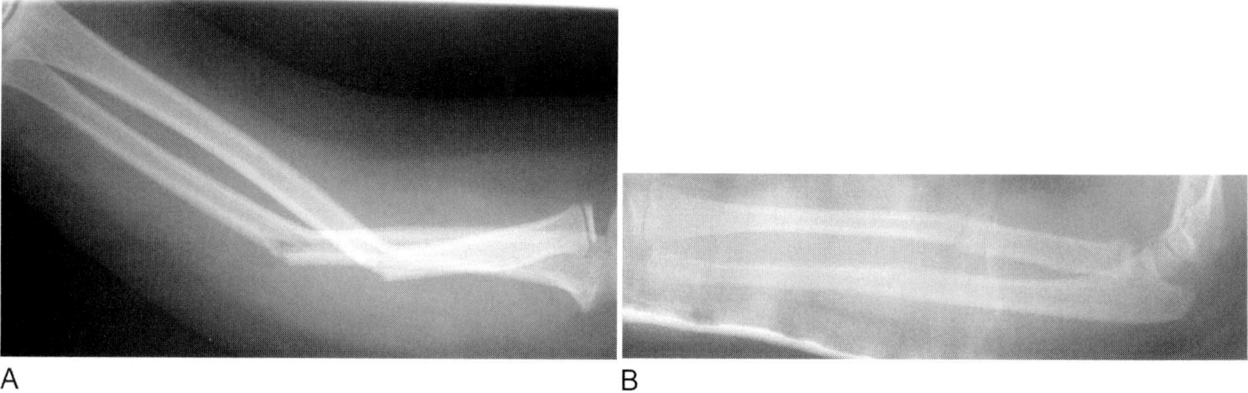

Figure 4–21: Closed reduction of a greenstick radius and ulnar fracture. (A) This radiograph demonstrates a diaphyseal forearm fracture that is difficult to manage. There is a midshaft greenstick fracture of the ulna and a closer greenstick fracture of the radius. (B) After proper closed reduction techniques, there is near-perfect anatomical alignment. This reduction was affected primarily by rotation. Understanding the rotational forces on the two fragments is critical to obtaining a proper reduction.

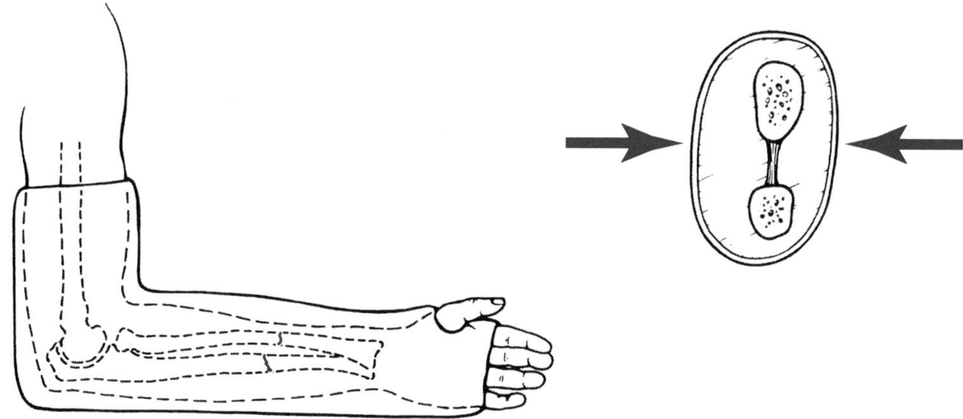

Figure 4–22: This schematic demonstrates the proper shape of a cast to hold a diaphyseal radius and ulna fracture. Redrawn from Green NE (1998) Skeletal Trauma in Children, 2nd edition. Philadelphia, WB Saunders.

Plastic Deformation of the Radius, Ulna, or Both

- In young children, especially those younger than 7, the radius and ulnar shafts can plastically deform rather than completely fracture. This occurs when the injury force exceeds the yield point—but not the failure point—of the bone.[12]
- In young children who have no cosmetic deformity and who have full range of motion, casting without reduction is acceptable. However, if the arm appears bowed or motion is lost, reduction should be attempted in the operating room.
  - A great amount of force is applied at a slow rate over a long period to correct the plastic deformation.
  - A long arm cast for 4-6 weeks can then be used.

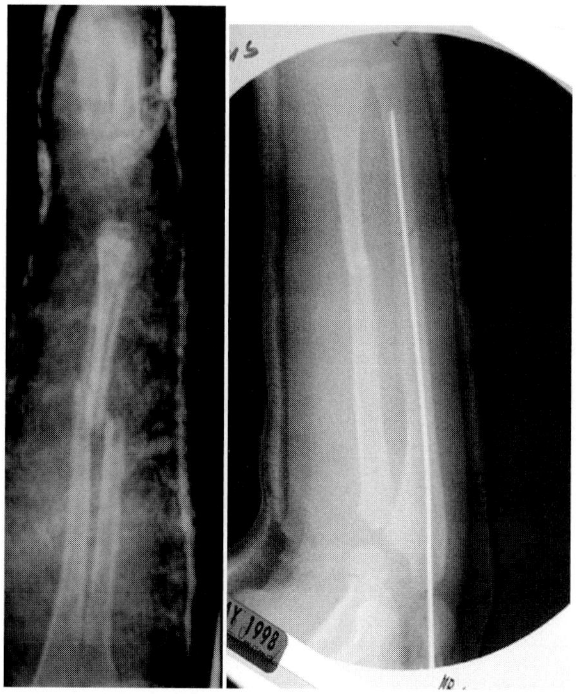

A B

Figure 4–23: Use of a single-bone fixation to manage a radius and ulna diaphyseal fracture. (A) This radiograph was taken after two attempts of closed reduction of a distal radius and ulnar fracture. (B) This intraoperative radiograph shows anatomical alignment of the radius and ulna. The ulna was held with an intramedually K-wire, then the radius was reduced and held by the cast.

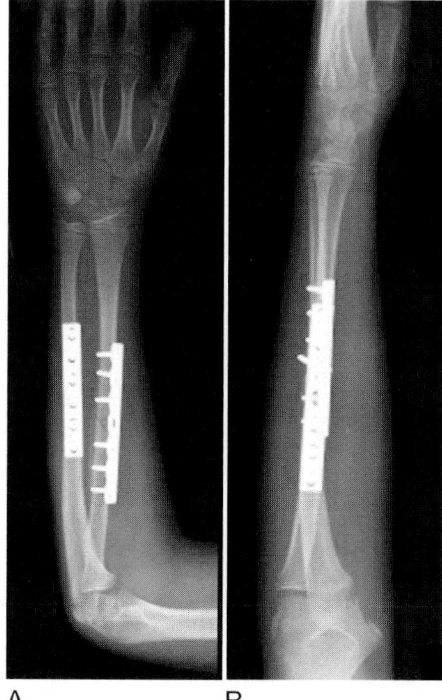

A B

Figure 4–24: This AP radiograph (A) and this lateral radiograph (B) shows a pediatric diaphyseal forearm fracture treated with internal fixation by plates after closed reduction failed. Note the use of the 2.7 dynamic compression plate (DCP). This is ideal for the smaller bone size in children. 3.5 DCPs are usually too large in this age group.

Monteggia Fractures

- The term *Monteggia fracture* describes a group of injuries with radial head subluxation or humeral dislocation and an ulnar fracture.
- Although these injuries represent less than 1% of all pediatric forearm fractures, they receive great attention because their recognition and treatment can be challenging.
- Most of these injuries occur in children younger than 10 years.
- Many isolated radial head dislocations discovered late were probably missed traumatic lesions rather than congenital dislocations.
- A commonly accepted classification of Monteggia fractures was described by Bado[13] (Figure 4–25).
- Type I fractures involve anterior dislocation of the radial head, type II fractures include posterior dislocation of the radial head, type III fractures involve lateral dislocation of the radial head, and type IV fractures are segmental radius fractures with dislocation of the radial head. In each case, the ulna angulates in the direction of the radial head dislocation.
- There are also a large number of Monteggia equivalents, which involve various fracture combinations of the proximal ulna, radial neck, and physis.
- Most fractures occur because of a fall on an outstretched hand with extreme pronation of the forearm caused by the weight of the body over the planted hand. This will dislodge the radial head anteriorly.
- With the same trauma and severe supination, a type II lesion is produced.
- Type III lesions may be caused by a fall with a varus force, fracturing the ulna and dislodging the radial head laterally.
- Type IV fractures are usually caused by pronation during a fall onto an outstretched hand.
- High-quality radiographs are mandatory to manage Monteggia fractures successfully.
  - Views of the whole forearm and isolated elbow radiographs should be obtained.
  - The radial head should point toward the center of the capitellum on all views (Figure 4–26).
- The treating physician should persist until a true lateral radiograph of the elbow is achieved. Without such a view, it is easy to miss subtle, anterior radial head subluxation.
- A careful neurological examination is essential because up to 20% of Monteggia fractures appear as a nerve palsy.[13,14] The most common finding is a posterior innerousus nerve palsy associated with Bado III lesions.
- Treatment involves an initial attempt at closed reduction with conscious sedation or general anesthesia.
- The reduction maneuver varies with the fracture type.
  - Type I fractures (Figure 4–27) are reduced with forearm supination and complete elbow flexion.
    1. The observant physician will detect a clunking sensation when the radial head relocates.
    2. A well-molded long arm cast is then applied for 4-6 weeks.

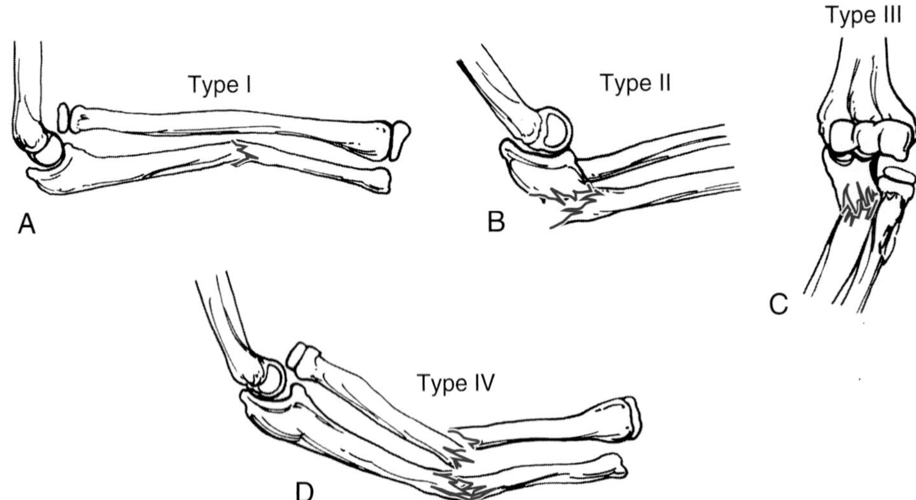

Figure 4–25: A schematic of the different types of Monteggia fractures. **(A) Type I Monteggia fracture with anterior angulation of the ulna and anterior dislocation of the radiocapitellar joint. (B) Type II Monteggia fracture with posterior angulation and radial head dislocation. (C) Type III Monteggia fracture with a greenstick fracture of the ulna and lateral subluxation of the radial head. (D) Type IV Monteggia fracture with complete fracture of the radius and ulna distally and an anterior dislocation of the radial head. Redrawn from Rockwood C, Wilkins K, Beaty J (1996) Fractures in Children, 4th edition. Philadelphia, Lippincott-Raven.**

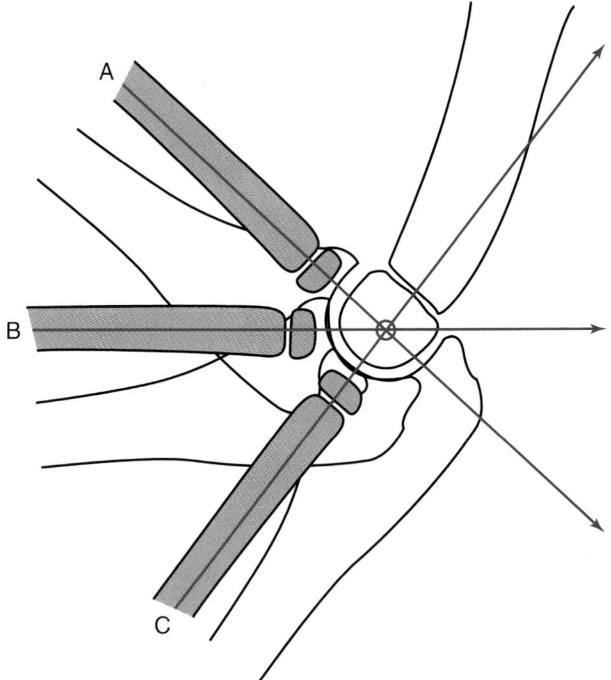

Figure 4–26: In all views, a line drawn down the center of the radial shaft should intersect the center of the capitellum. **Redrawn from Rockwood C, Wilkins K, Beaty J (1996) Fractures in Children, 4th edition. Philadelphia, Lippincott-Raven.**

- Type II fractures, more common in older children and adolescents, are reduced with forearm extension.
  1. Maintaining a reduction may be difficult in a long arm cast with the elbow flexed.
  2. If this is the case, K-wire fixation of the ulna is a relatively simple way to hold reduction and treat the injury in a long arm cast.
- Type III fractures require correction of the varus angulation to reduce the radial head.
  1. This can be challenging because the orthopedist needs to fight the deforming force of a greenstick proximal ulna fracture to keep the radial head reduced.
  2. Again, failure of simple closed techniques can be addressed with K-wire fixation of the proximal ulna in the operating room after reduction under fluoroscopic guidance.
- Type IV fractures are difficult to treat with a simple closed reduction. Often, the radial shaft fracture must be internally fixed with a plate or wires to successfully reduce the radial head.

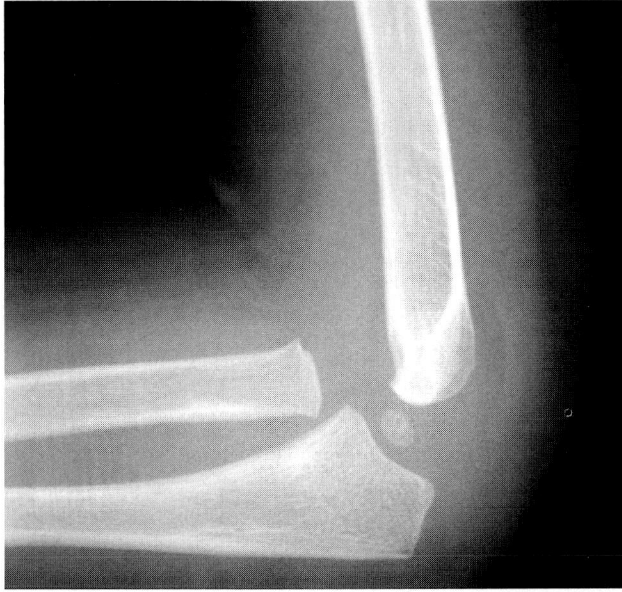

Figure 4–27: This lateral radiograph of the elbow depicts a dislocated radial head associated with an ulnar fracture. **This is a Bado I Monteggia fracture. Note the posterior fat pad associated with this elbow injury.**

- Vigilance by the treating surgeon in the postreduction period is essential.
  - Follow-up examination and radiographs once or twice in the first 3 weeks should assure that the radial head remains reduced.
  - If there is any question about whether the radial head has remained reduced, the surgeon should remove the cast and repeat the radiographs until the issue is clarified.
- It is better to repeat the reduction lost because of cast removal then to discover weeks later that the radial head has redislocated and that the ulna fracture has healed.
- Fixation of the ulna is sometimes necessary to achieve the stability required to keep the radial head reduced.
- Complications include failure of recognition, failure of reduction, loss of reduction, nerve injury, late stiffness, radial head avascular necrosis, and radial ulnar synostosis.
- If a Monteggia fracture is missed, late reconstruction involves the restoration of the ulnar length and alignment and an open reduction of the radial head, often with angular ligament reconstruction.
- Results of late reconstruction become poor more than 6-12 months after injury.

Fractures of the Proximal Radius and Ulna

Proximal Radius Fractures

- The so-called radial head fracture is a fairly common childhood injury (Figure 4–28).
- Many fractures are minimally displaced.
- In children, a displaced intra-articular fracture is rare.
- Because the radial head's relationship with the capitellum is critical in maintaining forearm rotation, optimal reduction of angulation—and more importantly, translation—offers the best chance of a good functional result.
- Evaluation at the time of injury should include a search for associated injuries and radiographs that show the forearm, the wrist, and the elbow anatomy.

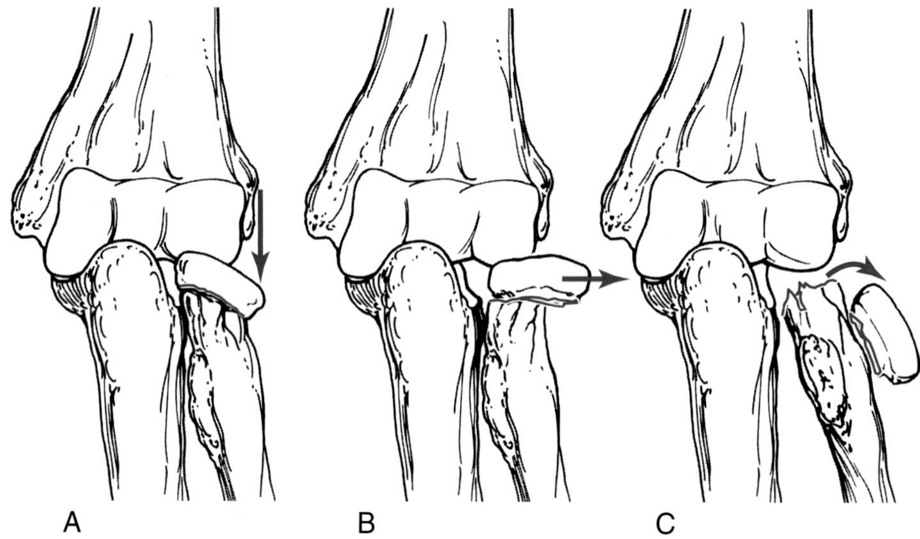

Figure 4–28: Three types of radial neck fractures. (A) Angulation of the radial neck. (B) Translocation of the radial neck. (C) Total displacement of the proximal radial fragment. Redrawn from Rockwood C, Wilkins K, Beaty J (1996) Fractures in Children, 4th edition. Philadelphia, Lippincott-Raven.

- The neurovascular examination should focus attention on the radial nerve.
- An attempt should be made to reduce all displaced fractures with conscious sedation or general anesthesia. This can be aided by injecting a local anesthetic into the radiocapitellar joint and evacuating the hematoma before reduction.
- After an attempt at closed reduction, up to 30 degrees of angulation but minimal translation can be accepted. If there is more than 30 degrees of angulation, a repeat reduction should be attempted.
- If reduction under conscious sedation fails, additional attempts should be made with fluoroscopic guidance in the operating room.
- Several maneuvers can help to reduce a radial head fracture.
  - With the elbow extended, a valgus force can be placed directly over the radial head to achieve a reduction.
  - If this fails, the flexion pronation technique is valuable.
    1. With pressure over the radial head, the elbow extended, and the forearm in supination, pronate the forearm while fully flexing the elbow (Figure 4–29).
    2. Even 100% radial head dislocations can be reduced closed with this maneuver.
  - When all closed measures fail, a small K-wire or awl can be introduced through a small and lateral incision to push the fractured fragment back into position.
- Complications after radial head fracture are more common than generally appreciated. Loss of motion is the most common complication. Therefore, immobilization should be for no more than 3-4 weeks in children.
- Avascular necrosis of the radial head and heterotopic ossification have also been described.

Proximal Ulna Fractures

- Olecranon fractures are uncommon in children.
- These fractures may occur from a fall onto an outstretched hand or a direct blow to the elbow.
- Most are minimally displaced metaphyseal fractures.
- Avulsion fractures have also been described in children with osteogenesis imperfecta.[15,16]
- Displaced intra-articular fractures are managed with open reduction and internal fixation using a tension band technique or compression fixation with an interfragmentary screw.
- In children, the tension band can be strong suture rather than wire and the K-wires can be left percutaneous. This technique obviates the need to return to the operating room for hardware removal.

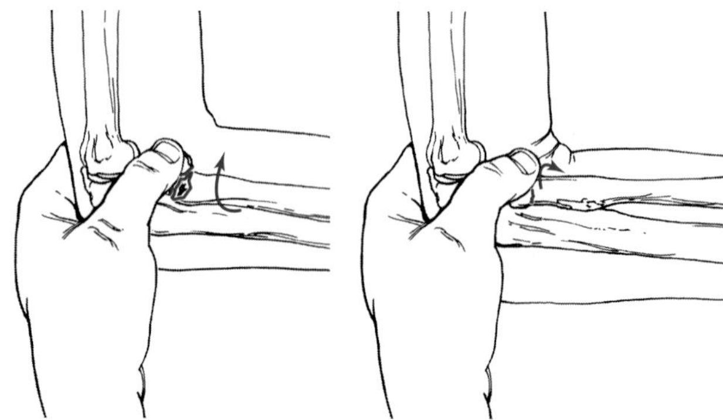

Figure 4–29: This schematic depicts the flexion–pronation technique of reducing a proximal radius fracture. Redrawn from Rockwood C, Wilkins K, Beaty J (1996) Fractures in Children, 4th edition. Philadelphia, Lippincott-Raven.

Fractures of the Elbow

General Principles

- Although elbow fractures are less common than forearm and wrist fractures, many pediatric elbow fractures receive more attention because more aggressive management is necessary to receive a good result.[17]
- Improper management of elbow injuries remains a common source of disability and malpractice litigation.
- Many elbow injuries are intra-articular, involve the physeal cartilage, or may result in rare pediatric malunions and nonunions with permanent functional loss.
- As the distal humerus develops, a series of ossification centers appear; these ossification centers can be mistaken for fractures by an inexperienced physician.
- The capitellar ossification center (Figure 4–30) appears first between 6 months and 2 years, followed by the medial epicondyle, the trochlea, and the lateral epicondyle.
- The medial epicondyle is the last to fuse to the distal humerus, usually in the midteenage years.
- The vascular supply around the elbow is good (Figure 4–31). This explains the rapid healing of metaphyseal fractures and the rich collateral network that allows profusion of the hand even when the distal brachial artery is occluded at the time of a severe supracondylar humerus fracture.
- Careful radiographic evaluation is an essential part of diagnosing and managing pediatric elbow injuries.
- The elbow has an anterior and posterior fat pad (Figure 4–32).
- The entire distal humerus is intra-articular.

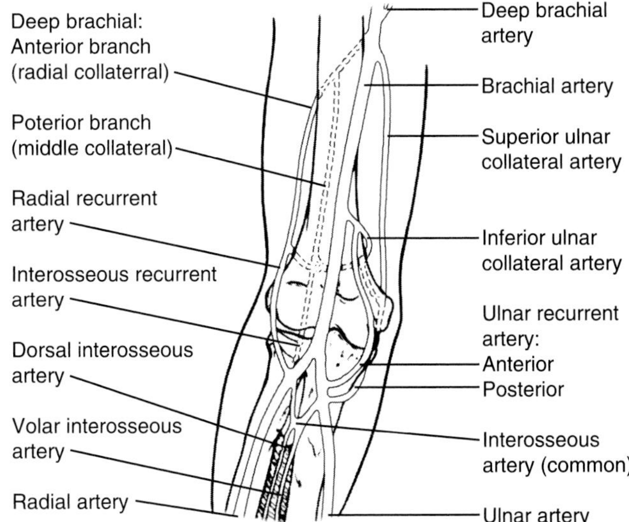

Figure 4–31: This schematic depicts the abundant vascular supply around the elbow. **Redrawn from Green NE (1998) Skeletal Trauma in Children, 2nd edition. Philadelphia, WB Saunders.**

- A distal humeral fracture will cause a hemarthrosis and elevate the fat pads.
- The posterior fat pad is the most important sign of an occult fracture. When the posterior fat pad sign is seen, there is a 70% chance of a fracture.[18]
- Several lines or radiographic relationships are important in evaluating elbow injuries in children.
  - On the AP view, Baumann's angle (Figure 4–33) is measured from the intersection of a line down the center of the humeral shaft and a line through the

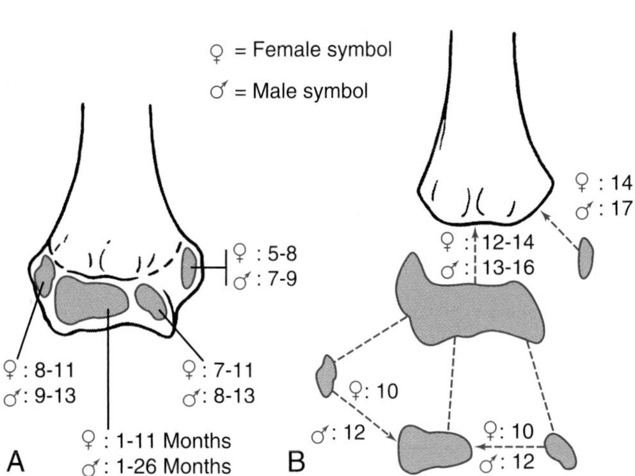

Figure 4–30: This schematic depicts the appearance (A) and the closure (B) of the ossification centers around the elbow in both boys and girls. **Redrawn from Green NE (1998) Skeletal Trauma in Children, 2nd edition. Philadelphia, WB Saunders.**

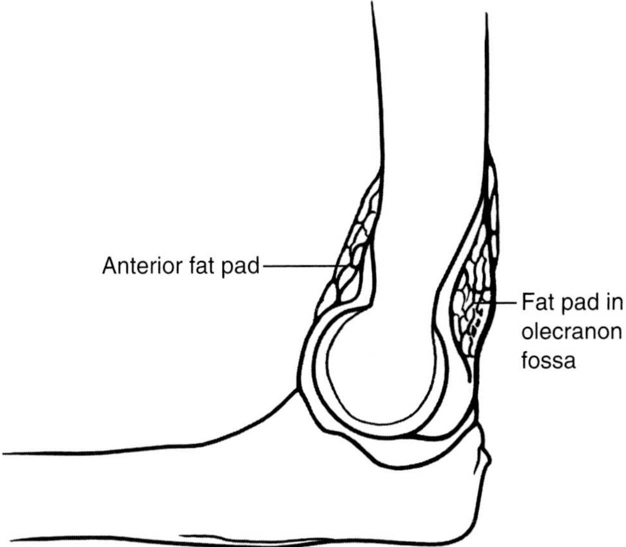

Figure 4–32: This schematic depicts the fat pads around the elbow. **Redrawn from Rockwood C, Wilkins K, Beaty J (1996) Fractures in Children, 4th edition. Philadelphia, Lippincott-Raven.**

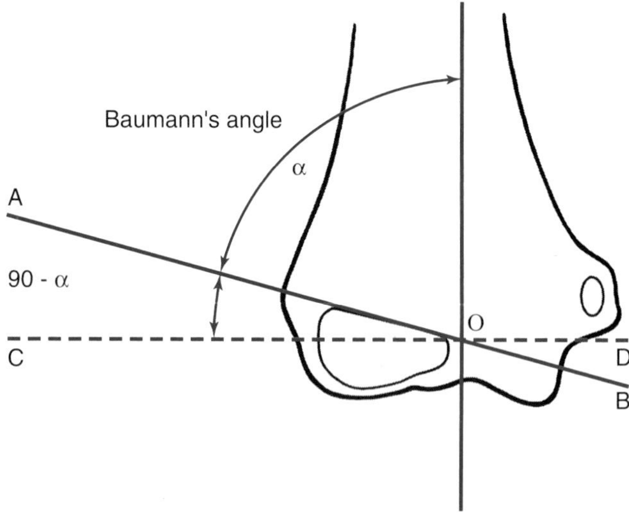

Figure 4–33: This schematic demonstrates a Baumann's angle. Redrawn from Rockwood C, Wilkins K, Beaty J (1996) Fractures in Children, 4th edition. Philadelphia, Lippincott-Raven.

capitellar physis. This should be within a few degrees of the opposite, uninjured side.
  - On a lateral view, a line drawn along the anterior humerus is valuable in assessing the amount of extension of a supracondylar fracture. Generally, the anterior humeral line should bisect the capitellum (Figure 4–34).

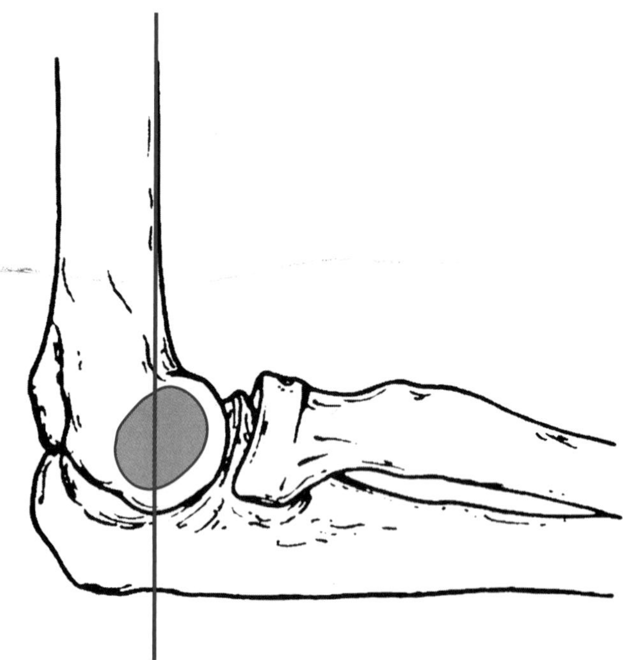

Figure 4–34: This schematic demonstrates the anterior humeral line. This line should intersect the capitellum. If the capitellum is behind this line, closed reduction pinning of an extension type supracondylar humerus fracture is indicated. Redrawn from Rockwood C, Wilkins K, Beaty J (1996) Fractures in Children, 4th edition. Philadelphia, Lippincott-Raven.

  - A humeral line that is anterior to the entire capitellum confirms an important extension of the distal humeral fracture fragment.

Supracondylar Fractures

- Supracondylar fractures occur most frequently in children younger than 8 years.
- Many young, ligamentously lax children can hyperextend their elbows. As they fall on an outstretched hand, this elbow hyperextension allows the olecranon to act as a wedge in the olecranon fossa, placing a tension force across the anterior humerus. If this force is sufficient, the anterior cortex is disrupted and a type I supracondylar fracture is produced.
- With further force, the fracture can partially or completely displace, producing a more significant injury.
- The distal humerus is a narrow area of rapidly remodeling bone in the young child, making this region particularly vulnerable to injury. The narrow width of the distal humerus also limits the bony stability necessary to hold a closed reduction of a displaced injury.
- Thus, before pinning was popularized, the completely displaced supracondylar humerus fractures treated in a cast would often rotate and angulate into varus, creating the so-called gunstock deformity.
- Many supracondylar humerus fractures are severe injuries in children and require careful evaluation and operative management.
  - At the time of the evaluation, the integrity of the skin should be assured and the neurovascular status should be checked carefully.
  - Nerve injuries occur in 10-15% of all supracondylar fractures (Figure 4–35).
  - The most common nerve injury is of the anterior interosseous nerve. This is evaluated by checking flexion of the thumb and index finger distal phalanx (Figure 4–36).
  - The radial nerve is most commonly injured when the distal fragment displaces in a posterior–medial direction.
  - Ulnar nerve injury is less common than median and radial nerve injuries but should be assessed carefully because pinning sometimes affects the ulnar nerve and documentation of the preoperative status is a valuable aid in managing this potential complication.
- Extension-type supracondylar humerus fractures are the most common source of fracture associated vascular injury in children.
- In an emergency room setting, the physician should assess the color and viability of the hand and the presence or absence of a radial pulse. The compartments of the forearm should be assessed carefully, especially in the presence of a possible vascular injury.
- Traditionally, the Wilkins modification of the Gartland classification has been used to describe supracondylar humerus fractures in children.

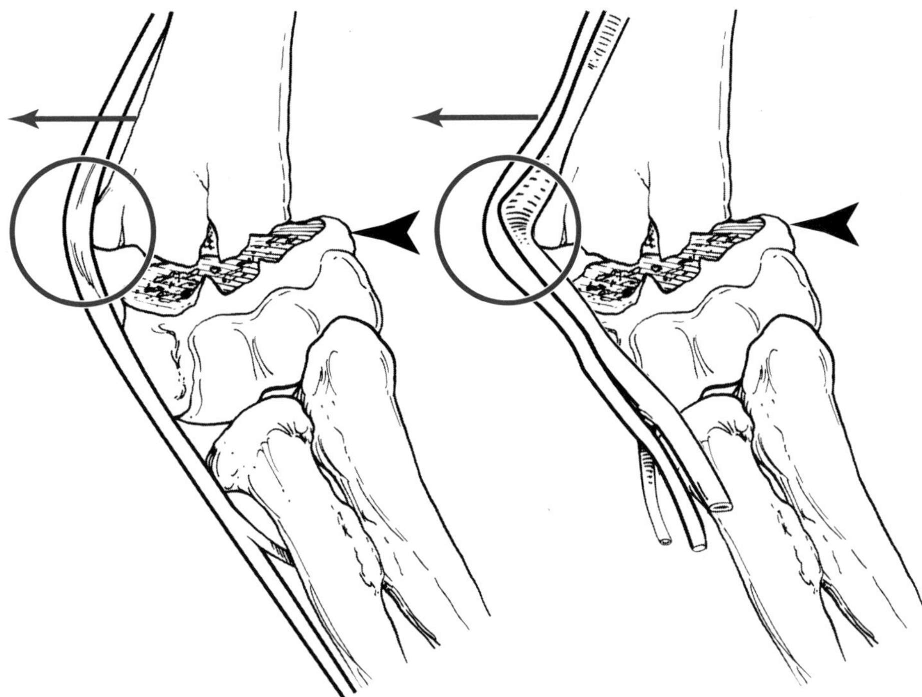

Figure 4–35: This schematic demonstrates how posterior–medial and posterior–lateral supracondylar humerus fractures can place tension on adjacent neurovascular structures. Redrawn from Rockwood C, Wilkins K, Beaty J (1996) Fractures in Children, 4th edition. Philadelphia, Lippincott-Raven.

- Type I fractures are nondisplaced, type II fractures are angulation with an intact posterior cortex, and type III fractures describe complete displacement of the distal humeral fragment.
- In Type III fractures, the humeral metaphysis often will tear through the brachialis muscle and can be palpated directly beneath the skin.
- The presence of ecchymosis and the puckering of the skin at the fracture site indicate a severe injury.

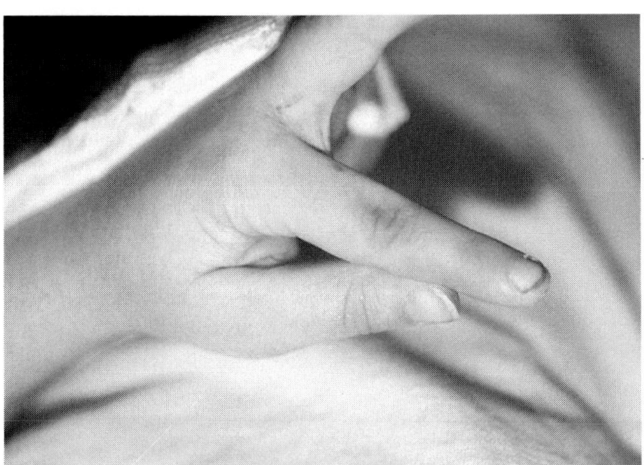

Figure 4–36: This clinical photograph demonstrates a child with anterior interosseous nerve palsy. The child was asked to flex the thumb interphalangeal joint and the index DIP joint but could not do so because of the nerve injury.

- Although the standard classification is valuable as a radiographic description, it may be easier to think of two types of supracondylar fractures: those that can be casted and those that need closed reduction and pinning.
  - Fractures in which the anterior humeral line intersects the capitellum and in which there is no collapse of the medial column can be treated with a cast for 3 weeks.
  - All other fractures are treated with closed reduction and pinning.
- In fractures with unacceptable extension or with medial collapse, simple evaluation and splinting should be performed in the emergency room. No reduction should be attempted.
- In more severe fractures, closed reduction and pinning are generally performed within 24 hours after injury.
  - With the child asleep and the elbow prepped, the fracture is reduced by correcting varus and valgus and then flexing the elbow fully, using the posterior periosteum to hold the distal humerus in position as pins are placed (Figure 4–37).
  - Two lateral pins, crossed medial and lateral pins, or two lateral pins and a medial pin are the most commonly used fixation strategies.
  - Evidence is increasing that lateral-entry pins only are the best way to avoid ulnar nerve injury and stabilize the fracture.[19] However, the technique is more demanding than crossed pins. Often three lateral pins are needed for type III fractures, and the surgeon must assure that all three engage both fragments securely (Figure 4–38).

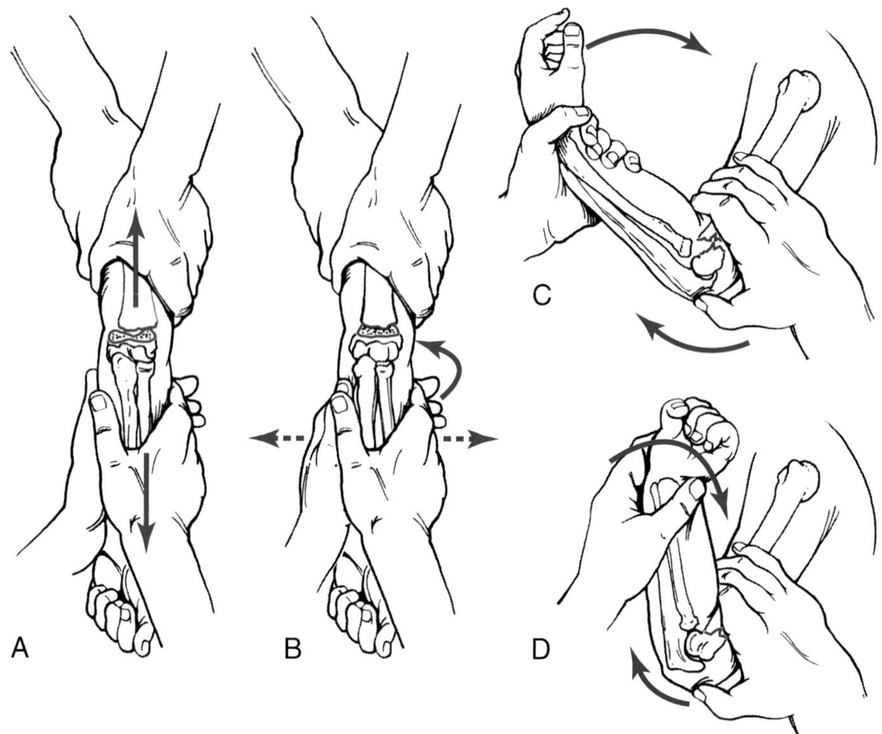

Figure 4–37: This schematic depicts the closed reduction maneuvers for a supracondylar humerus fracture. A, Gentle traction is first applied to the elbow and extension with the forearm supinated. B, Any varus or valgus angulation is corrected. C, The extension of the fracture is then reduced by pressure over the olecranon as the forearm is flexed. D, Pronation of the forearm further holds the fracture reduction in most cases.

  - If after pinning the hand is well perfused but a radial pulse cannot be felt, it is safe to observe the child closely rather than exploring the artery.
- Complications after supracondylar humerus fractures in children include loss of motion, cubitus varus, persistent neurological deficit, and avascular necrosis of the trochlea.
- Cubitus varus can be avoided by assuring that there is a satisfactory Bauman's angle after stable fixation is applied.
- Volkmann's ischemic contracture, fairly common when closed reduction alone was used, has been virtually eliminated.
- After pinning, the elbow can be immobilized in only 70–80 degrees of flexion, avoiding the forearm ischemia caused when the elbow was flexed above 90 degrees and the brachial artery was occluded because of arm position and swelling.

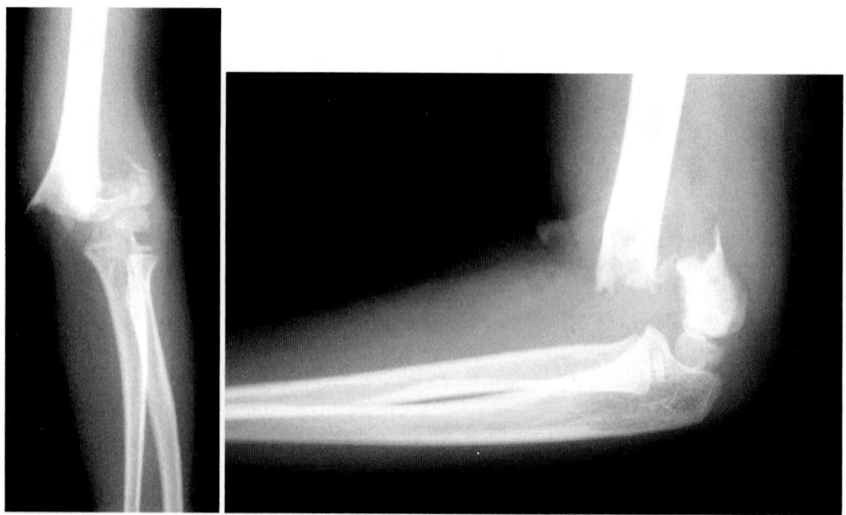

Figure 4–38: Pinning of a severe type III supracondylar humerus fracture. These AP (A) and lateral (B) radiographs show a completely displaced Type III supracondylar humerus fracture. These AP (C) and lateral intraoperative (D) radiographs demonstrate anatomical closed reduction and internal fixation using three widely divergent lateral pins. Fixation was stable, and the result was excellent.

Continued

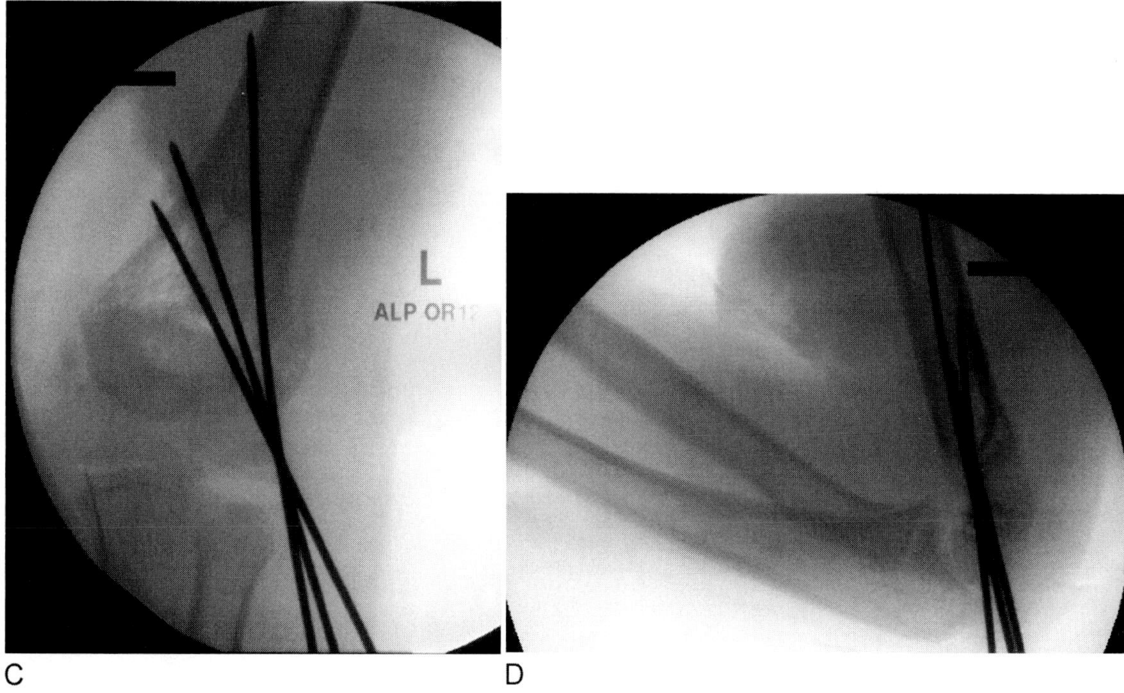

Figure 4–38, cont'd.

- Most nerve injuries associated with supracondylar fractures are neuropraxia that resolve without surgical intervention.
- Flexion-type supracondylar fractures are 50 times less common than extension-type supracondylar fractures. They generally occur when a child falls directly onto the elbow.
- Most displaced flexion supracondylar humerus fractures require internal fixation with pins.
- The most common nerve injury with flexion supracondylar fractures is to the ulnar nerve.
- A rare fracture is the distal humeral epiphyseal separation. It generally occurs in children younger than 5 years who fall on an outstretched hand and sustain an extension injury to the elbow.
- Reduction and treatment is similar to displaced supracondylar fractures with one exception: reduction after 3 days is not recommended because it risks causing a growth arrest of the distal humeral physis.

Lateral Condyle Fractures

- Fractures of the lateral condyle of the distal humerus are the second most common elbow fractures in children. These fractures can be caused by avulsion, by a varus force transmitted to the distal humerus during a fall on the outstretched hand, or by a direct blow on the capitellum by the humeral head through a fall on an outstretched hand.
- The Milch classification (Figure 4–39) is most commonly used to describe these injuries.
  - The type I fracture is a Salter-Harris IV fracture that passes from the metaphysis through the capitellar ossification center into the joint. The elbow is usually stable in these injuries.
  - In a Milch II fracture, the fracture line passes medial to the capitellum into the trochlear grove of the distal humerus. This is a Salter-Harris II fracture.
  - The Milch II fracture is more common than the Milch I and can be associated with elbow subluxation.
- A second classification, more valuable to surgeons, describes the stages of displacement.
  - A type I fracture is nondisplaced with an intact cartilaginous epiphyseal hinge.
  - A type II fracture is complete but not rotated.

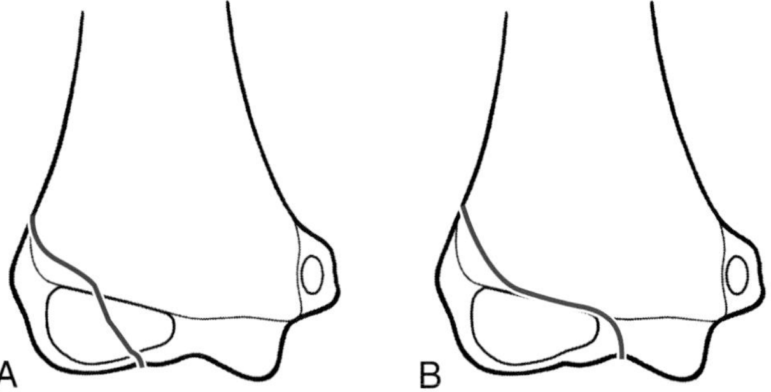

Figure 4–39: The Milch classification of a lateral condylar fracture. **A, The Milch I is a Salter-Harris IV fracture. B, The Milch II fracture is a Salter-Harris II fracture. Redrawn from Rockwood C, Wilkins K, Beaty J (1996) Fractures in Children, 4th edition. Philadelphia, Lippincott-Raven.**

- A type III fracture is completely displaced with the capitellum rotated out of the radiohumeral joint.

- Using this classification, some type I fractures can be treated with a cast whereas all other types are treated with either closed or open reduction and pinning.
- Evaluation at the time of injury includes a careful examination for other injuries and AP and lateral radiographs of the elbow.
- An oblique radiograph of the elbow often shows the greatest displacement of the fracture.
- Most lateral condyle fractures are treated surgically.
  - Lateral condyle fractures with less than 2 mm of displacement can be treated in a long arm cast for 4-6 weeks. X-rays should be taken 1 and 2 weeks after injury to assure that late displacement does not occur. It is wise to remove the cast for every radiograph to assure a quality image that will aid good decision making. If the fracture is so unstable that it moves at cast removal, then it should be pinned anyway.
  - Fractures with more than 2 mm of displacement are evaluated fluoroscopically in the operating room.

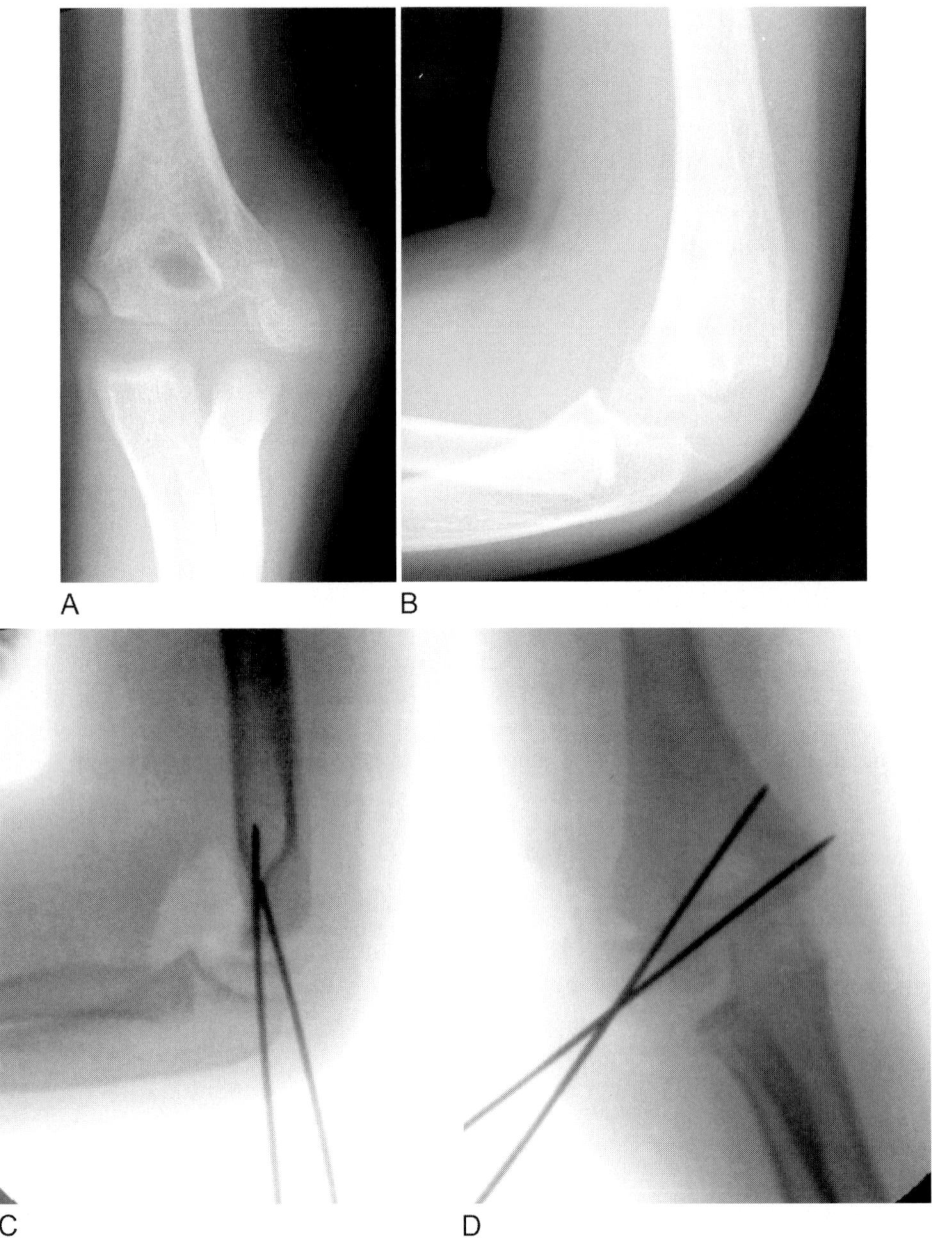

Figure 4–40: A displaced lateral condylar fracture treated with open reduction and internal fixation. This AP radiograph (A) and this lateral radiograph (B) demonstrate a widely displaced Milch type II lateral condyle fracture. This intraoperative lateral image (C) and this intraoperative AP image (D) were taken immediately after anatomical open reduction and internal fixation with two smooth K-wires.

  - Most require open reduction and internal fixation. Two K-wires are used to secure fixation after anatomical reduction (Figure 4–40).
  - Occasionally, a fresh, minimally displaced lateral condyle fracture can be satisfactorily treated with closed reduction and percutaneous pins.
- There are several important complications to remember when treating lateral condyle fractures.
  - These injuries are one of the rare pediatric fractures that can proceed to nonunion.
  - Because the fracture fragment is bathed in synovial fluid, is largely cartilage, and has a relatively tenuous blood supply, nonunion will occur in displaced, neglected fractures.
  - Late treatment of a neglected nonunion involves observation or open reduction, stable compression fixation, and bone grafting.
  - Cubitus valgus may occur with nonunion. This cubitus valgus may be associated with a tardy ulnar nerve palsy.

Medial Epicondyle Fractures

- Most medial epicondyle fractures occur in adolescent boys. The injury is thought to be caused by a valgus force combined with contraction of the forearm flexors–supinator complex.
- This same combination of forces will also cause an elbow dislocation. Therefore, the evaluating physician should never forget the association of medial epicondyle fractures with elbow dislocations.
  - These injuries occur together in nearly 50% of the cases.
  - The neurovascular status, particularly the status of the ulnar nerve, should be evaluated and other associated injuries should be ruled out.
  - The physician should study the AP and lateral radiographs of the elbow to determine the degree of displacement of the medial epicondyle.
- These injuries can be particularly subtle in younger children in which the medial epicondyle is minimally ossified.
- Remember, the medial epicondyle is a fairly posterior structure and may be difficult to appreciate on a lateral radiograph.
- The treatment of nondisplaced fractures involves cast immobilization for 3 weeks and then range of motion exercises.
- Less immobilization may be wise in children with an elbow dislocation because immobilization may be associated with greater stiffness after casting.
- The treatment of displaced medial epicondyle fractures is controversial.
  - If the fracture is displaced only 2-5 mm, most authors recommend cast immobilization for 3 weeks.
  - In fractures with more than 5 mm of displacement, internal fixation is standard treatment by most pediatric orthopedists, especially in the dominant arm of an athlete (Figure 4–41).
- Although several studies have documented high levels of function with nonoperative treatment of widely displaced medial epicondyle fractures, most surgeons fix these injuries. Families are generally not satisfied with the

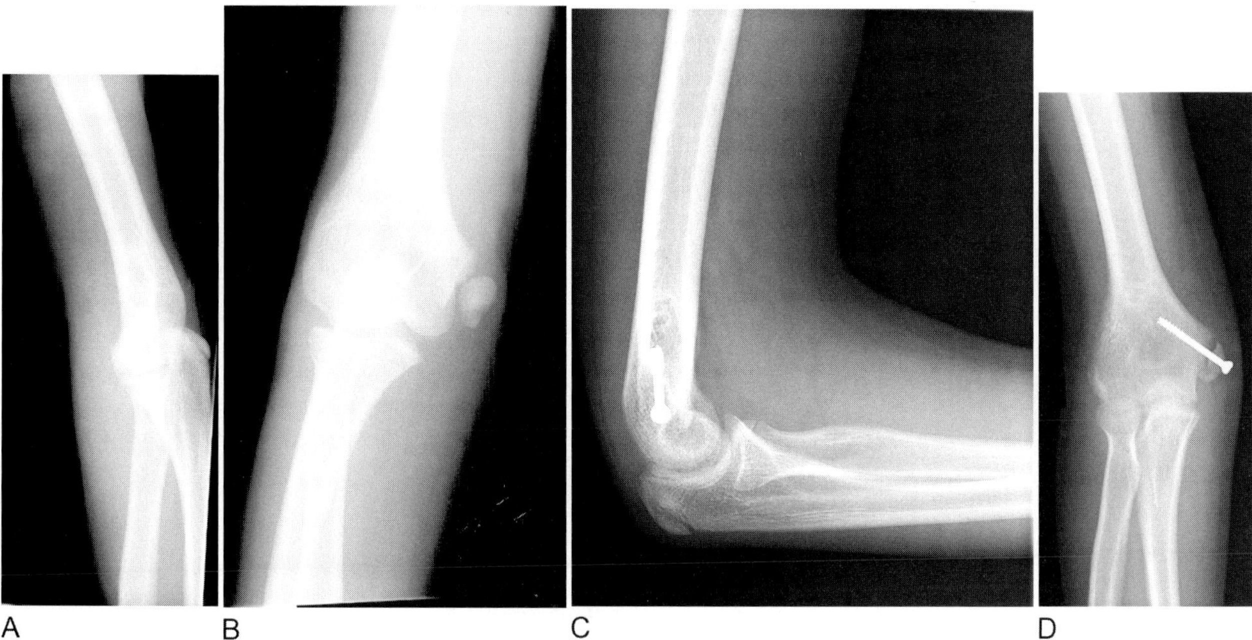

Figure 4–41: A displaced medial epicondyle fracture in an athlete treated with open reduction and internal fixation. This lateral radiograph (A) and this AP radiograph (B) show a completely displaced and rotated medial epicondyle fracture in a teenage baseball pitcher. This lateral radiograph (C) and this AP radiograph (D) were taken after open reduction and internal fixation of the fracture with a screw. Early mobilization was allowed.

fibrous nonunion that would be expected without treatment, even if it will eventually become asymptomatic.

- The main complication with medial epicondyle fractures is a loss of terminal elbow extension.
- This is particularly common if there has been an associated elbow dislocation or immobilization for an extended period.

Elbow Dislocations

- Although elbow dislocation is a rare injury in young children, it is seen with some frequency in adolescents. The same mechanism that will produce a supracondylar fracture in a 5- or 6-year-old produces an elbow dislocation in a teenager.
- Elbow dislocations are the result of the proximal radius and ulna being driven posteriorly from a force directed through the forearm, usually after a fall on the outstretched hand.
- The dislocation may occur with elbow flexion or extension.
- If there is a valgus component to the force, avulsion of the medial epicondyle may occur.
- Because the medial epicondyle may become incarcerated in the joint or maybe subtle, remembering the relationship between elbow dislocation and medial epicondyle is extremely important.
- In a child with a suspected elbow dislocation, the initial evaluation should include a careful neurovascular examination, the palpation of the upper extremity for other injuries, and an assessment of skin integrity.
- AP and lateral radiographs of the elbow and forearm should be assessed for the direction and extent of the dislocation, the presence of an incarcerated medial epicondyle fracture, and the presence of other associated injuries.
- The treatment of an elbow dislocation in children involves a prompt reduction of the dislocation under conscious sedation.
  - The reduction is generally easy, so general anesthesia is rarely required.
  - Reduction is through a traction maneuver or by pushing posteriorly over the olecranon (Figure 4–42) to reduce the displacement of the ulnar and radius onto the humerus.
  - In cases in which there is lateral displacement in addition to posterior displacement, correcting the lateral displacement first will avoid entrapment of the median nerve within the joint at the time of reduction. The reduction should be performed with the forearm supinated.
  - A satisfying "clunk" at the time of reduction is usually felt.
  - The elbow should then be taken through a gentle range of motion to assess stability.
  - Postreduction radiographs are essential. This AP and lateral of the elbow should be assessed for the congruency of the radial and ulnar articulations with the humerus and for the possible presence of an incarcerated medial epicondyle in the joint.

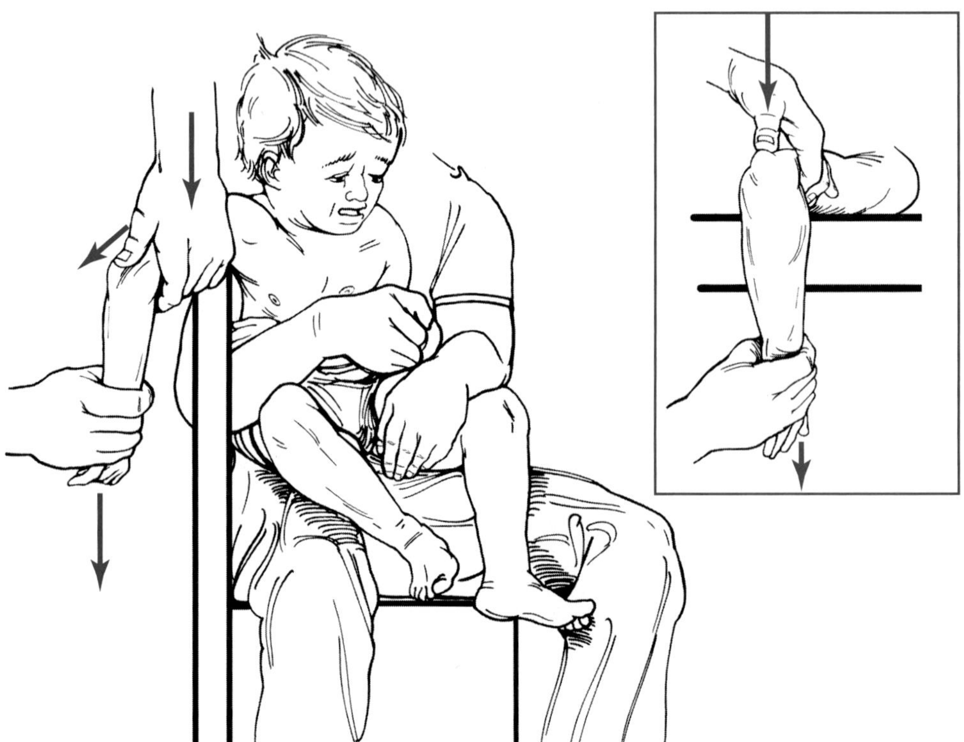

Figure 4–42: This schematic depicts a closed reduction technique for an elbow dislocation in a young child. Redrawn from Flynn JM, Nagda S (2004) Upper extremity injuries. In: Requisites in Pediatrics: Pediatric Orthopaedics and Sports Medicine (Dormans J, ed). Philadelphia, Mosby.

- The most common cause of an incongruent joint relationship is interposed tissue at the time of reduction.
- This usually involves the medial ligament and muscle-attached medial epicondyle.
- If this is noted, it is generally best to proceed to the operating room for general anesthesia and an open reduction to remove the interposed soft tissue.
- The postreduction assessment should also include an evaluation of nerve function.
- There are several alarming reports of an entrapped median nerve at the time of elbow reduction.

- Significant soft tissue disruption occurs at the time of an elbow dislocation. However, the greatest risk after these injuries is elbow stiffness rather than recurrent dislocation. Therefore, immobilization should occur for only 2-3 weeks followed by a supervised return to motion.
- In general, full terminal extension is avoided until 4-6 weeks after injury (depending on the stability).
- The authors generally prefer a cast for immobilization because splints and ace wraps are more likely to cause skin problems and become malpositioned during recovery.
- Complications from elbow dislocation include loss of motion, neurovascular injury, and recurrent dislocation.
- A careful assessment of stability and a return to early range of motion are the best ways to prevent elbow stiffness.
- The family should be counseled that terminal extension may be slow to return.
- Ulnar and median nerve injuries have been reported in several series of elbow dislocations. Some injuries occur at the time of injury, but median nerve injury can occur through entrapment at the time of reduction.
- As mentioned previously, recurrent dislocation is a rare problem after this elbow injury in children.
- If recurrent dislocation does not respond to immobilization, surgical reattachment or reconstruction of the elbow stabilizing ligaments may be required.

Nursemaid's Elbow

- These injuries are most common in young children, usually before the age of 4.
- They may occur into the early school-age years.
- Recurrence after the initial injury is common.
- The physician may encounter a worried parent who notes several "elbow dislocations" in their preschool child over the course of a year.
- It is important to understand the pathophysiology of this injury.
  - Nursemaid's elbow does not involve a dislocation of the radial head. Instead, it involves the entrapment of a portion of the annular ligament between the radial head and the capitellum (Figure 4–43).
  - After the initial injury, there is a small tear in this annular ligament and it is stretched, explaining the frequency of that recurrent injury.
- The mechanism of injury is generally pronation of the forearm with traction.
  - Typically this occurs when an adult is holding the child's hand or forearm and the child pulls away.
  - It can also occur when the child falls with pronation of the forearm.
- Initial assessment after injury should focus on a localization of the area of tenderness, a search for other injuries along the upper extremity, and a standard neurovascular examination.
- Good quality AP and lateral radiographs of the elbow should be studied carefully to ensure that other injuries are not present.
- In children with recurrent nursemaid's elbow whose diagnosis is assured by history and examination, reduction may be performed by the parent or physician without repeat x-rays.
- Reduction of a nursemaid's elbow involves full supination of the forearm and maximal flexion of the elbow. A child's supinated hand should oppose the anterior surface of the shoulder with maximal flexion.
- The most common reason for an unsuccessful nursemaid's elbow reduction is failure to maximally flex the elbow during initial reductions.
- Once the nursemaid's elbow reduction has been performed, the child should be observed for a few minutes to be certain that full use of the injured arm has begun.
- In nursemaid's elbow reductions done soon after injury, the child will rapidly adopt full use of the arm and show no signs of residual symptoms.
- In cases of missed nursemaid's elbow or multiple attempts at reduction over several days, inflammation of the annular ligament may cause the child to have symptoms for a day or so after the reduction. Rest in a splint for 2-3 days is helpful.
- In longer cases or in cases in which a complete reduction cannot be assured in an anxious child who is difficult to examine, an elbow ultrasound can reassure the parents and the physician that there is no longer any interposed tissue and that there are no other occult injuries masquerading as a nursemaid's elbow. Unless there is a radiologist with experience in elbow ultrasound, interpretation may be challenging.
- Complications after nursemaid's elbow are rare.
- The most common problem is recurrence.
- Recurrence generally ceases to be a problem as the child becomes older than 6 years and the annular ligament thickens and strengthens, thus resisting injury.

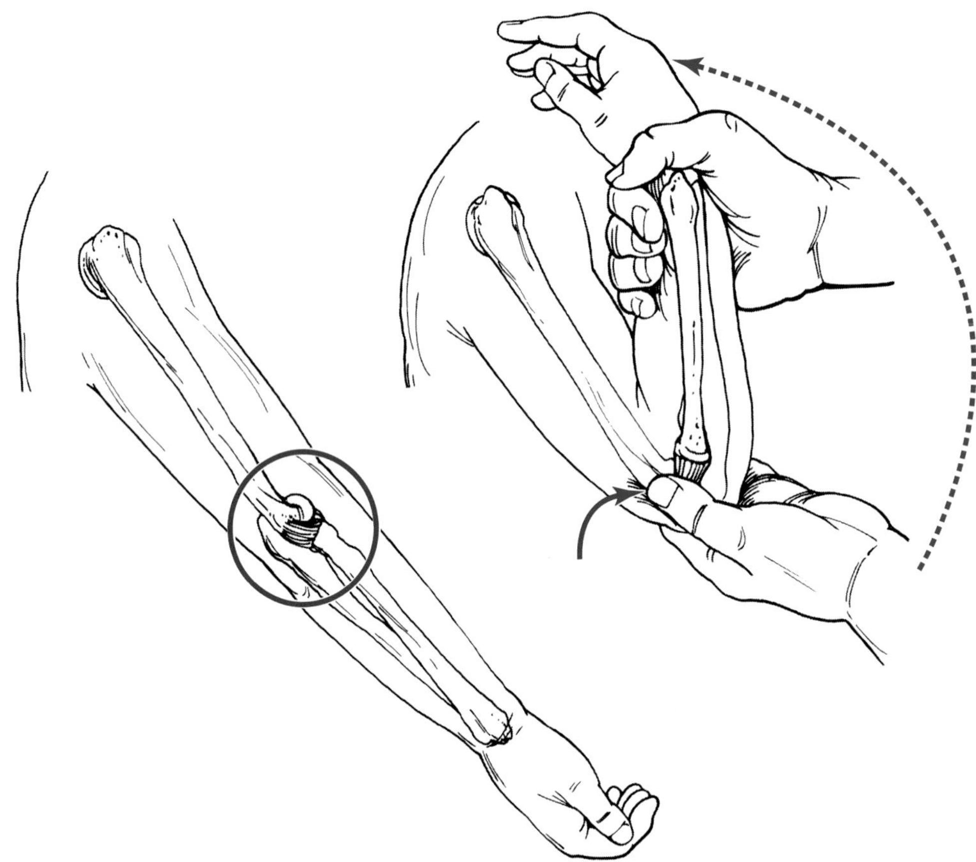

Figure 4–43: This schematic depicts a nursemaid's elbow with the orbicular ligament interposed between the radial head and the capitellum. The nursemaid's elbow is reduced and this ligament is freed by supination of the forearm and extreme flexion of the elbow. Redrawn from Rockwood C, Wilkins K, Beaty J (1996) Fractures in Children, 4th edition. Philadelphia, Lippincott-Raven.

Rare Elbow Injuries

- There are a few rare pediatric elbow injuries worthy of mention without detailed description or treatment guidelines.
  - T-condylar distal humerus fractures are seen occasionally in older children and teenagers.
    1. A fall includes a direct blow to the elbow.
    2. The ulna is driven up into the distal humerus, splitting the humerus longitudinally, in addition to a transverse or spiral fracture more proximally.
  - Most of these injuries are displaced and require operative reduction and fixation.
  - In widely displaced fractures in older children, a combination of plates and screws is used to obtain stable fixation and allow early motion of the injured elbow (Figure 4–44).
- Articular fractures of the capitellum and trochlea are rare in children.
  - Generally, the biomechanics of the condylar epiphysis dictate that force applied in this region will cause a lateral condyle or supracondylar fracture rather than a cartilaginous shear fracture of the capitellum or trochlea.
  - These injuries generally require open reduction and fixation or debridement with drilling.
- Medial condyle fractures are extremely rare injuries.
  - A major children's hospital that admits thousands of fractures per year may see a medial condyle fracture once every year or two.
  - Treatment of displaced medial condyle fractures involves open or closed reduction and pinning.
- A lateral epicondyle fracture is rare.
  - It generally involves an avulsion of the lateral epicondyle and attached soft tissues.
  - A short period of cast immobilization is generally a satisfactory treatment.

Fractures of the Humerus and Shoulder Region

Humeral Shaft Fractures

- Fractures of the humeral shaft account for about 2-5% of all fractures in children.[20]
- Their incidence is highest in children younger than 3 and older than 12 years.

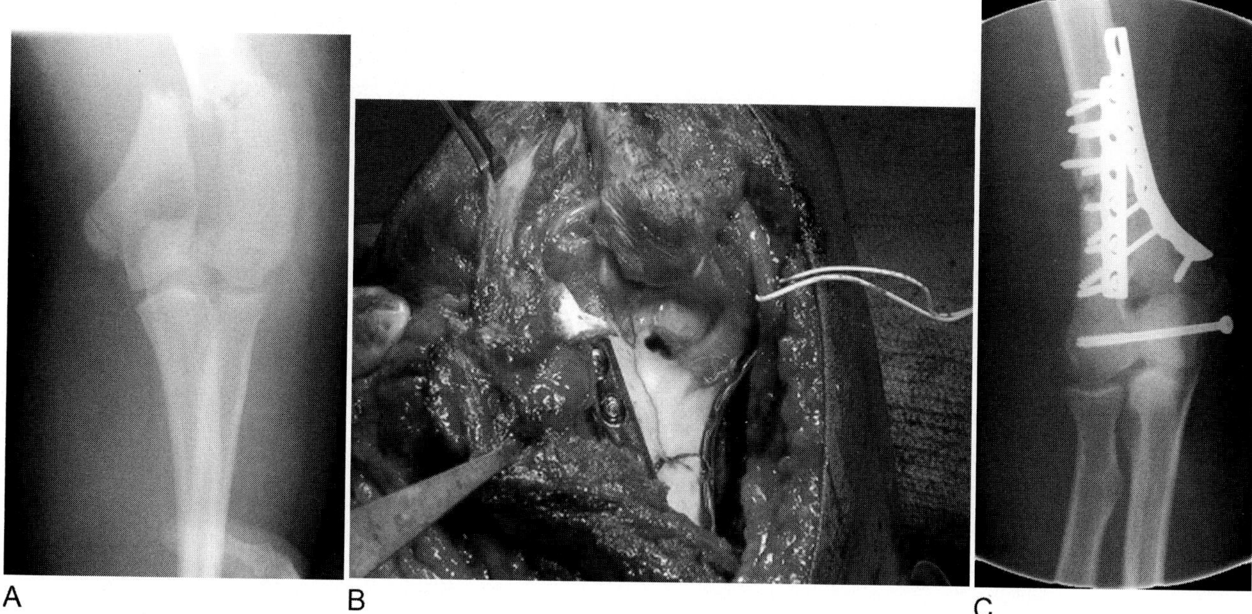

Figure 4–44: Treatment of a T-condylar humerus fracture in a teenager. A, An AP radiograph depicts a T-condylar humerus fracture. Note that there is no intra-articular comminution, as is often seen in older adults. B, This intraoperative photograph shows the fracture after anatomical reduction and fixation with two plates. Note that no olecranon osteotomy has been performed. Instead, a sleeve of periosteum has been taken down from the ulna. The ulna nerve is in a loop. C, Radiograph of the fracture after fixation.

- Transverse or short oblique fracture patterns usually occur as a result of a direct blunt. Spiral fracture patterns, however, can occur as a result of a twisting mechanism and may be suggestive of child abuse.
- Assessment of a patient with trauma to the arm should include an inspection to look for open fractures.
- This should be followed by a thorough neurovascular examination.
  - The radial nerve is especially vulnerable to injury with humeral shaft fractures.
  - Nerve injuries with humeral shaft fractures are usually a result of traction, and most resolve within 3-6 months.
- The brachial artery should also be evaluated by assessing distal pulses.
- The shoulder and the elbow should be included in the x-ray evaluation.
- A child's humerus has a great deal of remodeling potential. This allows for a wide range of acceptable deformity.
- Children under age 5 can tolerate 70 degrees of angulation and total displacement, children 5-12 can tolerate 40-70 degrees of angulation, and children older than 12 can tolerate 40 degrees of angulation and 50% apposition[21] (Figure 4–45).
- Shortening of 1-2 cm is acceptable because bony overgrowth will occur.
- A thorough neurological examination is especially important if reduction of the fracture is undertaken to appose the fracture fragments. A nerve that was previously intact but is compromised after the reduction is an indication for surgical exploration.
- Immobilization using a coaptation splint or a functional brace (often referred to as a Sarmiento brace) is valuable to maintain the alignment of the fracture fragments.
- Fracture in a newborn can be managed by splinting the arm to the chest wall. This can often be done using a simple safety pin connecting the sleeve to the shirt.
- Children with humeral shaft fractures usually do well with nonoperative treatment.
- Complications following humeral shaft fractures include the previously mentioned nerve palsies. Most resolve within 3-6 months.
- Vascular injuries can be devastating, and a high index of suspicion and prompt treatment are vital in preventing complications.
- Malunion or nonunion of a fracture are uncommon problems in children.
- Compartment syndrome is a rare complication; however, it has been reported.[22] A small limb length discrepancy is common but is usually less than 1 cm, and patients tolerate it well.

Proximal Humerus Fractures

- Fractures of the proximal humerus are relatively uncommon injuries, accounting for less than 5% of all fractures in children.[8] They usually result from a fall onto an outstretched arm.

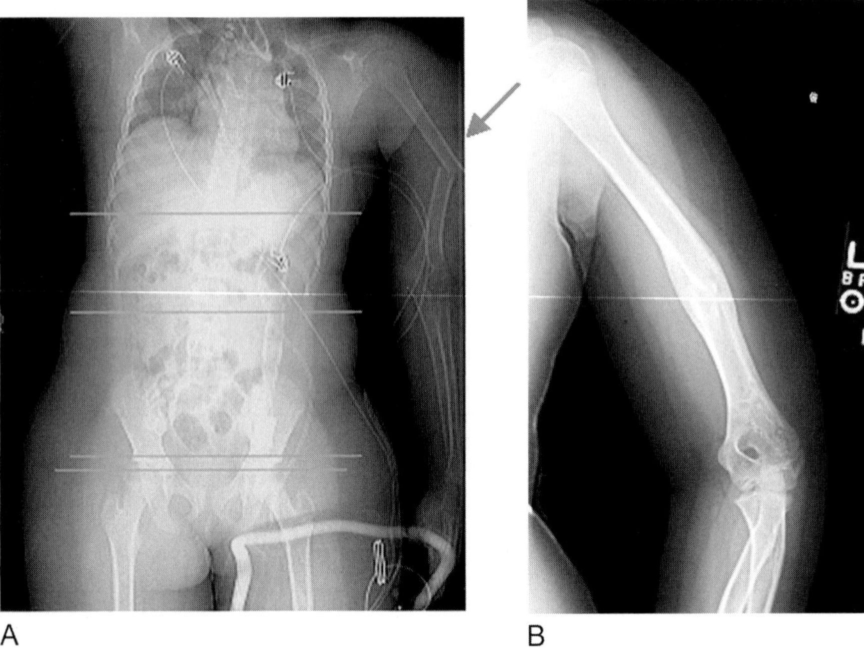

Figure 4–45: Healing and remodeling of a humeral shaft fracture in a multitrauma victim. A, This 11-year-old girl was struck by a car and sustained a femoral shaft fracture, a left humerus fracture, and a splenetic disruption. B, The humerus fracture 8 months after injury with excellent remodeling. The girl had no notable functional deficits.

- Neonatal fractures can occur during birth and can appear as a pseudoparalysis. This is usually a result of an excessive hyperextension and external rotation force during delivery.
- Fracture patterns tend to vary depending on the age group.
  - Neonates and children younger than 5 usually sustain Salter-Harris I fractures.
  - Children between 5 and 10 years of age usually have metaphyseal fractures. These are usually transverse or short oblique fractures.
  - Children older than 11 usually have Salter-Harris II fracture patterns.[23]
- Examination of the involved extremity should include a thorough neurological examination, including evaluation of the axillary nerve.
- Good quality plain x-rays should include an axillary view to rule out an associated dislocation.
- Children with Salter-Harris I fractures require no reduction. There is excellent remodeling potential, and immobilization in a sling and swathe for 2-3 weeks is usually sufficient for healing.
- Metaphyseal fractures in the 5- to 10-year-old patient usually require no reduction. If the fracture is angulated more than 50 degrees, a closed reduction is recommended to improve the alignment.
- Salter-Harris II fractures with less than 20-30 degrees of angulation and less than 50% displacement can be managed in a sling without reduction.
  - Reduction is usually accomplished by externally rotating, abducting, and forward flexing the arm.
  - This reduction often will require operative fixation to secure the fragments (Figure 4–46).
- The fractures usually are healed by 4-6 weeks, and some light activity can be permitted.
- Patients with severe angulation may lose some range of motion but will still be functional.
- Limb length inequalities are usually minimal, and nerve injuries usually resolve with 3-6 months.

Glenohumeral Joint Subluxation and Dislocation

- The shoulder joint is a ball-and-socket articulation. Although the glenoid functions as the socket, its relatively flat surface allows increased range of motion at the expense of stability.
- The shoulder capsule and rotator cuff muscles are the main providers of stability at this joint.
- Fortunately, shoulder dislocations in children are rare.
  - Most occur in adolescence near skeletal maturity.
  - In one series of 500 dislocations, only 8 were in children younger than 10 years.[24] Most traumatic dislocations are anterior.
- The mechanism of injury is usually from a force that abducts and externally rotates the outstretched arm.
- Posterior dislocations are rare and usually result from seizures.
- Atraumatic dislocations can result from inherent ligamentous laxity, such as in patients with Ehlers-Danlos

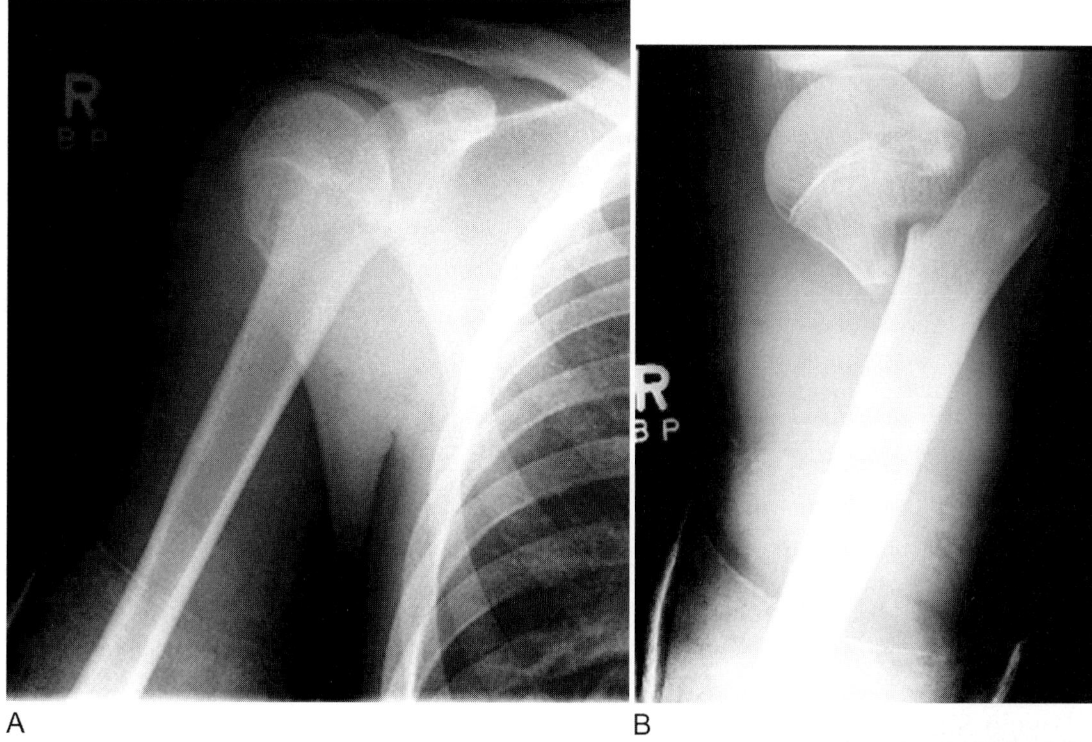

Figure 4–46: Displaced proximal humerus fracture requiring internal fixation. This AP view (A) and this axillary view (B) show a badly displaced proximal humerus fracture in a teenager who is nearly skeletally mature. This AP radiograph (C) after anatomical reduction and fixation with pins shows excellent overall alignment.

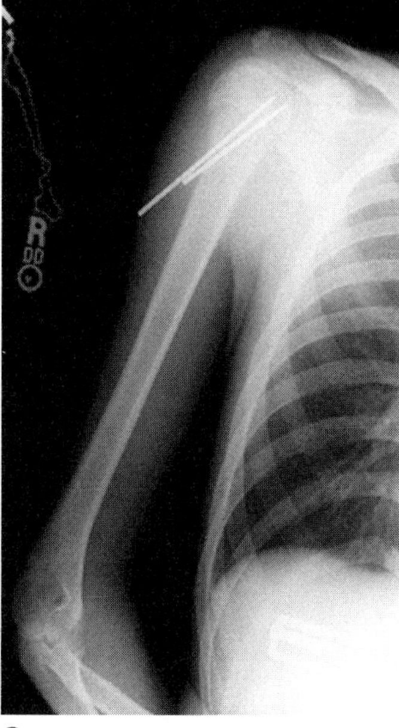

syndrome. This should be suspected when there is no clear-cut traumatic event.

- Physical examination should include a thorough neurovascular examination with special interest focused on axillary nerve function.
- X-ray evaluation is important even when the diagnosis is obvious.
  - A complete shoulder series should be obtained; the axillary view is the most important for diagnosis.
  - Prereduction x-rays are important to document any associated fractures that may be present before any reduction is undertaken.
  - Postreduction films should also be obtained.
- Prompt closed reduction of a traumatic dislocation should be undertaken using one of the many accepted techniques.
  - The key to any reduction is conscious sedation and possibly muscle relaxation.

  - The traction–countertraction method uses a sheet placed in the affected axilla and around the patient for countertraction.
  - The affected extremity is then gently distracted in line with the deformity until the muscles are fatigued and the humeral head relocates.
  - Improper technique can result in iatrogenic fractures of the glenoid or humeral head.
- Postreduction x-rays should document proper location of the head.
- The patient should be immobilized in a sling for 2-3 weeks before activity is restarted.
- The most common complication is recurrent dislocation, which can occur 50-100% of the time and is more common in younger patients.
  - Recurrent dislocations may require surgical reconstruction.
  - Axillary nerve injury can also occur. Most of these are neuropraxic injuries that resolve with time.
- Most patients with atraumatic dislocations will do well with vigorous rehabilitation and strengthening of the musculature around the joint.

Clavicle Shaft Fractures

- The clavicle is an S-shaped bone that articulates with the thorax medially and the shoulder joint laterally. It is the most commonly fractured bone in neonates and in childhood.[25] Neonatal fractures occur as a result of direct trauma during birth, most often as result of a tight birth canal. They can often be missed initially and can appear with pseudoparalysis of the affected extremity or a bump over the fracture 7-10 days after the injury.
- Childhood fractures are usually the result of a fall on the affected shoulder or direct trauma to the clavicle during sports.
  - The child will often hold the affected arm with the opposite arm and tilt the head toward the fracture.
  - Tenderness over the clavicle will make the diagnosis fairly easy.
- As always, a thorough neurovascular examination is important to diagnose any brachial plexus injuries.
- X-ray evaluation is useful and is usually all that is required.
- X-ray evaluation can help differentiate fracture from congenital pseudarthrosis of the clavicle.
  - This is a rare entity that is usually on the right side.[26]
  - Evaluation of the radiograph by an experienced observer may be necessary to differentiate the two.
- Most midshaft clavicle fractures, even with significant displacement, can be treated in a figure eight splint.
- A sling is an acceptable option either with or without the figure eight splint.
- Open fractures, or significant tenting of the skin from a fracture fragment, require surgical management.
- Clavicle fractures of birth can be treated with a safety pin attaching the sleeve to the infant's clothing as a sling. Most fractures in neonates will heal well without complications, and some may heal before they are ever diagnosed.
- In most children, deformity will remodel over time. In older children, a residual deformity manifested as a bump may remain. This rarely affects function.
- Complications include malunion, brachial plexus injuries, and vascular injuries.

Injuries around the Acromioclavicular Joint

- Injuries to the lateral end of the clavicle account for 10-12% of all clavicular fractures.[8]
- Unlike in adults, these injuries are less likely to be acromioclavicular (AC) dislocations and more likely to be pseudodislocations represented by distal clavicular fractures.
- The immature clavicle has a thick periosteum, and the coracoclavicular and AC ligaments attach to this periosteum (Figure 4–47).
- Injuries are usually fractures of the bone, which tends to slip out of this periosteum.
- Adolescent patients nearing skeletal maturity are more likely to sustain true AC joint dislocations.
- The injuries are usually from a direct blow to the lateral end of the clavicle or from a fall with the child landing on the affected shoulder.
- The patient will usually have pain and swelling over the AC joint. More severe injuries may show a deformity over the area.
- The child will usually support the affected arm with the other arm.
- The examination should include palpation of the rest of the clavicle, the shoulder, and the entire upper extremity.
- Radiographic evaluation with shoulder films may be sufficient.
  - However, x-rays centered over the AC joint are often required for proper evaluation.
  - Views of the contralateral AC joint may also be helpful.
  - A Stryker notch view is helpful in demonstrating fractures of the coracoid.
- Distal clavicular injuries are classified based on the severity.
  - Less severe injuries are managed nonoperatively.
  - Open fractures will require immediate attention.
- Most fractures in children younger than 16 will likely heal well with nonoperative management in a sling. This is because of the thick periosteum that is still intact and attached to the ligaments.
- Older children with true AC joint dislocations should be managed as adults when treating the injury.
- Outcomes are excellent with healing usually complete by 4-6 weeks.

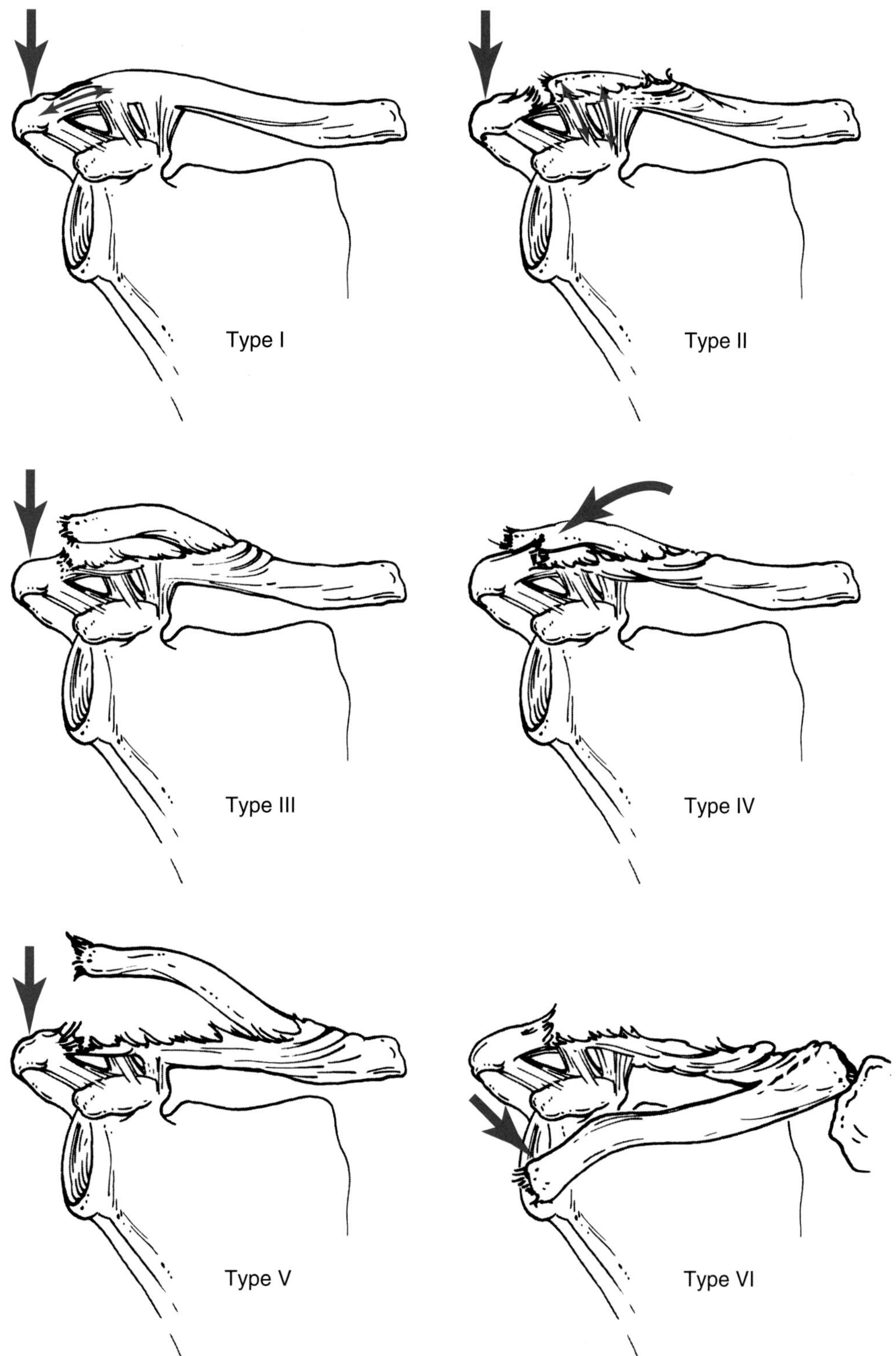

Figure 4–47: This schematic depicts types of injuries at the AC joint in children. Note the importance of the periosteum to the injury. Redrawn from Rockwood C, Wilkins K, Beaty J (1996) Fractures in Children, 4th edition. Philadelphia, Lippincott-Raven.

Rare Injuries about the Shoulder

- Injuries to the medial end of the clavicle and sternoclavicular (SC) joint are rare in children and represent only about 5% of clavicular fractures.[27] The mechanism is usually from lateral force applied to the shoulder.
- As with distal clavicular injuries, the lateral force produces a physeal injury rather than a pure dislocation of the SC joint.
- Occasionally the injury may result from a direct blow to the SC joint, in which case the displacement will be posterior.
- Posterior displacement should be evaluated promptly and carefully to assess for any neurovascular damage or injury to important mediastinal structures.
- Any complaints by the patient of trouble breathing or swallowing should be taken seriously.
- Pulses in the affected extremity should be carefully measured and compared with the contralateral side. Diminished or absent pulses suggest vascular injury.
- The patient will usually hold the affected arm across the chest and have pain with palpation over the SC joint.
- Chest x-ray evaluation with a may suffice.
- Signs of mediastinal injury should be excluded.
- A computerized tomography (CT) scan of the chest can provide an accurate assessment of injury and displacement.
- Fractures of the medial end of the clavicle have excellent healing and remodeling potential.
- Reduction is indicated only for posterior displacement.
- This should be done by an orthopaedic consultant and may need to be performed emergently.
- Surgical treatment is rarely indicated, and outcomes are excellent.
- Fractures of the scapula are extremely rare, comprising less than 1% of all fractures in children.[8] Fractures of the scapular spine and body are usually the result of a direct high-energy blow and often have associated injuries.
- Look for associated injuries.
- The scapular fractures are usually minimally displaced because the musculature surrounding the fragments often keeps them in place.
- Conservative treatment is usually indicated.
- Scapular neck fractures can be isolated or associated with clavicular fractures.
  - Isolated injuries are usually stable and require only conservative treatment.
  - Scapular fractures with clavicular fractures are unstable and may require internal fixation.
- Glenoid fractures are commonly associated with shoulder dislocations and should be ruled out in any patient with a dislocation.
  - They can range from small avulsion fractures to large intra-articular fragments causing severe disability and shoulder instability.
  - A CT scan may delineate the fracture pattern better than a plain radiograph.
- Scapular fractures, by themselves, usually have good outcomes.
  - However, the patient may have many other significant injuries with serious sequelae.
  - Most scapular fractures are treated nonoperatively with immobilization in a sling.

Summary

- Upper extremity injuries are common in children.
- Most can be treated with a cast or with reduction and pinning if cast treatment does not confer satisfactory stability to the injured bone or joint.
- Careful history and physical examination, followed by proper imaging, provide the key starting point for successful management.

References

1. Flynn JM, Nagda S (2002) Upper extremity fractures. In: Requisites in Pediatrics: Orthopaedics and Sports Medicine (Dormans J, ed). Philadelphia: Elsevier.

2. Flynn JM, Sarwark J, Waters P, Bae L, Lemke D (2002) The operative management of pediatric fractures of the upper extremity. J Bone Joint Surg 84A(11): 2078-2089.
   In the past 2 decades, surgical management of certain fractures (e.g., percutaneous pinning of displaced supracondylar fractures) has provided better results than closed management. Surgical management is clearly indicated for certain injuries, such as those requiring anatomical realignment of the physis or articular surface. Increasingly, however, surgical management is being used to maintain optimal alignment or to allow early motion.

3. Hastings H, Simmons BP (1984) Hand fractures in children: A statistical analysis. Clin Orthop Sep(188): 120-130.
   A retrospective review of 354 pediatric hand fractures was performed with a minimum follow-up period of 2 years. Although nondisplaced intra-articular fractures uniformly healed without malfunction, poor functional results were obtained from displaced intra-articular fractures. The following injuries presented particular problems: displaced intra-articular fractures, Salter-Harris I distal phalangeal fractures caused by crushing injuries, displaced subcondylar fractures, and open fractures.

4. Brighton C (1974) Clinical problems in epiphyseal plate growth and development. AAOS Intr Course Lect: 105-122.

5. Green DP (1977) Hand injuries in children. Pediatr Clin N Am 24(4): 903-918.

6. Beatty E, Light TR, Belsole J, Ogden JA (1990) Wrist and hand skeletal injuries in children. Hand Clin 6(4): 723-738.
   Pediatric wrist and hand skeletal injuries described in this article include growth mechanism injury, fractures and

dislocations, nail bed injuries, fingertip injuries, burns, and frostbite.

7. Crock HV, Chari PR, Crock MC (1981) The blood supply of the wrist and hand bones in man. Philadelphia 1: 335-349.

8. Graham TJ, Waters PM (2001). Fractures and dislocations of the hand and carpus in children. In: Fractures in Children, 5th edition (Beaty JH, Kasser JR, eds). Philadelphia: Lippincott-William & Wilkins Publishers. pp 269-380.

9. Christensen JB (1964) A study of the interosseous distance between the radius and the ulna during rotation of the forearm. J Bone Joint Surg 46B: 778-779.

10. Flynn JM (2002) Pediatric forearm fractures: Operative indications, techniques, and complications. AAOS Instr Course Lect 51(39): 355-360.

11. Flynn JM, Waters P (1996) Single-bone fixation to treat diaphyseal both-bone forearm fractures in children. J Pediatr Orthop 16(5): 655-659.

    Fixation of either the radius or the ulna was used to treat 17 children with diaphyseal both-bone forearm fractures for which closed reduction had failed. Results in all children were excellent; all had a full return of motion except 2 who lacked 5 degrees of pronation.

12. Mabrey JD, Fitch RD (1989) Plastic deformation in pediatric fractures: Mechanism and treatment. J Pediatr Orthop 9(3): 310-314.

    The plastic deformation often observed in children's long bone fractures is largely because of the complex nature of the molecular and histological aspects of pediatric bone. An algorithm and technique for treatment of plastic deformation of the radius and ulna, the two most commonly involved bones in plastic deformation, are reviewed.

13. Bado JL (1967) The Monteggia lesion. Clin Orthop 50: 71-86.

14. Olney BW, Menelaus MB (1989) Monteggia and equivalent lesions in childhood. J Pediatr Orthop 9(2): 219-223.

    The authors review 102 children with acute Monteggia lesions treated over 25 years. Using the Bado classification system, type 1 (53%) and type 3 (26%) fractures were the most common. The type 1 equivalent injury associated with a proximal radius fracture is more common in children than previously reported. Most injuries could be treated with closed reduction except the type 1 equivalent lesions, which required operative treatment in 10 of 14 children. Varus angulation of the ulna was the most common deformity after closed treatment. Nerve injuries occurred in 11% of the injuries and resolved in all cases without operative treatment.

15. DiCesare PE, Sew-Hoy A, Krom W (1992) Bilateral isolated olecranon fractures in an infant as presentation of osteogenesis imperfecta. Orthopedics 15(6): 741-743.

    Children with osteogenesis imperfecta may be prone to olecranon fractures. The authors recommend operative treatment for displaced fractures, and propose that the high rate of bilateral injury suggests that children with osteogenesis imperfecta who sustain this fracture should be counseled regarding the risk of injury to the opposite extremity.

16. Mudgal CS (1992) Olecranon fractures in osteogenesis imperfecta: A case report. Acta Orthop Belg 58(4): 453-456.

17. Tamai J, Lou J, Nagda T, Ganley T, Flynn JM (2002) Pediatric elbow fractures: Pearls and pitfalls. U Penn Orthop J 15: 43-51.

18. Skaggs DL, Mirzayan R (1999) The posterior fat pad sign in association with occult fracture of the elbow in children. J Bone Joint Surg Am 81(10): 1429-1433.

    This prospective study demonstrated that the posterior fat pad sign was predictive of an occult fracture of the elbow following trauma in 34 (76%) of 45 children who had no other evidence of fracture on AP, lateral, and oblique radiographs after the injury. The results of Skaggs and Mirzayan support the practice of managing children who have a history of trauma to the elbow, an elevated posterior fat pad, and no other radiographic evidence of fracture as if they have a nondisplaced fracture about the elbow.

19. Cluck M, Kay R, Mostafi A, Flynn J, Skaggs D (2004) Lateral-entry pin fixation in the management of supracondylar fractures in children. J Bone Joint Surg 86A(4): 702-707.

    In this large, consecutive series without selection bias, the use of lateral-entry pins alone was effective for even the most unstable supracondylar humeral fractures. There were no iatrogenic ulnar nerve injuries, and no reduction was lost. The authors outline the important technical points for fixation with lateral-entry pins.

20. Cheng JC, Shen WY (1993) Limb fracture pattern in different pediatric age groups: A study of 3350 children. J Orthop Trauma 7(1): 15-22.

    The fracture patterns of 3350 children with 3413 limb fractures admitted to one center from 1986 to 1990 were analyzed retrospectively. The overall boy-to-girl ratio was 2.7:1, rising to 5.5:1 in the adolescent group. Distal radius fracture was the most common fracture (19.87%) followed by supracondylar fracture of the humerus (16.64%) and forearm shaft fracture (13.36%).

21. Beaty JH (1992) Fractures of the proximal humerus and shaft in children. AAOS Instr Course Lect 41: 369-372.

22. Mubarak SJ, Carroll NC (1979) Volkmann's contracture in children: Aetiology and prevention. J Bone Joint Surg Br 61B(3): 285-293.

    A review was conducted of the records of 55 children between 1955 and 1975 with a diagnosis of Volkmann's contracture in 58 limbs. Of 10 patients with established ischemia after Bryant's traction for a fractured femur, all had a poor outcome. Volkmann's contracture affecting the superficial posterior compartment had been treated in 13 other cases with a fixed Thomas's splint and a Bradford frame after fractures of the femoral shaft. Supracondylar fractures of the elbow resulting in Volkmann's contracture frequently had both an arterial injury and a compartment syndrome. Most of the 55 children reviewed here had not had early appropriate treatment.

23. Dameron TB Jr, Reibel DB (1969) Fractures involving the proximal humeral epiphyseal plate. J Bone Joint Surg Am 51(2): 289-297.

24. Rowe CR (1956) Prognosis in dislocations of the shoulder. J Bone Joint Surg 38A: 957-977.

25. Stanley D, Trowbridge EA, Norris SH (1988) The mechanism of clavicular fracture: A clinical and biomechanical analysis. J Bone Joint Surg Br 70(3): 461-464.
A consecutive series of 150 patients with clavicular fractures was studied. In 81%, detailed information regarding the mechanism of the injury was available; of these, 94% had fractured their clavicle from a direct blow on the shoulder and only 6% had fallen on the outstretched hand. This finding, at variance with commonly held views regarding the mechanism of this injury, was further investigated by biomechanical analysis of the forces involved in clavicular fractures. The biomechanical model supported the clinical findings.

26. Kite JH (1968) Congenital pseudarthrosis of the clavicle. S Med J 61(7): 703-710.

27. Browner BD, Jupiter JB, Levine AM, Trafton PG, Lampert R, eds (1992) Skeletal Trauma: Fractures, Dislocations, Ligamentous Injuries, 2nd edition. Philadelphia: WB Saunders.

Trauma Related to the Lower Extremity

Lawrence Wells* and Jennifer E. Millman†

*MD, Assistant Professor of Orthopaedic Surgery, University of Pennsylvania School of Medicine, Philadelphia, PA; Attending Physician, The Children's Hospital of Philadelphia, Philadelphia, PA
†BA, Clinical Research Coordinator, Division of Orthopaedic Surgery, The Children's Hospital of Philadelphia, Philadelphia, PA

Introduction

This chapter provides an overview of common injuries sustained to the lower extremity in children. Various fracture patterns of the hip, femur, knee, tibia, foot, and ankle are described with suggested classification systems to guide diagnosis and treatment. Complications including avascular necrosis (AVN), limb length inequality, and fracture malunion are described. Age-specific treatment options for femoral diaphyseal fractures are also explained and illustrated.

Hip Injuries

General Principles

- Hip fractures in children account for less than 1% of all children's fractures[1,2] (Figure 5–1).
- These injuries result from high-energy trauma and are frequently associated with injury to the chest, head, or abdomen.
- Treatment of hip fractures in children entails a complication rate of up to 60%, an overall AVN rate of 50%, and a malunion rate of up to 30%.[1]
- The unique blood supply to the femoral head accounts for the high rate of AVN seen with these injuries.
- In infancy, the femoral head blood supply is derived from metaphysical vessels originating from the medial and lateral femoral circumflex arteries.
- These vessels transverse the proximal femoral physis and vascularize the proximal femoral epiphysis.[3]
- By 2 years, however, with normal growth and development of the proximal femoral physis, these vessels involute and the cartilaginous physis of the proximal femur becomes a barrier to blood flow to the femoral head. At this point, the blood supply to the proximal femoral epiphysis derives from the lateral epiphyseal vessels, the terminal vessels arising from the medial femoral circumflex artery.
- These posterosuperior and posteroinferior retinacular vessels lie on the femoral neck and are vulnerable to injury during fracture of the hip.[3] It is believed that damage to these vessels at the time of injury leads to AVN of the femoral head. This is underscored by the AVN rate of pediatric hip fractures, which is generally related to degree of fracture displacement and fracture location.
- Pediatric hip fractures are classified according to the system of Delbet.[4] The system classifies hip fractures into four types according to their location (Table 5–1).
- Management principles for pediatric hip fractures include urgent treatment of these injuries, anatomical reduction (either open or closed), stable internal fixation (avoiding the physis if possible), and spica casting.[2]
- A capsulotomy to decompress the hip joint is also recommended in an attempt to minimize tamponade of the retinacular blood vessels by the fracture hematoma.

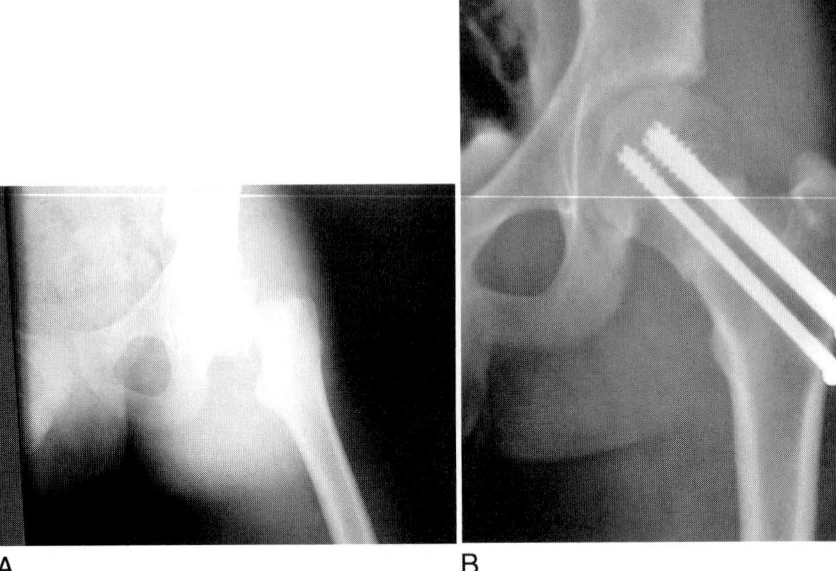

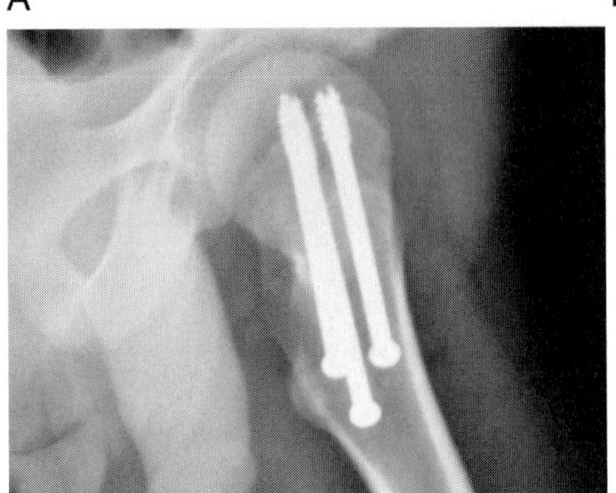

Figure 5–1: A, Type II femoral neck fracture in a 12-year-old boy. B and C, Fracture after closed reduction and internal fixation with cannulated screws.

- Type I fractures are uncommon, representing only about 8% of hip fractures.
  - They usually occur in infants and young children. In infants they can be secondary to birth trauma.
  - About 50% of such fractures will have an associated dislocation of the proximal femoral epiphysis.[4]
  - Type I fractures require an urgent reduction; frequently, an open reduction will be needed.

Table 5–1: Delbert Classification

TYPE	DESCRIPTION	AVN RATE (%)
I	Transphyseal separations	80
II	Fractures occur in the femoral neck and are known as transcervical fractures	50
III	Cervicotrochanteric fractures	25
IV	Intertrochanteric fractures	<10

  - Smooth pins should be used to stabilize the fracture, because threaded pins should not be used across a physis, and the pin fixation should be supplemented with a spica cast.
  - Type I fractures in children older than 2 years have an 80% AVN rate. In younger children, particularly with fractures secondary to birth trauma, the AVN rate is lower, most likely because these are low-energy injuries.
- Type II fractures are the most common hip fractures in children and account for many of the complications.[2,4]
  - They should be treated by an anatomical reduction (open if necessary) followed by screw or pin fixation.
  - Screw threads should avoid the physis if possible, so smaller children may require fixation with smooth transphyseal pins.
  - The AVN rate for type II fractures is 50%.
- Type III fractures, or cervicotrochanteric fractures, occur at the base of the femoral neck. They are the second most

common type of hip fracture in children and are analogous to adult basicervical hip fractures.
  - Like type II fractures, cervicotrochanteric hip fractures should be treated by urgent, anatomical reduction; stable internal fixation with smooth pins or screws (crossing the physis if necessary); and a spica cast.
  - Type III hip fractures have an AVN rate of 25% in displaced fractures.[4]
- Type IV, or intertrochanteric, hip fractures have the best prognosis.
  - These are frequently stable, and in children at least 8 years old, these fractures can be treated by a hip spica cast alone.
  - Displaced fractures in children younger than 8 years are best treated with open reduction and internal fixation. Type IV fractures have an AVN rate of less than 10%.[4]
- Complications of hip fractures in children include malunion, nonunion, and AVN.
- Recent studies have suggested that these can be minimized by early anatomical reduction, internal fixation, and spica cast immobilization.[2]
- Malunion usually results in a coxa vara and is secondary to a poor-quality reduction. Open reduction should be performed if an adequate closed reduction cannot be obtained.
  - Small degrees of coxa vara will remodel; larger malunions may require a femoral osteotomy for correction.
  - Nonunions typically result from a combination of a malreduction and inadequate fracture stabilization.
  - Varus malunion results in shear forces across the fracture site, which contributes to the nonunion.
- Treatment should consist of a valgus femoral subtrochanteric osteotomy (to convert the shear forces across the fracture site to compression), bone grafting, internal fixation, and spica casting.
- The incidence of nonunion and malunion seems to be decreasing with the use of anatomical reduction and internal fixation of these injuries.
- AVN is related to both fracture location and displacement. There is no simple, reliable treatment for postfracture AVN of the femoral head. Children younger than 8 years can be treated in abduction bracing (similar to treatment for Legg-Calve-Perthes disease). An early vascularized fibula strut graft may be or value in older children to promote healing of the avascular bone and to prevent femoral head collapse.

Specific Fractures of the Hip

Fractures of the Acetabulum

- In younger children, with an open triradiate cartilage, fractures of the acetabulum can be categorized according to the Salter-Harris classification (Figure 5–2).

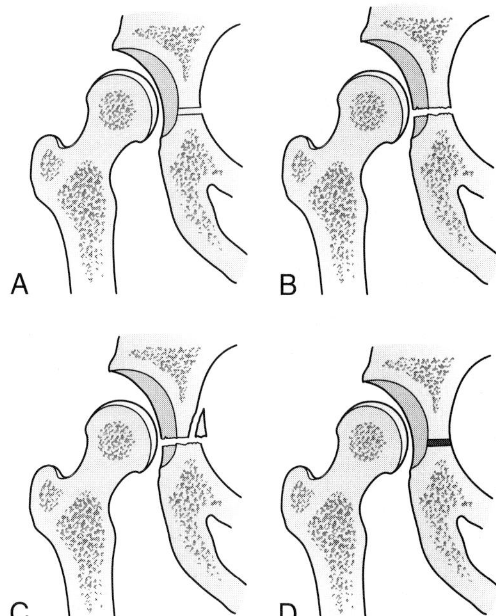

Figure 5–2: Salter-Harris classification of acetabular fractures. **A, Normal configuration of the triradiate cartilage. B, Salter-Harris I fracture. C, Salter-Harris II fracture. D, Salter-Harris V injury to the triradiate cartilage.**

- Most of these fractures will be Salter-Harris I, II, and V injuries.
- In older children and adolescents, with a closed triradiate cartilage, the classification system devised by Letournel and Judet can be used[5] (Figure 5–3).
- Children should be evaluated with plain radiographs and computerized tomography (CT).
- Stable fractures with less than 2 mm of intra-articular displacement can be treated nonoperatively if the patient does not bear weight until the fracture heals.
- Fractures with more than 2 mm of displacement or unstable fractures should be treated with open or closed reduction and internal fixation.
- Patients with a central fracture–dislocation require prompt reduction with skeletal traction and open reduction and internal fixation.
- Complications of acetabular fractures in younger children primarily occur from premature closure of the triradiate cartilage. This produces a shallow dysplastic acetabulum and may lead to hip subluxation.
- Acetabular fractures that heal with an articular incongruity may develop post-traumatic arthrosis of the hip, and AVN of the femoral head may develop after fractures of the hip accompanied by hip dislocation.

Fractures of the Pelvis

- Avulsion fractures typically occur secondary to athletic injuries involving running and jumping.

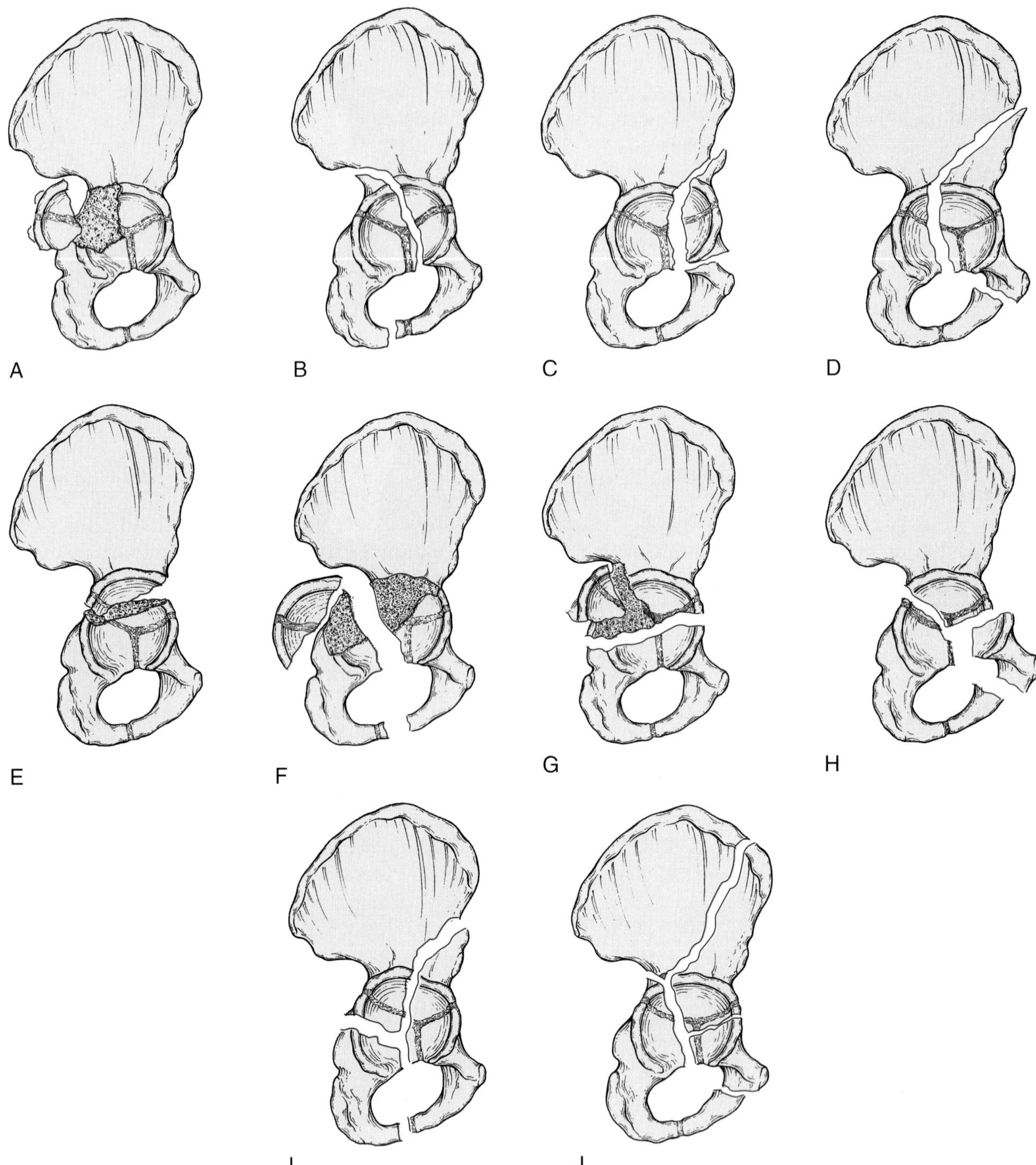

Figure 5–3: Letournel and Judet acetabular fracture classification. A, Posterior wall fracture, often associated with impaction on the intact side of the fracture margin. B, Posterior column fracture. C, Anterior wall fracture. D, Anterior column fracture. E, Transverse fracture pattern. F, Associated posterior column and posterior wall fractures. G, Associated transverse and posterior wall fractures. H, T-shaped fracture. I, Associated anterior column and posterior hemitransverse fractures. J, Both-column fracture. From Swiontkowski MF (2003) Fractures and dislocations about the hips and pelvis. In: Skeletal Trauma in Children (Green NE, Swiontkowski MF, eds), Volume 3. Philadelphia: Saunders, p 376, Figure 12-4.

- The most common mechanism of injury is an eccentric contraction of a muscle causing a traction injury to a cartilaginous apophysis.[6]
- The location of muscle origins about the pelvis determines the site of these injuries.
  - The direct head of rectus femoris muscles arises from the anterior–inferior iliac spine (AIIS) (Figure 5–4).
  - The sartorius originates from the anterior–superior iliac spine (ASIS).
  - The hamstring and adductor muscles originate from the ischial tuberosity.
- Violent contraction of the sartorius, particularly when the muscle is elongated (such as when the hip is extended and the knee flexed) can lead to ASIS avulsion fractures.
- Eccentric hamstring contractions can lead to ischial avulsion fractures, and tension injuries of the rectus femoris can lead to avulsion fractures of the AIIS.
- Patients frequently describe a history of a "pop" with a sudden onset of pain and difficulty bearing weight.
- Physical examinations reveal point tenderness over the affected region.
- Diagnosis may be confirmed with radiographs or CT.
- Treatment of fractures with less than 2 cm of displacement is symptomatic, consisting of restricted ability to bear weight and physical therapy.
- Fractures with more than 2 cm of displacement are best treated with open reduction and internal fixation.

Soft Tissue Injuries of the Hip

- Hip dislocations may occur in children without an associated acetabular or femoral fracture (Figure 5–5, *A*).
- Most of these are posterior, and 75% of hip dislocations occur secondary to high-energy injury.[7]
- In children younger than 10 years, however, ligamentous laxity often leads to hip dislocations from low-energy trauma.

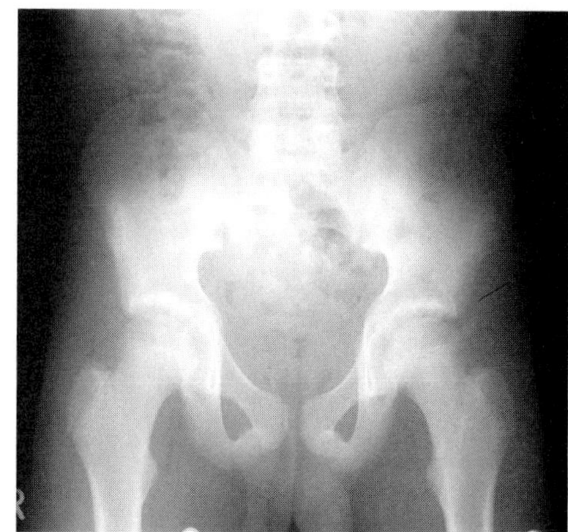

Figure 5–4: Anterior–inferior iliac spine.

- Reduction within 6 hours of injury is recommended to help minimize AVN of the femoral head.
- Adequate relaxation is required when reducing a dislocated hip to prevent physeal damage or fracture during reduction.
- Hip dislocations in younger children can generally be reduced in the emergency department under conscious sedation; dislocations in older children should have a reduction under a general anesthetic.
- After reduction, plain radiographs or a CT scan should be carefully evaluated for any hip joint incongruity (Figure 5–5, *B*), which may indicate soft tissue incarceration within the hip joint.
- After a satisfactory closed reduction, a spica cast or hip abduction pillows and limited weight should be applied to the involved leg for 3-6 weeks to allow soft tissue healing.
- Indications for open reduction of a dislocated hip include dislocations irreducible by closed methods, late-presenting

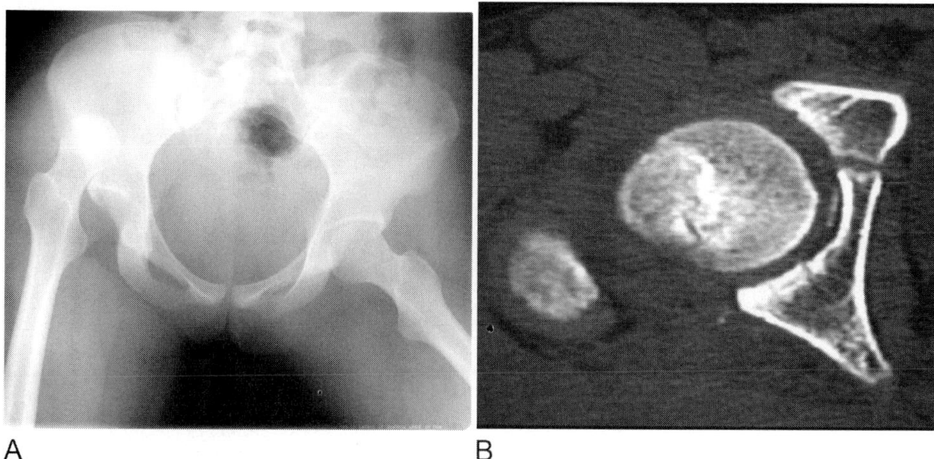

Figure 5–5: A, Traumatic hip dislocation in an 11-year-old girl who was struck by a car. B, Postreduction CT scan showing a bony fragment trapped in the hip joint, which required an arthrotomy for treatment.

dislocations, and soft tissue interposition in the hip joint preventing a congruous reduction.
- Complications from hip dislocations in children include AVN (8%), myositis ossificans, redislocation, neurovascular injury, and post-traumatic arthrosis of the hip.[7]

Femur Injuries

General Principles

- Fractures of the femur in children are common. All age groups, from early childhood to adolescence, can be affected.
- The mechanisms of injury vary from low-energy twisting-type injuries (seen in falls from playground equipment) to high-velocity injuries (seen in motor vehicle accidents in which the femur fracture is one of several injuries)[8] (Tables 5–2 and 5–3).
- Additional injuries can include life-threatening head, chest, and abdominal trauma that often take priority over the management of the femur fracture.
- Fracture patterns and epidemiology can be categorized by age group: 0-2, 3-5, 6-10, and older than 11 years.
  - With each age group there is a particular subset of issues that needs to be addressed when management and treatment plans are formulated.
  - Treatment algorithms based on age, fracture pattern, associated injuries, social economic factors, and family dynamics are the guiding principles by which fractures are managed today; such algorithms continue to evolve with new technology.
- Most femur fractures result from low-energy events, such as falls from playground equipment or mishaps on rollerblades or skateboards, and from contact sports, such as football (Figure 5–6). These low-energy injuries are primarily in the 6- to 10-year age group.
- Femur fractures in children under 2 years should raise the concern for child abuse. In the absence of an underlying metabolic or neurological disease process such as myelomeningocele (MM), muscular dystrophy (MD), osteogenesis imperfecta (OI), or cerebral palsy (CP), child abuse or endangerment should be considered (Figure 5–7).

Table 5–2: Common Injury Mechanisms

INJURY MECHANISM	PERCENTAGE OF CASES
Motor vehicle injury	46
Biking or sports-related injury	24
Injury resulting from a fall	27
Miscellaneous (e.g., stepping into a hole)	3

From Anglen J (2002) Percutaneous Plate Fixation of Pediatric Femur Fractures. American Academy of Orthopaedic Surgeons: Rosemont, IL

Table 5–3: Injury Mechanism and Fracture Pattern

INJURY MECHANISM	FRACTURE PATTERN
Torsion	Spiral pattern
Direct blow	Transverse
High energy	Comminuted, compound, or open

From Staheli LT (1984) Fractures of the shaft of the femur. In: Fractures in Children. (Rockwood C, Wilkins K, King R, eds). Philadelphia: JB Lippincott.

- Injury patterns are not specific. Fractures can vary in location from proximal to midshaft or distal with or without metaphyseal corner involvement. They can be transverse from a direct blow or can be spiral or oblique from a twisting mechanism (Figure 5–8).
- By obtaining a thorough history and conducting a complete physical examination, a skeletal survey, and a social services evaluation, the examiner can recognize the pattern of abuse and minimize the risk of repeat events that can often result in fatalities.
- Playground or sports-related fractures are usually isolated injuries and have a specific history with timely recruitment of medical attention. Mechanism of injury can be varied, but it is usually consistent with a fall during sport.
- Although underlying primary bone disease (MM, MD, OI, or CP), weakened bones because of osteopenia, or pathological fracture (Figure 5–9) secondary to tumor should be ruled out, the usual scenario is that the bone quality is normal.

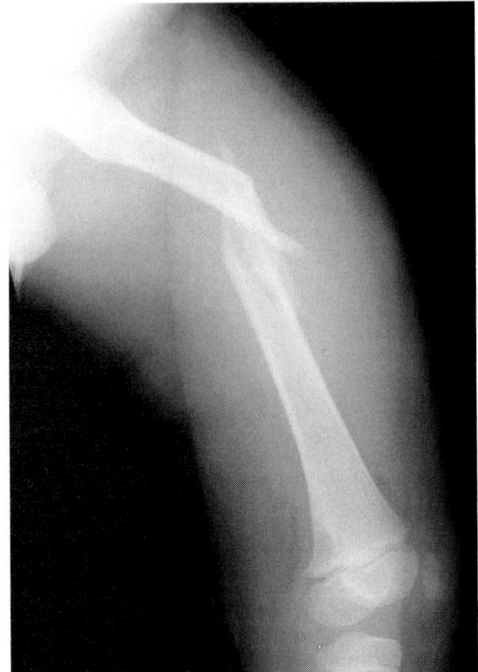

Figure 5–6: Most femur fractures are caused by low-energy accidents.

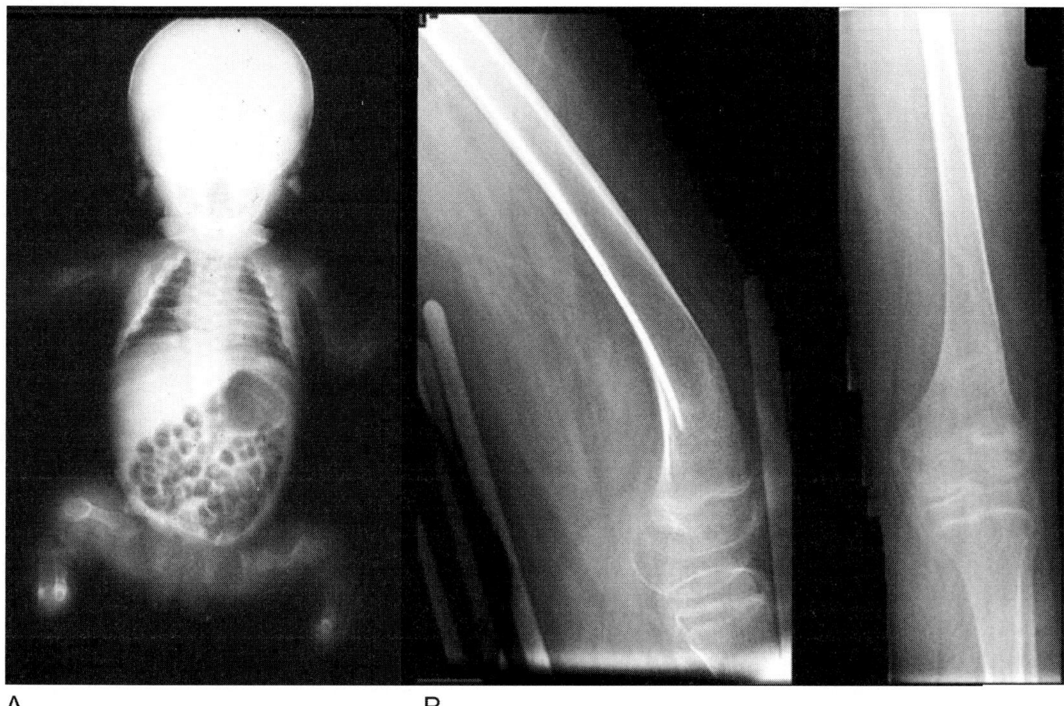

Figure 5–7: Distal femur fracture because of OI (A) and MD (B).

- High-energy fractures usually result from motor vehicle accidents or pedestrians struck by automobiles.
  - For example, Waddell's triad shows a femur fracture resulting from a car bumper striking the thigh, a chest or thoracic injury from the hood impact, and a head injury from being thrown by the initial impact (Figure 5–10).
  - All terrain vehicles and motorcycle injuries also contribute to high-energy trauma, particularly in the adolescent age group.

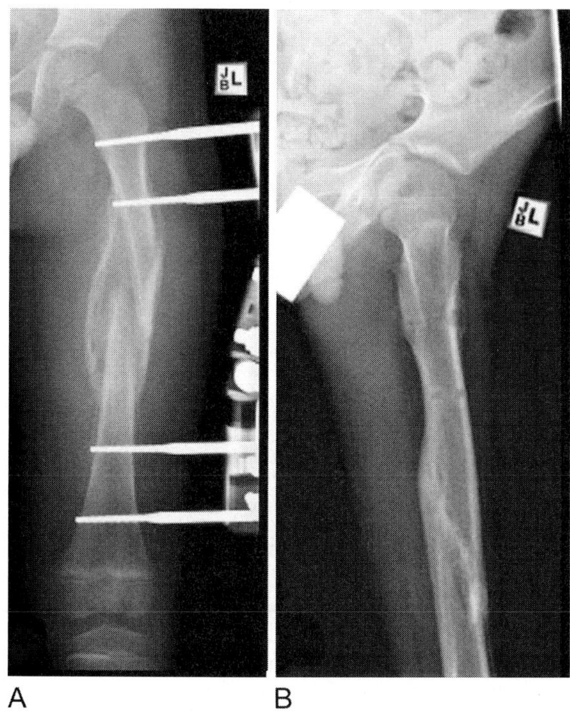

Figure 5–8: Spiral oblique femur fracture interval healing (A) and healed (B).

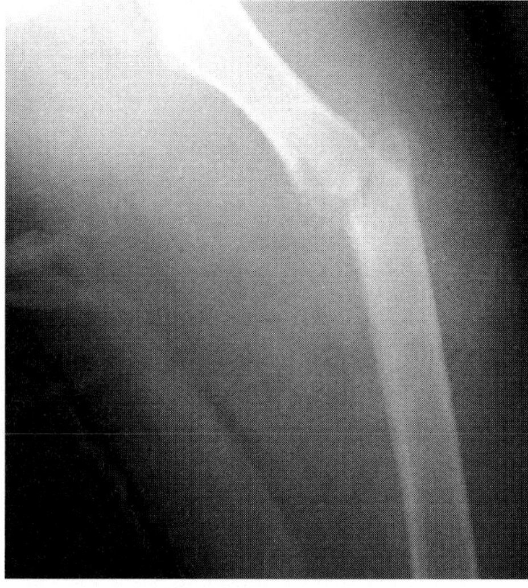
Figure 5–9: Cystic lesion leading to pathological femur fracture.

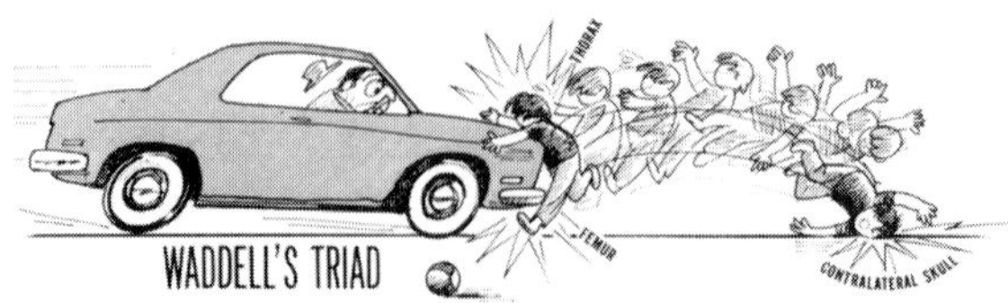

Figure 5–10: Wadell's triad of femur, chest, and head injuries. From Rang M (1981) Fractures in special circumstances. In: Beaty JH, Kasser JR (2002) Rockwood, Green, and Wilkins' Fractures in Children, 2nd edition. Philadelphia: Lippincott Williams & Wilkins, p 63, Figure 5-15.

Evaluation

- The initial evaluation begins with obtaining a history of the events leading up to the accident or injury. These details can be helpful when determining a high- versus low-energy mechanism and can prompt a search for additional injuries.
- The physical examination starts with making note of the patient's general appearance followed by checking the ABCs—airway, breathing, and circulation.
  - A complete musculoskeletal examination from head to toe should follow with emphasis on the neck, spine, and pelvis before examining the injured limb. Once satisfied, the examiner should check for obvious deformity, swelling, tenderness, open wounds, and neurological dysfunction.
  - Vital signs and serial hematocrits should be obtained.
  - Signs of hemodynamic instability should prompt the examiner to look for other sources of bleeding because it is rare that an isolated or even bilateral femur fracture results in significant blood loss that would cause hypotension.[9]

Management

- As with any fracture, the initial management includes splinting the limb in the field.
  - There are a variety of commercially available splinting materials; however, if unavailable, rolled-up newspaper, cardboard, or even wooden materials can serve as a temporary support.
  - Bandaging both lower limbs together also can be an effective temporary splint.
  - The primary purpose of splinting is to minimize pain; the secondary purpose is to prevent potential neurovascular injury from unstable fracture ends.
- Historically, definitive management of femur fractures has included a period of hospitalization, skin or skeletal traction to allow early fracture callus formation, followed by a spica body cast (Figure 5–11).
  - The cast covers the lower torso, pelvis, involved leg, and uninjured leg down to the knee.
  - Although this treatment plan is well tolerated by patients younger than 5 years with an isolated injury, it becomes less ideal for patients with multiple trauma involving the head, chest, and abdomen.
  - Furthermore, a spica cast is not well tolerated by older patients for whom assisted mobility is not available or by patients with preexisting bone demineralization—OI, MM, MD, or CP.
  - The treatment team often requires access to the chest and torso for frequent examinations, which can be limited by the cast. Moreover, subsequent radiographic studies such as CT or magnetic resonance imaging (MRI) scans can be unobtainable because of an inability to position the patient in the scanner.
  - For older or larger patients, cast immobilization presents challenges to the caretaker, particularly with difficulties in bed-to-chair transfers and ambulation.

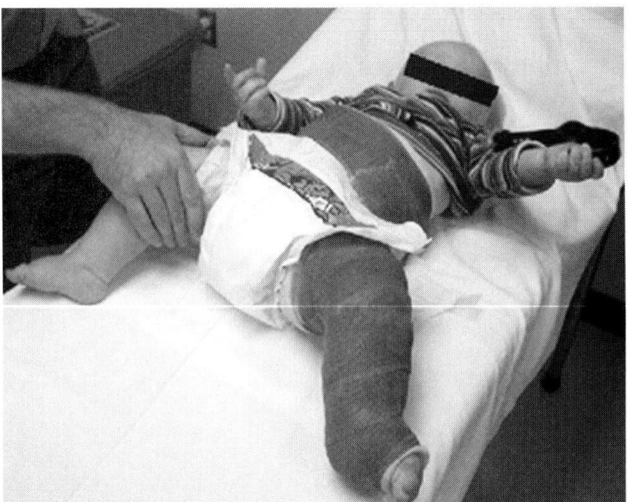

Figure 5–11: Spica cast.

- The parent and child are typically homebound for an additional 8-10 weeks (after 2-3 weeks hospitalization), making school and employment obligations issues.
- For a child with preexisting neurological or metabolic disease, the antigravity effect of the cast contributes to further disuse osteopenia and contributes to additional weakening of the bone.

Treatment

- Treatment varies with age group (Table 5–4).

Younger than 5 Years with an Isolated Injury

- The average hospital stay for patients with early spica casting is 11 days with a range 5-29 days.[10] The stay includes cast application, home care, and transportation planning. Most have uneventful healing with cast removal within 6-8 weeks. Outcomes are

Table 5–4: Treatment Options by Age (Femoral Shaft Fracture)

TREATMENT OPTIONS	0-2 YEARS	3-5 YEARS	6-10 YEARS	>11 YEARS	CLOSED GROWTH PLATE
Spica cast	X	X			
Traction and spica cast		X	X	X	
Intramedullary rod					
Single leg spica		X	X		
TEN		X	X		
Trochanteric antegrade nails				X	
Retrograde					X
External fixator		X *	X *	X *	
Screw or plate		X†	X‡	X	

*Proximal/Distal open (P/D)
†Proximal/Distal (P/D)
‡Subtrochanteric proximal distal supracondylar

excellent with low rates of leg length inequality, rotatory, or angular malunion.[11]

5-10 Years

- Treatment includes hospitalization with traction for 2-3 weeks (Figure 5–12) followed by casting. This method is low risk for the patient and provides good healing potential. However, there are many disadvantages to this treatment modality, such as psychosocial or body image issues related to the cast; missed school; a required caretaker in the hospital (nurses or parents) and at home (parents, extended family, or hired help); necessary family leave with job preservation but no pay; and arrangements with the school for a home tutor, lesson plans, etc. Outcomes are good but, for some, healing is a long, protracted course with many psychological and social issues.
- Many options exist for operative management. All facilitate earlier fracture stabilization without the need for callus formation. In the 5- to 10-year age group, treatment options include elastic intramedullary nails (Figure 5–13, *A*), plates and screws, and external fixators (Figure 5–13, *B*). All of these devices facilitate early mobilization and ambulation with crutches and wheelchairs without need for specialized vehicle transportation home and around the community. Most patients are able to return to school with limited assistance.

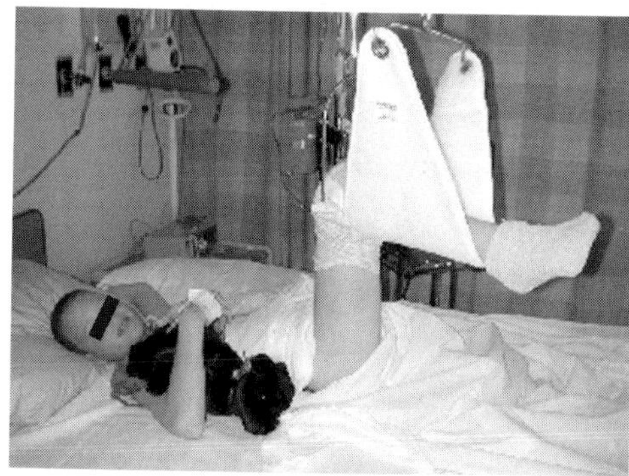

Figure 5–12: 90-90 skeletal traction.

Older than 11 Years

- Operative options are the mainstay of treatment and are thought to result in better long-term results than traditional traction and casting methods. In the older adolescent age groups, traditional reamed intramedullary nails are favored for their rigid fixation.
- Trochanteric antegrade nails are favored rather than piriformis fossa entry-point nails to minimize risk of AVN incurred with injury to femoral neck blood supply (Figure 5–14).
- The immediate stability allows early weight-bearing ability and return to function. A patient generally can expect the fracture to heal within 8-12 weeks and can expect to return to full activity within 6-12 months.

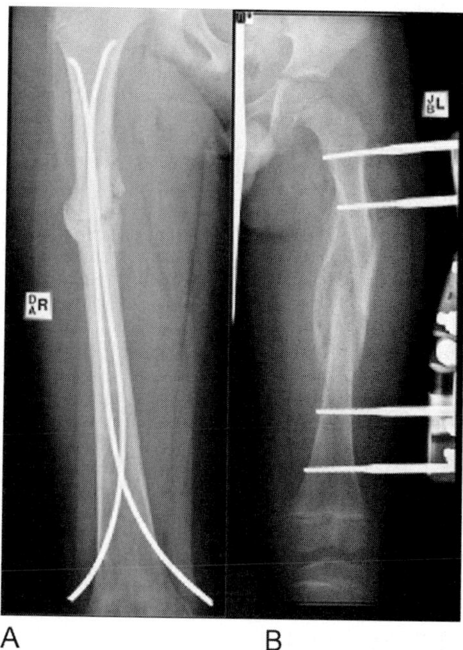

Figure 5–13: Operative management options include elastic intramedullary nails (A) and external fixators (B).

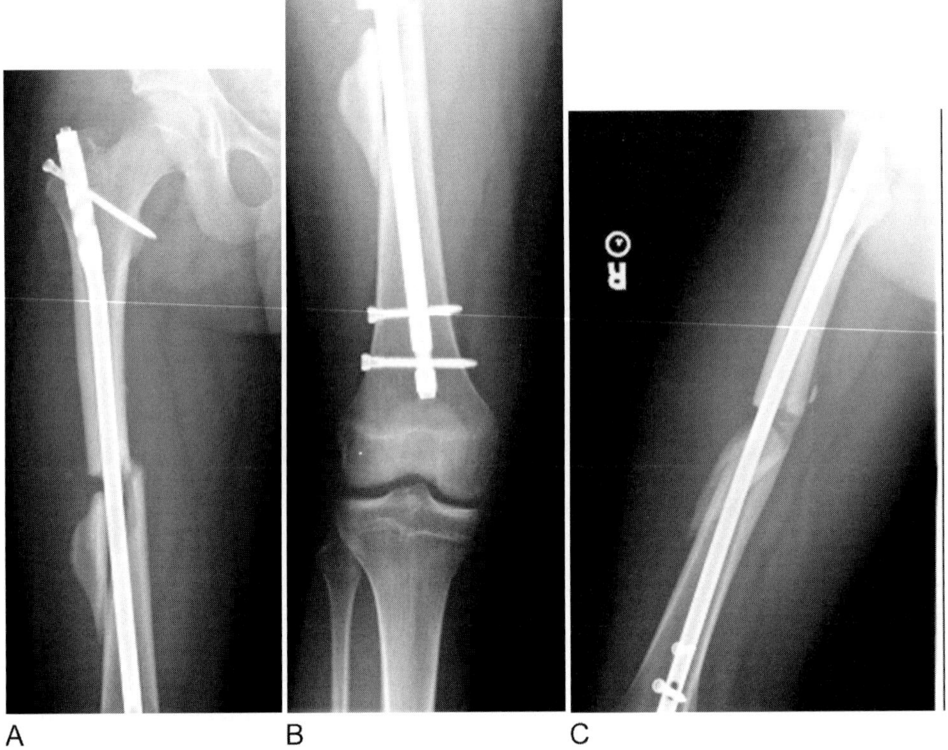

Figure 5–14: Trochanteric antegrade nails minimize risk of AVN. Femur fracture status post-intramedullary rodding (A), AP views (B), and a lateral view (C) are shown.

Knee Injuries

Knee Fractures

- Distal femur—Growth plate fractures are mostly Salter-Harris I and II. On occasion they are Salter-Harris III and IV. Salter-Harris V is rare (Figure 5–15).
- Treatment requires open reduction and internal fixation versus closed reduction and casting. Most are treated with cross-pin fixation and long leg cast or cannulated screw fixation if metaphyseal fragment is large enough to accommodate two screws.
- Long leg cast treatment alone requires close follow-up. Beware of later fracture displacement with cast treatment alone. These fractures also need a lengthy follow-up because of the high incidence of growth disturbance.

Specific Fractures of the Knee

Fractures of the Tibial Spine

- Avulsion fractures of the tibial spine are not common. They are reported most commonly in the 8- to 14-year age group, and the incidence is estimated to be 3 per 100,000.[12]
- These injuries are pediatric equivalents of anterior cruciate ligament (ACL) injuries and are thought to result because the incompletely ossified tibial spine of a child fails before the ACL. In addition, despite the avulsion fracture of its tibial attachment, the ACL is stressed and is often attenuated in these children.[13]
- The mechanism of injury is hyperextension of the knee and occurs with sports and bicycle injuries. This injury has been associated with collateral ligament and meniscal damage.

Classification

- Tibial spine avulsion fractures are described according to the Myers and McKeever classification system[14] (Figure 5–16).
- The difficulty in reducing tibial spine avulsion fractures has received attention in the literature.
- Interposition of different soft tissues may explain the irreducibility of these fractures.
  - The medial or lateral meniscus can be interposed between completely displaced fragments and may block reduction.
  - The lateral meniscus is more commonly involved than the medial meniscus.[15] The transverse meniscal ligament has also been found to block reduction.
  - Other observers discount the interposition theory and propose that the tibial spine fragment, which is attached to both the ACL and the anterior horn of the lateral meniscus, is pulled simultaneously by these

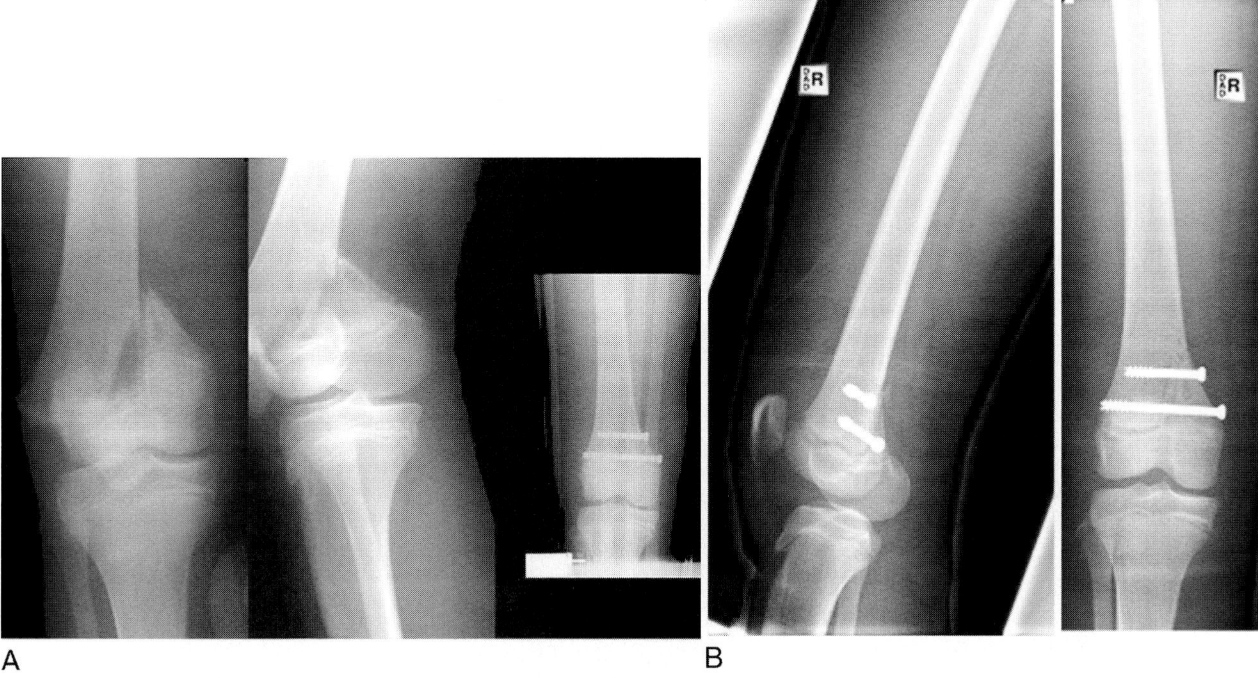

Figure 5–15: Displaced Salter-Harris II distal femur fracture (A) and Salter-Harris II distal femur fracture (B) following operative fixation.

ligaments in different directions and therefore cannot be reduced by manipulation.[14]

Evaluation

- The affected knee will have a large effusion, will be tender to palpation, and will be painful on manipulation. An acutely injured knee is difficult to examine. If the patient is sufficiently relaxed, the Lachman's test can be performed with the knee in about 15 degrees of flexion. Pulling the tibia anterior to the femur in this position tests the integrity of the ACL. The uninjured knee should be compared because individual variability in ligamentous laxity exists. More anterior displacement of the tibia compared with the contralateral knee suggests injury to the ACL or its attachment. The examiner should rule out any other ligamentous or physeal injuries.

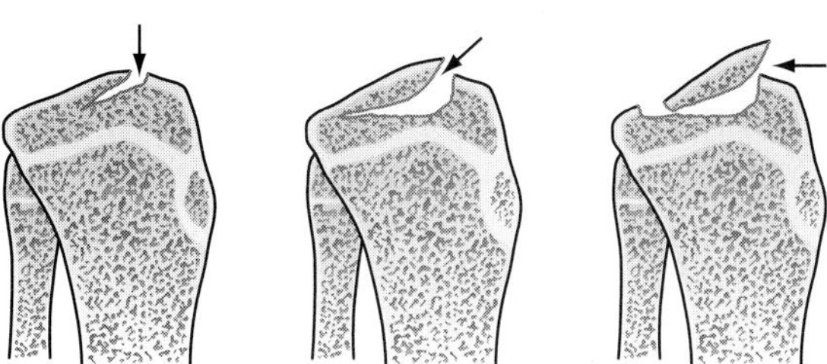

Figure 5–16: Myers and McKeever classification. Type I: Minimal or no displacement of the anterior margin of the fracture. Type II: Elevation of the anterior portion of the anterior tibial spine with an intact posterior hinge. Type III: Avulsed fragment is completely displaced. From Green NE, Swiontkowski MF, eds (1998) Skeletal Trauma in Children, Volume 3. Philadelphia: Saunders, p 454.

- AP and lateral radiographs of the knee are usually sufficient. MRI of the knee may be helpful in determining the presence of any additional intra-articular pathology.

Management

- Type I and II nondisplaced injuries can often be managed without an operation.
  - Sterile knee aspiration can relieve the bloody effusion. Injection of anesthetic at the same time can improve patient comfort and help the physician to position the knee appropriately.
  - Some children will not tolerate a knee aspiration without sedation.
  - Position of the knee for immobilization is controversial.
  - Some believe that placing the knee in full extension or hyperextension effectively reduces the avulsion fracture by allowing the femoral condyles to push the wide base of the avulsed tibial spine down to its original position.
  - Caveat—Hyperextension of the knee can cause increased stretch on ACL and popliteal vessels, which may compromise fracture reduction and blood supply to leg (i.e., compartment syndrome).[38]

- Others contend that the knee should be immobilized in 10 to 20 degrees of flexion to place the ACL in the most relaxed position, thereby allowing the fracture fragment to heal without undue traction.
- Immobilization in an above-knee cast or a cylinder cast for 3-4 weeks is sufficient for healing type I and II fractures (Figure 5–17*A* through *E*).

• Type II injuries that cannot be reduced with closed manipulation can be reduced arthroscopically or with open reduction. The meniscus or clot may be blocking the reduction.

• Type III and IV fractures will require reduction of the fragment and fixation (Figure 5–18). Both can usually be accomplished arthroscopically.

• An open reduction may be necessary.
  - The meniscus may be trapped in the fracture site and block reduction.
  - The frequency of this occurrence is under debate.

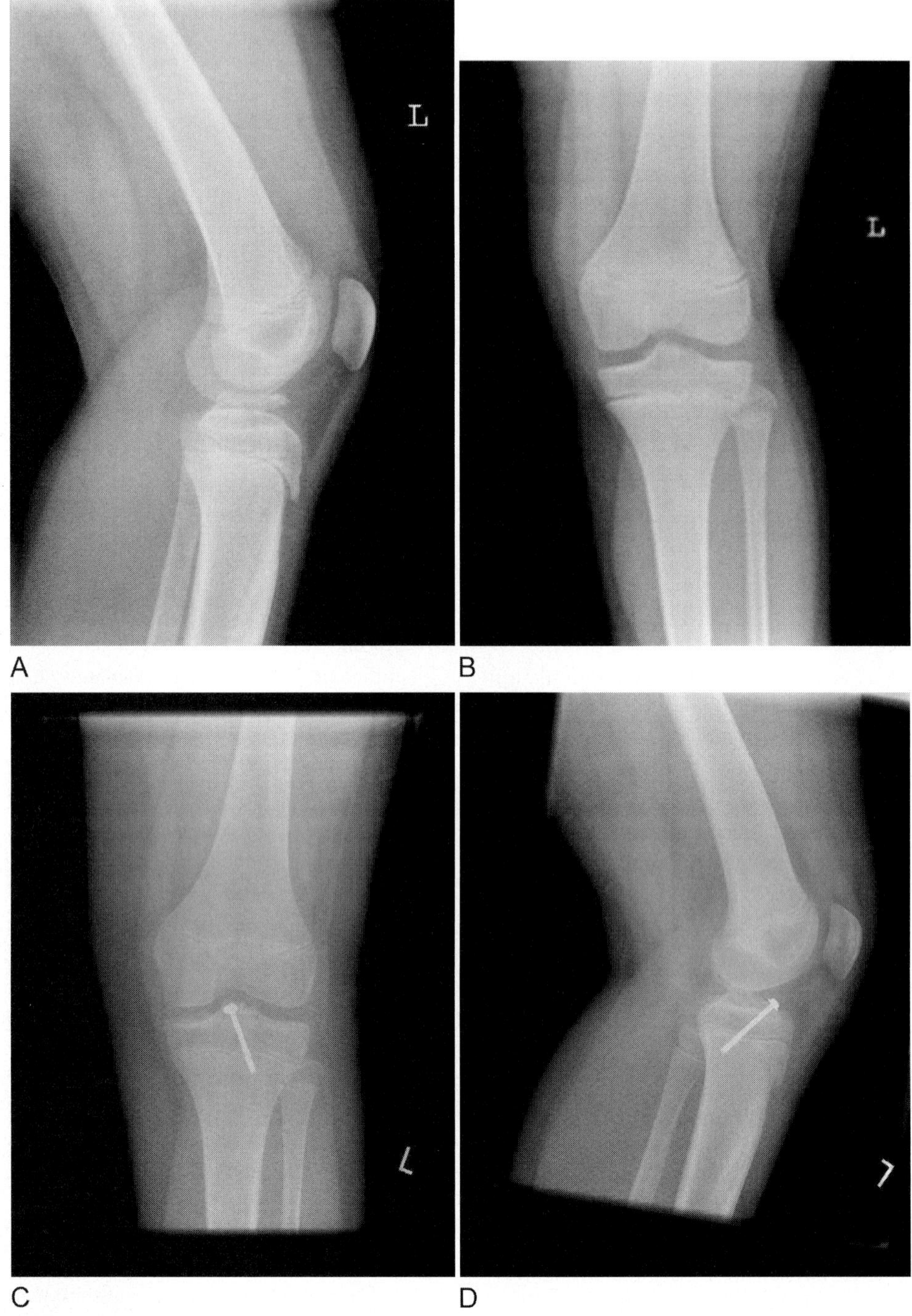

Figure 5–17: Tibial spine avulsion fracture. A and B, AP and lateral radiographs of the knee of this 12-year-old boy show the displacement of the tibial spine. C and D, Arthroscopic-assisted reduction and screw fixation was performed.

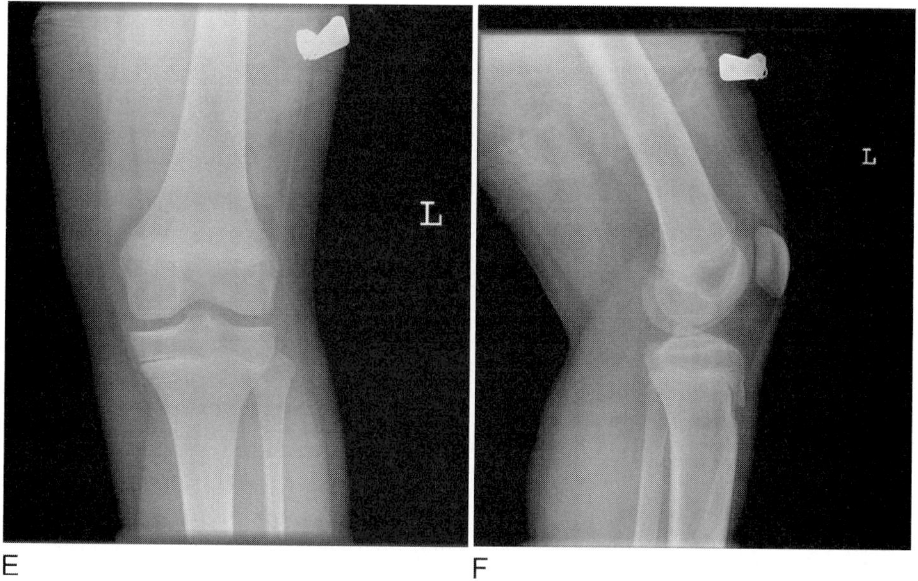

Figure 5–17, cont'd: E and F, One year later, the screw was removed. Courtesy Eric J. Wall, MD.

  - New literature suggests that the tibia is displaced anteriorly, thus effectively stopping tibial spine from reducing back in its proper position.
- Fixation can be performed by a variety of methods and with an array of commercially available devices.
  - Sutures can be placed through the mostly cartilaginous fragment and secured through small drill holes to the anterior tibial metaphysis.
  - Wires may serve the same purpose. A small, cannulated screw can also be placed through the tibial spine fragment and secured in the cancellous bone.
  - Effort should be made to avoid crossing the physis. These implants can be either bioabsorbable or metal.
  - Proper tensioning of the ACL should be performed, possibly even by countersinking the tibial spine fragment.

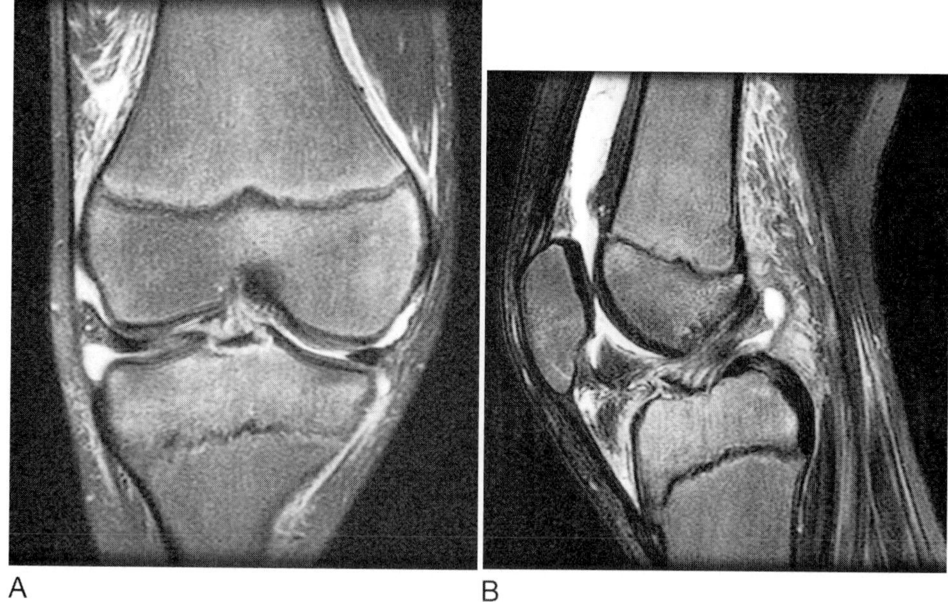

Figure 5–18: Tibial spine avulsion fracture. The knee MRI of an 11-year-old boy shows a hinged tibial spine avulsion fracture. He was treated with immobilization in an above-knee cast. He had asymptomatic residual laxity of his knee on the Lachman's test.

- Protection in a hinged knee brace will allow early exercises to assist range of motion.
- Prolonged immobilization has been associated with retropatellar chondromalacia.
- In general, with appropriate treatment, results are good and nonunions are rare. Mild symptomatic laxity is often present, but complaints of subjective instability are rare.[16]
  - Pathological knee laxity was not correlated to poor subjective knee function.[17] Anterior tibial spine injuries do not appear to be less severe in younger children. Furthermore, young children do not appear to have a greater capacity for reducing laxity of the ACL by further growth.[17]

Complications

- Arthrofibrosis, an excessive scarring of the joint, is a known complication of this injury and its treatment. Prolonged immobilization may increase the risk of developing this debilitating stiffness of the knee. Malunion of type III and IV fractures can cause impingement during knee extension. This can be treated with excision of the fragment and reattachment of the ACL.

Fractures of the Tibial Tubercle Avulsion

- Avulsion fractures of the tibial tubercle are uncommon.
- The incidence of these injuries is about 1% of epiphyseal injuries.
- The mechanism of injury involves athletic activities that include jumping and landing, such as basketball and football.
- In addition, many patients have had Osgood-Schlatter disease. The typical clinical presentation consists of a painful "pop" in the knee upon landing during a basketball game. Subsequently, the patient is unable to bear weight (Table 5–5).
- A classification method by Ogden describes the fracture in terms of the distance of the fracture from the distal tip of the tibial tubercle[18] (Figure 5–19).

Table 5–5: Outcomes Analysis of Knee Injury Mechanism

MECHANISM	POTENTIAL OUTCOMES
Twisting planted foot	Meniscal injury
Fall directly onto knee	Patella fracture
Valgus or varus stress	Collateral ligament injury
Sense of a "pop," immediate swelling, inability to continue activity participation	ACL injury patella dislocation
Sense of "giving up" or locking	Meniscal injury or chondral fracture
Pain with use of stairs or prolonged sitting or squatting	Patellofemoral chondromalacia

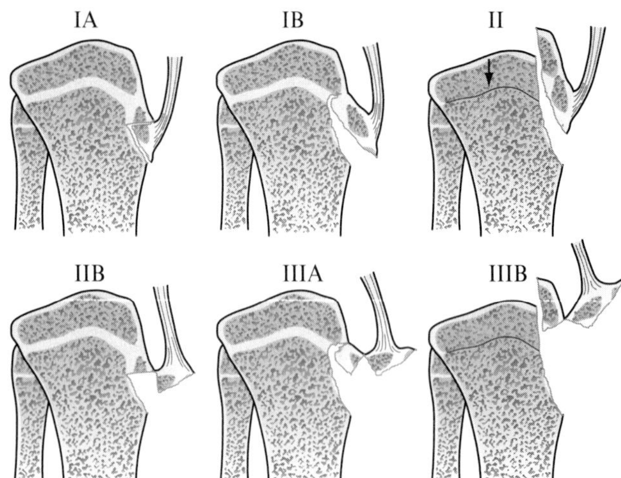

Figure 5–19: Ogden classification of tibial tubercle avulsion fractures. **Type IA: The fracture is distal to the normal junction of the ossification centers of the proximal end of the tibia and the tibial tubercle. Displacement is minimal. Type IB: The fragment is hinged (displaced) anteriorly and proximally. Type II: The primary fracture failure is at the junction of the ossification of the proximal end of the tibia and the tibial tubercle, essentially in line with a transverse continuation of the proximal tibial epiphysis. In type IIB, the tubercle fragment is comminuted, and the more distal fragment may be more proximally displaced. Type III: The fracture extends to the joint and is associated with displacement of the anterior fragment or fragments, leading to discontinuity of the joint surface. In type IIIA, the tubercle and the anterior aspect of the proximal tibial epiphysis are a composite unit. In type IIIB, the unit is comminuted, with the major site of fragmentation being the juncture of the ossification centers of the tubercle and proximal end of the tibia. From Green NE, Swiontkowski MF, eds (1998) Skeletal Trauma in Children, Volume 3. Philadelphia: Saunders, p 454.**

Physical Examination

- A large swelling is noted over the anterior knee, and the tibial tubercle is exquisitely tender to palpation.
- The patient is unable to perform an active straight leg raise, signifying disruption of the extensor mechanism.
  - This includes the entire quadriceps muscle group, the quadriceps tendon, the patella, the infrapatellar ligament, and the insertion into the tibial tubercle.
  - Injury to the tibial tubercle disrupts this chain at its most distal point.
  - Furthermore, the leg may be so swollen that compartment syndrome may ensue.

Imaging

- The lateral view of the knee is most helpful in this situation. The Ogden classification can be used to determine management. CT scans and MRIs are not necessary for diagnosis.

Management

- Immobilization in an above-knee cast is appropriate for all type I and nondisplaced type II and III fractures. Displaced type II and III fractures require open reduction and internal fixation through a longitudinal anterior incision and placement of cannulated screws (Figure 5–20). Periosteal sutures may also be used. The screw can be removed approximately 1 year later if the patient experiences subcutaneous irritation.
- Physeal arrest of the anterior portion of the proximal tibial physis can occur. The resulting asymmetric growth leads to a recurvatum deformity because the posterior aspect of the proximal tibial physis outgrows the anterior portion.

Fractures of the Patella

- Patella fractures are rare and account for 1% of all fractures that occur in children.[19]
  - Most injuries are caused by a direct blow to the patella that compresses it against the distal femoral condyles.
  - These injuries occur during falls and from impacts when patella strikes the dashboard in auto accidents.
  - Some injuries result from sudden forceful contraction of the quadriceps muscle upon a flexed knee during sporting events.
- Patients complain of pain directly over the patella, and physical examination reveals direct point tenderness over the injured area.
- A palpable defect overlying the patella signifies a disruption of the extensor mechanism. An inability to extend the knee against gravity (straight leg raise) also suggests an incompetent extensor mechanism.
- The fracture pattern can range from a sleeve avulsion at the superior or inferior pole, or it can occur in its midportion, either transverse or comminuted (Figure 5–21).
- In early childhood, the patella is primarily cartilaginous. It does not begin to ossify until 6 years.
- In young children, routine radiographs may not reveal a patella fracture because of its cartilaginous structure, which is not apparent on x-ray film. Lateral x-ray films (Figure 5–22) are best to evaluate the patella for fracture. Overlap of patella upon the distal femur often can obscure fracture lines in the AP radiograph. Careful analysis should also distinguish bipartite patella from a true fracture. Bipartite patellae are often bilateral and usually show a cleavage line in the superior lateral pole; although less common, other patterns can be present (Figure 5–23). A painful bipartite patella can indicate a fracture through its cartilaginous plate.
- All displaced fractures associated with disruption of the extensor mechanism should be treated with operative

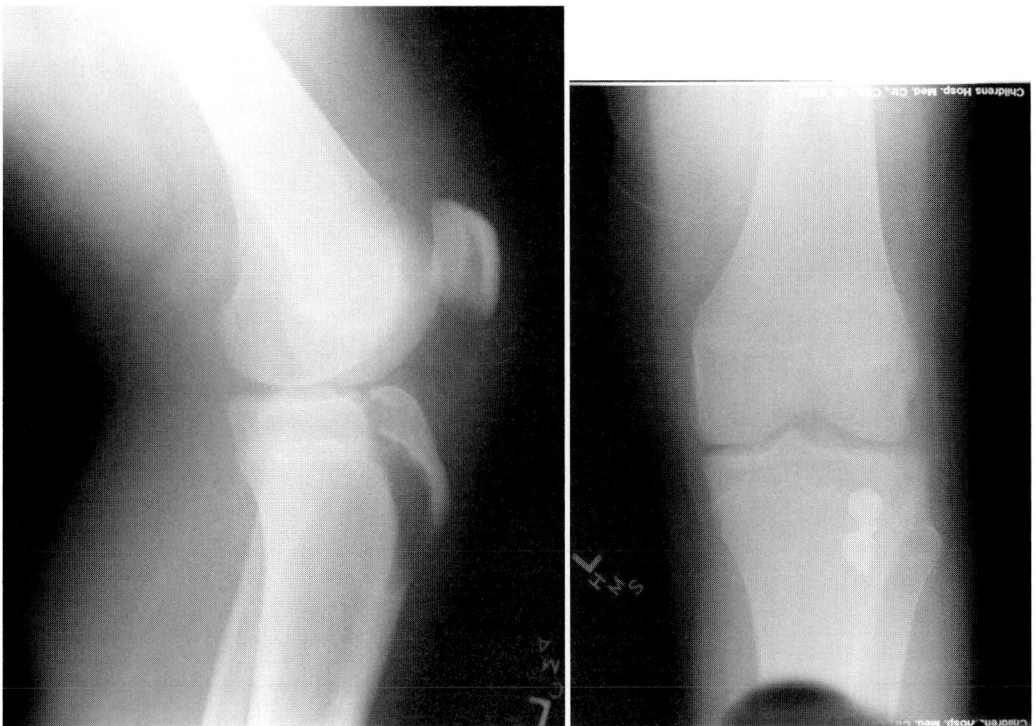

Figure 5–20: Tibial tubercle avulsion fracture. This 15-year-old boy sustained a type IIIA avulsion fracture of his tibial tubercle while playing basketball. He underwent open reduction and internal fixation. One year later, his only complaint was skin irritation from the screws. He subsequently had them removed. Courtesy Dennis Roy, MD.

Continued

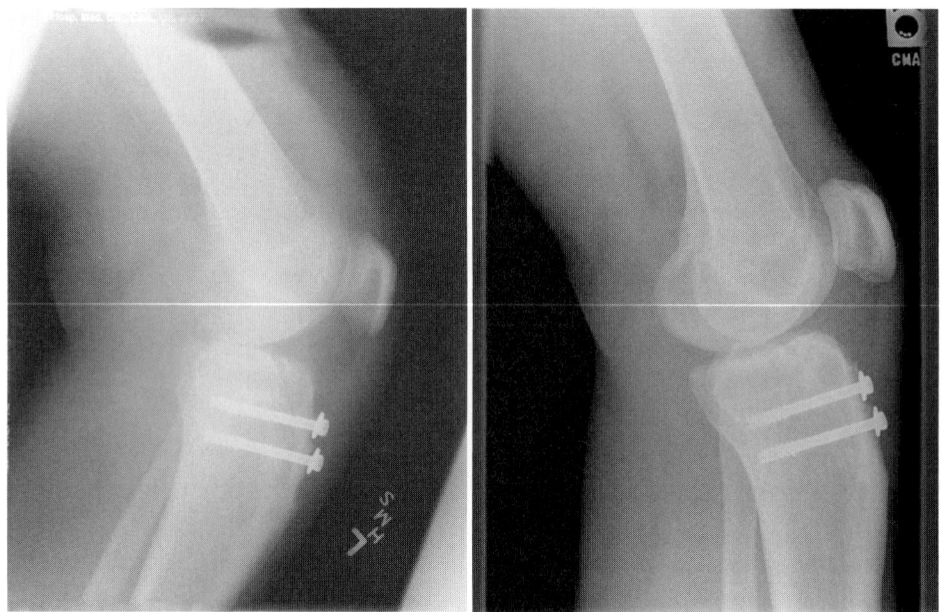

Figure 5–20, cont'd.

fixation techniques similar to those applied to adults (Figure 5–24). Nondisplaced fractures are treated with a cylinder cast or brace (Figure 5–25) until healing has occurred.

Ligament Injuries

Anterior Cruciate Ligament Injuries

- The patient complains of a painful popping sensation in the knee.
- This most commonly occurs in adolescents who participate in risky sports such as basketball, football, soccer, volleyball, and noncontact sports.[20]
- An inability to play sports is caused by immediate swelling.
- Treatment options range from nonoperative bracing to surgical reconstruction.
  - Functional bracing is useful for skeletally immature patients and especially for people who have instability

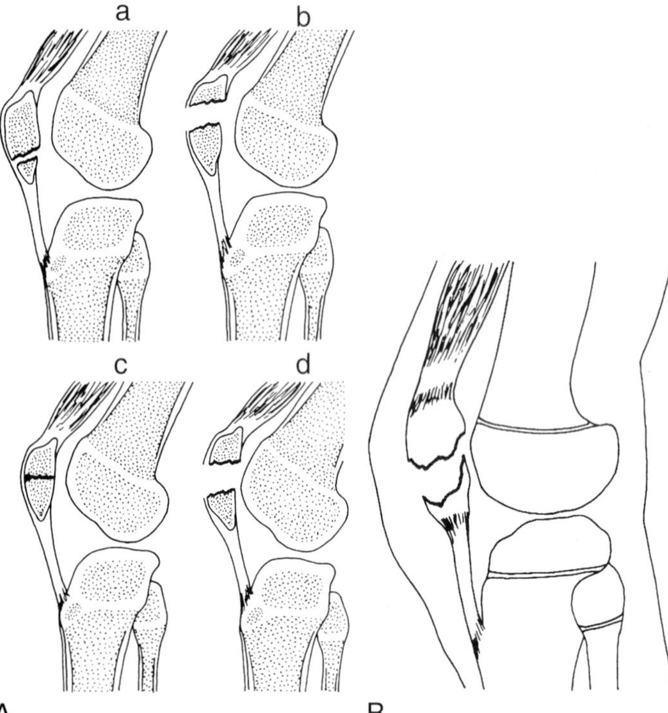

Figure 5–21: A, Types of patellar fractures: Inferior pole *(a)*, superior pole *(b)*, transverse undisplaced midsubstance *(c)*, and transverse displaced midsubstance *(d)*. B, From Houghton GR, Ackroyd CE (1979) Sleeve fractures of the patella in children. J Bone Joint Surg Br 61B(2): 165-168.

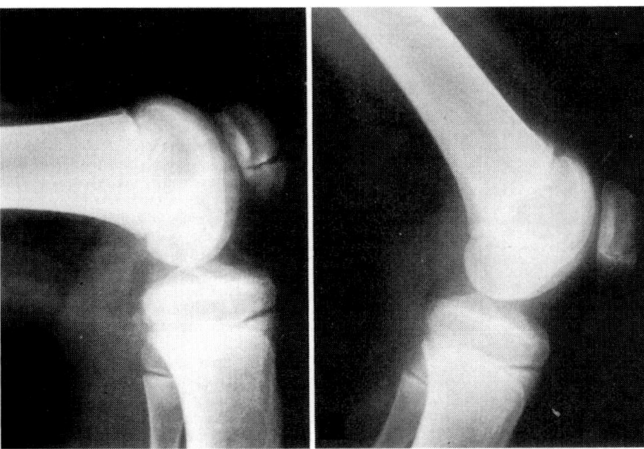

Figure 5–22: Fractures of the patella–transverse minimally displaced. From Tachdjian MO (1990) Pediatric Orthopaedics. WB Saunders, p 3285.

with simple activities of daily living, such as community ambulation.
 - Surgical reconstruction is preferred when a child is at or near skeletal maturity as defined by bone age—13 in females and 14 in males.[20]
 - Those who are unable to have surgery are advised to refrain from risky sports.
 - Physical therapy is advised with special attention to strengthening the hamstring musculature of the leg.

Posterior Cruciate Ligament Injuries

- Posterior cruciate ligament injuries are commonly caused by football tackles.
- Beware of knee dislocations.

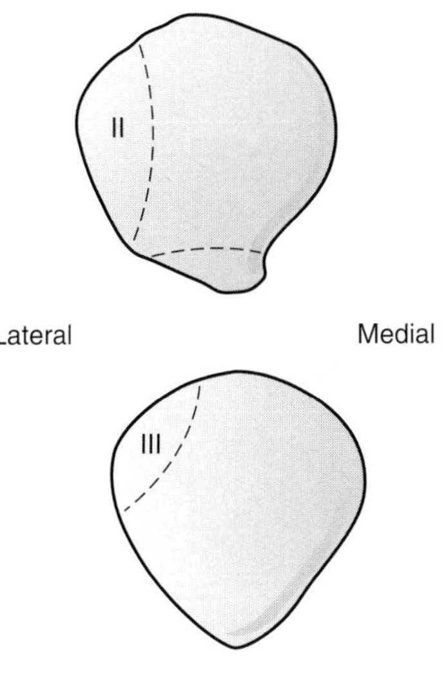

Figure 5–23: Saupe classification of bipartite patella. From Stanitski CL, Delee JC, Drez D Jr (1994) Pediatric and Adolescent Sports Medicine. WB Saunders, p 312.

- Nonoperative treatment emphasizes strengthening of the quadriceps muscles.
- Operative treatment seeks to reconstruct the posterior cruciate ligament.

Medial Collateral Injuries

- Patients have a history of valgus stress.
- They have tenderness at the inner aspect of the knee and the medial joint line.
- Brace treatment should be carried out for 4-6 weeks.

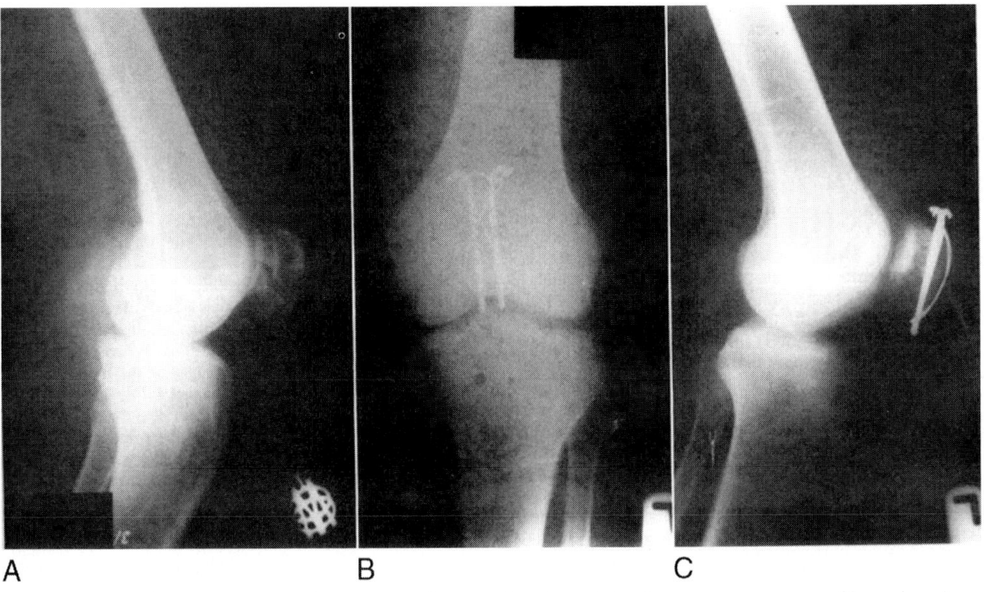

Figure 5–24: A, Displaced transverse fracture of the patella. B and C, Postoperative x-ray films showing modified tension band internal fixation using two anterior wire loops and two longitudinally directed Kirschner wires. From Campbell W (1987) Operative Orthopaedics. CV St. Louis: Mosby, p 1669.

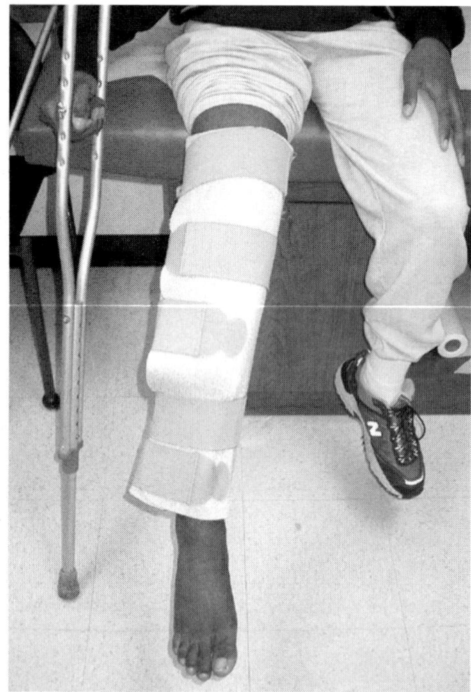

Figure 5–25: Immobilizer brace.

Lateral Collateral Injuries

- There is a history of tenderness over the lateral joint line.
- Varus stress requires a hinged brace for 4 weeks.
- Beware of peroneal nerve function.

Meniscal Injuries

- Meniscal injuries often appear with joint line tenderness extending from the midportion of the knee in the coronal plane posteriorly behind the femoral condyle.
  - Tender crepitance along the joint line with flexion–rotation (McMurray test) or compression–rotation maneuvers (Appley test) suggest a meniscal tear.
  - Severely displaced menisci often found in bucket handle-type tears can limit full knee motion, especially extension.

Patellofemoral Injuries

- Painful crepitance and tenderness along the medial or lateral parapatellar retinaculum are signs of patellofemoral injury. Malalignment is determined by measuring the Q angle, which is formed by the intersection of a line drawn along the long axis of the thigh and a line drawn from the midpoint of the patella to the tibia tubercle.

Proximal Tibia Metaphyseal Fractures (Cozen Fractures)

- Fractures involving the proximal tibia metaphysis commonly occur between the ages of 2 and 10.[21]
  - This fracture is relatively uncommon but has become clinically important because of the post-traumatic development of progressive valgus deformity.
  - This phenomenon was initially reported by Cozen in 1953; therefore, this fracture is sometimes referred to as the *Cozen fracture,* and the post-traumatic angulation is known as the *Cozen effect*. This deformity occurs after proximal tibial metaphyseal fractures in up to half of such cases.
- The etiology for this deformity has been debated in the literature and is intimately tied to the treatment method. It is imperative to inform the parents and caregivers of the injured child that post-traumatic valgus deformity of the tibia can occur with any form of treatment and that its development is unpredictable.
- Some factors are under the control of the treating orthopaedic surgeon. These include obtaining an adequate reduction, removal of soft tissue interposition, and close clinical follow-up with parental education.
- Inadequate reduction of the fracture initially angulated by trauma has been implicated as the cause of the tibia valga deformity.
  - Oftentimes, the child is placed in a bent-knee long leg cast, which does not adequately control varus and valgus angulation (Figure 5–26). Cast application with the knee fully extended allows the surgeon to better mold the cast to obtain an adequate reduction.
  - Furthermore, anatomical reduction can be lost because of a loosening of the cast. These children, therefore, never have the valgus angulation adequately corrected before fracture healing.
- If there is no associated fibula fracture, the connections between the lateral aspect of the tibia and fibula at the proximal tibiofibular joint near the knee and the distal tibiofibular joint at the ankle remain intact.
  - Thus, the growth stimulation, which normally occurs after children's fractures, may occur preferentially on the medial side, leading to a progressive valgus angulation.
  - However, this deformity occurs even when the fibula is fractured.[21]
- Another theory suggests that unequal growth between the medial and the lateral physis occurs because of an asymmetric vascular response.[21]
  - This factor cannot be controlled by the surgeon but may explain the progressive deformity phenomenon.
  - Technetium bone scans have shown increased uptake at the proximal tibial growth plate compared with the contralateral unaffected limb, with proportionally greater uptake on the medial side.
  - This suggests that the valgus deformity was caused by a relative increase in vascularity and consequent overgrowth of the medial portion of the proximal tibial physis.[22]

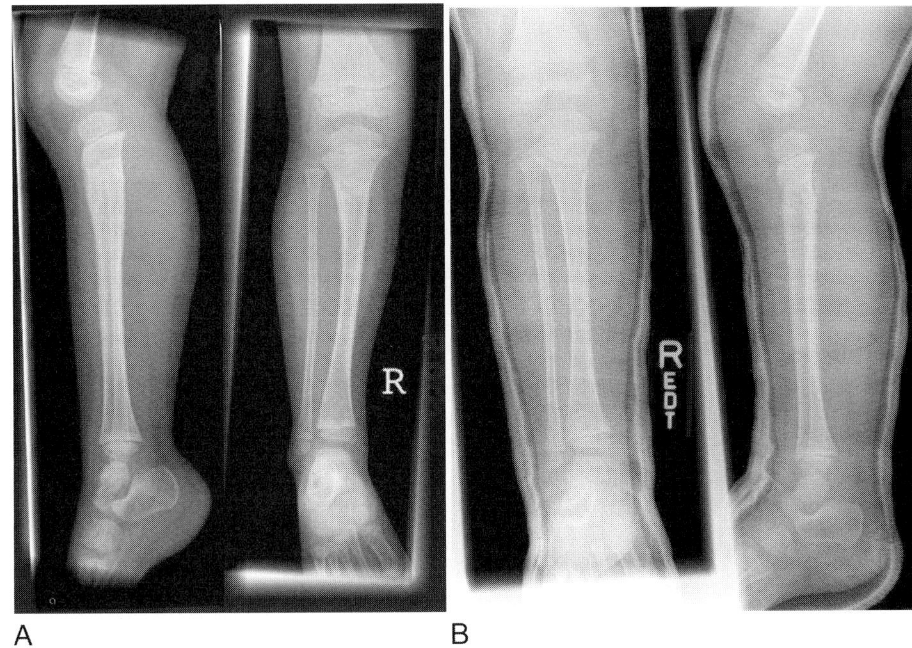

Figure 5–26: Cozen fracture. A post-cast healing film (A) and a casted injury (B).

- Once a valgus deformity develops, the treatment of choice is observation.
  - Most of the deformity will correct spontaneously, although this may take up to 3 years.[23]
  - The valgus deformity will progress most rapidly in the first year and can continue to progress over 20 months after injury.
- Reminding the parents of the nature of this condition at each office visit will be helpful. The parents may assign blame for the deformity and may pressure the surgeon to surgically correct the angulation.
- Results after nonoperative and operative treatment have been compared and showed no difference, making surgical correction of the valgus deformity unwarranted in the first 2 to 3 years after injury.[23]
- Should clinically significant valgus deformity persist after 2 to 3 years, surgical options include proximal tibial osteotomy and proximal tibial hemiepiphysiodesis. Proximal tibial osteotomy acutely corrects the valgus deformity.
  - Beware of peroneal nerve injury with large acute correction.
  - Consider techniques that allow gradual correction with large deformities.
  - The proximal tibia is cut and angulated into varus and held together with screws or staples.
  - This method, however, has been associated with recurrence of the valgus deformity and has not been found to change the clinical course of this condition.[23]
  - The valgus deformity is thought to recur because the osteotomy recreates the conditions of the initial fracture.
  - Proximal tibial hemiepiphysiodesis involves the surgical retardation or cessation of growth through the proximal tibial physis.
- In a young patient with years of growth remaining, staples placed across the medial proximal tibial physis slow growth through this area.
- Once adequate correction is achieved because of preferential growth of the lateral portion of the physis, the staples can be removed, allowing the growth on the medial side to resume. In this way, the deformity can be corrected without permanent closure of the medial physis.
- In an older patient with little growth remaining, the medial physis can be surgically ablated, leading to cessation of growth. The remaining lateral portion of the physis will continue to grow to correct the valgus deformity until closure of the physis at skeletal maturity.

Proximal Tibia Physeal Fractures

- Physeal fractures of the proximal tibial can result from either direct or indirect mechanisms of injury.
  - Most of these injuries can be classified as Salter-Harris I or II.
  - The most important aspect of this injury is to recognize a vascular injury because this is the pediatric equivalent of a traumatic knee dislocation (Figure 5–27).
  - The patient is in severe pain with this injury.
- A thorough neurovascular examination is particularly critical in this injury. In the presence of a vascular injury, assessment of the limb for compartment syndrome is also mandatory.

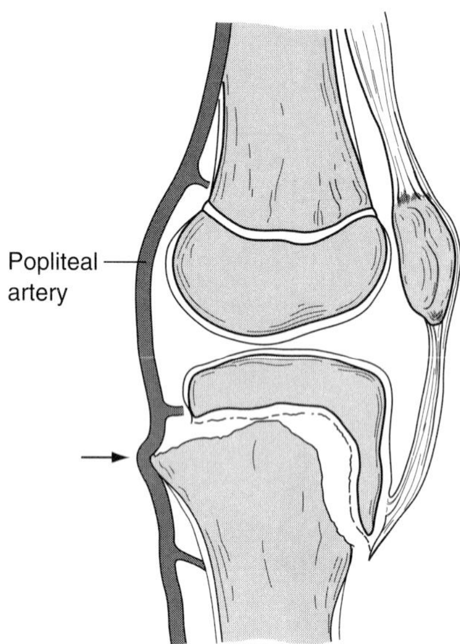

Figure 5–27: Proximal tibial physeal injury. **A displaced proximal tibial physeal injury can be associated with arterial injury because of the proximity of the proximal tibial physis to the popliteal artery. From Green NE, Swiontkowski MF, eds (1998) Skeletal Trauma in Children. Philadelphia: Saunders, p 460.**

  - Doppler and arteriogram studies are important.
  - Beware of late vascular compromise caused by an intimal flap injury.
  - If vascular repair is necessary, prophylactic fasciotomies of leg should be done to prevent compartment syndrome after revascularization.
- AP and lateral radiographs of the knee are usually sufficient to diagnose this injury. Recognition of a nondisplaced fracture may require clinical suspicion. MRI is usually not indicated.
- Nondisplaced proximal tibial physeal fractures should be immobilized in an above-knee cast.
- Displaced fractures will require a closed reduction under general anesthesia. If the reduction is stable under fluoroscopic evaluation, an above-knee cast will suffice.
- Unstable fractures may require fixation with percutaneously placed Steinman pins and immobilization in an above-knee cast.
- Four weeks of immobilization without bearing weight is followed by removal of the pins and initiation of a rehabilitation program.
- Close clinical follow-up is necessary to look for evidence of growth arrest or the development of angular deformity.

Tibial and Fibular Shaft Fractures

- The tibia is the most commonly fractured bone of the lower limb in children.
- Fractures involving both the tibia and the fibula generally result from direct injury.
  - Most tibia fractures are associated with fibula fractures.[24]
  - The mean age at fracture is 8 years.
- The child will have pain, swelling, and deformity of the affected leg and will be unable to bear weight. Distal neurovascular examination must be performed.
- AP and lateral views of the tibia–fibula should include the knee and the ankle.
- Closed reduction and cast immobilization have been the standard methods of treatment.
- Most fractures remodel well, and children usually have excellent results (Figure 5–28). Deformities that do not remodel well include valgus angulation, apex posterior angulation (recurvatum), and rotations, particularly internal rotation.[25]
- Casting should address all of these components so that the child's limb will be in the best alignment possible.
- For children younger than 10 years, 15 degrees of varus angulation, 10 mm of shortening, 10 degrees of apex anterior angulation, and 15 degrees of external rotation have been well tolerated.
- In older children, the criteria for acceptable reduction of the tibia are more stringent. Less than 10 degrees of angulation has generally been the goal, although a long-term study of adult patients has shown that less than 5 degrees of angulation was associated with less degenerative changes.
- Indications for internal or external fixation of tibia fractures in children are limited to open fractures, unstable closed fractures, neurovascular injuries, multiple trauma, and soft tissue abnormalities.
- Open fractures need to undergo irrigation and debridement multiple times; therefore, the wound needs to easily accessible.
- Casting will cover the wound. Immobilization with internal fixation in open fractures with little soft tissue injury is acceptable.
- In cases with more severe soft tissue injury, external fixation will be more applicable.
- Neurovascular injuries associated with fractures require a stable bed of tissue for healing.
- Stable operative fixation of the bones accomplishes this without compressing the soft tissues or preventing wound care.
- Multiple-injury patients need surgical stabilization of long bone fractures to aid mobility.
- Younger patients can tolerate more cast immobilization.
- Older patients, particularly adolescents, are more difficult to care for if they are immobilized with multiple casts because of their greater size and weight. In addition, prolonged cast immobilization in older patients is associated with the development of joint stiffness and deep vein thrombosis.

Isolated Tibia Shaft Fractures

- Isolated tibial fractures with an intact fibula are common in children. These fractures result from an indirect

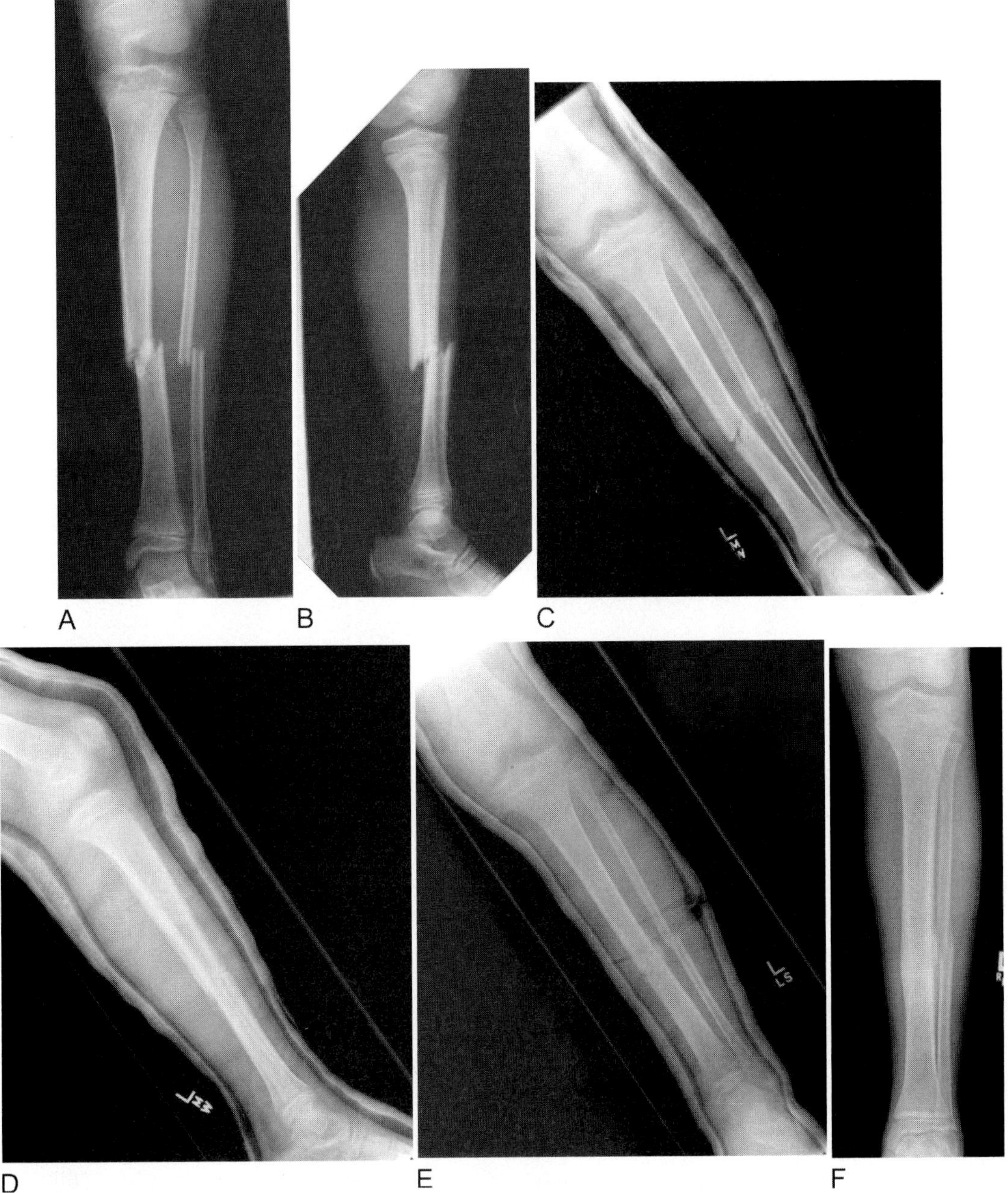

Figure 5–28: Tibia–fibula fracture. A and B, A 10-year-old boy sustained a displaced transverse fracture of the midshaft of his tibia and fibula. C, An above-knee cast was applied after a closed reduction. One month later, the tibia was noted to have valgus angulation. D, Cast wedging was performed to restore the alignment. E and F, Four months after the fracture, the tibia was healed in satisfactory alignment.

rotational twisting force and do not require as much energy to produce as the fractures involving both the tibia and the fibula. These fractures often occur at the distal third of the tibial shaft. Varus angulation occurred most commonly when the fracture line started distally on the anteromedial side of the tibia and progressed in an oblique or spiral manner to the proximal posterolateral aspect of the tibia. The posterior flexor muscle groups (the posterior tibialis and the toe flexors and extensors) are concentrated medially and therefore exert a varus-producing force.

- The physical examination findings are similar to those for tibia–fibula fractures.
- Tibia radiographs including the joint above and below the level of injury will suffice.
- The isolated tibial fracture with an intact fibula can be difficult to reduce and maintain in the anatomical position because of the splinting of the intact fibula.

- Recurrent deformities that drift into varus and posterior angulation are common within 3 weeks after initial injury (Figure 5–29).
- Immobilization of the fractures was best achieved with an above-knee cast, the knee flexed to 30 degrees, and the ankle in 15 degrees of plantar flexion to minimize varus forces.
- Varus and posterior angulation of greater than 10 degrees should be corrected because this deformity pattern has the least capacity to remodel.
- Premature physeal closure of the ipsilateral knee—at the level of the distal femur, the proximal tibia, or both—has been reported in adolescents after tibial diaphyseal fractures.[26]

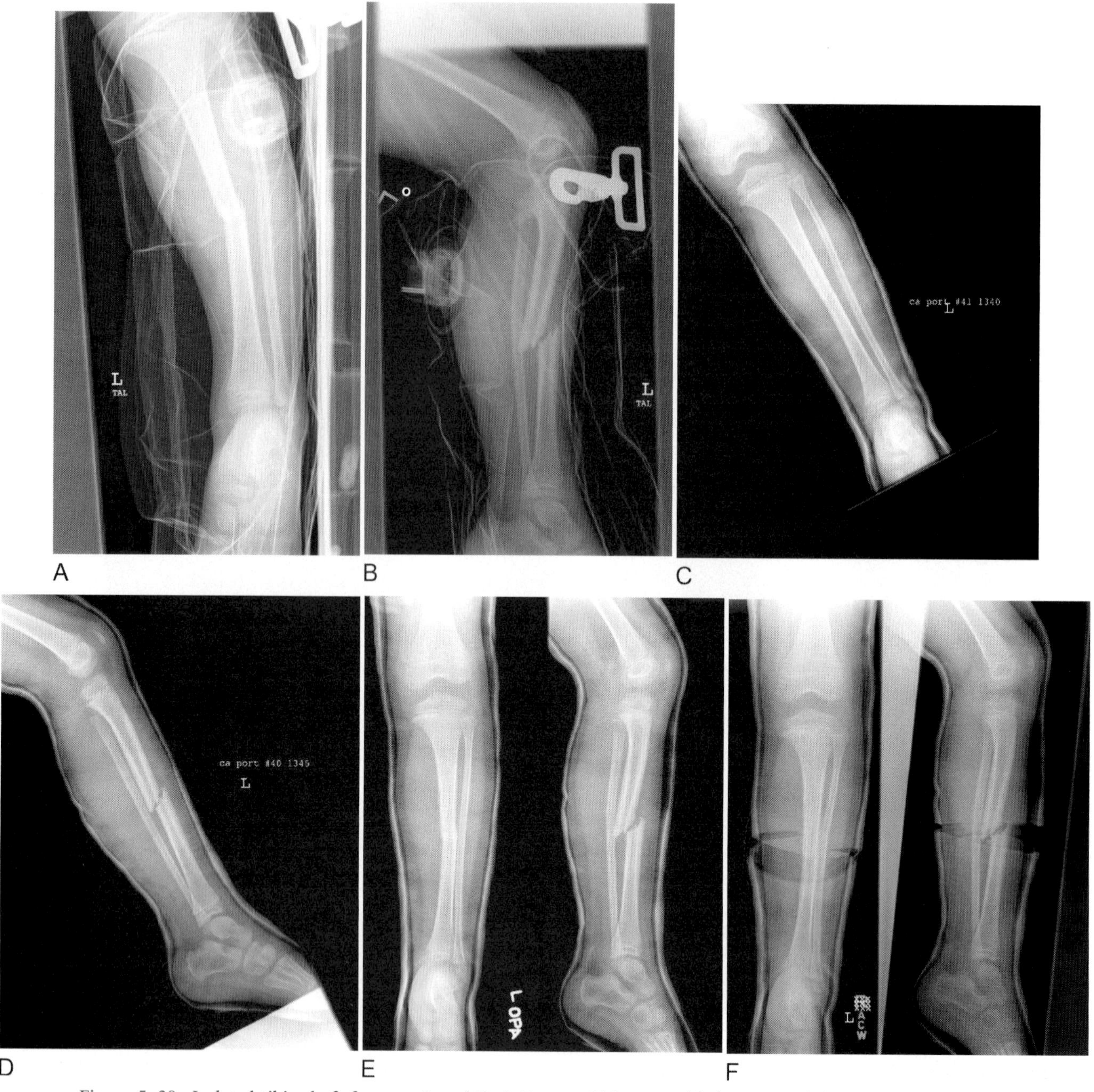

Figure 5–29: Isolated tibia shaft fracture. A and B, A 7-year-old boy was hit by a car while riding a scooter and sustained this displaced tibia fracture. C and D, Closed reduction in the operating room restored alignment with mild posterior translation. E, Two weeks later, the tibia had varus angulation. F, The cast was wedged to restore alignment.

Distal Tibial Transition Fractures

- Both triplane and Tillaux fractures (Figures 5–30 through 5–32) occur in the adolescent age group with incompletely fused or closed distal tibial physis.
- Closure usually occurs over a 19-month period during skeletal maturity. It begins in the central portion of the distal tibial physis, proceeds in a circular fashion medially, and ends at anterolateral quadrant of the tibial.
- The mechanism on injury is external rotation stress on planted foot.
- X-ray films—AP, lateral, and oblique views—of the tibia–ankle should be used in evaluation.
- Treatment calls for closed reduction, reversing the mechanism of injury, and long leg cast.
- Postreduction assessment necessitates x-ray films—AP, lateral, and mortise views of ankle. Perform a CT scan if the quality of reduction is questionable.
- Perform open reduction and internal fixation if an articular incongruity or diastasis greater than 2 mm exists.

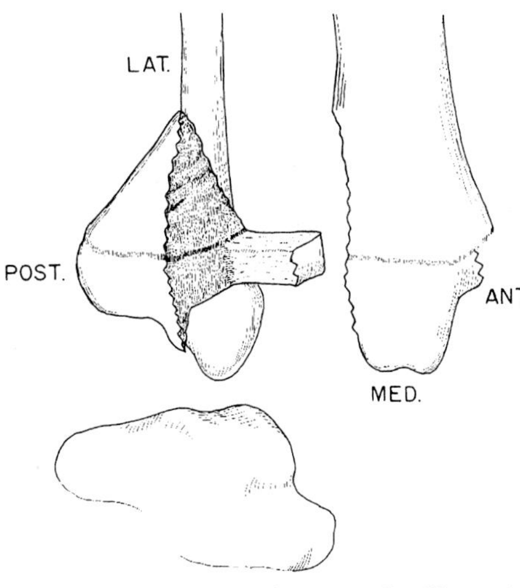

Figure 5–31: Triplane fracture diagram. **The illustration is a three-dimensional representation of the two-part triplane fracture shown in the previous images. From Cooperman DR, Spiegel PG, Laros GS (1978) Tibial fractures involving the ankle in children, J Bone Joint Surg 60A(8), Figure 2, *B*.**

Toddler's Fractures

- Toddler's fractures occur in young ambulatory children.
- The age range for this fracture is typically from around 1 to 4 years.

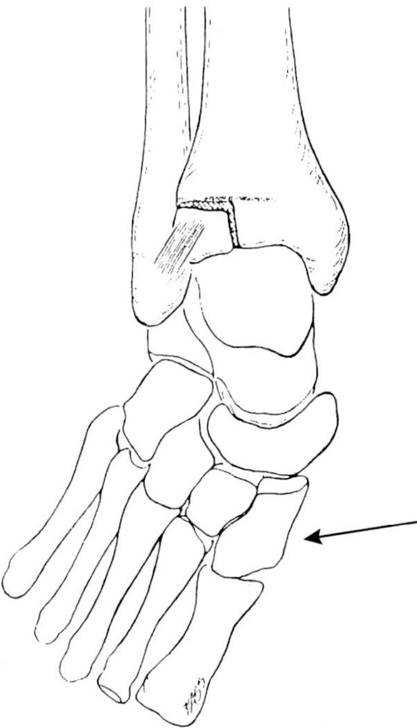

Figure 5–30: Tillaux fracture diagram. **Note the external rotation of the foot and the intact anterior tibiofibular ligament attached to the Tillaux fracture fragment. From Dias LS, Giegerich CR (1983) Fractures of the distal tibial epiphysis in adolescence, J Bone Joint Surg 65A(4): 438-444.**

- The injury often occurs after a seemingly harmless twist or fall and is frequently unwitnessed.
  - The child may not complain of pain until forced to bear weight on the affected extremity.
  - Frequently, the child will either refuse to bear weight or walk with a limp.
- Children in this age group are usually unable to articulate the mechanism of injury clearly or to describe the area of injury well.
- The radiographs also may show no fracture; therefore, the diagnosis is made by physical examination.
- Examining a child in this age group can be challenging.
  - Refusal to bear weight can manifest as pulling up the affected leg or as a florid display of protest.
  - The most accurate way to assess the location of injury is thorough palpation of the affected lower extremity while the child is distracted.
- AP and lateral views of the tibia–fibula may show a nondisplaced spiral fracture of the distal tibial metaphysic (Figure 5–33).
  - An oblique view is oftentimes helpful because the fracture line may be visible in only one of three views.
  - Fracture lines may not be visible, and the diagnosis often relies on the clinical examination.
- Radiographs are helpful in excluding pathological and metabolic conditions. A three-phase technetium bone scan can be helpful in excluding infections such as septic arthritis and osteomyelitis.
- Clinical suspicion of a toddler's fracture is the key to diagnosis.
- A child with a history of an acute injury, the inability to walk or a limp, no constitutional signs, and negative

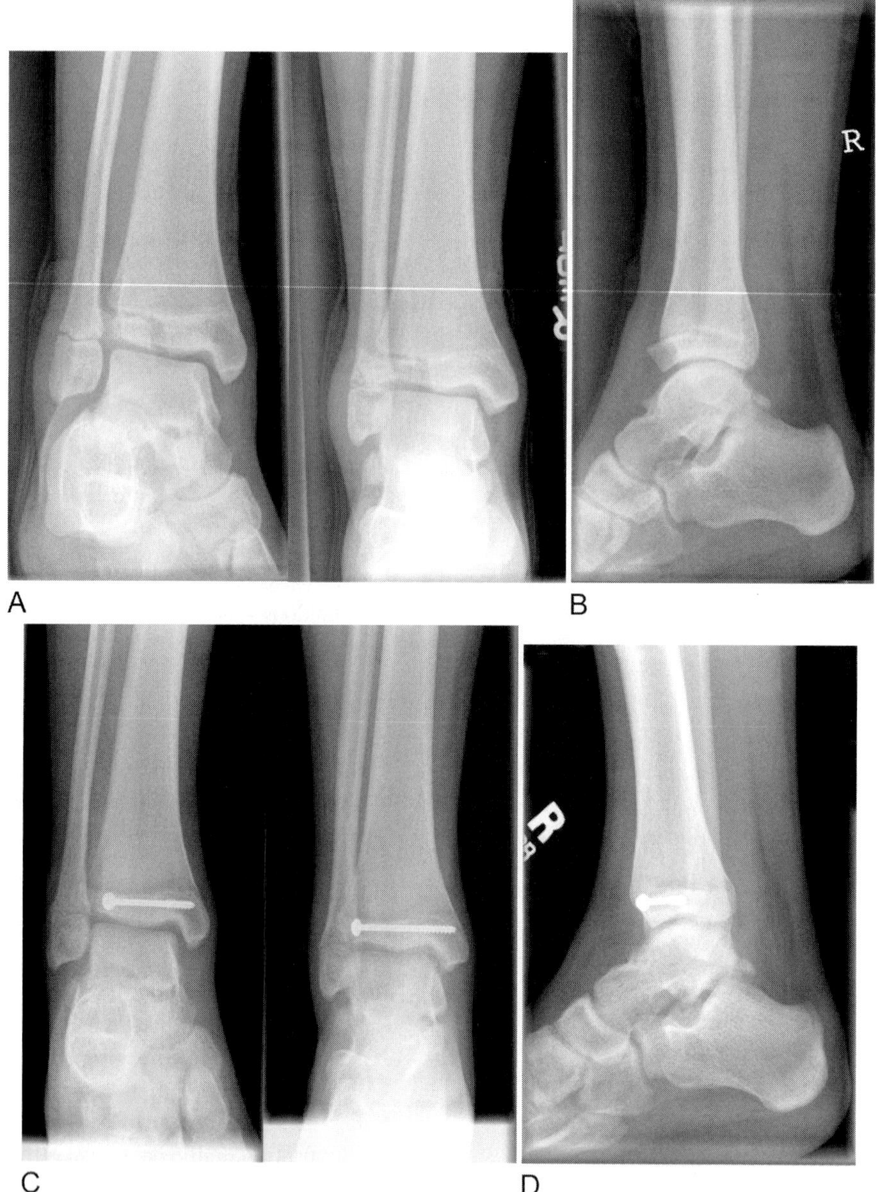

Figure 5–32: Tillaux fracture. Three views of the ankle of this 14-year-old boy show the avulsion fracture of the anterolateral portion of the distal tibial epiphysis. Mortise and AP views show the intra-articular component of the fracture. A and B, Lateral view shows the anterior displacement of the fragment. C and D, The patient underwent open reduction and internal fixation of the Tillaux fracture.
Courtesy Charles T. Mehlman, DO.

radiographs should be presumed to have a toddler's fracture.[27]

- The child with a toddler's fracture is immobilized in an above-knee cast for approximately 3 weeks.
- The portion above the knee helps to control rotation of the tibia and to keep the cast on the limb.
- The child may bear weight as tolerated.
- Once the cast is removed, the parents and caregivers are counseled about the postcast gait in which a child continues to walk as if still wearing the cast.
- While wearing the above-knee cast, the child is unable to move the knee or the ankle and therefore compensates by externally rotating the entire limb, including the foot. This adjustment allows the child to clear the ground effectively.
- Even after the cast is removed, this externally rotated gait persists for 1 to 2 months and becomes a major source of concern for some parents and caregivers, sometimes resulting in multiple doctor visits despite the child's painless mobility.

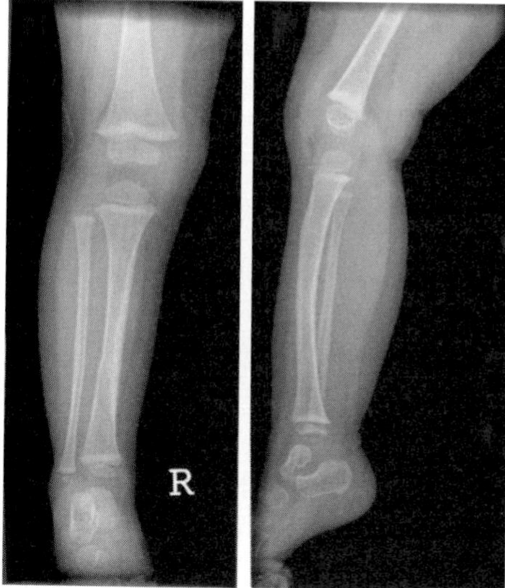

Figure 5–33: Toddler's fracture. Tibia radiographs of this 2-year–6-month-old child show the nondisplaced spiral metaphyseal fracture.

- Early counseling and reassurance is much more effective and less time consuming than explanations afterward.
- Toddler's fractures heal well without any adverse sequelae.

Stress Fractures

- Stress fractures are becoming increasingly common in adolescent athletes because of year-round sports and organized athletics at a younger age.
  - Stress fractures are commonly caused by sports that have an emphasis on repetitive running, such as cross country, basketball, track, soccer, and field hockey.
  - Stress fractures of the tibia and fibula appear as tenderness along the proximal medial tibia or distal fibula.
- Imaging—Bone scan or MRI can be diagnostic (Figure 5–34).
- The most essential component is rest.
- It is imperative that the patient avoids repetitive impact activities.
  - Generally, 6-8 weeks of rest are recommended.
  - Immobilization can be helpful. It is suggested that a return to sports should be gradual.
- Rehabilitation includes restoration of ankle motion, strength, and proprioception.
- Once the athlete has no tenderness to palpation and is able to perform exercises without pain, he or she may resume usual activities gradually.
- Special attention should be paid to adolescent female athletes.
  - Individuals with stress fractures may suffer from the female athlete triad, consisting of amenorrhea, anorexia, and osteoporosis (Box 5–1).
  - These patients usually do not volunteer information about their menstrual cycles or their eating habits; therefore, relevant questions need to be asked directly and discretely.
  - Goal-oriented, image-conscious adolescent girls may restrict food intake because they are too busy to eat or wish to lose weight.
  - In addition, carbonated beverages, which weaken bones, tend to be particularly popular in this age group compared with milk and soy products, which contain calcium.

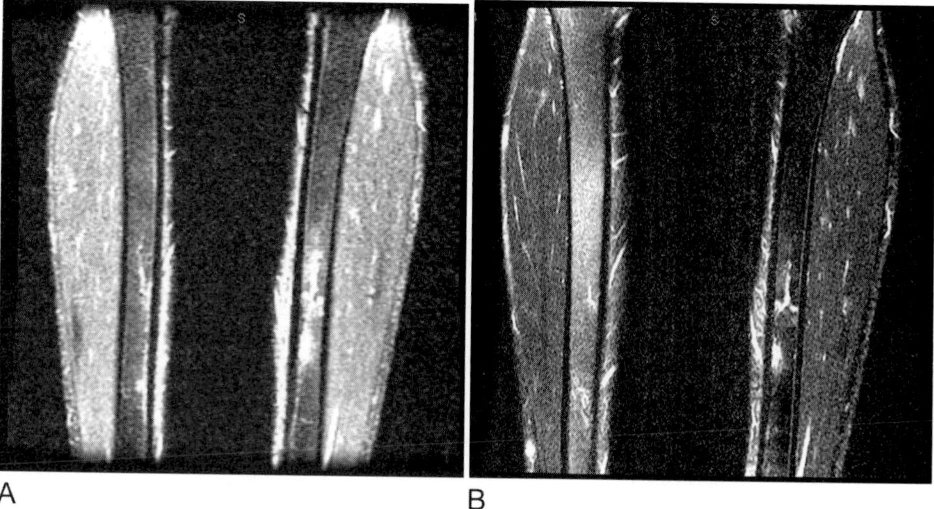

Figure 5–34: MRI of tibial stress fractures. White areas in T2 (A) and T1 (B) coronal images indicate stress fracture in bone.

Box 5–1 Female Athlete Triad

Amenorrhea
Anorexia
Osteoporosis

- All of these factors coupled with intense high-impact athletic activities create a situation in which calories and nutrients are not sufficient to keep up with the body's high energy requirements and mechanical demands.
- This leads to amenorrhea and osteoporosis, stress fractures or both.

Foot Injuries

General Principles

- Most foot fractures in children can be treated nonoperatively, and they have received relatively little attention in the orthopaedic literature.
- There are a large number of normal variations in the appearance of a child's foot. Familiarity with these is needed to avoid confusing a normal variant for a traumatic injury.
- In addition, the child's foot remains relatively unossified for a long period, making diagnosis of fractures on plane radiographs difficult.

Specific Fractures of the Foot

Fractures of the Talus

- Fractures of the talus are rare in children.
- Like adults, fractures of the talus can result in significant complications such as post-traumatic arthrosis and AVN because the talus has three articular surfaces and has a tenuous blood supply.
- Most fractures through the talus occur through the neck of the talus, and frequently these are only minimally angulated. Angulation less than 30 degrees can generally be accepted. Patients with angulation greater than 30 degrees should be treated with a closed or open reduction as needed, followed by long leg cast for 4 weeks.
- Long-term follow-up is recommended to detect any AVN that may occur.
- Older children and adolescents tend to have fracture patterns more in line with those seen in adults.
  - Displaced fractures in these age groups require open reduction and internal fixation as treatment.
  - Again, long-term follow-up is needed to carefully search for AVN subsequent to this injury.
- Fractures of the lateral process of the talus may occur in conjunction with a twisting ankle injury.
- Lateral process fractures seem particularly prevalent in snowboarders, and these injuries frequently require a CT scan for diagnosis.[28]
- Large displaced fractures should be treated by open reduction and internal fixation; small displaced fractures can be excised.[28]
- AVN following talus fractures occurs in children with a reported incidence in nondisplaced fractures as high as 29%.[29]
- After treatment for a talar neck fracture, radiographs should be observed for Hawkins sign or a radiolucent line beneath the dome of the talus.
  - This shows resorption of the subchondral bone beneath the talar dome, indicating an intact blood supply to the body of the talus, and carries a favorable prognosis regarding the development of AVN.[29]
  - If AVN does occur, treatment should be with long-term relief from bearing weight, typically with a patellar-tendon–bearing, molded-ankle foot orthosis with an articulating ankle.

Fractures of the Calcaneus

- Fractures of the calcaneus are less common in children than in adults.[30]
- Although most calcaneal fractures in children are isolated injuries, associated injuries, including spinal fractures, have been reported up to 1/3 of the time. A careful evaluation for associated injuries needs to be done in children with calcaneal fractures.[24]
- Treatment of calcaneal fractures varies with fracture extension and displacement.
- Nondisplaced or minimally displaced fractures can be treated with above-knee casts and non–weight-bearing status for 4-6 weeks.
- Displaced fractures should be treated with closed or open reduction as needed to restore the articular surface of the subtalar joint. Displaced fractures in adolescents are best treated as in adults, with open reduction and internal fixation.
- Most calcaneal fractures are accompanied by a large degree of soft tissue swelling, and this should be controlled before definitive treatment is initiated.

Fractures of the Midfoot

- Fractures of the navicular and cuboid also occur in children.
- Navicular fractures commonly are avulsion fractures that represent injury to the dorsal tarsal ligament.
  - These can be successfully treated with cast immobilization. Occult fractures of the cuboid and navicular may also occur and can be diagnosed with a Tc-99m bone scan.
  - CT may also be useful in evaluating these injuries because the fractures patterns may not be readily visible on standard radiographs.
- Displaced fractures may need surgical reduction and stabilization for treatment.
- Tarsometatarsal fractures (Lisfranc fractures) may occur in children.[31]

- They are best diagnosed by a combination of AP, lateral, and oblique radiographs and physical examination showing swelling and tenderness over the tarsometatarsal region.
- MRI may aid in the diagnosis.
- Treatment for these injuries consists of closed reduction for displaced injuries (with percutaneous pinning if unstable) without bearing weight in a short leg cast.

Fractures of the Metatarsals

- Metatarsal fractures account for most fractures in children.
  - They usually result from direct injury and most commonly involve the second metatarsal.
  - Most metatarsal fractures can be treated by closed methods with below-knee casts.
  - Displaced fractures may require closed or open reduction and internal fixation. Percutaneous, smooth Kirschner wires generally provide sufficient internal fixation for these injuries.
  - Multiple fractures and displaced fractures at the metatarsal base may be accompanied by large amounts of swelling.
- A high index for compartment syndrome of the foot must be maintained in these situations, and compartment pressures must be measured if indicated.
- The pressures in the central and intraosseous compartments of the foot should be measured because they are the most sensitive compartments showing increased pressure in a foot compartment syndrome.[32]
- Treatment for compartment syndrome of the foot is the complete release of all compartments in the foot followed by secondary closure or skin grafting.[32]

Fractures of the Phalanges

- Phalangeal fractures also commonly occur in children.
  - They can frequently be managed symptomatically with buddy taping and a hard-soled shoe.
  - Open phalangeal fractures may require irrigation, debridement, and stabilization. Smooth Kirschner wires may be needed for unstable injuries.
- Stubbed-toe injuries of the great toe, with bleeding from the nail margin, may indicate an occult open fracture of the physis of the distal phalanx of the great toe. This may result in osteomyelitis, so prophylactic antibiotics are recommended after this injury.

Special Considerations

Child Abuse

- Fractures are the second most common finding in child abuse.
- Soft tissue injuries are the most common.
- Of abused children, 25 to 50% with physical examination findings have fractures.
- Distinguishing child abuse from accidental trauma can be challenging.
- A high index for suspicion is necessary to make the diagnosis.
- Typically, the injuries are not witnessed and the descriptions by the parents and caregivers are vague.
- In addition, distinguishing child abuse from OI can be difficult.
- An abused child may have soft tissue injuries in various stages of healing, failure to thrive, and emotional problems because of deprivation and fear.
- Physical examination findings because of the fracture will vary with location and severity.
- Most tibia fractures in abused children are diaphyseal and transverse, not metaphyseal and spiral.
- A skeletal survey may be necessary to assess previous healing fractures and any evidence of subperiosteal new bone formation caused by blunt trauma.
- Closed reduction and immobilization are usually sufficient for most tibia fractures.
- Of paramount importance is identification of child abuse and prompt and appropriate intervention by a child abuse team. Additional red flags include a delay in seeking prompt medical attention or a history incompatible with injury (Box 5–2).
- In a study by Thomas et al., 22% of children younger than 5 years and 39% of children younger than 1 year at the time of fracture had been victims of child abuse.[33]

Multiple Trauma

- Operative treatment is favored in any child with multiple injuries.
- Uncontrolled spasms and emerging spasticity in the head of an injured child often worsen fracture alignment.
- Inadvertent manipulation of the unstable fracture causes pain that increases intracranial pressure and is undesirable.
- The goal of operative treatment is to stabilize the fracture and counteract the deforming muscle forces.
- Although there are many options for treatment, such as elastic intramedullary nails, percutaneous plating, and

Box 5–2 Child Abuse Red Flags

- Femur fractures in children less than walking age
- Delay in seeking prompt medical attention
- Metaphyseal corner fractures
- Rib fractures, multiple injuries, or both in different stages of healing

From Thomas SA, Rosenfield NS, et al. (1991) Long-bone fractures in young children: Distinguishing accidental injuries from child abuse. Pediatrics 88(3): 471-476. Also from Staheli LT (1984) Fractures of the shaft of the femur. In: Fractures in Children. (Rockwood C, Wilkins K, King R, eds). Philadelphia: JB Lippincott.

external fixation, the latter is favored for several reasons. It is minimally invasive and can be quickly applied with little blood loss or operative time.
- Furthermore, approximately 85% of head-injured children recover functional capabilities that allow ambulation; therefore, achieving an acceptable fracture alignment is necessary to minimize long-term functional deficit from a misaligned or foreshortened fracture.

Open Fractures

- All open or compound injuries require that the bone and wound be cleansed to minimize infection and osteomyelitis.
- Operative stabilization is usually done with an external fixator that allows access to the wound for frequent examination and dressing change.
- Fracture stability also enhances both bone and soft tissue wound healing.

Floating Knee

- Ipsilateral fractures of the femur and tibia are defined as a *floating knee* (Figure 5–35).
- These are high-energy injuries.
- Operative stabilization of the femur and often of both bones yields the best results.
- Length of hospitalization, time until unsupported ability to bear weight, and complications (excessive limb shortening and rotatory malunion) are lower with rigid internal fixation of both bones.[34]

Complications

Leg Length Inequality and Angular Deformity

- Limb length inequality is caused by either overgrowth or excessive shortening of the injured leg.

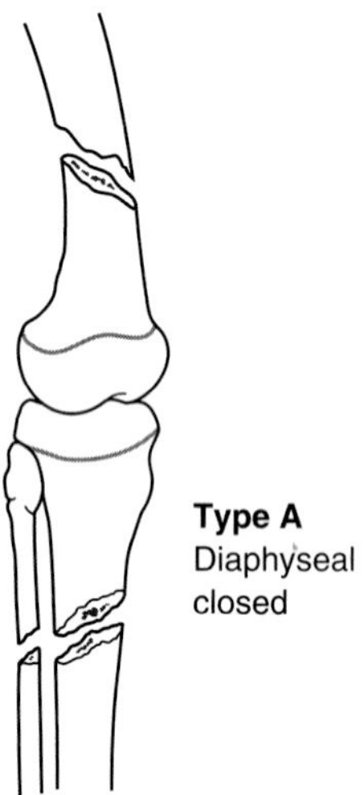

Figure 5–35: Floating knee fracture of the femur and ipsilateral tibia. **From Campbell W (1987) Operative Orthopaedics. St. Louis: CV St. Louis: Mosby, p 1196.**

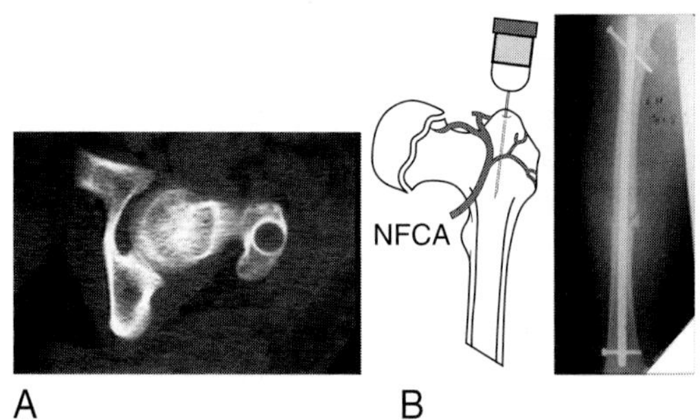

Figure 5–36: **A, Trochanteric femoral entry point for intramedullary femoral rodding. B, Guidewire placement to avoid iatrogenic AVN secondary to arterial injury in femoral rodding procedures. C, Intramedullary rod. From Townsend DR, Hoffinger S (2000) Intramedullary nailing of femoral shaft fractures in children via the trochanter tip. Clin Orthop, 376: 113-118, Figures 3 (A) and 2 (B).**

- At skeletal maturity, 2 cm of discrepancy is well tolerated.
- Greater limb discrepancies can be equalized with either involved or uninvolved limb shortening or lengthening procedures.

Avascular Necrosis

- AVN of femoral head is a serious complication that results from damage to blood supply to the proximal femur.
- It is generally an iatrogenic event secondary to antegrade intramedullary nail insertion (Figure 5–36) with additional injury to the peritrochanteric blood vessels in the piriformis fossa.
- This complication can be avoided by choosing alternate techniques such as placement through the greater trochanter, retrograde nailing, plating, or external fixator application.

References

1. Canale ST, Bourland WL (1977) Fracture of the neck and intertrochanteric region of the femur in children. J Bone Joint Surg Am 59(4): 431-443.

   Evaluations after an average follow-up of 17 years are reported in 61 cases (60 patients). The use of Knowles-pin fixation appeared to reduce the complications of nonunion and coxa vara when compared to complications in previously reported series. AVN caused most of the poor results. However, younger children with AVN obtained better results than older ones.

2. Flynn JM, Wong KL, Yeh GL, Meyer JS, Davidson RS (2002) Displaced fractures of the hip in children: Management by early operation and immobilization in a hip spica cast. J Bone Joint Surg Br 84(1): 108-112.

   The authors treated displaced fractures using early anatomical reduction, internal fixation, and immobilization in a spica cast to try to reduce these complications. They reviewed 18 patients under 16 who had a displaced nonpathological fracture of the hip. The authors' treatment of displaced hip fractures in children using early reduction, internal fixation, and immobilization in a spica cast gave reduced rates of complications compared with those of a large published series in the literature.

3. Chung SM (1976) The arterial supply of the developing proximal end of the human femur. J Bone Joint Surg Am 58(7): 961-970.
   The authors used perfusion studies to review 150 specimens from autopsied fetuses to analyze the arterial supply to the proximal end of the femur. The authors demonstrated that the epiphyseal plate constituted an absolute barrier to blood flow between the epiphysis and the metaphysis in all but 2 of the 124 barium sulphate-perfused specimens examined. This finding may be important for the etiology of Legg-Perthes disease.

4. Hughes LO, Beaty JH (1994) Fractures of the head and neck of the femur in children. J Bone Joint Surg Am 76(2): 283-292.

5. Judet R, Judet J, Letournel E (1964) Fractures of the acetabulum: Classification and surgical approaches for open reduction—Preliminary report. J Bone Joint Surg Am 46: 1615-1646.

6. Metzmaker JN, Pappas AM (1985) Avulsion fractures of the pelvis. Am J Sports Med 13(5): 349-358.

7. Hamilton PR, Broughton NS (1998) Traumatic hip dislocation in childhood. J Pediatr Orthop 18(5): 691-694.
   The authors reviewed 18 cases of traumatic dislocations of the hip in children under 15 years between 1985 and 1995. All but two patients were treated by closed reduction. On long-term follow-up of the 16 available patients (average length of follow-up was 5 years and 10 months with a range 17-132), there were no cases of AVN or early degenerative change.

8. Gray D (2002) Trauma to the hip and femur in children. Orthop Know Update 2: 81-91.

9. Lynch JM, Gardner MJ, Gains B (1996) Hemodynamic significance of pediatric femur fractures. J Pediatr Surg 31(10): 1358-1361.
   The author retrospectively reviewed 178 patients (182 femur fractures) to determine incidence of hemodynamic bleeding. Patients with multisystem injury and patients with femur fractures were included. Mean age of patients was 6.04 years (range of 1 month to 19 years).
   Hemodynamic instability or evidence of a declining hematocrit in the child should not be attributed to a closed femur fracture; other sources of blood loss must be found.

10. Wright JG (2000) The treatment of femoral shaft fractures in children: a systematic overview and critical appraisal of the literature. Can J Surg 43(3): 180-189.
    OBJECTIVE: The authors reviewed existing literature to determine whether a certain method of treatment was preferential to another for treatment of pediatric femoral shaft fractures. CONCLUSION: Early application of a hip spica cast had lower costs and malunion rates than traction.

11. Infante AF Jr, Albert MC, Jennings WB, Lehner JT (2000) Immediate hip spica casting for femur fractures in pediatric patients: A review of 175 patients. Clin Orthop (376): 106-112.
    Between 1988 and 1996, 190 immediate hip spica casts were placed on children with isolated femoral shaft fractures who weighed between 10 and 100 lb. The authors think that immediate closed reduction and placement of a well-molded hip spica cast is a safe and reliable treatment option for isolated, closed femur fractures in children from birth to 10 years who weigh less than 80 lb.

12. Skak SV, Jensen TT, Poulsen TD, Sturup J (1987) Epidemiology of knee injuries in children. Acta Orthop Scand 58(1): 78-81.
    The authors analyzed 91 consecutive metaphyseal fractures, physeal injuries, and ligament ruptures in children from 0 to 14 years. In the younger children, metaphyseal fractures dominated, whereas teenagers had ligament rupture associated with low-energy trauma and physeal injury with high-energy trauma.

13. Smith JB (1984) Knee instability after fractures of the intercondylar eminence of the tibia. J Pediatr Orthop 4(4): 462-464.
    The author reviewed 15 children with fracture of the intercondylar eminence of the tibia for a mean follow-up of 7 years. The authors conclude that the ACL probably stretches before its tibial attachment fractures. Even though the fracture heals in its normal position, mild degrees of ACL laxity often will result.

14. Lowe J, Chaimsky G, Freedman A, Zion I, Howard C (2002) The anatomy of tibial eminence fractures: arthroscopic observations following failed closed reduction. J Bone Joint Surg Am 84-A(11): 1933-1938.
    The author reviewed twelve patients who had had a failed manipulative reduction of a type III tibial eminence fracture who underwent arthroscopic reduction and fixation of the avulsed fragment. The authors concluded that the concept that avulsion fractures of the tibial insertion of the ACL cannot be reduced by manipulation because of soft tissue interposition was not supported by the findings of the study.

15. McLennan JG (1982) The role of arthroscopic surgery in the treatment of fractures of the intercondylar eminence of the tibia. J Bone Joint Surg Br 64(4): 477-480.
    35 patients with Type III fractures were followed for 2–7 years. The authors concluded that arthroscopic reduction and percutaneous pin fixation provided an effective treatment and significantly decreased the time spent in hospital and the morbidity experienced after alternative treatments.

16. Baxter MP, Wiley JJ (1988) Fractures of the tibial spine in children: An evaluation of knee stability. J Bone Joint Surg Br 70(2): 228-230.
    The authors reviewed 45 patients with fractures of the tibial spine 3 to 10 years after injury to determine the degree of residual laxity of the cruciate or collateral ligaments. After fractures that had been partially or completely displaced, some anterior cruciate laxity was evident even if patients were asymptomatic. It was also found that an anatomical

reduction did not prevent laxity or some loss of full extension of the knee.

17. Janarv PM, Westblad P, Johansson C, Hirsch G (1995) Long-term follow-up of anterior tibial spine fractures in children. J Pediatr Orthop 15(1): 63-68.
    In a long-term follow-up (mean 16 years) of 61 children with anterior tibial spine fractures, subjective knee function (Lysholm score) was excellent or good in 87% of the subjects and fair in 13%. Arthroscopy guiding or open reduction and internal fixation seems to be worthwhile procedures only in dislocated type III fractures.

18. Ogden JA, Tross RB, Murphy MJ (1980) Fractures of the tibial tuberosity in adolescents. J Bone Joint Surg Am 62(2): 205-215.

19. Maguire JK, Canale ST (1993) Fractures of the patella in children and adolescents. J Pediatr Orthop 13(5): 567-571.
    Between 1942 and 1987, 66 children with patellar fractures were treated. Overall results were good in 13, fair in 8, and poor in 3. Children with fractures of the ipsilateral femur, tibia, or both and those with comminuted, displaced fractures had the poorest results.

20. Johnston DR, Ganley TJ, Flynn JM, Gregg JR (2002) Anterior cruciate ligament injuries in skeletally immature patients. Orthopedics 25(8): 864-871; quiz 872-873.

21. Jordan SE, Alonso JE, Cook FF (1987) The etiology of valgus angulation after metaphyseal fractures of the tibia in children. J Pediatr Orthop 7(4): 450-457.
    The authors conducted a retrospective study of proximal metaphyseal fractures of the tibia in children who developed valgus deformities. They suggest that the most likely primary mechanism is an increased vascular response causing an asymmetric growth stimulation of the medial metaphysis of the proximal tibia.

22. Zionts LE, Harcke HT, Brooks KM, MacEwen GD (1987) Post-traumatic tibia valga: A case demonstrating asymmetric activity at the proximal growth plate on technetium bone scan. J Pediatr Orthop 7(4): 458-462.
    Post-traumatic tibia valga is a well-recognized complication following fracture of the upper tibial metaphysis in young children. The authors present the case of a child who developed a valgus deformity following fracture of the proximal tibia and fibula. Their findings suggest that the valgus deformity in their patient was caused by a relative increase in vascularity and consequent overgrowth of the medial portion of the proximal tibial physis.

23. McCarthy JJ, Kim DH, Eilert RE (1998) Post-traumatic genu valgum: Operative versus nonoperative treatment. J Pediatr Orthop 18(4): 518-521.
    The authors compared the results of operative and nonoperative treatment for post-traumatic genu valgum. They performed a retrospective chart and radiographic review of all patients diagnosed with post-traumatic genu valgum. In both groups, the valgus deformity improved at follow-up. There was no significant difference in the complementary physeal shaft and tibial femoral angles, between the groups at the time of injury, at maximal deformity, or at follow-up.

24. Schmidt TL, Weiner DS (1982) Calcaneal fractures in children: An evaluation of the nature of the injury in 56 children. Clin Orthop (171): 150-155.
    The authors retrospectively reviewed children with calcaneal fractures. The prognosis for a normally functioning calcaneus without the presence of post-traumatic arthrosis should be expected in most cases because of the nature of the fracture in children.

25. Shannak AO (1988) Tibial fractures in children: Follow-up study. J Pediatr Orthop 8(3): 306-310.
    117 children with tibial shaft fractures were treated by above-knee cast with or without traction depending on stability. All fractures united in an average period of 37 days. The author concluded that shortening can be compensated by growth acceleration and that varus deformities can undergo spontaneous correlation, whereas valgus deformity and posterior angulation partially persist and rotational deformities persist.

26. Navascues JA, Gonzalez-Lopez JL, Lopez-Valverde S, Soleto J, Rodriguez-Durantez JA, Garcia-Trevijano JL (2000) Premature physeal closure after tibial diaphyseal fractures in adolescents. J Pediatr Orthop 20(2): 193-196.
    Seven cases of premature physeal closure secondary to diaphyseal fractures of the tibia in adolescents between 12 and 15 years are presented. At the time of the accidents, there was no evidence of physeal lesion in any of the patients. Adolescents with diaphyseal fractures of the long bones should be monitored until they have stopped growing because of the risk of developing leg length discrepancy as a consequence of premature closure of one or more leg physis.

27. Halsey MF, Finzel KC, Carrion WV, Haralabatos SS, Gruber MA, Meinhard BP (2001) Toddler's fracture: presumptive diagnosis and treatment. J Pediatr Orthop 21(2): 152-156.
    The authors propose the presumptive diagnosis of toddler's fracture, despite negative radiographs, when the history and physical examination are consistent with the diagnosis. To avoid delay in the treatment of toddler's fracture, the authors recommend a long leg cast on those children with a history of an acute injury, the inability to walk or a limp, no constitutional signs, and negative radiographs.

28. Kirkpatrick DP, Hunter RE, Janes PC, Mastrangelo J, Nicholas RA (1998) The snowboarder's foot and ankle. Am J Sports Med 26(2): 271-277.
    The authors undertook a prospective study to determine the type and distribution of foot and ankle snowboarding injuries. Reports of 3213 snowboarding injuries were collected from 12 Colorado ski resorts between 1988 and 1995. There was no significant correlation between boot type (soft, hybrid, or hard) and overall foot or ankle injury rate. Diagnosis of this fracture pattern is paramount; the physician should be suspicious of anterolateral ankle pain in the snowboarder, where subtle fractures that may require surgical intervention can be confused with anterior talofibular ligament sprains.

29. Letts RM, Gibeault D (1980) Fractures of the neck of the talus in children. Foot Ankle 1(2): 74-77.
   A review of children with talar injuries treated at the Winnipeg Children's Hospital yielded 12 patients that had been treated for fractures of the neck of the talus between 1960 and 1978, inclusive. Three developed AVN of the body of the talus; two of these had their fractures recognized only after AVN had become radiologically evident. The children ranged in age from 1 year 7 months to 13 years 11 months at the time of the injury. Fracture of the neck of the talus occurs in children and may be associated with AVN of the body. This injury should be considered and the talus should be examined in all children sustaining trauma secondary to falls from a height or motor vehicle trauma.

30. Matteri RE, Frymoyer JW (1973) Fracture of the calcaneus in young children: Report of three cases. J Bone Joint Surg Am 55(5): 1091-1094.

31. Wiley JJ (1981) Tarsometatarsal joint injuries in children. J Pediatr Orthop 1(3): 255-260.
   Tarsometatarsal joint injuries do occur in the pediatric age group, and the mechanisms and patterns of injury are similar to the adult variety. Surgical reduction is indicated in those cases with obvious displacement. Unstable reductions are best managed by percutaneous pin fixation across the tarsometatarsal joint. The short-term results are generally good despite extensive disruption at the tarsometatarsal joint complex. Only long-range follow-up will reveal the realistic results of these injuries.

32. Silas SI, Herzenberg JE, Myerson MS, Sponseller PD (1995) Compartment syndrome of the foot in children. J Bone Joint Surg Am 77(3): 356-361.
   Seven children and teenagers were identified as having had compartment syndrome of the foot during a 5-year period. The average age at the time of the diagnosis was 10 years (with a range of 4 to 16 years). The cause of the compartment syndrome was a crush injury in six patients and a motor vehicle accident in one. Orthopaedists managing children who have a traumatic injury of the foot, especially a crush injury, should have a high index of suspicion for compartment syndrome, even in the absence of severe fracture.

33. Thomas SA, Rosenfield NS, Leventhal JM, Markowitz RI (1991) Long-bone fractures in young children: Distinguishing accidental injuries from child abuse. Pediatrics 88(3): 471-476.
   Based on medical record reviews, two clinicians and two pediatric radiologists rated the likelihood that a fracture was accidental or caused by child abuse. Long-bone fractures were strongly associated with abuse. This report focuses on the 39 children with either humeral or femoral fractures. Of femur fractions in infants younger than 1 year, 60% were caused by abuse. Although it is taught that femur fractures in young children are inflicted unless proven otherwise, in this study it was found that femur fractures often are accidental and that the femur can be fractured when the running child trips and falls.

34. Yue JJ, Churchill RS, Cooperman DR, Yasko AW, Wilber JH, Thompson GH (2000) The floating knee in the pediatric patient: Nonoperative versus operative stabilization. Clin Orthop (376): 124-136.
   The authors reviewed 29 consecutive patients with open physes (30 affected extremities). Based on the results of the study, operative stabilization of at least the femur fracture and, preferably, both fractures in the treatment of a child with a floating knee is recommended, even for younger children.

35. Anglen J (2002) Percutaneous Plate Fixation of Pediatric Femur Fractures. America Academy of Orthopaedic Surgeons: Rosemont, IL.

36. Staheli LT (1984) Fractures of the shaft of the femur. In: Fractures in Children. (Rockwood C, Wilkins K, King R, eds). Philadelphia: JB Lippincott.

37. Scherl SA, Miller L, Lively N, Russinoff S, Sullivan CM, Tornetta P 3rd (2000) Accidental and nonaccidental femur fractures in children. Clin Orthop (376): 96-105.
   A retrospective review of 207 patients younger than 6 years who sustained nonpathological diaphyseal femur fractures emphasized the characteristics of accidental versus nonaccidental injury. The authors' data show that although spiral fractures were less common than transverse fractures overall, and no more common in the cohort of patients in whom the results of the child abuse investigations were positive, they were overrepresented in the investigated cohort. This suggests that spiral fractures are viewed as particularly suspicious, which may lead to missed cases of nonaccidental injury in children with transverse fractures.

38. Wheeless CR Wheeless' Text book of Orthopaedics. *http://www.wheelessonline.com.*

CHAPTER 6

Spine and Pelvis Trauma

Lee S. Segal

MD, Associate Professor of Orthopaedics and Pediatrics, Chief, Division of Pediatric Orthopaedics, Department of Orthopaedics and Rehabilitation, Milton S. Hershey Medical Center, Pennsylvania State University College of Medicine, Hershey, PA

Introduction

- Trauma remains the leading cause of death and disability in children older than 1 year.
- Fractures and other traumatic injuries of the spine and pelvis in children are uncommon, most often occurring after high-energy trauma such as pedestrian–motor vehicle accidents (MVAs).
- The unique features of the child's spine and pelvis result in different patterns and responses to injury compared with those of adults.
- Treatment considerations must take into account the dynamic elements of growth and remodeling.

Unique Characteristics of the Pediatric Spine

Cervical Spine

- The anatomical and physiological characteristics of the pediatric cervical spine evolve over time, developing adult-like features after 8-10 years of age.
- At birth, the atlas (C1) is composed of three ossification centers, the axis (C2) has four ossification centers, and the lower cervical vertebrae (C3-C7) have three ossification centers. The synchondroses that unite the neural arches to the bodies fuse at different times for each of these vertebrae. Abnormalities in the ossification or development of these centers, and the presence of the synchondrosis before fusion, can easily be mistaken for fractures.[1]
- Children younger than 8 years demonstrate increased range of motion compared with adults. This is partly because of their relative ligamentous laxity, muscle weakness, incomplete ossification of the cervical spine, and horizontal orientation of the facet joints.[2]
- Two distinct groups of cervical spine injuries based upon age, with different patterns and mechanisms of injury, have been identified by McGrory et al.[3] (Box 6–1).

Thoracolumbar Spine

- Because of the well-hydrated intervertebral disks in children, the high energy sustained during spinal trauma can be dissipated over several levels and can result in injury to several contiguous and noncontiguous levels.[2]
- The increased elasticity of the ligamentous complex of the spinal column in response to high-energy trauma may result in traumatic spinal cord injury without radiographic abnormality (SCIWORA).[4] This occurs when a force applied to the flexible spine exceeds the tensile limits of the relatively inelastic spinal cord. Stretching of the spinal cord will occur under these conditions and result in a distraction or an ischemic injury to the spinal cord. No obvious fracture is identified on radiographs or computerized tomography (CT) scans. SCIWORA is associated with complete and incomplete lesions, is more common in younger children, and may be associated with a delayed presentation.[1,4]
- The presence of the ring apophysis contributes to the developing contour and width of the vertebral body during growth. Under certain single or repetitive axial loads, the apophysis can slip or separate into the spinal

Box 6–1 Patterns of Cervical Spine Injuries Based upon Age

1. In children younger than 11 years, injuries to the upper cervical spine (occiput to C3) predominate. These younger children have relatively horizontal facet joints, which offer little resistance to shear forces from trauma. The fulcrum of motion in the sagittal plane is closer in this age group at the C3-C4 level. With their disproportionately larger head size and ligamentous laxity, traumatic injuries to the upper cervical spine are common. These injuries tend to occur more often from falls, and the mortality rate is higher in this younger age group.
2. After the age of 10, the anatomy of the cervical spine develops adult-like characteristics; the injuries sustained by the older age group (11-15 years) are similar to adult fracture patterns of the cervical spine. The subaxial or lower cervical spine (C3-C7) has a greater rate of involvement, often occurring with sports or recreational activities, and carries a higher risk of permanent spinal cord injury.

From McGrory BJ, Klassen RA, Chao EY, Staeheli JW, Weaver AL (1993) Acute fractures and dislocations of the cervical spine in children and adolescents. J Bone Joint Surg 75A: 988-995.

canal and mimic the clinical findings of a herniated intervertebral disk.

Mechanisms of Pediatric Spine Injury

- Different mechanisms of injury predispose children to spinal trauma depending upon their age at the time of injury. Infants and toddlers are prone to spinal trauma after falls and MVAs. Adolescents sustain traumatic spinal injuries following sports and recreational activities such as diving.[3] Specific causes of spinal trauma are unique to children. These include child abuse, birth trauma, and the use of passive seat belt restraint systems.
- Several reports in the literature have increased awareness that spine trauma can occur as part of the spectrum of injuries in the battered child syndrome. In children, 3% of all spine fractures are the direct result of child abuse, and the average age of a child with a spine fracture because of child abuse was 22 months. Many of these spine injuries are not recognized initially because of the lack of neurological involvement and the absence of gross deformity. Most of these injuries occur at the thoracolumbar junction, and the presence of multiple spinous process fractures or multiple compression fractures on radiographs should raise the index of suspicion for child abuse. In suspected cases, a lateral radiograph of the thoracolumbar spine should be part of the routine skeletal survey.
- Trauma to the spine or spinal cord should be suspected in neonates after a difficult or traumatic delivery and unexplained hypotonia or delay in development. In the evaluation of the "floppy infant," consider magnetic resonance imaging (MRI) or somatosensory-evoked potentials. Injury to the upper cervical spine may occur in cephalic presentations and injury to the lower cervical spine and thoracic spine may follow breech deliveries.[2]
- The mandatory use of seat belt restraint systems has increased the incidence of flexion–distraction or Chance fractures of the lumbar spine in children. The unique characteristics of the child's small pelvis, higher center of gravity, and typical slouched posture prevents the normal or intended positioning of the lap belt across the pelvis.[5] At the time of frontal impact, the properly positioned lap belt is intended to dissipate the deceleration forces through the pelvis and the hips. Children tend to slide under the seat belt, and the lap belt improperly rides up to the level of the midlumbar spine. The lap belt then acts as an anterior fulcrum that generates the flexion–distraction mechanism of injury (Figure 6–1). In addition to the spinal injury, there may be associated injury to the spinal cord resulting in paraplegia and life-threatening visceral injury.[5,6]

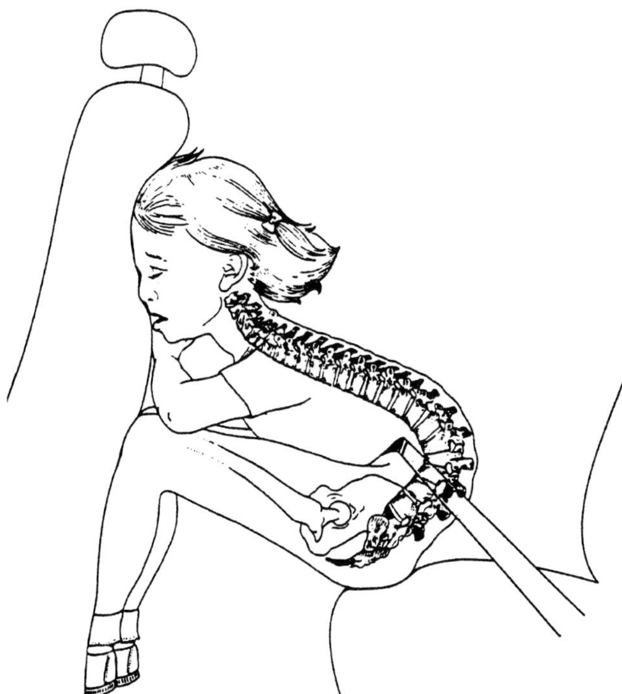

Figure 6–1: Lap belt injury in a child at impact. The lap belt rides up over iliac crests to create a bending moment at the midlumbar region and generate a flexion–distraction injury. From Johnson DL, Falci S (1990) The diagnosis and treatment of pediatric lumbar spine injuries caused by rear seat lap belts. Neurosurg 26(1): 438.

- Hoy and Cole[7] described the pediatric cervical seat belt syndrome in seven children wearing either three-point or four-point restraint systems. A range of injuries was noted in these children, including fractures and fractures–dislocations of the upper and lower cervical spine, spinal cord injuries, head injuries, and laryngeal fractures. Flexion of the neck over the poorly fitting sash in the three-point restraints riding up across the neck, and hyperflexion injuries in the properly fitting four-point systems produced by the deceleration forces on the disproportionately large head, were thought to be the mechanisms of injury with this syndrome.

Physical Examination

- Infants or children with suspected spine injuries should be properly immobilized to prevent motion that could cause injury to the spinal cord or other injuries. Children with a history of high-energy trauma such as a motor vehicle-related injury or a fall, loss of consciousness or altered mental status, complaints of neck pain or guarding, or associated head or facial trauma should be immobilized in a rigid cervical collar with sandbags on each side. Careful logrolling and other spinal precautions should be maintained until appropriate screening radiographs can be obtained.
- The disproportionate head size in young children during transport or immobilization on an adult backboard forces the neck into an undesirable position of flexion and anterior translation of the upper cervical spine. Modifications to the backboard have been recommended for children younger than 6 years to stabilize the child's cervical spine into a relatively neutral position. These include lowering the child's head with an occipital recess or raising the chest on a mattress pad such that the occiput is 1 to 2 inches below the level of the back.[8]
- The clinical examination of a child with a suspected spine injury can be extremely difficult. Often the child is quite young, frightened, and unable to communicate the location of pain.
- The physical examination must closely evaluate the upper cervical spine in young children because of their increased risk of injury to this area. Any signs of facial or head trauma demand careful evaluation of the upper cervical spine.
- Muscle spasm about the paraspinal or sternocleidomastoid muscles may be present. Torticollis may be an initial physical sign of C1-C2 rotary instability. There may be tenderness about the posterior neck along the interspinous process ligaments or along the thoracolumbar spine.
- Evaluation of the skin for any cutaneous signs such as abrasions or bruising is important. The presence of a band-like pattern of ecchymosis about the abdomen or iliac crest is described as a "seat belt" sign and may indicate an underlying lumbar spine fracture and associated visceral injuries (Figure 6–2).
- A thorough neurological examination should be performed to evaluate motor strength, sensation, reflexes, and proprioception. A rectal examination to evaluate for the bulbocavernosus reflex should be done in children with suspected acute spinal cord injury to determine when the period of spinal shock is over.

Radiologic Examination

- After appropriate immobilization of the cervical spine, radiographs of the cervical spine as part of the trauma series are obtained in the pediatric trauma patient. Other radiographs, including the thoracolumbar spine, should be taken as clinically determined. Anteroposterior (AP), lateral, and open-mouth views of the odontoid comprise the trauma series.
- It is mandatory that the C7-T1 junction be viewed on the lateral radiograph. If the cervicothoracic junction cannot be seen, additional views such as a Swimmer's view or a CT scan should be acquired.
- Like the physical examination, the radiographic assessment of a child's spine can be difficult. The plain radiographs alone can miss up to 50% of cervical spine injuries.[2]
- Unique characteristics of the pediatric cervical spine such as incomplete ossification and increased motion of the spine contribute to the variability of radiographic findings in the pediatric spine that can easily be mistaken for traumatic injuries of the spine[9] (Box 6–2).
- All of these normal radiographic variables must be interpreted with the physical examination findings. Rapid resolution of symptoms with the return of a full range of motion in a child is suggestive of a normal variant. On the other hand, continuous muscle spasm, limited range

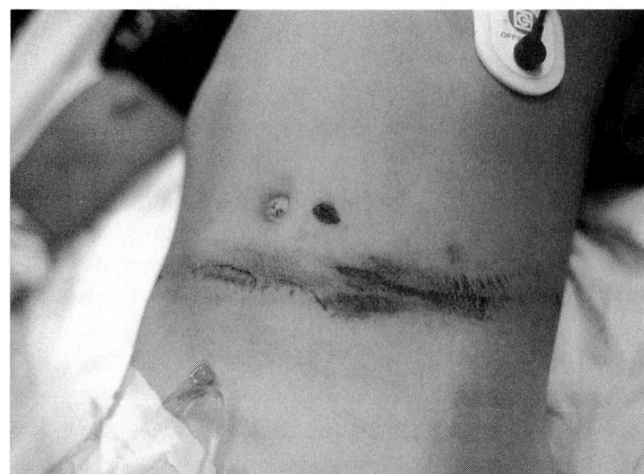

Figure 6–2: Lap belt sign in a child sustaining a Chance fracture of the lumbar spine. **A transverse band of contusion and ecchymosis caused by the lap belt.**

Box 6–2 Unique Characteristics of the Pediatric Cervical Spine

- Anterior angulation of the odontoid process (4%)
- Overriding anterior arch of C1 on the odontoid (20%)
- C1-C2 ADI up to 4-4.5 mm in normal children
- Decreased cervical lordosis (14%)
- C2-C3 and C3-C4 pseudosubluxation possibly misinterpreted for instability (20% in children up to 7 years)
- Basilar synchondrosis of C2 possibly mistaken for an odontoid fracture
- Tip of odontoid (ossiculum terminale) possibly confused with a fracture
- Neurocentral synchondroses and multiple ossification centers of C1 that may mimic fracture appearance
- Rounding of anterior vertebral bodies that may mimic compression fractures
- Secondary centers of spinous processes possibly mistaken for avulsion fractures
- SCIWORA (at both cervical and thoracolumbar [TL] levels)

of motion, or tenderness in a child warrants further investigation with other imaging studies.[9]

- Evaluation of the lateral radiographs should initially focus on the four lines that correspond to the anterior and posterior vertebral bodies, the spinolaminar line, and the tips of the spinous processes from the C1 through C7 vertebral bodies.[9] Each of these four lines should have a smooth contour (Figure 6–3).
- Because of the importance of the upper cervical spine in young children, increased attention should be directed at the C1-C2 level. In children younger than 8 years, the atlantodens interval (ADI), which is the space between the anterior arch of C1 and the anterior border of the odontoid, should not be greater than 4 mm. If these views are normal, then flexion–extension radiographs under physician guidance should be obtained if the child is alert and cooperative.

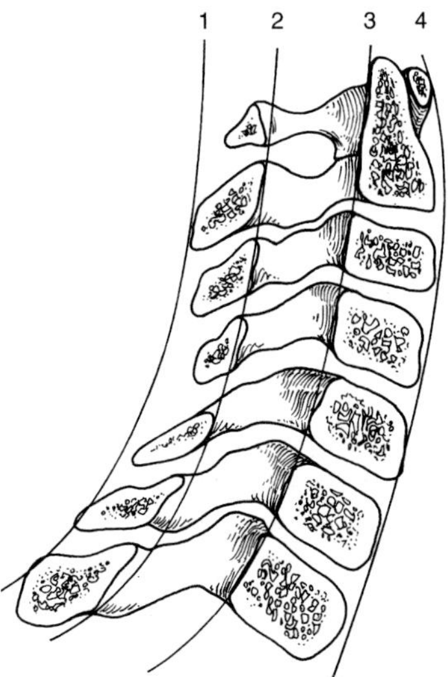

Figure 6–3: Four lines of the normal lateral cervical spine: 1, spinous processes; 2, spinolaminar line; 3, posterior vertebral body line; 4, anterior vertebral body line. From Copley LA, Dormans JP (1998) Cervical spine disorders in infants and children. J Am Acad Orthop Surg 6(4): 207.

- Soft tissue swelling should be evaluated on the lateral radiograph. Caution must be exercised in the interpretation of these studies in a crying child. The retropharyngeal space should be less than 7 mm and the retrotracheal space should be less than 14 mm in children[9]; these may be increased in a crying child.
- Indications for additional imaging studies in pediatric cervical spine trauma are described in Box 6–3.

Cervical Spine Injuries

Occiput-C1 Dislocations

- An Occiput-C1 dislocation is a rare injury frequently associated with severe head trauma and other injuries. This is often a fatal injury, but some children now survive this catastrophic injury as a result of rapid response and resuscitation in the field.
- Many of these children will be quadriplegic and require ventilator support, having complete spinal cord injuries below the level of the brainstem.
- Radiographs may miss this injury if the dislocation spontaneously reduces. Several radiographic parameters can be used to evaluate this injury. One of these is the Power's ratio, suggestive of possible dislocation at this level when the ratio is greater than 1:1.[9]
- MRI and CT are beneficial in confirming the injury. Early treatment by halo immobilization either alone or with posterior spine fusion (occiput to C3), by iliac crest or autogenous rib bone grafts, and by internal fixation (depending upon age) is recommended to mobilize these children into an upright position and to promote pulmonary care.

Atlas Fractures

- This is a rare injury in children caused by axial loads, and the specific pattern of the injury depends on the position of the head at impact. Disruptions of both the anterior and the posterior rings of the atlas, also known as Jefferson fractures, occur as the occipital condyles are forced into the lateral masses of C1.

Box 6–3 Indications for Additional Imaging in Pediatric Cervical Spine Trauma

1. Additional imaging may be necessary for children whose radiographs are equivocal and whose mechanism of injury and physical findings are highly suspicious for an underlying spine or spinal cord injury. An uncooperative child or an unconscious, intubated child requiring cervical spine clearance would also warrant other studies such as CT or MRI.[9]
2. CT scans can be helpful in delineating injuries such as fractures poorly appreciated on plain radiographs and may be confused with normal variants of the pediatric spine. Be aware that CT scans may miss a fracture if the orientation of the CT scan is in the same plane as a fracture. Three-dimensional CT scan reconstruction images have improved clinicians' abilities to evaluate difficult injuries of the pediatric cervical spine.
3. Dynamic CT scans should be considered in the child who has a painful torticollis and suspected atlantoaxial rotary instability.[11] CT scans are essential in the assessment of thoracolumbar spine fractures to determine the extent of an osseous injury such as canal compromise in burst fractures, the presence of an unrecognized posterior lamina or facet fracture, and the relative stability of a fracture pattern that may influence treatment decisions.
4. MRI is the imaging study of choice in children with a spine fracture and an associated neurological deficit. It is also warranted in a child with suspected SCIWORA to evaluate the location and extent of spinal cord injury. Advancements in the techniques of MRI have refined the evaluation of injuries to the spinal cord, the ligaments and other soft tissues, the intervertebral disks, and the cartilaginous or unossified pediatric spine. Most level I pediatric trauma centers routinely use MRI for clearance of the cervical spine in an intubated, unconscious child.[23] MRI also has an important role in the assessment of thoracolumbar fractures to accurately determine fracture pattern, fracture stability, and the degree of acute spinal cord injury if present.

- The presence of a persistent synchondrosis may result in only a single break in the rings in children.
- The incidence of spinal cord injury and nonunion of atlas fractures is extremely low. Rupture of the transverse atlantal ligament can be associated with this fracture pattern as the lateral masses are driven apart, which may subsequently result in atlantoaxial instability.
- CT scans best define the specific fracture patterns of the atlas (Figure 6–4).
- The recommended treatment for atlas fractures is either Minerva cast or halo vest immobilization.

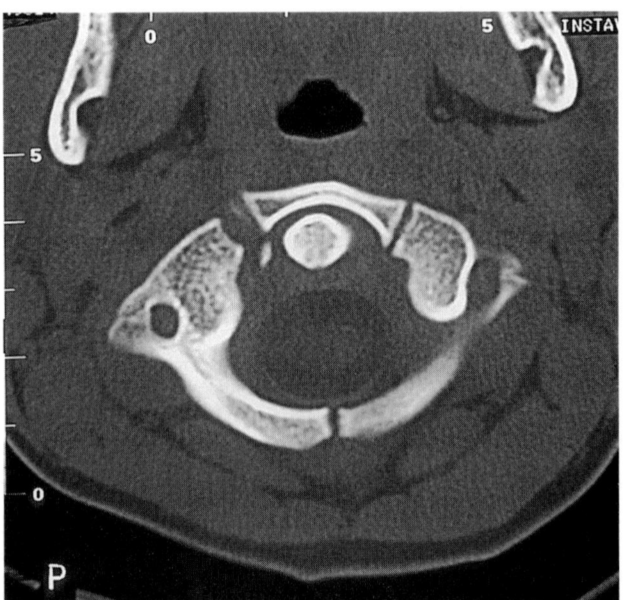

Figure 6–4: CT scan of an atlas fracture in a 5-year-old child. Note the "single break" in the posterior ring of C1 with the synchondrosis present.

Odontoid Fractures

- Often associated with head or facial trauma, odontoid fractures occur at an average age of 3 to 4 years (Figure 6–5). Most injuries occurred in an MVA.
- In children, odontoid fractures most often occur at the base within the body of the C2 vertebra and below the level of the facet joints. Normal variants of the cervical spine, as previously mentioned, can be mistaken for fractures of the odontoid process.
- These injuries are usually Salter-Harris type I physeal fractures through the synchondrosis.
- The risk of neurological injury is thought to be low with this injury.
- Displaced fractures are easily reduced in extension and posterior translation then immobilized with a Minerva cast or halo vest. An intact periosteal hinge at the base of the odontoid stabilizes the fracture and facilitates reduction.[2]
- Because of their location within the body of C2 and because they are physeal-type fractures, odontoid fractures typically heal rapidly, within 6-8 weeks, and have a low nonunion rate.
- Controversy exists about whether the cause of this entity is developmental or traumatic. Failure to identify and properly immobilize an odontoid fracture in children may be responsible for the development of an os odontoideum (Figure 6–6). With an os odontoideum, the fracture line is usually proximal to the body of C2. These may be asymptomatic or may result in neck pain or neurological symptoms. Posterior C1-C2 arthrodesis is indicated if instability is present radiographically.

C2 Spondylolisthesis

- These uncommon injuries are believed to result from hyperextension injuries. Also known as hangman's fractures,

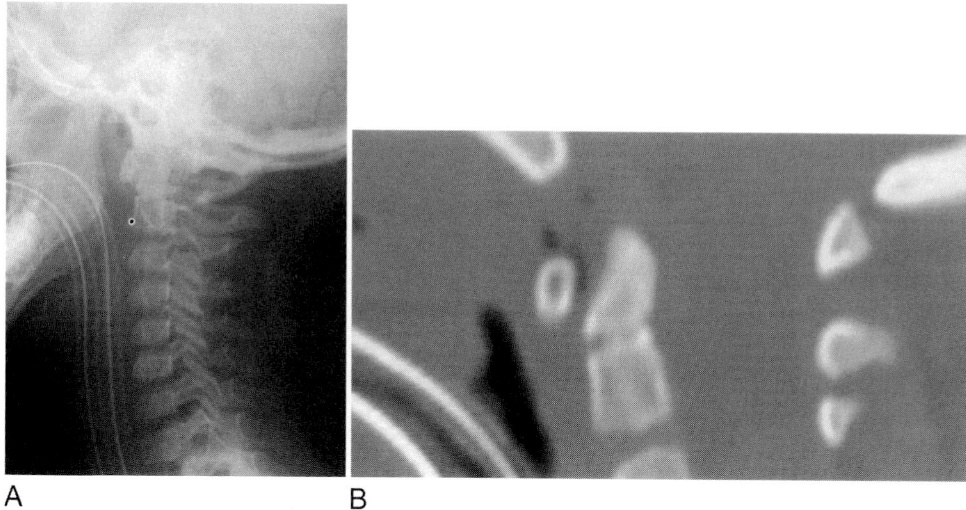

Figure 6–5: Odontoid fracture in a 4-year-old child. Concomitant closed head injury and occipital condyle fracture were also sustained in an MVA. A, Lateral cervical spine radiograph upon admission. B, CT scan of the cervical spine demonstrating angulation of the odontoid fracture. The child was treated in a Minerva brace.

they tend to be minimally displaced and will heal with cast or halo vest immobilization (Figure 6–7).

- Operative indications are only for delayed union with instability or for nonunion.

Atlantoaxial Instability

- Atlantoaxial instability may occur after a traumatic event, although it is more commonly seen in chronic progressive conditions such as in children with Down's syndrome, skeletal dysplasias, and juvenile rheumatoid arthritis.
- After obtaining a history of trauma, radiographs in flexion demonstrating an ADI greater than 5 mm are suggestive of C1-C2 instability. The ADI is measured from the anterior cortex of the dens to the posterior cortex of the anterior ring of C1.

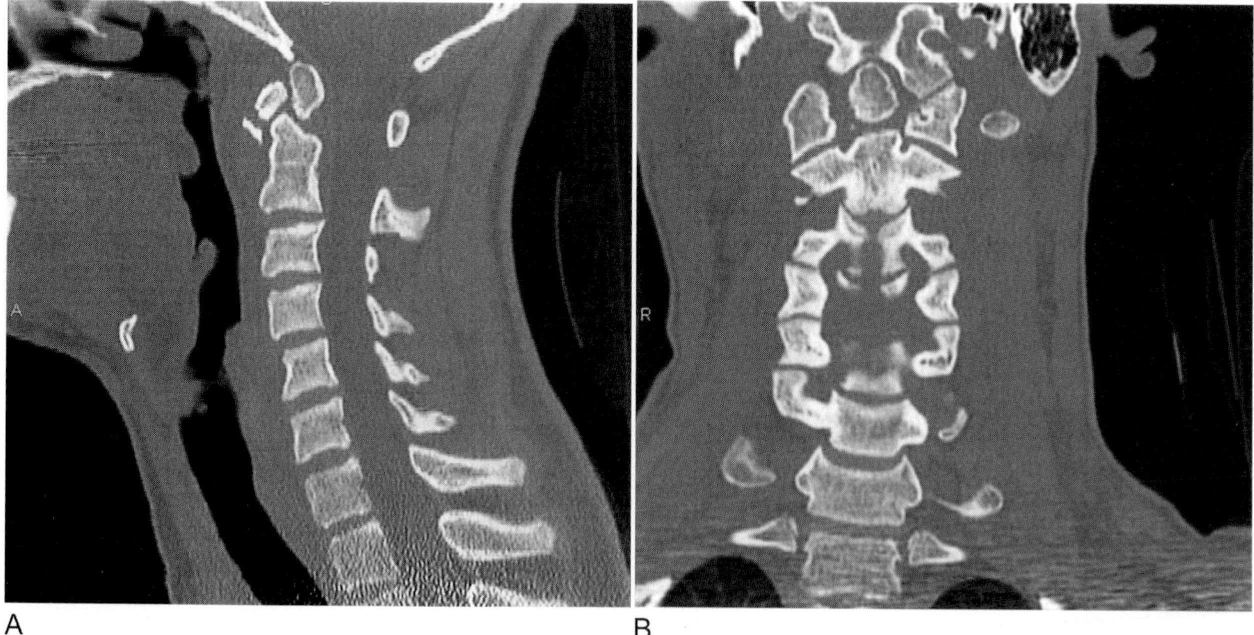

Figure 6–6: Os odontoideum in a 15 year old. At age 2, the patient fell off a bunk bed and wore a cervical collar for 1 month for neck pain. Radiographs were not obtained. The patient has an identical twin brother without radiographic evidence of an os odontoideum, supporting a traumatic cause. Sagittal reconstruction of osodontoideum (A) and AP reconstruction of osodontoideum (B) CT reconstruction images.

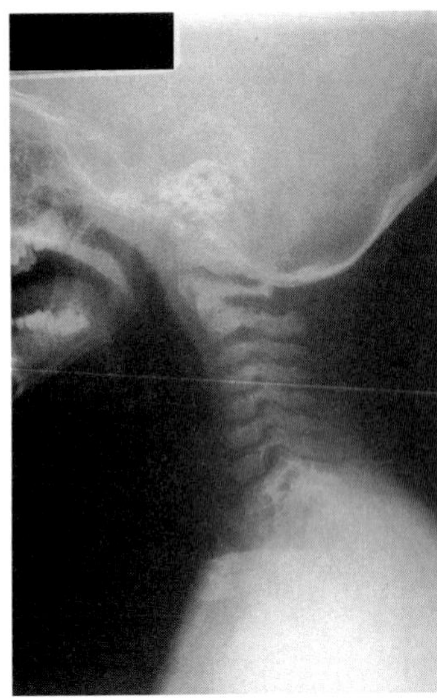

Figure 6–7: C2 fracture (Hangman's fracture) in a 2-year-old child.

- Atlantoaxial instability may occur after atlas fractures with disruption of the transverse atlantal ligament or with odontoid fractures.
- For acute injuries, recommended treatment is reduction in extension followed by C1-C2 posterior arthrodesis with halo brace or Minerva cast immobilization for 2-3 months.[1,2]

Atlantoaxial Rotary Instability

- An atlantoaxial rotary instability (AARI) patient has torticollis, pain, and limited range of motion of the neck. Although this condition can occur following trauma, it is more commonly seen after upper respiratory infections; ear, nose, and throat surgery; or other inflammatory conditions. There is often a delay in diagnosis. When the deformity persists, it results in resistant torticollis described as fixed AARI.
- Rarely, an associated clavicle fracture following a traumatic event can be seen with AARI.
- Four types of subluxation of increasing severity have been described (Table 6–1) depending on the degree and direction of displacement and reflecting the integrity of the C1-C2 ligaments.[10] The diagnosis is made by radiographs and dynamic CT scans, which demonstrate the fixed nature of the subluxation.[11]
- Treatment with head halter traction and cervical collar immobilization is often effective if symptoms last less than 1 month. Nonsteroidal anti-inflammatory drugs and muscle relaxants are also used with traction. Symptoms of longer duration may require posterior arthrodesis from C1-C2.
- The indications for surgery include neurological involvement, failure to achieve and maintain correction of a deformity present for longer than 3 months, and recurrence of the deformity after 6-8 weeks of nonoperative care.[11]

Table 6–1: Atlantoaxial Rotary Instability Classification

TYPE	DESCRIPTION
I	Simple rotary displacement without an anterior shift of C1
II	Rotary displacement with an anterior shift of 5 mm or less
III	Rotary displacement with an anterior shift greater than 5 mm
IV	Rotary displacement with a posterior shift

From Fielding JW, Hawkins RJ (1977) Atlantoaxial rotary fixation (fixed rotary subluxation of the atlantoaxial joint). J Bone Joint Surg 59A: 37-44.

Subaxial Cervical Spine Injuries

- Injuries of the lower cervical spine are more common in older children and adolescents, and fracture patterns take on adult-like characteristics.
- These fractures may include wedge- or compression-type fractures, facet dislocations, and fractures–dislocations.
- Ligamentous injury with instability may also occur in children. Pennecot and coauthors reported on 16 children with ligamentous disruption, 11 sustaining injuries at or below the C3 level.[12] The patients had a stiff neck and loss of lordosis, representing protective muscle spasm of the cervical spine. Radiographs showed widening of the interspinous process space, kyphosis at the disk space, and loss of parallelism of the facet joints. Surgery was indicated in those patients with persistent pain and progressive deformity.[12]
- Most pediatric cervical spine fractures can be treated in a closed fashion with cervical collar or halo immobilization.
- Compression fractures are thought to be the most common fracture type, occurring after flexion–axial load injuries. They are stable fractures, which can be associated with spinous process, laminar, and anterior teardrop fractures of the vertebral body. Flexion–extension radiographs should be obtained after 4-6 weeks of cervical collar immobilization to assess posterior ligamentous stability.
- Facet dislocations in the pediatric spine may be unilateral or bilateral and may be associated with a fracture of the facet (Figure 6–8). Prereduction MRI studies should be obtained to evaluate the status of the spinal cord and the intervertebral disks. Bilateral facet dislocations tend to be unstable and are associated with a greater risk of neurological involvement. Attempts at reducing the facet dislocation should be made initially closed with gentle guided traction. If the dislocations do not reduce easily, then open reduction and posterior fusion are indicated.

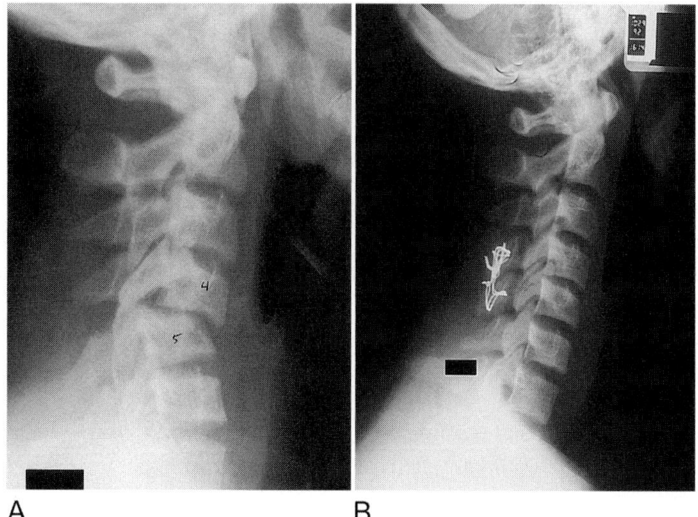

Figure 6–8: C4-C5 unilateral facet fracture–dislocation with incomplete neurological deficit in a 15 year old sustained while playing football. He underwent open reduction, was given a posterior arthrodesis with wire fixation, and had full neurological recovery.

- Fractures–dislocations of the cervical spine are often the result of high-energy trauma and are at high risk of having associated spinal cord injuries. The goal of treatment for these fractures is early reduction and operative stabilization. This will allow early mobilization, facilitate rehabilitation, and prevent late deformity.
- Physeal fractures through the vertebral endplates are unique pediatric cervical spine injuries. The inferior endplate is more frequently involved. Identification of this fracture can be difficult on radiographs because spontaneous reduction and normal realignment may occur. MRI may be used to identify this injury as well as SCIWORA if neurological deficits exist. These fractures are typically unstable and may require surgical stabilization.

Thoracolumbar Spine Injuries

Overview of Management

- The management of pediatric thoracolumbar fractures requires thoughtful consideration of the stability of the fracture pattern, coronal or sagittal plane deformities, neurological deficit if present, and associated injuries.
- The integrity or stability of the spinal column can be determined using several methods. The three-column concept of the spine, dividing the thoracolumbar spine into anterior, middle, and posterior columns, can be applied to pediatric spine fractures. The spinal injury is thought to be unstable if two or more columns of the spine are involved, particularly when there is ligamentous disruption.
- The mechanism of injury and direction of forces applied to the spine at the time of injury contribute to the specific fracture patterns identified on the radiographs and other imaging studies.
- In general, most these injuries are stable, the risk of spinal cord injury is low compared with the risk for adults, and most can be treated conservatively.
- In older children, the risk of neurological injury is highest in fractures–dislocations occurring at the thoracolumbar junction.
- The incidence of progressive spinal deformity after complete spinal cord injury approaches 100% in children. It is related to the age of the child, the degree of spasticity, and the level of the spinal cord injury. Treatment should be started for a progressive spinal deformity before it becomes severe.

Compression Fractures

- Compression fractures primarily occur in the thoracic spine because of flexion injuries. These fractures tend to be stable, involving only the anterior column of the spine. The thoracic rib cage provides inherent stability to these injuries.
- Wedging of the anterior vertebral bodies with less than 50% loss of anterior vertebral height is often noted.
- Multiple contiguous compression fractures can be found, resulting from the increased flexibility of the spine and hydration of the intervertebral disks, which enables the forces to be dissipated over several levels.
- The increased elasticity of the posterior ligamentous complex is thought to contribute to the increased

incidence of multiple compression fractures noted at the thoracolumbar junction and lumbar spine following lap belt injuries. Despite the flexion–distraction mode of injury, only the anterior column fails in flexion in skeletally immature individuals.[6]

- The ability of the skeletally immature spine to spread the traumatic forces over several vertebral levels minimizes the incidence of neurological injury.
- Most of these stable fractures can be treated nonoperatively, but the degree of kyphosis and wedging may influence treatment decisions. In younger children, reconstitution of anterior vertebral body height predictably occurs.
- In all children, child abuse or pathological causes must be considered when multiple compression fractures are seen.

Flexion–Distraction Injuries

- Also known as Chance fractures, flexion–distraction injuries are often associated with lap belt injuries.
- The management should address both the fracture and the potential for associated intra-abdominal injuries.
- Approximately two-thirds of these patients have intra-abdominal injuries that may be life-threatening (Figure 6–9). The most common injuries include tears or perforations of the small and large bowel, disruptions of the mesentery, and abdominal vascular structures.[5,6] Delayed diagnosis of these injuries because of the overlap of clinical signs with the spinal fracture is common.[6]
- The incidence of neurological injury is low because of the flexibility of the spine.
- Specific management of this spinal injury depends on the degree of deformity, stability of the fracture, associated injuries, and the presence or absence of a neurological deficit.
- Four types of flexion–distraction injuries have been described (Table 6–2) that define the distraction plane of injury through the ligaments, bone, or intervertebral endplates.[6]
- The fracture is thought to be stable when it extends through bone only in the posterior column of the spine and when it can potentially heal without operative intervention. Hyperextension casting or bracing is indicated in neurologically intact patients with stable fracture patterns.

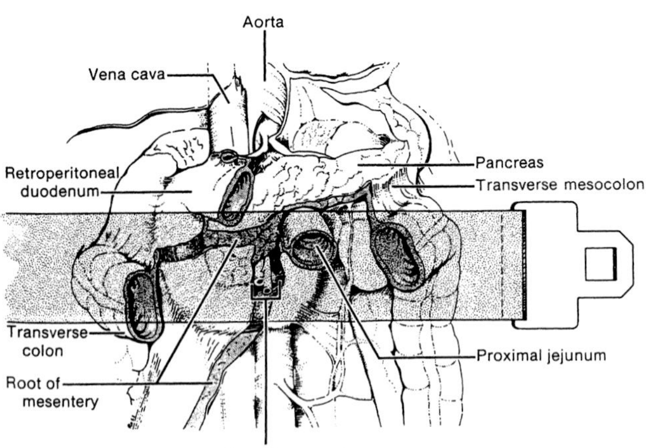

Figure 6–9: Intra-abdominal structures attached in the retroperitoneum at the midlumbar region vulnerable to a lap belt injury. **From Johnson DL, Falci S (1990) The diagnosis and treatment of pediatric lumbar spine injuries caused by rear seat lap belts. Neurosurg 26(1): 439.**

- Disruption of the posterior ligamentous complex usually results in an unstable fracture pattern that will not heal on its own. Surgery is indicated for patients with unstable fractures, significant kyphotic deformity, or neurological injury (Figure 6–10). Patients may also benefit from operative stabilization of the fracture when associated abdominal injuries require surgery, because hyperextension casting may not be possible and internal fixation of the fracture would promote early mobilization. Internal fixation depends on the age of the patient. In young children, interspinous process wiring and hyperextension casting is used. In older children and adolescents, segmental fixation with compression instrumentation is recommended.

Burst Fractures

- Burst fractures comprise only 10% of all pediatric thoracolumbar fractures and are more common in older children approaching skeletal maturity. The increased flexibility of the skeletally immature spinal column in younger children is able to dissipate the concentrated compressive forces that result in burst fractures.

Table 6–2: Flexion–Distraction Classification

TYPE	DESCRIPTION
A	Bony disruption of the posterior column extending just into the middle column
B	Avulsion of the posterior elements with facet joint disruption or fracture and extension into the apophysis of the vertebral body
C	Posterior ligamentous disruption with a fracture line entering the vertebra close to the pars interarticularis and extending into the middle column
D	Posterior ligamentous disruption with a fracture line traversing the lamina and extending into the apophysis of the adjacent vertebral body

From Rumball K, Jarvis J (1992) Seat belt injuries of the spine in young children. J Bone Joint Surg 74B: 571-574.

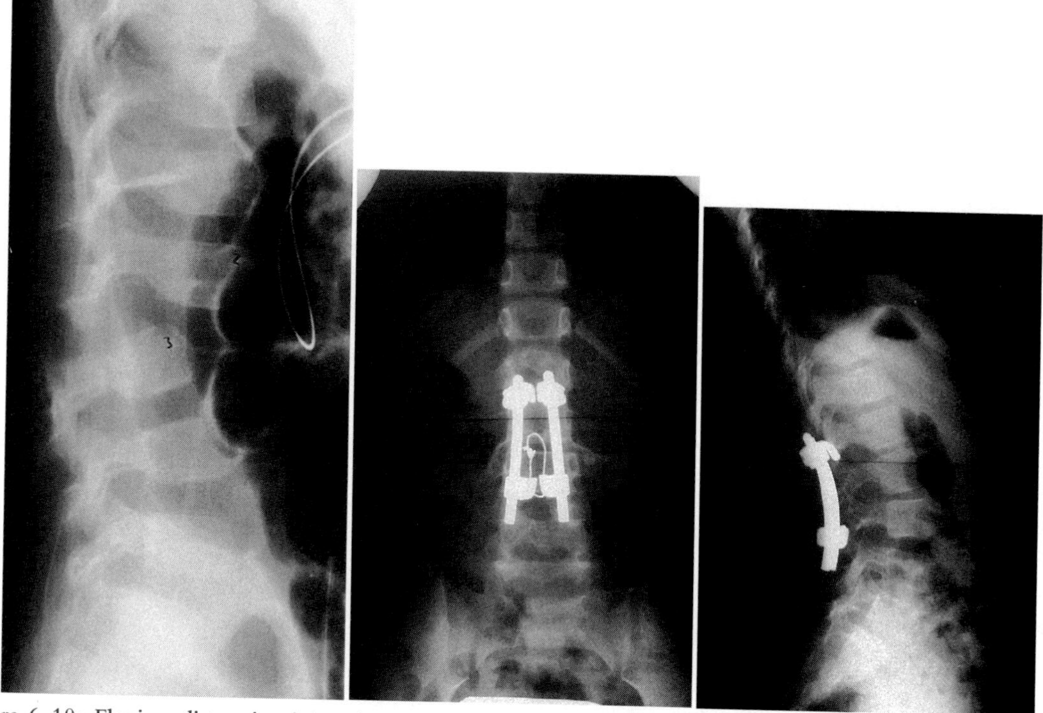

Figure 6–10: Flexion–distraction injury in a 4-year-old child restrained with a lap belt. **Despite the near dislocation of the spine at the L2-L3 level, the child had normal neurological function. Open reduction and posterior fusion with compression instrumentation were performed to stabilize the injury.**

- These fractures result from axial load and flexion forces applied to the spine. Failure of the middle column occurs as the vertebral endplate fails and the intervertebral disk is forced into the vertebral body, leading to retropulsion of bone into the spinal canal.
- Compared with adults, the spinal canal is larger relative to the spinal cord and cauda equina in children and a greater degree of canal compromise is tolerated without impingement of the cord or cauda equina. Burst fractures occurring far from the L1 level tend to also have a lower incidence of permanent neurological injury because the cauda equina is more tolerant of compression than the spinal cord.
- Hyperextension casting or bracing can be considered in a child (typically an adolescent) who is neurologically intact, has a stable fracture pattern, and has minimal kyphotic deformity.
- The degree of spinal canal compromise is usually not a factor in decision making for treatment of these fractures. In addition to the larger relative canal dimensions in children, resorption of the retropulsed bone fragments predictably occurs with remodeling.
- Operative decompression and stabilization with internal fixation are indicated for unstable burst fractures in patients with significant kyphotic deformity (often more than 20 degrees), with neurological deficits, or both (Figure 6–11). The individual fracture is addressed from an anterior or posterior approach.

Spinal Cord Injury Without Radiographic Abnormality

- Children may have a complete or incomplete spinal cord injury after a traumatic event despite having normal radiographs and CT images of their spine. This injury is defined as SCIWORA, as explained earlier, and is unique to the pediatric population.
- It is a consequence of a stretch or distraction injury to the relatively flexible spinal column that exceeds the tensile limits of the underlying spinal cord in a skeletally immature individual.
- Numerous theories have been proposed to explain the spinal cord injury, including stretch or traction injury, vascular compromise or ischemic injury, and transient disk herniation or endplate separation.
- The injury often occurs following a high-energy traumatic event such as a pedestrian–MVA or a fall from a significant height. These children require a thorough assessment of their neurological deficit and evaluation for associated injuries that frequently occur with SCIWORA.
- This unique injury is often noted in children 8 years or younger, commonly occurs at the cervicothoracic junction, and is more likely to be a complete spinal cord injury in these younger patients.[4]

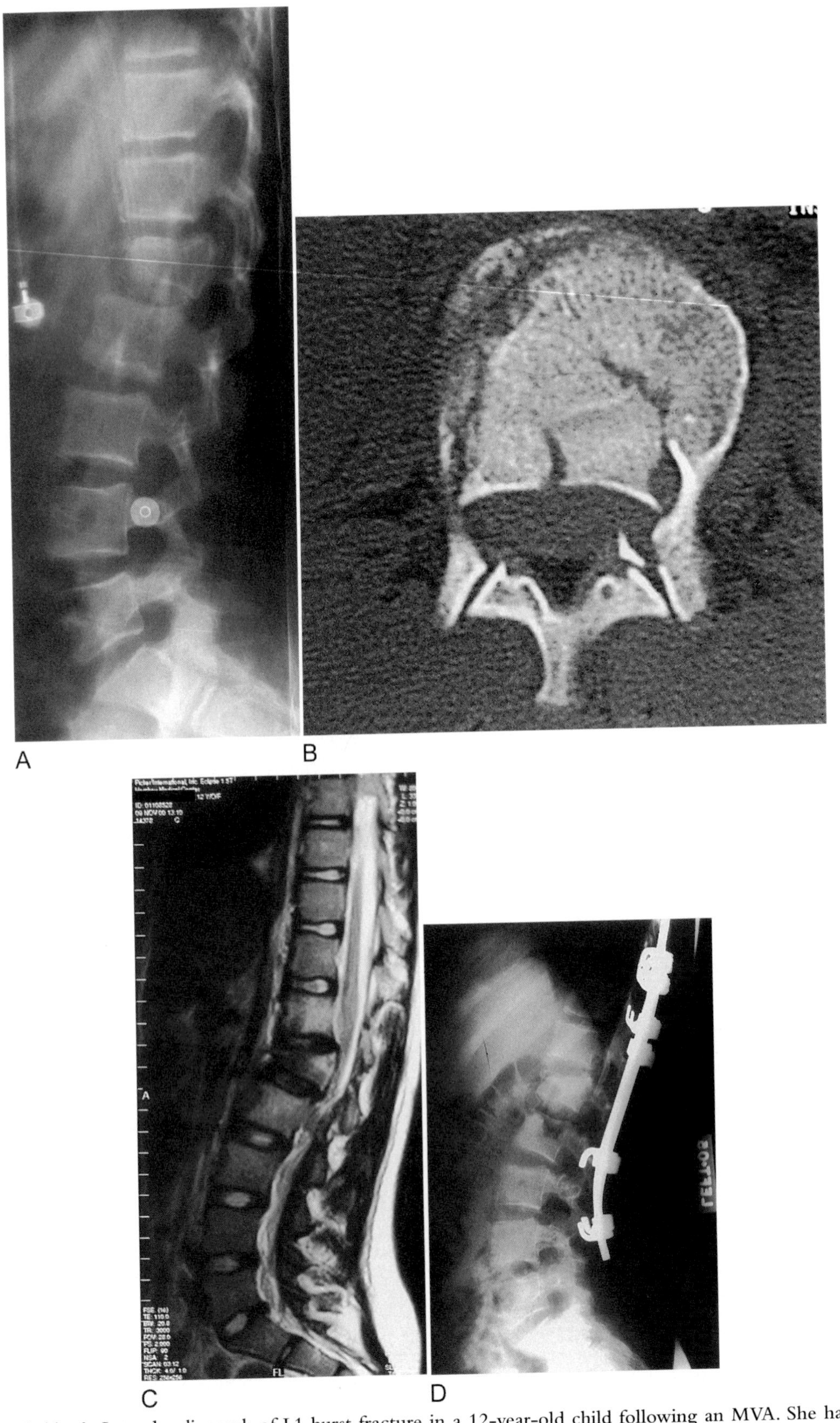

Figure 6–11: A, Lateral radiograph of L1 burst fracture in a 12-year-old child following an MVA. She had intact neurological function. B, CT scan demonstrates failure of the middle column with retropulsion of bone fragments into the spinal canal. C, MRI shows impingement of the spinal cord at the level of the conus. D, Lateral radiograph following posterior arthrodesis and instrumentation from T10-L3.

- Children with incomplete spinal cord injuries should be treated with the expectation of neurological improvement.
- MRI best defines the location and extent of injury to the cord, ligaments, and unossified cartilage (Figure 6–12).
- Management is guided by the stability of the spinal column injury and the severity of the injury to the spinal cord. The role of steroids for the management of progressive neurological deficits has not been defined. Fusion of the spine is indicated in children with unstable spine injuries or with progressive neurological deficits. The role of brace immobilization for all patients with "stable" spine injuries for 3 months, with reevaluation of spine stability with physician-guided radiographs, has recently been questioned. The neurological status of each patient should be followed closely, regardless of whether brace treatment is used, and operative stabilization of the spine should be performed if instability is noted on follow-up radiographs.
- A spinal cord rehabilitative program should begin for patients with complete or incomplete SCIWORA when other acute injuries permit. Children with spinal cord injuries are at risk for developing progressive spinal deformities such as scoliosis and require follow-up through skeletal maturity.

Traumatic Pelvis Injuries

Overview

- Fractures of the pelvis in children are uncommon injuries. The incidence of these fractures seen at major pediatric trauma centers ranges from 2-5%,[13] and most of these fractures are stable injuries that do not require intervention.
- Despite their relatively rare occurrence, the presence of a pelvis fracture in the trauma setting is often an indication of other potentially life-threatening injuries that take precedence over the skeletal injury.
- The mechanism of injury for pediatric pelvis fractures is different than that of adults. Most of these injuries are the result of a pedestrian–MVA trauma, often occurring as a child runs out into the street and is struck by an oncoming car. Most studies report this mode of injury to occur in 60% of pelvis fractures.[14] Pelvic fractures occur in 30% of cases in which the child or adolescent is either the passenger or the driver involved in an MVA. In contrast, this is the most common mode of injury in adults. Falls and other miscellaneous injuries account for the remaining 10% of injuries that cause pelvis fractures.

Anatomy

- The evaluation and management of traumatic injuries to the pelvis in pediatric patients must take into account several unique features. The skeletally immature pelvis is flexible and plastic because of the large percentage of cartilage and the porous nature of its cortical bone. The increased elasticity of the posterior sacroiliac joints and the anterior symphysis pubis enables the pelvis to absorb significant amounts of energy and to allow large amounts of displacement before a fracture occurs.[14,15]
- The pelvis can easily "bend but not break" in the face of significant forces that occur from high-energy trauma. Compared with adults, single breaks or fractures in the pelvic ring are seen in children, and most pelvic fractures are stable injuries.

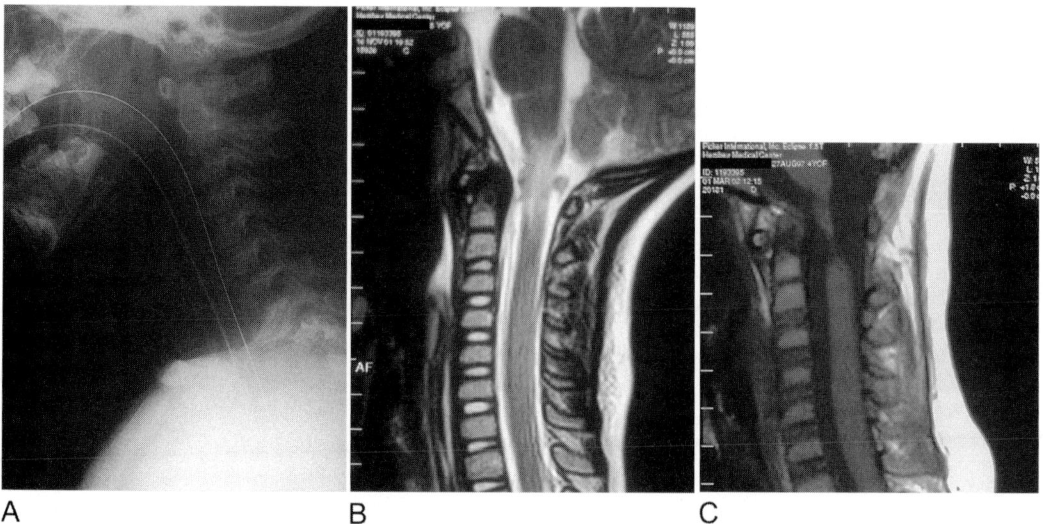

Figure 6–12: A 4-year-old child with SCIWORA following an MVA. A, A lateral radiograph of the cervical spine was taken on admission. No obvious fracture or dislocation was noted. B, MRI reveals contusion at the level of the brain stem and upper cervical spinal cord. C, Repeat MRI 4 months after injury demonstrates marked atrophy of the spinal cord at the craniocervical junction.

- The presence of cartilage within the pelvis can delay diagnosis of fractures involving the cartilage on radiographs and can therefore result in growth disturbances.
- The primary and secondary centers of ossification in the developing pelvis can easily be confused with fractures. The pelvis in a child consists of three primary ossification centers (the ilium, ischium, and pubis) that meet at the triradiate cartilage and fuse around the age of 16–18 years (Figure 6–13).
- The growth of the acetabulum involves the complex interaction of interstitial growth within the triradiate cartilage complex, appositional growth at the periphery of the cartilage, and periosteal new bone formation at the acetabular margins.[16] The concavity of the acetabulum forms from the direct mechanical response of a reduced spherical femoral head.
- The triradiate cartilage within the chondro-osseous complex of the acetabulum can prematurely close if injured, most often after a crush-type injury, resulting in a possible limb length discrepancy, progressive acetabular dysplasia, and possible hip subluxation.[17]
- The secondary centers of ossification include the anterior–superior and anterior–inferior spines, the iliac crest, and the ischial tuberosity. The age of appearance and fusion for each of these apophyses is different, and they can be pulled or avulsed off the pelvis by forceful muscle contractions.[18]

Physical Examination

- Children that sustain pelvic fractures often have multiple injuries that can be life threatening and require initial resuscitative measures in the field and the emergency room as established by the Advanced Trauma Life Support.

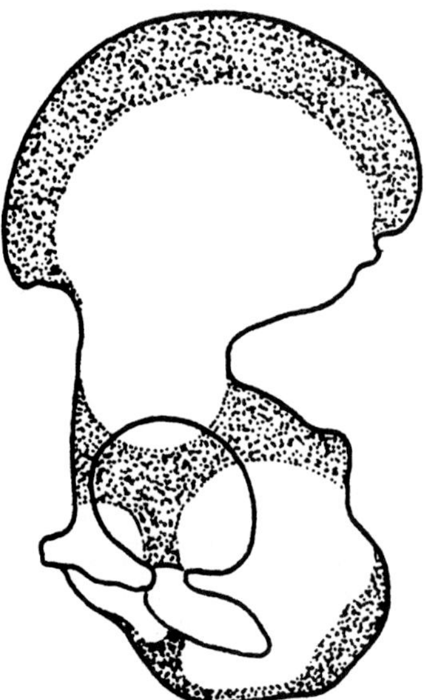

Figure 6–13: Confluence of the triradiate cartilage at the junction of the three pelvic bones and within the acetabulum. **From Bucholz RW, Ezaki M, Ogden JA (1982) Injury to the acetabular triradiate physeal cartilage. J Bone Joint Surg 64A(4): 600.**

- A history of the accident and the mechanism of injury should be obtained.
- The primary survey centers on the evaluation and treatment of these potentially life-threatening injuries and includes the ABCs of airway assessment, breathing or ventilation, and circulatory status. A brief neurological examination and exposure of the child is required to complete the primary survey.
- Detailed examination of the pelvis begins with inspection of the skin for any signs of contusion, ecchymosis, abrasions, or lacerations about the pelvis and perineum. The location of these cutaneous signs may often help to define the pattern of injury to the pelvis, such as a lateral compression injury. Any lacerations of the skin are suggestive of an open pelvic fracture and should be probed or explored to define the depth of the laceration and whether it communicates with a spike of bone from a pelvic fracture.
- The landmarks of the pelvis should be palpated for tenderness, symmetry, or abnormal motion. Lateral compression at the iliac crests and AP compression at the symphysis pubis helps to define instability or pain from a pelvic fracture.
- An apparent limb length discrepancy may represent an unstable pelvic fracture with a vertical shear component.
- Milch outlined three signs representative of pelvic fractures. Destot's sign is a superficial hematoma below the inguinal ligament or in the scrotum. Roux's sign is a decreased distance between the greater trochanter on the involved side and the pubic spine. Earle's sign is a bony prominence or hematoma on rectal examination.[19]
- Lacerations noted within the rectum are strongly indicative of an open pelvic fracture.
- A thorough neurological and vascular examination of the lower extremities should also be performed in the trauma bay. Traumatic injuries involving the sacroiliac joint can stretch or disrupt the lumbosacral plexus. A detailed evaluation of sensation and muscle strength of the lower extremities will determine whether a neurological deficit is present.

Imaging

- A screening AP radiograph of the pelvis, done without a gonadal shield, is routinely performed during the secondary survey of a pediatric trauma patient.
- Additional radiographs, including the inlet and outlet views, are obtained to evaluate specific injuries to the pelvic ring after the child is stabilized. The inlet view directed at an angle of 30–45 degrees caudad helps to define disruptions of the posterior pelvic ring such as the sacroiliac joints. The tangential view directed 40–45 degrees cephalad is used to evaluate anterior pelvic ring injuries.

- When fractures of the acetabulum are suspected on the screening radiographs, 45-degree oblique views (iliac and obturator oblique) described by Judet are obtained to better define the fracture.[19]
- CT scans are being used with increasing frequency when a pelvic fracture is noted or suspected on the screening radiograph. The CT scan of the pelvis can be readily obtained when other CT studies, such as abdominal or head studies, are requested on pediatric trauma patients. The pelvis can be scanned using 2- to 3-mm cuts extending from the L5 vertebra to the lower end of the pelvis. The use of soft tissue windows in addition to bone windows is helpful in defining the extent of pelvic hematoma. CT scans are important in defining the severity of injury to the posterior sacroiliac joints, occult posterior pelvic ring fractures of the ilium and the sacrum, posterior wall fractures of the acetabulum after fractures–dislocations of the hip, and intra-articular fragments within the hip joint after reduction of hip dislocations (Figure 6–14).
- Technetium bone scans can also be obtained to detect occult or nondisplaced fractures of the pelvis.
- Injuries to the lower urinary tract should be investigated in pelvic fractures that widely displace the anterior pelvic ring. Retrograde urethrograms are obtained before Foley catheter insertion to delineate traumatic bladder injuries, and intravenous pyelograms help to define renal or urethral anatomy and function.

Associated Injuries

- The presence of a pediatric pelvic fracture should alert the clinician that the child has experienced a significant high-energy trauma and may have other potentially life-threatening injuries.
- The incidence of associated injuries in children with a pelvis fracture is high. These may involve intra-abdominal injuries, neurovascular and other intrapelvic injuries, genitourinary injuries, and closed head injuries.
- Evaluation and treatment of these injuries takes priority over the obvious pelvic fracture seen on the screening radiograph taken as part of the trauma survey.
- Long-term morbidity in children with fractures of the pelvis is more often the result of the associated injuries rather than the skeletal injury.
- Numerous studies have evaluated the predictive risk of associated injuries occurring with pediatric pelvis fractures. These injuries may be difficult to diagnose in a child in the trauma setting. A child's age, noncompliance, or unconsciousness may limit his or her ability to communicate.
- Bond et al.[13] noted a 60% risk of concomitant abdominal injuries when multiple pelvis fractures are present.
- Unstable pelvic ring disruptions involving both the anterior and the posterior parts of the pelvis have been found to be associated with life-threatening hemorrhage and increased blood transfusion requirements. The presence of a pelvis fracture and an additional skeletal fracture are associated with a significantly higher incidence of head and abdominal injuries. A recent study reported associated nonpelvis fractures in 54% of patients.[14]
- The incidence of concomitant abdominal or visceral injuries occurring with fractures of the pelvis is 20%, often involving the spleen, liver, pancreas, or bowel.[13,14] The high costal margin of the rib cage and the poorly developed abdominal wall musculature contribute to the high incidence of these injuries in children.
- Chest trauma such as pulmonary contusions and pneumothorax occur concurrently in 12-20% of cases,

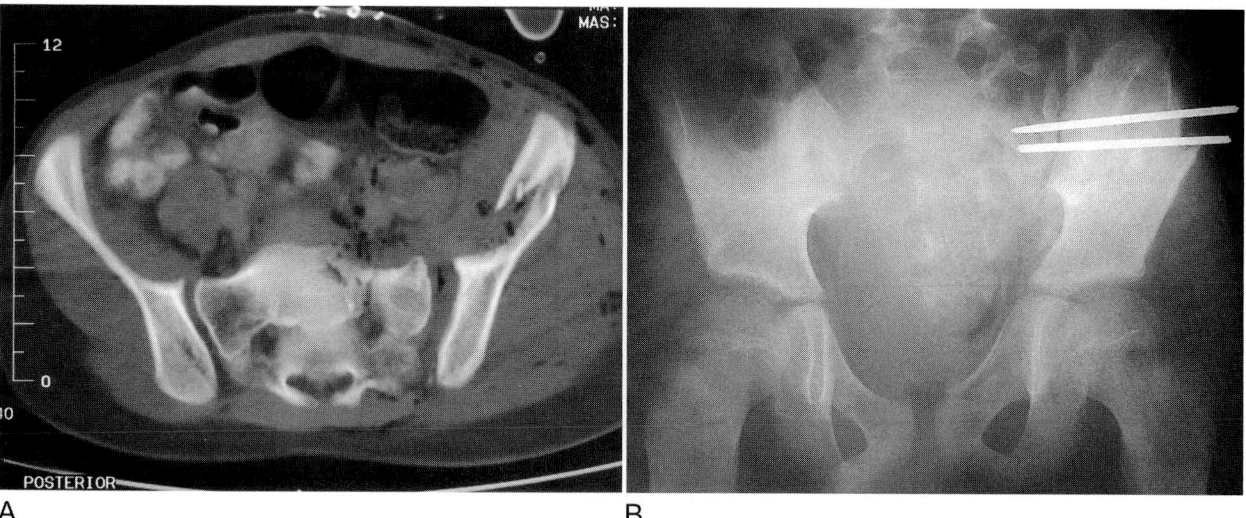

Figure 6–14: A, CT scan of a 10-year-old child demonstrating widening of the left sacroiliac joint with associated iliac wing fracture. B, Postoperative fixation of the left sacroiliac joint with pin fixation.

partly because of the increased compliance of a child's chest wall.[14]

- Children may be at less risk for urological injuries to the bladder and urethra compared with adults primarily because of the decreased incidence of "straddle" fractures (bilateral fractures of the superior and inferior pubic ramus) in children.[14]
- Closed head injuries occur frequently with pelvis fractures in children, ranging from 21-61%, and they are the most frequent cause of death in children with pelvis fractures.[14,20]
- The mortality of children following pelvic fractures has been reported in 2-12% of cases.[14,21] In contrast, adult pelvic fractures have a higher mortality rate (17%), and fatal exsanguination from the pelvic fracture is one of the leading causes of death in adults.
- The decreased rate of life-threatening hemorrhage after pelvis fractures in children may be the result of several contributing factors. As noted previously, pelvis fractures most commonly occur after pedestrian–MVA injuries, and a lateral compression fracture pattern results. A different mechanism of injury occurs in adults, usually the result of an anterior–posterior force leading to an "open book" fracture pattern that can lead to increased pelvic volume and the potential for fatal bleeding. Lateral compression fractures of the pelvis in children do not increase pelvic volume and consequently decrease the risk of life-threatening hemorrhage.[14] The thick periosteal sleeve of the pediatric pelvis may also limit the amount of displacement in a fracture, contributing to a more stable fracture pattern and minimize the potential for bleeding. In addition, children's vessels are thought to be more vasoreactive, which may also limit the amount of bleeding from these smaller vessels.[13]

Classification

- The use of classification methods for fractures in general is important to define the severity of the fracture and associated injuries, determine treatment, and allow assessment of outcomes of treatment. Factors critical in the analysis of pelvic fractures include stability, anatomical location, and mechanism of injury. Many classification systems have evolved in describing both pediatric and adult pelvic fractures (Box 6–4).
- Quimby classified pediatric pelvic fractures corresponding to the severity of the associated injuries, such as visceral injuries requiring operative exploration and those with significant hemorrhage. This classification represents a logical approach because these associated injuries can be life threatening and take precedence over most pelvic fractures in the initial evaluation and management of these patients. The major disadvantage of this system is the lack of defining the skeletal injury.[14]
- The Torode and Zieg classification method (Table 6–3) is frequently used for pediatric pelvis fractures.[14,21] This classification predicts the potential associated injuries and expected outcomes with four types of pelvic fracture patterns of increasing severity, taking into account the anatomical and physiological differences of a child's pelvis following high-energy trauma. In their series, Torode and Zieg found the greatest risk of growth disturbances, long-term disability, and mortality in type IV fractures (Figure 6–15).[21]
- The presence of an open triradiate cartilage defining a skeletally immature pelvis has recently been proposed as an important radiographic marker that differentiates pediatric from adult-like pelvic fracture patterns and outcomes observed in the older child and adolescent before skeletal maturity.[15] The incidence of unstable pelvic disruptions such as diastasis of the pubic symphysis or the sacroiliac joints was decreased in the skeletally immature patient. The increased elasticity of the sacroiliac joints and the pubic symphysis, as well as the plasticity

Box 6–4 Pediatric Pelvic Fracture Classifications

- Key and Conwell (1951)
- Quimby (1966)
- Watts (1976)
- Pennal and Tile (1980)
- Torode and Zieg (1985)

Table 6–3: Torode and Zieg Classification Pediatric Pelvic Fractures

TYPE	DESCRIPTION
I	Avulsion fractures of the pelvis that commonly occur through the cartilaginous apophyseal growth plates.
II	Involving the iliac wing and more common in children as isolated injuries than in adults. A laterally directed force against the pelvis in a pedestrian versus MVA is the most common mechanism of injury.
III	Defined as simple ring fractures. These can be pubic rami fractures or disruptions of the pubic symphysis (diastasis) that are stable injuries. Because of the plasticity of the pelvis and the elasticity of the joints, the posterior sacroiliac joint ligaments remain intact. These tend to be stable fractures, even with displaced fracture fragments present. These fractures can occur by AP compression, lateral compression, or vertical shear mechanisms of injury.
IV	Unstable pelvic fractures that include bilateral pubic rami or straddle fractures, fractures of the left or the right pubic rami (or the equivalent injury involving the pubic symphysis) and a disruption of the sacroiliac joint or fracture adjacent to the sacroiliac joint, and acetabular fractures. These fractures represent the most severe injuries with the highest incidence of associated injuries to other organ systems.

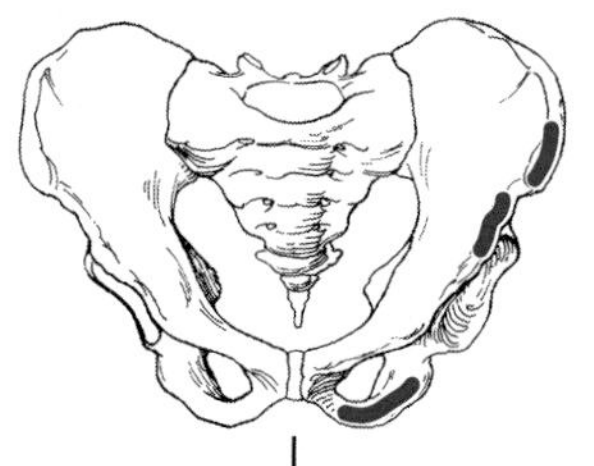

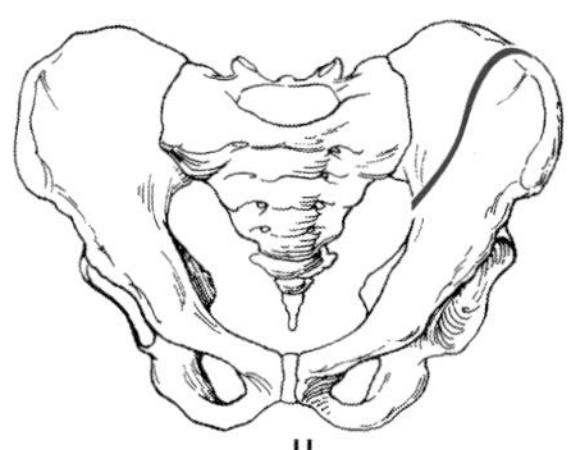

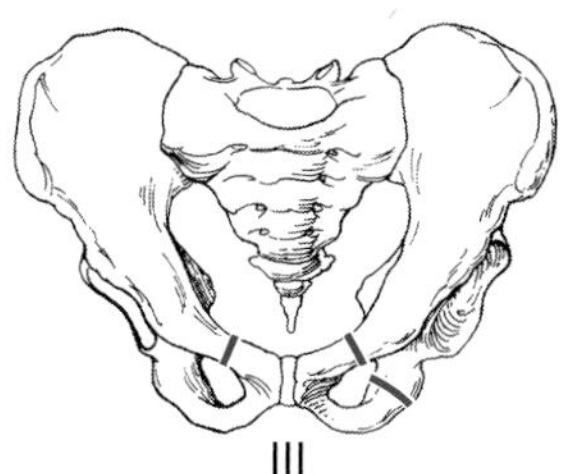

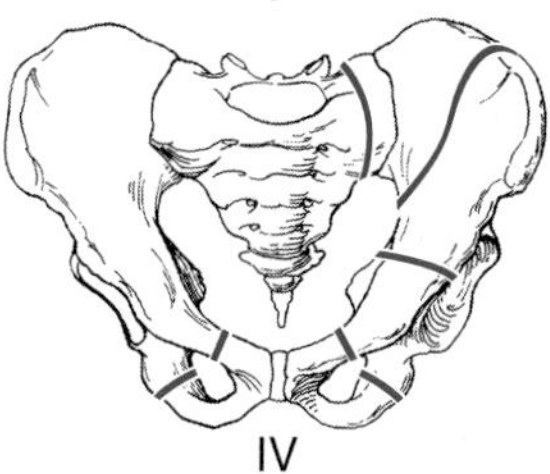

Figure 6–15: Torode and Zieg classification of pediatric pelvis fractures. From Torode I, Zieg D (1985) Pelvic fractures in children. J Ped Orthop 5: 77-79.

of the pelvis itself in the skeletally immature patient, accounts for these differences.

Stable Pelvic Ring Fractures

- Most pediatric pelvic fractures are stable injuries and require little more than a brief 4- to 6-week period of recumbency or without bearing weight to allow predictable healing.
- The thick periosteal sleeve of the pediatric pelvis provides inherent stability to most pelvic fractures. Even with mild fracture displacement, both healing and remodeling readily occur, and long-term morbidity with stable pelvic fractures is rare.
- Progressive efforts to bear weight are permitted when patients are comfortable with activities such as transfers, and as the associated injuries allow. Pain from the motion at the fracture site will diminish with early fracture healing and decreased motion of the fracture fragments. The patients are then rapidly mobilized, initially with crutches or a walker (partial ability to bear weight), then advancing to full and independent ability to bear weight.
- Some children may benefit from a hip spica cast to obtain pain control, painless mobility, and an earlier discharge from the hospital.

Unstable Pelvic Fractures

- The type IV fractures described by Torode and Zieg demand a more aggressive approach.[21] These fractures, often involving both the anterior and posterior pelvic ring, have the highest risk of long-term deformity and disability.
- Patients with these unstable fracture patterns also have the highest risk of associated abdominal or closed head injuries and, rarely, can be hemodynamically unstable.
- The goals for treatment of these severe fractures, often both rotationally and vertically unstable, are to prevent deformity, restore joint congruity, minimize growth disturbances, and obtain hemodynamic stability.
- Reduction of the fractures can be achieved by either closed or open methods. Older methods of closed reduction consist of the use of a pelvic sling for open-book–type injuries, with separation of the pubic symphysis of greater than 3 cm, and the use of distal femoral skeletal traction for vertical shear injuries.
- External fixation of pelvic fractures is still widely used, particularly with open-book fractures and disruption of the anterior sacroiliac joint ligaments (Figure 6–16). In the hemodynamically unstable child or adolescent, the application of an external fixation frame can rapidly close the pelvis and decrease pelvic volume, creating a tamponade effect and minimizing further hemorrhage from the fracture.
- On rare occasions, angiographic embolization is required to control life-threatening bleeding in a child.
- There are several indications for open reduction and internal fixation of pelvis fractures, and at times these are performed with external fixation of the anterior pelvic ring (Figure 6–17). Such instances include open displaced pelvic fractures, displaced and rotationally unstable pelvic fractures unable to be reduced by closed methods, displaced vertical shear fractures (with disruption of the posterior sacroiliac joint complex), and open-book–type fractures with more than 3 cm of separation between the symphysis pubis and the associated hemorrhage or exploratory laparotomy. Open reduction and internal fixation are thought to facilitate the care of the multiple-injury child.

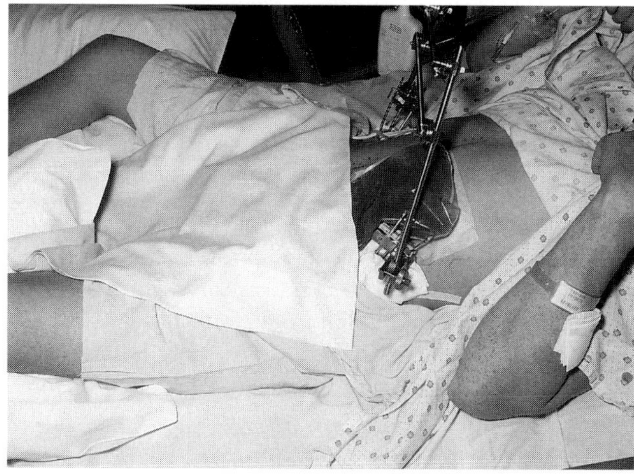

Figure 6–16: External fixation of the pelvis in a 14-year-old child following an open pelvis fracture. Note the diverting colostomy.

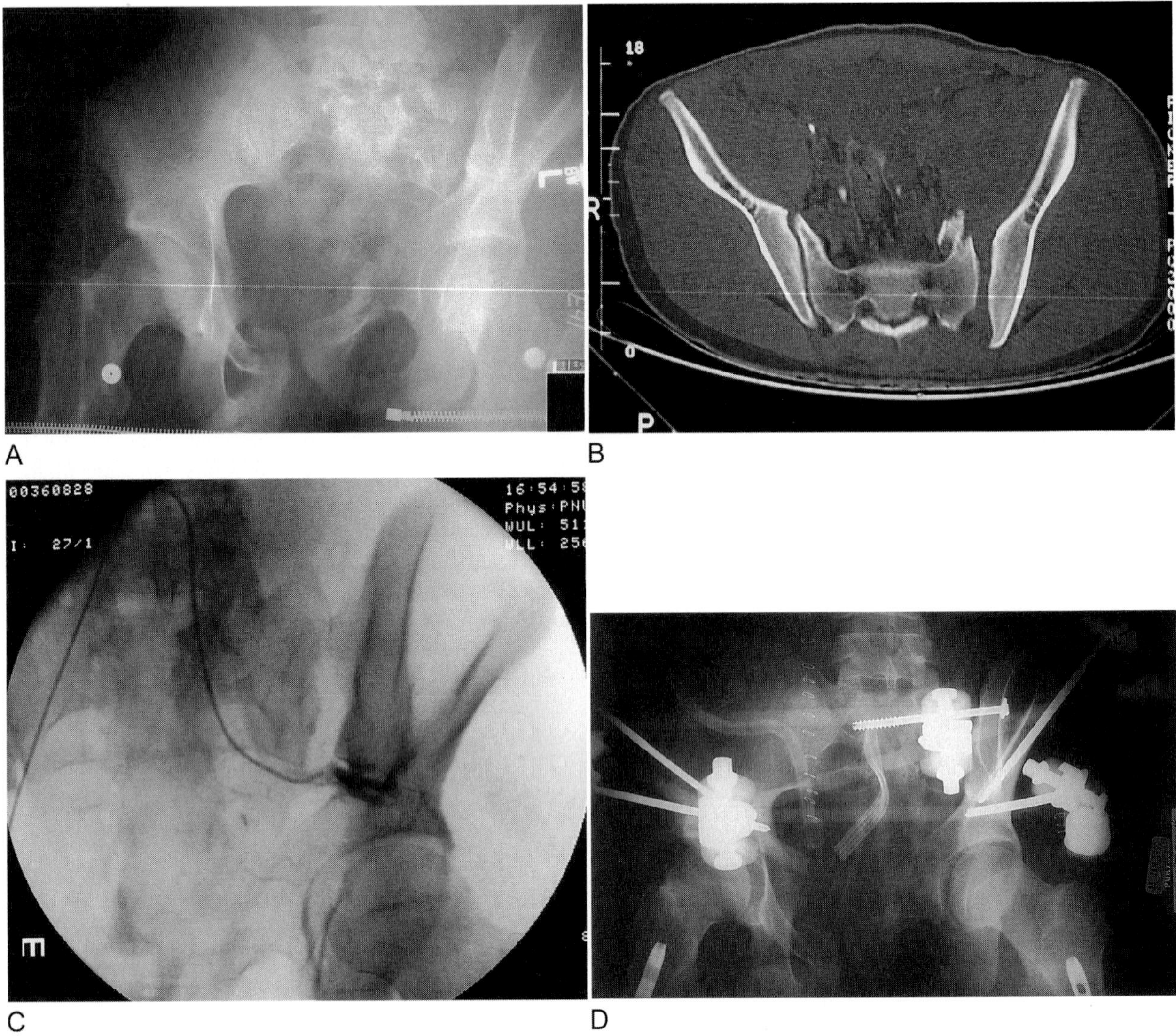

Figure 6–17: Torode and Zieg IV pelvis fracture in a 16-year-old patient following an MVA. The adolescent also sustained severe head and intra-abdominal injuries. A, AP radiograph of the pelvis demonstrating a straddle fracture of the anterior ring and disruption of the left sacroiliac joint. He was hemodynamically unstable upon admission. B, CT scan of the pelvis showing the left sacroiliac joint injury and an associated sacral fracture. C, Angiographic embolization performed to control life-threatening hemorrhage D, Stabilization of the anterior ring with external fixation, and internal fixation of the posterior ring with a left sacroiliac joint screw.

Avulsion Fractures

- The presence of apophyses about the pelvic ring in children often results in avulsion fractures, most often occurring in adolescents after competitive athletic events.
- The apophysis or the secondary center of ossification is located at the iliac crest, the anterior–superior iliac spine, the anterior–inferior iliac spine, and the ischium (Figure 6–18).
- The apophyses tend to appear and fuse later than the epiphyseal centers of long bones.
- Forceful concentric or eccentric contractures of large muscle groups can generate significant tension across an open pelvic apophysis to result in an avulsion fracture. Displacement of the avulsed fragment of bone depends on the specific avulsion fracture and can be limited by additional soft tissue attachments to the apophysis.[18]
- Most of these injuries can be treated nonoperatively. Early recognition of the injury, which often has a classic presentation, is important. Patients are often between 13-17 years, have a sudden onset of pain about the pelvic, and will often describe feeling a "pop" in their thigh or hip region. Palpation about the pelvis for areas of tenderness and resistance testing of specific muscle groups should localize the site of injury. Tenderness about the

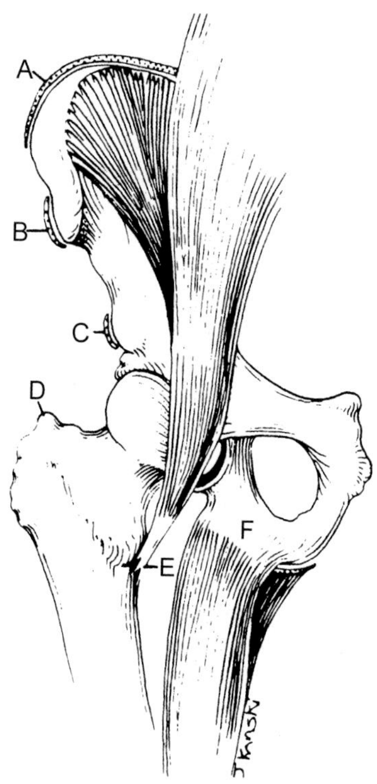

Figure 6–18: Sites of apophyseal avulsion fractures of the pediatric pelvis. A, Iliac crest. B, Anterior–superior iliac spine. C, Anterior–inferior iliac spine. D, Greater trochanter. E, Lesser trochanter. F, Ischial tuberosity. From Fernbach SK, Wilkinson RH (1981) Avulsion injuries of the pelvis and proximal femur. AJR 137: 582.

ischium and pain with knee extension because of the pull of the hamstring muscles on the ischial apophysis is suggestive of an avulsion injury to the ischial tuberosity.

- Radiographs of the pelvis will reveal and confirm the avulsion fracture, further diagnosed by history and clinical examination. The radiographs may also disclose avulsion injuries of the greater or lesser trochanter.
- When patients have not had a clear traumatic episode, infectious or neoplastic processes such as osteomyelitis or Ewing sarcoma may be evident from plain radiographs.
- Most of these injuries can be treated conservatively with a graduated rehabilitative program of partial or foot-flat ability to bear weight on crutches for 6 weeks until evidence of healing of the avulsion fracture is present; then, a progressive strengthening program should be initiated before returning to competitive activities.[18]
- Operative reattachment or excision for persistent disability of avulsion fractures is rarely required if properly treated.

Acetabular Fractures

- Fractures of the acetabulum in children are uncommon injuries, accounting for 12% of pediatric pelvic fractures.[17]
- The presence of an open triradiate cartilage in children distinctly changes the pattern of injuries, prognosis, and complications compared with those for adult acetabular fractures.
- The chondro-osseous complex involving the triradiate cartilage is formed by the confluence of the ischium, innominate, and pubic bones. Normal growth and development of the pediatric acetabulum occurs by interstitial and appositional growth.[16]
- Injuries to the acetabulum can occur by a shearing force resulting in a Salter-Harris I or II injury or by a crushing-type injury leading to a Salter-Harris V injury (Figure 6–19). The latter injury has a poorer prognosis, which may result in premature closure of the triradiate cartilage and subsequent growth disturbance. These crush injuries may often be missed on initial radiographs.
- In addition to the chondro-osseous injury, disruption of the blood supply to the germinal zone of the physis or growth plate of the triradiate cartilage may contribute to a growth disturbance of the acetabulum.[17]
- Prognosis depends on the age of the child at the time of injury and the extent of the chondro-osseous injury.[17,22]
- Premature closure of the triradiate cartilage in a young child will lead to a progressively shallow or dysplastic acetabulum. Over time, the growing femoral head will be displaced superiorly and laterally, resulting in eventual hip subluxation. Progressive acetabular dysplasia may not be noted until several years after the fracture occurred, and patients with suspected injury to the triradiate cartilage must be followed until skeletal maturity has been attained.[17,21,22]
- Evaluation of pediatric patients with acetabular fractures requires the three standard radiographic views of the pelvis: AP, internal oblique, and external oblique images (Judet views). These views help to define the extent and pattern (classification) of the fracture (Figure 6–20).

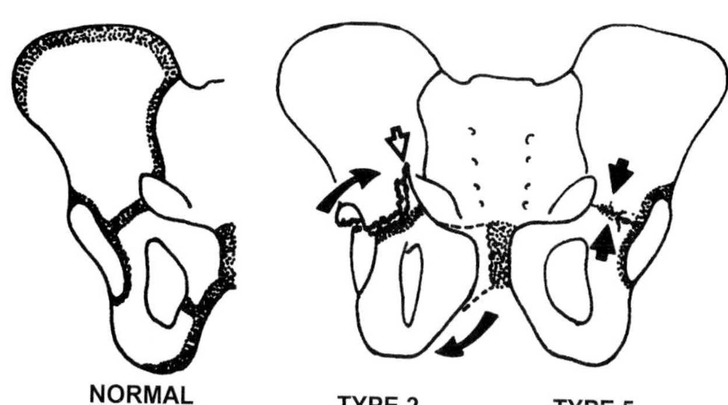

Figure 6–19: Salter-Harris II and V physeal fractures of the pediatric acetabulum. From Bucholz RW, Ezaki M, Ogden JA (1982) Injury to the acetabular triradiate physeal cartilage. J Bone Joint Surg 64A(4): 603.

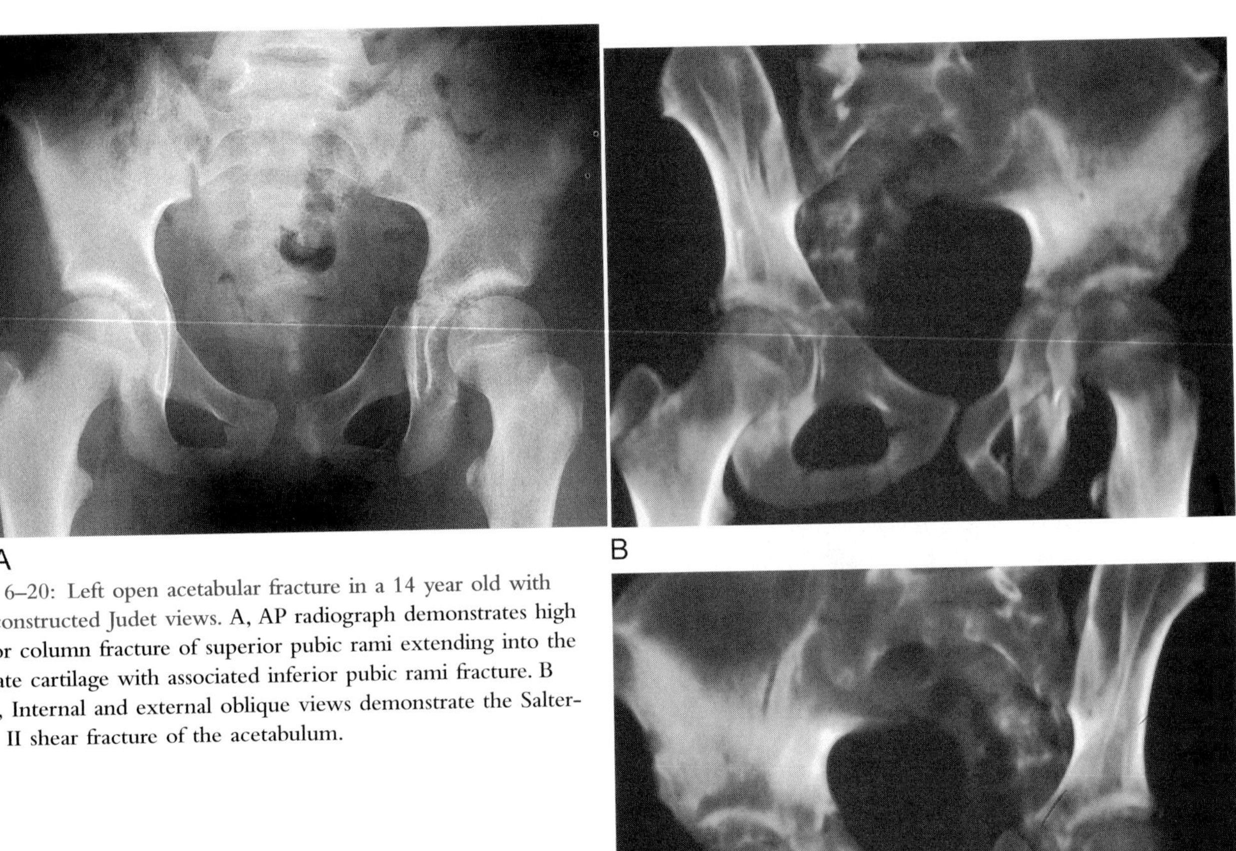

Figure 6–20: Left open acetabular fracture in a 14 year old with CT-reconstructed Judet views. A, AP radiograph demonstrates high anterior column fracture of superior pubic rami extending into the triradiate cartilage with associated inferior pubic rami fracture. B and C, Internal and external oblique views demonstrate the Salter-Harris II shear fracture of the acetabulum.

Determining roof arc angles may also determine stability of the fracture.

- The CT scan can be performed at the initial trauma evaluation in an effort to identify other injuries to the pelvic ring and to define the extent of the injury.
- CT scans are mandatory in the assessment of postreduction fractures–dislocations of the acetabulum, evaluating for joint space widening or joint incongruity. Loose cartilage fragments or inverted labrum preventing concentric reduction are easily missed on plain radiographs.
- Dislocations of the femoral head frequently occur with acetabular fractures, and urgent reduction of the dislocation is critical to decrease the risk of avascular necrosis to the femoral head.
- The management of acetabular fractures depends on the extent and severity of the injury. The goals of treatment are (1) to achieve and maintain anatomical alignment of the triradiate cartilage to minimize the risk of premature closure, growth arrest, and hip dysplasia; and (2) to achieve joint congruity and hip stability to decrease the risk of post-traumatic arthritis. Options for treatment include bed rest, non–weight-bearing status, skeletal traction, percutaneous internal fixation, and open reduction and internal fixation (Figures 6–21 and 6–22).
- The indications for open reduction and internal fixation are fractures that involve the major weight-bearing surface of the acetabulum with more than 2 mm of displacement and unstable posterior wall fractures–dislocations.[19]

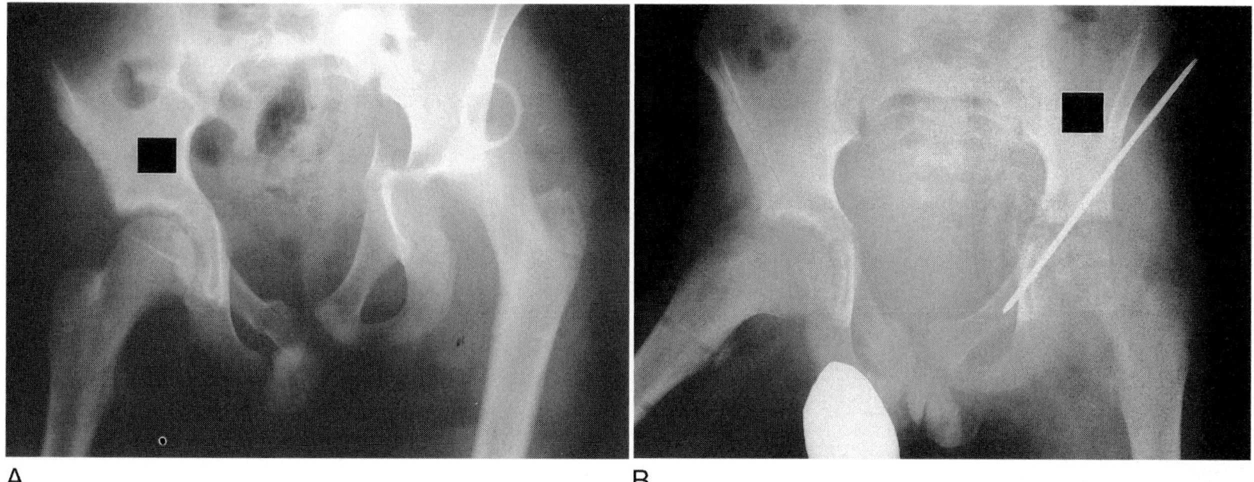

Figure 6–21: Left acetabular fracture–dislocation in an 11-year-old child following an MVA. He sustained multiple injuries including a closed head injury, a right forearm fracture, and a right femur fracture. A, AP radiograph demonstrating the left Salter-Harris II acetabular fracture and dislocation of the femoral head. B, Open reduction with pin fixation of the left acetabular fracture.

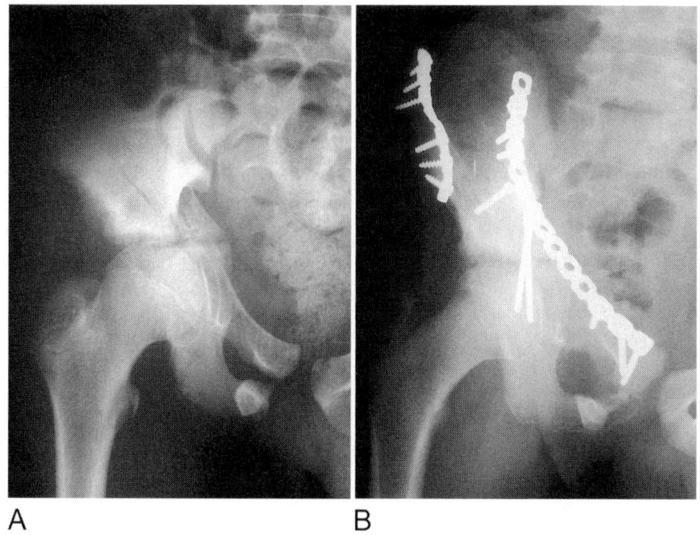

Figure 6–22: Right Salter-Harris II fracture of the acetabulum and associated iliac wing fracture in a 14-year-old following an MVA. A, AP radiograph of the right Salter-Harris II acetabular fracture. B, Open reduction and internal fixation of the right acetabular and iliac wing fractures.

References

1. Jones ET, Loder RT, Hensinger RN (1996) Fractures of the spine. In: Fractures in Children, 4th edition (Rockwood CA Jr, Wilkins KE, Beaty JH, eds). Philadelphia: Lippincott-Raven, pp 1023-1105.
   Excellent review of the normal growth and development and the unique patterns of injury of the pediatric spine. The evaluation and management of cervical and thoracolumbar spine fractures are extensively covered.

2. Flynn JM, Dormans JP (1998) Spine trauma in children. Semin Spine Surg 10(1): 7-16.
   Excellent review of the evaluation and management of pediatric spine trauma. The unique features of the cervical and thoracolumbar spine in skeletally immature patients that result in specific patterns of spine injury and management are underscored.

3. McGrory BJ, Klassen RA, Chao EY, Staeheli JW, Weaver AL (1993) Acute fractures and dislocations of the cervical spine in children and adolescents. J Bone Joint Surg 75A: 988-995.
   Two distinct age-dependent patterns of cervical spine injuries were noted in children and adolescents. Children younger than 11 years had a predominance of ligamentous injuries of the upper cervical spine, often the result of falls,

and a high rate of mortality secondary to spinal cord injury. Children and adolescents 11 to 15 years were more often injured during sports and recreational events, had injuries that involved the subaxial cervical spine, and had patterns of cervical spine injury similar to those found in adults.

4. Pang D, Wilberger JE (1982) Spinal cord injury without radiographic abnormalities in children. J Neurosurg 57: 114-129.
   This study before the use of MRI described spinal cord injury in children without evidence of fracture or dislocation on radiographs. The authors report a high incidence of severe SCIWORA in the upper cervical spine in children younger than 8 years because of the increased elasticity of the vertebral column in infants and young children.

5. Johnson DL, Falci S (1990) The diagnosis and treatment of pediatric lumbar spine injuries caused by rear seat lap belts. Neurosurg 26: 434-441.
   The authors report their experience with the "lap belt syndrome" in nine patients and the spectrum of injuries sustained, including life-threatening visceral injuries and paraplegia. The unique body proportions of a child do not conform to the principles and application of the lap belt restraint system, resulting in flexion–distraction fractures of the midlumbar spine and the predictable pattern of associated injuries. Three-point restraint systems for children were advocated to reduce the incidence of this injury.

6. Rumball K, Jarvis J (1992) Seat belt injuries of the spine in young children. J Bone Joint Surg 74B: 571-574.
   Four distinct patterns of seat belt injury of the lumbar spine are described in skeletally immature patients. The delay in diagnosis, the associated intra-abdominal injuries, the mechanism of injury, and the optimal use of restraints to prevent this injury are described.

7. Hoy GA, Cole WG (1993) The pediatric cervical seat belt syndrome. Injury 24: 297-299.
   The authors described a spectrum of injuries in seven children wearing three- or four-point seat belt restraint systems. These injuries included a fracture–dislocation of the upper cervical spine, spinal cord injuries at the level of the cervical spine, and laryngeal fracture or nerve injury.

8. Herzenberg JE, Hensinger RN, Dedrick DK, Phillips WA (1989) Emergency transport and positioning of young children who have an injury of the cervical spine: The standard backboard may be hazardous. J Bone Joint Surg 71A: 15-22.
   This retrospective review of 10 children with unstable injuries of the cervical spine demonstrated anterior translation, angulation, or both on radiographs taken with the child supine on a standard flat board. The disproportionately large head size in young children forces the neck into relative kyphosis. Modifications to the standard backboard during emergency transport and radiography are recommended to provide safer alignment of the cervical spine in young children.

9. Dormans JP (2002) Evaluation of children with suspected cervical spine injury (instructional course lecture). J Bone Joint Surg 84A: 124-132.
   Comprehensive review article on the evaluation and management of cervical spine injuries in children. A thorough description of the developmental anatomy of the cervical spine, physical examination, and the use of newer diagnostic imaging techniques provides the basis for understanding and treatment of unique types of pediatric cervical spine injuries.

10. Fielding JW, Hawkins RJ (1977) Atlantoaxial rotary fixation (fixed rotary subluxation of the atlantoaxial joint). J Bone Joint Surg 59A: 37-44.
   The authors report on 17 patients with irreducible atlantoaxial rotary fixation in this landmark study. Most patients had a delay in their diagnosis and persistent clinical and radiographic deformity. Of the patients, 13 underwent a C1-C2 arthrodesis.

11. Philips WA, Hensinger RN (1989) The management of atlantoaxial subluxation in children. J Bone Joint Surg 71A: 664-668.
   The use of dynamic CT scan is described in this retrospective review of 23 children to diagnose the presence of fixed atlantoaxial rotary subluxation. The success of closed reduction with traction and the length of hospitalization were found to be related to the duration of symptoms before treatment.

12. Pennecot GF, Leonard P, Peyrot Des Gachons S, Hardy JR, Pouliquen JC (1984) Traumatic ligamentous instability of the cervical spine in children. J Ped Orthop 4: 339-345.
   Retrospective review of 16 cases of traumatic dislocation or ligamentous disruption of the cervical spine in children. Of the patients, 11 had injury to the lower cervical spine. Diagnosis of ligamentous disruption included increased interspinous process distance, loss of parallelism between articular processes, and posterior widening of the disk spaces. The authors recommend operative intervention only with persistence of clinical and radiographic signs after a long period of immobilization.

13. Bond S, Gotshall C, Eichelberger M (1991) Predictors of abdominal injury in children with pelvic fractures. J Trauma 31: 1169-1173.
   The authors evaluated 54 children over a 4-year period admitted to a level I pediatric trauma center with a pelvic fracture, using contingency table and stepwise logistic analysis to determine the best predictors of abdominal injury. Children sustaining multiple fractures had a 60% risk of associated abdominal injury.

14. Silber JS, Flynn JM, Koffler KM, Dormans JP, Drummond DS (2001) Analysis of the cause, classification, and associated injuries of 166 consecutive pelvic fractures. J Ped Orthop 21: 446-450.
   This retrospective review of 166 consecutive pediatric pelvic fractures evaluated the mechanism of injury, fracture patterns, associated injuries, and mortality from a single, level I pediatric trauma center. Anatomical differences in the skeletally immature pelvis and the mechanism of injury account for the differences in fracture patterns, associated injuries, and outcomes compared with those of adults.

15. Silber JS, Flynn JM (2002) Changing patterns of pediatric pelvic fractures with skeletal maturation: Implications for classification and management. J Ped Orthop 22: 22-26.
In a related study, the authors identified two distinct fracture patterns of the pelvis depending on the triradiate cartilage. In patients with open triradiate cartilage (immature pelvis), the patients had a higher incidence of isolated pubic rami and iliac wing fractures. Patients with closed triradiate cartilage (mature pelvis) had a higher predilection for acetabular fractures and pubic or sacroiliac diastasis. The evaluation of the triradiate cartilage may be important in future classification methods of pediatric pelvic fractures.

16. Ponseti IV (1978) Growth and development of the acetabulum in the normal child: anatomical, histological, and roentgenographical studies. J Bone Joint Surg 60A: 575-585.
Classic paper on the normal developmental anatomy of the acetabulum and triradiate physeal cartilage. The acetabulum in a growing child normally develops in response to interstitial growth of the triradiate cartilage, appositional growth at the periphery of this cartilage, periosteal new bone formation at the acetabular margin, and the presence of a normal spherical femoral head.

17. Bucholz R, Ezaki M, Ogden J (1982) Injury to the acetabular triradiate physeal cartilage. J Bone J Surg 64A: 600.
This study describes two patterns of injury to the triradiate physeal cartilage. Type I or II Salter-Harris shearing injuries have a favorable prognosis for continued normal acetabular growth. Type V or crush injuries have a poor prognosis with premature closure of the triradiate cartilage. For either group of injuries, prognosis depends on the age of the patient at the time of injury and the severity of the chondro-osseous injury.

18. Metzmaker JN, Pappas A (1985) Avulsion fractures of the pelvis. Am J Sports Med 13: 349-358.
The authors retrospectively review their consecutive series of avulsion fractures of the pelvis in 27 patients. These injuries demonstrate a consistent pattern of mechanism of injury, age, symptoms, presentation, and x-ray film appearance. Early diagnosis and a directed and graduated rehabilitation program resulted in an excellent outcome in 26 cases.

19. Canale ST, Beaty JH (1996) Pelvic and hip fractures. In: Fractures in Children, 4th edition (Rockwood CA Jr, Wilkins KE, Beaty JH, eds). Philadelphia: Lippincott-Raven, pp 1109-1147.
Excellent review of the normal development, physical examination, diagnostic imaging, classification systems, and management and outcomes of fractures of the pelvis and acetabulum in a pediatric patient.

20. Rang, M (1983) Children's Fractures. 2nd edition. Philadelphia: JB Lippincott, pp 233-241.
Classic textbook on pediatric fractures.

21. Torode I, Zieg D (1985) Pelvic fractures in children. J Ped Orthop 5: 76-84.
The authors developed their classification of pediatric pelvic fractures from a retrospective review of 141 patients. Four patterns of pelvic fractures (I-IV) increasing in severity correlated with the incidence of associated injuries and expected outcomes from the fracture. Type IV fractures with pelvic ring disruption have the highest incidence of associated injuries, mortality, and complications, including nonunion and premature closure of the triradiate cartilage.

22. Heeg M, Klassen H, Visser J (1989) Acetabular fractures in children and adolescents. J Bone Joint Surg 71B: 418.
This study is a retrospective review of 23 acetabular fractures in children and adolescents up to 17 years old with average follow-up of 8 years. Open reduction and internal fixation were performed in 5 patients with either unstable posterior fractures–dislocations or irreducible central fractures–dislocations. Overall, good or excellent functional results were reported in 21 patients, and good or excellent radiographic results were found for 16. Two patients with type V injuries to the triradiate cartilage developed progressive hip subluxation after premature closure of the triradiate cartilage.

23. Flynn JM, Closkey RF, Mahboubi S, Dormans JP (2002) Role of magnetic resonance imaging in the assessment of pediatric cervical spine injuries. J Ped Orthop 22: 573-577.
This study assessed the role of MRI in the evaluation of suspected cervical spine injury in 237 children. MRI confirmed the findings on plain x-ray films in 66% of patients and changed the diagnosis in 34%. The authors found MRI to be useful in the obtunded child with equivocal plain radiographs.

CHAPTER 7

Pediatric Sports Medicine

Theodore J. Ganley*, Emily A. Kolze†, and John R. Gregg‡

*MD, Orthopaedic Surgeon, Division of Orthopaedic Surgery; and Orthopaedic Director, Sports Medicine and Performance Center, The Children's Hospital of Philadelphia, Philadelphia, PA; Assistant Professor of Orthopaedic Surgery, University of Pennsylvania School of Medicine, Philadelphia, PA
†Clinical Research Coordinator, Division of Orthopaedic Surgery, The Children's Hospital of Philadelphia, Philadelphia, PA
‡MD, Orthopaedic Surgeon, Division of Orthopaedic Surgery, The Children's Hospital of Philadelphia, Philadelphia, PA

- Childhood and adolescence are periods of rapid development, growth, and maturation.
- These features and an interest in varied physical activities make young athletes uniquely susceptible to injury.[1]
- Sports injuries account for nearly one quarter of all injuries in children and adolescents.
- Those caring for young athletes must be aware of the unique characteristics of injuries incurred on the field of play.
- The treating physician is in a position to counsel patients and families about prevention and can alleviate fears by offering prognosis and appropriate rehabilitation for return to activity following an injury.[2,3]

Soft Tissue Injuries

Sprain

- Sprains occur when forces placed on a ligament or joint capsule cause them to stretch or, in some cases, rupture.
- Injury depends on the amount of force applied and the rate of application of this force in accordance with the viscoelastic properties of these structures.
- In grade I sprains, the integrity of the ligament is intact, although tearing of some fibers occurs. There is no pathological laxity and generally no restriction of the range of motion in this injury.
- Grade II sprains involve damage to the ligament with incomplete tearing of fibers. Pathological laxity is noted, and some resistance occurs as a firm end point when anterior drawer ligamentous stress testing is performed.
- In grade III sprains, complete rupture is noted, demonstrating instability to ligamentous stress testing. Complete rupture of grade III severity is uncommon but possible in young athletes.

Strain

- Strains include injuries to the muscle and muscle–tendon unit as a result of muscle contraction.
- Specifically, eccentric contraction, which stretches a preloaded muscle, appears to play a substantial role in causing strains.
- The myotendinous junction is most often the site of muscle strains, although there is evidence that muscle strain can occur in the muscle fibers.[4]
- Muscles with a high content of fast-twitch muscle fibers (type II fibers) and muscles that cross two joints are most susceptible to strain.
- The hamstrings are at high risk for strain because of these two factors and the eccentric contractions that occur with running and deceleration in athletics.
- Strains are classified similar to sprains.
  - First-degree strains result in mild tenderness and pain with stretching.

- Second-degree strains involve partial tearing and subsequent muscle spasms.
- Third-degree strains result from complete tearing of the musculotendinous junction, at which point a palpable defect may be found through physical examination.

- With proper treatment, rapid recovery is expected and morbidity in young athletes is usually minimal.

Management

- Management of soft tissue injury includes rest, ice, compression, and elevation (RICE).
  - This first line of treatment should occur within the first 48-72 hours after the injury as it minimizes swelling and increases rate of recovery.
  - Resting protects the soft tissue structures from reinjury and helps to minimize swelling.
  - Ice helps to minimize swelling and discomfort and should be applied for 20 minutes intermittently throughout the day. Icing causes constriction, which diminishes bleeding and inflammation, helping to reduce edema and to relieve pain.
  - Compression controls edema by limiting compartment volume, increasing interstitial pressure, and reducing fluid transduction from the capillary bed.
    1. An elastic wrap or bandage should be applied from the end of the limb to well past the injured area.
    2. Ideally, the compression should be the most snug at the distal end of the limb and slightly less snug above the injury to enhance circulation.
    3. The fit should be not so tight that it causes swelling below the wrapped area.
  - Elevation assists in controlling edema by improving lymphatic and venous return from the injury site. The injured extremity should be elevated above the level of the heart until swelling resolves.
- Once soft tissues have responded to initial RICE, the rehabilitation phase of treatment is emphasized. Parents and coaches are counseled that although range of motion and strength are restored, the use of brief intervals of the RICE principles should be continued judiciously.

Chronic and Overuse Injuries Unique to Sports Medicine

- As sports specialization and competition has become more prevalent, training regimens have increased in intensity and duration with shorter rest periods during and between seasons. Although stress is normal for connective tissue development, excessive stress without intervening periods of rest can lead to soft tissue, chondral, and bone injuries.
- Injuries can occur in the unconditioned athlete with poor biomechanics of body alignment, technique, or both, and it can occur in the more highly conditioned athlete whose training regimen exceeds the limits of the musculoskeletal system.
- The patient's history of symptoms is essential in determining the cause of the injury. It is important to identify those factors leading to the development of symptoms, including training levels, environmental factors, and anatomical factors.
- Marked changes in the intensity, duration, or frequency of workouts may produce overuse syndromes.[5] Environmental factors such as equipment and playing surfaces should also be considered.
- Patients may describe pain with intensive activity, with lower levels of activity and training, or with activities of daily living.

Thrower's Shoulder

- The proximal humeral physis is susceptible to overstress, which may result in a fatigue fracture that widens the physis, called epiphysiolysis.[6]
- Although symptoms are frequently nonspecific, pain and aching with throwing is a common finding (Figure 7–1).

Imaging

- Radiographs are useful for imaging widening of the physis in fatigue-fractured shoulders.
- Using comparison views can prevent physicians from misreading the appearance of physeal widening in a normal shoulder as a result of projection.

Management

- Patients with tenderness at the proximal humeral physis but no physeal widening may be treated with 4 weeks of rest followed by strengthening and a gradual return to an activity program.
- Those with physeal widening on plain radiographs are recommended to refrain from throwing for 3 months.

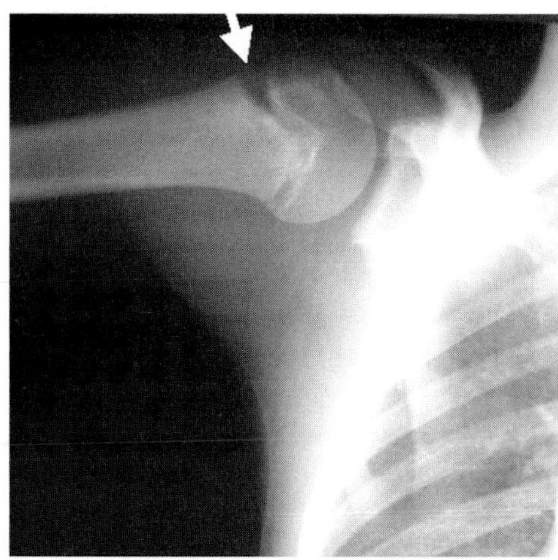

Figure 7–1: Shoulder radiograph of humeral epiphysiolysis as shown by the widened proximal humeral physis *(arrow)*.

- A progressive strengthening and interval-throwing program is then instituted.
- A study of thrower's shoulder demonstrated that 21 of 23 patients treated with an average rest of 3 months were subsequently asymptomatic.[7]
- Although some advocate limiting pitchers to no more than 6 innings per week with 3 days of rest between outings, others have advocated counting specifically the number of pitches per game and limiting players to 60-80 pitchers per game and 30-40 pitches per practice.
- Coaches and parents should also be advised to monitor players closely for changes in throwing mechanics, which may suggest fatigue.

Thrower's Elbow

- Thrower's elbow encompasses several conditions.
- It most commonly includes overstress of the medial elbow stabilizing structures and repetitive compression injury to the lateral radiocapitellar articulation.
- Overuse problems involving secondary ossification centers of the proximal ulna and distal humerus have been observed in throwing athletes.
  - Microtrauma to the medial chondral osseous structures is caused by repetitive forces on the medial aspect of the elbow resulting from the pull of the medial musculature.
  - This is manifest as a medial epicondyle apophysitis (inflammation of the developing chondroepiphysis) in the growing athlete. Medial epicondylitis (inflammation of the medial proximal flexor pronator mass) is found in the fully grown athlete.
  - Macrotraumatic acute fractures have also been demonstrated when adolescent athletes avulse part or all of the medial epicondyle.
- Repetitive compressive forces on a lateral side of the elbow may result in irregular fragmentation of the ossific nucleus of the capitellum in the form of osteochondritis dissecans (OCD) (Figure 7–2).
  - Physical findings include lateral pain and loss of motion.
  - Loose bodies from fragmentation of the capitellum may cause elbow joint locking.
- The forces experienced at the elbow during pitching have been described throughout each phase of the throwing motion.
  - Although there are several forces at work throughout the throwing motion, it has been observed that during the cocking phase significant tension is placed on the medial structures with compression laterally.
  - Although forces significantly neutralize during the acceleration phase, forearm pronation during a follow-through imparts both compression and sheering forces laterally with tension at the olecranon.
  - The repetitive force on the medial apophysis at the muscle insertion may produce subsequent inflammation.

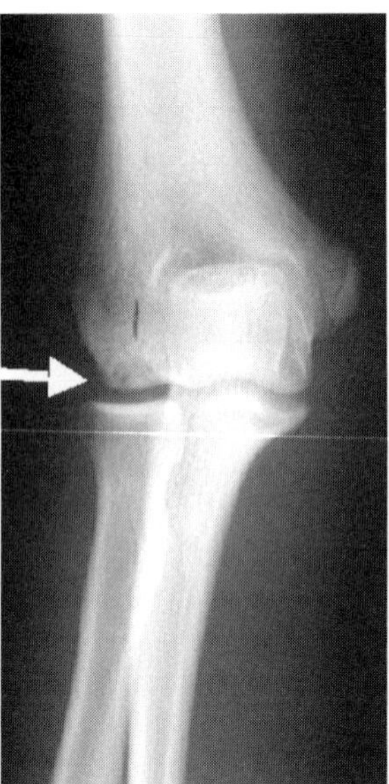

Figure 7–2: AP radiograph of the elbow radiolucency indicative of an OCD lesion *(arrow)* of the capitellum.

- Treatment of mild forms of medial epicondyle apophysitis consists of nonoperative measures, including splint use and rest.
- After 3 to 4 weeks of activity modification, a graduated rehabilitation program may be instituted followed by a throwing program after strength and flexibility have been restored.
- The most appropriate intervention for this and other overuse injuries in young athletes is prevention.

Gymnast's Wrist

- Chronic repetitive mechanical overload of the distal radius has been described in competitive gymnasts.
- The specific pathology ranges from discomfort without radiographic changes to disabling pain and mechanical symptoms secondary to altered anatomical and subsequent biomechanical changes at the wrist.
- Physeal damage may lead to permanent asymmetrical deformity at the wrist.
- Because approximately 80% of the compressive load across the wrist is transmitted through the radius, early recognition of this problem can allow treatment to decrease mechanical loads and thereby prevent physeal damage and deformity.
- Wrist pain and physeal damage correlates with the hours of training per week and the number of years of competition and level of competition.
- As competition and level of training increases, competitive gymnasts more frequently use their upper extremities to bear weight.
- Physeal injury at the distal radius may cause progression of radiographic changes including widening of the physes, with irregularity of metaphyseal margins, and haziness of the physis[8] (Figure 7–3).

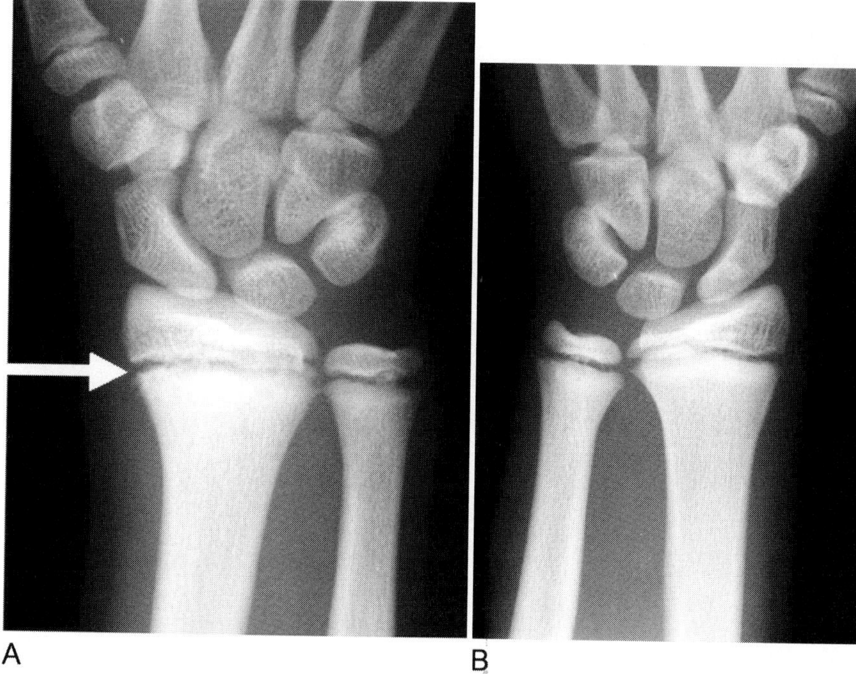

Figure 7–3: A, Physeal widening of the distal radial physis demonstrating a gymnast's wrist. B, Radiographic image of contralateral wrist with no physeal widening.

- Treatment consists of early recognition and activity modification to permit healing.
- Patients without radiographic changes have been noted to heal after 4 weeks. Those with radiographic changes have required 3 months of rest before becoming asymptomatic.[8]

Osgood-Schlatter Disease

- The most common overuse injury, which occurs at the knee of young athletes, is Osgood-Schlatter disease, an apophysitis at the anterior tibial tubercle.
- Although adults develop inflammation at the tendon, such as patellar tendonitis at the knee and lateral epicondylitis at the elbow, preteen and teenage athletes more commonly develop inflammation at the tendon–bone interface, such as the anterior tibial tubercle.
- Osgood-Schlatter disease commonly affects preteen girls and young teenage boys during periods of growth and can be noted bilaterally in some patients.
- Because 70% of the growth of the lower extremities occurs at the physis about the knee, young athletes can develop tight hamstrings and quadriceps.
- Symptoms include a painful prominence at the anterior proximal tibia and intermittent or constant pain with high-impact running or jumping sports, kneeling, and walking on stairs.
- Poor flexibility and high-impact sports are contributing factors for this condition.
- Osgood-Schlatter disease may significantly interfere with sports and, in more severe cases, activities of daily living.

Imaging

- Radiographs demonstrate fragmentation prominent at the anterior tibial tubercle, a consequence of the traction stress at this apophysis (Figure 7–4).

Management

- Patients are placed on a flexibility program to stretch the hamstrings and quadriceps, a straight leg raising exercise regimen to strengthen the quadriceps, and activity modification to eliminate sports when they are symptomatic. Patients are encouraged to follow a home regimen of daily maintenance stretching during their years of growth and development.
- This problem is almost universally resolved with growth plate closure. There are rare exceptions in patients who develop an ossicle at the anterior tibial tubercle, which may become symptomatic.
- Those rare skeletally mature patients with a persistently symptomatic ossicle at the tibial tubercle that has not responded to nonoperative measures, including activity modification and stretching, may have this fragment excised.

Sinding-Larsen-Johansson Syndrome

- Sinding-Larsen-Johansson syndrome is an apophysitis of the inferior pole of the patella, which is caused by chronic repetitive tension and overstress in the form of tension.
- Fragmentation in a small ossicle may be visualized at the inferior pole on anteroposterior (AP) and lateral radiographs.

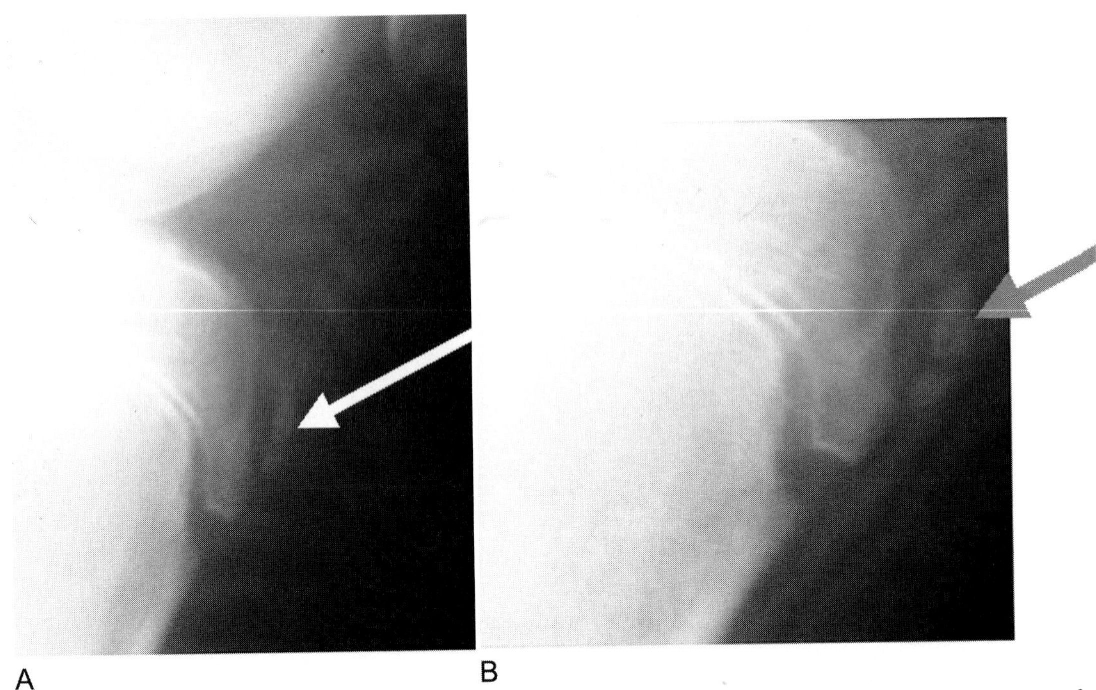

Figure 7–4: A, Plain radiograph. Fragmentation *(arrow)* is noted at the anterior tubercle. B, A closer view of Figure 7–4, *A*, showing the fragmentation *(arrow)* consistent with Osgood-Schlatter disease.

- The treatment of this condition is the same as that for Osgood-Schlatter disease.

Sever Disease

- Sever disease is an inflammation of the apophysis at the posterior aspect of the calcaneus (Figure 7–5).
- Patients with this condition tend to be younger than those with Osgood-Schlatter disease. These patients are primarily in the early phase of accelerated growth; they are most commonly 9 through 12 years but may be younger.
- Factors that contribute to Sever disease include a tight gastroc–soleus tendo Achillis complex and a tight plantar fascia. High-impact running and jumping sports such as basketball, soccer, and gymnastics that impart repeated loading on this growth center may cause pain in one or both heels.
  - Symptoms include swelling and tenderness at the insertion of the tendo Achillis into the posterior calcaneus and pain with running and jumping sports.
  - This pain tends to be most prominent during preseason and early season training, especially on hard playing surfaces in patients with poorly cushioned shoes.
  - Swelling and tenderness is limited to the location at the posterior heel and sometimes the distal aspect of the Achilles. These conditions are not associated with other pathological findings of the foot or ankle.
- Treatment recommendations include education and counseling about the nature and self-limiting condition of this process, activity modification including rest when symptoms appear, appropriate ice application, flexibility exercises, heel cushioning, and the use of a heel lift.
- Patients are encouraged to change their athletic footwear from cleats to turf shoes if they are playing on dry ground in an effort to eliminate a component of the sheering forces imparted on the posterior calcaneus.
  - Heel cups and other forms of shock absorbing insoles may be used to treat this condition.
  - Although insoles can secondarily help to improve patients' symptoms, of primary importance is activity modification and flexibility training.

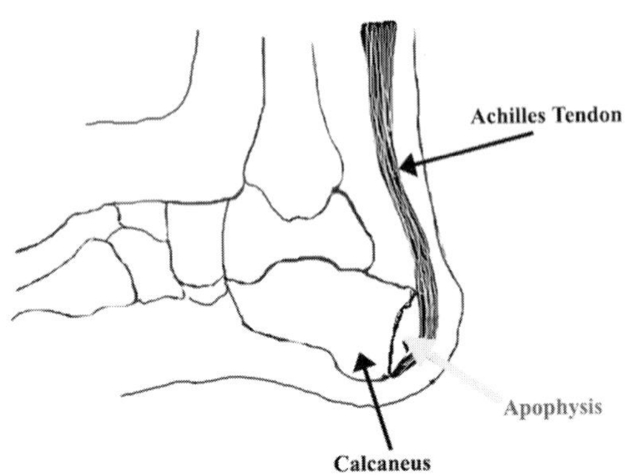

Figure 7–5: Ankle drawing demonstrating inflammation of apophysis *(gray arrow)* at the posterior aspect of the calcaneus results in Sever apophysitis.

- Symptoms usually resolve within a few weeks or occasionally months with appropriate treatment and without forms of immobilization. In those patients with refractory symptoms, several weeks of immobilization can relieve severe symptomatology, which can be followed by a formal therapy regimen.
- Radiographs are not required in routine cases but can be beneficial in ruling out other pathology, such as tumor, infection, or bone cyst at the ankle or the calcaneus in patients with refractory symptoms.
- Patients are also counseled about appropriate activities that they can continue to perform to maintain their fitness including, swimming, walking, and riding on a stationery bike. Patients are encouraged to maintain a home baseline stretching program after symptoms resolve to prevent recurrences, which can occur during periods of rapid growth.

Osteochondritis Dissecans

- OCD is an osteochondral lesion that affects the subchondral bone and overlying articular cartilage.
- With OCD, a fragment of bone or cartilage partially or completely separates from the joint surface (Figure 7–6, *A*).
- The fragment may stay in place in the bone in mild cases of OCD.
- However, in more severe cases, the fragment separates and falls into the joint.
- There are four stages of OCD describing the progression of the condition:
  - Stage I consists of a small area of subchondral edema.
  - Stage II consists of a partially detached fragment (Figure 7–7).
  - In stage III, a loose body is present.
  - By stage IV, the loose body is displaced.
  - This condition is most commonly found in teenagers ages 13-17, although it may occur in preteen and skeletally mature patients.
- OCD more commonly affects one joint, usually the knee, although multiple joint involvements have been reported.
- The elbow and ankle are less commonly affected followed by the shoulder, wrist, hand, and hip joints.
- The etiology of OCD is unknown, although trauma, interruptions in the local blood supply to the bone, uneven or excessive pressure, and genetic factors are all considered potential causes.
- OCD commonly occurs with generalized pain and sometimes swelling that increases with strenuous activity and twisting motions.
- The joint may become locked and the patient may complain of a sense of instability of the joint.

Imaging

- Radiographs may confirm the presence and location of OCD lesions (Figure 7–6, *B*).
- Magnetic resonance imaging (MRI) is useful for evaluation of the status of the overlying cartilage and the amount of subchondral edema, which helps the clinician to grade lesions and predict clinical outcome[9] (Figure 7–7).

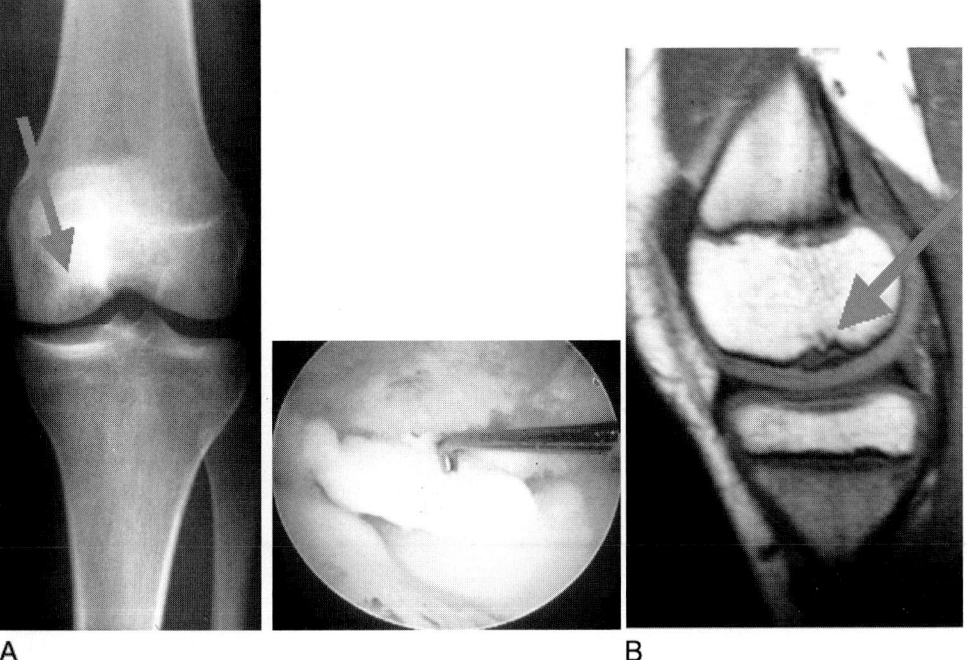

Figure 7–6: A, Plain radiograph *(arrow)* and arthroscopic picture showing full thickness defect in an OCD lesion. B, T1-weighted MRI showing a small intact OCD lesion *(arrow)*.

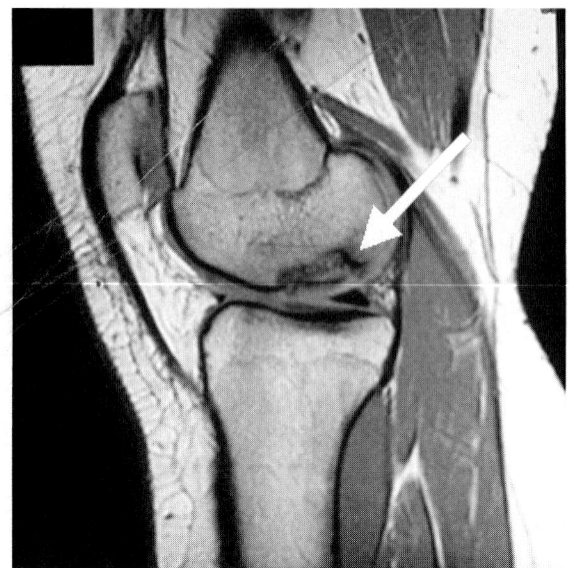

Figure 7–7: T1-weighted MRI of a femoral condyle OCD lesion.

Management

- OCD is usually treated by adjusting activity levels, which may include changing or stopping sports participation.
- Healing of OCD may be determined by follow-up x-ray films, at which point patients can return to normal activity levels.
- Older patients with closed growth plates tend to have worse prognosis.
- More severe cases may require immobilization with casts or braces.
- Patients that develop lesion fragmentation and mechanical symptoms, which do not improve or become worse despite nonoperative measures, may require surgical treatment to stimulate increased blood flow to the area or to remove or secure any loose pieces.
- Bone and cartilage grafting may be necessary in severe cases with loss of large fragments.[10]
- Following surgery, patients undergo a motion program and may or may not be allowed to return to preoperative activity levels.
- Treating OCD early and effectively often prevents recurrent symptoms in adulthood, although some severe lesions may be symptomatic later in life.

Acute Osteochondral Fractures

- Acute osteochondral fractures of the knee typically involved the medial or lateral femoral condyle or the patella.
- Like all acute sports injuries, there is an acute onset of symptoms with a well-defined event.
- According to Kennedy, there are two distinct mechanisms of injury, namely the exogenous and the endogenous.[11] A direct blow resulting in a shearing force to the femoral condyles is considered exogenous, and a flexion–rotation twist to the knee is deemed endogenous.
- Most pediatric patients with acute osteochondral fractures have a history of flexion–rotation injury consistent with patellar dislocation.
- A bloody effusion is almost always present.
- Tenderness to palpation in the medial or lateral femoral condyle or the medial patellar can be elicited.
- The knee joint is frequently held in slight flexion, and motion in any direction is restricted.

Imaging

- Osteochondral fractures can be difficult to identify on a plain film x-ray because a significant portion of the lesion is cartilage rather than calcified bone.
- Often, only a small defect is seen on a plain radiograph.
- A "tunnel" view may be helpful in evaluating the intercondylar notch.
- Arthrogram, computerized tomography (CT) scan, and MRI have also been used.

Management

- The treatment of these lesions is based on the size and origin of the fragment.
- In general, small fragments (<2 cm) at a non–weight-bearing area of the knee can be removed by an arthroscope.
- Fragments larger than 2 cm, especially when located at a weight-bearing area, may benefit from internal fixation.
- Small fragments from non–weight-bearing areas have the best prognosis.
- Potential complications include adhesions, quadriceps insufficiency, and hardware problems.

Stress Fractures

- Stress fractures following repetitive trauma are well documented in athletes such as runners, football players, gymnasts, and ballet dancers.
- Stress fractures have been described as spontaneous fractures of normal bone resulting from the summation of stresses, any of which by itself would be harmless[12] (Figure 7–8).
- The most common sites for a stress fracture in children are the proximal tibia followed by the distal fibula.[13]
- Sprints, hurdles, and jumps are associated with a significant number of injuries compared with those from other events.
- Professional female ballet dancers suffer most commonly from metatarsal fractures,[14] whereas ice skaters often suffer fractures in the distal fibula.
- Patients have localized pain during activity and may complain of dull aching, discomfort at rest, and tenderness at palpation of the affected area.

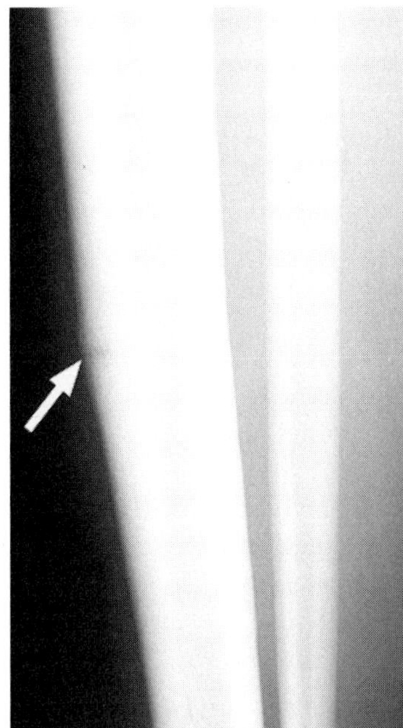

Figure 7–8: Cortical hypertrophy at the midanterior tibia with a horizontal radiolucency *(arrow)* indicative of a chronic tibial stress fracture.

Imaging

- Radiographs are helpful because they may demonstrate a radiolucent line suggestive of a stress fracture.
- A bone scan is usually most beneficial in obtaining a diagnosis in the extremities, and a single-photon emission CT scan is most precise when evaluating the spine.

Management

- Patients are typically treated with immobilization in a cast or brace followed by a progressive return to activity.
- The goal of treatment is to obtain complete healing by keeping patients pain-free for 2 to 3 months with immobilization followed by activity modification.

Acute Upper Extremity Injuries

Shoulder Dislocation

- Shoulder joint mobility allows the upper extremity to be moved correctly in space so that the hand can be in a desired location.
- Many static and dynamic mechanisms contribute to the stability of the glenohumeral joint.
- The bony constraint is limited to the shallow glenoid fossa, which is somewhat deepened by the labrum.
- The primary stabilizer is believed to be the capsular–ligamentous complex, and the four rotator cuff muscles serve as the dynamic secondary stabilizer that keeps the humeral head in place as the humerus moves through a full range of motion.
- In an anterior shoulder dislocation, the arm and shoulder are commonly forced into an abducted and externally rotated position as the humeral head is levered anteriorly over the glenoid.
- Posterior dislocations are much less common and probably represent about 2 to 4% of all dislocations.
- Immediately after the injury, there is pain and swelling around the shoulder.
- The humeral head can often be palpated anterior to the glenoid.
- The axillary nerve is most commonly injured. It provides sensory innervation to the lateral upper arm and motor function to the deltoid and the teres minor muscles.
- Generalized ligamentous laxity, if present, should be noted on clinical examination.

Imaging

- Radiographic assessment of shoulder dislocations in skeletally immature patients is similar to that made in the adult population (Figure 7–9).
- Although many radiographic techniques have been described, the basic trauma series should include a true AP view of the glenohumeral joint, the scapular Y-view, and an axillary view.
- An impression fracture at the posterolateral humeral head, commonly known as the Hill-Sachs lesion, can be seen with an internal rotation view of the proximal humerus.
- Should there be mechanical symptoms suggesting associated intra-articular pathology, such as a Hill-Sachs or labral injury with a shoulder dislocation or subluxation, further imaging should be performed.
- Arthrograms were commonly used in the past; however, they have been largely replaced by CT and MRI scans with cuts through the glenohumeral joint.

Management

- Acute dislocation of the shoulder should be reduced by one of the standard methods.

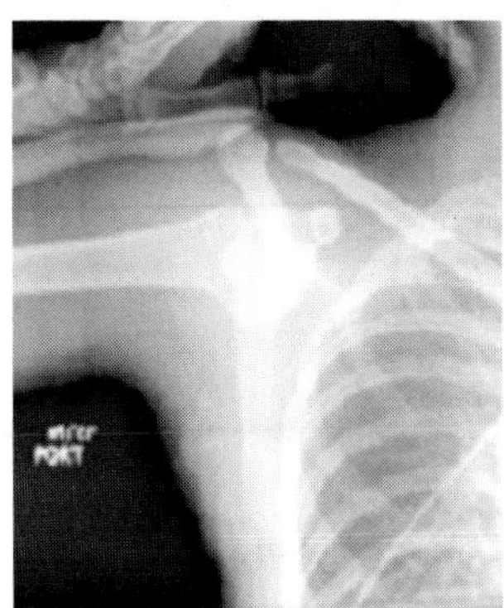

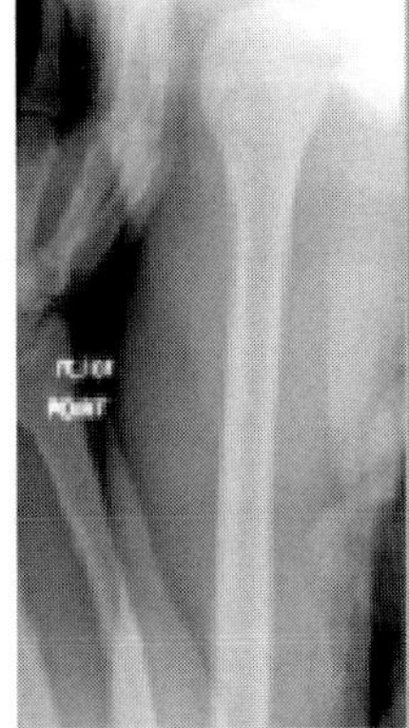

Figure 7–9: AP and axillary plain radiographs of a right shoulder anterior dislocation.

- Adequate sedation is essential for a successful closed reduction.
- Intra-articular injection of local anesthetic can be used as an adjunct and provides added postreduction analgesia.

- A commonly used technique involves traction and countertraction.[15]
  - An assistant pulling a sheet wrapped around the trunk of the patient at the level of the scapular body from the contralateral side provides countertraction while steady, continuous traction is applied to the affected arm.
  - As the muscle fatigues, spasms that lock the humeral head lessen allowing reduction of the shoulder joint with gentle manipulation.
  - The Stimson maneuver positions the patient prone with the ipsilateral arm hanging over the edge of the examination table.
  - Hanging weights from the affected upper extremity provide traction.
- Reduction then follows the principles described previously.
- After relocation, a plain film radiograph should be obtained to assess the adequacy of reduction.
- The arm is then placed in a sling for immobilization.
- The issue of operative intervention after an initial dislocation remains a topic of debate.
- Treatment should be tailored toward the individual patient and the goals of that patient in life.
- Similar to advances in knee surgery a decade ago, a greater understanding of the shoulder and its pathology has led to a refinement of surgical techniques and enthusiasm in minimally invasive operations.
- The incidence of recurrent dislocation after the first traumatic event is closely related to the energy of the initial insult, the soft tissue involvement, the age of the first dislocation, the activity level, and the overall ligamentous condition of the patient.
- Early range of motion prevents the formation of adhesion that compromises overall function of the upper extremity.
- Rehabilitation should also focus on scapular stabilization exercises and rotator cuff and deltoid strengthening to enhance the dynamic stabilizers of the shoulder joint.

Acromioclavicular Separation

- The acromioclavicular joint is a diarthrodial joint between the lateral clavicle and the acromion of the scapula.
- The primary stabilizer of the shoulder is the strong coracoclavicular ligament. In comparison, the acromioclavicular ligament is weaker and serves only as a secondary stabilizer.
- In sports activities, this joint can be injured during a violent fall.
- Typically, the scapula, and therefore the acromion, is driven inferiorly as the top of the shoulder strikes the ground.
- At the same time, the clavicle stays elevated and extended as the medial end remains attached to the sternoclavicular joint.
- The classification system of this injury is similar to the system used for adults.[15]
- Because of the thick periosteal sheath around the clavicle, dislocation in this area tends to split out of the periosteal tube, much like a banana being peeled out of its skin.
- Type I and II injuries may have only mild to moderate swelling and tenderness.
- The gross deformity is usually obvious with type III and V separation.
- Type IV injuries are probably the most frequently missed because the distal end of the clavicle can be buried inside the belly of the trapezius.
- Type VI injuries are rare, and the restriction in shoulder motion is usually remarkable.

Imaging

- Plain film radiographs are essential in determining correct diagnosis and eliminating associated fractures or dislocations.
- Stress views are obtained by hanging 5- to 10-lb weights to the injured upper extremity.
- Traction exaggerates any instability of the acromioclavicular joint in an AP view, and the contralateral side is filmed simultaneously for comparison.

Management

- In the pediatric population, type I, II, and III injuries can be expected to heal and remodel without major sequelae.
- Oftentimes, nothing more than a sling to support the weight of the upper extremity is required.
- Operative treatment with internal fixation is reserved for type IV, V, and VI injuries with gross displacement and deformity.
- After age 16, acromioclavicular separations may be true dislocations rather than periosteal splits and therefore may require more aggressive intervention in high-performance athletes.

Acute Lower Extremity, Sports-Specific Injuries

Pelvic Avulsion Fractures

- With an ever-increasing number of children and adolescents participating in sports activities, pelvic avulsion fractures are becoming more prevalent. These injuries are caused by sudden powerful contractions of a muscle pulling on a developing apophysis.
- Knowledge of the muscle origins and insertions around the pelvic area aids in the diagnosis.

- The sartorius muscle originates from the anterior–superior iliac spine, the direct head of the rectus femoris originates from the anterior–inferior iliac spine, and the hamstrings and adductors from the ischial tuberosity.
- Anterior–superior iliac spine avulsions and ischial avulsions are the most common, each accounting for about 30% of the total number of injuries[16] (Figure 7–10).
- Pulling of the sartorius, especially when it is stretched while the hip is extended and the knee is flexed, causes avulsion fractures of the anterior–superior iliac spine.
- Ischial avulsions are produced by contraction of the hamstrings in a similar manner.
- These injuries are commonly associated with gymnastics, football, and track.
- Although the apophyses of the ischium ossifies at age 15, it may not unite until age 25, making this diagnosis plausible even in young adults.
- Physical examination will elicit pain and localized swelling around the injured apophysis.

Imaging

- Although plain film radiographs may demonstrate gross displacement when present, more subtle changes can only be detected with comparison views of the contralateral side.[17]

Management

- Usually, the only treatment necessary for these injuries is a period of rest in the form of protected weight-bearing status.
- Positioning of the hip should limit stretching of the muscle involved, thus decreasing the amount of traction on the injured apophysis.

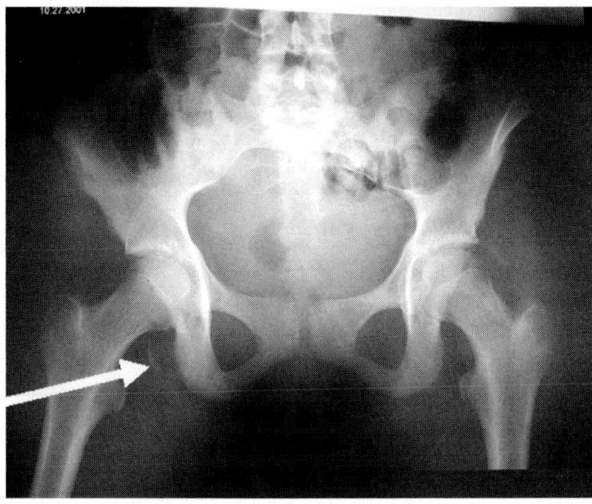

Figure 7–10: AP pelvis plain radiograph showing an ischial avulsion fracture *(arrow)*.

- The ability to bear weight is limited with crutches until appropriate callus is visible.
- Prognosis is usually excellent for a return to sports after complete healing and adequate rehabilitation.
- Occasionally, excessive callous formation that is symptomatic needs to be excised surgically.

Patellar Dislocation

- The patella is a sesamoid bone, which increases the mechanical advantage of the extensor mechanism of the knee joint.
- Because the quadriceps muscle pull is not perfectly in line with the tracking of the patella in the femoral grove, there is a tendency for the patella to displace laterally.
- Patellar dislocation is relatively common in children and is more common in females than in males.
- Patellar dislocation should be considered in all athletic injuries to the knee, especially if a sizable effusion is present.
- Pain is diffuse but typically severe at the medial side of the knee.
- Retinacular tear causes hemarthrosis, which can also be a result of an osteochondral fracture.

Imaging

- Radiographs should be obtained to delineate the exact location of the patella and to rule out osteochondral fractures.
- A merchant view reveals the position of the patella within the femoral groove when the knee is flexed 30 degrees.
- MRI can also reveal patellar dislocations (Figure 7–11).

Management

- Rarely seen is the acutely dislocated patella that remains in the displaced position.
- Usually, the patella reduces spontaneously with knee extension. The physician must reduce acute dislocations that do not reduce spontaneously.
- Under adequate sedation and analgesia, the hip is flexed to relax the quadriceps muscle.

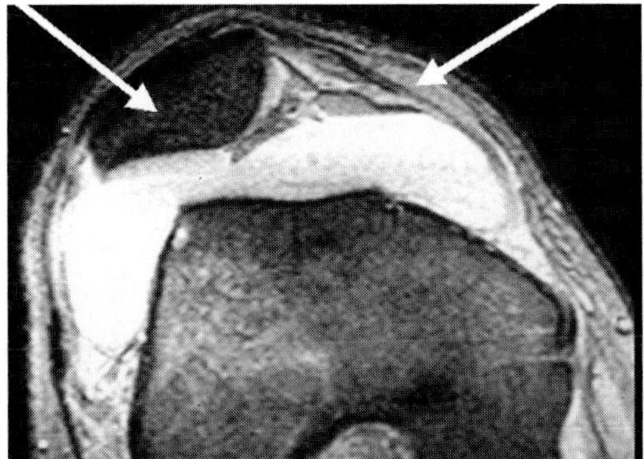

Figure 7–11: T2-weighted MRI of a knee following a patellar dislocation with a torn medial retinaculum *(right arrow)* and a lateral patellar tilt and translation *(left arrow)*.

- With the knee gradually extended, the patella can usually be pushed back in place.
- The knee is then usually immobilized by a cast or a knee immobilizer for 2 to 4 weeks.
- Surgical management should be reserved for children who fail nonoperative measures with debilitating subluxations or dislocations.
- Many procedures have been described for treatment of patellar instability. Most approaches use isolated or combined proximal or distal realignment, lateral releases, and medial reefing.
- Rehabilitation following an isolated dislocation or following surgery should focus on progressive strengthening of the quadriceps muscles, in particular the vastus medialis obliques, and on range of motion exercises.
- About one in six pediatric patellar dislocations develops into a recurrent dislocation.
- The first line of management is aggressive physical therapy after the initial inflammation and swelling subside.
  - Bracing with a neoprene knee sleeve and lateral patellar supports can be helpful.
  - Patients should also be counseled on activity modification.
  - High-risk activities include jumping, pivoting, and twisting sports.
  - More appropriate exercises include walking, biking, swimming, and light jogging.

Patellar Fractures

- Fractures of the patella after a direct blow to the patella rarely occur.
- A variant of patella fracture seen primarily in the pediatric patient is the sleeve fracture, in which the infrapatellar tendon avulses a fragment of bone from the inferior pole of the patella with articular cartilage.
- When displacement is minimal with a functioning extensor mechanism, patella fractures are typically treated nonoperatively with immobilization in extension.
- Displaced fractures and inability to actively extend the knee indicate a need for operative reduction and fixation using a tension band technique.

Meniscal and Ligament Injuries

Meniscal Injuries

- The menisci arise from the intermediate zone of mesenchyme between the distal femur and the proximal tibia.
- The semilunar appearance is formed by the tenth week of gestation.
  - As growth continues, the menisci increase in size but remain the same shape.
  - They primarily transmit and distribute loads across the articular surfaces.
- Meniscal tears are much less common in children than in adults.
- The mechanism of injury is typically rotation as the flexed knee is extended.
- Pain is present in most patients, and a knee effusion may be found.
- Positive physical findings may include a knee effusion, a joint line tenderness, and a painful click with knee flexion and circumduction maneuvers, such as the McMurray's test.[18]

Imaging

- Plain film x-rays should be obtained to rule out other occult pathology. MRI can be helpful in patients with equivocal findings (Figure 7–12, *A*).

Management

- Many techniques for meniscal repair have been described, such as open or arthroscopic-assisted partial resection or repair (Figure 7–13).
- Their success is largely based on the blood supply to the area, with peripheral vascular zone tears having a better prognosis than central tears.
- Repairable lesions are considered vertical tears through the meniscosynovial junction or in the most peripheral one third of the meniscus because the remainder of the meniscus is not sufficiently vascular to heal following repair.[19]
- Data suggests the development of degenerative changes after total meniscosynovial.
- Recommendations include cast immobilization for small peripheral tears (<1 cm), repair of large peripheral tears, and limited partial meniscectomy for tears that cannot be repaired, preserving as much healthy meniscus as possible.
- Knee motion should be restricted using a brace or a cast for 6 weeks after meniscus repair.

Discoid Lateral Meniscus

- Discoid lateral meniscus is a cause of "snapping knee" and, when torn, can be a cause of locking and knee pain in children.
- This is because of an abnormally thick meniscus covering a large percentage of the tibial surface, which is thought to be caused congenitally.
  - Its incidence varies from 1.5 to 15.5%, occurring almost exclusively in the lateral compartment of the knee.[20,21]
  - On rare occasions, the discoid meniscus may occur on the medial side of the knee.
- Watanabe's system classifies the discoid meniscus into three groups—complete, incomplete, and Wrisberg variant—based on the amount of tibial surface covered by

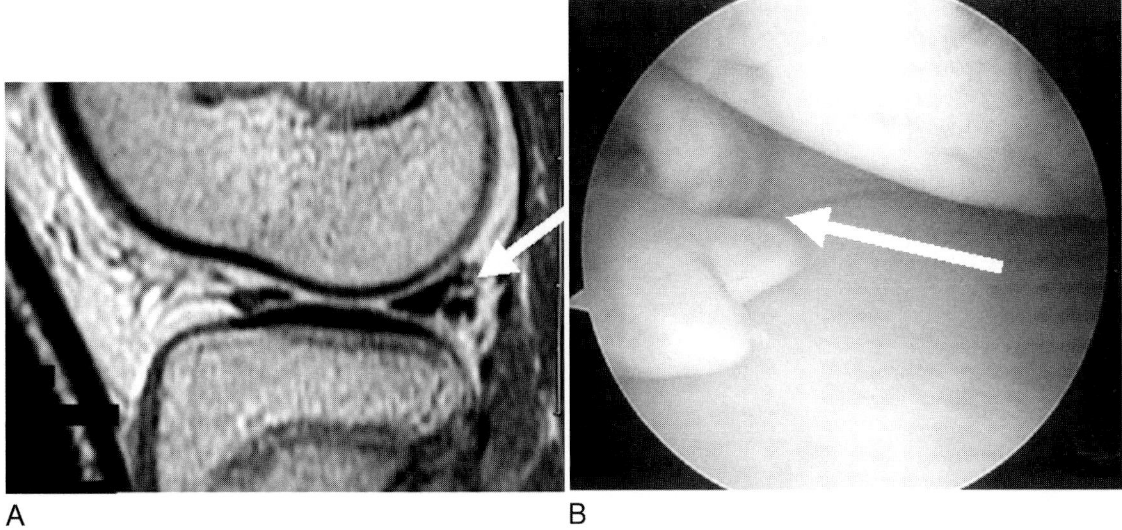

Figure 7–12: Photographs of medial meniscus tear. A, T1-weighted sagittal MRI demonstrating a meniscus tear *(arrow)*. B, Arthroscopic photograph of a meniscus tear *(arrow)*.

the meniscus and whether the meniscus has normal posterior horn attachments.

- Both the complete and incomplete types of discoid meniscus have normal posterior horn attachments.
- The complete type covers the entire tibial surface; the incomplete type covers only a portion of the tibial surface.
- The Wrisberg type lacks normal posterior horn attachments and is bounded posteriorly to the medial femoral condyle only by the meniscofemoral ligament, the ligament of Wrisberg.[20,21]

- In children and adolescents, the most common symptom is pain.

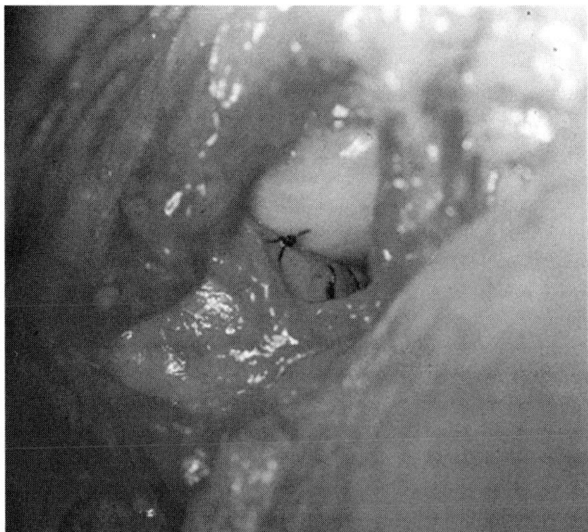

Figure 7–13: Photograph of a meniscus repair of the knee repaired through an open incision.

- The onset of knee pain may be associated with a traumatic event; more often it has an insidious onset.
- Children may describe mechanical symptoms such as locking, catching, clicking, or the knee giving way.

- The classic snapping knee usually appears in children and is associated commonly with the Wrisberg variant discoid meniscus.
  - Patients with the classic snapping knee describe an audible snap as the knee extends from a flexed position.
  - The symptoms are attributed to the trapped meniscus reducing with knee extension.
  - On physical examination, the patient has joint line tenderness.
  - There may be signs such as decreased range of motion, quadriceps atrophy, and knee effusion.
  - Provocative tests may reveal a positive McMurray test.[22]

Imaging

- Diagnostic imaging modalities useful in the evaluation of the discoid meniscus include plain radiographs—which are often obtained at initial patient presentation and usually appear normal in cases of discoid meniscus—and MRI.
- Occasionally, radiographs reveal widening of the lateral joint space and squaring of the lateral femoral condyle.
- MRI has become the imaging modality of choice for confirming a diagnosis of discoid meniscus (Figure 7–14).
- An MRI study that displays continuity between the anterior and the posterior meniscal horns on three consecutive sagittal images signifies a discoid meniscus.
- Other MRI characteristics seen in the presence of a discoid meniscus are a transverse diameter greater than 15 mm at the midbody and a difference between medial and lateral meniscal height of at least 2 mm.[23]

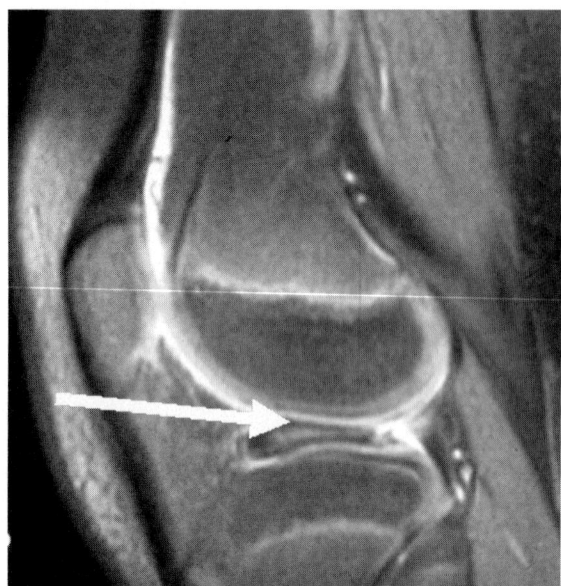

Figure 7–14: T2-weighted sagittal MRI of a discoid meniscus showing increased signal intensity indicative of intrasubstance degeneration and delamination.

Management

- The treatment approach varies according to Watanabe meniscal type and the presence of any coexisting knee pathology.
- Traditionally, an asymptomatic discoid meniscus requires no intervention as long as there is no clinical evidence suggesting meniscal pathology and there are no signs of meniscal hypermobility.
- The treatment approach for the discoid meniscus consists initially of rest, activity modification, and quadriceps and hamstrings strengthening.
- A complete or incomplete discoid meniscus with evidence of meniscal degeneration and meniscal tear or meniscal hypermobility that has failed conservative management requires surgery.
- Loose fragments of meniscus-causing symptoms necessitate removal with meniscoplasty performed along the remaining meniscal substance to form a more normal-appearing meniscal rim.
- Symptomatic complete and incomplete types are often treated with partial or total meniscectomy.
- Although total meniscectomy for the symptomatic Wrisberg variant has been advocated, peripheral reattachment for the symptomatic Wrisberg variant is recommended.

Anterior Cruciate Ligament Tear

- Children with anterior cruciate ligament (ACL) injuries constitute a unique patient population because of their open growth plates and differing ligamentous and bone strength.
- Significant attention is paid to this topic because damage to a child's open physes may potentially cause angular deformity, limb length inequality, condylar dysplasia, and subsequent functional limitations.
- Generalizations regarding all ACL injuries in the pediatric population should not be made because children grow at different rates. Therefore, one patient at a given age may be prepubescent with significant growth remaining and another at the same age may be nearing skeletal maturity.
- The ACL functions as a primary stabilizer to anterior tibial translation.
- The mechanisms of ACL injury in children and in adults are similar, resulting from knee twisting, a blow to the knee, or knee hyperextension when the foot is planted on the ground.
  - Usually, a "pop" is heard or felt by the patient and a hemarthrosis follows.
  - Giving way is a common presenting complaint, as are sudden swelling of the injured knee, knee hemarthroses, a feeling of knee instability, or inability to bear weight on the leg.
- Upon physical examination, increased anterior tibial translation can be appreciated by either the Lachman test (with the knee tested at 30 degrees of flexion) or the anterior draw test (with the knee tested at 90 degrees of flexion). It is important to ensure that the thigh muscles, especially the hamstrings, are relaxed during these provocative tests; false negatives can result because of tensed muscles that prevent movement of the tibia relative to the femur.
- Some children may have congenital ACL deficiencies, which may represent the absence of ACL or constitutional laxity. In addition, physiological laxity is often seen in the prepubescent knee, which can mislead the clinician. Therefore, it is essential that the uninvolved knee is examined in all children with knee laxity.

Imaging

- A plain film radiographic study including AP, lateral, tunnel, and patella radiographs can rule out tibial eminence fractures, osteochondral fractures, and other bony damage.
- MRI may delineate other internal derangement of the knee, such as occult fractures, and may determine the extent of soft tissue damage of the ACL and other supporting structures, including the menisci (Figures 7–12, *A,* and 7–15).

Management

- The treatment of ACL tears in the pediatric population revolves around the issue of skeletal age and how to address the open physis where approximately 65% of lower extremity growth occurs.
- To select a treatment plan for the pediatric patient, it is necessary for the examiner to accurately evaluate the

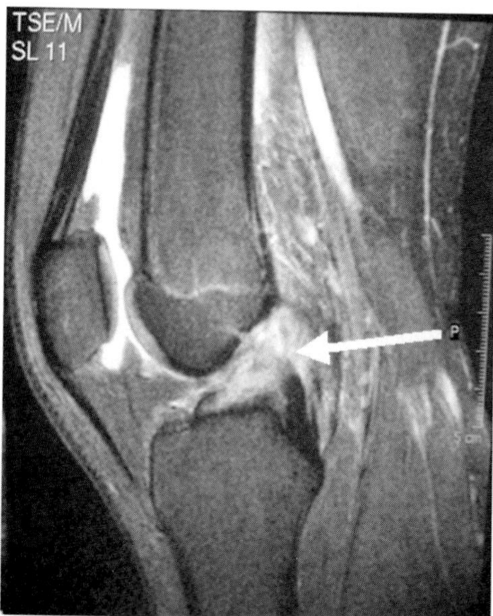

Figure 7–15: T2-weighted sagittal MRI of an ACL rupture (arrow).

child's skeletal age and remaining growth to avoid physeal and epiphyseal growth disturbances and subsequent angular deformity, leg length discrepancy, and condylar dysplasia.

- Several factors are helpful in determining skeletal age, including the following:
  - Bone evaluation by wrist radiographs according to Greulich and Pyle[24]
  - Secondary sex characteristics
  - Patient and familial height
  - Recent foot growth
- Based on these factors, an informed decision can be made by the physician regarding risk to the growth plates.
  - Nonoperative treatments include muscle strengthening, bracing, activity modification, and counseling.
  - Nonsurgical treatment of ACL tears in skeletally immature patients has characteristically led to recurrent instability and further meniscal damage, with a poor outlook for returning patients to previous athletic levels.[25-28] This is why extra-articular and intra-articular surgical options have received more attention recently.
  - In addition, because children may not comply with activity restrictions, understanding of the severity and nature of their injury may be lacking, or both, nonoperative management is less likely to be successful.
  - Bracing alone is not sufficient to allow patients to return to sports without restriction.
  - Complete ACL tears require surgery to reconstruct the ligament.
- The goal of operative reconstruction should include establishment of a stable joint, prevention of the internal soft tissue damage that results from recurrent instability, and return to sports activities.
- Intra-articular reconstruction with either an autograft (e.g., part of the patellar tendon or hamstring) or an allograft (e.g., the Achilles tendon) fixed in bone tunnels in the proximal tibia and distal femur is a common practice for skeletally mature adults.
- In patients with wide-open physis around this area, growth arrest becomes a concern with the adult technique. A debate remains regarding the age and maturity level at which it is safe to drill across open physes. Extraphyseal procedures aim at working around the open physis to produce knee stability and may have a role in treating skeletally immature patients. These procedures have achieved mixed results.[29]
- Patients with a nearly but not completely closed physis can be treated with an intra-articular soft tissue graft placed across the physis (Figure 7–16).
- Patients usually are able to return to an unrestricted activity level in approximately 6 months once the clinician determines that the knee is fully rehabilitated and strengthened.

Tibial Spine and Tibial Tuberosity Fractures

Tibial Spine (Eminence) Fractures

- In young children, bone fails before ligaments under tensile or shear stresses.
- This helps to explain why ACL injuries in children frequently involve a breach in the bone at the tibial spine (Figure 7–17), where the ACL inserts, as compared with a midsubstance tear in older adolescents.[29,30]

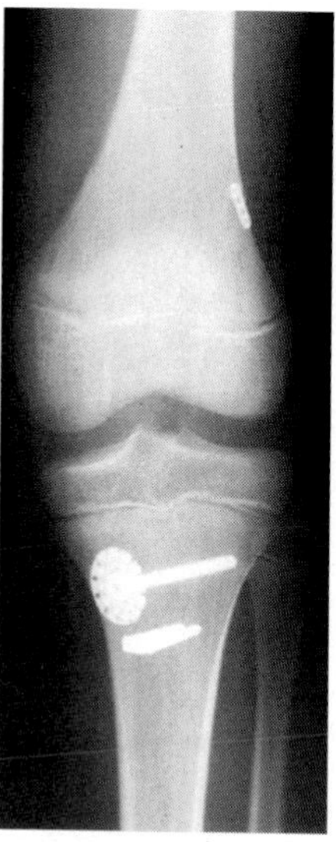

Figure 7–16: Plain AP radiograph of a transphyseal soft tissue ACL reconstruction with fixation near the femoral growth plate and far from the tibial growth plate.

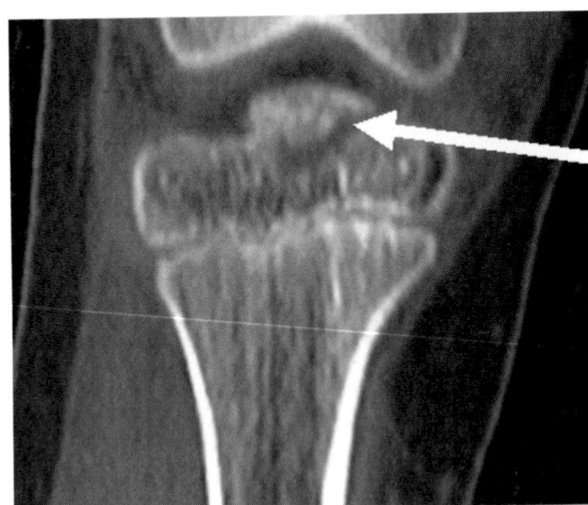

Figure 7–17: **Minimally displaced tibial spine fracture** *(arrow)*.

- The association of tibial eminence avulsion with collateral ligament and meniscal damage underscores the importance of a thorough examination and evaluation of all imaging studies.
- These fractures occur with valgus rotational stress on the knee or occasionally hyperflexion and result in an impressive hemarthrosis.
- The tibial eminence fracture may be nondisplaced, hinged, or displaced (Figure 7–18). Meyers and McKeever classified fractures of the intercondylar eminence into three types in 1970.[31]
  - Zaricznyj later added a fourth type to this classification system.[16]
  - Type I fractures have minimal or no displacement.
  - Type II fractures display a partially attached portion of the tibial eminence.

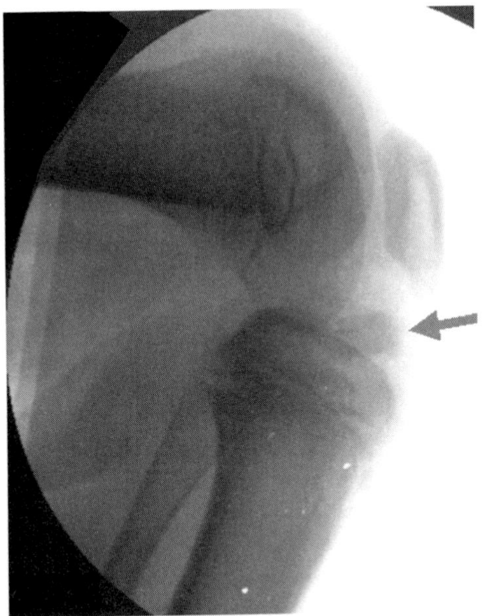

Figure 7–18: **Hinged displaced tibial spine fracture** *(arrow)*.

  - Type III fractures are characterized by complete displacement of a bony fragment that may be rotated.
  - Type IV fractures are comminuted.
- Anatomical reduction should be the goal of treatment.
- With type I and II injuries, reduction can usually be achieved by aspiration of the bloody effusion followed by casting of the knee in full extension.
- Postmanipulation x-ray films should be obtained to confirm the adequacy of reduction.
- Type III and IV fractures routinely require open reduction and internal fixation with metal pins, wires, or screws, depending on the preferences and level of comfort of the surgeon.[32]
- Even with perfect reduction and fracture healing, residual laxity can result because of plastic deformation or stretching of the ACL under excessive load before fracture of the bone occurs.

Tibial Tubercle Fractures

- Avulsion of the tibial tubercle at the attachment of the infrapatellar tendon is found primarily in patients 14–16 years old.
- Open reduction and internal fixation are necessary if the fracture is displaced or occurs at the level of the physis.
- Nondisplaced or minimally displaced fractures may be treated with a cast in extension.

Ankle Fractures and Sprains

Ankle Injuries of the Young Athlete

- The ankle is one of the most frequently damaged structures in adolescents.
- The ankle is the most commonly injured body part among athletes of all ages.
- In adolescents, the ankle is also the most common site of physeal injuries.
- The effect of these injuries may become more predominant as sport participation among young athletes increases.
- Structures important to lateral ankle stability include the peroneus longus and brevis tendons, which provide stability, and the calcaneal fibular (anterior and posterior) ligaments, which provide static support.
  - The primary medial stabilizing structure is the deltoid ligament with less contribution from the tibialis posterior, flexor digitorum longus, and flexor hallucis longus tendons.
  - Ankle morphology also contributes to ankle stability.
  - The wider anterior portion of the talus is well seated within the mortise when the foot is in dorsiflexion, providing stability in this position.
- Inversion injuries occur to the ankle more easily with the foot plantar flexion because the talus is narrower posteriorly.

- The anterior talar fibula ligament is taut during plantar flexion. It is, therefore, more susceptible to injury than the calcaneal fibular and posterior talar fibular ligaments.
- The patient should be asked about the position of the ankle and the direction of forces at the time of the injury. This history can provide information about the most likely type and location of injury.
  - A history of deformity, swelling or inability to bear weight immediately following an injury may be suggestive of a more severe ligamentous injury or fracture.
  - A history of underlying illnesses, previous ankle injuries, or underlying pathology of the foot and ankle—such as pes planus or cavus, tarsal coalition, or clubfoot—may influence the patient's evaluation and treatment. These should, therefore, be noted.
- An evaluation of lower extremity pain in skeletally immature patients should involve an evaluation of hip range of motion, which can prevent the examiner from missing a slipped capital femoral epiphysis or other disorders.[33]
- Severely limited and painful hip range of motion, especially restricted to one side, is an indication for AP and lateral hip radiographs.
- If examination of the hips, knees, and contralateral ankle is unremarkable, the examination can be focused on the affected ankle and lower leg.
- Deformity and location of swelling and ecchymosis at the ankle should be noted.
- The physis, located within 2 cm of the most distal tip of the tibia and fibula, should be palpated.
- An acute inversion injury strongly suggests a growth plate fracture if tenderness and swelling are noted over the physis.
- Lateral ankle sprain is a less common injury in more immature patients and is found in patients with a physical examination of severe isolated tenderness over the lateral ligamentous complex.
- Eversion injuries are rare secondary to the strength of the deltoid ligament and the bony configuration of the ankle and to the orientation of the foot at heel strike.
- Immediate tenderness and swelling, however, may occur following eversion injuries and can be associated with a fracture.
- Patients are encouraged to perform active range of motion including dorsiflexion, plantar flexion, inversion, and aversion.
- Because significant variability in motion and laxity is present in young patients, an evaluation of the contralateral ankle provides a basis for comparison.
- A helpful test to evaluate the status of the ankle's ligamentous structures, commonly positive in adolescents with closed physes, is the anterior drawer test.
  - This tests the ligamentous stability with the patient's knee in slight flexion and the ankle in 30 degrees of plantar flexion. The patient's heel is grasped, and a forward pull is placed on the foot while the tibia is maintained in a fixed position.
  - Significant side-to-side difference suggests a tear of the anterior talofibular ligament.
  - Patients experiencing severe discomfort that tends to come immediately or shortly after an inversion ankle injury may not tolerate passive range of motion testing or anterior drawer testing.

Imaging

- Several guidelines including Ottawa ankle rules are used to recommend radiographs if the patient feels pain in specific locations around the foot and ankle.
- These findings include pain and bone tenderness at the posterior edge of the lateral medial malleolus, midfoot pain with tenderness at the base of the fifth metatarsal, pain in the area of the midfoot, or an inability to bear weight.
- It should be noted that Ottawa ankle rules do not universally apply to patients with open physes.
- We recommend obtaining radiographs, including AP, lateral, and mortise views of patients with significant ankle pain, tenderness, and inability to bear weight or of patients who can bear weight but limp.[34]

Management

- Using the Salter-Harris classification of growth plate injuries, rapid healing following simple reduction is the rule in type I and II ankle fractures. This rapid healing is partly because of the thick periosteal sleeve found in patients with open physes.
- Type III and IV injuries are intra-articular.
- Open reduction and internal fixation are often indicated to restore a smooth joint surface.
- Surgery is also recommended to prevent displacement of the growth plate that can lead to physeal arrest or growth disturbance.[35]
- Ankle rehabilitation varies based on the severity of the injury.
  - Regardless of injury severity, a functional rehabilitation program is more efficient than early surgical intervention for restoring comfort, strength, and function.
  - Skeletally immature persons are permitted to progressively bear weight using lateral and medial stabilizing supports with a 48- to 72-hour period of RICE.
  - We recommend 2 weeks in a short leg weight-bearing cast for children with severe sprains with marked swelling and limited motion.
  - Protective weight-bearing status is followed by a rehabilitation program focusing on restoring ankle range of motion, strength, balance, agility, and endurance.

- Initially a general active and pain-free range of motion will help to reduce stiffness and pain.
- In patients with markedly diminished resistance, ankle exercises with elastic tubing and toe raises may be instituted.
- Rehabilitation is not complete until strength and proprioception are fully restored and sports-specific and functional activities have been completed.
- Bracing and taping may help patients in terms of comfort and may provide appropriate receptive feedback. However, these are no substitute for appropriate physical rehabilitation.
- Ultimately the rehabilitation program should focus on restoring ankle range of motion, strength, balance, agility, and endurance.

Tillaux and Triplane Fractures

- Tillaux and triplane fractures are seen in patients with partially closed growth plates. As the distal tibial physis closes from central to medial and then to lateral, there exists a transitional period during adolescence in which the growth plate is fused medially but not laterally, making this the only part vulnerable to injuries.
- The Tillaux fracture is a type III injury involving the anterolateral segment of the distal tibial epiphysis. In this injury pattern, the anterior tibiofibular ligament avulses the unfused lateral tibial epiphysis when the foot is externally rotated (Figure 7–19).
- Reduction is therefore achieved by internally rotating the foot relative to the tibia and applying direct pressure over the avulsed epiphyseal fragment.
- Open reduction with internal fixation would be indicated if an intra-articular step-off persists after closed means.
- CT scan is a valuable tool to evaluate the articular surface after manipulation. If the reduction is deemed adequate, it can be treated with a long leg cast for 3 weeks followed by a short leg walking cast for 3 weeks.
- The triplane fracture is so named because the injury has coronal, sagittal, and transverse components. It can be viewed as a Tillaux fracture with a Salter-Harris type II extension to the posterior distal metaphysis of the distal tibia.
- The typical radiographic hallmark of this injury has the appearance of a Salter-Harris type III injury on the AP view, as seen in Tillaux fractures, with the Salter-Harris type II component visible only on the lateral view (Figure 7–20).
- Copperman described a reduction technique by internally rotating the foot for a slightly displaced, two-part triplane fracture.[35]
- As with Tillaux fractures, CT scan should follow all closed reduction to delineate the extent of the joint involvement, and surgery is recommended if a residual articular step-off is found. Otherwise, it can be treated with a long leg non–weight-bearing cast for 3 to 4 weeks followed by a short leg cast for another 3 to 4 weeks.

Fifth Metatarsal Fractures and Midfoot Sprains

- Fifth metatarsal fractures are categorized into types based on whether the fracture is located at the tuberosity or within the metatarsal shaft (Figure 7–21).
- Older patients tend to suffer tuberosity fractures more than younger patients, who are more likely to have shaft fractures.

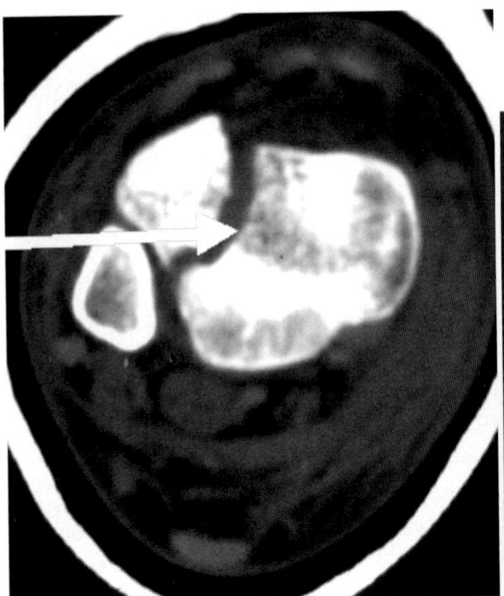

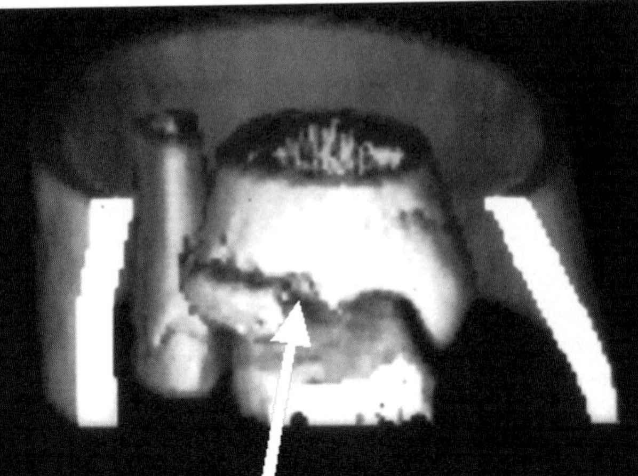

Figure 7–19: CT scans of a juvenile Tillaux fracture *(arrows)*.

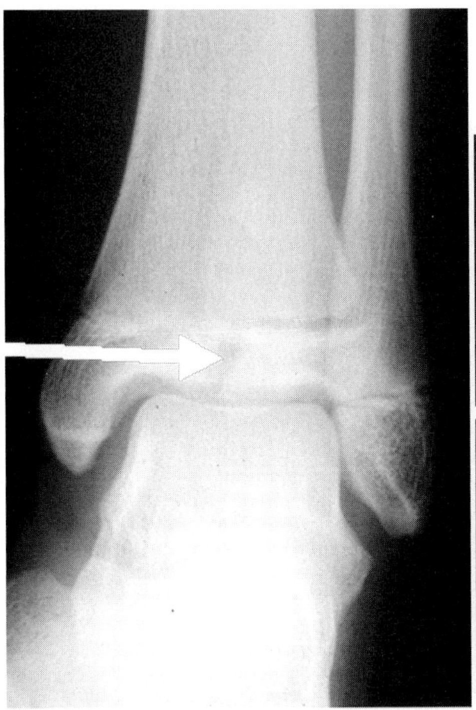
A

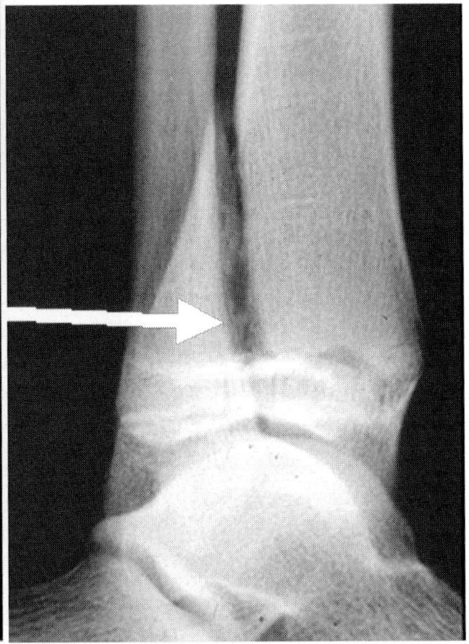
B

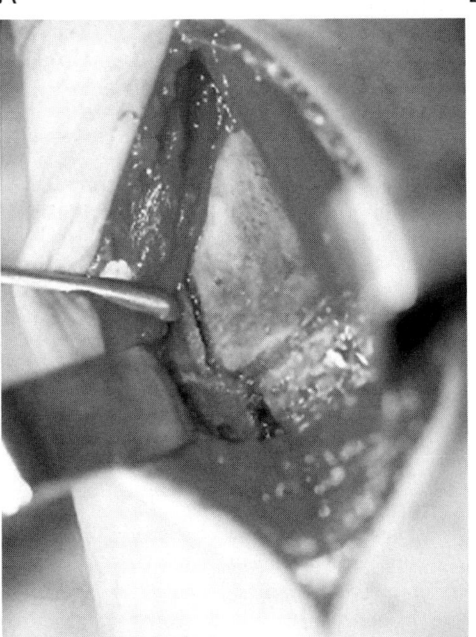
C

Figure 7–20: A, Plain AP radiograph of a triplane fracture. B, Plain sagittal radiograph of the triplane fracture. C, Operative picture of a triplane fracture through the growth plate.

- These injuries generally occur in patients 15 years or older.
- Patients younger than 15 years tend to sustain a proximal apophyseal separation rather than a true fracture.
- It is important to differentiate between a stress reaction as a result of trauma and an acute metatarsal fracture.[12]
- Nonoperative treatment is standard for most patients suffering fifth metatarsal fractures.

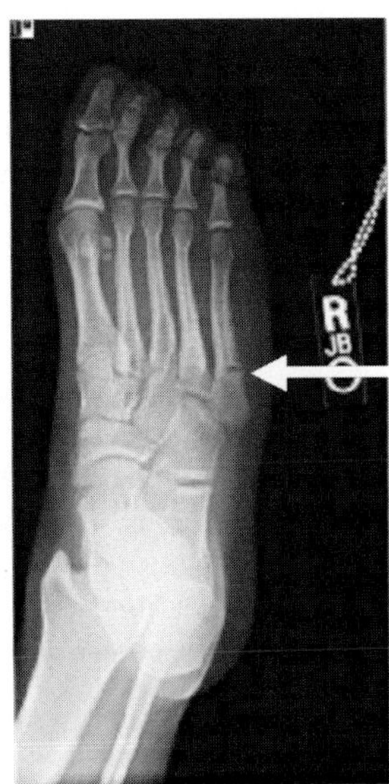

Figure 7–21: Oblique radiograph of a right foot Jones fracture *(arrow)* at the base of the fifth metatarsal.

- Most patients are immobilized in a short leg cast without bearing weight.
- If the patient does not show healing, operative treatment by percutaneous compression screw insertion is advised.
- Complications associated with this fracture type include delayed union, nonunion, and, rarely, refracture after union.[35]

Conclusions

- Exercise and athletic activity is beneficial to every child and adolescent. They facilitate the following:
  - Weight control
  - Strong bones
  - Improved cardiovascular risk factors
  - Mental health
- Athletic involvement is a sound and largely risk-free investment in the present and future health of children and adolescents.
- Sports instill the values of teamwork and lifelong habits of exercising.
  - Physicians must be aware of the injuries and injury patterns that often occur in young athletes and must recognize that various childhood sequelae may manifest as exertion and agility demands increase with higher levels of competition.
- The goal of practicing safe, enjoyable activities to promote a lifelong habit of good health and fitness is attainable for virtually all youngsters.

References

1. Ganley TJ, Pill SG, Flynn JM, Gregg JR (2001) Pediatric sports medicine. Curr Opin Ortho 12: 456-461.

2. Flynn JM, Lou JE, Ganley TJ (2002) Prevention of sports injuries in children. Curr Opin Pediatr 14(6): 719-722.
   Safety guidelines and protective equipment are crucial to minimizing pediatric recreational injuries. Combined with appropriate physical activity programs, nutrition is essential in battling, the increasing epidemic of childhood obesity. Specific training for the female pediatric athlete may have a preventive effect in halting the rising injury rates.

3. Lou JE, Ganley TJ, Flynn AJ (2002) Exercise and children's health. Curr Sports Med Rep 1(6): 349-353.
   This article describes current literature regarding exercise and its effects on children's health, including nutrition and cardiovascular issues. It also reviews the epidemiology and treatment of injuries in young athletes, including preventative measures.

4. Tidball JG, Chan M (1989) Adhesive strength of single muscle cells to basement membrane at myotendinous junctions. J Appl Physiol 67(3): 1063-1069.
   These findings suggest that, in muscle strain injuries that occur under conditions simulated here, failure occurs at myotendinous junctions unless the muscle has suffered previous compression injury leading to failure within the muscle.

5. Ganley, T (2000) Exercise and children's health: The pediatric athlete. Phys Sports Med 28(2): 85-97.

6. Ganley TJ, Spiegel DA, Gregg JR, Flynn JM (1998) Overuse injuries to the physes in young athletes: A clinical and basic science review. U Penn Orthop J II: 36-39.

7. Brighton CT (1978) Structure and function of the growth plate. Clin Orthop 136: 22-32.

8. Roy S, Caine D, Singer KM (1985) Stress changes of the distal radial epiphysis in young gymnasts. A report of twenty-one cases and a review of the literature. Am J Sports Med 13(5): 301-308.
   Between 1980 and 1983, 21 young, high-performance gymnasts with stress changes related to the distal radial epiphysis were treated and followed for a mean of 24 months (with a range of 6 to 42 months).

9. Pill SG, Ganley TJ, Milam RA, Lou JE, Meyer JS, Flynn JM (2003) Role of magnetic resonance imaging and clinical criteria in predicting successful nonoperative treatment of osteochondritis dissecans in children. J Pediatr Orthop 23(1): 102-108.
   The purpose of this study was to compare the value of MRI, plain radiographs, and clinical findings in predicting the success of nonoperative treatment of juvenile OCD lesions. Although no single factor was uniformly predictive of successful nonoperative treatment, younger, skeletally immature patients with no MRI criteria of instability were most amenable to nonoperative treatment.

10. Ganley TJ, Pill SG, Flynn JM, Gregg JR (2003) Treatment of massive osteochondritis dissecans lesions of the capitellum: Arthroscopic-assisted debridement and bone grafting for large, full-thickness defects. Arthroscopy 19(2): 222–225.

11. Kennedy J (1979) The Injured Adolescent Knee. Baltimore: Williams & Wilkins.

12. DeLee JC, Evans JP, Julian J (1983) Stress fracture of the fifth metatarsal. Am J Sports Med 11(5): 349-353.
    Stress fractures of the fifth metatarsal have been reported with increasing frequency, especially in athletes. Prolonged healing time and the risk of refracture following conservative treatment have led to recommendations for operative treatment including bone grafting of these fractures.

13. Devas MB (1963) Stress fractures in children. J Bone Joint Surg Br 45: 528-541.

14. Kadel NJ, Teitz CC, Kronmal RA (1992) Stress fractures in ballet dancers. Am J Sports Med 20(4): 445-449.
    The authors surveyed 54 female dancers in two professional ballet companies. A total of 27 fractures were reported in 17 dancers. (63%) followed by fractures of the tibia (22%) and spine (7%). Of the 17 dancers with stress fractures, only 1 had neither of these risk factors.

15. Dameron TB, Rockwood CA (1984) Fractures and dislocations of the shoulder. Philadelphia: Lippincott Williams & Wilkins.

16. Zaricznyj B (1977) Avulsion fracture of the tibial eminence: Treatment by open reduction and pinning. J Bone Joint Surg Am 59(8): 1111-1114.

17. Waters PM, Millis MB (1994) Hip and pelvic injuries in the young athlete. In: Pediatric and Adolescent Sports Medicine (Stantinski CL, DeLee JC, Drez D, eds). Philadelphia: WB Saunders, pp 279-293.

18. Ganley TJ, Wallach D, Dormans JP (2000) Bilateral knee pain of several months duration in a 12-year-old girl. In: Pediatrics: A Problem-Based Review (Burg F, Vaughn V, Nelson K, eds). Philadelphia: WB Saunders.

19. Ganley T, Arnold C, McKernan D, Gregg J, Cooney T (2000) The impact of loading on deformation about posteromedial meniscal tears. Orthopedics 23(6): 597-601.
    To simulate how partial ability to bear weight affects meniscal repair, full-thickness tears were produced in the posteromedial aspect of seven ACL-intact cadaveric knees.

20. Dickhaut SC, DeLee JC (1982) The discoid lateral-meniscus syndrome. J Bone Joint Surg Am 64(7): 1068-1073.
    The authors saw 12 patients with the so-called complete type of discoid lateral meniscus, with intact ligament attachments as an incidental finding at the time of arthroscopy. Of the 12 patients, 10 were without significant symptoms attributable to the meniscus; that is, they had no meniscal tears or laxity.

21. Washington ER 3rd, Root L, Liener UC (1995) Discoid lateral meniscus in children: Long-term follow-up after excision. J Bone Joint Surg Am 77(9): 1357-1361.
    The authors retrospectively reviewed the results for 15 patients, 8 girls and 7 boys, who had a total of 18 meniscectomies performed for a discoid meniscus.

22. Ganley TJ, Pill SG (2002) Discoid meniscus. In: The 5-Minute Pediatric Consult (Schwart WM, ed). Philadelphia: Lippincott Williams & Wilkins, pp 330-331.

23. Silverman JM, Mink JH, Deutsch AL (1989) Discoid menisci of the knee: MR imaging appearance. Radiology 173(2): 351-354.
    In approximately one third of the cases in which coronal images were obtained, the measurable height difference between the discoid and the opposite meniscus was greater than or equal to 2 mm. Arthroscopic correlation (obtained in 10 cases) revealed that 6 cases of discoid meniscus were diagnosed correctly with MRI, although 1 meniscus was considered discoid at MRI but was not considered discoid at arthroscopy. Of 3 discoid menisci seen to be torn at arthroscopy, 2 were seen to be torn at MRI.

24. Greulich WW, Pyle SI (1950) Radiographic Atlas of Skeletal Development of the Hand and Wrist. Stanford, CA: Stanford University Press.

25. Andrews M, Noyes FR, Barber-Westin SD (1994) Anterior cruciate ligament allograft reconstruction in the skeletally immature athlete. Am J Sports Med 22(1): 48-54.
    The purpose of this study was to evaluate ACL allograft reconstruction in skeletally immature athletes. Eight patients (with a mean age of 13 years, 6 months and a range of 10 to 15 years) with radiographic documentation of open growth plates had ACL repair and reconstruction with fascia lata or Achilles tendon allograft tissue. At follow-up, all patients showed closure of the growth plates.

26. Graf BK, Lange RH, Fujisaki CK, Landry GL, Saluja RK (1992) Anterior cruciate ligament tears in skeletally immature patients: meniscal pathology at presentation and after attempted conservative treatment. Arthroscopy 8(2): 229-233.
    The authors evaluated 12 skeletally immature patients with acute, intrasubstance tears of the ACL and open physes for meniscal pathology. After return to sports, all braced patients developed instability with multiple episodes of "giving way." The authors conclude that meniscal pathology is commonly associated with ACL tears in skeletally immature patients, and they recommend arthrography or arthroscopy to evaluate patients with suspected ACL tears.

27. Mizuta H, Kubota K, Shiraishi M, Otsuka Y, Nagamoto N, Takagi K (1995) The conservative treatment of complete tears of the anterior cruciate ligament in skeletally immature patients. J Bone Joint Surg Br 77(6): 890-894.
    The authors describe the results of conservative treatment for complete midsubstance tears of the ACL in 18 skeletally immature patients followed for a minimum of 36 months. The authors conclude that the results of nonoperative treatment for ACL injuries in this age group are poor and not acceptable.

28. Parker AW, Drez D Jr, Cooper JL (1994) Anterior cruciate ligament injuries in patients with open physes. Am J Sports Med 22(1): 44-47.
    From July 1988 to August 1989, six children with open physes and injuries to the ACL were treated operatively. Despite the overall clinical stability, MRI scans of the five patients consistently demonstrated areas of increased signal in the ACL grafts.

29. Aronowitz ER, Ganley TJ, Goode JR (2000) Anterior cruciate ligament reconstruction in adolescents with open physes. Am J Sports Med 28(2): 168-175.
    The purpose of this study was to evaluate ACL reconstructions performed in adolescents with open physes and a skeletal age of at least 14 years. This study demonstrates that ACL reconstruction using an Achilles tendon allograft is a viable treatment option for skeletally immature patients with a skeletal age of 14 years who have sustained midsubstance tears of the ACL.

30. Lo IK, Bell DM, Fowler PJ (1998) Anterior cruciate ligament injuries in the skeletally immature patient. Instr Course Lect 47: 351-359.
    ACL injury in the skeletally immature is becoming increasingly recognized and reported. In patients with significant growth remaining, however, surgical treatment carries much higher risks of physeal damage and subsequent deformity. Yet intra-articular reconstruction in truly skeletally immature patients using a soft tissue graft through a

transphyseal tibial tunnel of moderate or small diameter and the over-the-top position on the femur has not been shown to cause early physeal closure, limb length discrepancy, or angular deformity.

31. Meyers MH, McKeever FM (1970) Fracture of the intercondylar eminence of the tibia. J Bone Joint Surg Am 52(8): 1677-1684.

32. Flynn JM, Skaggs D, Sponseller P, Ganley TJ, Kay R, Leitch K (2003) Management of pediatric fractures of the lower extremity. AAOS Instr Course Lect 52: 647-659.
Most pediatric fractures of the lower extremity can and should be treated with closed reduction, immobilization, and close follow-up. However, there is an ongoing debate in the orthopaedic community regarding the role of surgical management in the treatment of pediatric fractures. Certain technical advances, such as the use of flexible intramedullary fixation and bioreabsorbable implants, have further increased enthusiasm for surgical management of pediatric fractures of the lower extremity.

33. Ganley TJ, Flynn JM, Pill S, Hanlon P (2000) Ankle evaluation in the young athlete: Fracture vs. sprain. J Musculoskel Med 17(6): 311-325.

34. Canale ST, Belding RH (1980) Osteochondral lesions of the talus. J Bone Joint Surg Am 62(1): 97-102.
In a retrospective study of 31 ankles in 29 patients with osteochondral lesions, the authors found that lateral lesions were associated with inversion or inversion–dorsiflexion trauma, were morphologically shallow, and were more likely to become displaced in the joint and to have persistent symptoms.

35. Ganley TJ, Flynn JM, Gregg JR (1998) Sports medicine of the adolescent foot and ankle. Foot Ankle Clin 3(4): 767-785.

Upper Extremity Disorders

Benjamin Chang* **and Scott H. Kozin†**

*MD, FACS, Plastic Surgeon, The Children's Hospital of Philadelphia; Assistant Professor of Surgery, Division of Plastic Surgery, University of Pennsylvania Medical School, Philadelphia, PA
†MD, Hand Surgeon, Shriners Hospital for Children, Philadelphia, PA; Associate Professor, Department of Orthopaedic Surgery, Temple University, Philadelphia, PA

Injury

- Initial assessment—History, physical examination, and x-ray evaluation
- Goal—Determine which structures have been injured
- Consider child's age and maturity—Obtain the necessary information without hurting or alarming the patient

History

- Interview the patient, parents, and other adult witnesses.
- The mechanism and circumstances of injury can provide important clues about what has been injured.

General History

- Age
- Sex
- Hand dominance
- Medical history—Last tetanus and major health problems
- Surgical history—Anesthetic or bleeding problems
- Medications
- Allergies

History of Injury

- Time since injury
- Mechanism—Sharp or blunt, clean or contaminated
- Symptoms—Pain, numbness, location, severity, and aggravating or ameliorating factors
- Functional deficits—Loss of mobility, dexterity, sensibility, or strength
- Previous injuries to the extremity—Old functional deficits
- Prior treatment
  - Local anesthesia—Interferes with sensory examination
  - Wound management—Cleansing, exploration, and closure
  - Skeletal reduction
- Associated injuries
  - Life-threatening injuries take priority.
  - Head and cervical spine injuries complicate anesthesia.

Physical Examination

Principles

- Purpose—Determine which structures have been injured.
- Examine the uninjured side first, then compare it with the injured side.
- Start the examination distally and work proximally. Functional deficits away from the zone of injury point to injured structures proximally.
- Test all structures within the zone of injury including all symptomatic areas and at least one joint proximal to and distal from the level of injury.
- Do the least invasive parts of the examination first:
  - *Observation*
  - Gentle *palpation*
  - Tests of *active motion*
  - *Exploration*—Perform only under adequate anesthesia; you can often gain all necessary information by testing the parts of the extremity distal to the level of injury without probing the wound.

- Examine the upper extremity *in the following order* (Table 8–1):
  - Circulation is most critical and can be checked with minimal discomfort.
  - Sensibility
  - Soft tissues
  - Skeleton
  - Motor function is tested last because it requires the patient's cooperation and depends on intact musculotendinous units, stable bones, and mobile joints.

Circulation

- *Color*—Fingertips and nail beds should be pink.
- *Temperature*—Compare temperature with that of the uninjured side.
- *Capillary refill*—Refill should be two seconds or less.
- *Pulses*—Radial and ulnar pulses should be easily palpable at the wrist unless there is proximal occlusion or vasoconstriction (e.g., from hypothermia).
- Adjuncts to physical examination—Doppler and pulse oximeter

Sensibility

- *Light touch*—Use your finger or cotton-tipped applicator, *not* a needle. "Look away and tell me which finger I am touching."
- *Static two-point discrimination*—Normal discrimination is 5 mm or less in the fingertips.
- Objective signs of denervation are as follows:
  - Anhydrosis of the skin
  - Lack of skin wrinkling with immersion in water[1]
  - Useful in young children
- Autonomous sensory zones in the hand correspond to the three major sensory nerves:
  - Index fingertip (median)
  - Small fingertip (ulnar)
  - Dorsum of the thumb–index web space (radial)

Soft Tissues

- Sketch the wound, including old scars.
- Observe any swelling, erythema, or other signs of infection.
- Palpate the muscles to make sure that a compartment syndrome is not overlooked.
- Explore open wounds only with anesthesia.
  - Do not use local anesthesia until after the sensory examination.
  - Look for exposed bone, joint, or tendon—if exposed, there is more urgency in closing the wound.
- Simple lacerations—Irrigate, debride, and close the wound in the emergency room within 8 hours.
- Complex wounds—Repair the following in the operating room:
  - Skin deficit
  - Devitalized areas
  - Extensive contamination

Skeleton

- Signs of skeletal injury
  - Obvious angular or rotational *deformity*—Dislocated joint or a displaced fracture
  - *Loss of mobility*
  - *Abnormal mobility*—"If you can move it, it's not broken" is utterly unreliable.
  - *Point tenderness* + swelling + bruising
- Obtain three-view radiographs of all injured hands.
  - Obtain posteroanterior, true lateral, and oblique radiographs.
  - The fracture may be visible in only one view.
  - Specify the part to be examined—if the long finger is injured, requesting a radiograph of the hand will invariably produce a lateral projection with overlapped fingers, thus obscuring the injured finger.

Treatment of specific upper extremity fractures is covered in Chapter 4.

Table 8–1: Upper Extremity Examination

PHYSICAL EXAMINATION	OBSERVATION	MANIPULATION	SPECIAL TESTS
Circulation	Color	Temperature Capillary refill Pulse	Doppler Pulse oximeter
Sensibility	Anhydrosis	Immersion test Light touch Two-point discrimination	Nerve conduction
Soft tissues	Open wounds	Exploration	
Skeleton	Deformity	Palpation Range of motion	X-ray film
Motor function	Spontaneous motion	Tenodesis effect Squeeze test Range of motion Strength	Nerve conduction Electromyography

Motor Function

- Observation
  - *Resting posture*—Normally, the fingers are held in slight flexion at rest because of the resting tone of the flexor muscles, which are stronger than the extensors. A complete flexor tendon laceration will disrupt the normal cascade; the injured digit will be more extended than the uninjured ones (Figure 8–1).
  - *Lack of spontaneous movement*—This indicates possible nerve, muscle, or tendon injury; however, painful injuries such as fractures, dislocations, sprains, lacerations, or even contusions can all cause guarding.
- Manipulation of younger or uncooperative patients
  - *Tenodesis effect*—Resting muscle tone will cause the fingers to flex as the wrist is passively extended and to extend as the wrist is flexed because the digital flexors cross the wrist joint (Figure 8–2).
  - *Squeeze test*—Direct compression of the finger and thumb flexors in the distal forearm tightens those tendons and will cause the digits to flex.[2]
- Manipulation of older, cooperative patients
  - Test each muscle group (Table 8–2) on the uninjured side first to make sure that the patient understands what to do.
  - Note any deficits in active or passive range of motion.
  - Compare the strength of the injured with that of the normal side.
- Nerve conduction studies and electromyograms (EMGs) can provide objective information regarding the level, severity, and chronicity of nerve injury.

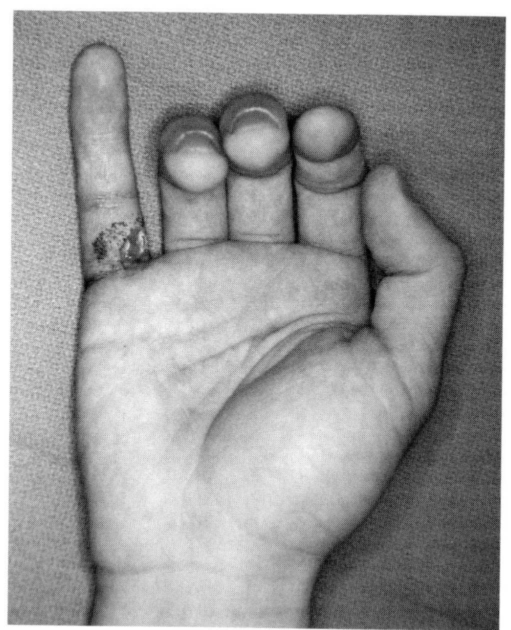

Figure 8–1: Complete flexor tendon laceration.

Soft Tissue Injury

Skin

- Simple lacerations
  - Lacerations may be mistaken for tissue avulsion because children have elastic skin. If irregularities along the two sides of the wound margin match up, it is likely that no skin has been lost.
  - Before closure, explore the wound to check that all structures within the zone of injury are intact and that there are no foreign bodies.

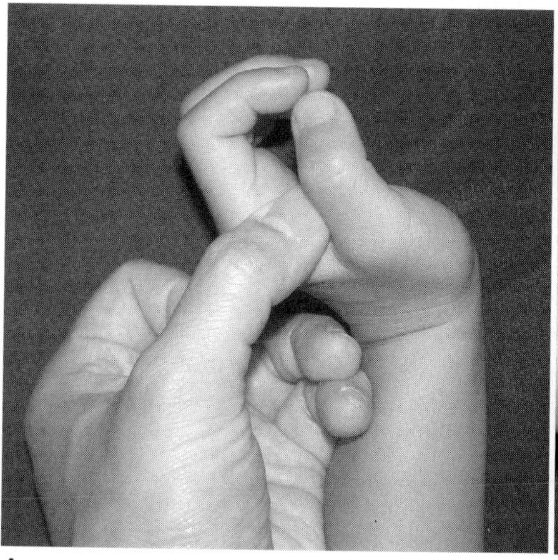

A

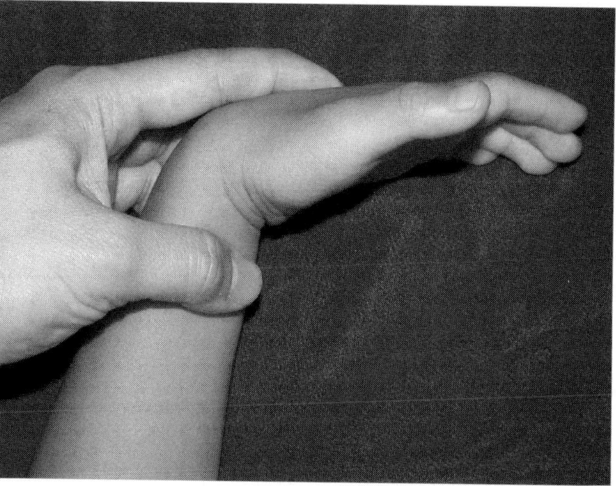

B

Figure 8–2: Tenodesis effect. A, Fingers passively flex with extension of the wrist. B, Fingers passively extend with flexion of the wrist.

Table 8–2: Upper Extremity Motor Function

	MUSCLES (PRIMARY)	NERVES	ROOTS
ACTION Elbow			
Flexion	Biceps brachii and brachialis	Musculocutaneous	C5-C6
	Brachioradialis	Radial	C6-C7
Extension	Triceps brachii	Radial	C6-C7
Wrist			
Flexion	Flexor carpi radialis	Median	C6-C7
	Flexor carpi ulnaris	Ulnar	C8-T1
Extension	Extensor carpi radialis longus	Radial	C6-C7
	Extensor carpi radialis brevis	PIN	C6-C7
	Extensor carpi ulnaris	PIN	C6-C7
Forearm			
Pronation	Pronator teres	Median	C6-C7
	Pronator quadratus	AIN	C8-T1
Supination	Biceps brachii	Musculocutaneous	C5-C6
	Supinator	PIN	C6-C7
Thumb			
Flexion	Flexor pollicis longus	AIN	C8-T1
Extension	Extensor pollicis longus	PIN	C6-C7
Abduction	Abductor pollicis longus	PIN	C6-C7
Adduction	Adductor pollicis	Ulnar	C8-T1
Palmar abduction	Abductor pollicis brevis	Median	C8-T1
	Opponens pollicis		
Finger			
PIP flexion	Flexor digitorum superficialis	Median	C7-C8
DIP flexion	Flexor digitorum profundus	AIN (index, long)	C7-C8
		Ulnar (ring, small)	C7-C8
MCP extension	Extensor digitorum communis	PIN	C6-C7
	Extensor indicis proprius	PIN	C6-C7
	Extensor digiti minimi	PIN	C7-C8
MCP flexion, IP extension	Interossei, lumbricals	Ulnar	C8-T1
	Lumbricals	Median	C8-T1
Abduction	Dorsal interossei	Ulnar	C8-T1
	Abductor digiti minimi	(small)	
Adduction	Volar interossei	Ulnar	C8-T1

AIN, anterior interosseous nerve, a branch of the median nerve; *DIP,* distal interphalangeal joint; *IP,* interphalangeal joint; *MCP,* metacarpophalangeal joint; *PIN,* posterior interosseous nerve, a branch of the radial nerve; *PIP,* proximal interphalangeal joint.

  - Radiographs can be helpful in identifying radiopaque foreign bodies and fractures.
  - Lacerations may be irrigated, debrided, and closed primarily if there are no injuries to underlying structures.
  - Lacerations that cross the digital flexion creases should be closed with a Z-plasty to avoid a flexion contracture after healing.
- Contaminated wounds—Delayed primary closure
  - Debride and apply moist saline dressings for 48 hours, changing twice daily, then close if there are no signs of infection.
  - Delayed closure is also useful when edema precludes primary closure without tension.
- Lacerations that create skin flaps
  - There is a risk of ischemia and necrosis of the flap, especially if closed under tension.
  - Narrow flap—Excise and close primarily.
  - Larger flaps—Close with V-Y advancement to reduce tension.
- Degloving injuries
  - Skin is undermined but not missing.
  - Debride any obviously nonviable skin and suture remaining skin to the underlying tissues *under no tension* to maximize the survival of the degloved skin.
  - Return to the operating room for a second look the next day. Excise any additional nonviable skin. Skin graft all remaining open areas.

   - Major degloving injuries—Harvest skin graft from the degloved skin with a dermatome on the day of injury and apply immediately to the open wound.
- Skin avulsion injuries—Choice of soft tissue coverage (Box 8–1) depends on the size of the defect and the nature of the wound bed.

Primary Wound Closure

- Use *absorbable* sutures—Removing nonabsorbable sutures can be as traumatic to the patient (and doctor) as putting them in!
- Fingers and palm—Use a single-layer closure with 5–0 plain gut.
- Use the following for the dorsum of the hand and proximal to the wrist:
   - Subcuticular closure with an absorbable monofilament suture such as Monocryl
   - Two-layer closure with buried interrupted sutures in the deep dermis to bring the wound edges together and a superficial running subcuticular suture to accurately align the skin edges

Local Flaps

- Formed by elevating and rearranging skin adjacent to the wound
- Distribute tension over a larger area
- Depend on the elasticity of skin adjacent to the wound
- Useful for smaller wounds that are too large to close primarily
- Can be advanced, transposed, or rotated into the wound
- V-Y advancement flap (Figure 8–3)—Particularly useful for closing fingertip defects

Box 8–1 Options for Soft Tissue Coverage

- Primary closure
- Local flap
- Skin graft
- Regional flap
- Distant flap
- Free flap

1. A V-shaped incision is made in the skin adjacent to the open wound with the wound at the top of the V.
2. The skin in the V is left attached to the subcutaneous tissues, from which it derives its blood supply.
3. Advancing the skin flap into the open wound closes the primary defect.
4. Suturing the skin together at the apex of the V to form a Y-shaped closure closes the donor defect.

Skin Grafts

- Skin grafts can close large wounds that have a well-vascularized bed and no exposed bone, tendon, or joint.
- *Full-thickness skin grafts* contain the full thickness of the epidermis and dermis.
   - *Advantages* over split-thickness grafts—Provide better quality skin coverage, contract less during healing, and are more durable and supple after healing
   - *Disadvantages*—Lower rate of survival ("take") and need to close the donor site
   - *Donor sites* for full-thickness skin grafts—lower abdomen, groin, elbow flexion crease, and wrist flexion crease in decreasing order of size

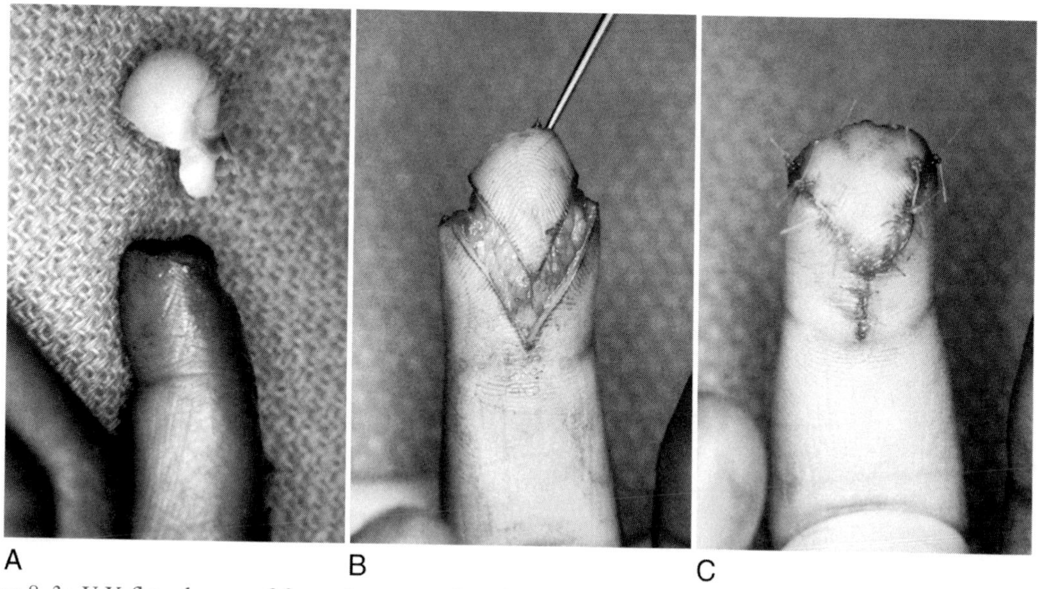

Figure 8–3: V-Y flap closure of fingertip amputation. A, Fingertip amputation. B, V-shaped advancement flap. C, Y-shaped closure.

- *Split-thickness skin grafts* contain the epidermis and a partial thickness of the dermis (can be adjusted with dermatome).
  - *Advantages*—Better take, larger area possible (donor site reepithelializes just like a second-degree burn)
  - *Disadvantages*—Poorer quality, donor site pain and scar

If a wound is too large for closure with local flaps and the bed is not suitable for skin grafting, you can chose a regional, distant, or free flap to close the wound. These flaps can contain skin and subcutaneous tissue, muscle, bone, nerve and even tendon. They provide soft tissue coverage and can restore function.

Regional Flaps

- Use tissue that is not immediately adjacent to the wound but can be transferred over to cover the wound while remaining attached to its blood supply.
- The radial forearm flap (Figure 8–4) is an example of a regional flap that can be used to cover defects from the MCP joints to the elbow based on its vascular pedicle, the radial artery, and veins.

Distant Flaps

- Use tissue from distant parts of the body.
- Distant flaps are attached to the hand recipient site to allow ingrowth of the blood supply for approximately 2 weeks then are divided from the distant donor site.
- The flap survives on its new blood supply entering the flap around its periphery, unlike the skin graft, which derives its blood supply from the wound bed under the graft.
- Distant flaps can be used to cover tissue not suitable for skin grafting, such as tendon or bone.
- The groin flap (Figure 8–5) can supply a fairly large area of skin and subcutaneous tissue and still allow primary closure of the donor site. It is useful for coverage of soft tissue defects in the hand and wrist.

Free Flaps

- Free flaps are the most versatile flaps for soft tissue coverage of the hand.
- They consist of an area of tissue with a single dominant artery and vein. The free flap is elevated with its artery and vein, then detached and transferred to the soft tissue defect where the vessels are anastomosed to suitable recipient vessels.
- *Advantages*—Can cover extensive soft tissue defects, do not rely on the wound bed for blood supply (like skin grafts), are not tethered to a limited "arc of rotation" (like regional flaps), and do not tie the hand to the donor area for 2 weeks (like distant flaps)
- *Disadvantage*—Are technically more demanding, especially in young children, because of the need to perform microvascular anastomoses
- Figure 8–6 shows a 4-year-old patient who was dragged by a car and suffered a deep abrasion injury to the arm, exposing the elbow joint. A scapular free flap was transferred from the back to cover the joint, and skin grafts covered the exposed muscle.

Vascular Injury

- Exsanguinating hemorrhage, although rare, is one of only two hand emergencies that can be life threatening (the other being necrotizing infection). Partial laceration of a major artery is almost always the source because a completely transected vessel will usually retract and thrombose.

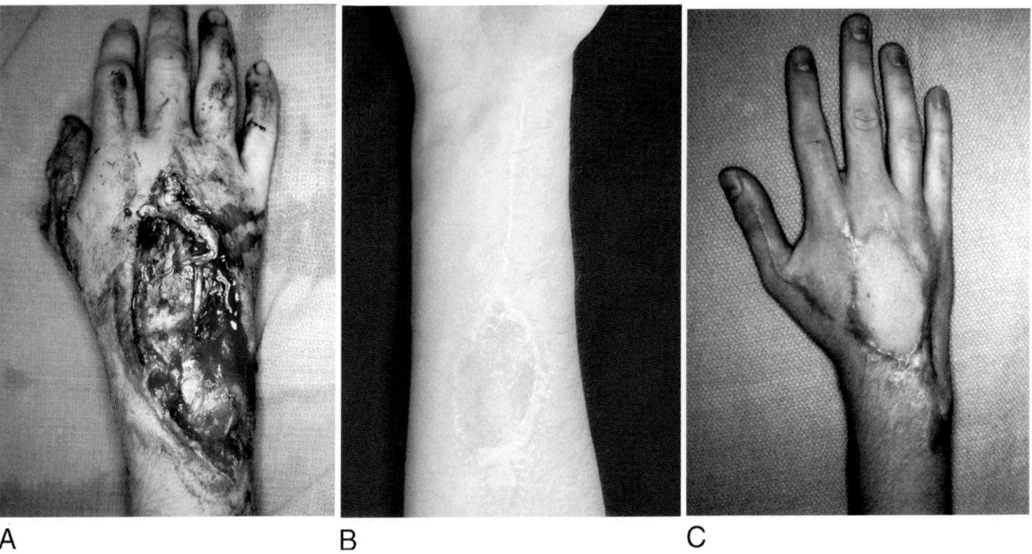

Figure 8–4: Radial forearm flap. A, Dorsal hand avulsion wound. B, Flap donor site covered with a skin graft. C, Healed flap.

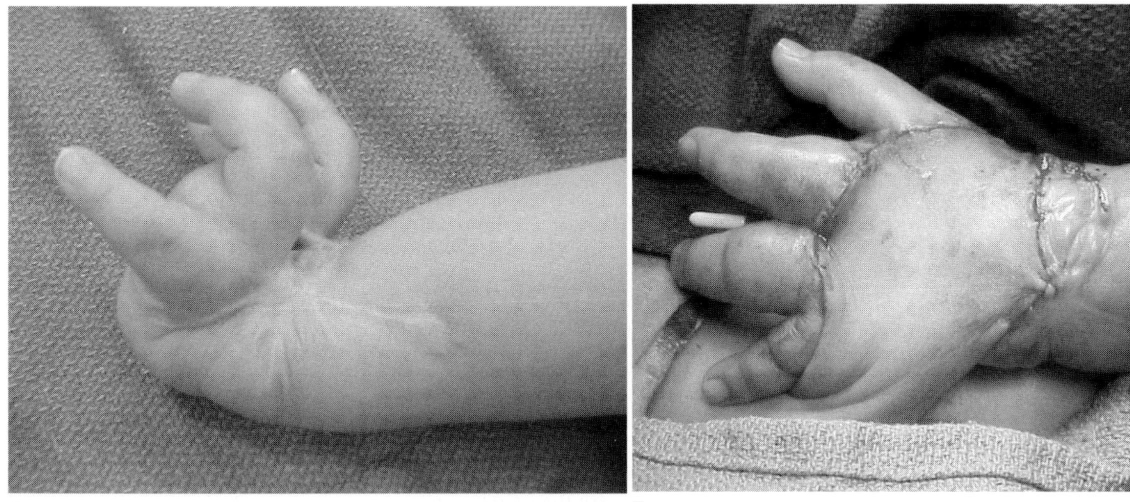

Figure 8–5: Groin flap. A, Wrist contracture from severe intravenous infiltration. B, First stage of groin flap. C, Healed flap.

- To control bleeding, elevate the extremity and apply direct pressure to the bleeding vessel with a gloved finger. Because of collateral circulation, both ends of the lacerated vessel need to be compressed. Most bleeding will stop after 10 minutes of *constant* pressure. If bleeding cannot be controlled by direct pressure, apply pressure to the brachial artery nearest the injury to diminish the arterial inflow and continue to apply direct pressure to the bleeding vessel.
- As a last resort, apply a pneumatic tourniquet near the bleeding vessel and rapidly transport the patient to the operating room for surgical control of the bleeding. Without anesthesia, most patients have unbearable ischemic pain after the tourniquet has been inflated for

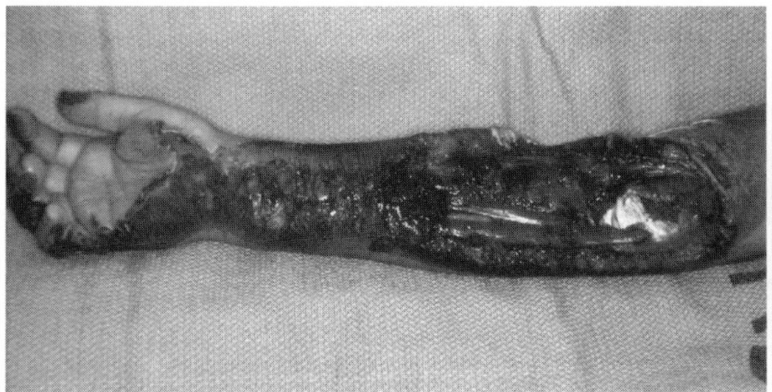

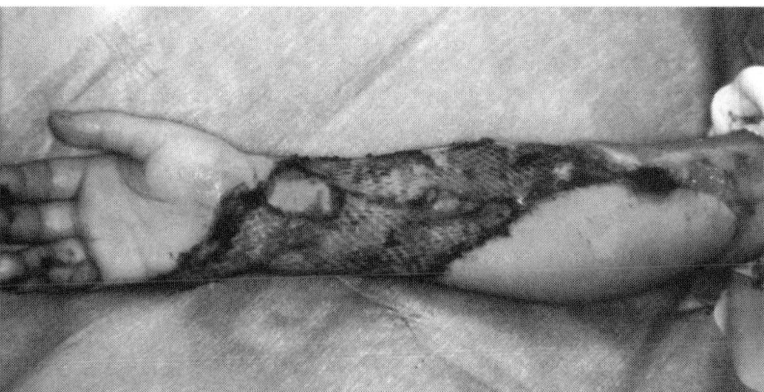

Figure 8–6: Scapular free flap. A, Deep abrasion injury with an exposed elbow joint. B, Joint covered with a scapular flap.

15 to 20 minutes and the tourniquet will have to be released for at least 5 minutes before reinflation. Exsanguinate the arm by elevation before inflating the tourniquet to 100 mm Hg above systolic pressure. A blood pressure cuff wrapped with tape can substitute for a pneumatic tourniquet.

- *Never* blindly clamp bleeding vessels because nerves accompany most major vessels.
- In addition to causing bleeding, vascular injuries can cause ischemia to the hand or arm. Collateral circulation is usually excellent in children, but occluding both digital arteries to a digit or both the radial and the ulnar arteries in the forearm can produce ischemia. If the palmar arch is incomplete, occluding either the radial or the ulnar artery can cause part of the hand to become ischemic. Because of collateral circulation, occluding the brachial artery may or may not cause ischemia depending on the length and location of the occluded segment. Once a lacerated artery has been identified and occluded, you can assess the distal perfusion and decide whether to repair or ligate the vessel.
- If distal perfusion is adequate, both proximal and distal cut ends of the artery should be ligated. Sometimes, the patient is no longer bleeding by the time he is examined but has a history of pulsatile bleeding immediately after injury. In this instance, you must still identify and ligate the injured artery to prevent delayed hemorrhage, arteriovenous fistulas, or pseudoaneurysm formation.
- If distal perfusion is inadequate, prompt restoration of perfusion is essential. Muscle will suffer permanent damage after 6 hours of warm ischemia. For most penetrating trauma, the patient should be taken directly to the operating room for exploration and repair of the injured vessel. A fractured limb with ischemia should be reduced and splinted to see whether perfusion improves with improved alignment.
- If the ischemia persists, the patient should undergo emergency angiography followed by operative repair. Usually you will find that the vessel is trapped in the fracture site or that the vessel has a segmental thrombosis from intimal damage. In the upper extremity, vascular injury is most common after a supracondylar humeral fracture, which can damage the brachial artery. The damaged segment of artery should be resected and replaced with an interposition vein graft. Prophylactic fasciotomy should be performed if ischemia time exceeds 6 hours.
- Radial artery cannulation for hemodynamic monitoring, especially if the patient is hypotensive or receiving vasopressors, can also cause hand ischemia. The initial treatment is to remove the cannula and improve cardiac output. Anticoagulation or thrombolytic therapy may be helpful if ischemia persists and threatens tissue loss. Surgical revascularization is another option, but many patients who require radial arterial lines for monitoring are not stable enough for a long microsurgical procedure.
- An Allen's test (Box 8–2) should be performed before placing a radial artery cannula to ensure that the ulnar artery will adequately perfuse the hand. If all digits do not promptly reperfuse with only the ulnar artery open, the palmar arch is incomplete and the thumb may become ischemic if a radial arterial line is inserted.

Nerve Injury

- Nerve injuries in children usually occur after penetrating trauma. Lacerations with broken glass seem especially prone to involving deep neurovascular and tendinous structures, even when the skin laceration appears small and innocuous.
- You should suspect a nerve laceration if there are motor or sensory deficits away from the level of injury or if there is an arterial injury, because many nerves travel with arteries in the upper extremity (Table 8–3).
- Nerve injuries from sharp penetrating trauma should be treated by exploration and repair. If there are associated injuries that require immediate exploration (e.g., vascular), nerve repair can be done at the same time. Otherwise, the wound can be irrigated and closed, and a delayed primary repair can be performed within 1 week.
- Lacerations to small, purely sensory nerves (e.g., digital nerves) can be delayed up to 3 weeks without compromising the final outcome. Nerve deficits after gunshot wounds are best observed for 3 weeks to see whether there is any spontaneous recovery of nerve function, which can occur if the nerve has not been directly transected by the bullet. If the nerve has been transected, the delay will allow clear demarcation of the zone of injury by fibrosis so that this segment of the nerve can be debrided before nerve repair (usually requiring nerve graft).
- Blunt trauma can cause nerve injury by direct crush, compartment syndrome, or traction. The degree of injury determines the potential for recovery.
  - *Neurapraxia* produces a localized conduction block with no Tinel's sign (tingling with percussion over a nerve) at the site of injury. Recovery should begin by 3 weeks and be complete by 3 months.
  - *Axonotmesis* produces axonal damage with loss of the axoplasm and myelin away from the injury (wallerian degeneration). The nerve regenerates 1 mm/day by axonal sprouting into the empty Schwann cell tubes. A Tinel's sign will be present at the site of injury and

Box 8–2 Allen's Test

1. Elevate and squeeze the hand to exsanguinate.
2. Compress radial and ulnar arteries at the wrist.
3. Release the radial artery with the hand open and check capillary refill.
4. Repeat steps 1 and 2, then release the ulnar artery and check capillary refill.

Table 8–3: Nerves Close to Arteries

ARTERY	ADJACENT NERVE
Axillary	Brachial plexus
Brachial	Median and ulnar
Ulnar	Ulnar
Digital	Digital

will advance with the regenerating nerve. Recovery is complete, but the time to recovery is determined by the distance between the site of injury and the end organ.

  - *Neurotmesis* is complete transection of the nerve. A neuroma forms at the end of the transected nerve and may cause dysesthesia. Nerve function does not recover without surgery, and repair of the transected nerve is the best way to avoid neuroma symptoms.
  - These specific degrees of nerve injury are discrete points along a continuum. Many nerve injuries will exhibit different degrees of injury in different parts of the same nerve.
- Electrodiagnostic testing can be a useful adjunct to clinical tests in determining the degree of injury and in following the progress of recovery. The presence of denervation changes on EMGs, such as fibrillations or positive sharp waves, signifies a degree of injury greater than neurapraxia. Nerve conduction studies can help to determine the degree and location of injury but may not identify partial nerve injuries.
- Good prognosis for recovery after nerve repair is associated with nerves with pure motor or sensory function, age below 10 years, sharp mechanism of injury, distal level of injury, and a delay of less than 6 months.
- With prolonged delay in nerve repair, recovery of motor and sensory function is limited by degeneration of the end organs. After denervation, muscle becomes atrophied by 2 months, fibrotic by 1 year, and fragmented by 3 years. The motor endplates are gone after 2 years; therefore, recovery of motor function is not expected after 2 years of denervation.
- With sensory function, there is no clear correlation between timing of repair and degree for recovery except that after 1 year you can expect recovery of only protective sensibility.
- The total delay in reinnervation is the sum of the delay in repair plus the time needed for the nerve to regrow from the point of injury to the end organ (roughly 1 month for each inch).

Tendon Injury

- Tendon injuries are primarily caused by penetrating trauma, and the diagnosis is usually clear from the history and physical examination. Common mechanisms in children include lacerations from broken glass and knives.
- Assume that any tendon deep to a skin laceration may have been injured and that every tendon in the zone of injury should be tested. Suspect a tendon injury if there is evidence of nerve or arterial injury in the hand because all three structures lie proximately.
- The level of the tendon injury may be different from the level of the skin laceration depending on the position of the hand during injury. For example, if a flexor tendon laceration occurs with the fingers in a fully flexed position, the tendon laceration will retract away from the skin laceration when the hand is examined in an open position.
- First observe the hand in the resting posture: all fingers should be in a gently flexed posture with the small finger most flexed and the index finger least flexed. A *complete* tendon laceration will cause that finger to fall outside of this normal cascade (Figure 8–1).
- Each tendon should then be tested by active motion both without and with resistance. A finger with a partial tendon laceration will have a normal resting posture and active motion, but resisted motion will produce pain.
- Young children may not cooperate with active motor testing because of anxiety, pain, or inability to understand the directions. Magnetic resonance imaging (MRI) and high-resolution ultrasound can demonstrate tendon lacerations but are currently not reliable for partial tendon lacerations. Surgical exploration may be the only way to determine whether a tendon or nerve has been injured.
- Exploration in the emergency room should be discouraged because visualization is usually inadequate because of poor lighting, instruments, anesthesia, and exposure.
- *Flexor tendon* injuries are divided into five zones (Figure 8–7). The level of the tendon injury with the finger extended determines the zone of injury, not the level of the skin laceration.
  - Zone 2 extends from the distal palmar flexion crease to the middle of the middle phalanx and is referred to as "no man's land" because results of repair are poorest in this area. The flexor digitorum superficialis (FDS) and profundus (FDP) tendons are enclosed in a tight flexor tendon sheath in zone 2 and tend to adhere to each other and to the surrounding sheath after repair.
  - Flexor tendon injuries are best explored and repaired within 1 week before the proximal end of the tendon retracts and the tendon sheath fills with scar tissue. If treatment is delayed, a primary repair may not be possible, necessitating a two-stage repair with tendon grafting that carries a much worse prognosis.
  - In addition to partial lacerations, flexor tendon injuries are most often missed in the palm (zone 3) and wrist (zone 5). The FDS lies superficial of the FDP in the palm and can be completely transected, leaving the FDP intact. The finger will still flex at all three joints,

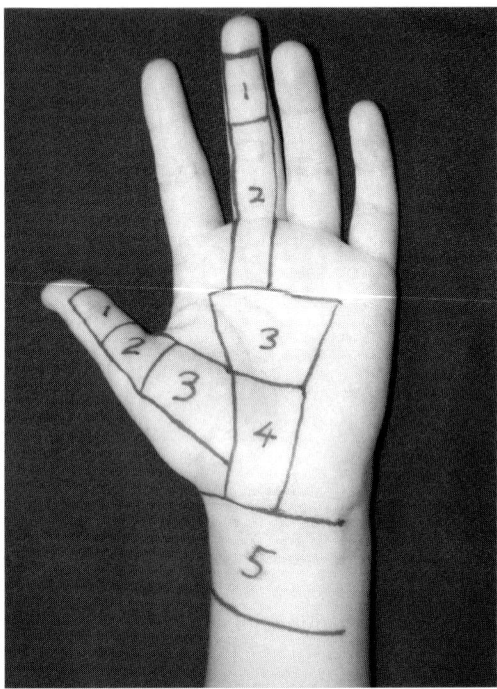

Figure 8–7: Zones of flexor tendon injury.

but flexion of the proximal interphalangeal (PIP) joint will be weak and cause pain.

  - The wrist flexors, flexor carpi ulnaris and flexor carpi radialis, are superficial and may be lacerated without injury to the deeper digital flexors. The wrist will still flex actively with just the digital flexors intact, but flexion against resistance will cause pain.
  - A flexor tendon injury can occur without laceration of the skin. The patient usually gives a history of grabbing an opponent's jersey while playing ball and feeling a sharp pain snapping sensation in the long finger. Afterward, he is unable to actively flex the distal interphalangeal (DIP) joint (Figure 8–8) and may attribute the injury to a sprain or dislocation. However, the injury is actually an avulsion of the FDP from its insertion on the distal phalanx *(jersey finger)* caused by forced flexion against resistance. The avulsed tendon may retract proximally into the palm and should be repaired within a week to prevent excessive shortening of the tendon–muscle unit and scarring of the tendon sheath.

- *Extensor tendon* injuries can cause flexion deformities of underlying joints if not recognized and repaired. The deformity may not be immediately apparent but may develop over time and may involve adjacent joints as the finely balanced extensor mechanism is thrown out of balance.
  - As with flexor tendon injuries, diagnosis is usually apparent on physical examination. Resisted extension is weak compared with the uninjured side and produces pain.

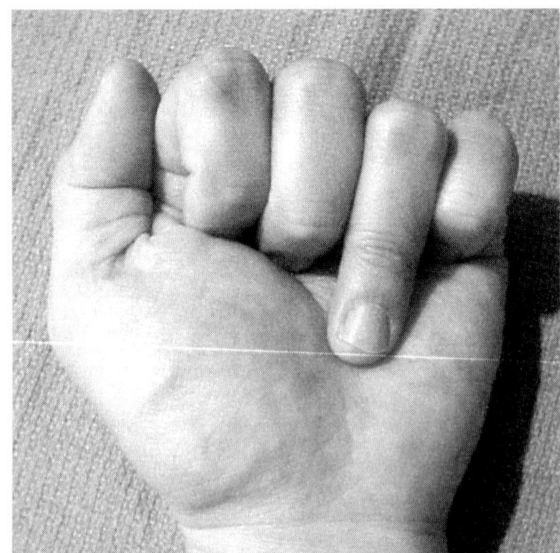

Figure 8–8: Jersey finger (FDP avulsion).

  - Extensor tendons usually do not retract as much as flexor tendons, and the cut ends may be clearly visible in the wound. If both ends are visible, repair the tendon in the emergency room. Otherwise, irrigate and close the wound and refer the patient to a hand surgeon for repair within 3 weeks.
  - Independent extensor tendons, such as the thumb extensors, extensor indicis proprius (index finger), and extensor digiti minimi (small finger), should be repaired within 1 to 2 weeks because they are not tethered to adjacent tendons through juncturae tendinum and tend to retract when lacerated.
  - Lacerations to dorsal radial and ulnar sensory nerves are common and should be repaired at the time of tendon repair.

- A *mallet finger* (inability to extend the DIP joint) develops after injury to the terminal portion of the digital extensor tendon (Figure 8–9).
  - The mechanism of injury can be a laceration of the tendon over the DIP joint or, more commonly, a blunt

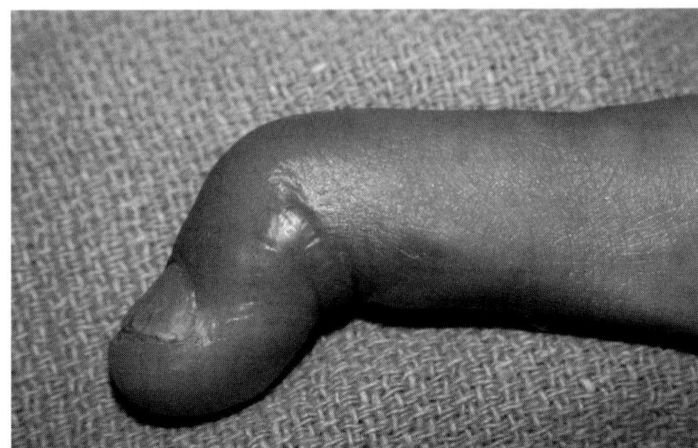

Figure 8–9: Mallet finger.

axial load injury to the end of the finger, causing avulsion of the tendon from its insertion at the base of the distal phalanx.
- The closed injury can cause avulsion of a fragment of bone from the distal phalanx articular surface; therefore, radiographs are essential. In the child, the fracture may involve the growth plate.
- Most closed mallet injuries, even with fracture, are best treated by 6 weeks of constant (24 hours a day) splinting in extension. You can use a straight, dorsal, padded aluminum splint secured by tape or a specially designed splint such as the Stack splint. The DIP joint should be kept in extension without hyperextension to avoid ulceration of the skin on the dorsum of the digit. Splinting can be used successfully to treat a mallet injury even if the patient has symptoms as late as 6 months after injury. The PIP joint is left free; active motion is encouraged at the PIP and metacarpophalangeal (MCP) joints to avoid stiffness.
- Displaced mallet fractures associated with subluxation of the DIP joint or involving more than one third of the articular surface on the lateral radiograph should be treated by anatomical reduction and internal fixation. Lacerations to the terminal extensor tendon should be repaired with suture and immobilized in extension for 4 weeks. Untreated terminal extensor injuries can lead to a fixed flexion deformity of the DIP joint and hyperextension at the PIP joint, the *swan neck deformity* (Figure 8–10).

- Injury to the extensor tendon over the PIP joint allows unopposed flexion at the joint by the FPS tendon and over time can lead to the *boutonnière deformity* (Figure 8–11): hyperextension of the DIP joint, fixed flexion of the PIP joint, and hyperextension of the MCP joint.
  - The portion of the extensor tendon over the PIP joint, the central slip, inserts dorsally at the base of the middle phalanx and can be injured by laceration or by dislocation of the PIP joint.
  - Central slip injury is often missed and should be suspected if the patient has pain and weakness on resisted extension of the PIP joint, even if the patient can actively extend the joint immediately after injury. The boutonnière deformity may not develop for several weeks after injury until the lateral bands on either side of the central slip subluxation palmar to the axis of the PIP joint and become flexors of the joint rather than extensors.
  - Treat central slip injuries by splinting in extension at the PIP joint for a minimum of 4 weeks, leaving the MCP and DIP joints free. Open central slip injuries should be sutured then splinted.

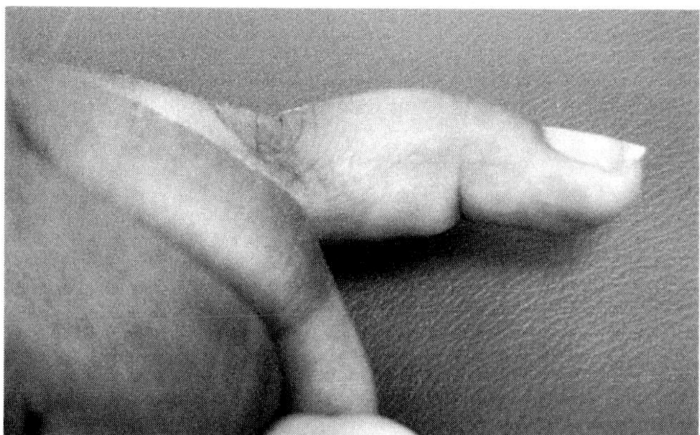

Figure 8–10: Swan neck deformity.

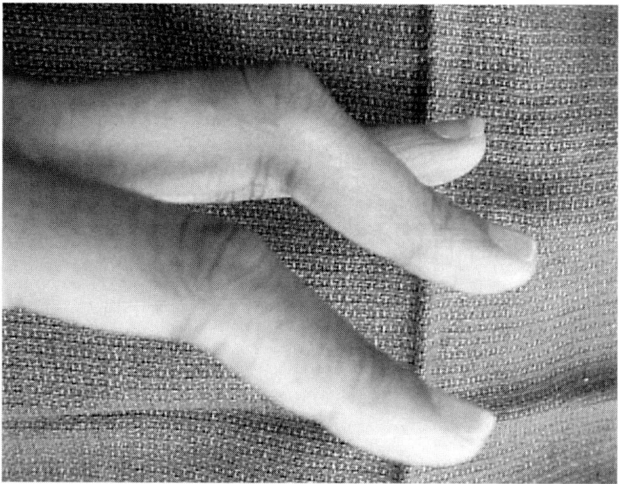

Figure 8–11: Boutonnière deformity.

- Laceration of the central extensor tendon will produce pain on resisted extension and an extensor lag at the MCP joint.
  - The extensor mechanism over the MCP joint is made of a thick central portion and a thin extensor hood that encircles the dorsum of the proximal phalanx.
  - Lacerations are typically partial but should be repaired by direct suture within 3 weeks. (The skin should be closed in the emergency room and placed in a volar splint.)
  - Lacerations over the MCP joint are often *fight bites* caused by a clenched fist striking an opponent's tooth and are at high risk for septic arthritis (described later in this chapter). These should not be closed.
  - Laceration of the extensor hood sagittal bands may lead to subluxation of the central extensor tendon to either the radial or ulnar side of the joint, making it difficult for the patient to initiate extension of the MCP joint from a flexed position.
- Overall, extensor tendon injuries have a better prognosis than flexor tendon injuries. It is imperative that flexor tendon injuries be recognized and repaired promptly because primary repair carries a much better prognosis.
- Prognosis is worse in tendon injuries associated with extensive soft tissue trauma, fracture, and neurovascular

injury. In these combined injuries, the priority for repair is revascularization, skeletal stabilization, then soft tissue coverage.

Compartment Syndrome

- One of the true emergencies in hand surgery, compartment syndrome is excessive pressure in the subfascial muscle compartments that results in irreversible loss of muscle and nerve function if left untreated.
- Causes include severe crush injuries, bleeding after arterial puncture, fractures, burns, muscle ischemia, and excessively tight casts. Any mechanism that causes swelling of the muscle increases compartment pressure, decreases venous outflow, and can initiate a positive feedback loop in which increased pressure decreases venous outflow, thus further increasing pressure within the tight fascial compartment, ultimately causing ischemic necrosis of the muscles and nerves within the compartment.
- Compartment syndrome may affect the volar or dorsal compartments of the forearm and the intrinsic muscle compartments (thenar, hypothenar, and interosseous) of the hand (Figure 8–12).
- Pain in the involved muscle compartment out of proportion to injury is usually the first symptom. Pain on passive stretch of those muscles is pathognomonic. The compartment becomes tense and painful to palpation. Compression of the nerves in the compartment causes paresthesias and later leads to paralysis. Pallor and loss of distal pulses are late findings and may not be present in all cases of compartment syndrome (Table 8–4).
- If left untreated, the muscles and nerves in the compartment undergo ischemic necrosis, leaving a paralyzed, contracted, and insensate extremity known as *Volkmann's contracture.*
- If the diagnosis of compartment syndrome remains equivocal after physical examination, the compartment pressure can be measured with an arterial line setup and an 18-gauge needle or a commercially available device specifically made for measuring compartment pressure. A pressure level greater than 30 mm Hg, or within 30 mm Hg of the mean arterial pressure in a hypotensive patient, warrants fasciotomy. Serial measurements of compartment pressure may be useful in obtunded patients. Compartment pressure measurement is contraindicated in coagulopathic patients and in patients with clear signs and symptoms of compartment syndrome.
- Treatment of compartment syndrome is urgent fasciotomy of all affected compartments and debridement of devitalized tissues. In severe cases, the wound may be left packed open until the swelling subsides then may be closed with skin graft. The carpal tunnel should also be decompressed, but the skin can be closed to protect the median nerve and flexor tendons. Consider prophylactic fasciotomy for obtunded patients who have had an appropriate mechanism of injury or for injuries that have caused a period of ischemia to the limb. Early hand rehabilitation is essential to restore maximal range of motion.
- Compartment syndrome is a problem that responds readily to early treatment and is irreversible when found late. The presence of compartment syndrome should be actively sought in every patient with a high-energy injury to the limb. If signs and symptoms are not present at the initial examination, they can appear later when swelling increases as a response to injury. Serial examinations are warranted until the swelling subsides. Complaints of increasing pain after application of a dressing or cast should prompt removal of the entire dressing or cast and examination for compartment syndrome. Missed diagnosis and late diagnosis are the main pitfalls associated with compartment syndrome.

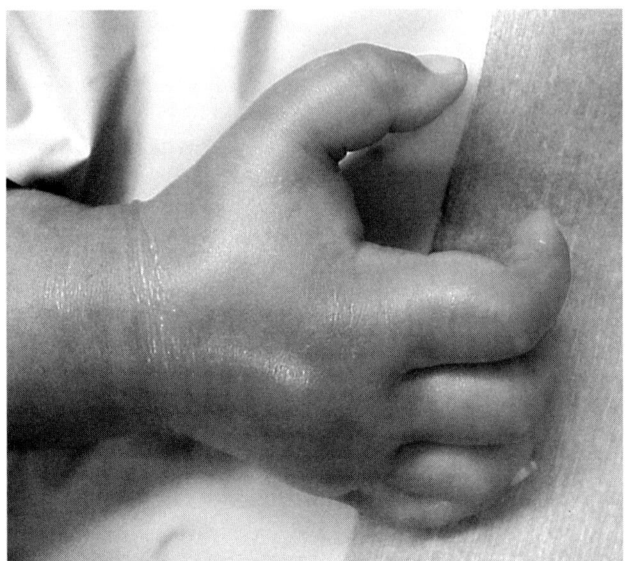

Figure 8–12: Compartment syndrome of the hand after a crush injury.

Table 8–4: Symptoms of Compartment Syndrome

TIMING	SYMPTOM
Early	Pain Paresthesias
Late	Paralysis Pallor Pulseless

Fingertip and Nail Injuries

- Fingertip injuries are common in children, mostly from being crushed in a door.
- Initial examination should note the level of injury, the presence of nail bed injury, and whether there is exposed

bone. If still attached, the distal tip color, capillary refill, and sensibility should be checked. Radiographs are essential.

- The level of injury determines the choice of treatment for complete amputations.
  - Amputation distal to the bone heals well with daily dressing changes. The parents must be reassured that fingertip amputation wounds less than 1 cm in diameter, with no exposed bone, heal better by secondary intention than by surgical closure.
  - Amputations through the distal phalanx require closure with a local fingertip flap or a thenar flap (Figure 8–13) to cover the bone and maintain length.
  - Amputations near the nail fold but distal to the DIP joint are best treated by shortening and primary closure. In children younger than 2 years, the fingertips are so small that amputated fingertips can survive as composite grafts if they are sutured back on with a few absorbable sutures to approximate the skin.
  - Amputations proximal to the DIP joint should be considered for replantation, which will be described in the following section.
- Incomplete amputations are often associated with nail bed lacerations and distal phalanx fractures (Figure 8–14). These injuries can usually be treated in the emergency room under sedation and digital nerve block. A Penrose drain is used as a digital tourniquet to provide a bloodless field. The nail plate should be dissected free of the nail bed with a fine hemostat or smooth periosteal elevator to fully expose the laceration. The nail bed is then repaired with 6–0 or 7–0 absorbable sutures, and the nail plate is replaced to protect the repair. Realignment and repair of the nail bed laceration is usually sufficient treatment for the underlying fracture as well. Lacerations to the adjacent skin can be repaired with 6–0 absorbable sutures.
- A laceration through the most proximal portion of the nail bed can be associated with an open Salter-Harris type I fracture of the distal phalanx growth plate (Seymour fracture). These fractures should be treated in the operating room with irrigation, reduction, and percutaneous pinning of the fracture (Figure 8–15). This will bring the nail bed laceration together without the need for suturing.
- Isolated subungual hematomas from a crush injury to the fingertip can be painful and can be drained by trephination of the nail plate with an ophthalmic cautery or heated paperclip. The nail plate should be removed and the nail bed should be explored if there is a displaced fracture of the distal phalanx, laceration to the skin adjacent to the nail, or displacement of the proximal portion of the nail plate from the nail fold. These three findings are more accurate predictors of nail bed laceration than the size of the hematoma.

Amputations

- Amputations in children are most often caused by a crush or avulsion mechanism such as a bicycle chain or spoke. Replantation of the amputated part is the ideal reconstruction because it restores both form and function without any donor site morbidity and maintains growth potential. By definition, *replantation* is reattachment of a completely amputated part, and *revascularization* is reattachment of an incompletely amputated part requiring vascular reconstruction (Figure 8–16). If there are no life-threatening injuries and replantation is technically feasible, all amputated parts should be replanted in children.
- Initial treatment for a child with an amputation begins with a complete trauma survey to identify other, potentially life-threatening injuries. An intravenous line is

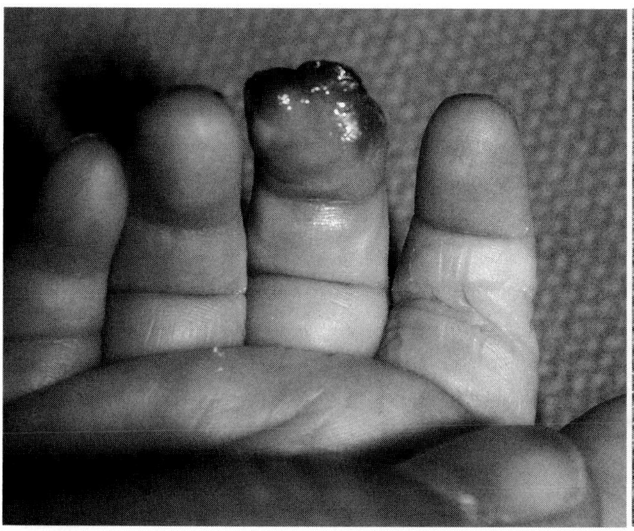

A

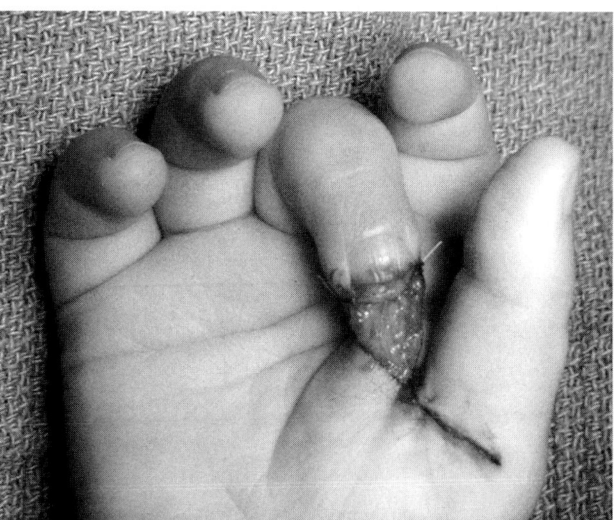

B

Figure 8–13: **A, Fingertip amputation with exposed bone. B, Thenar flap attached.**

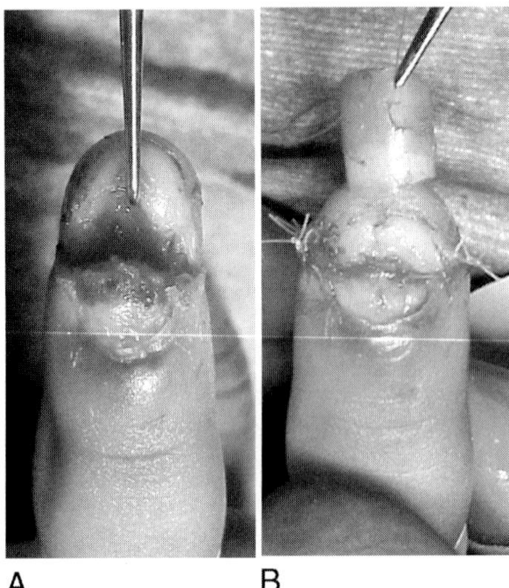

Figure 8–14: A, Nail bed laceration. B, Nail bed after repair.

established, cephalothin is administered, and tetanus prophylaxis is given.

- The amputation stump is irrigated, bleeding is stopped, and a sterile dressing is applied. Radiographs are obtained of the stump and the amputated part. The part is then irrigated, wrapped in moist saline gauze, and placed in a sterile watertight container. The container is placed in mixture of ice and water to cool the part, thus delaying the onset of ischemic necrosis.
- Partially amputated parts should be immobilized with a splint and cooled with an ice pack over the dressing. *Do not complete the amputation.* If the patient is stable, arrange prompt transfer to a replantation center.
- You should avoid the temptation to reassure the patient or family that the part can be replanted. Only the

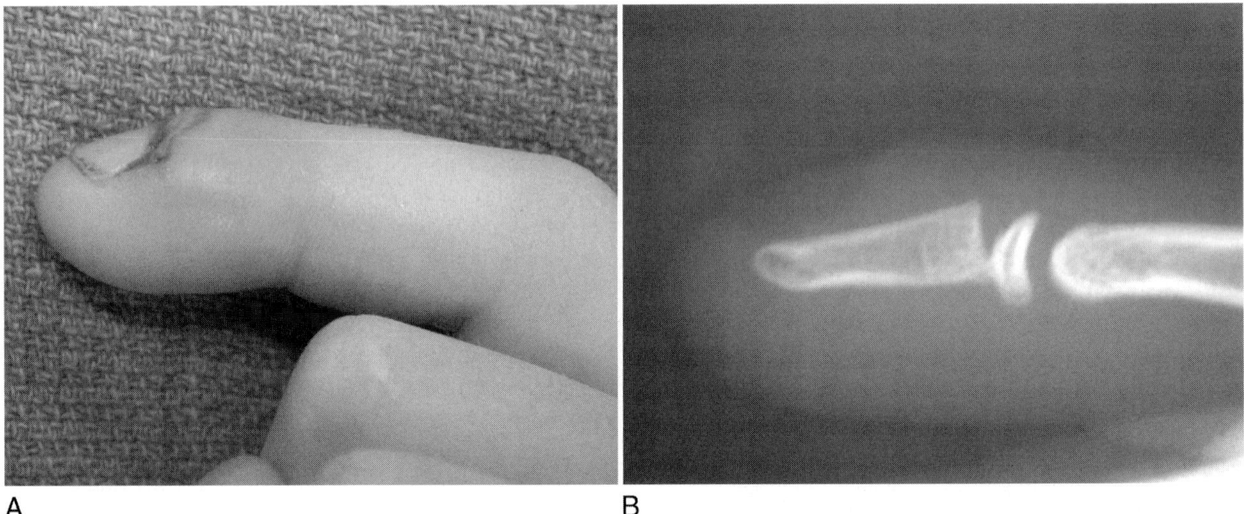

Figure 8–15: Seymour fracture. A, Gross appearance. B, Radiograph demonstrating growth plate fracture of the distal phalanx.

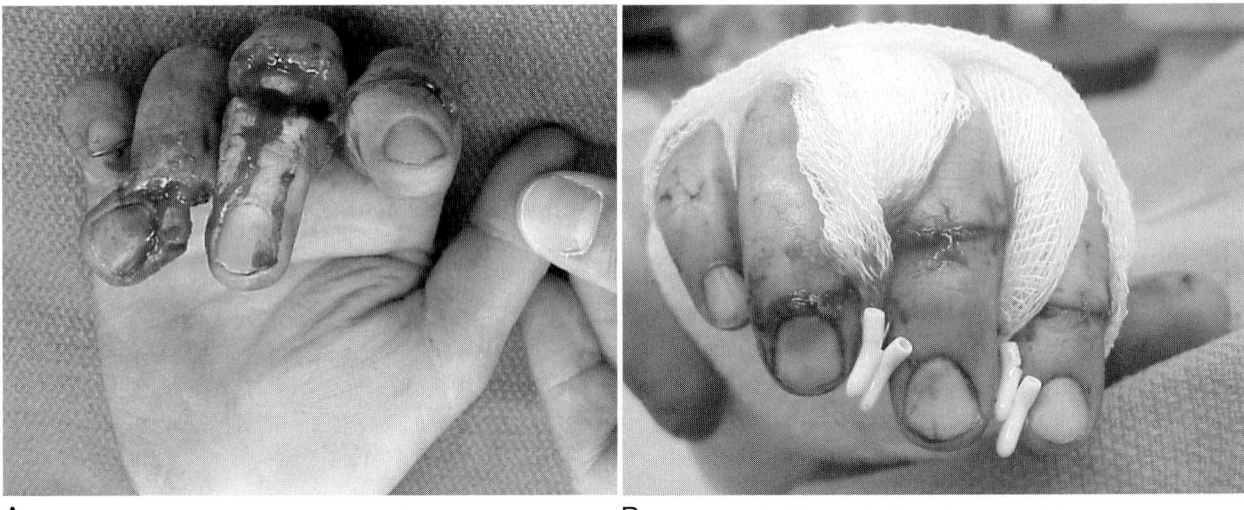

Figure 8–16: A, Partial amputation of digits from a crush injury. B, Digits after revascularization.

surgeon, after exploration in the operating room, can determine whether a part can be replanted.

- Contraindications to replantation include multilevel injury (Figure 8–17), prolonged ischemia time, and severe crush or avulsion.
- Replantation entails 4 to 8 hours of surgery for a single digit. The replanted part is monitored by continuous pulse oximetry and hourly checks of color and capillary refill for the first 48 to 72 hours after surgery. Any sign of decrease perfusion or venous insufficiency should prompt a return to the operating room for reexploration. The patient remains hospitalized for approximately 1 week after replantation. The hemoglobin level should be monitored; children are more likely to require transfusion after replantation than adults.
- Approximately 70% to 85% of pediatric upper extremity replantations survive, which is lower than in adults. However, children achieve better function, if the part survives, because of better nerve regeneration, bone healing, and joint mobility.
- Functional outcome after replantation is poorest for crush and avulsion injuries and is best for partial amputations. The functional outcome also depends on the level of the amputation: replantation at the upper arm or proximal forearm carries the worst prognosis, and replantation at the wrist, the palm, and the finger distal to the insertion of the FDS carries the best prognosis.

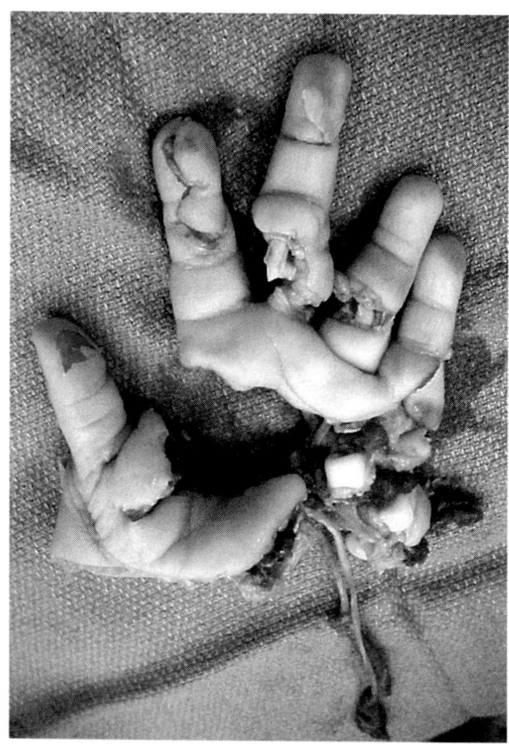

Figure 8–17: Multilevel meat grinder injury in a 4-year-old.

Burns

- Burns can be caused by thermal, mechanical, chemical, or electrical injury.
- In children, thermal injury is most common because most chemical and electrical burns are occupational. Direct contact with a hot surface, scalding, and an open flame can cause thermal burns. Typical examples include touching a fireplace glass enclosure, scalding from pulling down a hot pot of water, and burning clothes from a house fire.
- Scalding and contact burns on infants still unable to walk should raise the suspicion of child abuse.
- *Thermal burns* are classified by depth of injury.
  - First-degree burns produce erythema but no skin necrosis.
  - Second-degree burns exhibit painful blistering with loss of the epidermis and part of the dermis.
  - Third-degree burns involve the full thickness of the skin, leaving the skin dry, pale, and insensate.
- First- and second-degree burns will heal by reepithelialization from the skin appendages as long as infection and desiccation are avoided.
- Third-degree burns heal by scarring and contraction, which can restrict motion in the hand. A joint contracture develops if a third-degree burn crosses a flexion crease and is allowed to heal by scar contraction.
- First- and second-degree burns are treated by a topical antimicrobial ointment, usually silver sulfadiazine, which is soothing, minimizes the chance of infection, and keeps the wound moist. These more superficial burns typically reepithelialize in 1 week. If the burn crosses a joint flexion crease, the hand should be splinted with the involved joints in extension.
- Third-degree burns are best treated by early tangential excision and full-thickness skin graft to prevent joint contracture. The hand is then splinted in the "safe" position (MCP joints flexed and PIP and DIP joints extended). Range of motion exercises begin as soon as the grafts are adherent. Once the grafts are healed, custom compression gloves are fitted to reduce edema and the formation of hypertrophic scars.
- It may be difficult to differentiate a deep second-degree burn from a third-degree burn, but any hand burn that has not healed by 2 weeks is probably best treated by excision and skin graft.
- Exposed tendon or bone requires pedicled or free flaps for coverage.
- *Mechanical abrasions* from contact with a rough surface can occur from child versus motor vehicle collisions and from exercise treadmills. Many of these are equivalent to deep second- or third-degree thermal burns. Treatment is identical to that for thermal burns except that more extensive cleansing and debridement is usually necessary.

- Children can suffer *chemical burns* by coming in contact with household products containing strong acids (e.g., toilet cleaners) and alkalis (e.g., bleach). Initial treatment includes removal of all clothing contaminated by the chemical and copious irrigation of the affected skin with tap water for at least 20 minutes. Specific neutralizing agents may be indicated (e.g., calcium gluconate for hydrofluoric acid burns).
- *Electrical burns* in children are most often from a 110-volt household current that rarely causes problems associated with high-voltage (more than 1000 volts) injuries such as cardiac arrhythmias, renal failure, seizures, and compartment syndrome. Most burns occur when the child sticks a conductive object into an electric socket and suffers a flame burn to the hand from the electric arc. These injuries usually heal with topical silver sulfadiazine dressings.

Infection

- Infections of the hand in children often arise from traumatic wounds contaminated by skin flora or saliva. Diagnosis is evident from swelling, erythema, tenderness, and fluctuance.
- Infection may involve a variety of tissues and spaces: skin (cellulitis and paronychia), subcutaneous tissues (felon), bone (osteomyelitis), flexor tendon sheath (tenosynovitis), and joint space (septic arthritis).
- Early diagnosis, adequate drainage of purulent collections, and coverage with appropriate antibiotics are the keys to successful outcome. Undrained collections are the most common reasons for failure of antibiotic therapy.
- Purulent collections can usually be diagnosed by physical examination, but ultrasound and MRI may be needed to diagnose deep collections. Radiographs should be obtained to look for osteomyelitis in all cases of deep infection.
- Antibiotic coverage should be based on cultures and susceptibility whenever possible. Obtain material for cultures by incision or aspiration before beginning empiric antibiotic therapy (Table 8–5). Appropriate tetanus prophylaxis should be given.
- All animal and human bites to the hand require irrigation and prophylactic antibiotic coverage with amoxicillin–clavulanate (clindamycin and ciprofloxacin for the penicillin allergic). Common infectious organisms include gram-positive cocci, anaerobes, *Pasteurella multocida* (cat), *Eikenella corrodens* (human), and *Pasteurella canis* (dog).
- In general, bites should be left open for drainage to minimize chance of infection. Patients who suffer cat, dog, and wild animal bites should receive prophylactic rabies treatment with both antirabies globulin and the vaccine if the animal has not been immunized and cannot be observed for 10 days.
- Patients with cellulitis, felon, and paronychia can usually be treated as outpatients. Exceptions include patients who are immunocompromised, diabetic, unreliable, or have systemic signs of infection such as lymphangitis, leukocytosis, or fever.
- Patients with septic arthritis, flexor tenosynovitis, osteomyelitis, and human bites of the hand require admission for adequate drainage and at least a few days of intravenous antibiotics until clinical signs show improvement.

Paronychia

- An infection of the soft tissues around the nail is called a paronychia (Figure 8–18). The infection may start as a cellulitis and progress to a localized abscess. It may involve the nail fold (eponychial fold) or dissect under the nail, creating a subungual abscess.
- Untreated paronychia can evolve into osteomyelitis and septic arthritis.
- The infection is usually caused by *Staphylococcus aureus* but may be caused by oral flora in children who suck their fingers.
- Early infections in the cellulitis stage can be treated with oral antibiotics and hand washing with warm soaks several times a day.
- Palpable fluctuance signifies the presence of an abscess, which should be drained by incising the entire diameter of the abscess through the thinnest portion of the abscess wall. If the abscess extends under the nail, the nail should be elevated or partially excised for adequate drainage. All infected bone must be debrided.
- Wounds are left open and treated with soap and water washings and warm soaks several times a day to promote drainage. These procedures can usually be accomplished under digital block anesthesia.

Table 8–5: Empiric Antibiotic Therapy for Hand Infections

CLINICAL CONDITION	EMPIRIC TREATMENT	DURATION
Cellulitis, felon, paronychia	Dicloxacillin, cephalexin, or erythromycin	7-14 days
Septic arthritis, tenosynovitis	Nafcillin and third-generation cephalosporin or vancomycin and gentamicin	2-4 weeks
Osteomyelitis	Nafcillin and ciprofloxacin; ampicillin–sulbactam; or vancomycin, ciprofloxacin, and clindamycin	6 weeks
Human or animal bite	Ampicillin–sulbactam or clindamycin and ciprofloxacin	Depends on location

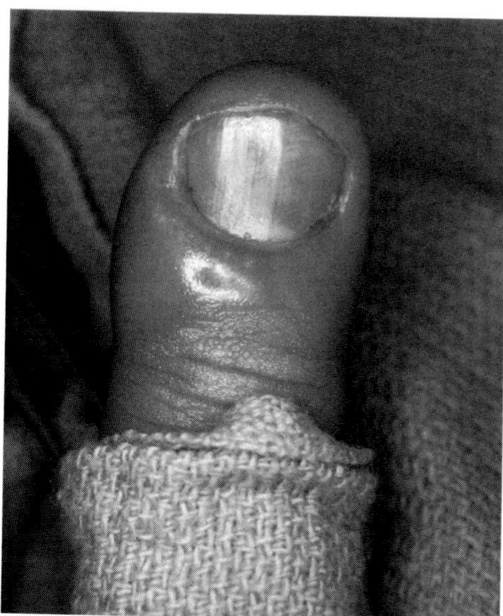

Figure 8–18: Paronychia in a nail biter.

- Antistaphylococcal antibiotics are used for 7 to 14 days depending on clinical improvement. Osteomyelitis requires 6 weeks of intravenous antibiotics.

Felon

- A felon is an infection of the volar subcutaneous tissues of the distal phalanx. The volar pad becomes tense, exquisitely tender, and erythematous. A felon can extend into the flexor tendon sheath, causing a suppurative tenosynovitis.
- Early infection may respond to antistaphylococcal antibiotics alone.
- Once an abscess cavity develops, it must be incised and packed open for a few days to promote complete drainage. The incision is best made in the thinnest portion of the abscess wall; any loculations created by the vertical fibrous septa should be drained by dividing the septa. All necrotic soft tissues and infected bone must be debrided.

Flexor Tenosynovitis

- A sheath extending from the distal palm to the distal phalanx encloses the flexor tendons. The potential space between the tendon and the sheath can become infected by penetrating trauma (Figure 8–19) or by hematogenous or contiguous spread.
- This is a true hand emergency. Delayed treatment will cause adhesions to form between the tendon and the sheath, impairing tendon gliding and range of motion. Left untreated, the infection will destroy the tendon and can track proximally into the palm and forearm along the bursae, which surround the tendons.
- The diagnosis of flexor tenosynovitis can usually be made by physical examination (Box 8–3). All of the four signs need not be present for the flexor tenosynovitis to be present. Conversely, a subcutaneous abscess or severe cellulitis can sometimes produce all four signs and masquerade as flexor tenosynovitis. If there is any question about the diagnosis, the tendon sheath should be explored in the operating room.

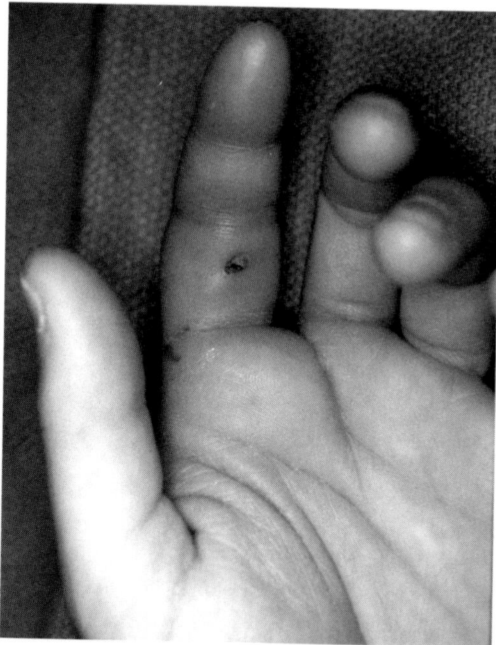

Figure 8–19: Flexor tenosynovitis after a cat bite.

- The treatment for suppurative flexor tenosynovitis is prompt incision, drainage, and irrigation of the flexor tendon sheath. Broad-spectrum antibiotic therapy should commence immediately after cultures are obtained. The tendon sheath is opened proximally in the palm, and an 18-gauge intravenous catheter is inserted into the flexor tendon sheath for postoperative irrigation. A counter incision is made in the distal sheath at the DIP flexion crease for egress of the irrigation fluid. The sheath is then irrigated while the patient is on the operating table until the fluid runs clear. The hand is placed in a bulky gauze dressing and waterproof splint.
- After surgery, the catheter is left in place for 48 hours and the sheath is irrigated with saline solution at 10 ml/hr using an intravenous pump. The catheter is then removed, and active range of motion exercises are begun under the supervision of a hand therapist. The most common complication of this infection is stiffness of the finger. The

Box 8–3 Kanavel's Signs of Flexor Tenosynovitis

1. Symmetrical swelling along the flexor tendon sheath
2. Tenderness and erythema over the flexor tendon sheath
3. Flexed position of the finger
4. Severe pain on passive extension

wounds are left open to heal by secondary intention. Hand washing and soaking in warm water twice daily help to keep the wounds clean and to promote drainage.

Septic Arthritis

- Infection of a joint usually arises from penetrating trauma. Delayed diagnosis and treatment can lead to devastating joint destruction, osteomyelitis, and ascending limb-threatening infection.
- You should suspect any laceration to the dorsum of the hand over a joint to be a human bite from a clenched fist striking an opponent's tooth (fight bite).
  - The MCP joint is most commonly injured by this mechanism. A radiograph should be obtained to look for fracture and foreign body (Figure 8–20).
  - The wound should be anesthetized, irrigated, and explored with the joint in flexion and extension to check for penetration into the joint. If the extensor tendon mechanism is punctured, it is likely that the joint space has been violated and the patient should be taken to the operating room for exploration and irrigation of the joint.
  - If the wound was indeed a human bite, it should be left open and the patient should be treated with amoxicillin–clavulanate to cover the common infective organisms (*Staphylococcus aureus, Streptococci, Eikenella corrodens,* and anaerobes).
  - More commonly, the patient does not seek treatment until there are signs and symptoms of established infection in the joint such as swelling, erythema, pain on passive motion, lymphangitis, or frank purulence. These patients should be taken to the operating room for arthrotomy and for the placement of an irrigation catheter into the joint. The wound is left open and the joint is continuously irrigated for 48 hours with saline at 10 ml/hr. The tendon is not repaired primarily; the wound is allowed to heal by secondary intention with early active motion to prevent joint stiffness. Intravenous ampicillin–sulbactam is given empirically until bacterial culture results are available. Antibiotic therapy is continued for 2 to 4 weeks depending on clinical response.

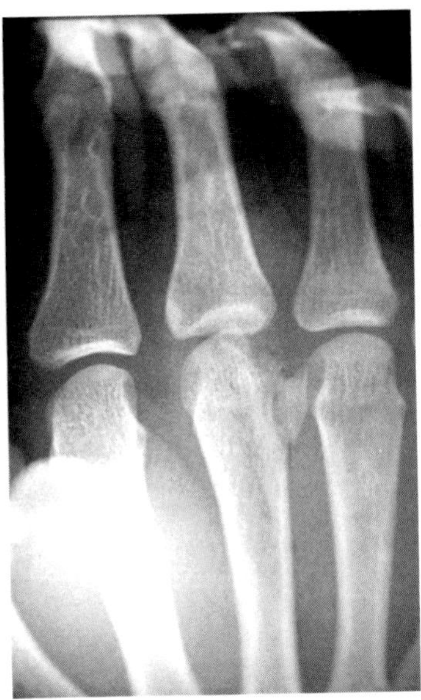

Figure 8–20: Metacarpal head fracture and septic arthritis after punching an opponent in the mouth.

- Septic arthritis not associated with penetrating trauma can arise from hematogenous spread (e.g., gonococcus) and contiguous spread from paronychia, felon or local abscess. Treatment is by aspiration or incision and drainage of the joint followed by empiric treatment with nafcillin and a third-generation cephalosporin (or vancomycin and gentamicin in those with penicillin allergy) until culture results are available.
- Rheumatoid arthritis, gout, and pseudogout should be considered in the differential diagnosis of septic arthritis.

Tumor

- Hand tumors in children are rare, and most tumors are benign[3] (Table 8–6).
- When faced with a child with a hand tumor, a careful history and physical examination can suggest a likely diagnosis.
- Imaging studies can be helpful with the diagnosis of bony tumors. Ultrasound can differentiate between cystic and solid tumors.
- If the diagnosis is still uncertain after obtaining the history, physical examination, and imaging studies, the mass should be excised for pathological examination. If the mass is large, an incisional biopsy may be performed first and definitive excision may be deferred until the pathological diagnosis is available. Pathological examination of the specimen is the only way to definitively exclude malignancy.

Table 8–6: Pediatric Hand Tumors

TUMOR	FREQUENCY (%)
Cysts	27
Foreign body	21
Vascular malformations	14
Enchondroma	9
Epidermal inclusion cysts	7
Fibrous tumors	6
Nodular tenosynovitis	3
Exostoses	3
Pseudoaneurysm	3
Glomus tumor	2
Lipoma	2
Malignant tumors	2

Adapted from Colon F, Upton J (1995) Pediatric hand tumors: A review of 349 cases. Hand Clin 11(2): 223-244.

History

- The *history* should include the following details regarding the tumor: duration, changes in size, changes in pigmentation for cutaneous lesions, antecedent trauma, pain, and functional problems.
- A long duration of existence with no growth favors a benign lesion but is insufficient to exclude malignancy.
- Changes in pigmentation or contour can signify malignant change in cutaneous nevi.
- A history of penetrating trauma before the onset of a tumor suggests a foreign body, pseudoaneurysm, or epidermal inclusion cyst as the likely diagnosis.
- Pain and functional impairment may be indications for excision.
- A family history should also be obtained because some conditions are inherited, such as multiple hereditary exostoses.

Physical Examination

- The size, location, presence of tenderness, texture, firmness, and fixation to surrounding tissues should be noted.
- A complete neuromuscular and vascular examination of the extremity should be performed.
- Functional impairments should be measured and recorded.

Diagnostic Imaging

- Plain radiographs should be obtained on all *bony tumors.*
- If there are any unusual radiographic or clinical features, additional imaging with MRI or computerized tomography (CT) can help to diagnose and stage the lesion.
- *Soft tissue tumors* that are not obviously ganglion cysts or vascular malformations should undergo MRI before excision unless they are small, superficial, and easily excised for diagnosis.
- Magnetic resonance angiography (MRA) and MRI can identify the extent and flow characteristics of vascular tumors such as malformations and pseudoaneurysm.

Benign Soft Tissue Tumors

Cysts

- Fluid-filled cysts are the most common soft tissue hand tumors in children; such cysts are more common in children than they are in adults.
- The most common locations are the wrist (ganglion cysts, Figure 8–21) followed by the flexor tendon sheath (retinacular cysts). Both types are firm and rubbery in consistency, fixed to the underlying joint or tendon sheath, and covered by normal, mobile skin.
- Tenderness may or may not be present; most are asymptomatic. If the appearance or location is atypical, an ultrasound can confirm the diagnosis.

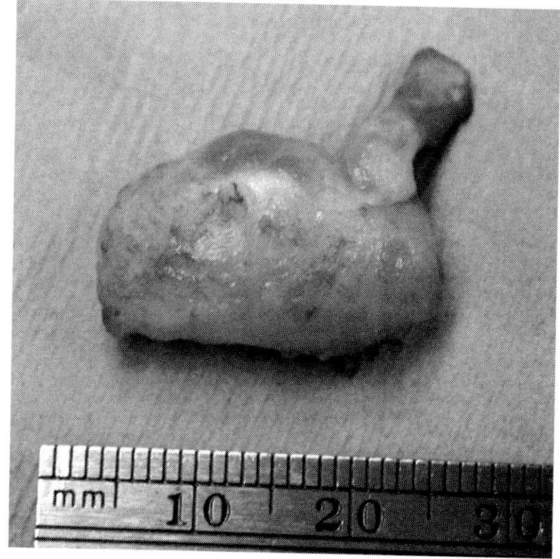

Figure 8–21: Ganglion cyst with a stalk.

- Wrist ganglion cysts arise from the joint, and retinacular cysts arise from the tendon sheath. Synovial cysts are the least common and arise from the extensor tendons on the metacarpal portion of the hand.
- Cysts may fluctuate in size, and some may spontaneously regress. Cysts may appear at any age from infancy to adolescence. Mucous cysts of the DIP joint are not found in children because they are caused by osteoarthritis.
- Immobilization, traumatic rupture, and aspiration are not recommended. Aspiration was effective in only 20% of Upton's cases.[3]
- Observation is the preferred treatment unless the cyst causes pain or functional impairment.
- Surgical excision includes removal of the entire cyst wall with a small portion of the wrist capsule or tendon sheath to prevent recurrence.

Foreign Body

- Foreign bodies are most often found in the palmar surface of the hand and should be suspected when there is a history of a puncture wound or the patient has a mass and infection unresponsive to antibiotics. Many younger children do not give a history of antecedent trauma.
- Imaging with plain radiographs can demonstrate metal, stone, and some glass foreign bodies. Radiolucent foreign bodies such as splinters or pencil lead can be detected by ultrasound, but this is not mandatory.
- Treatment is removal of the foreign body and curettage of the cavity. The incision should be left open if there is any evidence of infection.

Vascular Tumors

- Vascular tumors represent nearly 20% of tumors in the upper extremity. Hemangiomas and vascular malformations are the most common pediatric vascular tumors and occur with equal frequency in the upper extremity. Other vascular tumors include pyogenic granuloma, pseudoaneurysm, and glomus tumor (in descending order of frequency).

- *Hemangiomas* (Figure 8–22) can arise anywhere on the hand and are the most common vascular tumors in children. They rapidly proliferate during the first 2 years of life and spontaneously involute by 5 to 7 years of age. Therefore, surgery is rarely necessary.
- *Vascular malformations* are usually present at birth, grow proportionately with the patient, and do not involute.[4] Prognosis is strongly determined by whether the malformation is a slow- or fast-flow type.
  - Slow-flow malformations have a good prognosis and are further categorized as capillary, venous, or lymphatic (Figure 8–23).
  - Fast-flow malformations have a palpable pulsation or thrill (Figure 8–24). They contain arteriovenous fistulae, which progressively enlarge and can produce a distal vascular steal.
  - Initial treatment in all malformations is use of compression garments, although these are not well tolerated in many patients.
  - Surgical indications include pain, excessive bulk, functional impairment, bleeding, and vascular steal. MRI and MRA should be obtained before surgery to define the extent and flow characteristics of the malformation.
  - Low-flow malformations and some high-flow malformations can be debulked in stages.
  - High-flow malformations that exhibit vascular steal are the most difficult to treat and progress to amputation in 90% of cases.[5] Selective embolization has been used instead of surgery or before surgery in the high-flow type. Surgery is reserved for the specific indications listed previously and is not done prophylactically.
- *Pyogenic granulomas* (Figure 8–25) are rapidly growing polypoid tumors composed of highly vascular granulation tissue that bleeds easily. They arise from small wounds that fail to heal. In the hand, they are most often found on the palm and palmar side of the digits. Small pyogenic granulomas may resolve with silver nitrate cautery. Larger granulomas should be excised, and the defect should be closed. Curettage or shave excision frequently results in recurrence.
- *Pseudoaneurysms* (Figure 8–26) of the upper extremity present as slowly enlarging pulsatile masses weeks to months after a puncture wound. Typically, pulsatile bleeding was noted at the time of injury and stopped with direct pressure. MRA or Doppler confirms the diagnosis. If distal perfusion is adequate, the pseudoaneurysm can simply be excised and the can be artery ligated. Revascularization with vein graft is necessary if there are signs of ischemia after excision of the pseudoaneurysm.
- *Glomus tumors* are rare but can be the source of unexplained pain in the hand. If the pain is worse with

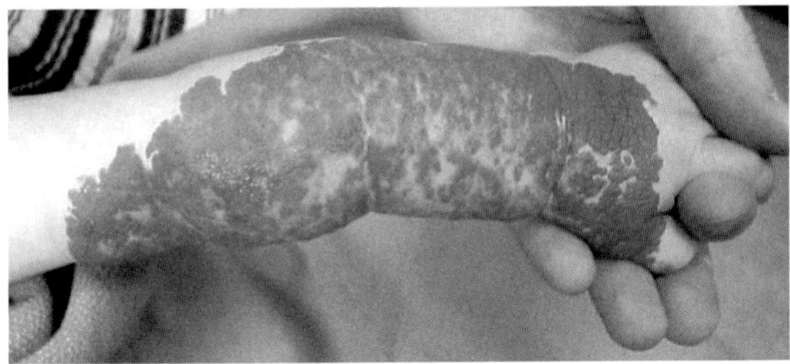

Figure 8–22: Hemangioma with areas of regression.

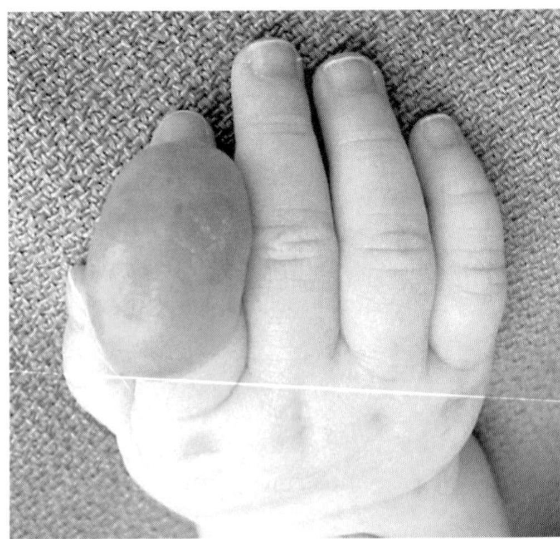

Figure 8–23: Low-flow lymphatic–venous vascular malformation.

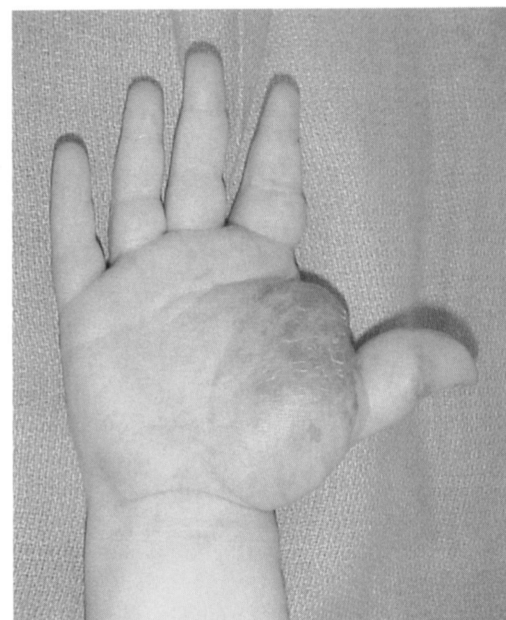

Figure 8–24: High-flow arteriovenous malformation.

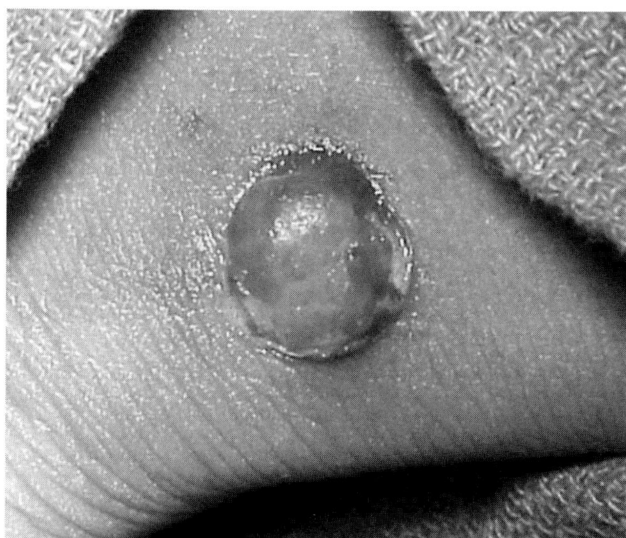

Figure 8–25: Pyogenic granuloma.

exposure to cold or with pressure, you should suspect a glomus tumor. They can be visible as small bluish tumors and are most often found on the glabrous surface of the hand or in a subungual location. The glomus tumor may be hard to palpate because of its small size. MRI can aid in the diagnosis but is usually not necessary. Treatment is complete excision.

Epidermal Inclusion Cyst

- This firm, fixed, nontender mass is most frequently found in the palm and the volar pads of the fingers. It follows an episode of penetrating trauma by months to years, but the history of trauma may not be elicited in every case.
- Fragments of epithelium or germinal matrix are left in the subcutaneous tissue after the penetrating trauma and continue to produce keratin, forming a cystic collection. The cyst grows slowly and can erode the underlying distal phalanx; thus radiographs may aid in the diagnosis.
- Complete excision is curative. The cysts can recur if part of the cyst wall remains.

Fibrous Tumors

- Fibrous tumors are rare but create anxiety in parents because they are hard, are immobile, and grow.
- *Infantile digital fibroma* is found in young children on the sides or dorsal surfaces of the ulnar three digits. It grows rapidly and can infiltrate the skin.
- *Juvenile aponeurotic fibroma* is usually found in the palm. Stippled calcifications are present on radiographs.
- Fibromas can be found in other locations, such as between the extensor tendon and the proximal phalanx.
- Treatment for all fibromas is complete excision. Recurrence rates are high because complete excision is often impossible.

Nodular Tenosynovitis

- Like fibromas, these tumors are hard, immobile, immobile, and expansile, but they are multilobulated (Figure 8–27). Other names for nodular tenosynovitis are giant cell tumor and xanthoma. These tumors are yellowish brown, multilobulated, and encapsulated, and they can extend into joints and around tendons. They occur more frequently in adolescents than in young children. Complete excision is curative.

Lipoma

- Lipomas appear as large, soft, painless masses in the palm. They are much less common in children than in adults.

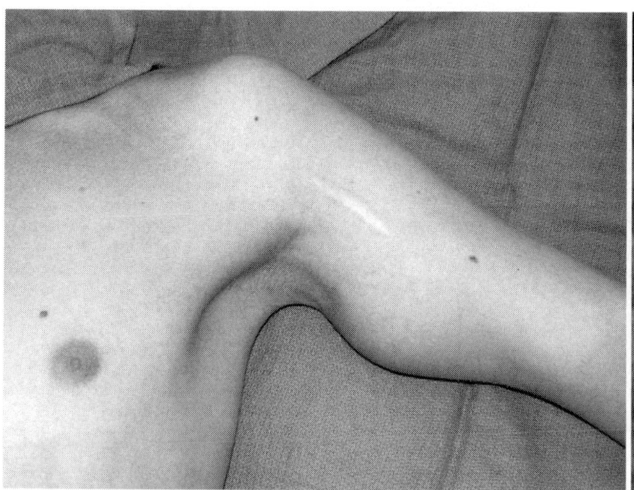

A

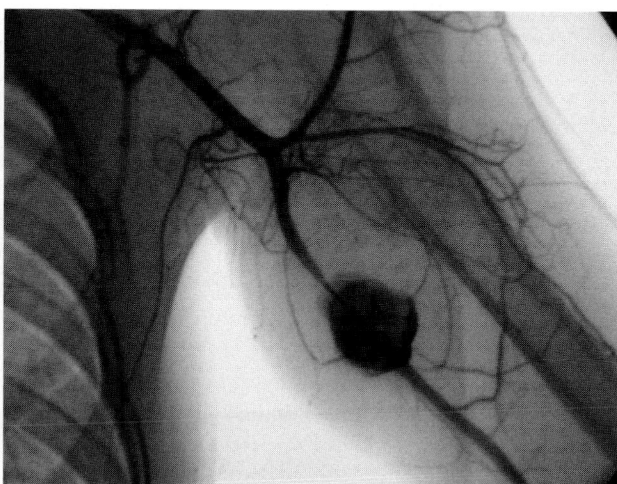

B

Figure 8–26: A, Pseudoaneurysm of a brachial artery 13 years after excision of an osteochondroma. B, Angiogram of pseudoaneurysm.

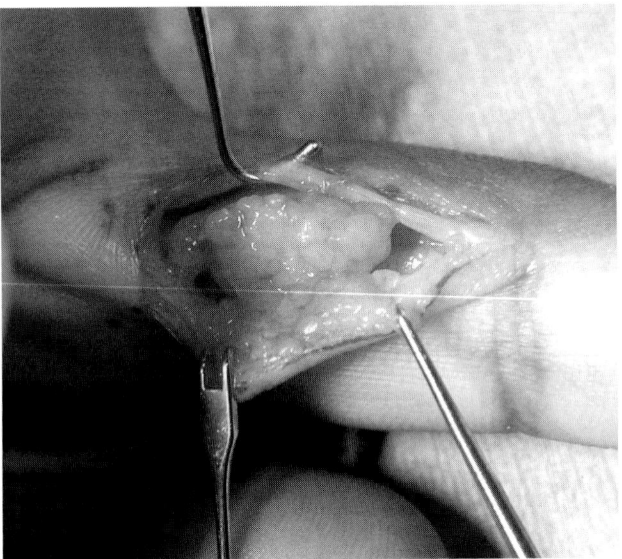

Figure 8–27: Nodular tenosynovitis of the digit with a hook retracting the digital nerve.

- Surgery is reserved for symptomatic lipomas. They are encapsulated and usually shell out easily. Recurrence is rare.

Benign Bone Tumors

Enchondroma

- In children, enchondromas are the most common primary bone tumor and are frequently associated with Ollier's disease (multiple enchondromatosis) or Maffucci's syndrome (multiple enchondromas and vascular malformations).
- The proximal phalanges are most frequently involved.
- Radiographs show thinning of the cortex and replacement of the cancellous bone by a radiolucent mass containing calcifications.
- Enchondromas usually appear in adolescence and young adulthood as pathological fractures. The fracture is reduced and allowed to heal before curettage of the enchondroma and cancellous bone grafting.

Osteochondroma (Exostosis)

- Osteochondromas are benign outgrowths from a bone and are capped by cartilage (Figure 8–28). Most osteochondromas of the hand in pediatric patients are found in patients with multiple hereditary exostoses.
- Osteochondromas are excised only if they cause symptoms such as pain, nerve impingement, restriction of joint motion, or angulation of the underlying bone.

Malignant Hand Tumors

- Malignant pediatric hand tumors are exceedingly rare, representing only 2% of the cases in Upton's series.[3]

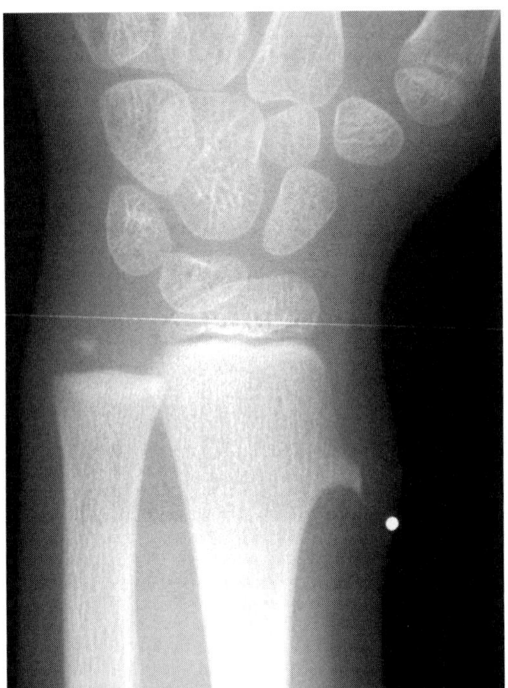

Figure 8–28: Osteochondroma of the distal radius.

- The most common soft tissue malignancies are sarcoma (Figure 8–29) and melanoma. The most common skeletal malignancies are osteosarcoma and Ewing's sarcoma.
- The key to treatment of malignancies is tissue diagnosis. Incisional biopsy is preferred for large lesions; small tumors can be excised as long as the incision is oriented

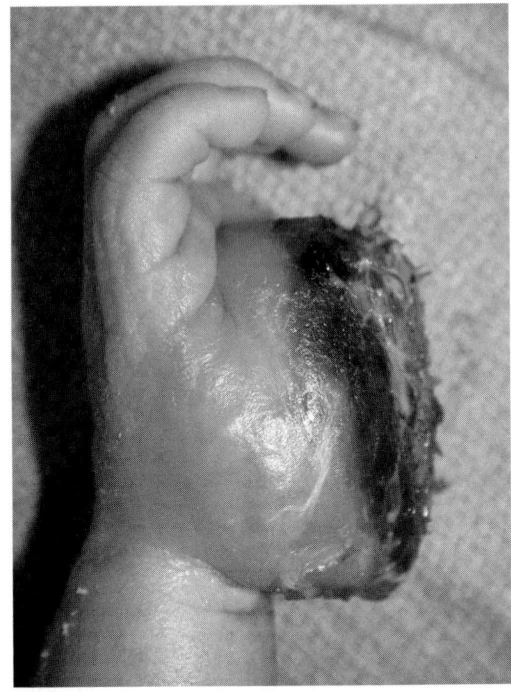

Figure 8–29: Infantile fibrosarcoma in a newborn.

so that the biopsy site can be completely excised at the time of definitive resection without compromising the chances for limb salvage.

- Complete staging of the tumor to define the extent of local invasion and the presence of metastases is mandatory *before* definitive treatment. MRI, bone scan, and CT of the chest are frequently used for staging.
- For some tumors, limb-sparing surgery combined with radiation or chemotherapy produces survival rates comparable with amputation alone and preserves hand function.

Congenital Anomalies

- Congenital anomalies affect 1 to 2% of newborns, with approximately 10% of the anomalies occurring in the upper extremity.[6]
- Anomalies require an accurate diagnosis and communication of relevant information to the family.
- Certain upper extremity anomalies occur in isolation; others are associated with systemic conditions. These associated ailments often take precedence over the limb anomaly; therefore, they must be attended to before the limb condition is treated.

Embryology

- Embryogenesis of the upper extremity commences with formation of the upper limb bud on the lateral wall of the embryo 4 weeks after fertilization.
- Eight weeks after fertilization, embryogenesis is complete and all limb structures are present.
- Most congenital anomalies of the upper extremity occur during embryogenesis (fourth to eighth week).
- Three signaling centers have been discovered that control different aspects of limb development. These are referred to as the apical ectodermal ridge (AER), zone of polarizing activity formation (ZPA), and the wingless type (Wnt) signaling center[7] (Table 8–7).
  - The AER, a thickened layer of ectoderm that condenses over the limb bud, is required for limb development in a proximal to distal direction. It is also responsible for interdigital necrosis, which separates the webbed hand.
  - The ZPA resides within the posterior margin of the limb bud and regulates anterior to posterior (radioulnar) limb development.
  - The Wnt signaling center resides in the dorsal ectoderm and mediates the development of dorsal to ventral axis configuration.
  - The AER, ZPA, and Wnt pathway all function in a coordinated effort to ensure proper limb patterning and growth during embryogenesis. Abnormalities within one center indirectly affect functioning of the remaining signaling centers and alter limb formation.
- Additional organ systems are developing and maturing during embryogenesis. The error in limb formation often occurs simultaneously with additional organ system defects. Many of these conditions are more consequential than the limb anomaly (e.g., cardiac anomalies) and require timely and accurate evaluation to prevent life-threatening problems.

Classification of Limb Anomalies

- There are numerous classification systems for upper extremity limb anomalies based on embryology, teratological sequencing, anatomy, or a combination of these.
- The most widely used classification of congenital limb anomalies is based on embryonic failure during development and relies on clinical diagnosis for categorization. Each limb malformation is classified according to the most predominant anomaly and placed into one of seven categories (Box 8–4). Different clinical presentations of similar categories of embryonic failures are explained by varying degrees of damage within the organization of the limb mesenchyme.

Radial Deficiency

- Radial deficiency (preaxial) is the classic anomaly often associated with systemic conditions (Figure 8–30).
- The degree of preaxial deficiency can range from mild thumb hypoplasia to complete absence of the radius (Table 8–8).
- Irrespective of the degree of expression, all forms warrant systemic evaluation for syndromes or associations. Holt-Oram syndrome, thrombocytopenia-absent-radius syndrome, VACTERL association (vertebral abnormalities, anal atresia, cardiac abnormalities, tracheoesophageal fistula, esophageal atresia, renal defects, radial dysplasia, lower limb abnormalities), and Fanconi anemia are the primary concerns.

Table 8–7: Signaling Pathways During Embryogenesis

SIGNALING CENTER	RESPONSIBLE SUBSTANCE	ACTION	ANOMALY
Apical ectodermal ridge	Fibroblast growth factors	Proximal to distal limb development or interdigital necrosis	Transverse deficiency or syndactyly
Zone of polarizing activity	Sonic hedgehog protein	Radioulnar limb formation	Mirror hand
Wnt pathway		Ventral and dorsal limb axis	Nail patella syndrome

Box 8–4 Embryologic Classification of Congenital Anomalies

I. Failure of formation of parts
    A. Transverse deficiencies
    B. Longitudinal deficiencies
        1. Phocomelia
        2. Radial
        3. Central
        4. Ulnar
II. Failure of differentiation
    A. Synostosis
    B. Radial head dislocation
    C. Symphalangism
    D. Syndactyly
    E. Contracture
        1. Soft tissue
            a. Arthrogryposis
            b. Pterygium
            c. Trigger
            d. Absent extensor tendons
            e. Hypoplastic thumb
            f. Clasped thumb
            g. Retroflexible thumb
            h. Camptodactyly
            i. Windblown hand
        2. Skeletal
            a. Clinodactyly
            b. Kirner's deformity
            c. Delta bone
III. Duplication
    A. Thumb
    B. Triphalangism–hyperphalangism
    C. Polydactyly
    D. Mirror hand
IV. Overgrowth
    A. Limb
    B. Macrodactyly
V. Undergrowth
VI. Congenital constriction band syndrome
VII. Generalized skeletal abnormalities

- Principal systems involved in these syndromes are cardiac, renal, and hematological. Children with VACTERL association can also have vertebral, tracheoesophageal, and anal problems (Table 8–9).

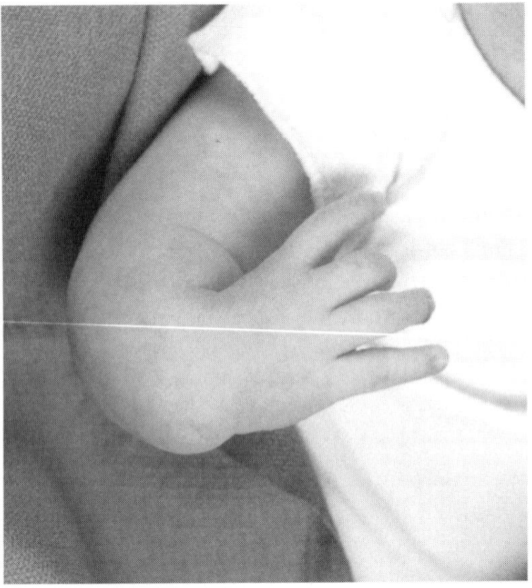

Figure 8–30: A 6-month-old child with absent radius and thumb. Wrist positions into radial deviation.

- Evaluation for radial deficiency and associated systemic conditions necessitate coordination with the child's pediatrician and referral to subspecialists.
- Auscultation and echocardiography is used to assess for cardiac anomalies. Ultrasound is performed to evaluate the renal system. Blood count and peripheral blood smear are obtained to judge platelet status.
- The most devastating associated condition is Fanconi anemia. Children with Fanconi anemia lack signs of bone marrow failure at birth. Therefore, the diagnosis requires a high index of suspicion. A chromosomal challenge test, however, is available that allows detection of the disease before the onset of bone marrow failure. Because the disease is autosomal recessive and bone marrow transplant is the only cure for Fanconi anemia, this prefatory diagnosis is crucial for the child and affected family.
- Children with VACTERL association warrant additional evaluation for spinal abnormalities, such as congenital scoliosis, and require x-ray evaluation of the spinal column.
- The basic goals of treatment are to (1) correct the radial deviation of the wrist, (2) balance the wrist on the

Table 8–8: Global Classification of Radial Longitudinal Deficiency

TYPE	THUMB ANOMALY	CARPAL ANOMALY*	DISTAL RADIUS	PROXIMAL RADIUS
N	Absent or hypoplasia	Normal	Normal	Normal
0	Absent or hypoplasia	Absence, hypoplasia, or coalition	Normal	Normal, radioulnar synostosis, or radial head dislocation
1	Absent or hypoplasia	Absence, hypoplasia, or coalition	>2 mm shorter than ulna	Normal, radioulnar synostosis, or radial head dislocation
2	Absent or hypoplasia	Absence, hypoplasia, or coalition	Hypoplasia	Hypoplasia
3	Absent or hypoplasia	Absence, hypoplasia, or coalition	Physis absent	Variable hypoplasia
4	Absent or hypoplasia	Absence, hypoplasia, or coalition	Absent	Absent

Adapted from James MA, McCarroll HR, Manske PR (1999) The spectrum of radial longitudinal deficiency: A modified classification. J Hand Surg 24A: 1145-1155.
* Carpal anomaly implies hypoplasia, coalition, absence, or bipartite carpal bones. Hypoplasia and absence are more common on the radial side of the carpus, and coalitions are more frequent on the ulnar side. X-ray films must be of children older than 8 years to allow ossification of the carpal bones.

Table 8–9: Syndromes Associated with Radial Deficiency

SYNDROME	CHARACTERISTICS
Holt-Oram	Heart defects; most commonly cardiac septal defects.
TAR	Thrombocytopenia absent radius syndrome. Thrombocytopenia is present at birth but improves over time.
VACTERL	Vertebral abnormalities, anal atresia, cardiac abnormalities, tracheoesophageal fistula, esophageal atresia, renal defects, radial dysplasia, and lower limb abnormalities
Fanconi anemia	Aplastic anemia is not present at birth but develops around 6 years of life. It is fatal without a bone marrow transplant. A chromosomal challenge test is now available for early diagnosis.

forearm, (3) maintain wrist and finger motion, (4) promote growth of the forearm, (5) reconstruct thumb deficiency, and (6) improve the function of the extremity.

- The radial deviation deformity is corrected by a combination of nonoperative and operative management that begins shortly after birth. Passive stretching and splinting of the taut radial structures are initiated in the infant.
- Centralization or radialization combined with tendon transfer is indicated in radial deficiency types II, III, and IV with severe radial wrist deviation and insufficient support of the carpus. Thumb hypoplasia is usually addressed at a second stage after wrist centralization.
- Contraindications for surgical intervention are mild deformity with adequate support for the hand (type I), elbow extension contractures that prevent the hand from reaching the mouth, severe hand defects, and adults who have adjusted to their deformity.
- Despite numerous technical modifications to preserve alignment, some recurrence of the radial deficiency is universal. Prolonged maintenance of the carpus on the end of the ulna without sacrificing wrist mobility or stunting forearm growth remains a daunting task.

Ulnar Deficiency

- Ulnar deficiency is 4 to 10 times less common than radial deficiency and affects the postaxial border of the limb.
- Ulnar deficiencies are not associated with systemic conditions as seen in children with radial deficiency.
- Ulnar deficiencies are associated with other musculoskeletal abnormalities that warrant careful physical examination supplemented by x-ray evaluation (e.g., congenital scoliosis).
- Classification of this deficiency is based on the amount of ulna remaining and the degree of deformity (Table 8–10).
- The forearm is difficult to manage, and treatment should be individualized. Treatment depends on forearm stability, available elbow motion, and function. Unfortunately, surgery cannot restore motion for synostosis across the elbow, forearm, or both.
- Ulnar deficiencies can have thumb anomalies, ranging from a narrow web space to an absent thumb (Table 8–11). These radial-sided deficiencies do not transform an ulnar anomaly into a radial deficiency and thus do not warrant systemic evaluation.
- Hand deformities are the major predictor of function in ulnar deficiency. Ulnar-sided syndactyly is common, and separation with web space reconstruction is indicated. In addition, the thumb deficiency limits prehensile activities. The thumb is treated according to similar principles for isolated thumb hypoplasia.

Central Deficiencies

- Cleft hand results from a longitudinal deficiency of the central rays of the hand (index, long, and ring).
- There are two types of cleft hand (typical and atypical) that possess distinct features and require discrimination from each other (Table 8–12).
- The differences between the typical and atypical cleft hand (a form of symbrachydactyly) are major and may warrant placement of the two conditions into different categories of embryologic malformation (Table 8–12).

Table 8–10: Classification of Ulnar Deficiencies

TYPE	GRADE	CHARACTERISTICS
I	Hypoplasia	Hypoplasia of the ulna with distal and proximal ulnar epiphysis and minimal shortening Slight ulnar deviation of the hand Minimal bowing of the radius
II	Partial aplasia	Absence of the distal or middle one third of the ulna Possible distal ulna anlage causing progressive ulnar deviation Stable elbow Progressive radial bowing
III	Complete aplasia	Total agenesis of the ulna Unstable elbow Relatively straight radius Commonly severe deficiencies of the hand and carpus
IV	Synostosis	Fusion of the radius to the humerus creating stable elbow Possible distal ulna anlage causing progressive ulnar deviation

Table 8–11: Classification of Ulnar Deficiency According to First Web Space Abnormality

TYPE	GRADE	CHARACTERISTICS
A	Normal	Normal first web space and normal thumb
B	Mild	Mild first web deficiency and mild thumb hypoplasia with intact opposition and extrinsic tendon function
C	Moderate to severe	Moderate to severe first web deficiency and similar thumb hypoplasia with malrotation into the plane of the digits, loss of opposition, and dysfunction of the extrinsic tendons.
D	Absent	Absence of the thumb

Adapted from Cole RJ, Manske PR (1991) Classification of ulnar deficiency according to the thumb and first web space. J Hand Surg 22A: 479-488.

- The typical cleft hand has a V-shaped defect with a varying degree of long ray absence. Most commonly, the phalanges are missing and the metacarpal is present (Figure 8–31).
- Typical cleft hand is often bilateral and is usually inherited as an X-linked dominant trait with incomplete penetrance. There may be syndactyly of the ring–small or thumb–index web space, and other associated conditions include cleft lip and palate.
- Atypical cleft hand is a form of symbrachydactyly and involves the central three digits (index, long, and ring).
- Symbrachydactyly is a spectrum of hand deficiencies ranging from small fingers (brachydactyly) that may be connected (syndactyly) to absence of the central three fingers to complete absence of all digits, similar to a transverse deficiency.
- In atypical cleft hand, the index, long, and ring finger rays are absent and the metacarpals are present. This deficiency creates a U-shaped cleft instead of the V-shaped configuration associated with typical cleft hand.
- Atypical cleft hand is not associated with systemic conditions and is not inherited. This deficiency is usually unilateral, sporadic, and without foot involvement.
- All forms of symbrachydactyly (including atypical cleft hand) can be associated with Poland's syndrome, characterized by an ipsilateral chest wall deficiency. Absence of the sternocostal portion of the pectoralis major muscle is the most common chest wall finding, although absence of additional muscles and breast underdevelopment may be found.
- The degree of hand deficiency does not correlate with the extent of chest wall abnormality. Therefore, even when a patient has mild symbrachydactyly, a complete evaluation of chest wall integrity is required.

Transverse Deficiencies

- Congenital transverse deficiency is classified according to the last remaining bone segment.
- A short, below-the-elbow–type amputation is the most common transverse deficiency of the upper extremity.
- The residual limb is usually well cushioned with rudimentary nubbins or dimpling, often found on the end (Figure 8–32).
- These anomalies are usually unilateral, sporadic, and rarely associated with other anomalies.
- A less common level of transverse deficiency is through the hand or metacarpals. The long residual limb length

Table 8–12: Characteristics of Cleft Hand

	TYPICAL CLEFT HAND	ATYPICAL CLEFT HAND
Clinical Features		
Involvement	Bilateral	Unilateral
Inheritance	Familial	Spontaneous
Syndactyly	Common	Rare
Associated with Poland's syndrome	No	Yes
Cleft lip or cleft palate	Yes	No
Anatomical Findings		
Arterial supply	Three digital arteries possible on ring finger	Vestigial supply to central digits
Tendon	Commonly dual tendons to ring	Minimal
Skeleton	Hypertrophy adjacent to cleft	Hypoplasia
Classification	Failure of differentiation or abnormal number of digits	Failure of formation

Adapted from Miura T, Suzuki M (1984) Clinical differences between typical and atypical cleft hand. J Hand Surg 9B: 311-315.

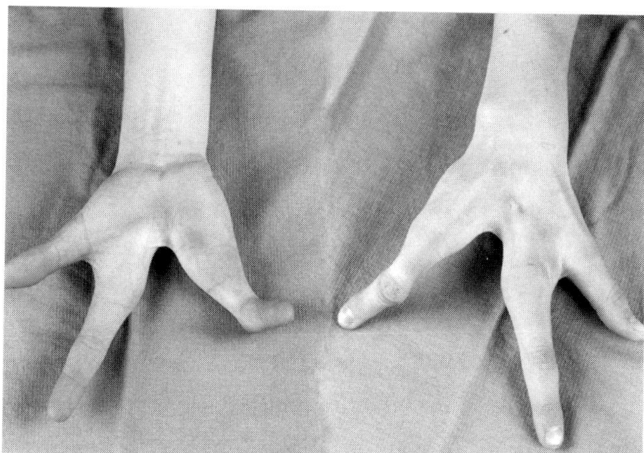

Figure 8–31: A 10-year-old child with bilateral central deficiencies and a V-shaped cleft.

dissuades the child from accepting a prosthesis and promotes use of this limb as a sensate helper.

- Phocomelia represents a longitudinal failure of formation with an absent intervening segment of the extremity (intercalary aplasia). The missing segment can be the arm, forearm, or both with the hand attached directly to the shoulder.
- Phocomelia is uncommon except for a marked increased prevalence (60%) associated with thalidomide taken during the first trimester of pregnancy.
- Surgery is rarely indicated for phocomelia, and prosthetic fitting is beneficial, especially in bilateral cases.

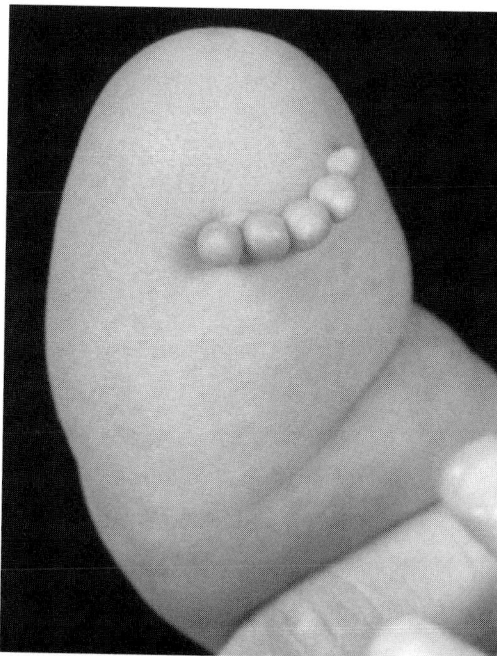

Figure 8–32: Short, below-the-elbow transverse deficiency with residual nubbins.

Syndactyly

- Syndactyly is defined as an abnormal interconnection between adjacent digits and is described according to the magnitude and extent of the linkage (Figure 8–33).
- The interconnection may encompass the entire length of the adjacent digits (complete) or may discontinue before the fingertip (incomplete).
- The syndactyly may involve only skin and fibrous tissue (simple) or may include bone (complex). Syndactyly that occurs with other anomalies (e.g., Apert's syndrome) is referred to as complicated syndactyly.
- Syndactyly is a common congenital anomaly that occurs in 2 to 3 per 10,000 live births. It tends to occur in families and has an autosomal dominant mode of transmission with variable expressivity and incomplete penetrance.
- Syndactyly can also occur sporadically and is not ordinarily associated with systemic conditions.
- Simple syndactyly of any considerable degree warrants surgical reconstruction of the web space for improved function and appearance. The timing of release and technique of separation are both controversial but abide by certain guidelines (Table 8–13).
- Border digits (thumb–index and ring–small web spaces) have marked differences in their respective lengths and should be separated within the first few months of life. This allows the thumb to participate in prehensile function and prevents tethering of the longer digit, which develops a flexion contracture and rotational deformity over time.
- In contrast, the long and ring fingers are relatively equal lengths and separation can be deferred until the child is older (between 12 and 18 months of age). This delay facilitates surgical reconstruction and has a

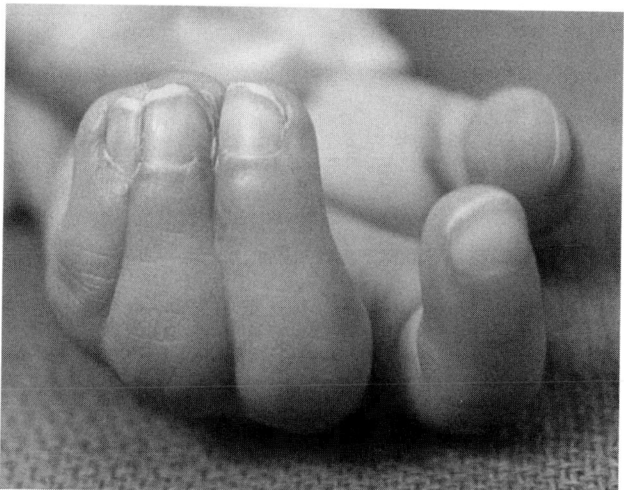

Figure 8–33: An 8-month-old child with complete syndactyly of the long–ring and ring–small web spaces.

Table 8–13: Surgical Guidelines for Syndactyly

Timing	Observe border digits, digits of unequal length early (3 to 6 months), or both
Commissure reconstruction	Avoid skin graft
Number of digits separated	Never operate on both sides of a digit during a single setting
Skin graft	Always need to perform except with incomplete syndactyly
Dressings	Apply bulky dressings above the elbow reinforced with plaster

lower incidence of complications and unsatisfactory results (e.g., web creep).

- Skin graft is almost needed during release of complete syndactyly, which should never be placed within the commissure to avoid interdigital contracture and motion limiting scar. This requires the creation of a flap to re-create the commissure, which is usually based along the dorsum of the connected digits.
- Syndactyly of three or four adjacent digits creates additional difficulty and requires staged surgical procedures. Surgical reconstruction should only include one side of an affected digit at a time to avoid ischemia of the skin flaps, digit, or both.
- Complex syndactyly is associated with an increased incidence of neurovascular anomalies and is more challenging to treat, especially as the quantity of bony union intensifies. In addition, fusion of the distal phalanges creates a combined fingertip with a coalescence of the nail bed, which is hard to reconstruct. Similar surgical principles are used during separation of adjacent digits.

Polydactyly

- Polydactyly can occur on the preaxial (radial) or postaxial (ulnar) side of the limb.
- Preaxial polydactyly is more common in whites, and postaxial polydactyly is more common in blacks.
- Postaxial polydactyly in a white individual is uncommon and is often indicative of an underlying syndrome (e.g., chondroectodermal dysplasia or Ellis-van Creveld syndrome) (Figure 8–34).
- Postaxial polydactyly is frequently inherited through an autosomal dominant pattern but has a variable penetrance pattern. The supranumery digit is either well developed (type A) or rudimentary and pedunculated (type B).
- A small nubbin or scrawny postaxial element (type B) is commonly removed by tying the base in the nursery, allowing it to turn gangrenous and fall from the hand. A residual bump or nubbin is the most common complication of this method of treatment and can be avoided by excising the duplicate under local anesthesia.

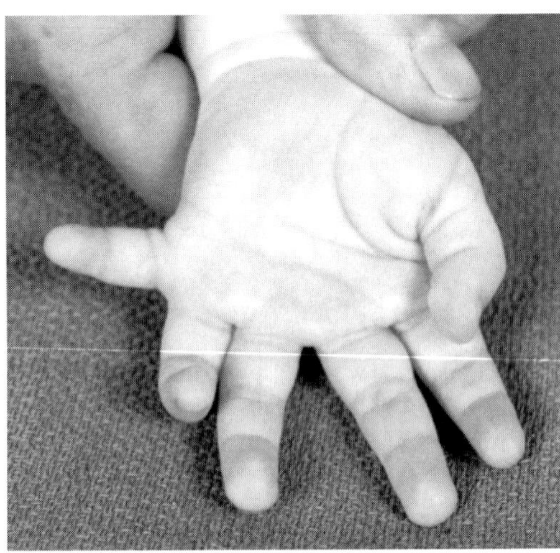

Figure 8–34: A 6-month-old white child with postaxial polydactyly that warrants evaluation for associated syndromes.

- A large or near-normal digit (type A) requires operative ablation. The extra digit is removed, and any important functional parts (e.g., ulnar collateral ligament and abductor digiti quinti) are transferred to the adjacent finger.
- Preaxial thumb duplication is usually unilateral, sporadic, and without systemic problems. Further subdivision into various categories has been performed and depends on the degree of skeletal replication (Figure 8–35, Table 8–14).
- The most common type of preaxial polydactyly involves duplicated proximal and distal phalanges that share a common articulation with a bifid metacarpal head.

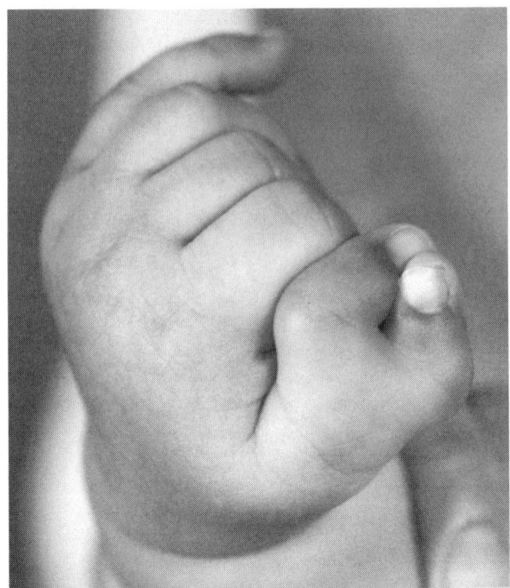

Figure 8–35: A 3-month-old child with unilateral preaxial thumb duplication.

Table 8–14: Classification of Duplicated Thumbs

TYPE	DUPLICATED ELEMENTS
I	Bifid distal phalanx
II	Duplicated distal phalanx
III	Bifid proximal phalanx
IV	Duplicated proximal phalanx*
V	Bifid metacarpal phalanx
VI	Duplicated metacarpal phalanx
VII	Triphalangeal component

Adapted from Wassel HD (1969) The results of surgery for polydactyly of the thumb: A review. Clin Orthop 125: 175-193.
* Most common type.

- Treatment often requires using portions of each component (so-called spare parts) to construct a properly aligned and functional thumb.

Camptodactyly

- Camptodactyly is a painless flexion contracture of the small finger PIP joint that is usually gradually progressive (Figure 8–36).
- The MCP and DIP joints are not affected, although they may develop compensatory deformities.
- Camptodactyly is believed to occur in less than 1% of the population, although most cases are asymptomatic and many do not seek medical attention.
- Camptodactyly is bilateral in approximately two thirds of cases, although the degree of contracture is usually not symmetrical.
- Other digits can be affected, but the incidence decreases toward the radial side of the hand.
- Camptodactyly has been divided into three categories (Table 8–15).
- Treatment is difficult and surgery is reserved for flexion deformities greater than 30 degrees that impair function.
- Surgical approach consists of a combination of release of tight and anomalous structures along with tendon transfer to augment PIP joint extension.

Clinodactyly

- Clinodactyly typically affects the small-finger middle phalanx and produces an angulation of the DIP joint. The deviation is usually in a radial direction.

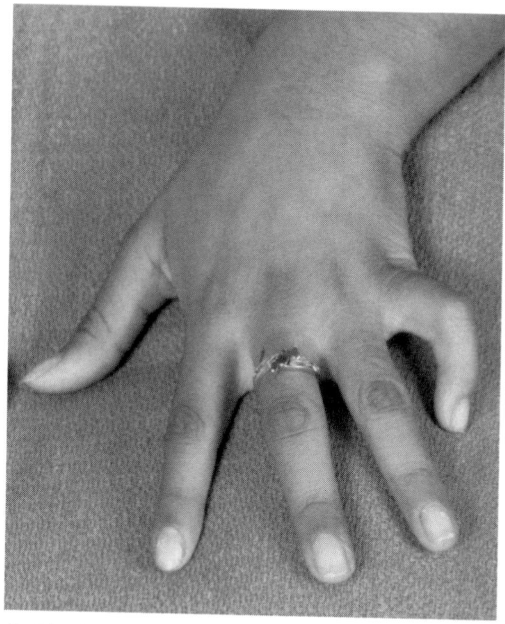

Figure 8–36: A 12-year-old female with camptodactyly of the small finger.

- Occasionally, clinodactyly can involve several digits and is usually related to one or more Δ-shaped middle phalanges.
- Clinodactyly can be inherited and is considered an autosomal dominant trait with variable expressivity and incomplete penetrance.
- Familial clinodactyly is usually not associated with systemic conditions.
- Many genetic syndromes and chromosomal abnormalities, however, have clinodactyly as a physical finding, most notably Down's syndrome. Thumb clinodactyly is a prominent feature of Apert's syndrome, Rubinstein-Taybi syndrome, diastrophic dwarfism, and triphalangeal thumbs.

Macrodactyly

- Macrodactyly represents overgrowth of all structures of the involved digit and is different from an isolated enlargement of the bone (e.g., enchondroma) or vessels (e.g., hemangiomas).

Table 8–15: Types of Camptodactyly

TYPE	CATEGORY	DESCRIPTION
I	Congenital	Apparent during infancy. Usually limited to the fifth finger.
II	Preadolescence	Develops between the ages of 7 and 11. Does not improve spontaneously. May progress to a severe flexion deformity of 90 degrees.
III	Syndromic	Multiple digits of both extremities. Associated with a variety of syndromes (e.g., craniofacial disorders, short stature, and chromosomal abnormalities).

Adapted from Benson LS, Waters PM, Kamil NI, Simmons BP, Upton J (1994) Camptodactyly: Classification and results of nonoperative treatment. J Pediatr Orthop 14: 814-819.

- Macrodactyly can affect one digit or multiple fingers (Figure 8–37). The radial fingers are more commonly involved than the ulnar fingers.
- Macrodactyly usually occurs as an isolated abnormality but can occur with neurofibromatosis or Klippel-Trenaunay-Weber syndrome (limb hypertrophy, hemangiomas, and varicose veins).
- The etiology remains unknown; both static and progressive forms exist.
- Static macrodactyly consists of an enlarged digit that is present at birth and that grows proportionately over time. Serial debulkings and epiphysiodesis to stunt longitudinal growth are the mainstays of treatment.
- Progressive macrodactyly is more common and begins in childhood. The involved digit or digits enlarge throughout growth and stiffen during enlargement. Progressive growth persists until skeletal maturity and physeal closure. Amputation is often required.

Synostosis

- *Synostosis* is a generic term that indicates an osseous union between bones that are normally separate.
- Synostosis most commonly involves the elbow. The synostosis can be isolated or associated with a radial head dislocation.
- A delay in diagnosis of radioulnar synostosis is common. Shoulder and wrist motion are able to compensate for lack of forearm rotation during many activities of daily childhood. The lack of forearm rotation becomes evident as the complexities of daily activities amplify, such as catching a ball or eating soup.
- Mild degrees of fixed pronation or supination are well tolerated and require no treatment.
- Extremes of position create functional handicaps and may require rotational osteotomy through the fusion mass to a more functional position.

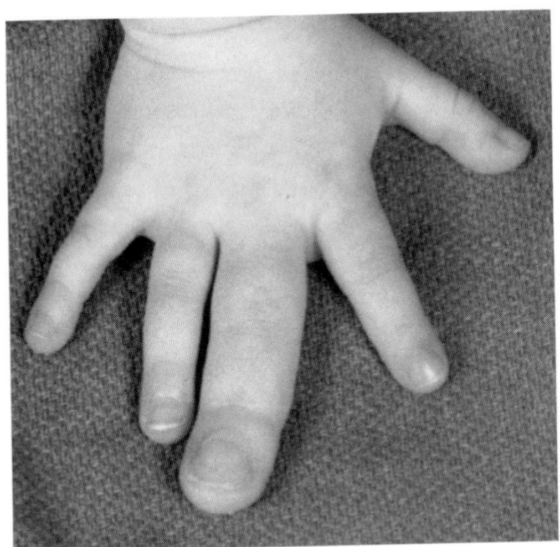

Figure 8–37: A 1-year-old with isolated macrodactyly of the right long finger.

- Synostosis can also occur in other parts of the upper extremity. A radiohumeral joint synostosis can occur as part of ulnar deficiency. Metacarpal transverse synostosis occurs most commonly between the ring and small fingers and is frequently bilateral (60 to 80%).

Thumb Hypoplasia

- Thumb hypoplasia occurs in varying grades and most commonly is part of radial deficiency.
- The underdeveloped thumb (Figure 8–30) has been classified into five types, which guide treatment recommendations (Table 8–16).
- The main distinction between a thumb that can be reconstructed and a thumb that requires ablation is the presence or absence of a stable carpometacarpal joint.
- A stable carpometacarpal joint provides a foundation for thumb reconstruction. An absent carpometacarpal joint negates the possibility of thumb reconstruction and is best treated by ablation and pollicization.
- Pollicization is the procedure of choice for types IIIB, IV, and V hypoplasia.
- Pollicization is a complex procedure that involves neurovascular transposition of the index digit to the thumb position with reconstruction of the intrinsic muscles of the thumb (Table 8–17). The index digit must be rotated at least 120 degrees to attain proper orientation of the new thumb.
- Results after pollicization are directly related to the status of the transposed index digit and surrounding musculature. A mobile index finger transferred to the thumb position will provide stability for grasp and mobility for pinch (Figure 8–38). In contrast, a stiff index finger will provide a stable thumb for gross grasp but will not participate in pinch.
- Early good results have been shown to persist into adulthood.

Neuromuscular Disorders

Cerebral Palsy

- Cerebral palsy is an irreversible, static, perinatal brain injury that affects the musculoskeletal system.

Table 8–16: Thumb Deficiency Classification

TYPE	FINDINGS	TREATMENT
I	Minor generalized hypoplasia	Augmentation
II	Absence of intrinsic thenar muscles First web space narrowing UCL insufficiency	Opponensplasty First web release UCL reconstruction
III	Similar findings as type II Extrinsic muscle and tendon abnormalities Skeletal deficiency A—Stable carpometacarpal joint B—Unstable carpometacarpal joint	A—Reconstruction B—Pollicization
IV	Pouce flottant or floating thumb	Pollicization
V	Absence	Pollicization

UCL, Ulnar collateral ligament.

Table 8–17: Reconstruction During Pollicization

STRUCTURE	POLLICIZATION FUNCTION
Distal interphalangeal joint	Interphalangeal joint
Proximal interphalangeal joint	Metacarpophalangeal joint
Metacarpophalangeal joint	Carpometacarpal joint
First dorsal interosseous	Abductor pollicis
First volar interosseous	Adductor pollicis
Extensor indicis proprius	Abductor pollicis longus
Extensor digitorum	Extensor pollicis longus

- The extent and degree of involvement is extremely variable. Cerebral palsy can affect one side of the body (hemiplegia) or all four limbs (quadriplegia). The motor effect can range from flaccidity to spasticity to athetosis.
- Sensibility of the affected part is usually diminished, and the intelligence of the patient is unpredictable.
- The wide variation in presentation complicates the formulation of a generalized treatment plan and the assessment of a uniform outcome measurement.
- Early treatment is primarily therapy to achieve developmental milestones. Therapy modalities are also useful to prevent joint contractures, and splints provide functional benefits.
- In appropriate candidates, surgery is performed during childhood and adolescence.
- Surgery is most beneficial in children that are less affected and have mild to moderate spasticity.

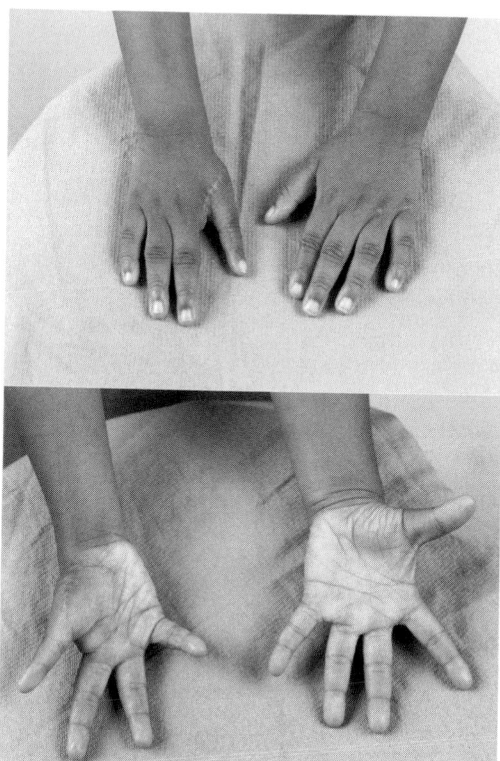

Figure 8–38: A 2-year-old after right index finger pollicization with good position and motion.

- Surgery is least helpful in children with severe involvement, uncontrollable spasticity, and athetosis.
- Realistic preoperative goals are paramount because surgery is reparative and is not curative.
- The typical posture of the extremity is shoulder internal rotation, elbow flexion, forearm pronation, wrist flexion, fingers flexion, and thumb positioned within the palm.
- The goal of surgery is to rebalance the extremity using a combination of joint stabilization procedures, tendon lengthening techniques, and tendon transfers.
- The physical examination remains the guide to surgical treatment. The evaluation includes a determination of joint position and an inventory of muscle activity. The deforming forces (i.e., agonists) and antagonists about each deformity require assessment.
- Each muscle is assessed for volitional action, spasticity, and phasic activity.
- Muscles that exhibit continuous firing and scarce purposeful recruitment are not candidates for transfer and are better treated by release or lengthening.
- Muscles that possess volitional activity, have mild spasticity, and are expendable represent potential donor candidates for tendon transfer.
- Adjunctive methods are available to supplement the physical examination before surgical reconstruction. Dynamic EMGs are useful to identify spastic and flaccid muscles. The timing of muscle contracture during certain activities can also be delineated by electromyography. Temporary neuromuscular blockade of the agonists with botulinum toxin, phenol, or an anesthetic agent can provide additional information regarding the status of the antagonists.
- Surgery is indicated to expand function, enhance hygiene, and improve appearance.
- Shoulder position is usually not a limiting factor with regards to function. In severe cases, lengthening of the subscapularis and pectoralis major muscles can be performed to correct an internal rotation contracture.
- The elbow often lacks extension, which decreases the available workspace and is detrimental to function. The amount of elbow flexion tends to increase during ambulation, which augments underlying problems with balance. Treatment is directed at lessening the elbow flexion tone by lengthening the elbow flexors.
- The forearm is positioned in pronation, which creates problems with feeding, perineal care, and bimanual activities. Surgical options are aimed at reducing the pronation force by a flexor–pronator slide or direct manipulation of the pronator teres and quadratus (lengthening, releasing, or rerouting).
- Wrist flexion deformity directly impairs finger function and the ability to grasp and release. The wrist is treated by redirection of a flexion force to act as an extensor

moment. Transfer of the flexor carpi ulnaris to the extensor carpi radialis is a common procedure, and concomitant transfer of the extensor carpi ulnaris to the midline can add extension.

- When the wrist is placed into extension and passive digital extension is not possible in this position, concomitant lengthening of the finger flexors (FDP, FDS, or both) is necessary to allow sufficient release of objects.
- If active finger extension is not present, additional tendon transfer to the finger extensor tendons may be necessary.
- The thumb-in-palm deformity is extremely difficult to correct. An inventory of the thumb muscles often reveals spasticity of the intrinsic muscles (thenar and adductor pollicis muscles) and deficiencies within the extensor mechanism. Release of the thenar and adductor pollicis muscles from their origins allows these muscles to slide and diminishes their force. Augmentation of thumb extension and abduction is achieved by rerouting of the extensor pollicis longus tendon through the first dorsal compartment or by arranging other tendon transfers.

Pediatric Brachial Plexus Palsy

Introduction

- Brachial plexus birth palsy has a reported incidence between 0.38 and 1.56 per 1000 live births. The quality of obstetrical care available and the average birth weight in different geographic areas may explain the variable incidence.
- Perinatal risk factors for brachial plexus palsy include fetal macrosomia, prolonged labor, multiparous pregnancies, previous deliveries resulting in brachial plexus palsy, breech delivery, vacuum or forceps usage, and difficult deliveries.
- Delivery by caesarian section does not exclude the possibility of birth palsy.
- Shoulder dystocia in vertex deliveries and difficult arm or head extraction in breech deliveries increases the risk of brachial plexus palsy.
- The right upper limb is more commonly involved because of the more frequent left occiput anterior vertex presentation.
- Brachial plexus palsy most commonly involves the upper trunk (C5-C6) with or without an injury to C7. Less often, the entire plexus (C5-T1) is injured.
- Nerve injuries vary in severity. Classification systems have been developed to grade the extent of nerve injury and reflect the prognosis. Seddon's classification is most commonly employed and provides a basis for treatment[8] (Table 8–18). The gradation of nerve injury begins with neurapraxia, extends to axonotmesis, and culminates in neurotmesis.
- A neurapraxia is a segmental demyelination with maintenance of intact nerve fibers and axonal sheath. Demyelination causes a temporary conduction block without axonal damage and wallerian degeneration; electrodiagnostic studies demonstrate a decrease in nerve conduction without electromyographic changes of denervation within the muscle. Complete recovery occurs over the ensuing days to weeks while remyelination is completed.
- An axonotmesis is a disruption of nerve fiber integrity with preservation of the axonal sheath and framework. Wallerian degeneration and nerve fiber regeneration are necessary for recovery.
- Wallerian degeneration is characterized by the proliferation of Schwann cells that phagocytose myelin and axon debris. The axons distal to the injury degrade from lack of nutrition and loss of blood supply. Electrodiagnostic studies exhibit a decrease in nerve conduction and electromyographic changes of muscle denervation (insertional activity, fibrillations, positive sharp waves, and reduction in amplitude of motor-evoked potentials). These electromyographic changes are apparent 1 to 3 weeks after injury.
- The regeneration rate after wallerian degeneration is approximately 1 mm/day or 1 inch/month. This regeneration process is slow, delays return of function, and often results in incomplete recovery. In addition, prolonged muscle denervation longer than 18 to 24 months results in irreversible motor endplate degradation and muscle fibrosis. This irreversible motor endplate demise prevents continued muscle reinnervation.
- A neurotmesis is a disruption of both nerve fiber and axonal sheath integrity. Transection is the classic example of neurotmesis, but severe traction or contusion can produce a similar injury with severe intraneural scarring. Electrodiagnostic studies exhibit a loss of nerve conduction and subsequent electromyographic changes of

Table 8–18: Seddon's Classification of Nerve Injury

TYPE	DEFINITION	OUTCOME
Neurapraxia	Interruption of nerve conduction, some segmental demyelination, and intact axon continuity	Reversible
Axonotmesis	Disrupted axon continuity and intact neural tube	Wallerian degeneration and incomplete recovery
Neurotmesis	Complete disruption of nerve continuity and loss of axons and neural tubes	No spontaneous recovery but required surgery

Adapted from Seddon HJ (1972) Surgical Disorders of Peripheral Nerve Injuries, 2nd edition. Edinburgh: Churchill-Livingstone.

denervation 1 to 3 weeks after injury. The prognosis is bleak without surgical resection of the intervening scar and nerve coaptation by direct repair or graft interposition.

- Brachial plexus injuries are also classified according to the anatomical site. The nerve injury can be at the root level, which disrupts the rootlet connection with the spinal cord and is called an *avulsion* injury. This separates the motor cell body in the spinal cord from its axons, whereas the sensory cell body located in the dorsal root ganglion remains connected to its axons (Figure 8–39). Subsequently, the motor portion of the nerve undergoes wallerian degeneration with degradation of the axons and myelin sheaths. In contrast, the sensory fibers are spared from wallerian degeneration but have been irreversibly detached from the spinal cord.
- An avulsion injury causes a clinical motor and sensory loss, whereas electrodiagnostic studies reveal absent motor conduction with intact sensory conduction.
- An injury distal to the root can affect the trunks, divisions, cords, branches, or a combination of these. Complete disruption along these segments is a *rupture,* in which both motor and sensory cell bodies are separated from their axons. This results in motor and sensory wallerian degeneration and in disruption of both motor and sensory nerve conduction.
- The differentiation between avulsion and rupture is an important element in the treatment algorithm of brachial plexus traction injuries. Avulsion injuries are irreparable, although experimental work is being performed in root reimplantation. Ruptures along the brachial plexus can be treated by a variety of surgical techniques to reestablish nerve continuity.
- The most prevailing theory regarding the etiology of brachial plexus palsies is that of mechanical stretching of the plexus during the birthing process. There are, however, rare reports of possible *in utero* causes of birth palsy attributed to abnormal *in utero* forces on the posterior shoulder region as the fetus passes over the sacral promontory. Increased *in utero* pressure and traction have also been proposed as a cause for brachial plexus injury in an anomalous uterus, such as a bicornuate or fibroid uterus.

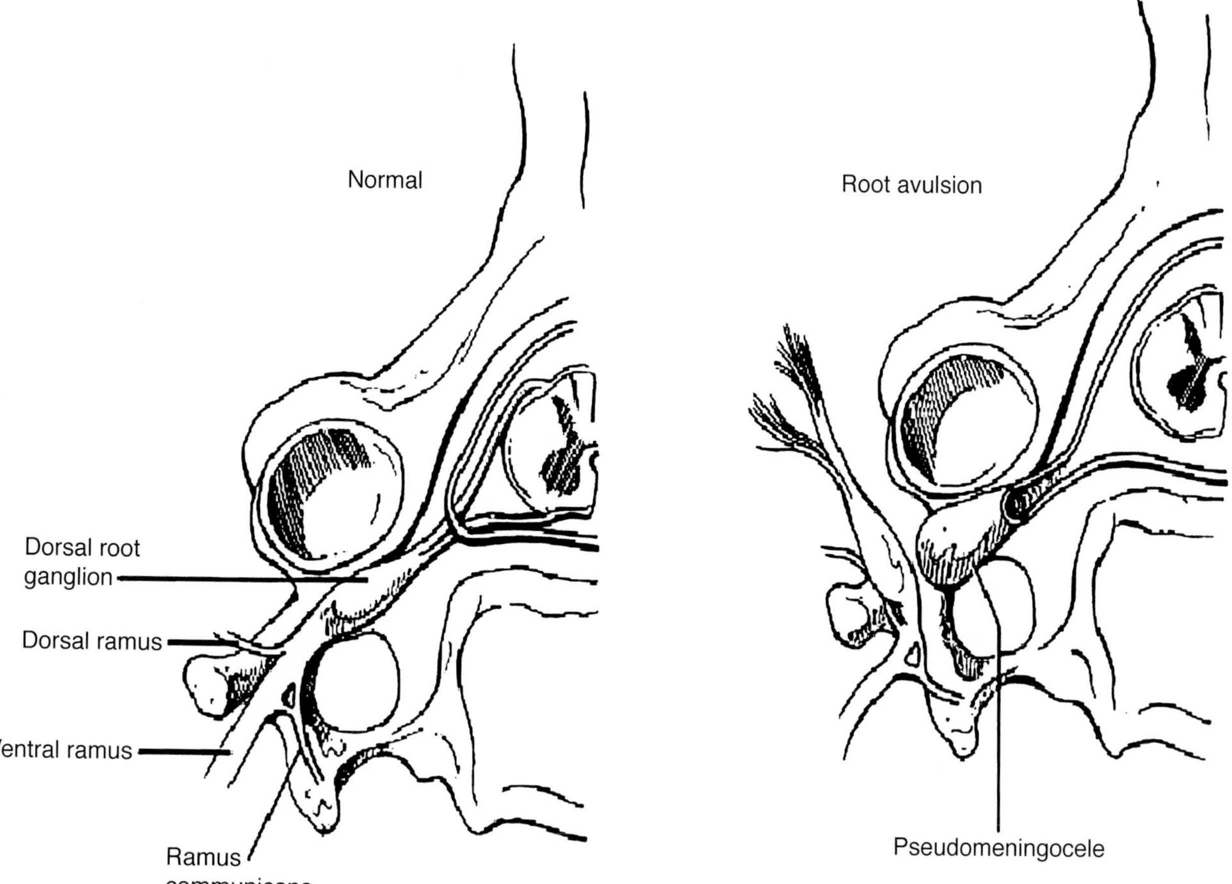

Figure 8–39: Diagram of a root avulsion injury illustrating disruption of the rootlet connection with the spinal cord and separation of the motor cell body in the spinal cord from its axons. The dorsal root ganglion (sensory cell body) remains connected to its axons.

Diagnosis

- Diagnosis is primarily by physical examination.
- Differential diagnosis is limited to pseudoparalysis as the result of fracture (clavicle or proximal humerus), central nervous system or cervical spinal cord injury with peripheral paralysis, or congenital anomaly of the upper limb with limited motion and strength.
- Concomitant fracture of the clavicle or humerus can occur with birth palsy. Clinical suspicion requires x-ray evaluation.
- The diagnosis of brachial plexus palsy is usually readily apparent. The clinical presentation depends on the extent of neural injury. Observation of limb posture, notation of spontaneous movement, use of neonatal reflexes, and stimulation of motor activity are all necessary for accurate examination. Patience is required to obtain a reliable examination in an infant. Serial examinations every 1 to 3 months during infancy are necessary to forecast outcome and indications for surgical intervention.
- Brachial plexus palsies have been categorized into four groups (Table 8–19). The mildest clinical group (I) represents a classic Erb's palsy (C5-C6) with initial absence of shoulder abduction and external rotation, elbow flexion, and forearm supination. Wrist and digital flexion and extension are intact. Successful spontaneous recovery is reported as high as 90% in this group.
- Group II includes involvement of C7 with the additional absence of wrist and digital extension and with C5-C6 impairment. Prognosis is poorer with C5-C7 involvement.
- Group III is a flail extremity without a Horner's syndrome.
- Group IV is a flail extremity with a Horner's syndrome (ptosis, myosis, enopthalmos, and anhydrosis). These infants may have an associated phrenic nerve palsy with an elevated hemidiaphragm, which increases the probability an avulsion injury has occurred and decreases the chances of spontaneous recovery.
- An isolated Klumpke's paralysis (isolated C8-T1) is rare.
- Most brachial plexus injuries involve the upper trunk. The level of this injury is usually postganglionic and not an avulsion. When the lower plexus is also injured, it is more common to have a preganglionic avulsion of C8-T1.
- The exception to this generalization is an upper trunk lesion after a breech delivery. These injuries tend to be preganglionic C5-C6 avulsions from the spinal cord.[9]
- To assess the location of injury, a careful examination of nerves that originate from the proximal portion of the brachial plexus is performed. Injury proximal to a preganglionic nerve or nerves implies avulsion of that segment. Specifically, a Horner's syndrome (sympathetic chain), an elevated hemidiaphragm (phrenic nerve), a winged scapula (long thoracic nerve); and the absence of rhomboid (dorsal scapular nerve) and latissimus dorsi (thoracodorsal nerve) function all raise considerable concern about a preganglionic lesion.
- Preganglionic lesions can only be reconstructed by bypassing the injury, usually using nerve transfers. This is most commonly accomplished with thoracic intercostals or a branch of the spinal accessory nerve. Postganglionic ruptures are reconstructed by excising the neuroma and nerve grafting the defect.

Management

- The upper trunk supplies innervation to the biceps and brachialis muscles. Consequently, the evaluation of elbow flexion is a key indicator of nerve regeneration across the injured segment.
- In addition to clinical examination, myelography, myelography with CT scans, and MRI scans have all been used to distinguish between avulsion and ruptures. There are false-negative and false-positive rates associated with these imaging studies, which has led to limited acceptance. Often, the final decision regarding the presence or absence of an avulsion injury is made at the time of surgery.
- Electrodiagnostic studies with EMGs and nerve conduction velocities can help to diagnose the severity of the neural lesion. The presence of normal sensory nerve

Table 8–19: Patterns of Brachial Plexus Injuries

PATTERN	NERVE ROOTS INVOLVED	PRIMARY DEFICIENCY
Erb-Duchenne lesion Upper brachial plexus	C5 and C6	Shoulder abduction and external rotation; elbow flexion
Extended Erb's lesion Upper and middle plexus	C5 through C7	Shoulder abduction and external rotation; elbow flexion and extension; finger extension
Dejerine-Klumpke lesion Lower brachial plexus	C8 and T1	Hand intrinsic muscles; finger flexors
Total or global lesion Entire brachial plexus	C5 through T1	Entire extremity

conduction in the absence of motor nerve conduction is diagnostic of root avulsion. Unfortunately, the presence of motor activity in a muscle has not been accurate in predicting the degree of motor recovery.

Natural History

- Most brachial plexus palsies are transient. Those infants that recover partial antigravity upper trunk muscle strength in the first 2 months of life usually have a full and complete recovery over the first 1 to 2 years of life.
- Infants that do not recover antigravity bicep strength by 5 to 6 months of life are candidates for microsurgical reconstruction because successful surgery will result in a better outcome than natural history alone.
- Infants with partial recovery of C5-C7 antigravity strength during the first 3 to 6 months of life will have limitations of motion and strength about the shoulder, elbow, and forearm. Children with incomplete recovery consistently develop an internally rotated and adducted shoulder. The limited glenohumeral motion leads to a compensatory increase in scapulothoracic motion.
- The muscle imbalance of external rotation and abduction weakness and of relatively normal internal rotation and adduction strength leads to a contracture and subsequent glenohumeral joint deformity that appears early in infancy and is progressive (Figure 8–40).

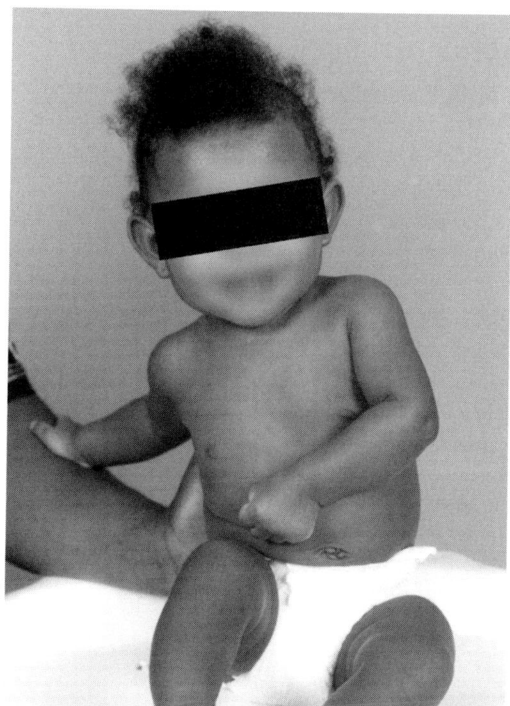

Figure 8–40: An 8-month-old child with left brachial plexus palsy and incomplete recovery. The shoulder is in a position of internal rotation and adduction and often develops a contracture over time.

- The glenoid becomes more retroverted and changes configuration. As the deformity advances, the normal concavity becomes flat then bilobed, and eventually a pseudoglenoid forms.
- The position of the humeral head also alters over time. The humeral head subluxates in a posterior direction, and the neck becomes more retroverted.
- Many children develop a mild elbow flexion contracture. Usually this is less than 30 degrees and is associated with limited functional consequence. Children with marked weakness of the triceps develop a more severe contracture that can interfere with activities of daily living.
- Avulsion of the lower plexus yields profound permanent loss of hand and wrist function. Microsurgery offers the best alternative, although limited functional recovery is the rule.

Microsurgery

- The role and timing of microsurgery are controversial issues.
- The spectrum of nerve surgery includes neurolysis, neuroma resection, nerve grafting, and nerve transfers.
- Direct repair is rarely performed because of the extensive nature of the lesion and inability to obtain a repair without tension.
- Neurolysis has been performed extensively. There is little data to suggest that neurolysis alone enhances outcome.
- The present microsurgical approach is resection of the neuroma and sural nerve grafting in postganglionic ruptures. In the upper trunk rupture, sural nerve grafts are performed from the C5 and C6 roots to the most proximal healthy nerve tissue of the upper trunk and the suprascapular nerve.
- In the case of avulsions at one or more levels, a combination of nerve grafting across the ruptured segments and nerve transfers around the avulsed sections is performed using the thoracic intercostals (T2-T4), a branch of the spinal accessory nerve (cranial nerve XI), or both.
- Entire plexus avulsions can only be reconstructed by nerve transfers. Options included the intercostals, a spinal accessory, the phrenic, the cervical plexus, a portion of the ulnar nerve, the contralateral C7, and even the hypoglossal nerve.
- The timing of microsurgery is still debatable. The range varies between 3 and 9 months of age. Earlier surgery is indicated for lower trunk involvement to allow time for reinnervation before muscle endplate demise. Later surgery is appropriate for upper trunk lesions because the reinnervation distance is shorter.

Shoulder Weakness and Deformity

- Shoulder weakness, contracture, and joint deformity are frequent in infants and children with residual brachial plexus palsies. Initially, the newborn should possess full passive motion as the contracture develops over time. A newborn without passive external rotation implies infantile posterior head dislocation and requires urgent attention.

- The shoulder assessment involves observation of spontaneous activity, neonatal reflex activity, and stimulated activity with and without gravity assistance. Passive glenohumeral motion is assessed with scapular stabilization to separate glenohumeral from scapulothoracic motion.
- Initial physical therapy is designed to maintain supple joint motion and prevent joint contracture. Full glenohumeral range with scapular stabilization is the goal. Abduction and external rotation splints have been used to improve or maintain range of motion.
- Most commonly, abduction and external rotation weakness ensues secondary to incomplete neuromuscular recovery. Over time, an internal rotation and adduction contracture develops, which results in underlying joint deformity.
- Failure to recover external rotation strength leads to functional consequences, including hand to mouth activity and placing the hand to the nape of the neck and the top of the head.
- Failure to recover overhead reach will limit workspace and decrease the ability to reach objects.
- Plain x-ray films are of limited value to assess glenohumeral joint deformity. The secondary centers of ossification are not present from birth to 6 months of life, and most the glenoid and humeral head are still cartilaginous.
- Ultrasound can be used in infancy to evaluate the glenohumeral joint and to assess joint position and congruency during internal and external rotation.
- Arthrograms provide a better depiction of the joint and bony development than plain x-ray films or ultrasound.
- MRI provides the best resolution using axial imaging and cartilage sensitive techniques.
- Treatment of shoulder dysplasia varies with the age of the child and the degree of the deformity. Failure to maintain joint motion should raise concerns regarding joint formation and should require imaging (preferably MRI).
- Young children (less than 3 years) with mild deformity can be treated by rebalancing the joint by lengthening the tight musculotendinous structures (subscapularis ± pectoralis major) with or without tendon transfer of the latissimus dorsi and teres major muscle. These tendons are transferred to the posterior rotator cuff to restore external rotation and abduction.
- Older children (3 to 8 years) with mild to moderate deformity can be treated by a similar rebalancing but always require tendon transfer. In addition, an anterior capsular release (open or arthroscopic) should be considered to allow better passive external rotation.
- Children older than 8 years with moderate to severe deformity have limited capacity to remodel. This group is best treated by external rotational osteotomy of the humerus to reposition the limb.
- Children that fail to regain elbow flexion are severely hampered. Reconstructive options include tendon transfer or free muscle transfer. Local muscles that can be transferred include the latissimus dorsi, pectoralis major, triceps, and flexor–pronator group (Steindler flexorplasty). Free muscle transfer usually uses the gracilis muscle and is reinnervated by intercostal nerves or spinal accessory.
- Limitation of forearm supination is commonplace after residual brachial plexus palsy. Restoration of shoulder external rotation often improves supination as the long head of the biceps is better positioned.
- Persistent deficiency in supination is usually not treated because most activities of daily life are accomplished in a position of pronation.
- On occasion, persistent C7 or middle trunk deficit will result in the lack of pronation and will inhibit certain tasks. A supple deformity can be treated by rerouting of the biceps to restore some pronation. A fixed deformity may require osteotomy of the radius ± ulna.
- Persistent hand dysfunction secondary to deficits in lower trunk recovery is difficult to treat. Each patient must be carefully assessed for function. Tendon transfers may be an option as long as sufficient donor tendons are available.

Conclusion

- The hand is important for mechanical interaction with the environment by both adults and children. In children, it also plays a critical role in brain development and sensory input.
- When treating children with upper extremity disorders, you must pay particular attention to their functional requirements and growth potential. Conditions that interfere with function or are worsened by growth should be corrected early.
- Diagnosis may be made more difficult by the patient's inability to report symptoms or cooperate with examination.
- Children generally have better recovery potential than adults because of their superior wound healing and adaptability.

References

1. Seiler JG, ed (2002) Essentials of Hand Surgery. Philadelphia: Lippincott Williams & Wilkins.
   This handbook covers the essentials of hand anatomy, examination, and common problems in hand surgery in a single, paperback volume.

2. Smith P (2002) Lister's The Hand, 4th edition, London: Churchill Livingstone.
   This excellent single-volume textbook covers the diagnosis of hand problems and indications for surgery in detail. Specifics on surgical procedures are not covered.

3. Colon F, Upton J (1995) Pediatric hand tumors: A review of 349 cases. Hand Clin 11(2): 223-244.
   In this large review of pediatric hand tumors, the authors found that cysts, foreign bodies, and vascular tumors accounted for nearly 66% of the tumors and malignant tumors accounted for only 2%.

4. Fleming ANM, Smith PJ (2000) Vascular cell tumors of the hand in children. Hand Clin 16(4): 609-624.
   This review article on pediatric vascular tumors of the hand covers classification and treatment. The comparison of hemangiomas with vascular malformations, as well as the subclassification of vascular malformations, is particularly lucid.

5. Upton J, Coombs C (1995) Vascular tumors in children. Han Clin 11(2): 307-336.
   This article presents indications and guidelines for surgery on pediatric vascular tumors. Useful algorithms are presented for management of slow- and fast-flow malformations.

6. McCarroll HR (2000) Congenital anomalies: A 25-year overview. J Hand Surg 25A: 1007-1037.
   This article provides an overview of the major advances in the treatment of congenital hand anomalies over the past 25 years. It describes principles of treatment of the more common anomalies, such as syndactyly and radial deficiency. It also provides a glimpse into future treatment regimens, such as genetic engineering of joints and the field of fetal surgery.

7. Daluiski A, Yi SE, Lyons KM (2001) The molecular control of upper extremity development: Implications for congenital hand anomalies. J Hand Surg 26A: 8-22.
   This is a general review of the various signaling pathways and molecular tracks that control limb development. The article correlates aberrations of normal limb development with anomalies of the upper extremity. It provides an update of syndromes attributed to defined molecular abnormalities.

8. Seddon HJ (1972) Surgical Disorders of Peripheral Nerve Injuries, 2nd edition. Edinburgh: Churchill-Livingstone.

9. Al-Qattan MM (2003) Obstetric brachial plexus injuries. J Am Soc Surg Hand 3: 41-54.
   This article provides an overview of the assessment and management of children with brachial plexus palsies. It describes the differential diagnosis and assessment after birth. It also explains the factors for spontaneous recovery, the role of early and late surgery, and the outcome after reconstruction.

Bibliography

Benson LS, Waters PM, Kamil NI, Simmons BP, Upton J (1994) Camptodactyly: Classification and results of nonoperative treatment. J Pediatr Orthop 14: 814-819.

Clarke HM, Curtis CG (1995) An approach to obstetrical brachial plexus injuries. Hand Clin 11: 563-580.
   This article details the assessment of children with brachial plexus palsies. It explains the method to obtain a pertinent history, motor and sensory assessment, and use of ancillary studies. The natural history of brachial plexus palsies and indications for surgery are highlighted.

Cole RJ, Manske PR (1991) Classification of ulnar deficiency according to the thumb and first web space. J Hand Surg 22A: 479-488.

James MA, McCarroll HR, Manske PR (1999) The spectrum of radial longitudinal deficiency: A modified classification. J Hand Surg 24A: 1145-1155.
   A global classification system is proposed for radial deficiency that includes the spectrum of pathology affecting the radial side of the extremity, including deficiency of the radius, carpal abnormalities, and hypoplastic thumbs. Type N has a normal length radius and a normal carpus with thumb hypoplasia, type O has a normal length radius and radial side carpal abnormalities, type 1 has a shortening of the radius greater than 2 mm, type 2 has a hypoplastic radius, type 3 has a partial radius without the distal physis, and type 4 lacks the radius.

Kozin SH, Weiss AA, Webber JB, Betz RR, Clancy M, Steel HH (1992) Index finger pollicization for congenital aplasia or hypoplasia of the thumb. J Hand Surg 17A: 880-884.
   The authors evaluated 14 hands (10 patients) after index finger pollicization. Patients with unilateral pollicization averaged 67% grip strength, 60% lateral pinch, 56% palmar pinch, and 39% three-point pinch compared with the normal contralateral hand. Manual dexterity averaged 70% efficiency compared with normal standards.

Kozin SH (2001) Syndactyly. J Am Soc Surg Hand 1: 1-13.
   The author reviews syndactyly, including inheritable, spontaneous, and syndromic forms. He details the established principles for timing, technique, and postoperative management. He also provides a classification system to guide management.

Lourie GM, Lins RE (1998) Radial longitudinal deficiency: A review and update. Hand Clin 14: 85-99.
   This review of radial deficiency covers the gamut, including pathoanatomy, demographics, diagnosis, and treatment. Recent contributions to the management of radial deficiency are included.

Miura T, Suzuki M (1984) Clinical differences between typical and atypical cleft hand. J Hand Surg 9B: 311-315.

Pearl ML, Edgerton BW (1998) Glenoid deformity secondary to brachial plexus birth palsy. J Bone Joint Surg 80A: 659-667.
   The authors detail the association between internal rotation contracture secondary to brachial plexus palsy and deformity and posterior dislocation of the glenohumeral joint. Twenty-five children, ranging in age from 1.5 to 13.5 years, had an operation to release an internal rotation contracture secondary to brachial plexus palsy; 11 had a latissimus dorsi transfer to augment external rotation power. Arthrograms were made intraoperatively to clarify the

pathological changes that occur in the glenohumeral joint. Seven children had a concentric glenohumeral joint (the humeral head was well centered in the glenoid fossa). The remaining 18 children (72%) had a deformity of the posterior aspect of the glenoid with posterior subluxation of the humeral head.

Van Heest AE, House J, Cariello C (1999) Upper extremity surgical treatment of cerebral palsy. J Hand Surg 24A: 323-330.
This article describes an upper extremity approach in children with cerebral palsy. An individualized approach with joint stabilization, tendon lengthening, and tendon transfer is detailed. Enhanced limb function is reported even in children with diminished sensibility.

Wassel HD (1969) The results of surgery for polydactyly of the thumb: A review. Clin Orthop 125: 175-193.

Waters PM, Smith GR, Jaramillo D (1998) Glenohumeral deformity secondary to brachial plexus birth palsy. J Bone Joint Surg 80A: 668-677.
This prospective study evaluates the association among persistent brachial plexus palsy, musculoskeletal deformity, and functional limitations. In this study, 94 patients were entered; 42 had either CT or MRI to assess the glenohumeral joint. The degree of retroversion of the glenoid on the affected side was −25.7 degrees compared with −5.5 degrees on the unaffected side. Of the 42 shoulders, 26 (62%) had evidence of posterior subluxation of the humeral head, with a mean of only 25% (and a range of 0 to 50%) of the head being intersected by the scapular line. Progressive deformity was found with increasing age.

Watson BT, Hennrikus WL (1997) Postaxial type B polydactyly: Prevalence and treatment. J Bone Joint Surg 79A: 65-68.
A prospective screening program of 11,161 newborns identified 21 infants who had postaxial type B polydactyly (a prevalence of 1 in 531 live births). Of the infants, 16 (76%) had bilateral postaxial type B polydactyly. Eighteen infants (86%) had a family history of the anomaly. The racial prevalence was 1 in 143 live births of black infants and 1 in 1339 live births of white infants. The duplicated small fingers were treated in the newborn nursery with suture ligation at the base of the pedicle. No major complications occurred. A residual bump was the most common sequelae, although all parents were satisfied with the cosmetic result.

Pediatric Lower Limb Disorders

David M. Wallach* and Richard S. Davidson†

*MD, Orthopaedic Surgeon, the Milton S. Hershey Medical Center, Hershey, PA; Assistant Professor, Orthopaedics and Rehabilitation, Pennsylvania State University
†MD, Orthopaedic Surgeon, The Children's Hospital of Philadelphia and Shriners Hospital, Philadelphia, PA; Associate Professor, University of Pennsylvania School of Medicine, Philadelphia, PA

Introduction

- General and pediatric orthopaedists frequently evaluate childhood lower extremity alignment and foot morphology.
- An understanding of normal limb development and the ability to recognize pathological deviations are essential to the care of these young patients.

Rotational Abnormalities

- Parents' concern regarding their child's foot or leg pointing "in" (internal–medial rotation) or "out" (external–lateral rotation) during gait is a common reason for orthopaedic referral.
- Limb position is determined by the sum of dynamic (muscle function and ligamentous laxity) forces and static (osseous) forces.
- During normal gait, muscles contract concentrically (shorten) or eccentrically (lengthen) in a well-defined sequence.
- Muscle function that is too vigorous, weak, absent, prolonged, or rapid will cause an abnormal gait.
- In neuromuscular conditions (e.g., cerebral palsy) persistent activity of the medial hamstrings and adductors cause the limb to internally rotate.
- Excessive intra-articular motion may occur in children with ligamentous laxity (e.g., Ehlers-Danlos).
- For "normal" children, dynamic factors, although important to limb rotation, do not play a role as central as that of static (skeletal) factors.

Hip Rotation

- The hip joint forms by the eleventh gestational week.
- The proximal femur and acetabulum continue to develop until physeal closure in adolescence.
- At birth, the femoral neck is rotated forward an average of 40 degrees.
- Hip orientation is referred to as femoral anteversion when facing forward and retroversion when facing backward.
- During gait, the limb is automatically positioned to ensure full and concentric seating of the femoral head within the acetabulum.
- Anteversion of the hip leads to internal rotation of the leg; the converse is true with retroversion.
- In the absence of a neuromuscular abnormality, femoral version decreases to between 15 and 20 degrees by 8 to 10 years of age (Figure 9–1).
- In the first year of life, the effect of femoral anteversion is masked by an external hip rotation contracture. The contracture spontaneously resolves once the child begins walking.

Tibial Rotation

- Infants may have as much as 30 degrees of internal rotation of the tibia.
- Internal rotation corrects until 4 years of age, when the tibia assumes its permanent alignment.
- External tibial rotation deformities, however, do not tend to correct with growth.

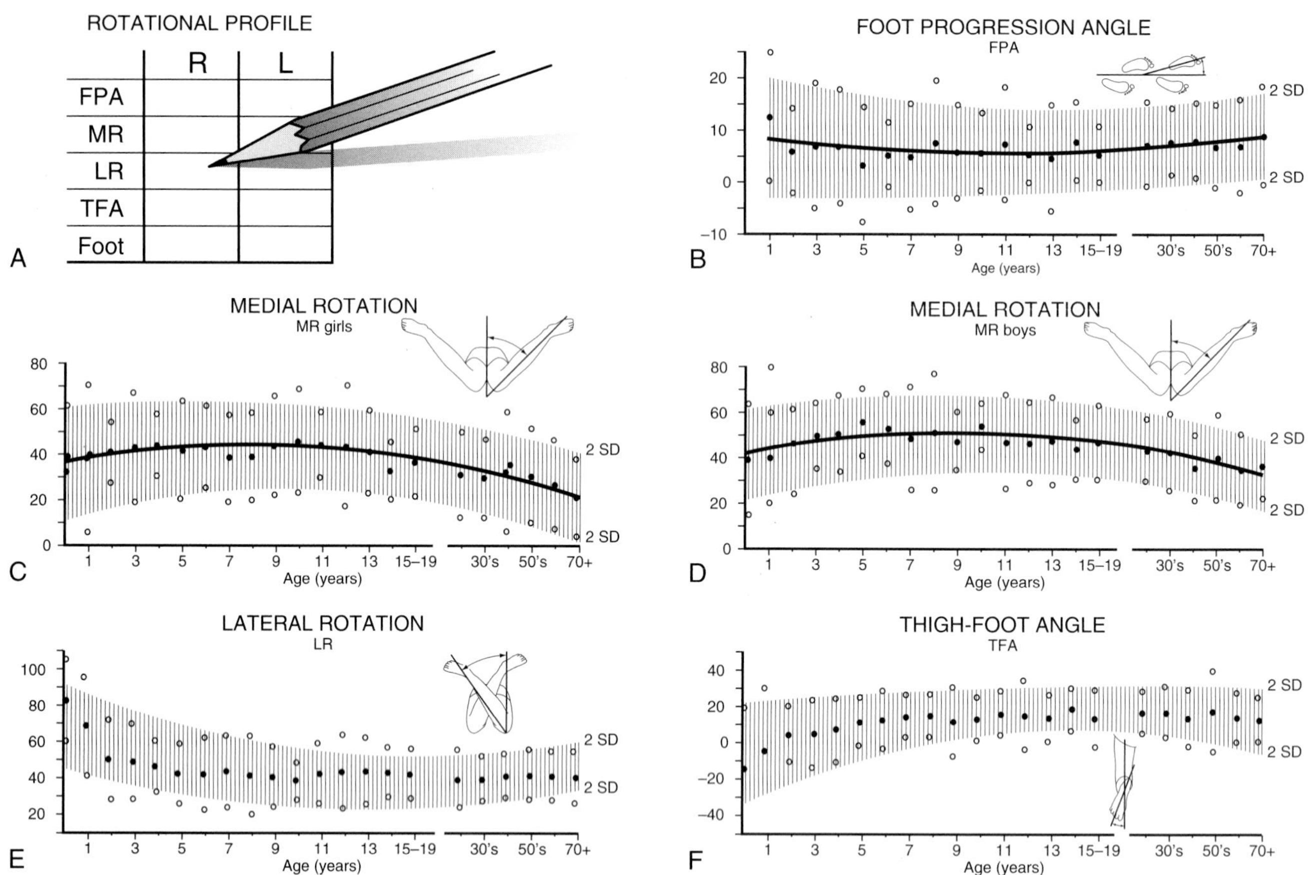

Figure 9–1: The rotational profile from birth to maturity is depicted graphically. **All graphs include two standard deviations from the mean for FPA, femoral medial and lateral rotation (for boys and girls), and the thigh–foot angle. From Morrissy, RT, Weinstein, SL, eds (1990) Lovell and Winter Pediatric Orthopaedics, 3rd edition. Philadelphia: Lippincott Williams & Wilkins.**

- At maturity, the normal range of tibial alignment is from 5 degrees medial to 15 degrees lateral rotation.
- Excessive medial rotation is referred to as medial, or internal, tibial torsion (MTT), and external rotation is known as lateral, or external, tibial torsion (LTT).
- Either MTT or LTT can be unilateral.

Metatarsus Adductus

- Abnormal foot adduction occurs with metatarsus adductus (MA), metatarsus primus varus, clubfoot, and skewfoot
- Abnormal foot abduction is seen with the planovalgus foot, congenital vertical talus (CVT), and calcaneovalgus foot.

Physical Examination of Limb Rotation

- Limb position during gait is expressed as the foot progression angle (FPA). The FPA is the summation of femur, tibia, and foot rotation.
- The FPA is formed from the longitudinal axis of the foot during single-leg stance compared with the direction the child is walking.
- A foot parallel to the line of gait progression has an FPA of 0 degrees.
- Internal rotation of the foot is assigned the label "negative," and external rotation is assigned the designation "positive."
- Children with femoral anteversion are able to sit in the W position (Figure 9–2) and have patellae that face medially during both stance and gait (squinting patellae sign).
- The standard method of measuring hip rotation is with the child prone. The hips are adducted and in neutral extension–flexion while the knees are flexed to 90 degrees (Figure 9–3). By convention, 0 degrees of rotation is with the tibia perpendicular to the table. Rotating the leg toward the ipsilateral side of the body is medial rotation. Rotating the leg toward the contralateral side of the body is lateral rotation.
- Tibial rotation is measured using the transmalleolar angle. This angle is derived from a line along the longitudinal

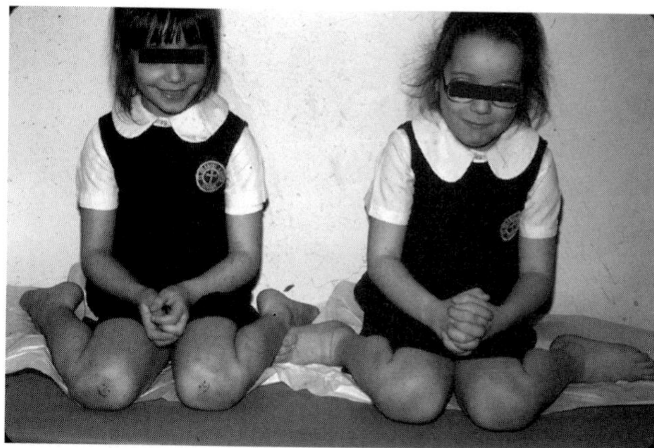

Figure 9–2: Photo of children sitting in the W position. From Wallach DM, Davidson RS (2004) Pediatric lower limb disorders. In: Pediatric Orthopaedics and Sports Medicine (Dormans JP, ed). Philadelphia: Mosby.

axis of the thigh compared with a line perpendicular to the axis of the medial and lateral malleolus.

- In the absence of a foot deformity, however, it is easier to measure the thigh–foot angle. This angle is measured with the child lying prone. The longitudinal axis of the thigh is compared with the longitudinal axis of the foot. Normative age adjusted values for hip and tibial rotation are available based on the work of Staheli et al.[1]
- Foot adduction and abduction are evaluated using the heel–bisector line (HBL). The HBL is derived from the distal extension of a line that divides the plantar heel in half along its longitudinal axis. The HBL in a "normal" foot bisects the second toe. The abducted foot has a HBL lying medial to the second toe. Conversely, an adducted foot has the HBL lateral to the second toe[2] (Figure 9–4)
- Radiographs of the tibia and feet are not needed during the initial evaluation of tibial and foot rotation. It is reasonable, however, to obtain an anteroposterior (AP) pelvis radiograph to rule out hip dysplasia.
- Femoral retroversion has been associated with slipped capital femoral epiphysis.
- The natural history of femoral anteversion and tibia torsion is benign. Femoral anteversion and tibial torsion do not cause arthritis of the hip, knee, or ankle.
- In the absence of a neurological disorder, there is no evidence that children with either medially or laterally rotated limbs are at increased risk for falling.
- The initial treatment for rotational abnormalities is observation and reassurance.
- Physical therapy, braces, custom shoes, or a combination of these do not alter limb alignment.
- Severe tibial malrotation that does not correct by 4 years and femoral malrotation that does not correct by 8 years is treated with corrective osteotomy.
- Femoral anteversion may be measured with a limited computerized tomography (CT) scan through the hip and knee.[3] More than 50 degrees of femoral anteversion is excessive.
- Proximal (subtrochanteric) and distal (supracondylar) osteotomies to "derotate" the femur have been described with similar success rates.[4,5]
- Fixation may be achieved with crossed pins, a plate, an external fixator, and—in the skeletally mature—an intramedullary device.
- Relative indication for a tibial osteotomy is greater than 15 degrees of internal rotation or 30 degrees of external rotation.
- The osteotomy is best performed in the supramalleolar region (versus a proximal tibial region) to decrease the risk of peroneal nerve injury and compartment syndrome
- Adequate derotation of the tibia can often be achieved without division of the fibula. An intact fibula increases lower extremity stability in the postoperative period and may protect the peroneal nerve against traction.[6]

Coronal Limb Abnormalities (Frontal Prone)

- Genu varum (bowed legs) and genu valgum (knock knees) are common pediatric deformities.
- An infant's legs are varus at birth.
- Varus persists until 2 years when the legs straighten.
- The limbs then overcorrect and become maximally valgus between 3 and 4 years.
- By 6 to 7 years, a mature knee alignment is achieved with 5 to 7 degrees of valgus[7] (Figure 9–5).
- Spontaneous resolution occurs for physiological genu varum and genu valgum.
- The differential diagnosis of pathological genu varum is trauma, skeletal dysplasia (e.g., achondroplasia), rickets, fibrous dysplasia, and Blount disease.

Trauma

- Trauma can produce deformities acutely from angulation–translation, partial growth arrest, or both following physeal injury.
- The distal femoral physis is especially prone to growth arrest.
- A complete or partial arrest occurs 50% of the time following physeal fracture of the distal femur.
- Harris-Park growth arrest lines form asymmetrically when a partial growth arrest is present[8] (Figure 9–6). The line is found closer to the physis in a region of diminished growth and further from more normal growth.
- Deformities causing or predicted to cause mechanical dysfunction are treated surgically.
- Factors to consider during surgical planning include the location of physeal arrest, the percentage of physeal involvement, the degree of angular deformity, and the amount of growth remaining.

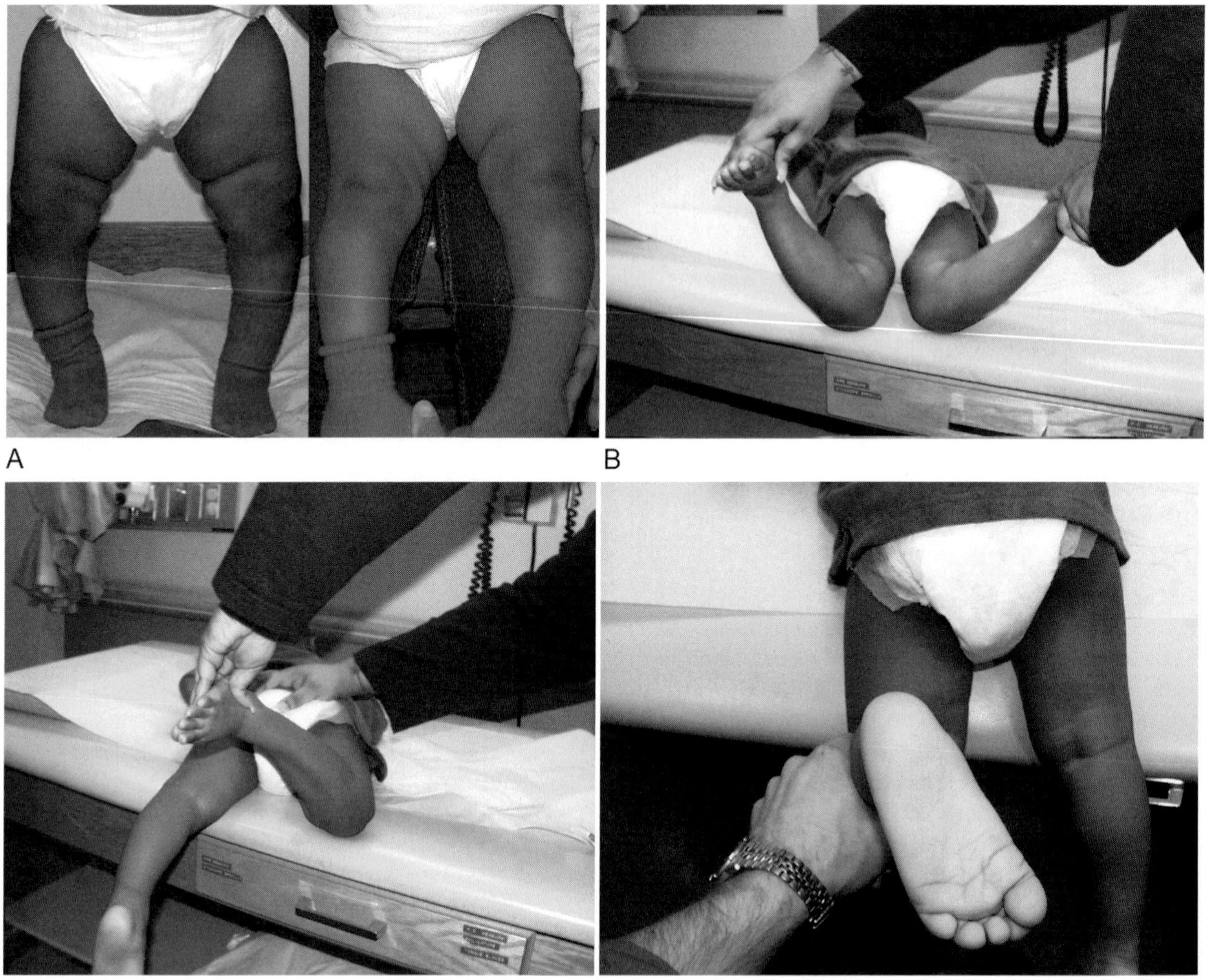

Figure 9–3: Clinical method of static rotational profile in a child. A, First picture: Pseudo–bow legs in child with tibial torsion. Note the feet forward and the patellae lateral and flexed. Second picture: The same child with legs turned so that the patellae are forward, the knees are extended, and the feet are crossed. Note that the legs are now straight. X-ray films must be taken in same position. B, Measurement of medial rotation of the hip. C, Measurement of lateral rotation. Note that the pelvis is maintained in neutral. D, The thigh–foot angle is seen. The medial rotation of the tibia in this child accounts for the appearance of the patellae in *panel* A.

- Surgical options include physeal bar excision, physeal closure, redirectional osteotomy, and limb equalization procedures.
- Resection of a physeal bar is appropriate when at least 2 years of growth remain and the bar involves less than one third of the plate.
- Interpositional substances include fat, silastic, and methyl methacrylate.
- Concomitant osteotomy with resection is indicated when unacceptable angulation is present.
- Observation and timely intervention are required to address physeal bar recurrence following resection procedures.

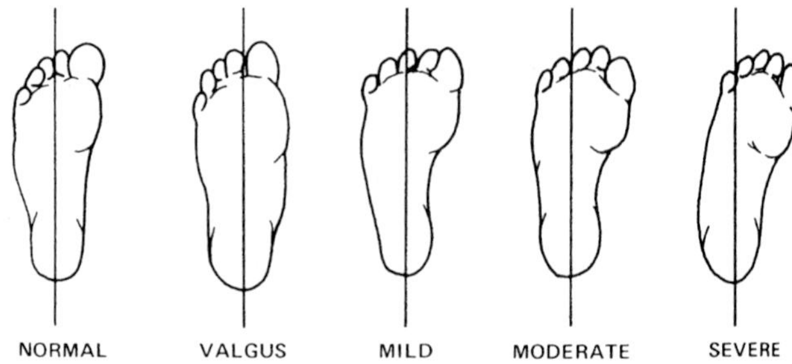

Figure 9–4: The HBL is demonstrated schematically. Deviation of the foot laterally is abduction, and deviation medially is adduction. From Bleck EE (1982) Developmental orthopaedics: III—Toddlers. Dev Med Child Neurol 24(4): 533-555.

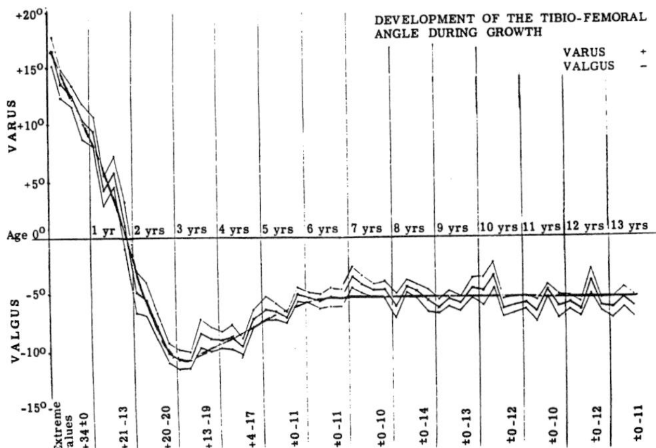

Figure 9–5: The normal coronal alignment of the knee plotted for age. From Salenius P, Vankka E (1975) The development of the tibiofemoral angle in children. J Bone Joint Surg Am 57: 259-261.

- Patients with less than 2 years of growth, large physeal arrests, or both are treated with an epiphysiodesis (possibly bilateral) with or without an osteotomy.[9]

Skeletal Dysplasias

- Genu varum associated with short stature (height less than the 5th percentile for the age) is seen with skeletal dysplasias.
- Many of these conditions have a characteristic facial appearance and body habitus. For example, achondroplasia is associated with frontal bossing, trident hand, and rhizomelic dwarfism.
- Most lower limb deformities seen with skeletal dysplasias are merely observed.
- In this population, the indication for surgical correction of limb malalignment is based on the presence of associated symptoms (e.g., ankle or knee pain).

Metabolic Disease

- Rickets, like skeletal dysplasias, is associated with short stature.
- Limb deformities may occur on multiple planes (Figure 9–7, *A*).
- The physeal regions are enlarged secondary to a deficiency in mineralization in the zone of provisional calcification.
- In severe cases, the wrists appear swollen and chest wall abnormalities are present *(rosary ribs)*.
- These changes are secondary to a widened physis (Figure 9–7, *B*).
- Medical management is the first line of treatment.
- Spontaneous realignment may occur once the metabolic abnormality is addressed.
- Surgical intervention is considered in patients once there has been a plateau in limb correction following medical stabilization of their disease.

Blount Disease

- Blount disease is an idiopathic, nonphysiological form of genu varum.
- Classification by age of presentation divides Blount disease into infantile (0 to 4 years old), juvenile (5 to 10 years old), and adolescent (11 years old to maturity) types.
- Risk factors for infantile Blount disease are early ambulation and weight greater than the 95% for the age.
- Blount disease can also occur in thin people.

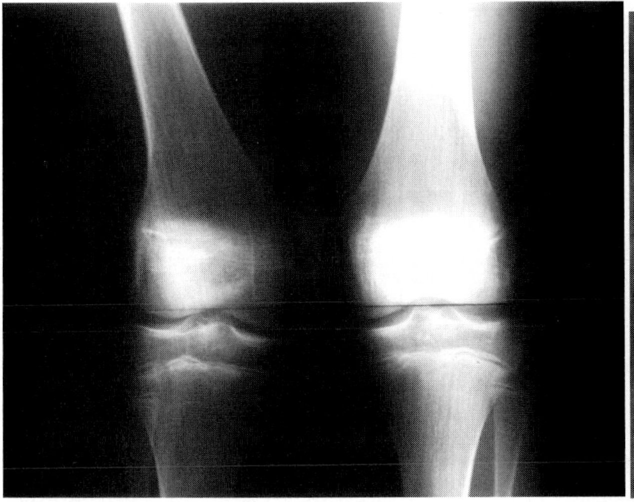

A

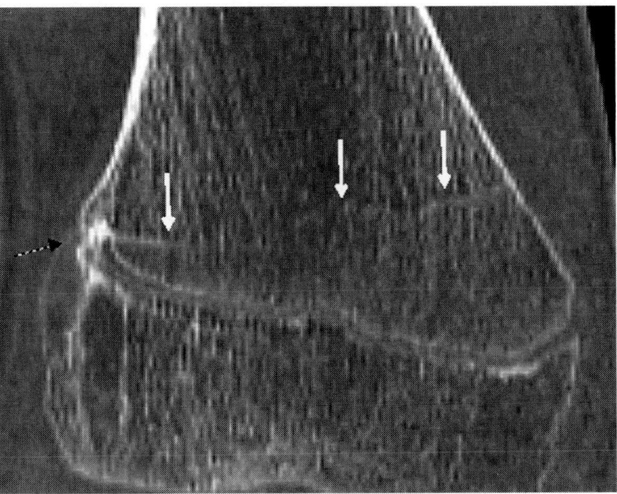

B

Figure 9–6: A, Genu valgum of the right distal femur following a lateral physeal injury. B, Reconstruction of a CT scan demonstrating a lateral physeal bar *(black arrow)* and an angled Harris-Park growth arrest line *(white arrows)*.

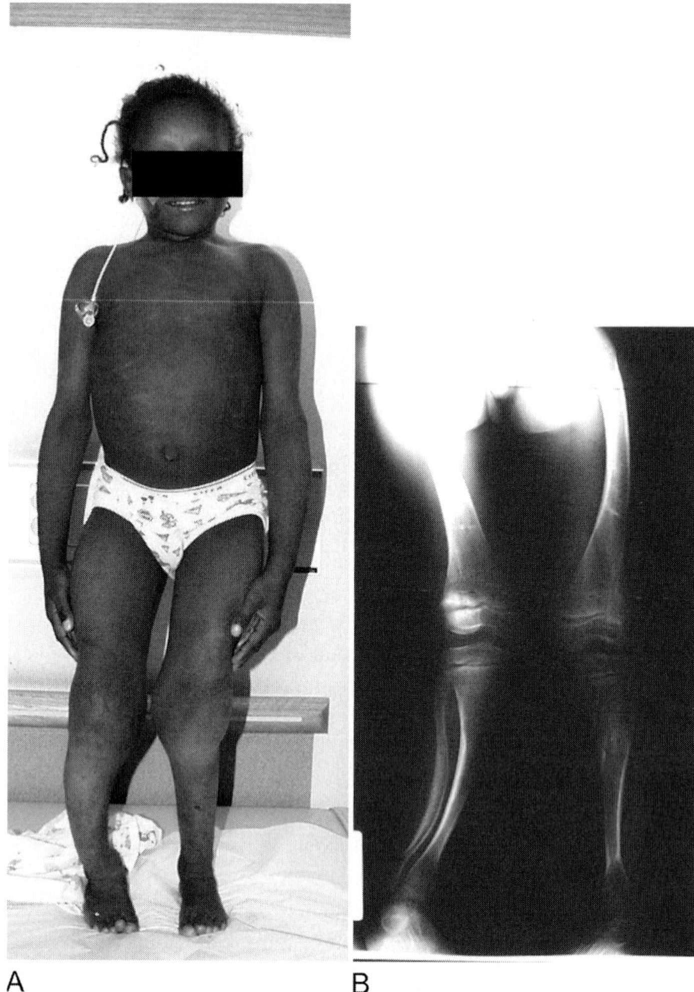

Figure 9–7: A, Clinical appearance of a child with bow legs secondary to rickets; recurrent deformity 6 years after surgical correction. B, X-ray film of an infant with rickets. Note the thickened physis and the widened and cupped metaphysis.

- Knee angulation is measured both clinically and radiographically by the tibiofemoral angle. The tibiofemoral is formed by the longitudinal axis of the femoral and tibial shafts.
- Concomitant MTT increases apparent genu varum; therefore, the tibiofemoral should be measured with the patellae and not with the feet facing forward.
- Distinguishing physiological genu varum from Blount disease is a difficult task in patients under 2 years.
- Physical findings associated with physiological genu varum include a smooth angular deformity with contributions from both the femur and the tibia.
- Infantile Blount disease, in contrast, has an angular deformity isolated to the proximal tibia (no femoral involvement) and, unlike the physiological condition, is often associated with lateral knee thrust (Figure 9–8).
- Radiographic changes associated with infantile Blount disease were described and divided into six stages by Langenskiöld[10] (Figure 9–9).
- The stages, which typically appear after the second birthday, are characterized by progressive medial physeal inclination of the proximal tibia with physeal bar presence in stage 6.
- Levine and Drennan described the metaphyseal–diaphyseal angle (MDA), a measurement taken from an AP knee radiograph that predicts the likelihood of a given limb developing infantile Blount disease[11] (Figure 9–10).
- Although Levine and Drennan advocated a predictive threshold of 11 degrees, Feldman and Schoenecker have proposed that MDAs of 9 degrees and 16 degrees (a 95% confidence interval) be used to predict the future absence and presence of Blount disease, respectively.[12]
- Observation is the mainstay of treatment for infantile Blount disease in children under 3 years.
- A brace is prescribed before 3 years in the presence of a lateral thrust.
- In the absence of spontaneous correction, a valgus-producing knee–ankle–foot orthosis is worn.
- Surgery is recommended following brace failure or for children who failed to respond to conservative treatment by their fourth birthday.
- Correction is achieved surgically with a proximal tibial realignment osteotomy.
- Recurrence is common in procedures performed after 4.5 years.

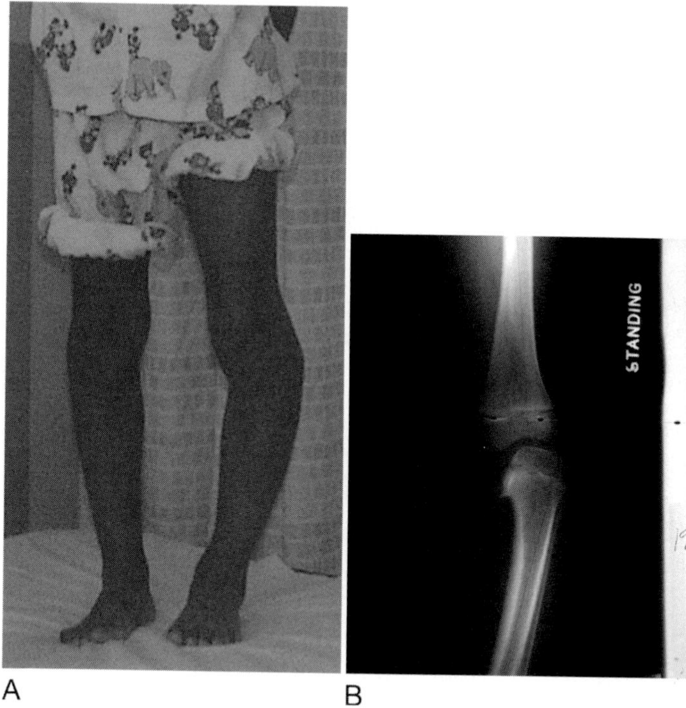

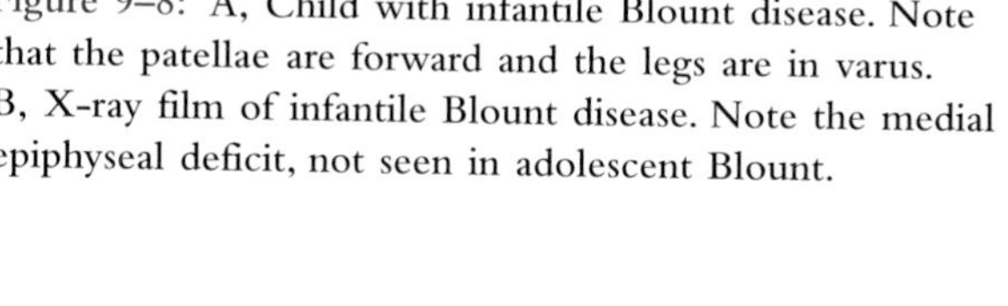
Figure 9–8: A, Child with infantile Blount disease. Note that the patellae are forward and the legs are in varus. B, X-ray film of infantile Blount disease. Note the medial epiphyseal deficit, not seen in adolescent Blount.

Adolescent Blount Disease

- Late onset Blount disease shares a common pathophysiology with early onset Blount disease even though they are different diseases.
- The prevailing theory is that excessive loads produced by the patient's body weight and preexisting genu varum inhibit proximal medial physeal growth.
- The proposed etiology is an application of the Hueter-Volkmann principle.
- As in early onset Blount disease, a lateral thrust may be present.
- In contrast to early onset disease (infantile and juvenile), the distal femur may be angulated (in valgus). Unilateral limbs are affected more often, and MTT is present less often.
- Medial physeal and epiphyseal hypoplasia with proximal tibial angulation are evident on AP radiographs.
- The treatment for late onset Blount disease is surgical, consisting of proximal tibial osteotomies, lateral physeal hemiepiphysiodesis (selective closure of half of the growth plate to allow the contralateral portion of the physis to correct with growth), or both.

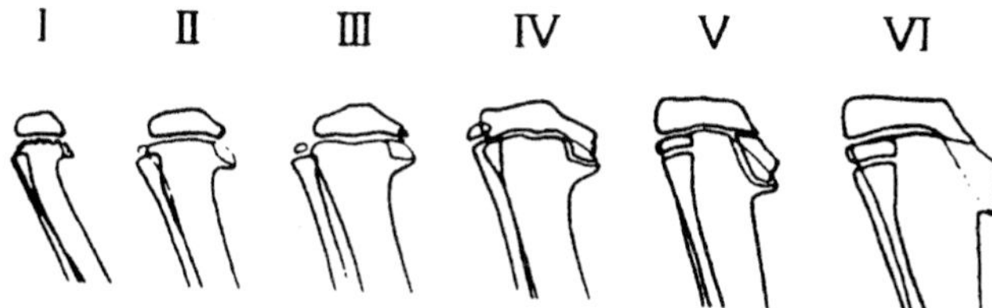

Figure 9–9: Depiction of the stages of infantile Blount disease. From Langenskiöld A (1952) Tibia vara (osteochondrosis deformans tibiae): A survey of 23 cases. Acta Chir Scand 103: 1.

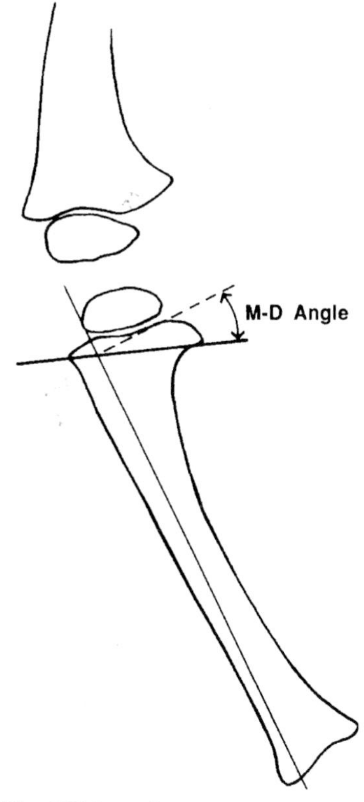

Figure 9–10: The MDA to diagnose Blount disease. Draw a line on the radiograph through the proximal tibial physis. Draw another line along the lateral tibial cortex. Lastly, draw a line perpendicular to the shaft line at the level of the physeal line. A knee with an angle less than 9 degrees is unlikely to progress to Blount disease. An angle greater than 16 degrees is likely to become Blount disease. From Morrissy, RT, Weinstein, SL, eds (1990) Lovell and Winter Pediatric Orthopaedics, 3rd edition. Philadelphia: Lippincott Williams & Wilkins.

Genu Valgum

- As for genu varum, trauma, skeletal dysplasia, and metabolic disorders are all potential causes of genu valgum.

Multiple Hereditary Exostoses

- Multiple hereditary exostoses (MHE) or osteochondromatosis is an example of a skeletal dysplasia that produces genu valgum.
- MHE has autosomal dominant genetics.
- Multiple firm subcutaneous masses are characteristic.
- Most osteochondromas are painless; however, pain will occur when there has been contusion, neurovascular compression (from the mass), or malignant transformation.
- Rare in children, malignant transformation is believed to occur in less than 1% of adult patients.
- Reasons given for surgical intervention include persistent pain, restricted motion, neurovascular compression, limb length discrepancy, and progressive limb deformity.
- Ankle and knee valgus, two common conditions seen with MHE, are produced by a relative hypoplasia of the fibula with resultant tethering of the lateral tibial physis.
- Treatment of the angular deformity is based on the degree of malalignment and the expected growth of the limb.
- Removal of the osteochondroma is performed with metaphyseal osteotomies, complete epiphysiodesis or hemiepiphysiodesis, or a combination of these (Figure 9–11).
- The ankle can be treated with a similar technique using a medial malleolar screw to obtain a hemiepiphysiodesis, or it can be treated with a corrective angular osteotomy.[13]

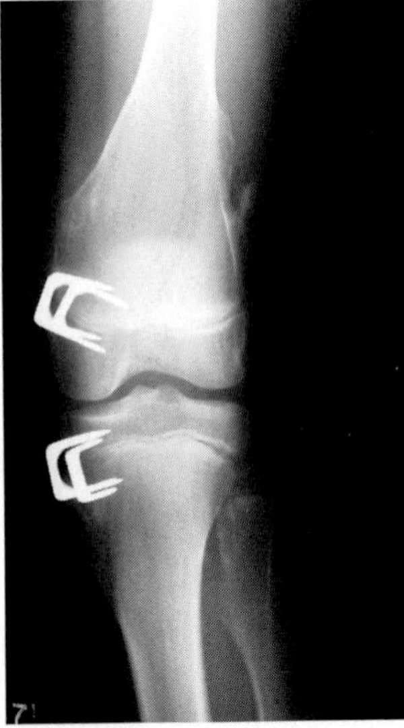

Figure 9–11: Radiograph of knee with genu valgum secondary to MHE. Staples placed medially are correcting the limb.

Idiopathic Genu Valgum

- The diagnosis of idiopathic genu valgum is one of exclusion.
- Patients with severe valgum complain of pain, instability, or both.
- The angular deformity is measured clinically and radiographically.
- CT may be needed to rule out a physeal bar.
- Treatment is operative, with a medial hemiepiphysiodesis performed when adequate lateral physeal growth remains to level the physis.
- A medial hemiepiphysiodesis of the distal femur or proximal tibia will on average cause a 7- or 5-degree/year correction, respectively.[14]
- When inadequate growth remains, a realignment osteotomy is performed.

Tibial Bowing

- Lower extremity bowing can occur in oblique plains.
- The apex of the deformity defines the direction of bowing.
- Posterior medial bowing is associated with a calcaneovalgus foot deformity.
- Anterolateral deformity is associated with congenital pseudarthrosis of the tibia.
- Anterior bowing is associated with fibula hemimelia.

Congenital Pseudarthrosis of the Tibia

- Congenital pseudarthrosis of the tibia is a structural defect within the tibia that is susceptible to fracture and resistant to healing.
- Pseudarthrosis may occur in any bone, although the tibia is the most common.
- Typically the lesion is diaphyseal, located at the junction of the middle and distal third.
- Neurofibromatosis is the most common associated condition, accounting for almost 50% of the cases.
- Other associated conditions include Ehlers-Danlos and amniotic band syndrome.
- With rare exception, the natural history of the condition is that of limb angulation, repeated fracture, and limb length discrepancy.
- Diaphyseal narrowing and sclerosis are evident on radiographs. The medullary cavity may have cysts at the apex of the deformity or may be completely ablated.
- Early treatment, before fracture and the development of significant angular deformity, consists of a full-contact clamshell ankle–foot orthosis or knee–ankle–foot orthosis with regular orthopaedic follow-up.
- Fracture, progressive bowing, or both are indications for surgical intervention.
- No single treatment has emerged has clearly superior.

- An intramedullary nail that crosses the ankle joint is the procedure most often recommended in North America.[15]
- Three unsuccessful attempts to maintain limb alignment is a relative indication for a Syme or Boyd amputation.
- Although neither amputation heals the pseudarthrosis, each allows better prosthetic application, facilitating ambulation.

Fibula Hemimelia

- Fibula hemimelia is a longitudinal deficiency of the lateral portion of the lower limb in which part or all of fibula may be missing.
- The foot commonly is missing its lateral rays, and the ankle may be unstable with severe equinus and valgus deformities.
- Absence of the cruciate ligaments makes the knee unstable.
- Fibula hemimelia can occur in isolation or with a longitudinally and structurally deficient femur, acetabulum, or both.
- Treatment is directed at producing a sound limb for ambulation.
- Limb equalization procedures have a role when there is less than 30% shortening of the limb.
- Although substantial length can be gained with distraction osteogenesis, it is important to weigh the benefits of length versus potential complications and years of lost childhood spent in an external fixator.

Toe Walking

- Developmental milestones are achieved in a predictable and orderly fashion.
- Children gain head control followed by sitting balance, cruising, and finally ambulation.
- Ambulation for 95 percent of children begins between 10 and 17 months.
- A toddler's gait has a short stride length, rapid cadence, and broad base.
- The gait lacks both side-to-side symmetry and consistent cadence.
- An adult gait pattern is achieved by 7 years.[16]
- Toe walking, or equinus gait, can be a normal gait pattern in children until their third year.
- After 3 years, toe walking is considered abnormal.
- The term *equinus* comes from the Latin *equus,* which means horse-like; these children, like horses, walk on their toes.
- Acute (recent toe walkers who formerly walked plantigrade) can be divided by the presence or absence of pain.
- Causes of acute painful toe walking include recent trauma (calcaneal fractures) and the presence of a foreign body (e.g., glass, splinter, or thorn) in the plantar aspect of the foot.
- Acute painless toe walking suggests a neuromuscular differential diagnosis such as muscular dystrophy or spinal cord lesion (e.g., tumor, syringomyelia, or tethered cord).
- Duchenne muscular dystrophy occurs in males. It is characterized by calf pseudohypertrophy, a positive Gower's sign (indicative of proximal muscle weakness), and—in 65% of cases—a positive family history for the condition.
- Spinal cord pathology may be associated with upper motor neuron lesions (e.g., hyperreflexia—clonus or Babinski sign); sensory abnormalities; and bowel, bladder, or both types of dysfunction.
- Chronic toe walking is seen with limb length inequality, congenital limb anomalies (e.g., proximal femoral focal deficiency and fibula hemimelia), and neuromuscular conditions such as cerebral palsy.
- Spastic hemiplegia a type of cerebral palsy is commonly associated with toe walking. (Cerebral palsy is discussed in greater detail in Chapter 17.)
- Hand dominance before 1 year is suggestive of hemiplegia because children are ambidextrous during their first year.
- Lower extremity spasticity produces ankle equinus with or without an associated foot drop (absence of active ankle dorsiflexors) in the involved leg.
- Concomitant hindfoot varus when present is secondary to overactivity of the tibialis posterior tendon (TPT), tibialis anterior tendon, or both.
- Gastrocnemius–soleus lengthening with posterior or anterior tendon lengthening or transfer is effective in treating equinus and foot varus.
- The diagnosis of idiopathic, also known as habitual, toe walking is one of exclusion.
- A family history of idiopathic toe walking may be present.
- The technique of examining an ankle with an equinus deformity involves inversion of the subtalar joint before ankle dorsiflexion. Inversion locks the tarsal joints, preventing dorsiflexion through the midfoot. Midfoot dorsiflexion gives a false impression of normal ankle motion.
- Ankle motion is measured based on the angle formed among the shaft, the tibia, and the lateral border of the foot.
- Normal ankle dorsiflexion measures 10 to 15 degrees.
- Toe walking secondary to a fixed ankle contracture may be distinguished by physical examination from dynamic toe walkers with good ankle motion.
- A fixed ankle contracture is treated initially with physical therapy to stretch the gastrocnemius–soleus complex.
- If therapy fails to correct the contracture, serial casting, botulinum toxin injections, or both should be prescribed.
- All of these treatments temporarily weaken the gastrocnemius–soleus complex.

- Casting is preferred in children who will not tolerate an injection (unless anesthetized) or who have failed botulinum toxin.
- Seasonal considerations (snow sports in the winter and swimming in the summer) may influence families' refusal of casting.
- The failure of conservative treatment is the indication for surgical lengthening of the Achilles tendon.
- The same conservative measures are recommended for dynamic toe walking.
- Surgery on dynamic toe walkers carries the risk of overlengthening the Achilles tendon with a resultant crouch gait.

Foot Deformities

- A description of a given deformity must include the location and plane of the abnormal rotation, translation, or both.
- The foot is divided into the forefoot (metatarsals and phalanges), midfoot (cuboid, navicular, and cuneiforms), and hindfoot (talus and calcaneus).
- In the hindfoot, coronal rotation produces heel varus (medial) and valgus (lateral). Axial rotation of the hindfoot is coupled with varus (internal) and valgus (external) rotation of the subtalar joint. Sagittal plane rotation of the hindfoot (equinus and calcaneus) primarily occurs at the ankle joint; however, it may occur between the talus and the calcaneus.
- Coronal rotation of the midfoot and forefoot is described as adduction or abduction as it relates to medial or lateral deviation of the foot, respectively. Pronation and supination are axial rotations through the midfoot and the midfoot–forefoot articulation. Pronation is a plantar flexion, and supination is a dorsiflexion of the medial column of the foot as it relates to the position of the hindfoot.
- The toes may rotate through the sagittal (flexion and extension), axial (abduction and adduction), and coronal (pronation and supination) planes.

Metatarsus Adductus

- The three primary conditions producing foot adductus are MA and clubfoot, which are common, and skewfoot, which is not.
- MA is a medial deviation of the forefoot at the level of the midtarsal joints.
- In MA, the hindfoot is in neutral to valgus alignment (never in varus), and the forefoot may be in a variable amount of supination.
- The clubfoot, in contrast, has ankle equinus, hindfoot varus, midfoot cavus (pronation of midfoot), and adduction.
- Skewfoot, also known as serpentine or Z foot, is an MA, midfoot abduction (+/− lateral translation), and hindfoot valgus.
- MA is the most common congenital foot deformity, present in 1 per 1000 live births.
- The etiology of MA is not completely understood; it is theorized to result from abnormal mechanical intrauterine forces applied to the foot.
- Both twin births and oligohydramnios, two conditions with decreased room available for the fetus, predispose the child for the development of MA.
- Conditions such as MA, torticollis, and hip dysplasia are considered *packing abnormalities,* having this shared etiology, and should be ruled out during all routine infant examinations.
- A deep medial crease and convex lateral border produces the "bean shaped" (kidney bean) foot characteristic of MA (Figure 9–12, *A-B*).
- The HBL is valuable in measuring and documenting the deformity.
- The medical record should state which toe or web space the heel bisector crosses.
- Obtaining photocopies of the soles of the child's feet is an easy pictorial technique to record foot adduction[17] (Figure 9–12, *C*). To avoid breaking the copier and injuring the child, never place the child's entire weight on the glass surface.
- A flexible foot can be corrected beyond the midline (second web space), a moderately flexible foot can be corrected to the midline, and a severe foot cannot be corrected to the midline.[18]
- Radiographs are rarely necessary for the initial evaluation of MA.
- In the largest natural history study of this condition, 179 feet were followed in patients from 3 to 11 years old. At study completion, 86% were normal or had a mild deformity, 10% had a moderate deformity, and 4% had a severe deformity.[19]
- Ponseti and coworkers found that 88% of patients with MA have complete resolution of their deformity without treatment.[20] The remaining 12% (44 patients) underwent manipulation and casting. Of the feet treated in plaster, 5% had significant residual deformity.
- The foot that corrects beyond the midline when the lateral border of the foot is stroked should be observed for spontaneous resolution.
- A flexible foot that only corrects to the midline may be treated with a home stretching program.
- The technique of stretching is as follows: While facing the child, cup the heel of the foot with your left hand for right foot MA (the alternate hands are used for left foot MA). Keep the heel in varus with that hand while abducting the foot with the contralateral hand. Apply pressure *gently* across the metatarsals; proof of gentle pressure is a quiet, relaxed child.
- A foot that does not correct to the midline or has not responded to stretching should be casted prior to the child's eighth month of life.

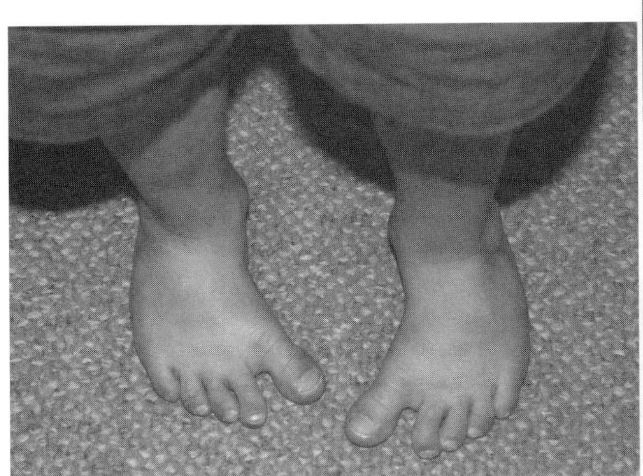

A

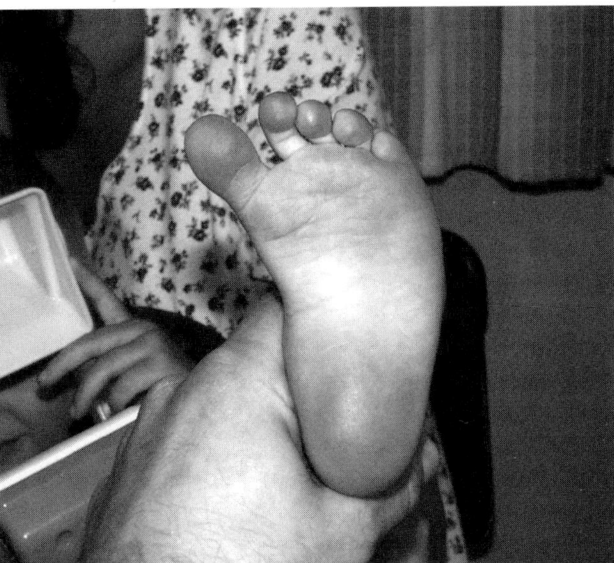

B

C

Figure 9–12: A, Clinical photograph of the dorsal aspect of the feet of a child with MA. B, The same child's feet but viewed from the plantar aspect. C, A photocopy taken directly from the feet of a child with MA for documentation.

- Serial casts are applied every 1 to 2 weeks.
- Cast results are best when instituted before 8 months of age.
- Surgery is indicated when casting is unable to produce a foot that is pain free, plantigrade, shoeable, and flexible.
- Surgery is not considered before 4 years to allow for spontaneous resolution.
- Capsulotomies of the metatarsal–tarsal joints were once recommended; however, the procedure lost favor secondary to an unacceptably high rate of recurrence.
- Multiple metatarsal osteotomies through the bases of the metatarsals may correct the foot deformity; care must be taken not to damage the proximally located first metatarsal's growth plate.
- The double tarsal osteotomy, a cuboid shortening and medial cuneiform lengthening osteotomy, has been used with excellent results without the preceding risks.[21]

Skewfoot

- Skewfoot is distinguished from MA by the presence of abduction (+/− lateral translation) of the midfoot and valgus of the hindfoot (Figure 9–13).
- Skewfoot occurs primarily from neuromuscular disease and iatrogenically following improper casting for MA.
- Without treatment, the condition leads to pain and difficulty wearing shoes.
- The manipulation and casting technique used is the same as that described for MA.
- Failure of conservative care with the inability of the foot to accommodate a standard shoe is an indication for surgery.
- Numerous procedures have been recommended.
- Early soft tissue procedures may be effective; however, in the older child, lengthening the medial midfoot with an

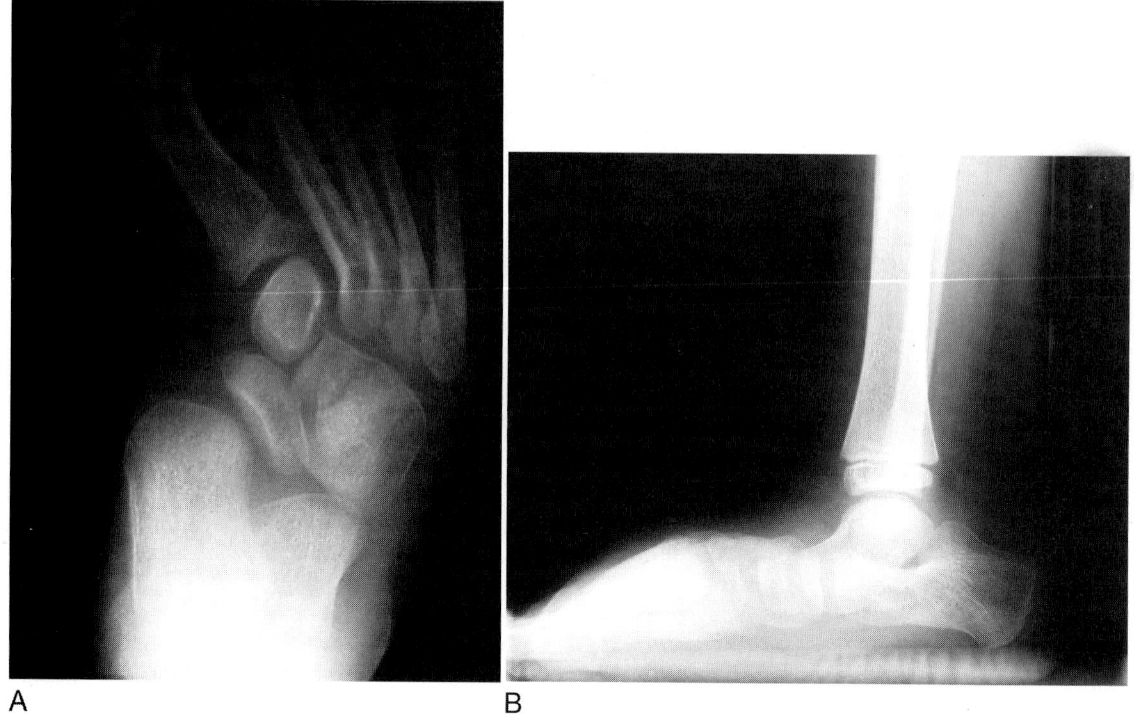

Figure 9–13: Radiograph of a skewfoot. A, On the AP radiograph, note the forefoot adduction, hindfoot abduction lateral translation, and hindfoot valgus. B, Lateral radiograph demonstrates the collapse of the arch.

opening wedge osteotomy and shortening the lateral midfoot with a cuboid closing wedge osteotomy is preferred. Hindfoot valgus may correct with a calcaneal osteotomy.[22]

- Fusions are reserved for severe foot deformity in mature patients.

Clubfoot

- The term *clubfoot* was initially applied to any deformity of the foot in equinus.
- More recently the term is only applied to the foot deformed in hindfoot equinus, midfoot varus, and forefoot adductus or talipes equinovarus (Figure 9–14).
- The deformity has been further divided into congenital and acquired deformities with the latter secondary to neuromuscular diseases, such as cerebral palsy, myelomeningocele, and polio, or external forces, such as amniotic band syndrome.
- The etiology of clubfoot remains unknown and is most likely a combination of genetic and environmental factors.
- An increased risk of acquiring clubfoot with a positive family history suggests a genetic influence. Siblings have up to 30 times the risk of clubfoot deformity. Clubfoot affects both siblings in 32.5% of monozygotic twins but in only 2.9% of dizygotic twins.
- The incidence of clubfoot varies widely by race and sex.
- The incidence among different races varies from 0.39 per 1000 among Chinese to 1.2 per 1000 among whites and 6.8 per 1000 among Polynesians.
- Males are affected twice as often as females.
- Histological anomalies have been reported in every tissue in the clubfoot (muscle, nerve, vessels, tendon insertions, ligaments, fascia, and tendon sheaths).[23]

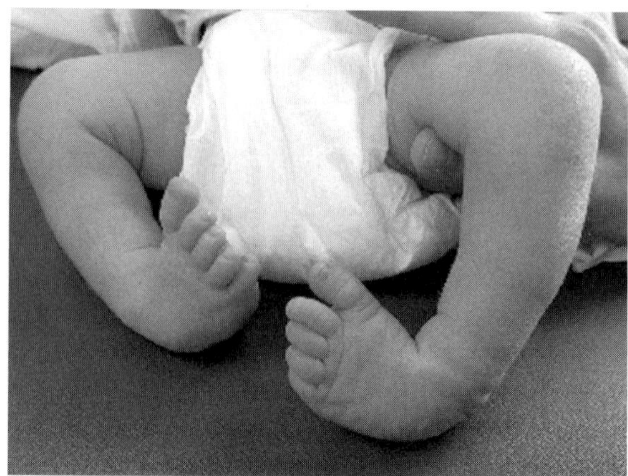

Figure 9–14: Clubfoot. Note the foot in hindfoot varus, hindfoot equinus, and forefoot varus. From Wallach DM, Davidson RS (2004) Pediatric lower limb disorders. In: Pediatric Orthopaedics and Sports Medicine (Dormans JP, ed). Philadelphia: Mosby.

- Defects have been found that suggest the following etiologies:
  - Germ plasma
  - Growth disturbances
  - Mechanical effects
  - Soft tissue contractures
  - Nerve supply imbalance
  - Anomalous muscles
  - Viral causes
- Farrell and coworkers reported a clubfoot rate of 1.1%, about 10 times more than with a live birth risk (0.1%).[24] They postulated that some occurrence during early amniocentesis with fluid leakage interrupted the normal development of the foot.
- Anatomically clubfoot varus is caused by talar deformity with medial neck angulation and medial tilting and rotation of the body of the talus. Varus is also the result of medial tilting and rotation of the calcaneus. The varus deformity of the hindfoot leads to the supination of the forefoot.
- Congenital talipes equinovarus feet are positioned in hindfoot equinus, hindfoot varus, midfoot adduction, and often midfoot cavus.
- Feet vary greatly in the amount of stiffness, bone deformity, muscle involvement, and response to treatment.
- A standardized examination of the clubfoot should be performed initially and after each manipulative casting to assess progress of treatment and, eventually, to help to determine the need for surgery.
- Physical and radiographic examinations, although not accurate or reproducible, can provide significant information about severity, improvement with treatment, and need for surgery.
- Associated anomalies of the upper extremities, back, legs, abnormal reflexes, etc., can provide information about etiology and the likelihood of successful treatment.
- Distinguishing gastrocnemius from soleus–capsular (ankle) contractures is accomplished by dorsiflexing the ankle in flexion and extension, respectively.
- The posterior os calcis must be palpated carefully in measuring the equinus of clubfoot because the bone is located proximally away from the heel pad (Figure 9–15).
- The talar head is palpated dorsolaterally at the midfoot. The talar head usually is lined up with the patella but plantar flexed. Manipulation to reduce the forefoot onto the talar head will indicate the amount of midfoot stiffness.
- Radiographic examination, although used widely to determine foot deformity and response to treatment, has several problems. The images are hard to reproduce, evaluate, and measure because of difficulty in positioning the feet, lack of ossification, failure to define the "true shape" of the bones (based on the secondary centers of ossification), and presence of rotation.

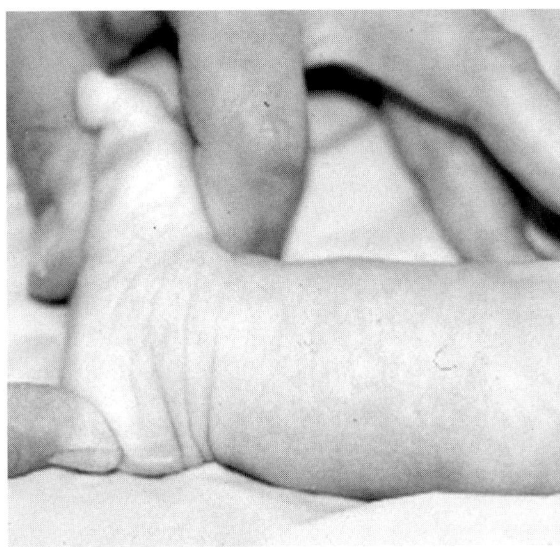

Figure 9–15: The foot appears to be corrected to neutral, but the heel pad is empty and the calcaneus is in equinus. The foot should dorsiflex at least 20 degrees. From Wallach DM, Davidson RS (2004) Pediatric lower limb disorders. In: Pediatric Orthopaedics and Sports Medicine (Dormans JP, ed). Philadelphia: Mosby.

- In the older clubfoot patient, radiographic evaluation can help to identify deformity, degenerative changes, stress changes, and fractures.
- To optimize the radiographic studies, the feet should be held in the position of best correction: a weight-bearing or, for infants, a simulated weight-bearing position.
- Because the AP and lateral talocalcaneal angles are the most commonly measured angles (Kite's angles[25]), the x-ray beam should be focused on the hindfoot (about 30 degrees from the vertical for the AP; the lateral should be transmalleolar with the fibula overlapping the posterior half of the tibia to avoid rotational distortion).
- In the older child, it may be useful to focus the x-ray beam on the midfoot. This view will assess dorsolateral subluxation and narrowing of the talonavicular joint. Lateral dorsiflexion and plantar flexion views may be useful to assess ankle motion (as with flat top talus), abutting of the anterior tibia against the talar neck, or hypermobility in the midfoot.
- Three radiographic observations are made based on the AP view:
  1. For the AP–talocalcaneal angle, lines are drawn through the long axes of the talus and the os calcis (when it is difficult to outline the os calcis, a line can be drawn parallel to the lateral border). The AP talocalcaneal angle typical for clubfoot is less than 20 degrees (Figure 9–16).
  2. For the talar–first metatarsal angle, lines are drawn through the long axes of the talus and the first metatarsal. In the normal foot, this angle is from mild

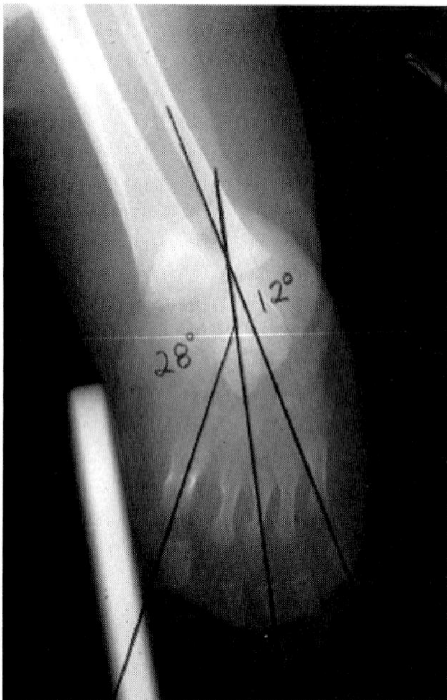

Figure 9–16: AP x-ray film of a clubfoot. Note that the talocalcaneal angle is reduced to 12 degrees (normal is 30 to 55 degrees). The talar first metatarsal angle is varus (normal is valgus). From Wallach DM, Davidson RS (2004) Pediatric lower limb disorders. In: Pediatric Orthopaedics and Sports Medicine (Dormans JP, ed). Philadelphia: Mosby.

valgus to about 30 degrees; in the clubfoot, it is from mild to severe varus.

3. Medial displacement of the cuboid ossific center on the os calcis axis can be determined on the AP view. This apparent displacement may represent angular deformity of the calcaneus or medial subluxation of the cuboid on the calcaneus.

- For the lateral view, the foot should be held in maximum dorsiflexion with the foot laterally rotated but without pronation. The x-ray beam should be focused on the hindfoot. The foot should be positioned with the x-ray plate laterally against the posterior half of the foot. The foot is bean shaped, and placement of the x-ray plate medially will force the foot to be laterally rotated in the x-ray beam.
- Two observations should be made:
  1. For the talocalcaneal angle, lines are drawn through the long axis of the talus and the inferior margin of the os calcis. The resulting angle for clubfoot demonstrates hindfoot equinus and is typically less than 25 degrees (Figure 9–17).
  2. For the talar–first metatarsal angle, lines are drawn through the long axes of the talus and the first metatarsal. Plantar flexion of the forefoot on the hindfoot indicates contracted plantar soft tissues or midtarsal bone deformity (triangular navicular).
- As children, patients with a clubfoot can walk and run surprisingly well; however, with age and increased body

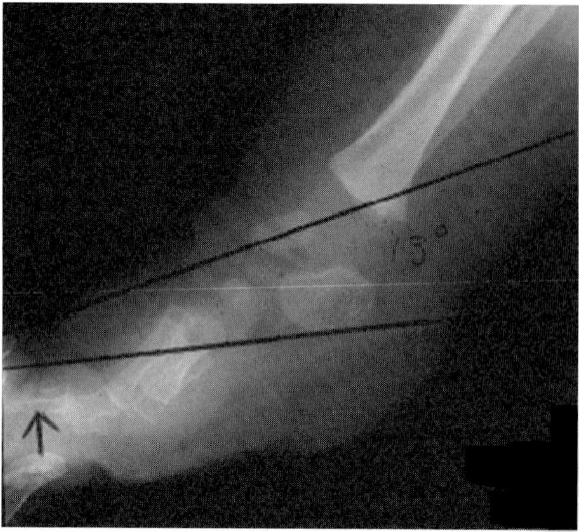

Figure 9–17: Lateral x-ray film of a clubfoot. Note that the talocalcaneal angle is reduced (normal is 25 to 55 degrees). From Wallach DM, Davidson RS (2004) Pediatric lower limb disorders. In: Pediatric Orthopaedics and Sports Medicine (Dormans JP, ed). Philadelphia: Mosby.

weight, the foot (lateral forefoot) develops a thickened callus, which becomes painful. Ordinary shoe wear becomes difficult.

- The stigma of the deformity may cause the child to be shunned in certain societies.
- As treatment is relatively easy for the infant, treatment should be begun as early as is reasonable.
- Hippocrates described the earliest known treatment of clubfoot around 400 BC. He described manipulating the deformed foot and wrapping bandages to maintain the correction. He reported that when the correction was begun in infancy, and the deformity was not too severe, treatment was successful, and surgery was not necessary.
- With the development of mechanical devices in the seventeenth through nineteenth centuries, many physicians developed gradual correcting turnbuckle devices to stretch clubfeet over years.
- Plaster of Paris bandages, developed in 1838, soon supplanted these devices because of their ease of use.
- Inadequate compliance with treatment led to many failures.
- With continued failure, tenotomy of the Achilles tendon became popular in the first quarter of the nineteenth century.
- Pain and gangrene were dreaded complications until the development of anesthesia in 1846 and antisepsis in 1865.
- With the development of anesthesia and antisepsis, surgeons developed increasingly complex surgical treatments.
- Over the last decade there has been a reemergence of a less invasive approach to the clubfoot. The Ponseti's method is a program of approximately 4 to 6 weekly foot

manipulations and castings followed by a percutaneous tenotomy (90% of patients)[26] (Figure 9–18). A program of full time bracing (3 months) is followed by 2 to 4 years of nighttime Denis-Browne Bar usage. Of patients treated, 30% will eventually require transfer of the tibialis anterior tendon laterally to better balance the foot. Failure by this technique may require additional surgery.

- A tremendous number of surgical techniques have been described for the treatment of clubfeet, none of which have achieved dominance.
- Regardless of the specific technique, an à la carte principle is reasonable, addressing only components abnormal for a given foot.
- Equinus is addressed with Z lengthening of the Achilles and a posterior tibiotalar and talocalcaneal capsulotomy.
- Hindfoot varus is corrected with a posteromedial talocalcaneal capsulotomy alone (moderate deformity) or with a complete subtalar release (severe deformity). The lateral subtalar joint may be reached through a separate lateral incision[27] or through a Cincinnati incision.[28]
- Midfoot adduction is corrected by releasing the abductor hallucis and talonavicular joint. Severe adduction may require release of the calcaneal cuboid joint or decancellation of the cuboid (lateral column shortening).
- Lastly, cavus deformity is corrected with a plantar fascia release.

Flatfoot (Planovalgus)

- The "flat" or planovalgus foot is a common deformity consisting of hindfoot valgus, with compensatory midfoot supination and abduction.
- The arch increases in height with maturity as the fatty tissue along the sole of the foot decreases.[29]
- The true incidence of planovalgus feet is unknown. Depending upon the criteria used to define the condition, it may be present in as much as 23% of the adult population, most of which is asymptomatic.
- Foot flexibility and pain are the central issues to consider when evaluating the child with planovalgus feet.
- Patients with flexible flat feet should be reassured and instructed to return only if a problem develops.
- In contrast, stiff feet, even without pain, are concerning and require investigation. Such feet frequently become painful once body weight increases with maturity.
- The differential diagnosis for a planovalgus foot is flexible flatfoot, calcaneovalgus, accessory navicular, tarsal coalition, CVT, and flatfoot secondary to a neuromuscular disease (e.g., cerebral palsy).
- A thorough history and physical will provide most of the information needed to make the diagnosis.
- The history also serves to better understand parental concerns.
- The role of radiographs is to confirm a diagnosis and to help to plan treatment.
- Pain when present should be localized and characterized.
- Inciting, aggravating, or alleviating activities are elicited from the interview.
- Birth and developmental history are helpful in uncovering a neuromuscular origin for the foot deformity (e.g., spastic diplegic cerebral palsy).
- Physical examination begins with observation of the standing child. When looking at the child from the rear, the hindfoot will be in significant valgus and the "too many toes" sign may be present, resulting from significant midfoot abductus.
- The arch (instep) is reduced.
- Genu valgum causes the patient to stand on the medial aspect of the foot.
- A flexible foot with a functioning posterior tibial tendon will invert the hindfoot and reconstitute the arch (Figure 9–19) when the patient actively plantar flexes the foot.
- The presence of an arch can also be demonstrated with the Jack test. The test is performed by passively dorsiflexing the first metatarsal–phalangeal joint. With this maneuver, the plantar fascia raises the arch by shortening the distance between the metatarsal heads and the fascial origin of the calcaneus, the so-called windlass mechanism.
- The feet should be palpitated for tenderness.
- Free and unrestricted motion should be present when moving the heel into varus and valgus and when everting and inverting the midfoot.
- Examine the ankle for a contracted gastrocnemius–soleus as was described for idiopathic toe walking.

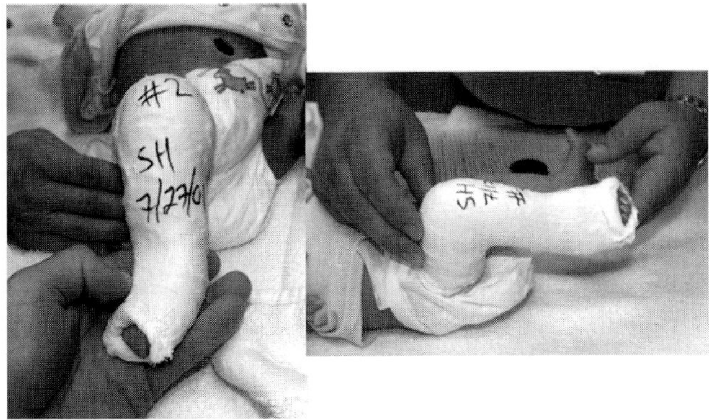

Figure 9–18: Ponseti-type casting of a clubfoot. The foot is spun laterally around the talus with pressure applied to the talar head. The long leg cast with the knee flexed 90 degrees helps to control rotation. The forefoot is supinated slightly. From Wallach DM, Davidson RS (2004) Pediatric lower limb disorders. In: Pediatric Orthopaedics and Sports Medicine (Dormans JP, ed). Philadelphia: Mosby.

Flexible Planovalgus Foot

- Reassurance is all that is required with a flexible, painless flatfoot in the absence of a tight Achilles tendon.
- There is no evidence that a flatfoot is a pathological condition or a condition that predisposes a patient to foot pain as an adult.

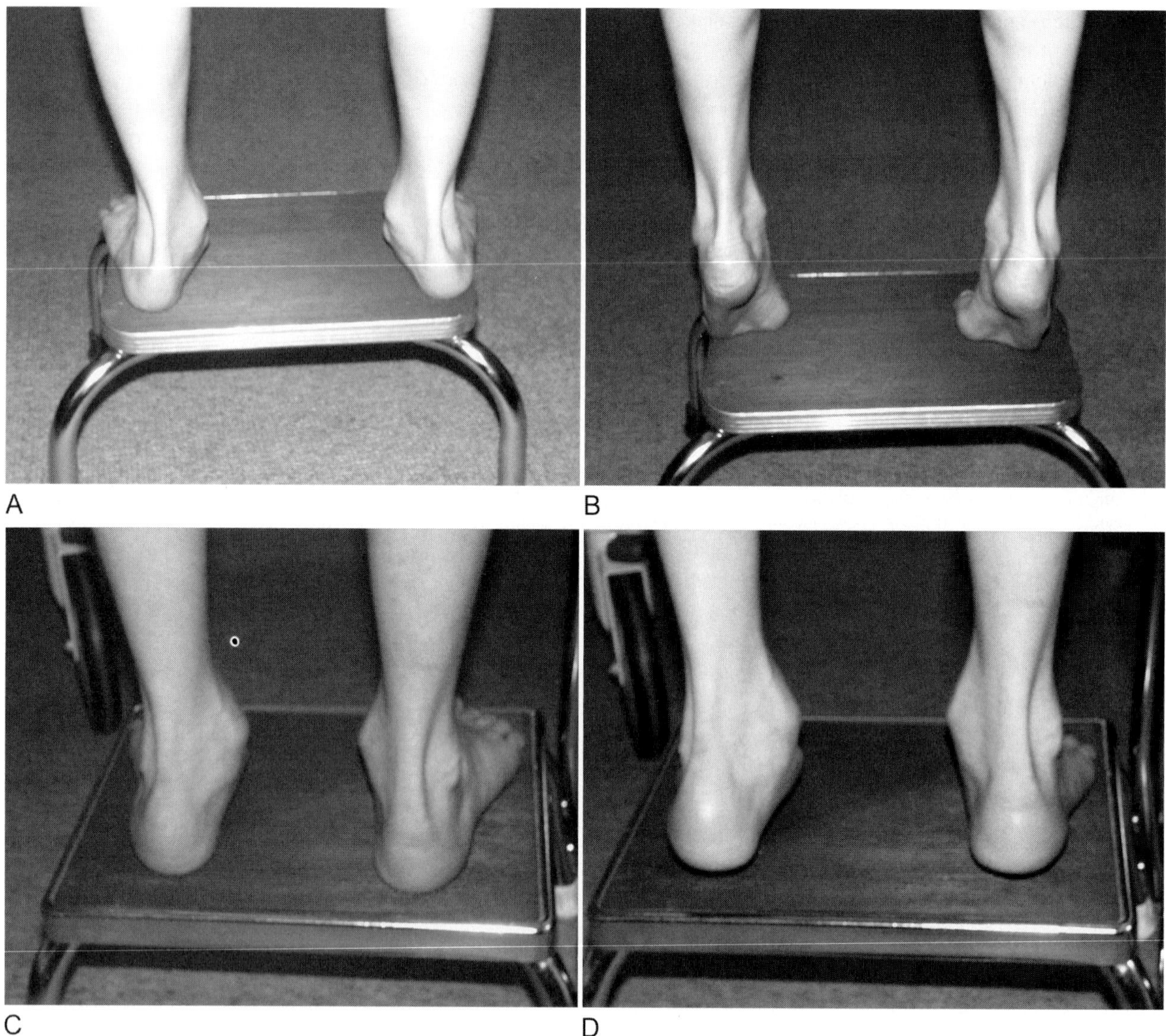

Figure 9–19: A, Flexible flatfoot. B, Hindfoot inversion of same foot with ankle plantar flexion. C, Photograph of another child with a stiff flatfoot secondary to a tarsal coalition whose hindfoot remains in valgus. D, The patient's hindfoot does not invert with ankle plantar flexion.

- Orthotics with a custom instep are expensive, need to be replaced with wear and growth, and have never been shown to alter arch development.[30]
- Shoe wear with a well-formed arch support is recommended in the adolescent–adult who has a flexible flatfoot and midfoot pain after prolonged walking–standing. A custom orthotic is prescribed if the off-the-shelf cushion is inadequate.
- Pain may also occur in the flexible foot with an associated contracture of the gastrocnemius–soleus. A limitation of ankle dorsiflexion results in hindfoot valgus and midfoot dorsiflexion with resultant pain.
- A course of physical therapy with an emphasis on Achilles tendon stretching is the first line of treatment.
- Serial casting and botulinum toxin injections may also be useful.
- Surgical lengthening of a contracted gastrocnemius–soleus is reserved for those patients with persistent ankle equinus.
- Procedures that correct hindfoot valgus include subtalar arthrodesis, arthrorisis, medial displacement osteotomy, and lateral column lengthening.
- In the past, a subtalar fusion was the preferred treatment for hindfoot valgus; however, as a result of poor long-term results, arthrodesis has a role currently only in the foot associated with arthrosis.
- Arthrorisis is technique involving the placement of a staple across the subtalar joint, thereby correcting

hindfoot valgus without a fusion.[31] Only short-term results have been reported with this technique (good to excellent results in 85% of 48 cases); therefore, it has not been universally adopted.

- Although both arthrodesis and arthrorisis correct hindfoot valgus, neither procedure restores the arch and both restrict hindfoot motion.
- Medial displacement calcaneal osteotomy is a method of directly correcting hindfoot valgus by translating the tuberosity into a varus position using an extra-articular osteotomy.
- Although a secondary deformity is created in the foot, motion is maintained and the subtalar joint is not violated.
- Correction of midfoot abduction is achieved with an opening wedge osteotomy of the cuboid,[32] and plantar flexion of the first ray is addressed with a superiorly based opening wedge osteotomy of the medial cuneiform.
- An alternative procedure is a lateral column lengthening of the calcaneus.[33] A trapezoidal opening wedge osteotomy through the calcaneus between the anterior and the medial talocalcaneal facets corrects the foot at the site of deformity.
- The long-term effect of intra-articular violation of the talocalcaneal facets is unknown.
- Medial midfoot capsular plication (talonavicular joint) and cuneiform osteotomy may be needed to fully correct the foot deformity.

Congenital Vertical Talus

- CVT is an anomaly characterized by a stiff "rocker bottom" foot[34] (Figure 9–20, *A*).
- The appearance is secondary to a dorsal dislocation of the navicular onto the head of the talus.
- Although idiopathic CVT occurs, CVT with other conditions is more common.
- Examples of associated abnormalities include arthrogryposis multiplex congenital (AMC), myelomeningocele, congenital myopathy, and intraspinal lesions (e.g., syringomyelia).
- Idiopathic CVT is a diagnosis of exclusion.
- The history and physical is the first and usually the best method of detecting these potentially underlying conditions.
- For example, children with AMC will have had decreased fetal motion. Many if not all limbs will be stiff, and there will be a noticeable absence of flexion creases in affected extremities.
- Foot examination reveals an equinus hindfoot and a dorsiflexed abducted midfoot.
- The deformity is rigid, and the talonavicular dislocation is not reducible.
- The talar head, which is not normally a weight-bearing structure, is palpable along the plantar surface of the foot.
- Over time, pressure on the talus leads to pain, callus formation, and ultimately a foot that will not permit standing.
- Radiographs are helpful in confirming the diagnosis of CVT.
- The dorsal dislocation cannot be directly observed on an infant's radiograph because the navicular does not ossify before 4 years.
- The position of the navicular is inferred because it is in line with the first metatarsal on a lateral radiograph.
- When the talonavicular joint is reduced, a line can be drawn through the talus and shaft of the first metatarsal on a lateral forced plantar flexion radiograph of the foot.
- Because the talonavicular dislocation of CVT is irreducible, the talus never lies in the plane of the first metatarsal (Figure 9–20, *B-E*).
- Without treatment CVT leads to progressive foot pain in all sensate ambulators.
- Patients unable to feel pain develop plantar decubitus and Charcot joints.
- Nonambulators are treated with shoes that accommodate their deformity.
- Although manipulation and casting techniques can "stretch" the skin, making wound closure easier at the time of surgery, they are ineffective in reducing the dislocation.
- The only corrective treatment for CVT is surgery.
- Best results occur when children undergo operative intervention before 2 years of age.
- As with clubfoot surgery, numerous surgical techniques have been described. Few studies are available with adequate patient volume and length of follow-up to prove the superiority of any technique.

Calcaneovalgus Foot

- Calcaneovalgus foot deformity is a condition that may be mistaken for a congenital rocker bottom foot (CVT).
- The condition is another example of a deformity resulting from an intrauterine packing abnormality.
- The fetal foot is maintained in extreme dorsiflexion against the uterine wall, resulting in an ankle dorsiflexion contracture.
- In severe cases, the dorsal aspect of the foot rests against pretibial skin.
- The tibia may also bow with a posterior medial apex.
- The natural history of a calcaneovalgus foot is one of spontaneous correction with some loss of ankle plantar flexion.
- Stretching is of debatable efficacy.
- Ankle motion improves over several weeks.
- Tibial bowing takes several years to resolve, and correction may be incomplete.
- With unilateral involvement, the affected leg may be from 1 to 5 centimeters shorter and may require a limb equalization procedure (e.g., epiphysiodesis or distraction osteogenesis).

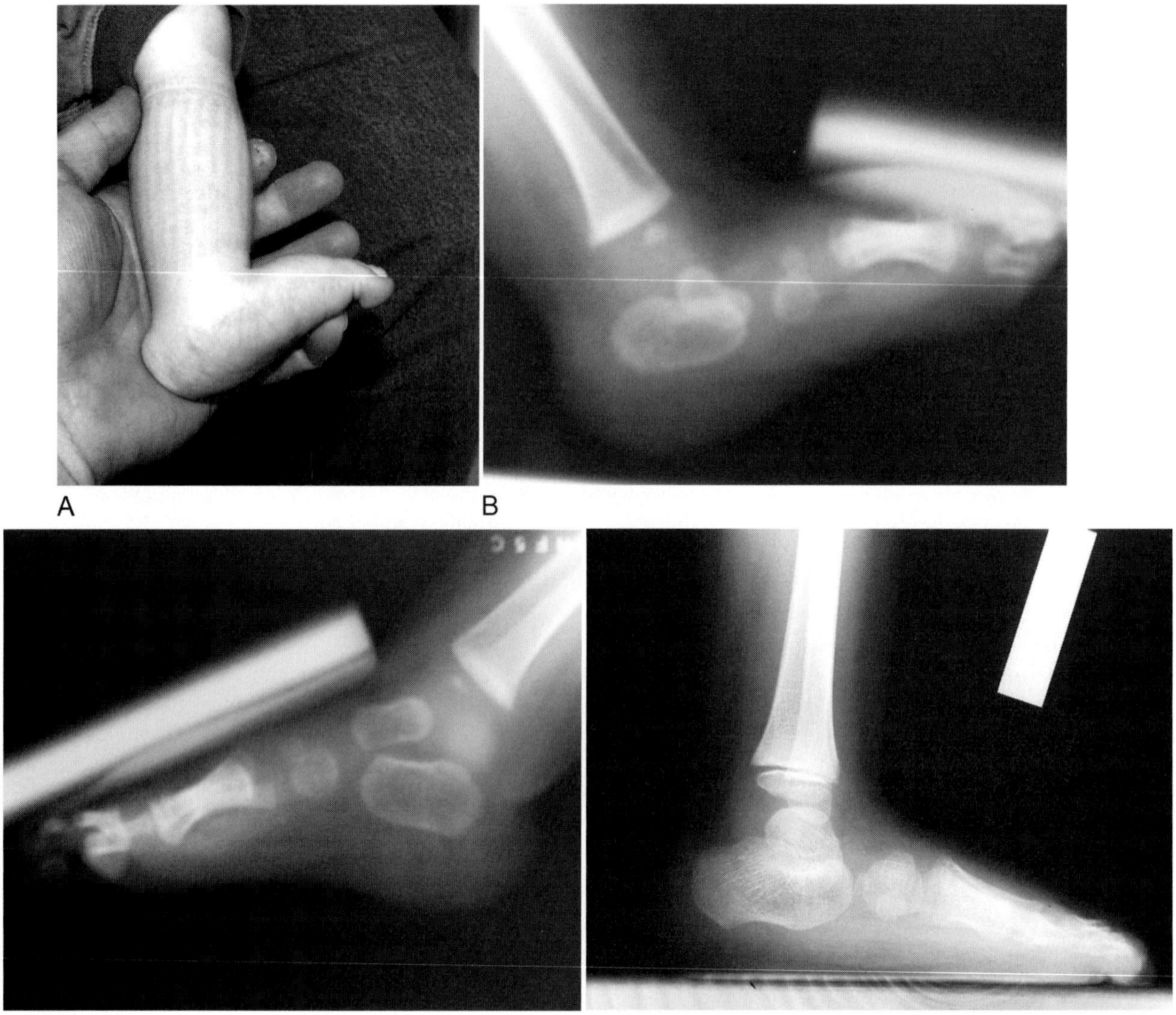

A B

C D

Figure 9–20: A, CVT with a rocker bottom foot. B, Plantar flexion lateral radiograph demonstrating the inability to reduce the navicular on the talus. C, A normal foot with the hindfoot, midfoot, and forefoot well aligned. D, An "oblique talus" with apparent plantar flexion of talus. E, Reduction of the oblique talus with the plantar flexion view distinguishing the condition from CVT.

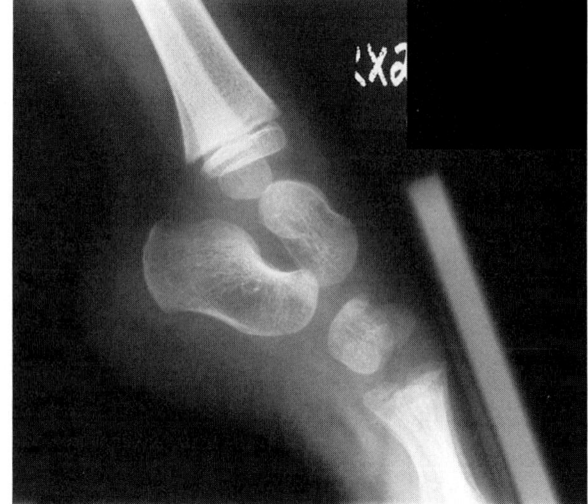

E

Tarsal Coalition

- Tarsal coalition is a failure of segmentation between adjoining tarsal bones.
- The abnormal joint has greatly reduced motion.
- Coalitions may be fibrous (syndesmosis), cartilaginous (synchondrosis), or osseous (synostosis) tissue.
- Motions between the tarsal bones produce pain in some patients.
- The subtalar joint is typically maintained in valgus, although a varus deformity has been described.
- Subtalar motion allows the foot to accommodate walks on uneven terrain.
- A child with a stiff hindfoot may give a history of frequent ankle sprains, fractures, or both.
- Coalitions may exist between all of the tarsal bones, but talocalcaneal and calcaneonavicular (CNC) coalitions are the most common.
- Pain from a talocalcaneal coalition is located in the medial hindfoot by the sustentaculum tali, a prominence just distal and anterior from the medial malleolus.
- Patients with CNC have pain in the sinus tarsi, a depression anterior to the tip of the fibula.
- With both talocalcaneal and CNC, lateral heel pain is common from fibula impingement on the valgus calcaneus.
- Subtalar motion is limited or absent.
- Normal active subtalar motion can be demonstrated by observing hindfoot inversion.
- The calcaneus assumes a varus position with ankle plantar flexion, best seen from behind patients when they rise up onto the balls (metatarsal heads) of their feet.
- In the presence of a coalition, the hindfoot stays in valgus and does not shift into varus with ankle plantar flexion (Figure 9–19).
- Passive subtalar inversion and eversion may also be assessed with patients lying prone with their ankles plantigrade and knees flexed to 90 degrees.
- The presence of a tarsal coalition is confirmed by standing weight-bearing AP, lateral, Harris-Beath and oblique radiographs (Figure 9–21).
- Evidence of a talocalcaneal is seen on the lateral radiograph with the C sign.[35] If there is any question, a Harris-Beath radiograph should be obtained.
- On a lateral radiograph, the "anteater nose" is a sign of a CNC.[36] The CNC is, however, best appreciated on the oblique view of the foot (Figure 9–21, *D*).
- CT is used to identify multiple coalitions and to assess the coalition location and percentage of joint involvement.
- Initial treatment consists of a 1-month period of immobilization in a short leg walking cast.
- Once symptoms subside, the patient is placed in a custom orthosis from University of California at Berkeley laboratories in an attempt to decreased painful subtalar motion.
- Resection and arthrodesis are the two surgical procedures available for patients who fail conservative care.
- Patients with a small talocalcaneal (less than 50% of the subtalar joint) or CNC undergo coalition resection with fat, muscle, or tendon interposition.
- Extensive or multiple coalitions are best treated with an arthrodesis.

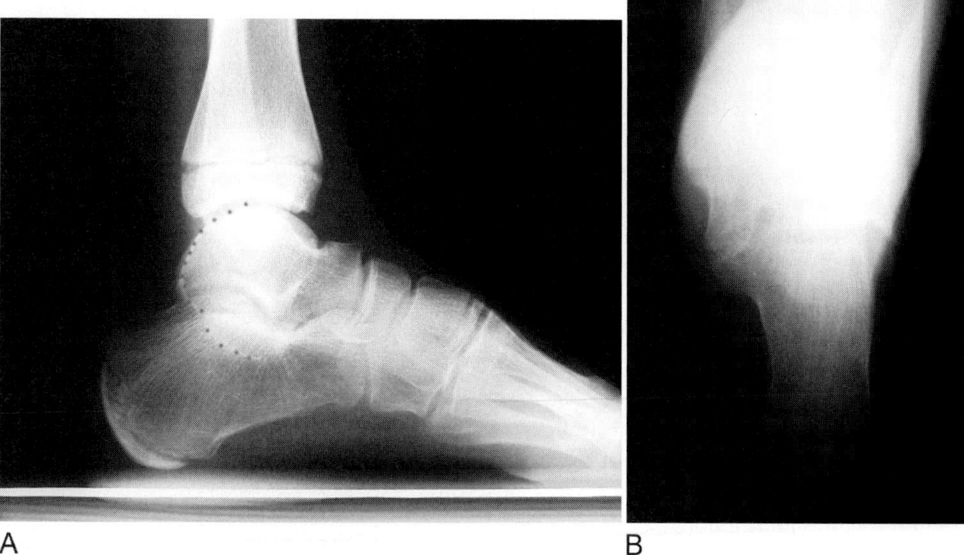

Figure 9–21: A, Lateral radiograph of a foot with talocalcaneal coalition. The C sign is outlined. B, Harris view demonstrating narrowing of the subtalar joint.

Continued

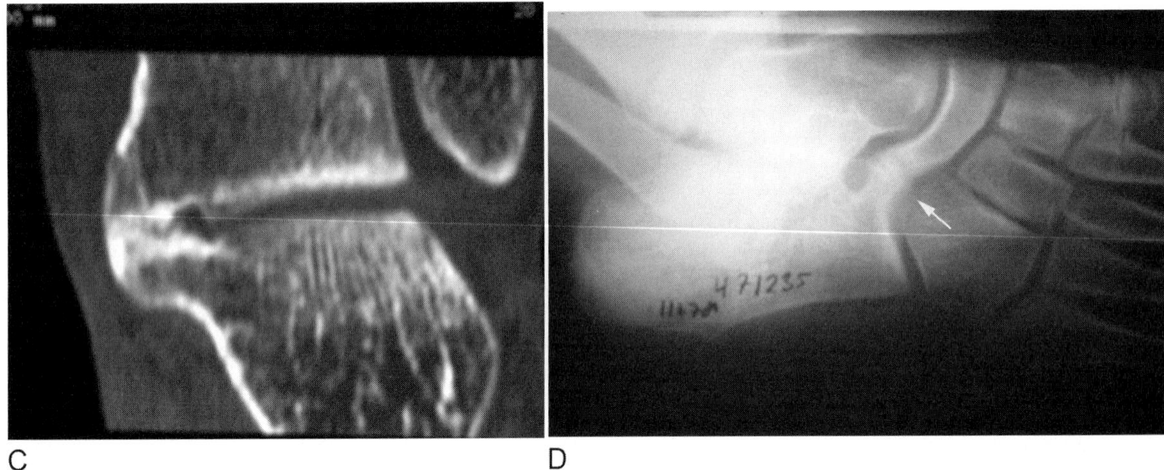

Figure 9–21, cont'd: C, CT scan demonstrating an osseous coalition of the talocalcaneal joint. D, An oblique radiograph of the foot with a calcaneonavicular coalition.

Accessory Navicular

- Accessory as the word implies refers to an "extra" bone known as an *os*.
- The accessory bone may be a located within a tendon, as is the case with os peronei, or as a separate bone, such as the os trigonum.
- These ossicles are common and usually asymptomatic.
- The os navicular is present in 12% of the population and is located within the TPT.
- The TPT is a dynamic contributor to the maintenance of the arch.
- Contraction of the TPT, which occurs during active ankle plantar flexion, causes the hindfoot inversion.
- An accessory navicular is one of the causes of a painful planovalgus foot.
- Pain, when present, is along the medial–plantar aspect of the navicular.
- The diagnosis is confirmed with AP and oblique standing foot radiographs.
- The accessory navicular has three morphologic types:[37]
  - Type I is a small oval to round ossicle within the tendon of the TPT (Figure 9–22).
  - Type II is a larger lateral projection from the medial aspect of the navicular with a clear separation from the base of the navicular.
  - Type III is a connected, "horn shaped" prominence.
- Pain is most common with type II lesions.
- The causes of pain include midfoot dorsiflexion stresses in a planovalgus foot, direct pressure on the prominence, and motion through the navicular–accessory navicular pseudarthrosis.
- Treatment is directed toward pain relief.
- A short leg walking cast is applied for 4 weeks.
- Following successful cast treatment, a custom orthosis with a pressure reducing relief is fashioned.
- Persistent pain is an indication for surgery.
- Surgery involves removal of the accessory navicular through a split made in the TPT.
- Plicating the TPT in an attempt to restore the midfoot arch is rarely effective (also known as the Kidner procedure) and is unnecessary for pain relief.

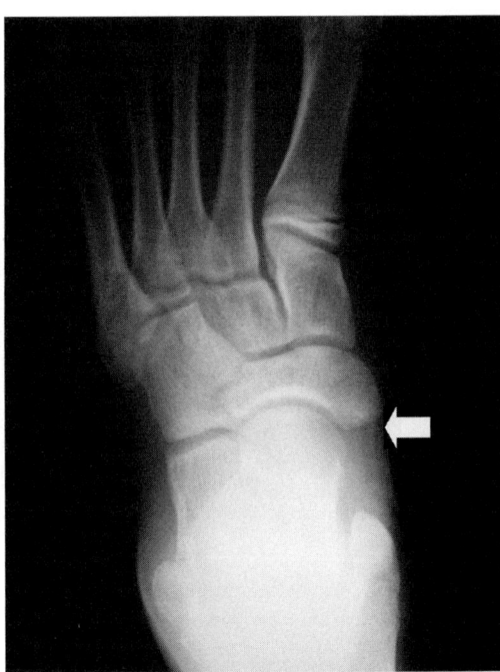

Figure 9–22: AP radiograph of a type I accessory navicular.

Foot Cavus

- A cavus foot has a "high arch," the opposite deformity of a planovalgus foot (Figure 9–23).
- Elevation of the arch is caused by plantar flexion of the medial metatarsals.
- The forefoot is thus pronated in relation to the hindfoot.
- The foot acts as a stable tripod with bases composed of the first and fifth metatarsals heads and the calcaneal tuberosity.[38]
- Depression (plantar flexion) of the first ray causes the calcaneus to assume a varus position to maintain tripod stability.
- As plantar flexion of the first ray increases, the patient bears more weight on the lateral aspect of the foot, increases the likelihood of ankle inversion injuries, and develops a painful callus along the lateral border of the fifth metatarsal.
- Initially, the subtalar joint is mobile and passively correctable; with time, however, heel varus becomes fixed.
- Foot rigidity is a function of plantar fascia, tibialis anterior and posterior contractures, and osseous adaptations.
- Cavus is the result of a peripheral neuropathy that affects the foot intrinsics and peroneals, especially the peroneal longus.
- Intrinsic weakness can lead to clawing of the toes.
- Conditions that cause a cavus foot are idiopathic, Charcot-Marie-Tooth disease, myelomeningocele, Fredrick's ataxia, and spinal cord lesions (e.g., syringomyelia and tumors).
- Mobility of the hindfoot is assessed with the Coleman block test[39] (Figure 9–24). The test is performed with the patient standing with the lateral border of the foot on an elevated surface. In this position, the unsupported first metatarsal will drop below the sole of the foot. The heel will assume a neutral to valgus alignment when the hindfoot is flexible. A rigid hindfoot, in contrast, stays in varus.
- Treatment begins with appropriate tests and referrals to confirm and manage any underlying disease.
- Patients with diminished plantar sensation must be instructed about appropriate foot care and encouraged to perform frequent self-examination.
- An orthosis will not retard disease progression but is valuable in treating a foot drop.

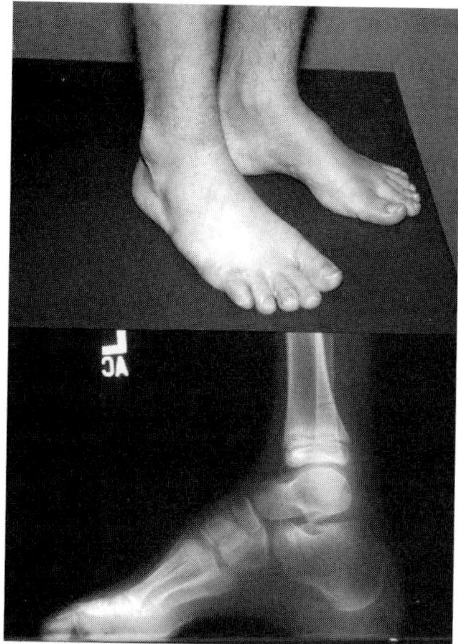

Figure 9–23: Clinical picture and x-ray film of a cavus foot with the pathognomonic elevated arch.

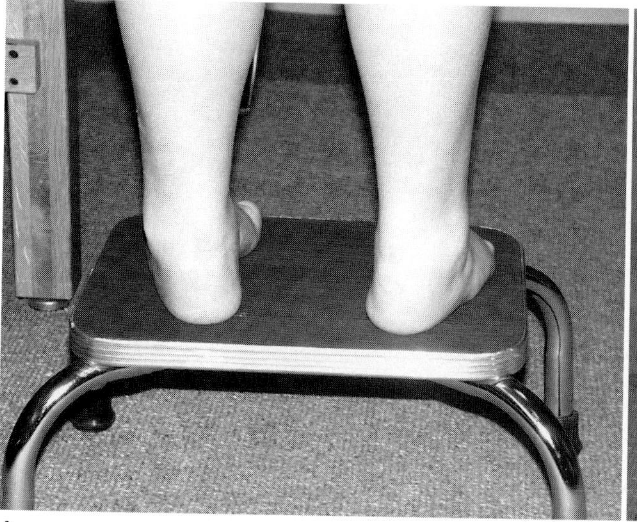

A

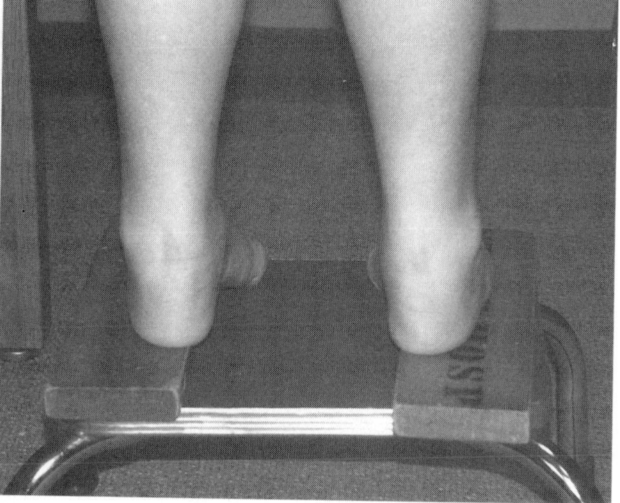

B

Figure 9–24: Demonstration of the Coleman block test. A, Hindfoot in varus with weight bearing upon a flat surface. B, The hindfoot is neutral once the first ray is allowed to hang free. This foot thus has a flexible hindfoot.

- Foot surgery is indicated in the presence of deformity progression and/or pain.
- Tendon transfers, plantar releases, and first metatarsal dorsiflexion osteotomies are reserved for the flexible foot.
- Calcaneal osteotomies are for patients with fixed hindfoot deformity.
- Arthritis, recurrent deformity, or both are treated with realignment and arthrodesis.[38]

Foot Pain

- Nonmechanical foot pain may be divided into inflammatory, infectious, vascular, neoplastic, and traumatic etiologies.
- Systemic symptoms, multiple joint involvement, morning stiffness, positive family history, and positive serum markers are evidence of an inflammatory arthropathy such as juvenile rheumatoid arthritis.
- The presence of fever, chills, and malaise are seen with an infectious etiology, although at times differentiating infectious and inflammatory arthritis can be challenging.
- Neoplasms may appear with or without associated pain. The lesion itself may be discovered as an incidental finding following trauma, or it may be the locus of a pathological fracture.
- Köhler disease and Freiberg infraction are examples of painful osteochondrosis of the foot.[40]
- Köhler disease involves the navicular, and Freiberg infraction involves the metatarsal head.
- It has been theorized that the etiology is one of vascular embarrassment following repetitive microtrauma to the immature foot.

Köhler Disease

- Patients with Köhler disease are typically younger than 6 years with sudden onset of foot pain.
- Pain is worse with activities and improves with rest and oral analgesics.
- Radiographs reveal fragmentation of the navicular bone (Figure 9–25).
- Eight weeks of short leg immobilization is the initial treatment.
- Ultimately, the condition will resolve without reports of long-term problems.

Freiberg Infraction

- In contrast, outcomes of patients with Freiberg infraction are not always favorable.
- The condition occurs in adolescence, frequently in running athletes.
- The patients complain of pain under a metatarsal head, with the second metatarsal being the most commonly affected.
- An antalgic gait is observed, and the metatarsal is tender.
- Radiographs taken early in the disease demonstrate increased metatarsal head density.
- With disease progression, the subchondral bone collapses, producing a crescent ("C") sign.
- Following collapse of the articular surface, a period of fragmentation and finally reformation ensues.
- Non–weight-bearing status is prescribed until symptoms resolve.
- Metatarsal pads reduce weight-bearing contact pressure on the involved bone, providing some relief.

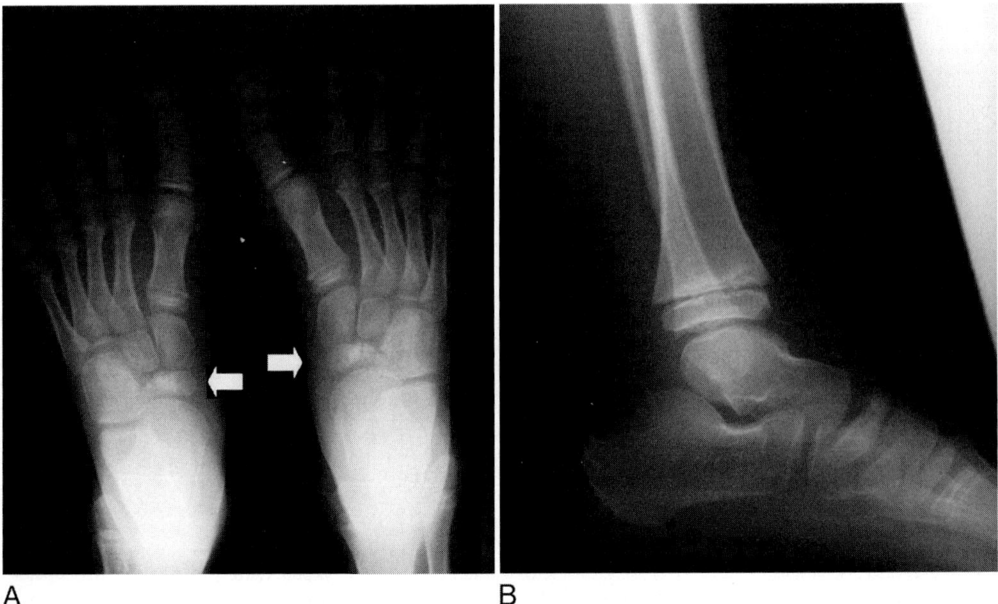

Figure 9–25: **A, AP radiograph of bilateral Kohler's disease. B, Lateral radiograph of Kohler's disease.**

- Persistent pain is addressed with decompression and bone grafting.
- Metatarsal resection and arthrodesis are salvage procedures reserved for severely involved metatarsals.

Sever's Disease

- Sever's disease is an enthesopathy of the calcaneus.[41]
- The condition is etiologically related to Osgood-Schlatter's disease.
- Sever's disease occurs in children with contracted gastrocnemius–soleus complexes.
- The condition can also be part of an inflammatory arthropathy such as spondyloarthropathy.
- On examination, the child has pain involving the plantar calcaneus and reduced ankle dorsiflexion.
- Treatment consists of rest, anti-inflammatories, heel pads, and Achilles tendon stretches.
- The condition resolves over weeks to months with conservative care and rarely needs surgical intervention.

Juvenile Bunion

- Hallux valgus is a deformity of the first ray characterized by abduction of the first metatarsal, with adduction and pronation of the great toe (Figure 9–26).
- The prominence formed by the medial aspect of the first metatarsal is known as a *bunion*.
- Both extrinsic (e.g., improper shoes) and intrinsic factors (e.g., hereditary factors and hindfoot valgus) lead to the development of hallux valgus, with intrinsic issues more common in children.
- Patients with a valgus hindfoot walk on the medial border of the first ray during toe-off. Laterally deviating stress produced during gait promotes the formation of bunions.
- Although bunions can be painful, most are not.
- It is important to identify and council those patients with unrealistic expectations.
- Inspect the shoes for inadequate toe box width.
- Bunion tenderness, swelling, redness, and blistering occur when the shoe rubs and compresses the prominence.
- Pain with dorsiflexion of the metatarsal phalangeal joint is consistent with arthrosis, incongruence, or both of the first metatarsal phalangeal joint.
- Treatment begins with shoe modifications. Patients should wear a shoe with a wide toe box or even sandals (weather permitting).
- Hindfoot valgus and Achilles tendon contracture are predisposing conditions and must be identified and treated with stretching and arch support. Failure to correct the hindfoot is a cause of bunion recurrence.
- Fixed hindfoot deformity or an Achilles tendon that remains "tight" should be addressed surgically.
- The goal of surgery is a painless, shoeable foot. Many patients will not be able to wear "fashionable" shoes (e.g., narrow-toed, high-heeled shoes) following surgery and should be so informed before surgery.
- The surgical treatment of juvenile bunions has a higher recurrence rate then that seen with adults.
- Patient education includes information concerning the possibility of chronic pain following surgery secondary to

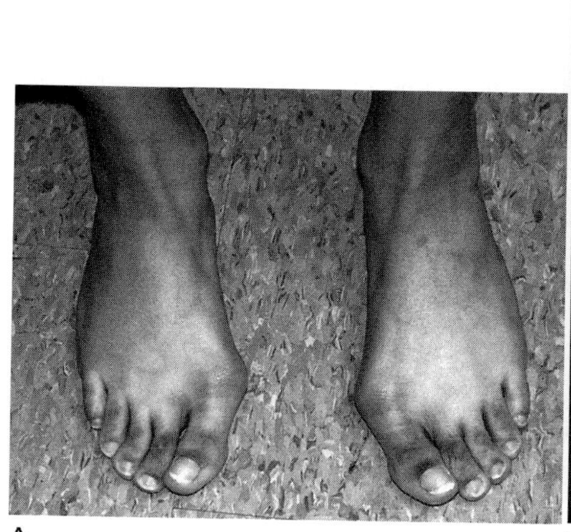

A

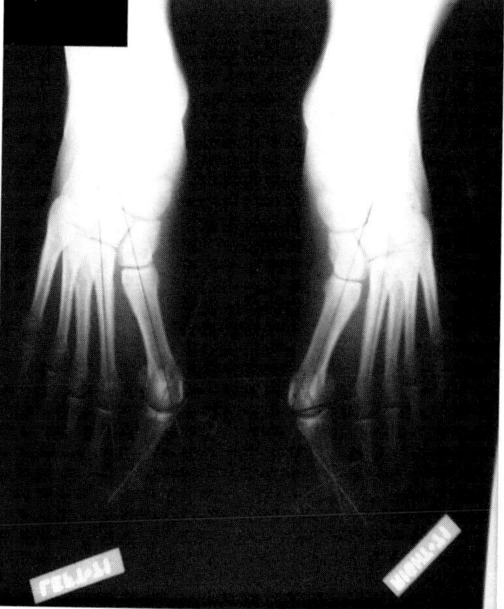

B

Figure 9–26: A, Clinical image. B, Radiographic appearance of feet with hallux valgus.

avascular necrosis, infection, neuroma, arthrosis, and metatarsal growth disturbance (secondary to violation of the proximal physis).
- Treatment consists of a first metatarsal single (distal) or double (proximal and distal) osteotomy with the addition of capsular plication for the subluxated metatarsal–phalangeal joint.[42]

Lesser Toe Deformities

Curly Toe

- Curly toe is a nonprogressive flexion deformity of a lesser toe. The main etiology of curly toe is idiopathic.
- Curly toe is to be distinguished from claw toe, a dorsiflexed metacarpophalangeal joint, and plantar-flexed interphalangeal joints.
- Clawing of the toes is a progressive deformity associated with spinal cord pathology (e.g., myelomeningocele and syringomyelia) or a hereditary motor sensory neuropathy such as Charcot-Marie-Tooth disease.
- The fourth and fifth toes are the most common digits to be affected by curling.
- The deformity is initially flexible and painless.
- Pain does not appear until the child begins to wear shoes.
- Shoes with a low toe box rub the dorsal skin, leading to a painful callous.
- Taping and stretching are not effective.
- Spontaneous resolution is common, making observation and shoe modifications the initial mode of treatment.
- Persistent pain or difficulties with shoe wear are the indications for surgery.
- Surgical correction consists of lengthening the toe flexors and removing redundant skin.

Syndactyly

- Syndactyly is a failure of segmentation of the digits (toes and fingers).
- Syndactyly can be partial (a portion of the toe) versus complete (the entire toe) and simple (skin only) versus complex (involving osseous connections).
- Syndactyly is usually of no clinical significance because few humans need their feet for fine motor function (e.g., writing).
- There are thus few indications for separation of the toes without a coexisting condition such as polydactyly.

Polydactyly

- Polydactyly is an error of duplication.
- The extra digit can be preaxial (medial to the first toe), postaxial (lateral to the fifth toe), or central.
- Patients with foot polydactyly may also have extra digits on their hands.
- The toe may be rudimentary (without osseous structures) or a complete digit with its own metatarsal.
- Isolated polydactyly is more commonly postaxial in children with a positive family history and among blacks.
- Indications for an amputation are pain, trouble wearing shoes, and cosmetic abnormalities.
- Rudimentary digits can be "tied off" in the newborn nursery.
- More complete digits require surgical excision, especially when they are fused to neighboring digits.

Macrodactyly

- Macrodactyly is a digital enlargement.
- Causes of macrodactyly include Proteus syndrome, neurofibromatosis, vascular anomalies (Klippel-Trenaunay-Weber), and lymphangioma.
- Difficulties with shoe wear are found more commonly with macrodactyly than with any other toe condition.
- The foot or toe can be debulked by excision of associated fat, debridement of the vascular structures, or both.
- The length of the digit can be reduced by a timely epiphysiodesis. Physeal arrest although decreasing longitudinal growth does not affect transverse growth.
- In severe cases, partial toe or foot amputation may be required to allow normal shoe wear.

Ingrown Toenail

- An ingrown toenail is largely a preventable condition.
- The causes of an ingrown toenail are improper nail trimming and tight shoes or socks that rub the ends of the toes.
- Dancers *on pointe* are particularly at risk for this condition.
- The toenail should be cut squarely and not too short.
- When too much nail is removed, the nail grows into, under, or into and under the paronychium, the medial and lateral nail folds.
- Irritation from the toenail under the paronychium causes the toe to become painful, swollen, and red.
- With time, the toe may become secondarily infected, most commonly with *Staphylococcus aureus*.
- The treatment of an ingrown toenail begins with cleaning and soaking the foot to address the infection and soften the nail plate. The skin is subsequently pushed off the edge of the nail with a clean cotton tip applicator. A small piece of cotton is left under the corner of the nail to keep the skin from falling back over the edge of the nail.
- Treatment continues until the nail "grows out."
- The process is time consuming and at times painful.
- Failure of conservative treatment may require partial or complete nail ablation.
- Incomplete ablation is a common reason for recurrence and the need for revision procedures.
- Infected ingrown toenails are best treated with antibiotics and drainage.
- Hospital admission with administration of intravenous antibiotics is indicated when there are systemic symptoms, lymphangitic streaking, or lymphadenopathy.

References

1. Staheli LT, Corbett M, Wyss C, King H (1985) Lower extremity rotational problems in children: Normal values to guide management. J Bone Joint Surg Am 67: 39-47.
   This is the classic paper evaluating the normal rotational profile of the growing child.

2. Bleck EE (1982) Developmental orthopaedics: III—Toddlers. Dev Med Child Neurol 24(4): 533-555.
   This is an excellent review of torsional disorders in children. The paper includes age of expected resolution and guidelines for treatment.

3. Ruwe PA, Gage JR, Ozonoff MB, DeLuca PA (1992) Clinical determination of femoral anteversion: A comparison with established techniques. J Bone Joint Surg Am 74(6): 820-830.
   The paper describes an effective clinical method of measuring femoral anteversion in children who have not undergone prior surgery. The technique was compared with CT scan, Magilligan radiographs, and intraoperative examination (gold standard) in 91 hips. The clinical method was found to be within 4 degrees of the anteversion found at the time of surgery.

4. Payne LZ, DeLuca PA (1994) Intertrochanteric versus supracondylar osteotomy for severe femoral anteversion. J Pediatr Orthop 14(1): 39-44.
   In this retrospective review, there was a 14.7% complication rate in the 17 patients treated with a supracondylar femoral osteotomy for the treatment of femoral anteversion. No complications were reported in the 16 patients treated with a proximal femoral osteotomy treated with a blade plate. Additional merits of the proximal technique include improved accuracy of correction (patient treated in prone position) and minimal use of postoperative immobilization.

5. Mazzocca AD, Thomson JD, Deluca PA, Romness MJ (2001) Comparison of the posterior approach versus the dorsal approach in the treatment of congenital vertical talus. J Pediatr Orthop 21(2): 212-217.
   This retrospective study examined CVT patients treated with a posterior approach (25 feet) or a dorsal approach (8 feet). The dorsal technique was faster to perform with less complication and superior postoperative clinical results.

6. Manouel M, Johnson LO (1994) The role of fibular osteotomy in rotational osteotomy of the distal tibia. J Pediatr Orthop 14(5): 611-614.
   After either dividing the fibula or leaving it alone, 35 patients were prospectively and randomly treated with a tibial derotation. No statical difference was found in the ability to rotate the tibia or in the time to union. There were more complications in the division group, but study power was inadequate for statical significance.

7. Salenius P, Vankka E (1975) The development of the tibiofemoral angle in children. J Bone Joint Surg Am 57: 259-261.
   This is the classic paper of normal coronal (genu varum and genu valgum) alignment in children.

8. Hynes D, O'Brien T (1988) Growth disturbance lines after injury of the distal tibial physis: Their significance in prognosis. J Bone Joint Surg Br 70: 231-233.
   In this retrospective study of 26 fractures, 5 patients developed growth injuries, all of which were associated with irregular growth disturbance lines.

9. Birch JG, Herring JA, Wenger DR (1984) Surgical anatomy of selected physes. J Pediatr Orthop 4(2): 224-231.
   A cadaveric study of a 5-year-old provided information concerning surgical approaches needed for the treatment of physeal arrests of the radius, tibia, fibula, and femur.

10. Langenskiöld A (1952) Tibia vara (osteochondrosis deformans tibiae): A survey of 23 cases. Acta Chir Scand 103: 1.
    This paper is the classic article describing the six stages of infantile Blount disease.

11. Levine AM, Drennan JC (1982) Physiologic bowing and tibia vara: The metaphyseal–diaphyseal angle in the measurement of bowleg deformities. J Bone Joint Surg Am 64: 1158-1163.
    The method of measuring the MDA is described. The MDA's prognostic value for developing infantile Blount disease is demonstrated.

12. Feldman MD, Schoenecker PL (1993) Use of the metaphyseal–diaphyseal angle in evaluation of bowed legs. J Bone Joint Surg Am 75: 1602-1609.
    The authors analyzed the MDA in 106 children, achieving a 95% confidence interval in predicting the occurrence of Blount disease by raising the threshold to 16 degrees.

13. Stevens PM, Belle RM (1997) Screw epiphysiodesis for ankle valgus. J Pediatr Orthop 17(1): 9-12.
    In this study, 50 valgus ankles were treated with a medial screw hemiepiphysiodesis. Correction of the deformity was noted without unintended physeal closure following screw removal.

14. Bowen JR, Torres RR, Forlin E (1992) Partial epiphysiodesis to address genu varum or genu valgum. J Pediatr Orthop 12: 359-364.
    The authors developed and demonstrated the value of a chart that predicts the timing of partial epiphysiodesis in corrective varus and valgus knee deformities. The chart and the method are described in detail.

15. Anderson DJ, Schoenecker PL, Sheridan JJ, Rich MM (1992) Use of an intradedullary rod for the treatment of congenital pseudarthrosis of the tibia. J Bone Joint Surg Am 74: 161-168.
    Union of congenital pseudarthrosis of the tibia was achieved in 9 of 10 patients with an intramedullary rod and bone grafting. Three of 5 patients had additional surgery to treat a refracture. All were able to walk without pain.

16. Sutherland DH, Olshen RA, Cooper L, Woo SL (1980) The development of mature gait. J Bone Joint Surg Am 62: 336-353.
    This paper describes the sequence and character of gait in the child during normal development.

17. Smith JT, Bleck EE, Gamble JG, Rinsky LA, Pena T (1991) Simple method of documenting metatarsus adductus. J Pediatr Orthop 11(5): 679-680.
    A practical method using a photocopy machine is described for recording MA.

18. Bleck EE (1983) Metatarsus adductus: Classification and relationship to outcomes of treatment. J Pediatr Orthop 3(1): 2-9.
   This study of 160 children with MA found that starting cast treatment before 8 months of age was the most significant predictor of a good outcome. Neither flexibility nor severity was found to influence the outcome.

19. Rushforth GF (1978) The natural history of hooked forefoot. J Bone Joint Surg Br 60: 530-532.
   The paper is a retrospective study of 130 untreated feet with MA. At the study's conclusion (after 7 years), only 4% were symptomatic and misshapen.

20. Ponseti IV, Becker JR (1966) Congenital metatarsus adductus: The results of treatment. J Bone Joint Surg Am 48: 702-711.
   The article describes the method (different from that for clubfeet) of manipulation and casting of feet with MA.

21. McHale KA, Lenhart MK (1991) Treatment of residual clubfoot deformity—the "bean shaped" foot—by opening wedge medial cuneiform osteotomy and closing wedge cuboid osteotomy: Clinical review and cadaver correlations. J Pediatr Orthop 11(3): 374-381.
   The technique corrected all seven feet with residual MA following clubfoot surgery. The method allows continued foot growth by keeping soft tissue and osseous violation to a minimum.

22. Mosca VS (1993) Skewfoot deformity in children: Correction by calcaneal neck lengthening and medial cuneiform opening wedge osteotomies. J Pediatr Orthop 13: 807.
   The author applies a modification of the Evans calcaneal lengthening to address the specific deformities of the skewfoot.

23. Ippolito E, Ponseti IV (1980) Congenital clubfoot in the human fetus: A histological study. J Bone Joint Surg Am 62(1): 8-22.
   Postmortem histological and gross examination was made of eight clubfoot specimens. Findings were used to support the theory of "retracting fibrosis" as the cause of the clubfoot shape.

24. Farrell SA, Summers AM, Dallaire L, Singer J, Johnson JA, Wilson RD (1999) Clubfoot, an adverse outcome of early amniocentesis: Disruption or deformation? (Canadian Early and Mid-Trimester Amniocentesis Trial). J Med Genet 36(11): 843-846.
   This paper links clubfoot with amniocentesis and describes a theoretical reason for the connection.

25. Kite JH (1972) Nonoperative treatment of congenital clubfoot. Clin Orthop 84: 29-38.
   The paper describes Kite's nonoperative method and the technique used to measure the clubfoot radiographically.

26. Ponseti IV (1996) Congenital Clubfoot: Fundamentals of Treatment. Oxford: Oxford University Press.
   The book describes the anatomy of the clubfoot. The Ponseti method is explained in detail, and long-term clinical and radiographic results are given.

27. Carroll NC, Gross RH (1990) Operative management of clubfoot. Orthopedics 13(11): 1285-1296.
   This point–counterpoint discussion examines the surgical technique advocated by the two authors. Anatomical considerations are presented as rational for the various methods.

28. McKay DW (1983) New concept of and approach to clubfoot treatment: Section II—correction of the clubfoot. J Pediatr Orthop 3(1): 10-21.
   The author provides a description and the rational for a method that advocates an extensive release and correction of the clubfoot deformity.

29. Staheli LT, Chew DE, Corbett M (1987) The longitudinal arch: A survey of eight hundred and eighty-two feet in normal children and adults. J Bone Joint Surg Am 69(3): 426-428.
   This is the classic paper evaluating the normal arch development in children.

30. Gould N, Moreland M, Alvarez R, Trevino S, Fenwick J (1989) Development of the child's arch. Foot Ankle 9(5): 241-245.
   The paper reported a prospective study of 125 toddlers followed over 5 years to assess arch development. Arch development occurred in all children whether or not they wore orthosis.

31. Crawford AH, Kucharzyk D, Roy DR, Bilbo J (1990) Subtalar stabilization of the planovalgus foot by staple arthrorisis in young children who have neuromuscular problems. J Bone Joint Surg Am 72(6): 840-845.
   The paper describes the technique of staple arthrorisis of the subtalar joint. After examinations of 48 feet followed for 4.1 years, 85% were considered excellent to good. In only 3 feet were the authors unable to maintain hindfoot alignment.

32. Rathjen KE, Mubarak SJ (1998) Calcaneal–cuboid–cuneiform osteotomy for the correction of valgus foot deformities in children. J Pediatr Orthop 18(6): 775-782.
   This is a retrospective review of 24 feet treated for hindfoot valgus with an extra-articular medial displacement osteotomy of the calcaneus. Midfoot and forefoot abduction are addressed with cuboid shortening and medial cuneiform lengthening osteotomies. A well-balanced foot was achieved in 23 of 24 feet. The advantage of the procedure is the maintenance of motion without violating the subtalar joint.

33. Mosca VS (1995) Calcaneal lengthening for valgus deformity of the hindfoot: Results in children who had severe, symptomatic flatfoot, and skewfoot. J Bone Joint Surg Am 77(4): 500-512.
   A modification of the Evans calcaneal lengthening procedure was effective in treating 31 symptomatic valgus feet. The technique carries the advantage of preserving motion.

34. Drennan JC (1996) Congenital vertical talus. Instr Course Lect 45: 315-322.
   This is an excellent review article of the conditions of anatomy and treatment.

35. Lateur LM, Van Hoe LR, Van Ghillewe KV, Gryspeerdt SS, Baert AL, Dereymaeker GE (1994) Subtalar coalition: Diagnosis with the C sign on lateral radiographs of the ankle. Radiology 193(3): 847-851.

The paper describes the C sign. The sign was present in 18 cases of known subtalar coalition and was found prospectively in 13 of 15 cases.

36. Oestreich AE, Mize WA, Crawford AH, Morgan RC, Jr. (1987) The "anteater nose": A direct sign of calcaneonavicular coalition on the lateral radiograph. J Pediatr Orthop 7(6): 709-711.
    The paper describes the utility of the anteater nose radiographic sign. The sign was present in all 30 feet (over 8 years of age) with CNC coalition and was absent in normal subjects.

37. Grogan DP, Gasser SI, Ogden JA (1989) The painful accessory navicular: A clinical and histopathological study. Foot Ankle 10(3): 164-169.
    For this study, 25 feet with accessory navicular were treated operatively by excision of the accessory bone (no Kidner procedure) with a 100% success rate. Postoperative microscopic findings were consistent with inflammation and attempted repair of microfracture in the synchondrosis.

38. Paulos L, Coleman SS, Samuelson KM (1980) Pes cavovarus: Review of a surgical approach using selective soft tissue procedures. J Bone Joint Surg Am 62: 942-953.
    The paper is a short-term (a minimum of a 2-year follow-up) retrospective study of the surgical treatment of 39 cavovarus feet. Of the results, 85% were judged "acceptable." The role of soft tissue and osteotomy procedures were outlined.

39. Coleman S, Chesnut W (1977) A simple test for hindfoot flexibility in the cavovarus foot. Clin Orthop 123: 60-62.
    The paper explains the block test used to distinguish a flexible hindfoot varus deformity from a fixed deformity.

40. Sever J (1912) Apophysitis of the os calcis. NY Med J 95: 1025.
    This is the original paper describing calcaneal apophysitis.

41. Ippolito E, Ricciardi Pollini PT, Falez' F (1984) Kohler's disease of the tarsal navicular: Long-term follow-up of 12 cases. J Pediatr Orthop 4: 416-417.
    This paper is a long-term follow-up (33 years) of 12 patients with a history of Kohler's disease treated conservatively. All patients were asymptomatic and without evidence of arthritis.

42. Peterson HA, Newman SR (1993) Adolescent bunion deformity treated with double osteotomy and longitudinal pin fixation of the first ray. J Pediatr Orthop 13(1): 80-84.
    Here, 15 pediatric bunions were corrected with a proximal medial opening and distal closing wedge osteotomy transfixed with a Steinmann pin. A low rate of recurrence and technical ease were additional reasons advocated for this procedure.

Bibliography

Morrissy, RT, Weinstein, SL, eds (1990) Lovell and Winter Pediatric Orthopaedics, 3rd edition. Philadelphia: Lippincott Williams & Wilkins.

Freiberg A (1914) Infraction of the second metatarsal bone: A typical injury. Surg Gynecol Obstet 19: 191.
    This is the original paper describing the condition.

Rubinovitch M, Said SE, Glorieux FH, Cruess RL, Rogala E (1988) Principles and results of corrective lower limb osteotomies for patients with vitamin D-resistant hypophosphatemic rickets. Clin Orthop (237): 264-270.
    This is a retrospective study of 44 legs deformed by rickets treated by osteotomy. Compartment syndrome in one patient was the only acute complication. The need for good metabolic control of the disease was stressed to optimize results and minimize recurrence (27% of patients).

Wallach DM, Davidson RS (2004) Pediatric lower limb disorders. In: Pediatric Orthopaedics and Sports Medicine (Dormans JP, ed). Philadelphia: Mosby.

CHAPTER 10

Hip Disorders

Bülent Erol[*] and John P. Dormans[†]

[*]MD, Attending Surgeon, Department of Orthopaedic Surgery, The Hospital of University of Marmara, Marmara University School of Medicine, Istanbul, Turkey
[†]MD, Chief of Orthopaedic Surgery, The Children's Hospital of Philadelphia, Philadelphia, PA; Professor of Orthopaedic Surgery, University of Pennsylvania School of Medicine, Philadelphia, PA

- Hip disorders are common in the pediatric population.
- A limp or an abnormal gait may be the initial symptoms. Alternatively, the child may complain of knee rather than hip pain.
- This chapter provides an overview of taking the history of and physically examining the pediatric hip; this overview is followed by detailed descriptions of the principal orthopaedic hip disorders of childhood (Box 10–1).

Box 10–1 Hip Disorders in Children

- DDH
- LCPD
- SCFE
- Idiopathic chondrolysis of the hip
- Coxa vara
- Femoral anteversion

History

- Careful attention should be paid to any reported changes in gait. A description of the severity and the time course for the gait change, as well as the activities that worsen it, is essential.
- Pain is the most common presenting complaint in older children with a hip disorder.
  - The severity, location, time course, and frequency of the pain should be noted.
  - Exacerbating and mitigating factors should also be elucidated.
- The clinician must inquire about previous episodes of pain and the presence of a similar condition on the other side (including both the knee and the hip).

Physical Examination

Observation and Inspection

- A careful observation of the patient's posture can detect hyperlordosis of the spine, which may accompany bilateral hip dislocations.[1]
- Having the patient stand on one foot forces the hip abductors to work to keep the pelvis level. A patient with a hip disorder may exhibit a positive *Trendelenburg sign* in which the abductors of the affected hip fail to keep the pelvis level so that the contralateral hip is lower than the affected hip (Figure 10–1).
- To assess gait, the clinician should have the patient walk in the examination room or the hallway.
  - A patient with a unilateral hip disorder may have *Trendelenburg gait* in which the child leans over the affected hip with each step to compensate for weak hip abductors.
  - A patient with pain in one hip or lower limb may exhibit *antalgic gait* in which the stance phase is shorter for the affected limb to unload that side more quickly; the unaffected limb appears to be taking quicker steps.
- Neurological examination of both lower extremities should be performed.
- All children with a hip disorder should be screened for deformity.

Palpation and Manipulation

- During the examination, the clinician should ensure that the patient is in the most comfortable position possible.
- The patient or caregiver should be asked to help localize the area of pain or discomfort by pointing to it with one finger.
- Gentle palpation should be used to search for effusion, spinal disease, or masses of the extremity and trunk.
- The clinician must be careful to isolate each joint during range of motion manipulation.
  - For example, the knee can be isolated from the hip by holding the thigh securely and allowing the leg to hang over the edge of the examination table. Moving the knee in this position will prevent inadvertent movement of the hip, thereby helping to distinguish between knee pain caused by a knee problem and referred pain caused by a hip disorder.
  - Hip pain can be elicited by the log-roll test in which the examiner gently rolls the supine patient's entire lower limb (internal and external hip rotation) by holding the thigh. The log-roll test effectively isolates the hip by preventing irritation of the knee and back during the movement.

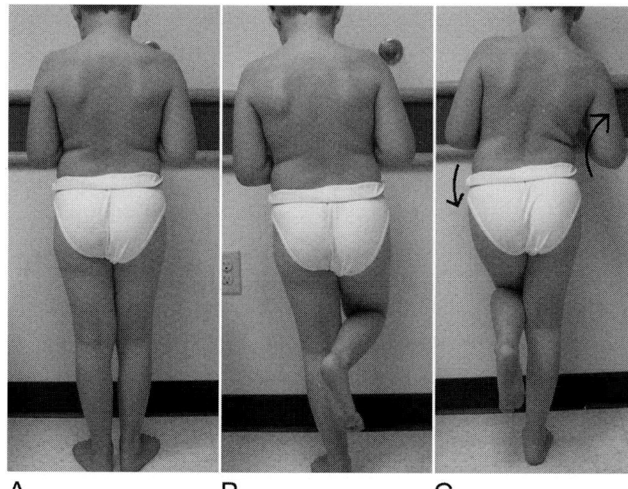

Figure 10–1: Trendelenburg sign. In a patient with a hip disorder, the abductor muscle mechanism of the affected hip is not able to keep the pelvis stable when the patient stands only on the affected limb. A, When the patient stands on both feet, the shoulders and pelvis are level. B, When the patient stands on the unaffected left limb, the level positions of the shoulders and pelvis are maintained. C, However, when the patient stands on the affected right limb, the pelvis tilts down to the left *(arrow)* and there is compensatory leaning (to the right) of the trunk *(arrow)* over the affected hip to maintain balance. From Dormans JP, ed (2004) Pediatric Orthopaedics and Sports Medicine. Philadelphia: Mosby.

Developmental Dysplasia and Dislocation of the Hip

- Developmental dysplasia of the hip (DDH) is a spectrum of disorders of development of the hip that occur in different forms at different ages.
- DDH is a disorder that evolves over time. The structures that make up the hip are normal during embryogenesis and gradually become abnormal for a variety of reasons, chiefly fetal position and presentation at birth and laxity of the ligamentous structures about the hip joint.
- About 2.5 to 6.5 infants per 1000 live births develop hip dysplasia, and a significant percentage of these are not evident on neonatal screening examinations.[1,2]
- Because the pathological processes leading to hip dysplasia may not be present or identifiable at birth, periodic examination of the infant's hip is essential at each routine, well-baby examination until the child is 1 year old.
- Teratological dislocation of the hip is a distinct form of hip dislocation that usually occurs with other disorders, such myelodysplasia and arthrogryposis.[3] These hips are dislocated before birth, have limited range of motion, and are not reducible on examination.

Pathophysiology

Normal Hip Development

- For normal hip joint growth and development to occur, there must be a genetically determined balance of growth of the acetabular and the triradiate cartilages and a well-located and centered femoral head.[4]
- The hip joint begins to develop about the seventh week of gestation, when a cleft appears in the mesenchyme of the primitive limb bud. These precartilaginous cells differentiate into a fully formed cartilaginous femoral head and acetabulum by the eleventh week of gestation.
- At birth, the neonatal acetabulum is composed of cartilage, with a thin rim of fibrocartilage called the *labrum*.
  - The cellular hyaline cartilage of the acetabulum is continuous with the triradiate cartilages, which divide and interconnect the three osseous components of the pelvis (the ilium, ischium, and pubis).
  - The surface of the acetabular cartilage, which abuts the bone of the pelvis, is made up of epiphyseal cartilage in the shape of a hemisphere and functions as a major growth plate. Growth of this physis is essential for acetabular development, and any damage to the periacetabular area may induce a growth disturbance.[3,4]
- Experimental studies have demonstrated that the development of the acetabulum depends on the geometrical pattern within it during growth.[2,3]
  - The concave shape of the hip joint is determined by the presence of a spherical femoral head.

- In addition, several factors determine acetabular depth, including interstitial growth within the acetabular cartilage, appositional growth under the perichondrium, and growth of adjacent bones (the ilium, ischium, and pubis)

- In the neonate, the entire proximal femur is a cartilaginous structure in the shape of a femoral head and greater and lesser trochanters.
  - The three main growth areas are the physeal plate, the growth plate of the greater trochanter, and the femoral neck isthmus.
  - Development of the proximal femur occurs through a combination of appositional growth on the surfaces of the upper femur and epiphyseal growth at the juncture of the cartilaginous upper femur and the femoral shaft.[2]
  - Between the fourth and seventh months, the proximal femoral ossification center (in the center of the femoral head) appears.[2,3]

    1. This ossification center continues to enlarge, with its cartilaginous anlage, until adult life, when only a thin layer of articular cartilage remains.
    2. During the period of growth, the thickness of the cartilage surrounding this bony nucleus gradually decreases, as does the thickness of the acetabular cartilage.

  - The growth of the proximal femur is affected by muscle pull, the forces transmitted across the hip joint by weight-bearing ability, normal joint nutrition, circulation, and muscle tone. Any alterations in these factors may cause profound changes in the development of the proximal femur.[2]

Hip Development in Developmental Dysplasia of the Hip

- DDH is a gradually progressive disorder associated with distinct anatomical changes, many of which are initially reversible. It is a malformation of anatomical structures that developed normally during the embryological period.
- In the normal hip at birth, there is a tight fit between the femoral head and the acetabulum. The femoral head is held in the acetabulum by the surface tension created by the synovial fluid. In DDH, this tight fit is lost and the femoral head spontaneously slides into and out of the acetabulum.[3]
- Most abnormalities in DDH are on the acetabular side. Changes on the femoral side are secondary to anteversion and pressure changes on the head from the acetabulum or ilium associated with subluxation or dislocation.[2] With growth and development, acetabular growth is affected by the primary disease, and any growth alterations incurred from secondary acetabular procedures.
- At birth, the pathological findings in DDH range from mild capsular laxity to severe dysplastic changes.
  - The most common pathological change is a hypertrophied ridge of acetabular cartilage in the superior, posterior, and inferior aspects of the acetabulum.

    1. This ridge, or *neolimbus,* as described by Ortolani, is composed of cellular hyaline cartilage.[4]
    2. It is over this ridge that the femoral head glides in and out of the acetabulum, producing the palpable sensation known as the *Ortolani sign.*

  - In most newborns with DDH, the labrum is everted.
- Hips that remain dislocated develop secondary barriers to reduction.[2]
  - In the depths of the acetabulum, the fatty tissue known as *pulvinar* thickens and may impede reduction.
  - The ligamentum teres elongates and thickens, and it may take up valuable space within the acetabulum.
  - The transverse acetabular ligament is often hypertrophic and may impede reduction.
  - The inferior capsule of the hip assumes an hourglass shape, eventually presenting an opening smaller in diameter than the femoral head.
- If the hip remains dislocated, the acetabular roof becomes progressively more oblique, the concavity gradually flattens and presents a convex surface, and the medial wall of the acetabulum thickens.
- In adults, the fully dislocated femoral head may lie well above the acetabular margin in a markedly thickened hip capsule, the so-called high-riding dislocation.

Etiology, Incidence, and Risk Factors

- The etiology of DDH is multifactorial, involving both genetic and intrauterine environmental factors.[2]
- The results of newborn clinical screening programs estimate that 1 in every 100 newborns examined has evidence of some hip instability (i.e., positive Ortolani or Barlow sign), although the true incidence of dislocation is reported to be between 1 and 1.5 cases per 1000 live births.[3]
- There is marked geographical and racial variation in the incidence of DDH.[1]
  - Some areas of the world have a high endemic incidence; in other areas, the condition is virtually nonexistent. The reported incidence based on geography ranges from 1.7 per 1000 babies in Sweden to 75 per 1000 in Yugoslavia to 188.5 per 1000 in a district of Manitoba, Canada.
  - The incidence of DDH in Chinese and African newborns is almost 0%, whereas it is 1% for hip dysplasia and 0.1% for hip dislocation in white newborns.[1]
  - These differences may be caused by environmental factors, such as child-rearing practices, rather than to genetic predisposition.

1. African and Asian caregivers have traditionally carried babies against their bodies in a shawl so that a child's hips are flexed, abducted, and free to move. This keeps the hips in the optimum position for stability and for dynamic molding of the developing acetabulum by the cartilaginous femoral head.
2. On the other hand, children in Native American and Eastern European cultures, which have a relatively high incidence of DDH, have historically been swaddled in confining clothes that bring their hips into extension. This position increases the tension of the psoas muscle–tendon unit and may predispose the hips to displace, and eventually dislocate, laterally and superiorly.

- Risk factors for DDH are well documented[1-3] (Box 10–2).
  - A positive family history for DDH may be found in 12 to 33% of affected patients.
  - DDH is more common among female patients (80% of cases). This is thought to be because of the greater susceptibility of girls to maternal relaxin hormone, which increases ligamentous laxity.
  - Although only 2 to 3% of all babies are born in breech presentation, the rate is 16 to 25% for patients with DDH. This is probably related to the strong hamstring forces on the hip that result from knee extension. The increased tension on the hamstrings pushes the femoral head out of the acetabulum, destabilizing the hip.
  - Any condition that leads to a tighter intrauterine space and, consequently, less room for normal fetal motion may be associated with DDH. These conditions include oligohydramnios, large birth weight, and first pregnancy.
  - The high rate of association of DDH with other intrauterine molding abnormalities, such as torticollis and metatarsus adductus, lends some support to the theory that the "crowding phenomenon" plays a role in the pathogenesis (Figure 10–2).
  - The left hip is the most commonly affected hip; in the most common fetal position, this hip is usually forced into adduction against the mother's sacrum.
  - Other children with a higher incidence of DDH are infants delivered by cesarean section and those cared for in special care units after birth.

Box 10–2 High-Risk Factors for Developmental Dysplasia or Dislocation of the Hip

- Breech position
- Female gender
- Positive family history or ethnic background (e.g., Native American)
- Lower limb deformity
- Torticollis
- Metatarsus adductus
- Oligohydramnios
- Significant persistent hip asymmetry (e.g., abducted hip on one side and adducted hip on the other side)
- Other significant musculoskeletal abnormalities

Clinical Presentation

Neonate

- DDH in a neonate is diagnosed by eliciting the Ortolani or the Barlow sign or from significant changes in the sonographic morphology of the hip.[2]
- Physical examination must be carried out with the infant unclothed and placed supine in a warm, comfortable setting on a flat examination table.

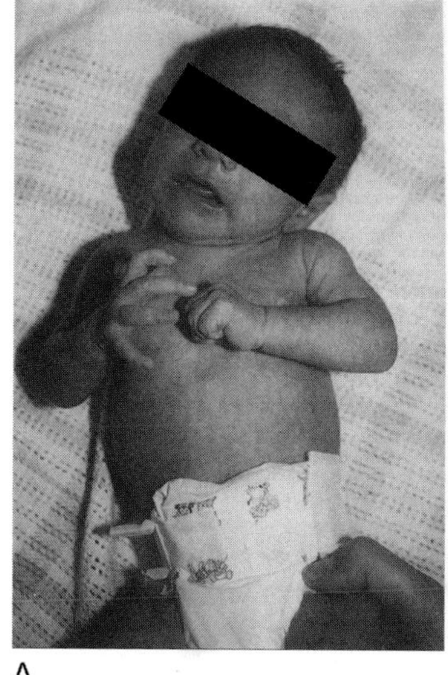
A

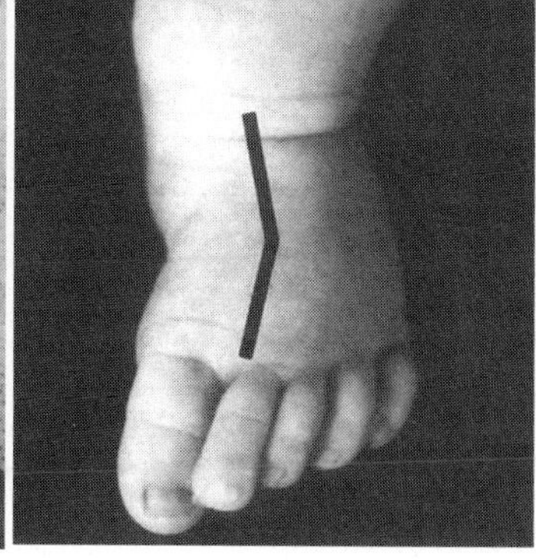
B

Figure 10–2: There is a high rate of association of DDH with other intrauterine molding abnormalities, such as torticollis (A) and metatarsus adductus (B).

- Both the Barlow and the Ortolani tests begin with the hips and knees flexed to 90 degrees.
  - The Barlow provocative maneuver assesses the potential for dislocation of a nondisplaced hip.
    1. The examiner adducts the flexed hip and gently pushes the thigh posteriorly in an effort to dislocate the femoral head (Figure 10–3).
    2. In a positive test, the examiner will feel the hip slide out of the acetabulum. As the examiner relaxes the proximal push, he or she will feel the hip slip back into the acetabulum.
  - The Ortolani test (*signo della scotto* in Italian, or "sign of the ridge") is the reverse of the Barlow test: the examiner attempts to reduce a dislocated hip (Figure 10–4).
    1. The examiner grasps the child's thigh between the thumb and index finger and, with the fourth and fifth fingers, lifts the greater trochanter while abducting the hip.
    2. When the test is positive, the femoral head will slip into the socket with a delicate "clunk" that is palpable but usually not audible. It should be a gentle, nonforced maneuver.
  - The examiner should repeat this sequence four or five times to be certain of the findings, alternating the Barlow test and the Ortolani test in a gentle arc of motion.

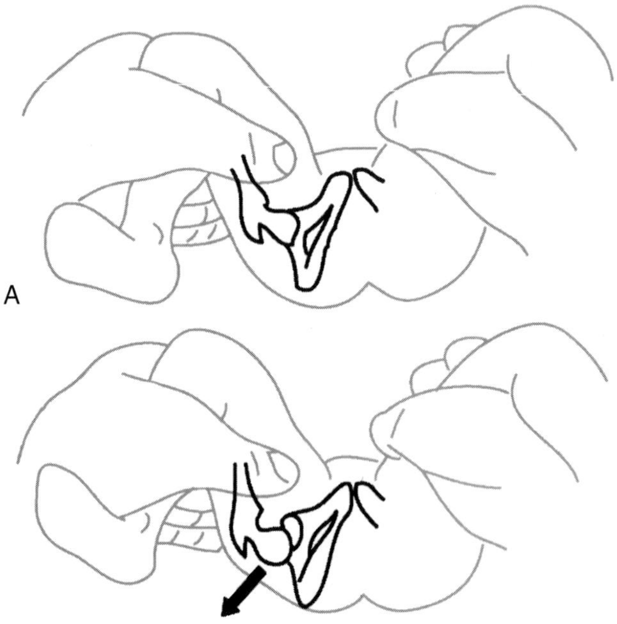

Figure 10–3: The Barlow test (provocative maneuver demonstrating dislocation of the hip) is performed with the patient's hips and knees flexed. A, Holding the patient's limbs gently, with the thigh in adduction, the examiner applies a posteriorly directed force. B, This test is positive in a dislocatable hip.

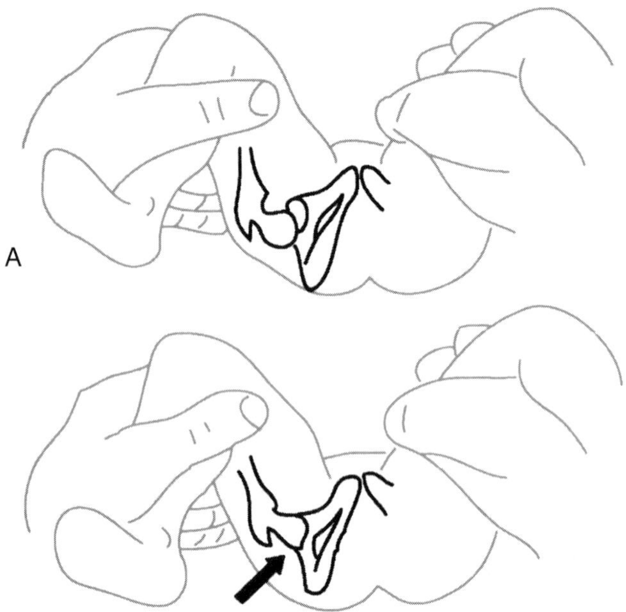

Figure 10–4: A, In the Ortolani maneuver (sign of the ridge ball of femoral head moving in and out of the acetabulum), the examiner holds the patient's thighs and gently abducts the hip while lifting the greater trochanter with two fingers. B, When the test is positive, the dislocated femoral head will fall back into the acetabulum with a palpable (but not audible) "clunk" as the hip is abducted.

- A *hip click* is the high-pitched sensation felt at the end of abduction during testing for DDH with the Barlow and the Ortolani maneuvers.
  - Classically, a hip click is differentiated from a *hip clunk,* which is heard and felt as the hip goes in and out of joint.[1]
  - Hip clicks usually originate in the ligamentum teres or occasionally in the fascia lata or psoas tendon. They do not indicate a significant hip abnormality.

Infant

- As a baby enters the second and third months of life, other signs of DDH appear.
- When the hip is no longer reducible, specific physical findings appear, including limited hip abduction, apparent shortening of the thigh, proximal location of the greater trochanter, asymmetry of the gluteal or thigh folds, and pistoning of the hip.[1]
  - Limitation of abduction is the most reliable sign of a dislocated hip[3] (Figure 10–5).
    1. A unilateral dislocation produces a visible reduction in abduction on the affected side compared with the normal side.
    2. Limited abduction is a clinical manifestation of the various degrees of adductor longus shortening associated with hip subluxation or dislocation.

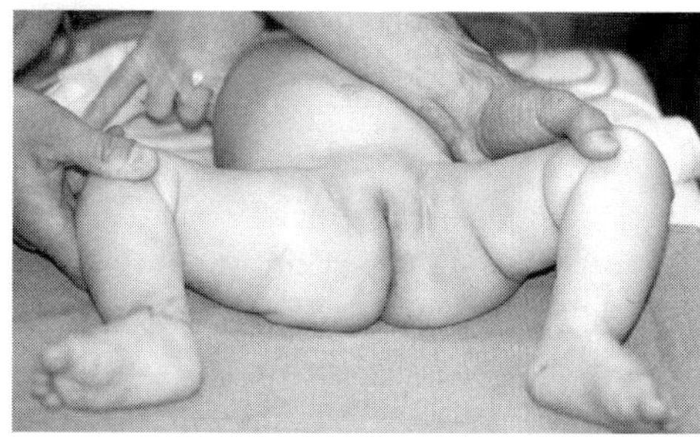

Figure 10–5: Decreased abduction of the left hip in an older child is indicative of left hip dislocation.

- Shortening of the thigh, the *Galeazzi sign,* is best appreciated by placing both hips in 90 degrees of flexion and comparing the height of the knees, looking for asymmetry (Figure 10–6).
- Asymmetry of thigh and gluteal skin folds may be present in 10% of normal infants but is suggestive of DDH (Figure 10–7). A short thigh with multiple skin folds on the medial thigh is consistent with proximal migration of the skeletal structures in a patient with a unilateral dislocated hip.
- The perineum on the side of the dislocation may be broadened because of the lateral displacement of the femoral head.

• Children with bilateral dislocation have no asymmetry on abduction and have flexed knees at the same level.
  - Combined abduction is limited, but this is difficult to detect because the limitation is symmetrical.
  - A helpful test is the *Klisic test* in which the examiner places the third finger over the greater trochanter and the index finger of the same hand on the anterior superior iliac spine (Figure 10–8).

    1. In a normal hip, an imaginary line drawn between the two fingers points to the umbilicus.

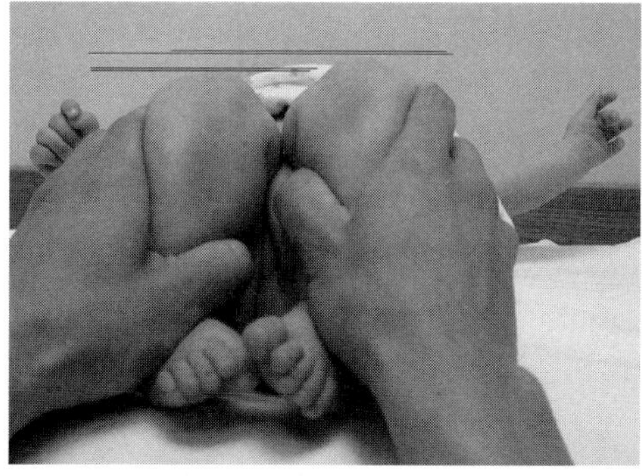

Figure 10–6: The Galeazzi test is performed with the patient's hips and knees flexed at right angles. **The patient must be placed supine on a flat, firm surface. An asymmetry in the apparent knee height indicates a difference in the length of the femur or a dislocation of one of the hips. The result would be negative for a patient with bilateral dislocation of the hips. A Galeazzi test performed on this patient shows that the right knee is lower than the left, indicating right hip dislocation. From Dormans JP, ed (2004) Pediatric Orthopaedics and Sports Medicine. Philadelphia: Mosby.**

    2. In the dislocated hip, the trochanter is elevated, and the line projects halfway between the umbilicus and the pubis.

Walking Child

• A walking child with previously undetected DDH often comes to the physician after the family has noticed a limp, a waddling gait, or a limb length discrepancy.[1]
  - The affected side appears shorter than the normal extremity, and the child will toe walk on the affected side.
  - The Trendelenburg sign is positive in these children, and a Trendelenburg gait is usually observed.

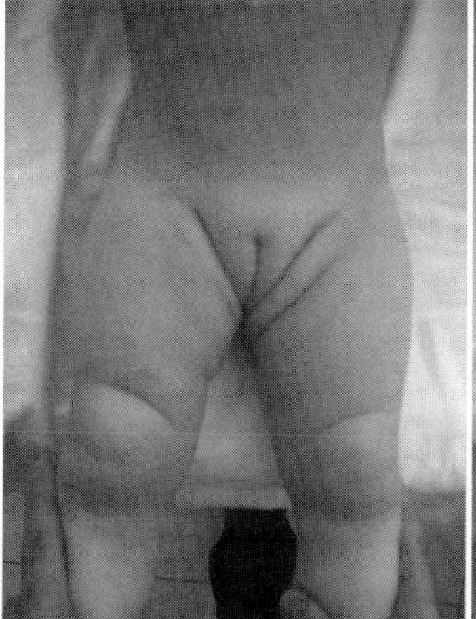

A

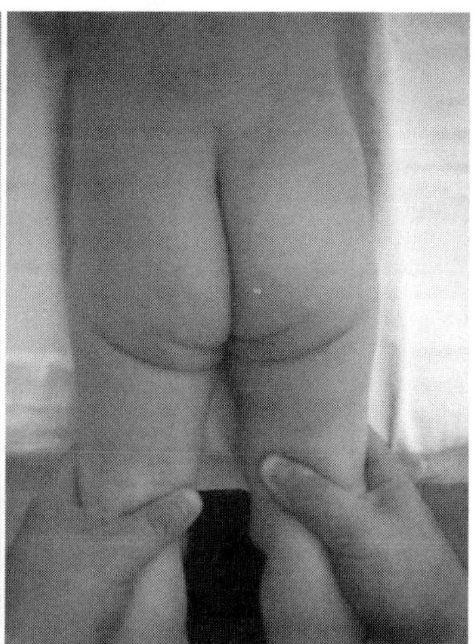

B

Figure 10–7: Asymmetrical skin folds suggest proximal migration of the underlying skeletal structures. **Note the difference in the proximal thigh folds anteriorly (A) and posteriorly (B).**

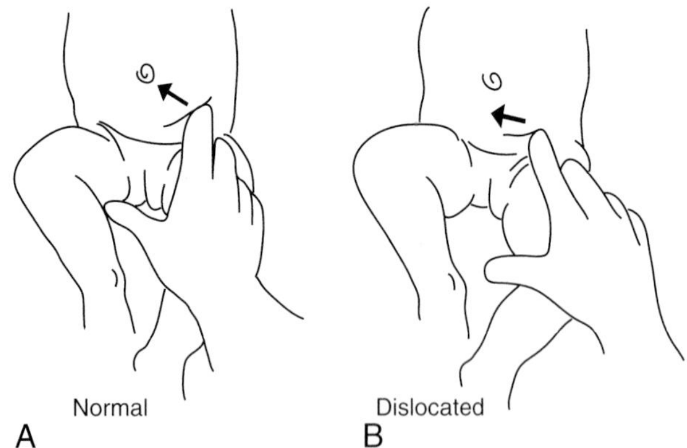

Figure 10–8: Klisic test. **A, In a normal hip, an imaginary line drawn through the tip of an index finger placed on the patient's iliac crest and the tip of the long finger placed on the patient's greater trochanter should point to the umbilicus. B, In a dislocated hip, the imaginary line drawn through the two fingertips runs below the umbilicus because the greater trochanter is abnormally high.**

- As in a younger child, there is limited abduction on the affected side and the knees are at different levels when the hips are flexed (the Galeazzi sign).
- Excessive lordosis, which develops secondary to hip flexion contracture, is common and is often the presenting complaint.
- In patients with bilateral dislocations, clinical findings include a waddling gait and hyperlordosis of the lumbar spine.

Radiographic Findings

Ultrasound

- In infants younger than 6 months, the acetabulum and proximal femur are predominantly cartilaginous and thus not visible on plain radiographs.
- In this age group, these structures are best visualized with ultrasound.
- In addition to morphological assessment, ultrasound provides dynamic assessment of the stability of the hip joint[1] (Figure 10–9).
- The morphological assessment, as pioneered by Graf, focuses primarily on critical evaluation of the anatomical characteristics of the hip joint.
  - This is accomplished by measuring two angles on the ultrasound image: the α angle, which is a measurement of the slope of the superior aspect of the bony acetabulum, and the β angle, which evaluates the cartilaginous component of the acetabulum.
  - The hip is classified into four types and several subtypes according to various factors.

    1. In their simplest form, type I hips are normal, type II hips are either immature or somewhat abnormal, type III hips are subluxated, and type IV hips are dislocated (Figure 10–10).
    2. Type I hips need no follow-up; type III and IV hips usually require treatment.
    3. Type II hips form the group in which the degree of abnormality and the need for treatment are less clear.

  - Some authors treat all type II hips with abduction devices; the others treat only those hips with clinical instability, regardless of ultrasound findings.
- The ultrasound examination can be used to monitor acetabular development, particularly of infants in Pavlik harness treatment; this method can minimize the number of radiographs taken and may allow the clinician to detect failure of treatment earlier.[1]
- The disadvantages of using ultrasonography are high cost, limited availability, and a paucity of expert ultrasonographers and qualified test interpreters. Moreover, the test may be limited by inadequate specificity and sensitivity, resulting in both overtreatment of benign conditions and failure to lower the incidence of late diagnosis.[2,3]

Radiography

- Radiographs are recommended for an infant once the proximal femoral epiphysis ossifies, usually between 4 and 6 months.
- In infants this age, the radiographic examination has proved more effective, less costly, and less operator dependent than ultrasound examination.[2]
- An anteroposterior view of the pelvis can be interpreted through several classic lines drawn on it (Figure 10–11).
  - *Hilgenreiner's line* is a horizontal line drawn through the top of the triradiate cartilage (the clear area in the depth of the acetabulum).
  - *Perkins's line,* a vertical line through the most lateral ossified margin of the roof of the acetabulum, is perpendicular to Hilgenreiner's line.
  - The ossific nucleus of the femoral head should be located in the medial lower quadrant of the intersection of these two lines.
  - *Shenton's line* is a curved line drawn from the medial aspect of the femoral neck to the lower border of the superior pubic ramus.

    1. In a child with normal hips, this line is a continuous contour.
    2. In a child with DDH, this line consists of two separate arcs and therefore is described as "broken" (Figures 10–11 and 10–12).

  - The *acetabular index* is the angle formed between Hilgenreiner's line and a line drawn from the depth of the acetabular socket to the most lateral ossified margin of the roof of the acetabulum. This angle measures the development of the osseous roof of the acetabulum. In a newborn, the acetabular index can be up to 40

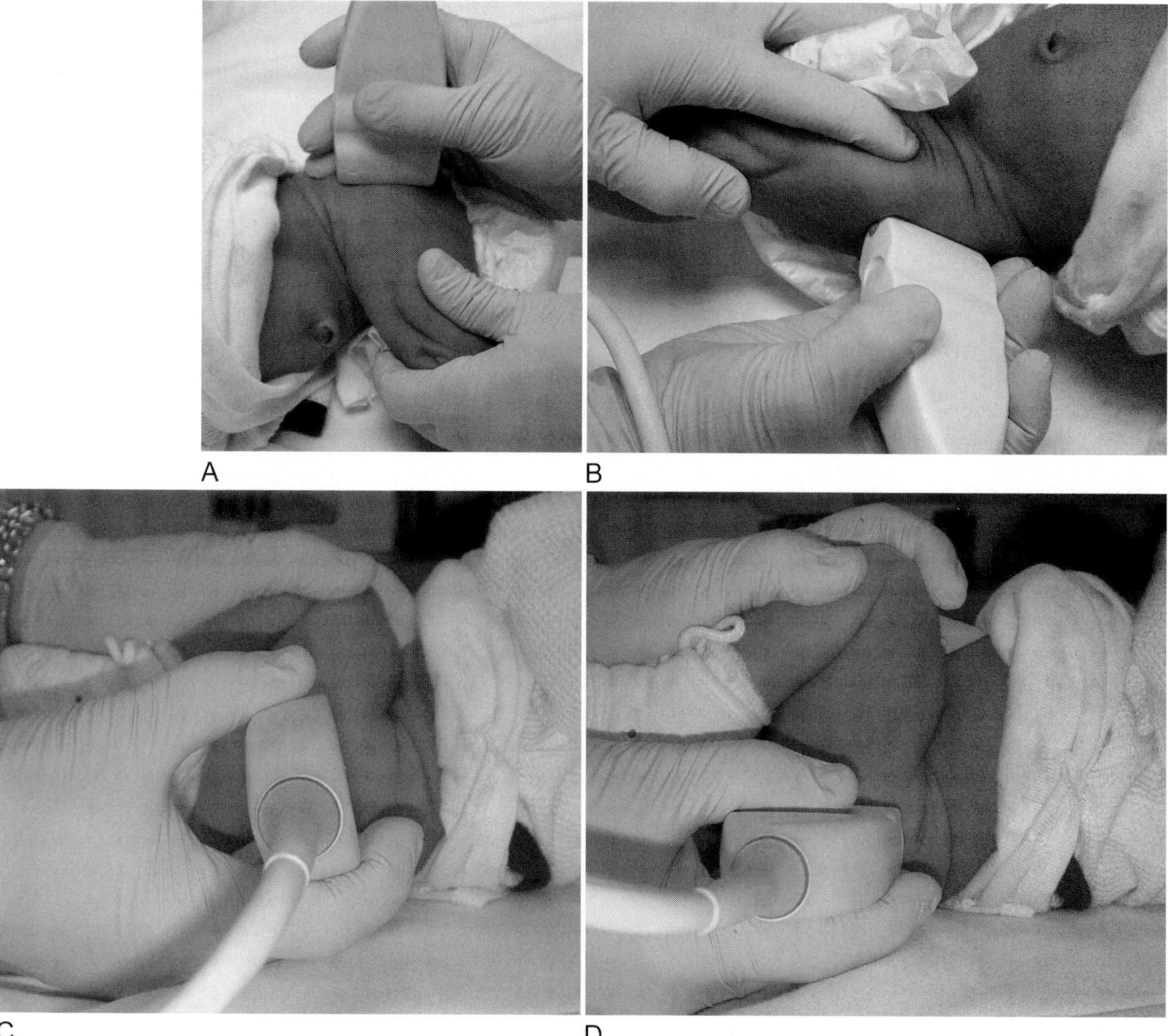

Figure 10–9: A-D, In a newborn child, an ultrasound examination by an experienced ultrasonographer is the most accurate method of detecting hip dysplasia. Ultrasound images can provide dynamic information when the ultrasonographer performs a Barlow test. The femoral head can be visualized sliding in and out of the acetabulum. From Dormans JP, ed (2004) Pediatric Orthopaedics and Sports Medicine. Philadelphia: Mosby.

degrees; by 4 months in a normal infant, it should be no more than 25 degrees (Figures 10–11 and 10–12).
  - In an older child, the *center–edge angle* is a useful measure of hip position. This angle is formed at the juncture of Perkins's line and a line connecting the lateral margin of the acetabulum to the center of the femoral head. In children 6 to 13 years old, an angle greater than 19 degrees has been reported as normal. In children at least 14 years old, an angle greater than 25 degrees is considered normal.
- Radiographs of the hip in abduction and internal rotation should also be obtained because these views show whether the hip is reducible.

Magnetic Resonance Imaging

- Magnetic resonance imaging (MRI) has been used for the diagnosis and evaluation of DDH and for the documentation of femoral head acetabular relationships after closed and open reduction.
- The need for anesthesia for pediatric patients limits the utility of this modality.

Screening Criteria

- All neonates should have a clinical examination for hip instability. Beyond that recommendation, there is lack of consensus about further screening criteria.

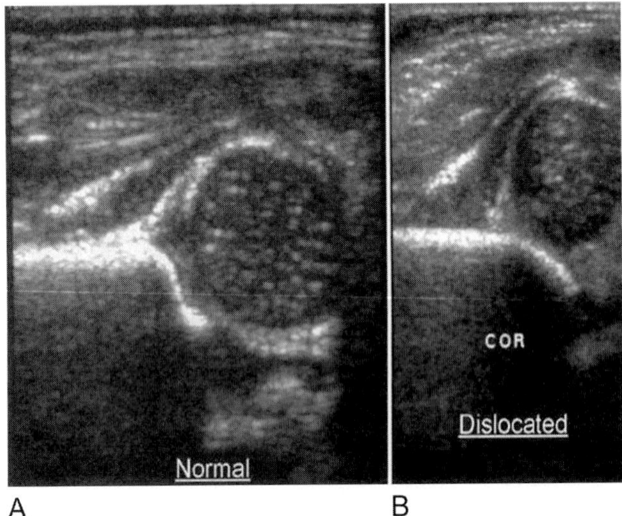

Figure 10–10: A, An ultrasound image in the coronal plane of a normal hip shows a femoral head well reduced in the acetabulum. B, A similar image from another patient shows the femoral head displaced proximally out of a shallow acetabulum.

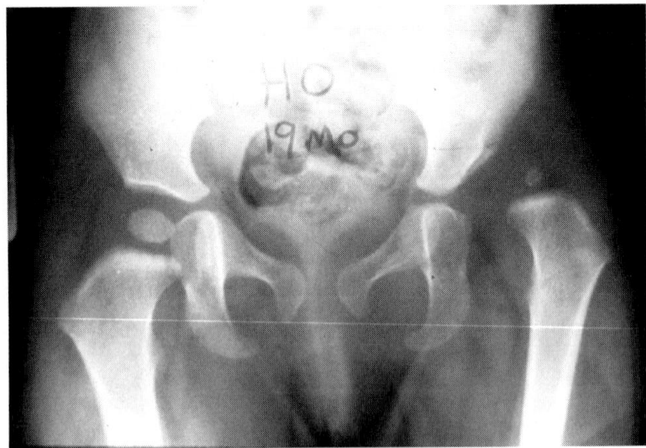

Figure 10–12: A 19-month-old child with developmental dysplasia of the left hip. Note that the ossific nucleus is displaced to lateral upper quadrant of the intersection of Hilgenreiner's and Perkins's lines. Shenton's line on the dysplastic left hip is broken. The acetabular index, which measures the slope of the ossified acetabular roof, is larger on the dysplastic side.

- Babies with risk factors associated with DDH (i.e., a positive family history, breech presentation, torticollis, metatarsus adductus, or oligohydramnios) should receive more careful screening, at least an examination by an experienced examiner, and possibly an ultrasound.[2]

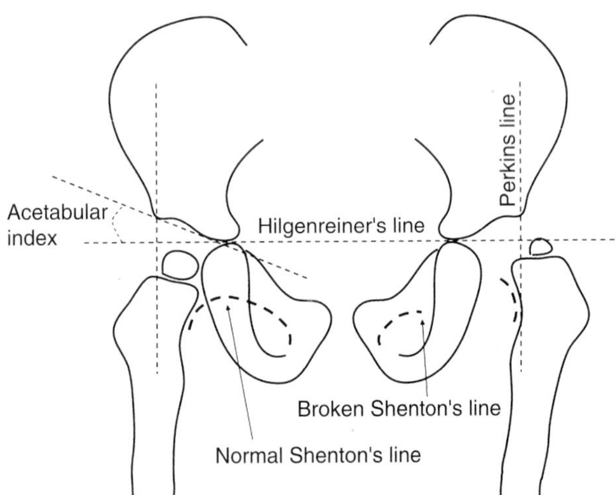

Figure 10–11: Radiographic measurements are useful in evaluating DDH. Hilgenreiner's line is drawn through the triradiate cartilages. Perkins's line is drawn perpendicular to Hilgenreiner's line at the lateral edge of the acetabulum. The ossific nucleus of the femoral head should be located in the medial lower quadrant of the intersection of these two lines. Shenton's line curves along the femoral metaphysis and connects smoothly to the inner margin of the pubis. In a child with DDH, this line consists of two separate arcs and therefore is described as broken. The acetabular index is the angle between a line drawn along the margin of the acetabulum and Hilgenreiner's line; in normal newborns, it averages 27.5 degrees and decreases with age.

- Screening with ultrasound remains controversial.
  - Some authors recommend ultrasound and clinical examination for all babies with risk factors.
  - Others, however, have found a low yield of significant abnormalities in the absence of clinical findings, even in hips at risk.

Natural History

- DDH is a progressive condition in which the hip structures fail to develop adequately. The spectrum of abnormalities involving the growing hip includes dysplasia, subluxation, or dislocation.[3]
  - The term *dysplasia* has an anatomical and radiographic definition.
    1. Anatomical dysplasia refers to inadequate development of the acetabulum, the femoral head, or both.
    2. Radiographic findings include increased obliquity and loss of concavity of the acetabulum with an intact Shenton's line.
  - The term *subluxation* is used when the femoral head is not in full contact with the acetabulum. In hip subluxation, Shenton's line is disrupted and the femoral head is superiorly, laterally, or superolaterally displaced from the medial wall of the acetabulum.
  - The term *dislocation* specifies that the femoral head is not in contact with the acetabulum.
  - Both subluxated and dislocated hips will have dysplastic changes.

- The natural history of hip subluxation is clear; degenerative joint disease will develop in all patients, usually in the third or fourth decade.[4]
- Although it is more difficult to predict the natural history of untreated dysplasia in adults, there is good evidence that dysplasia, particularly in females, leads to degenerative joint disease.[2]
- The natural history of untreated complete dislocations depends on two factors: bilaterality and development or lack of development of a false acetabulum.[4]
  - Patients with bilateral, untreated, high dislocations without a false acetabulum have a good range of motion and no pain. Hyperlordosis and low-back pain may develop over time.
  - If the completely dislocated femoral head articulates with the ilium and the patient has a false acetabulum, secondary degenerative arthritis will develop in the false acetabulum.
  - A patient with an untreated unilateral complete dislocation may have limb length inequality, ipsilateral valgus knee deformity, an abnormal gait, and postural scoliosis.

Treatment

- The goal in the management of DDH is to obtain and maintain a concentric reduction of the femoral head within the acetabulum to provide the optimal environment for the normal development of both the femoral head and the acetabulum.
  - The acetabulum has the potential for development for many years after reduction as long as the reduction is maintained.
  - The femoral head and femoral anteversion can remodel if the reduction maintained.
- The later the diagnosis of DDH, the more difficult it is to achieve these goals, the less potential there is for acetabular and proximal femoral remodeling, and the more complex the required treatments.

Newborns and Infants Younger than 6 Months

- The diagnosis of DDH ideally should be made in the newborn nursery.
- Triple diapers or abduction diapers have no place in the treatment of DDH in a newborn; they are usually ineffective and give the family a false sense of security.[3]
- The Pavlik harness is used for all degrees of hip dysplasia in otherwise normal newborns.[2,3] Although other braces are available (e.g., von Rosen splint and Frejka pillow), the Pavlik harness remains the most commonly used device worldwide.
- Infants between 1 and 6 months with hip dysplasia, subluxation, or dislocation also are readily managed with the Pavlik harness.
- Use of Pavlik harness is contraindicated when there is major muscle imbalance, as in myelomeningocele; major stiffness, as in arthrogryposis; or ligamentous laxity, as in Ehlers-Danlos syndrome.[5]
- The Pavlik harness consists of a chest strap, shoulder straps, and anterior and posterior stirrup straps that maintain the hips in flexion and abduction and restrict extension and adduction (Figure 10–13).
- This device does not rigidly immobilize the hips; therefore, it allows dynamic molding of the acetabulum by the cartilaginous femoral head
- By maintaining the Ortolani-positive hip in a Pavlik harness on a full-time basis for 6 weeks, hip instability resolves in 95% of cases.[2,3] After 6 months, the failure rate for the Pavlik harness is greater than 50% because it is difficult to maintain the increasingly active and crawling child in the harness.[3]
- Success of Pavlik harness treatment is likely if the patient is otherwise normal and the caregivers are both well educated about DDH and compliant with use of the harness.
- Frequent examinations and readjustments are necessary to ensure that the harness is applied correctly.
  - The patient is examined weekly, and reduction is evaluated by clinical and ultrasound examinations. With appropriate adjustment of the harness, hip stability usually is achieved 1 to 3 weeks after initiation of treatment.[5]
  - The harness should be continued about 6 weeks after stability is established.
  - When harness treatment is completed, some clinicians elect to place the child in an abduction splint for several months.
  - As the harness is discontinued, radiographs are obtained to assess hip reduction and acetabular development.

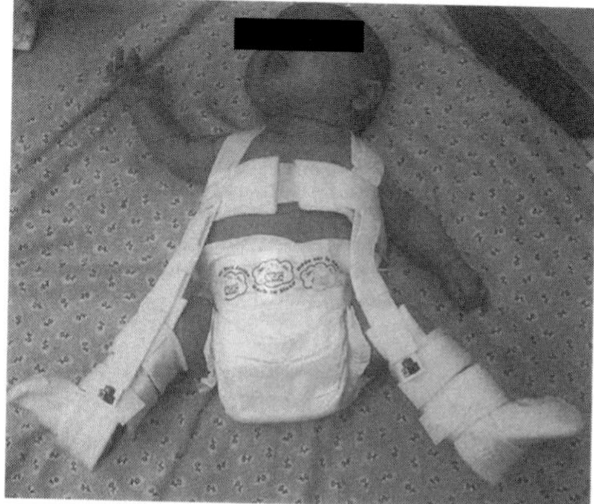

Figure 10–13: The Pavlik harness is applied to keep the hips flexed and abducted. Diaper changes can be performed without removing the device. Care must be taken to set the lengths of the straps properly and to check them regularly. Note that the child is free to move the hips and knees within the harness.

- If reduction is not obtained within 3 to 4 weeks, the harness should be discontinued and other treatment options should be considered.[2,3]
- Problems associated with the Pavlik harness include avascular necrosis (AVN) (because of excessive hip abduction), failure of hip reduction, and femoral nerve palsy (because of excessive hip flexion).[2]
  - The most common and sometimes most serious complication is AVN. This is usually secondary to forced abduction in the harness or cast or to persistent use of the harness despite the failure of guided reduction in a complete dislocation.
  - Inferior dislocations may occur with prolonged excessive hip flexion (>120 degrees).
  - Hyperflexion may also lead to femoral nerve palsy. Careful monitoring of the femoral nerve function (active quadriceps function) is essential.
  - Brachial plexus palsy may occur from compression by the shoulder straps, and knee subluxations may occur from improperly positioned straps.
  - Skin maceration may result when any immobilization device is not clean and dry at all times.

Children 6 Months to 2 Years

- The principle goals in the treatment of the late-diagnosed patient are to obtain and maintain reduction of the hip without damaging the femoral head.
- *Traction* followed by closed or open reduction is recommended by some for treatment of older infants with a dislocated hip for which attempted reduction with the Pavlik harness has failed or for children older than 9 months.[3,5]
  - This sequence of treatment may decrease muscular contracture and allows a safer, gentle closed reduction.
  - Generally, 2 to 3 weeks of skin traction, which can be performed at home with the proper setup, is sufficient.
- *Closed reductions* are performed in the operating room under general anesthesia (Figure 10–14).
  - The hip is gently manipulated into the acetabulum by flexion, traction, and abduction.
  - After a palpable reduction is felt, the hip is moved to determine the range of motion in which it remains reduced. This is compared with the maximum range of motion to construct a "safe zone"[6] (Figure 10–15). If the zone is relatively wide, the reduction is considered stable. On the other hand, if wide abduction or more than 10 to 15 degrees of internal rotation is required to maintain reduction, the reduction is considered unstable.
  - An open or percutaneous adductor tenotomy usually is necessary because of secondary adduction contracture and to increase the safe zone.
  - An arthrogram obtained at the time of reduction is helpful in evaluating the depth and stability of the reduction (Figure 10–14, *A*).
- The reduction is maintained in a well-molded plaster cast (Figure 10–14, *B*).
  - The "human position" of moderate flexion and abduction is the preferred position. Some internal rotation, no more than 10 to 15 degrees, may be used.
  - Wide, forced abduction or forced abduction with internal rotation should be avoided because these approaches are associated with an increased incidence of proximal femoral growth disturbance and AVN.[2]
  - The most experienced person should hold the hip in proper position while the cast is applied.
- After the cast is applied, an intraoperative radiograph is obtained (Figure 10–14, *C*). After the procedure, single-cut computerized tomography (CT), MRI, or ultrasound may be used to confirm the reduction.
- Twelve weeks after closed reduction, the plaster cast is removed and replaced by an abduction orthotic device to be used full time for 2 months until acetabular development is normal (Figure 10–16).
- Failure to obtain a stable hip with a closed reduction indicates the need for an *open reduction*. Failure may be evident at the time of the initial closed reduction, or it may become apparent if or when a hip redislocates in the cast.
- Open reduction has been described by Weinstein et al. as one of several medial approaches or from an anterior approach.[5]
  - Key steps during open reduction include removal of the ligamentum teres and the fibrofatty pulvinar with division of the transverse acetabular ligament and the iliopsoas tendon to allow the femoral head to seat deeply into the dysplastic, shallow acetabulum.
  - The most commonly used surgical approach is the *anterolateral* Smith-Petersen approach with a modified "bikini" incision.[2]

    1. This is a standard approach to the hip joint and is familiar to most surgeons.
    2. The anterior Smith-Petersen approach affords a good exposure and allows the surgeon to perform a capsulorrhaphy.
    3. If the surgeon thinks that a secondary procedure, such as pelvic osteotomy, is necessary, it can be accomplished through the same surgical approach.
    4. The disadvantages of anterior approach may include greater blood loss than with the various medial and anteromedial approaches, possible damage to the iliac crest apophysis and the hip abductors, and post-operative stiffness.
    5. If this approach is used in bilateral cases, the procedures usually are staged at 2- to 6-week intervals.

  - The various *medial* approaches have the advantage of approaching the hip joint directly over the site of the

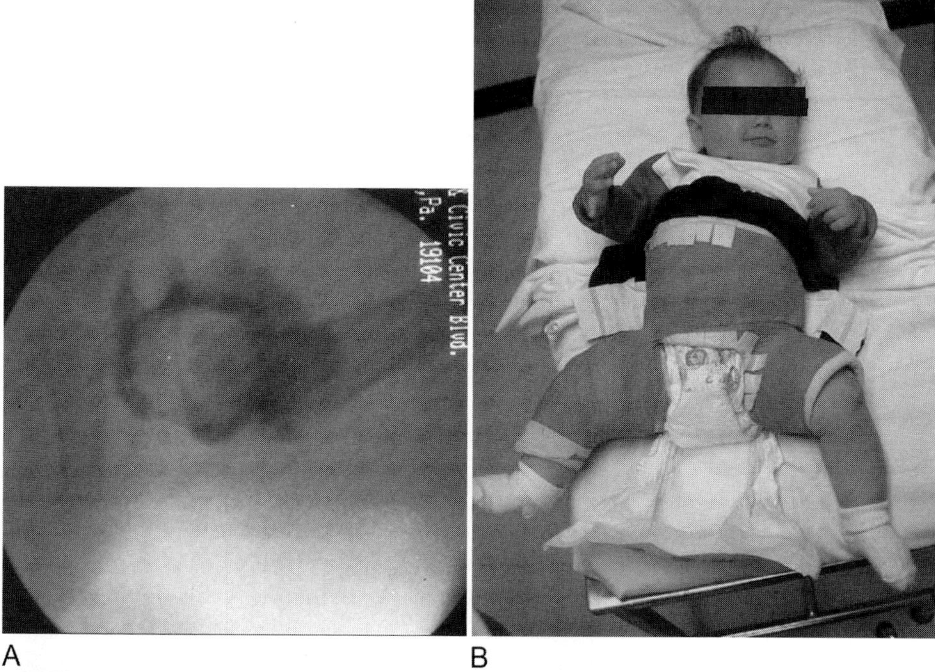

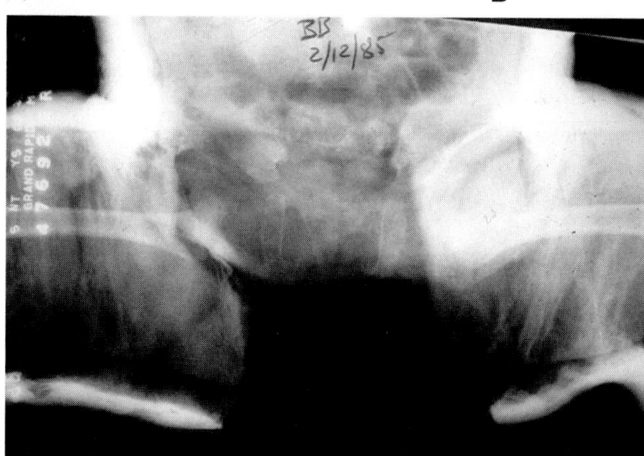

Figure 10–14: A and B, A spica cast is applied in the operating room after an examination of the hip under general anesthesia, an adductor tenotomy, a closed reduction, and an arthrogram. C, After closed reduction and application of the cast, a postreduction radiograph is taken. *B* from Dormans JP, ed (2004) Pediatric Orthopaedics and Sports Medicine. Philadelphia: Mosby.

obstacles to reduction. The disadvantages of the medial approach are a limited view of the hip, possible interruption of the medial femoral circumflex artery, and inability to perform a capsulorrhaphy.

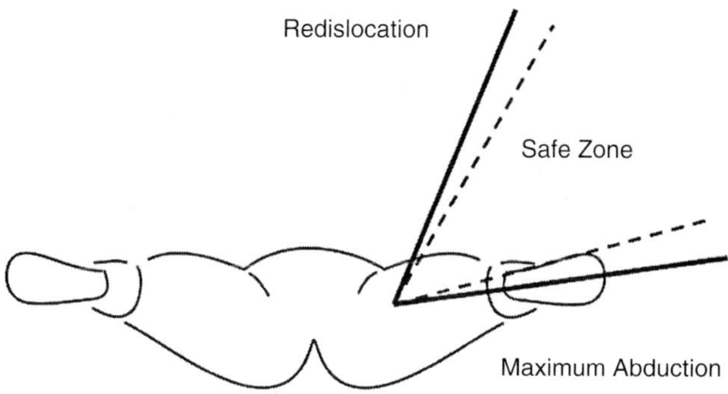

Figure 10–15: The safe zone of Ramsey.

- After the open reduction (performed with an anterior or medial approach), the child is placed in a spica cast for 12 weeks. Reduction should be confirmed by a radiograph intraoperatively and a single-section CT scan postoperatively.
- Some clinicians use abduction splinting for another 3 to 6 months depending on the development of the acetabulum; however, the need for further splinting remains controversial.

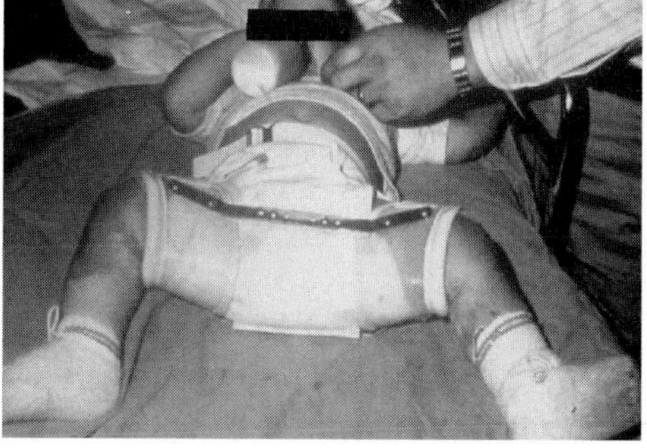

Figure 10–16: Abduction bracing. Once the spica cast is removed, the patient can be placed in an abduction brace to keep the hip in a stable position. From Dormans JP, ed (2004) Pediatric Orthopaedics and Sports Medicine. Philadelphia: Mosby.

- In patients younger than 2 years, a secondary acetabular or femoral procedure is rarely required.[2,3] The potential for acetabular development after closed or open reduction is excellent and continues 4 to 8 years after the procedure.

Children Older than 2 Years

- Treatment of children between 2 and 6 years with hip dislocation is more challenging.
- In a child older than 2 years, open reduction is usually necessary.
- Femoral shortening is an essential part of management in older children, and with higher dislocations, greater shortening is necessary.[2]
  - In children older than 3 years, femoral shortening to avoid excessive pressure on the proximal femur gives far lower rates of proximal femoral growth disturbance than preliminary traction followed by open reduction.
  - The age range of 2 to 3 years is considered a "gray zone," with some surgeons advocating preliminary traction before open reduction and others performing concomitant femoral shortening.
- For children between 2 and 3 years, because the potential for acetabular development is markedly diminished, a concomitant acetabular procedure is recommended with the open reduction.[3]
  - In this age range, the surgeon should evaluate the stability of the hip during the open reduction.

    1. If the acetabular coverage is insufficient, a pelvic osteotomy should be performed.
    2. If good stability is evident, acetabular development can be observed for the next few years.

- Children older than 3 years at reduction usually need an acetabular procedure to adequately cover the femoral head.[2,3]
- In this age group, the most common procedure accompanying open reduction is innominate osteotomy as described by Salter or by Pemberton.[2]
  - Salter innominate osteotomy redirects the entire acetabulum in an anterolateral direction and provides coverage of the femoral head by acetabular articular cartilage (Figure 10–17).
  - The Pemberton osteotomy repositions the acetabulum to improve anterior and lateral coverage of the femoral head.

Sequelae and Complications

Residual Acetabular Dysplasia

- Following reduction of a dislocated hip, the acetabulum begins to remodel in response to the pressure exerted by the femoral head. Many times, however, this process is incomplete, the acetabulum will remain shallow, and the roof will be inclined.
- If acetabular dysplasia persists 2 to 3 years after closed or open reduction and the patient has residual anteversion, proximal femoral varus–derotational osteotomy should be considered.[2]
- There is good evidence that if acetabular obliquity is still present at 5 years, after treatment of the dislocation, further acetabular development will be inadequate. If significant dysplasia persists through 5 years, a pelvic osteotomy should be performed to ensure adequate development of the hip.[2,3]

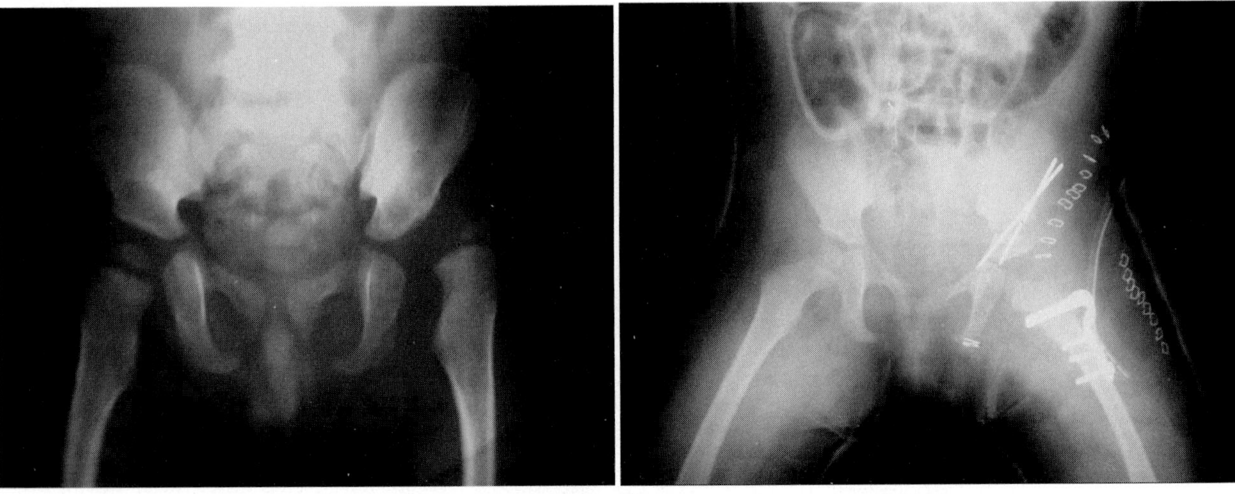

Figure 10–17: A and B, A 3-year-old child with dislocation of the left hip was treated by open reduction, Salter innominate pelvic osteotomy, and proximal femoral varus osteotomy. This child did not require femoral shortening.

Avascular Necrosis

- AVN is a major cause of long-term disability after the treatment of DDH.
- It is a problem directly associated with the treatment and is almost always preventable.
- AVN occurs when excessive pressure is applied for an extended period to the femoral head.
  - The most common cause is immobilization in a position that places excessive pressure on the femoral head, such as extreme abduction or internal rotation.[2]
  - AVN can be prevented by avoiding abnormal positions and by performing femoral shortening when reduction is too tight.
- AVN is diagnosed when the femoral head fails to ossify or to grow within 1 year after reduction.
- Some of the anatomical effects of AVN can be altered by appropriate intervention.[2] Procedures include trochanteric epiphysiodesis, trochanteric advancement, intertrochanteric double osteotomy, and lateral closing wedge valgus osteotomy with trochanteric advancement.
- The painful hip in the teenager with residual AVN and dysplasia may be caused by a torn labrum.[3] The diagnosis can be made using CT or MRI, and treatment may require open repair or excision.
- Early degenerative joint disease is another cause of hip pain.
  - It should be treated by the methods to correct residual subluxation and dysplasia.
  - Hip fusion or early total joint arthroplasty may be considered in severe cases.

Legg-Calve-Perthes Disease

- Legg-Calve-Perthes Disease (LCPD) is a femoral head disorder of unknown etiology.
- It involves temporary interruption of the blood supply to the bony nucleus of the proximal femoral epiphysis, impairing the epiphyseal growth and increasing bone density.
- The dense bone is subsequently replaced by new bone, flattening and enlarging the femoral head. Once new bone is in place, the femoral head slowly remodels until skeletal maturity.[2,3]

Etiology

- The etiology of LCPD remains unknown: infection, trauma, and transient synovitis have been proposed but unsubstantiated.
- Current theories center on disruption of blood flow to the capital femoral epiphysis (CFE).[3,7] Various factors have been proposed, including:
- An increase in blood viscosity.
- Disturbances in the clotting mechanism, and abnormal venous drainage of the femoral head and neck.
  - Factors leading to thrombophilia, an increased tendency to develop thrombosis and hypofibrinolysis, and a reduced tendency to lyse thrombi have been identified as disturbances in the clotting mechanism.
  - Factor V Leiden mutation, protein C and S deficiency, lupus anticoagulant, anticardiolipin antibodies, antitrypsin, and plasminogen activator may play a role in the abnormal clotting mechanism.
- A contrasting theory to disruption of the blood supply to the proximal femur is that the disorder may be a reflection of an underlying systemic disorder.[7]
  - Children with LCPD have delayed skeletal maturation and are shorter than normal.
  - Abnormalities of thyroid hormone and insulin-like growth factors have been reported.
- Other associated factors include hyperactivity or attention deficit disorder, hereditary influences, and environmental influences (including nutrition).
- Histological findings in the CFE reveal various stages of bone necrosis and repair.[3,7] Two possible pathways for the bone necrosis have been proposed: the vascular changes may be the primary event or events, or there may be a primary disorder of epiphyseal cartilage with collapse and necrosis as a result.

Pathogenesis of Deformity

- The deformity can occur by four mechanisms in LCPD.[7]
  - The first is a growth disturbance in the CFE and physis; a central arrest of the physis leads to a short neck (coxa breva) and trochanteric overgrowth, whereas a lateral physeal arrest tilts the head externally and into valgus with trochanteric overgrowth.
  - The second mechanism for deformity involves the repair process; the deformity can occur related to the asymmetrical repair process and the applied stresses on the femoral head.
  - The third mechanism for deformity is related to the disease process. The superficial layers of articular cartilage continue to "overgrow" as they are nourished by the synovial fluid. The deeper layers are, however, devitalized by the disease process, leading to epiphyseal trabecular collapse and deformity.
  - The fourth mechanism is iatrogenic and is caused by trying to contain, either nonsurgically or surgically, a noncontainable femoral head.

Patterns of Deformity

- Four patterns of residual deformity result from LCPD: coxa magna, premature physeal arrest patterns, irregular head formation, and osteochondritis dissecans.[3]
  - Coxa magna develops because of ossification of the hypertrophied articular cartilage and reactivation of the physeal plate along the femoral neck.

- Premature physeal plate closure generally leads to one of two patterns of arrest: central or lateral.
    1. In the central arrest pattern, the femoral neck is short and the epiphysis is relatively rounded. There is trochanteric overgrowth and mild acetabular deformity.
    2. In the lateral arrest pattern, the femoral head is tilted externally. There is trochanteric overgrowth and an oval epiphysis with corresponding acetabular deformity.

Epidemiology

- The overall incidence of LCPD in the United States is about 1 in 1200 children.[3]
- LCPD is more common in boys than in girls by a ratio of 4 or 5 to 1.
- The peak incidence of the disease is between 4 and 8 years; however, LCPD has been reported in patients from 2 to 12 years.
- Bilateral involvement may be seen in about 10% of the patients, but the heads are usually in different stages of collapse.

Clinical Presentation

- The most common presenting symptom is a painless limp for varying periods.
- Pain, if present, is usually activity related and may be localized in the groin or referred to the anteromedial thigh or knee region. Failure to recognize that thigh or knee pain in a child may be secondary to hip pathology and may further delay the diagnosis.
- Less commonly, the onset of the disease may be more acute and may be associated with a failure to ambulate.
- Parents often report that symptoms were initiated by a traumatic event.

Physical Examination

- An antalgic or Trendelenburg gait may be observed. Antalgic gait may be particularly prominent after strenuous activity at the end of the day.
- Hip motion, primarily internal rotation and abduction, is limited. Early in the course of the disease, the limited abduction is secondary to synovitis and muscle spasm in the adductor group; however, with time and the subsequent deformities that may develop, the limitation of abduction may become permanent.[3]
- A mild hip flexion contracture of 10 to 20 degrees may be present.
- Atrophy of the muscles of the thigh, calf, or buttock from disuse secondary to pain may be evident.
- There might be an apparent lower extremity length inequality because of an adduction contracture or from true shortening on the involved site because of CFE collapse.
- The classic portrait of a child with LCPD is a small, thin, extremely active child who is always running and jumping.[1]
- Laboratory studies generally are not helpful in LCPD, although they may be necessary to rule out other conditions.

Radiographic Findings

- Routine plain radiographs are the primary imaging tool for LCPD.
    - Anteroposterior and frog-leg lateral (Lauenstein) views are used to diagnose, stage, provide prognosis, follow the course of the disease, and assess results.
    - It is most important in following the course of the disease that all radiographs are viewed sequentially and compared with previous radiographs to assess the stage of the reparative process and to determine the constancy of the extent of epiphyseal involvement.
- Additional radiographic or imaging studies are rarely necessary but may be helpful in the initial assessment and follow-up of the condition.
- In the absence of changes on plain radiographs, particularly in the early stages of the disease, radionuclide bone scanning with technetium-99m may reveal the avascularity of the CFE.[7] Periodic technetium-99m bone scans have also been used for prognosis and to follow the course of the disease.
- MRI is sensitive in detecting infarction but cannot yet accurately portray the stages of healing. Its role in the management of LCPD has yet to be defined.
- Arthrography may demonstrate any flattening of the femoral head and the hinge abduction phenomenon with abduction of the leg.
    - Arthrography is most useful for assessing head shape and the relation to the acetabulum that would be necessary for treatment decisions; with severe flattening of the femoral head, it is useful in determining containability before any treatment, whether it will be Petrie casts, bracing, or surgery.[3]
    - Arthrography is also useful in determining the best position of containment, such as internal or external rotation and abduction or adduction, if surgical management is considered.

Radiographic Stages

- LCPD has been divided into four radiographic stages: initial, fragmentation, reossification (or repair), and residual (or healed) (Table 10–1).
    - In the initial stage, the radiographic changes include a decreased size of the ossification center, lateralization of the femoral head with widening of the medial joint space, a subchondral fracture, and physeal irregularity (Figures 10–18 and 10–19).
    - In the fragmentation stage, the epiphysis appears fragmented, and there are areas of increased radiolucency and radiodensity (Figure 10–20).

Table 10–1: Radiographic Stages of Legg-Calve-Perthes Disease

STAGE	FINDINGS
Initial (osteonecrosis)	*Early signs*—Lateralization of the femoral head and smaller ossific nucleus *Later signs*—Subchondral fracture, increased density of the femoral head, and metaphyseal lucencies
Fragmentation	Lucent areas appear in the femoral head Segments of femoral head are demarcated Increased density resolves Acetabular contour is more irregular
Reossification (healing)	New bone formation occurs in the femoral head Lucencies are replaced by new (woven) bone
Residual	Femoral head is fully reossified Gradual remodeling of the head shape occurs until skeletal maturity Acetabulum remodels

- During the reossification stage, the bone density returns to normal by new (woven) bone formation.
- The residual stage is marked by the reossification of the femoral head, gradual remodeling of head shape until skeletal maturity, and remodeling of the acetabulum (Figure 10–21).

Classification Systems

- *Catterall* (1971) proposed a four-group classification, based on the amount of CFE involvement and a set of radiographic head-at-risk signs, with a high degree of interobserver variability.[8]
  - Catterall group I hips have anterior CFE involvement of 25%, no sequestrum, and no metaphyseal abnormalities.
  - Catterall II hips have up to 50% involvement with a clear demarcation between involved and uninvolved segments. Metaphyseal cysts may be present.
  - Catterall III hips display up to 75% involvement with a large sequestrum.
  - In Catterall IV, the entire femoral head is involved.
- *Salter and Thompson* (1984) reported a two-group classification based on the extent of the subchondral fracture, which corresponded to the amount of subsequent resorption.[9]
  - In Salter-Thompson A, less than half of the femoral head is involved (Catterall I and II); in Salter-Thompson B, more than half of the femoral head is involved (Catterall III and IV).
  - The major determining factor between Salter-Thompson A and Salter-Thompson B is the presence or absence of a viable lateral column of the epiphysis. This intact lateral column (i.e., Catterall II, Salter-Thompson group A) may shield the epiphysis from collapse and subsequent deformity.
  - A disadvantage of the Salter-Thompson classification is that not all patients are diagnosed early during the phase of the subchondral fracture. However, this classification has good interobserver reliability.
- The *Herring* (1992) lateral pillar classification is the newest and the most widely used radiographic classification

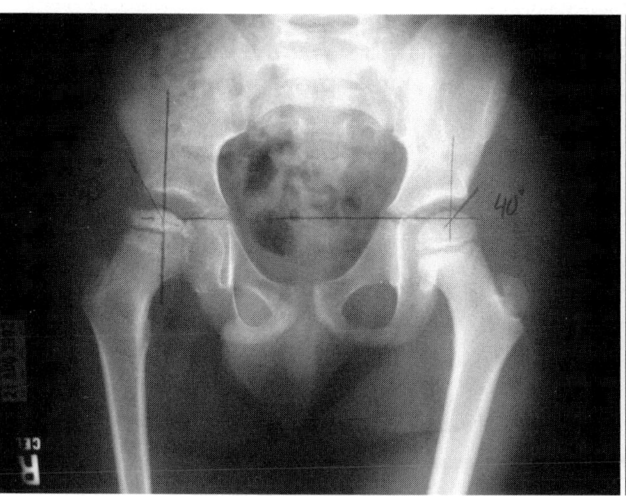

A

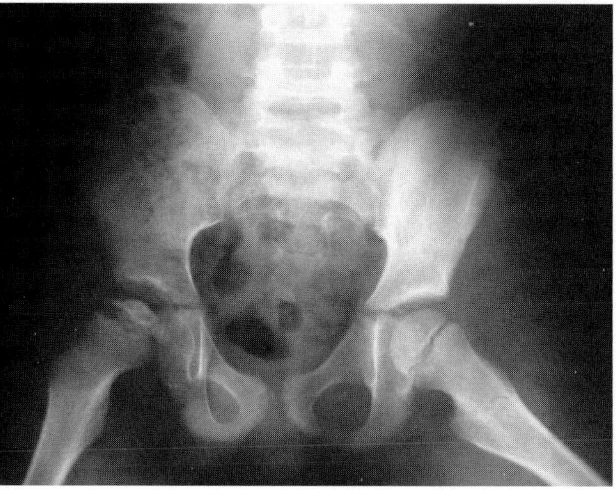

B

Figure 10–18: Anteroposterior (A) and frog-leg lateral (B) radiographs of a child with LCPD of the right hip. Note the lateralization of the femoral head and smaller ossific nucleus, which are the early signs of the initial phase. From Dormans JP, ed (2004) Pediatric Orthopaedics and Sports Medicine. Philadelphia: Mosby.

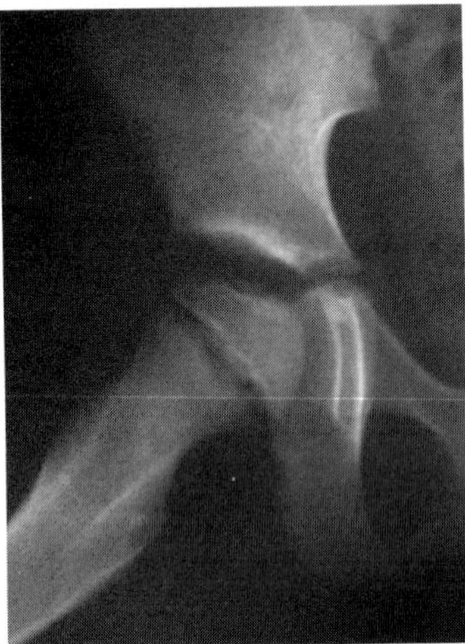

Figure 10–19: An 8-year-old boy with LCPD of the right hip. The frog-leg lateral view demonstrates subchondral fracture and increased density of the femoral head, which are the later signs of the initial phase.

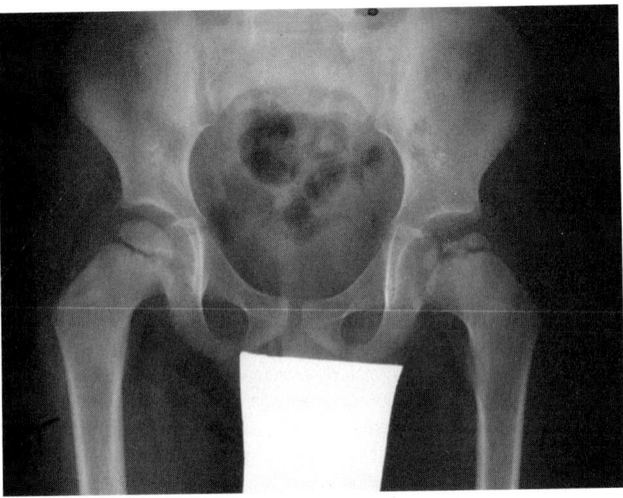

Figure 10–20: Anteroposterior radiograph of the pelvis shows epiphyseal fragmentation in the left hip, characteristic of the fragmentation phase of LCPD. From Dormans JP, ed (2004) Pediatric Orthopaedics and Sports Medicine. Philadelphia: Mosby.

system for helping to determine treatment and prognosis during the active stage of the disease (Table 10–2).[10]

- Classification is based on several radiographs taken during the early fragmentation stage. The radiograph with the greatest involvement of the lateral pillar is used for classification.
- The lateral pillar classification system for LCPD evaluates the shape of the femoral head epiphysis on anteroposterior radiograph of the hip.
  1. The head is divided into three sections or pillars. The lateral pillar occupies the lateral 15 to 30% of the head width, the central pillar about 50% of the head width, and the medial pillar 20 to 35% of the head width.
  2. The degree of involvement of the lateral pillar can be subdivided into three groups. In group A, the lateral pillar is radiographically normal. In group B, the lateral pillar has some lucency but greater than 50% of the lateral pillar height is maintained. In group C, the lateral pillar is more lucent than in group B and less than 50% of the pillar height remains (Figure 10–22).

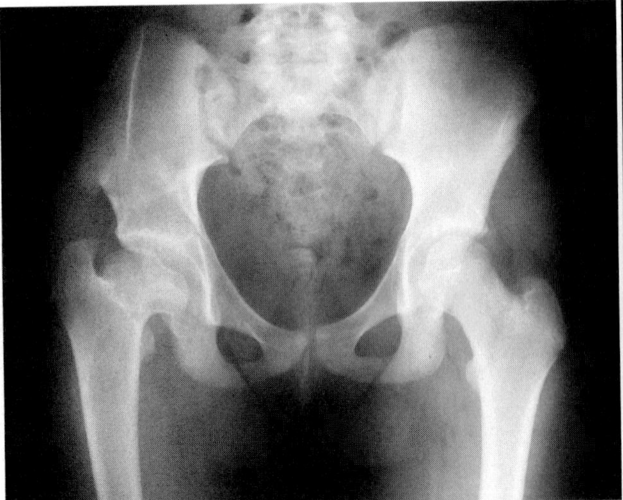

A

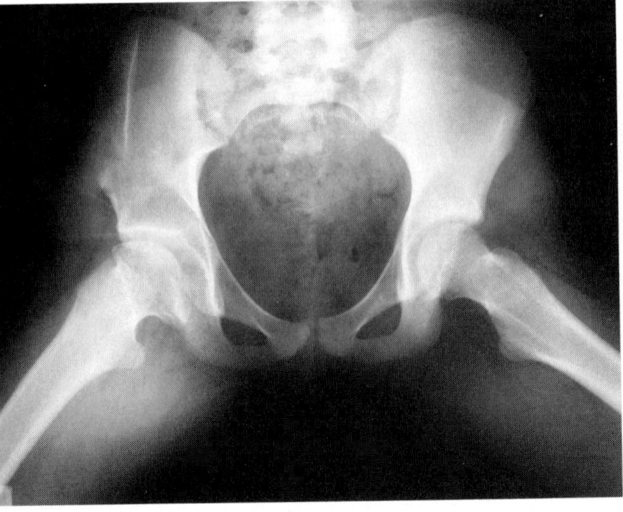

B

Figure 10–21: Anteroposterior (A) and frog-leg lateral (B) radiographs showing long-term follow-up of a 12-year-old girl with LCPD of the right hip, 5 years after an acetabular realignment procedure. Though the right hip is deformed, the patient is active and asymptomatic. From Dormans JP, ed (2004) Pediatric Orthopaedics and Sports Medicine. Philadelphia: Mosby.

Table 10–2: Lateral Pillar Classification

GROUP	FEATURES
A	No involvement of the lateral pillar; lateral pillar is radiographically normal Possible lucency and collapse in the central and medial pillars, but full height of the lateral pillar is maintained
B	Greater than 50% of the lateral pillar height is maintained Lateral pillar has some radiolucency with bone density maintained between 50 and 100% of the original height of the lateral head
C	Less than 50% of lateral pillar height is maintained Lateral pillar becomes more radiolucent than in type B, and any preserved bone is less than 50% of the original height of the lateral pillar

From Herring JA, Neustadt JB, Williams JJ, Early JS, Browne RH (1992) The lateral pillar classification of Legg-Calve-Perthes disease. J Pediatr Orthop 12(2): 143-150.

This classification has been found easy to apply during the active stage of the disease and has a correlation in predicting the amount of flattening of the femoral head at skeletal maturity.

When combined with age at onset, it can be used to predict the natural history of the disease.

1. Hips classified as group A had spherical femoral heads at skeletal maturity.
2. Outcomes for children with group B hips were better for those younger than 9 at the onset of disease.
3. In group C, most femoral heads became aspherical at skeletal maturity.[2]

Prognostic Factors

- Catterall identified certain radiographic signs, known as *at-risk signs,* associated with poor results (Box 10–3).[8]
- Radiographic at-risk signs include the following:
  - Gage sign—A radiolucency in the lateral epiphysis and metaphysis
  - Calcification lateral to the epiphysis
  - Lateral CFE subluxation
  - A horizontal physis

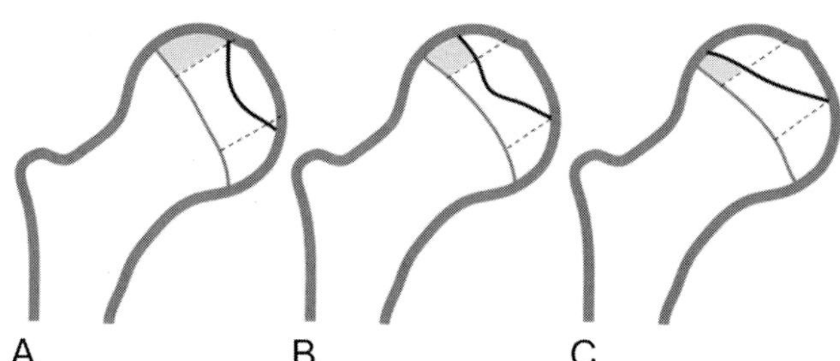

Figure 10–22: Lateral pillar classification for LCPD. **A, In group A, there is no involvement of the lateral pillar. B, In group B, more than 50% of the lateral pillar height is maintained. C, In group C, less than 50% of the lateral pillar height is maintained.**

Box 10–3 Catterall's Radiographic At-Risk Signs

- Gage sign—Radiolucency in the lateral epiphysis and metaphysis
- Calcification lateral to the epiphysis
- Lateral CFE subluxation
- Horizontal physis

- Gage sign and calcification are indicative of early ossification in the enlarged epiphysis. They are present only when the head is deformed. These signs are present when the changes are reversible with treatment.
- The value or accuracy of these head-at-risk signs remains controversial.

Classification of Radiographic Results

- Once the patient is skeletally mature, the shape of the femoral head can be measured by two radiographic techniques.
- *Mose* used a radiolucent template, with concentric circles placed over the femoral head on anteroposterior and lateral radiographs, and measured the sphericity.[11] A good result was one in which the femoral head sphericity did not deviate more than 1 mm, a fair result was within 2 mm, and a poor result was 3 mm or more of deviation.
- *Stulberg* and associates developed a system that correlates radiographic appearance of the femoral head and acetabulum in the healed stage of the disease to the long-term risk for degenerative arthritis (Table 10–3).[12] This classification has five classes.
  - Classes I and II are spherically congruent and have a good long-term prognosis (i.e., Mose's good and fair results).
  - Classes III and IV are aspherically congruent and have an intermediate prognosis (i.e., Mose's poor results).
  - Class V hips are aspherically incongruent and are destined to early degenerative joint disease.
  - This classification method has been shown to have poor interrater and intrarater reliability.

Differential Diagnosis

- The patient history, physical examination, and plain radiographs are usually sufficient to make a diagnosis of LCPD.
- Diagnosis early in the initial phase of the disease must be differentiated from conditions such as septic arthritis, whether primary or secondary to proximal femoral osteomyelitis, and toxic synovitis[1,3] (Box 10–4).
  - A complete blood count, including white cell differential, erythrocyte sedimentation rate, C-reactive protein, hip joint aspiration, and analysis of the fluid, may be necessary to rule out infection.
  - All laboratory studies of LCPD generally are normal, although the erythrocyte sedimentation rate may be slightly elevated.

Table 10–3: Stulberg Classification

CLASS	RADIOGRAPHIC FEATURES	CONGRUENCY	LONG-TERM PROGNOSIS
I	Normal hip	Spherical	Good
II	Spherical femoral head Same concentric circle on anteroposterior and frog-leg lateral views but with one or more of the following: coxa magna, shorter-than-normal neck, or abnormally steep acetabulum	Spherical	Good
III	Ovoid, mushroom-shaped (but not flat) head, coxa magna, shorter-than-normal neck, and abnormally steep acetabulum	Aspherical congruent	Intermediate
IV	Flat femoral head and abnormalities of the head, neck, and acetabulum	Aspherical congruent	Intermediate
V	Flat head and normal neck and acetabulum	Aspherical incongruent	Early osteoarthritis

From Stulberg SD, Cooperman DR, Wallansten R (1981) The natural history of Legg-Calve-Perthes disease. J Bone Joint Surg Am 63(7): 1095-1108.

- The differential diagnosis of LCPD includes conditions that can produce osteonecrosis, such as hemoglobinopathies, leukemia, lymphoma, idiopathic thrombocytopenic purpura, or hemophilia.
- In bilateral symmetrical cases, a skeletal dysplasia, such as multiple or spondyloepiphyseal dysplasia, or endocrinopathies, such as hypothyroidism, should be considered (see Chapters 14 and 15). Patients with bilateral involvement, particularly those with atypical radiographic features, must have obtained a careful family history, measurements of height and weight, and a bone survey to rule out a skeletal dysplasia or a metabolic condition.
- Some genetic syndromes, such as trichorhinophalangeal syndrome, may have LCPD-like changes.

Natural History and Prognosis

- No long-term natural history studies of LCPD have been published.

Box 10–4 Differential Diagnosis of Legg-Calve-Perthes Disease

- Inflammatory or infectious diseases
  - Toxic synovitis
  - Septic arthritis
  - Juvenile arthritis
- Other known causes of osteonecrosis
  - Sickle cell anemia
  - Thalassemia
  - Hemophilia
  - Idiopathic thrombocytopenic purpura
  - Leukemia
  - Gaucher's disease
- In bilateral symmetrical cases
  - Skeletal dysplasias (e.g., multiple or spondyloepiphyseal dysplasia)
  - Endocrinopathies (e.g., hypothyroidism)
  - Genetic syndromes (e.g., trichorhinophalangeal syndrome)

  - Catterall reported on 95 untreated patients with a mean short-term follow-up of 6 years.[8] In this study, 92% of Catterall I and II hips had a good result, whereas 91% of Catterall III and IV hips had a poor result.
  - McAndrew and Weinstein presented the results of 32 untreated patients with a mean long-term follow-up of 48 years.[13] Of these patients, 40% had an Iowa hip rating of greater than 80 points (92% of the same patients had Iowa hip ratings above 80 points at an average follow-up of 36 years), 40% had undergone an arthroplasty, and 10% were awaiting an arthroplasty.
- From a prognostic standpoint, long-term follow-up studies of patients with LCPD show that most hips do well until the fifth decade of life. Most of the patients are active and pain free, and they maintain a good range of motion.
- The deformity and congruency at maturity and the age at onset are main prognostic factors for LCPD.[2,3,7]
  - Children who develop signs and symptoms before 5 years tend to recover without residual problems.
  - Patients older than 9 years at presentation usually have a poor prognosis.
  - The remodeling potential is higher in younger children; the shape of the femoral head can improve significantly until maturity.
- The extent of CFE involvement and the duration of the disease process are additional factors associated with poor prognosis. Hips classified as Catterall III and IV, Salter-Thompson B, and lateral pillar group C are at risk for a poor prognosis.

Treatment

- The goal of treatment in LCPD is to create a spherical, well-covered femoral head with hip range of motion that is normal or close to normal.
- The two main principles of treatment are (1) maintenance of range of motion and (2) acetabular

containment of the femoral head during the active period of the process.
- The methods of treatment include observation or no treatment, intermittent symptomatic treatment, containment, late surgery for deformity, and late surgery for osteoarthritis.[7]

Nonoperative Treatment

- Abduction devices have been used to keep the femoral head contained in the acetabulum.
  - Most abduction orthoses are based on the Petrie abduction cast principle (Figure 10–23).
  - The most widely used abduction arthrosis is the Atlanta Scottish Rite orthosis or a modification thereof.[7] These devices were thought to provide for containment solely by abduction without fixed internal rotation. For the Scottish Rite orthosis to function satisfactorily, the affected hip must be able to be abducted in extension to between 40 and 45 degrees.
  - Abduction orthosis may be used while the patient either is bearing weight or is restricted from bearing weight. Weight-bearing abduction orthoses are not effective in changing the natural history of severely involved hips.
  - The use of the orthosis is continued until subchondral reossification is demonstrated on the anteroposterior radiograph. Generally, the active phase of the disease that requires an orthosis is 9 to 18 months.
- The two primary means of treating pain are bed rest and traction.
- A traction apparatus can be set up in the home.
- Nonsteroidal anti-inflammatory drugs and crutches (to reduce the need to bear weight) may also be helpful in minimizing pain.
- Once the patient is comfortable, physical therapy, with an emphasis on maintaining range of motion, is a crucial element of LCPD management.
- An alternative nonoperative treatment option is activity restriction without the use of braces or casts. The clinician follows the patient regularly and watches for any clinical or radiographic changes.

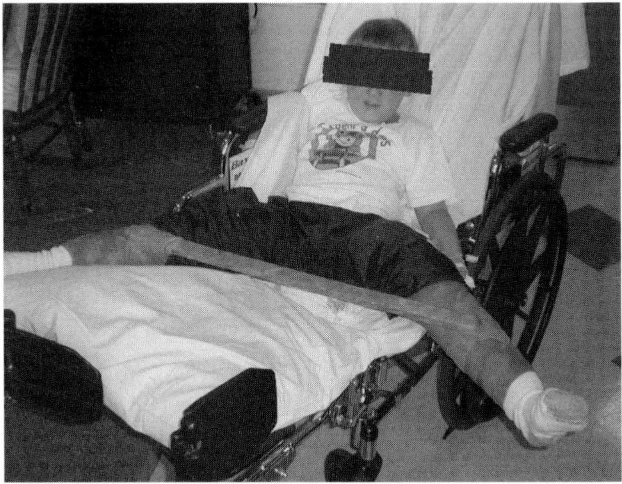

A

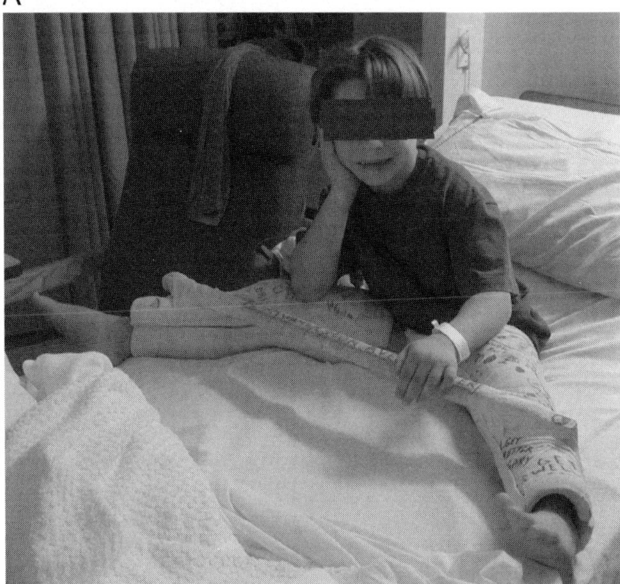

B

Figure 10–23: A and B, A Petrie cast consists of two cylinder casts connected by an abduction bar to maintain hip abduction. After the initial phase of treatment, the cylinder casts can be bivalved (split longitudinally) to serve as removable braces that the patient wears only in bed. From Dormans JP, ed (2004) Pediatric Orthopaedics and Sports Medicine. Philadelphia: Mosby.

Operative Treatment

- Surgical containment may be approached from the femoral side, the acetabular side, or both sides of the hip joint.
- *Proximal femoral osteotomy* has been widely used in the surgical treatment of LCPD.
- A *varus osteotomy* of the proximal femur is the most common proximal femoral procedure. This procedure is an effective method of containment in the early and fragmentation stages of the disease process. It can prevent femoral head deformity and restore spherical congruity, provided that the femoral head can be contained in the acetabulum and that growth remains to allow femoral head remodeling.
- Proximal femoral varus osteotomy has some advantages.[7]
  - Prerequisites for proximal femoral varus osteotomy are not as strict as the pelvic osteotomy; it can be performed when there is flattening or incongruity of the femoral head and when mild to moderate limitation of motion is present.

- The procedure is done on the affected side of the hip joint.
- It is said to decrease the venous congestion of the femoral head and neck.

• The potential disadvantage of proximal femoral varus osteotomy is that failure of remodeling may result in persistent varus angulation, trochanteric prominence, and lower extremity length inequality.[3] These are more likely to occur in older children with excessive varus angulation.
• Three prerequisites for successful containment by proximal femoral osteotomy are as follows:
  - The child must be in the early or fragmentation stage of disease.
  - A fair to good presurgical range of hip motion is required.
  - Containment must be possible without hinge abduction.
• The neck–shaft angle (the angle formed between the line of the femoral neck and the femoral shaft on the anteroposterior view) must be reduced enough to contain the femoral head without creating excessive varus. This angle should not be reduced below 105 degrees.
• Several types of internal fixation have been successful for maintaining alignment. The 90-degree fixed-angle blade plate allows medial displacement of the distal fragment more easily than other devices.
• Derotation at the time of surgery is not recommended. With an isolated femoral osteotomy, derotation will affect only the position of the distal fragment in a manner similar to a fracture reduced with the distal fragment externally rotated. This can lead to an external rotation gait without achieving additional containment of the femoral head.[7]
• *Hinge abduction* occurs in later stages of LCPD when the extruded, deformed femoral head impinges on the lateral margin of the acetabulum during abduction of the hip. This prevents containment and causes the medial surface of the femoral head to pull from the medial wall of the acetabulum during attempted abduction.
  - Clinical symptoms include increasing pain, limp, and restriction of movement during the fragmentation or resorption stages.
  - Arthrography under general anesthesia can confirm the presence of hinge abduction.
  - The presence of hinge abduction indicates a poor prognosis unless treatment is initiated. In the early stages of hinge abduction, it may be possible to restore motion and contain the femoral head as long as the disease process is still in the fragmentation stage and there is potential for remodeling.

    1. In these stages, the child may benefit from preliminary traction, adductor tenotomy, iliopsoas recession, and medial capsulotomy to reduce the femoral head into the acetabulum.
    2. The femoral head is then maintained in the acetabulum by Petrie casts for 2 to 4 months followed by surgical procedures, such as proximal femoral varus osteotomy, Salter osteotomy, or both.

  - When the hinge abduction is fixed, the options are a shelf acetabuloplasty, Chiari osteotomy, or proximal femoral valgus extension osteotomy.
• *Pelvic osteotomies* in LCPD are divided into three categories: acetabular rotational osteotomies, shelf procedures, and medial displacement or Chiari osteotomies.
• Any of these procedures can be combined with a proximal femoral varus osteotomy when severe deformity of the femoral head cannot be contained by a pelvic or proximal femoral varus osteotomy alone.[2,3,7]
• The *Salter acetabular rotational osteotomy* is the most commonly performed osteotomy.
  - The Salter innominate osteotomy and the other rotational osteotomies are designed to gain anterior and lateral coverage of the femoral head by acetabular rotation.
  - Prerequisites for this procedure include restoration of a full range of motion, a round or almost round femoral head, and joint congruency demonstrated arthrographically.
  - The disadvantage of Salter innominate osteotomy is that the procedure is performed on the normal side of the joint.
  - Satisfactory anatomical results from this procedure range from 69 to 94%.[7]
• *Shelf arthroplasty* is a common method of treatment of LCPD.
  - This procedure provides a congruous extension of the acetabulum by bone grafting the anterolateral, lateral, and posterolateral aspects of the acetabulum and prevents subluxation and lateral overgrowth of the epiphysis.
  - Shelf arthroplasty can be used as a primary method of management in children older than 8 years with Catterall II-IV disease with or without at-risk signs, lateral pillar groups B and C disease, and Salter-Thompson B disease; if subluxation is present, it must be reducible on a dynamic arthrogram.
• *Medial displacement osteotomy,* also known as *Chiari osteotomy,* is an extra-articular domed osteotomy at the capsular attachment of the acetabulum along the anterolateral, lateral, and posterolateral margins. It is done primarily for salvage of a deformed femoral head.
  - Chiari osteotomy increases the volume of the acetabulum to contain an enlarged, deformed femoral head.
  - Significant remodeling of the femoral head can be anticipated with growth.
• No long-term results of the Chiari osteotomy in LCPD have been published.

- The *combined procedures* usually are a Salter osteotomy and a proximal femoral varus derotation osteotomy.
- The combined procedures have the theoretical advantage of maximizing femoral head containment and avoiding the complications of either procedure alone.
  - The femoral osteotomy directs the femoral head into the acetabulum, theoretically reducing any increasing joint pressure or stiffness that would result from pelvic osteotomy.
  - The coverage provided by the innominate osteotomy reduces the degree of correction needed from the femoral osteotomy, thereby minimizing the complications of excessive neck–shaft varus, associated abductor weakness (Trendelenburg gait), and limb shortening.
- The disadvantages of this combined procedure include those mentioned for varus osteotomy and innominate osteotomy alone.
- Satisfactory anatomical results from this combined procedure are reported in up to 78% of patients.[2,7]
- Patients in the later stages (reossification) of the disease who have deformity, those with noncontainable deformities, and those who have lost containment, after either surgical or nonsurgical containment, present a management problem.
- These patients have an extremely poor prognosis without additional treatment.
- The salvage procedures to be considered include Chiari osteotomy, lateral shelf arthroplasty, cheilectomy, and abduction extension osteotomy.

Slipped Capital Femoral Epiphysis

- Slipped capital femoral epiphysis (SCFE) is a well-known hip disorder that affects adolescents, most often between 12 and 15 years, and involves the displacement of the CFE from the metaphysis through the zone of hypertrophy layer of the physeal plate.
- The term *slipped capital femoral epiphysis* is a misnomer because the femoral head is held in the acetabulum by the ligamentum teres; thus, the femoral neck comes upward and outward and the head remains in the acetabulum.

Classification

- SCFE may be classified temporally, according to onset of symptoms (acute, chronic, or acute on chronic); functionally, according to patient's ability to bear weight (stable or unstable); or morphologically, as the extent of displacement of the femoral epiphysis relative to the neck (mild, moderate, or severe), as estimated by measurement on radiographic or CT images.
- An *acute SCFE* has been characterized as one occurring in a patient with prodromal symptoms for 3 weeks or less.
  - The children with an acute slip usually have a sudden, severe, fracture-like pain in the upper thigh after trauma.
  - Radiographs demonstrate little or no femoral neck remodeling changes typical of chronic SCFE.
  - An acute SCFE should be distinguished from a purely traumatic separation of the epiphysis in a previously normal hip, that is, a true Salter-Harris I fracture.[2]

    1. The patient with an acute slip will usually have some prodromal pain in the groin, thigh, or knee and will usually report a relatively minor injury (a twist or fall), which normally is not sufficiently violent to produce an acute fracture of this severity.
    2. A true type I epiphyseal fracture, on the other hand, occurs in an otherwise completely normal patient without prodromal symptoms, is usually the result of severe trauma, is often associated with concomitant traumatic hip dislocation, and has an extremely high rate of subsequent osteonecrosis of the capital epiphysis.

- Osteonecrosis is a significant and frequent complication of acute SCFE, with a reported incidence of 17 to 47%.[2,3]
- *Chronic SCFE* is the most frequent form of presentation.
  - Typically, an adolescent has a history of a few months of vague groin, upper thigh, or lower thigh pain and a limp.
  - Radiographs show a variable amount of posterior migration of the femoral epiphysis and remodeling of the femoral neck in the same direction; the upper end of the femur develops a "bending of the neck."
- The children with *acute-on-chronic SCFE* may have features of both ends of the spectrum.
  - Prodromal symptoms have been present for more than 3 weeks with a sudden exacerbation of pain.
  - Radiographs demonstrate femoral neck remodeling and further displacement of the capital epiphysis beyond the remodeling point of the femoral neck.
- The stability classification separates patients based on their ability to ambulate. This classification has proved more useful in predicting prognosis and establishing a treatment plan.
  - The SCFE is considered "stable" when the child is able to walk with or without crutches.
  - A child with an "unstable" SCFE is unable to walk with or without crutches.
  - Patients with unstable SCFEs have a much higher prevalence of AVN (up to 50%) compared with those with stable SCFEs (nearly 0%).[14] This is most likely because of the vascular injury caused at the time of initial displacement.

- SCFE may also be categorized by the degree of displacement of the CFE on the femoral neck.
  - Southwick recommended measuring the femoral head–shaft angle on anteroposterior or frog-leg lateral views[15] (Figure 10–24).
    1. The head–shaft angle difference is less than 30 degrees in mild slips, between 30 and 60 degrees in moderate slips, and more than 60 degrees in severe slips compared with the normal contralateral side.
    2. When the contralateral hip is affected or not assessed, the femoral head–shaft angle of the affected hip is calculated from normal values for this angle: 145 degrees on anteroposterior view and 10 degrees posterior on the frog-leg lateral view.
  - Some authors, because of the three-dimensional nature of the deformity, recommended measuring the head–shaft and head–neck angles from either true lateral radiographs or from specifically positioned, modified lateral radiographs (Billing's or Dunlap's technique).[2]
  - The head–neck angle can be determined most accurately and reproducibly on CT scans of the head and neck, but this method is not routinely employed because most patients do not undergo CT to assess the deformity or to facilitate management.

Etiology

- The etiology of SCFE is unclear.
- Several hypotheses, mechanical and endocrine, have been proposed, but it is likely that true etiology is a combination of factors.
- Mechanical factors created by relative or true femoral neck retroversion; orientation of the capital epiphysis and the physis on the femoral neck; and alteration of the mechanical strength of the physis, periosteum, and perichondral ring during adolescence have all been conjectured to play a role in the etiology of SCFE.[1,3]
  - A decrease in normal femoral anteversion, a retroversion of the femoral neck, or a more oblique orientation of the physeal plate during adolescence have all been associated with increased shear force generation at the proximal femoral physeal plate and could be factors associated with physeal plate fatigue. Obese children often have retroverted femoral necks directed more posteriorly than those of other children.
  - The physeal perichondral ring, which functions as a stabilizer of the physeal plate, decreases in strength during the growth years. Physiological forces at the proximal femur generated by normal activities in obese patients can be of adequate magnitude to cause physeal fatigue if the perichondral ring is adequately weakened.
- An endocrinological etiology for SCFE has been suspected, based on the common association of this condition with obesity and, at least in boys, with hypogonadal features. The condition most frequently manifests during the adolescent growth spurt, which would suggest such an etiology.[3]
- Additional evidence for an association with endocrine dysfunction is suggested by the frequent association of SCFE with primary and secondary hypothyroidism,

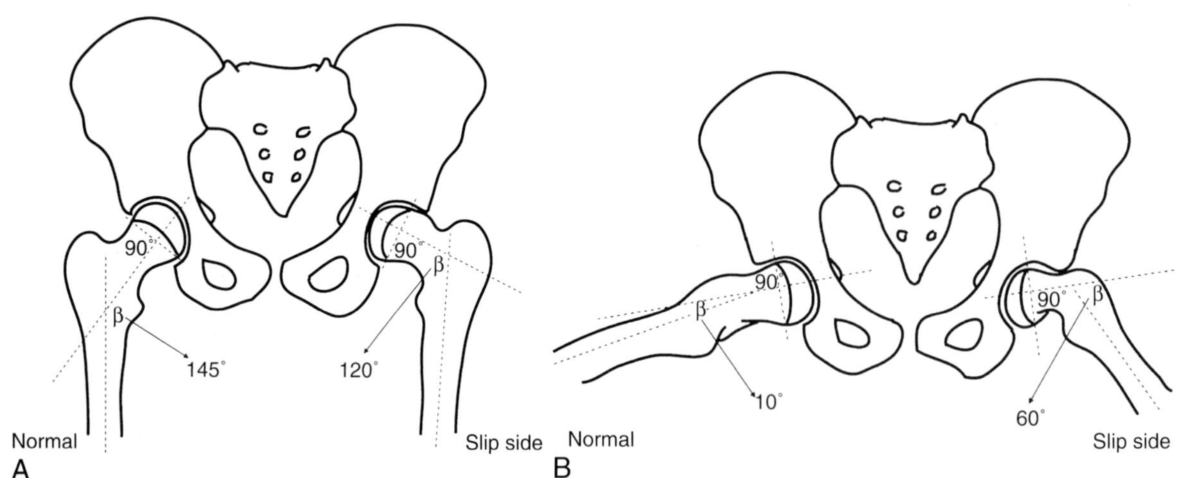

Figure 10–24: Southwick method of measuring the head–shaft angle to assess the severity of SCFE. A, Lines are drawn corresponding to the axis of the femoral shaft and the base of the CFE. The head–shaft angle is the angle between the axis line of the femoral shaft and the perpendicular line to the base of the epiphysis. Normally this angle is 145 degrees. B, Similar lines may be drawn on the frog-leg lateral radiographs. Mild slips have less than 30 degrees of displacement, moderate slips have 30 to 60 degrees of displacement, and severe slips have more than 60 degrees of displacement compared with the contralateral normal side.

panhypopituitarism, hypogonadal conditions, renal osteodystrophy, and growth hormone therapy (Box 10–5). During puberty, growth hormone increases the physiological activity of the physis, leading to rapid longitudinal growth of the physis and a widened and weakened proximal femoral growth plate.

Epidemiology

- The annual incidence of SCFE has been reported to average 2 per 100,000 in the general population. Globally, incidence has ranged from 0.2 per 100,000 in eastern Japan to 10.08 per 100,000 in the northeastern United States.[16]
- The African-American and Polynesian populations have been reported to have an increased incidence of SCFE.
- Obesity is the most closely associated factor in the development of SCFE; about two thirds of the patients are over the 90th percentile in weight-for-age profiles.[1]
- There is a definite predilection for males to be affected more often than females and for the left hip to be affected more often than the right. These predilections appear to be decreasing in studies.
- SCFE is related to puberty, as evidenced by 78% of cases occurring during the adolescent growth phase. The age range at presentation in boys is most often between 10 and 16 years (an average of 13.5 years), and in girls it is between 9 and 15 years (an average of 12.1 years).[2,3]
- A delay in skeletal maturation commonly seen in patients with SCFE; skeletal age has been found to be as much as 20 months behind chronological age in up to 70% of affected individuals.
- Seasonal variation in the presentation of patients with SCFE has been identified to some extent; an increased frequency in onset of symptoms in summer has been reported in some studies.
- Bilaterality has been reported in as many as 60% of cases; in nearly half of these, it may be present at the initial presentation.[1]
  - Involvement is usually not symmetrical.
  - A high degree of clinical suspicion should be maintained not only at the initial presentation but throughout the follow-up period.
  - Younger patients are particularly at risk for developing a slip on the contralateral hip because more time will elapse before closure of the proximal femoral physis.[17]

Box 10–5 Systemic Abnormalities Associated with Slipped Capital Femoral Epiphysis

- Hypothyroidism
- Hyperthyroidism
- Hypogonadism
- Panhypopituitarism
- Rickets or renal osteodystrophy
- Radiation exposure

Clinical Presentation

- Patients with SCFE usually have complaints of pain in the affected hip or groin, a change in hip range of motion, and a gait abnormality. Infrequently the patient will complain only of medial knee pain, which may be referred to the knee through the obturator and femoral nerves.
- The symptoms and physical findings vary according to whether the symptoms are chronic, acute-on-chronic, or acute; whether the slip is stable or unstable; with the severity of the resultant deformity; and with the coexistence of the complications of osteonecrosis or chondrolysis.
- In *stable, chronic SCFE,* the patient describes intermittent pain in the groin, the medial thigh, or the anterior suprapatellar region of the knee.
  - The pain is typically described as dull and vague and is exacerbated by physical activity such as running or sports.
  - The onset of pain may last several weeks or months.
  - The patient remains ambulatory but shows an antalgic gait with an associated limp.
  - The affected limb positions itself in an externally rotated and mildly shortened arrangement (Figure 10–25).
  - Thigh atrophy may be present in unilateral cases secondary to longstanding symptoms and disuse.
  - Physical examination of the affected hip reveals a restriction of internal rotation, abduction, and flexion.
    1. The amount of limitation depends on the severity of slip.
    2. Mild to moderate pain is noted with motion of the hip, particularly at the extremes of motion.
  - Commonly, the examiner will note that as the affected hip is flexed the thigh tends to rotate into progressively external rotation and that flexion is limited (Figure 10–26).
  - The presence of hip flexion contracture should alert the physician to the possibility of chondrolysis.
- Patients with either unstable acute or acute-on-chronic SCFE will characteristically report the sudden onset of severe, fracture-like pain in the affected hip region, usually as the result of a relatively minor fall or twisting injury.
  - The *acute-on-chronic* presentation is associated with an acute increase in severity from a previous, milder, chronically displaced pattern.
  - The *acute form* manifests by the sudden onset of severe pain and hip dysfunction in a patient who was previously asymptomatic.
  - Physical examination demonstrates that the affected limb is externally rotated and shortened with the patient refusing to bear weight.
  - Severe pain will result from any movement of the limb.

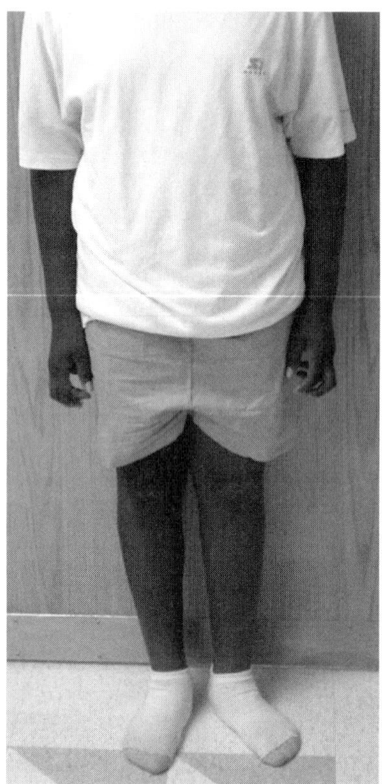

Figure 10–25: This 13-year-old boy with SCFE has the typical body habitus. Note the lateral rotation of the affected left lower extremity. From Dormans JP, ed (2004) Pediatric Orthopaedics and Sports Medicine. Philadelphia: Mosby.

- Patients with chondrolysis complicating SCFE will tend to have a history of more continuous pain and greater interference with daily activities because of the loss of hip range of motion.
- Because approximately 25% of patients will have evidence of contralateral slip on initial presentation, the contralateral hip must always be carefully assessed both clinically and radiographically by the treating physician.

Radiographic Findings

Radiographs

- Plain radiography in anteroposterior and lateral views is the primary and often the only imaging study needed to evaluate SCFE.
- Common radiographic findings include the following:
  - Widening and irregularity of the physis
  - A decrease in epiphyseal height in the center of the acetabulum
  - A crescent-shaped area of increased density in the proximal portion of the femoral neck, with the "blanch sign of Steel" corresponding to the double density created from the anteriorly displaced femoral neck overlying the femoral head
- In an unaffected patient, *Klein's line*—a straight line drawn along the superior cortex of the femoral neck on anteroposterior radiograph—intersects the lateral capital

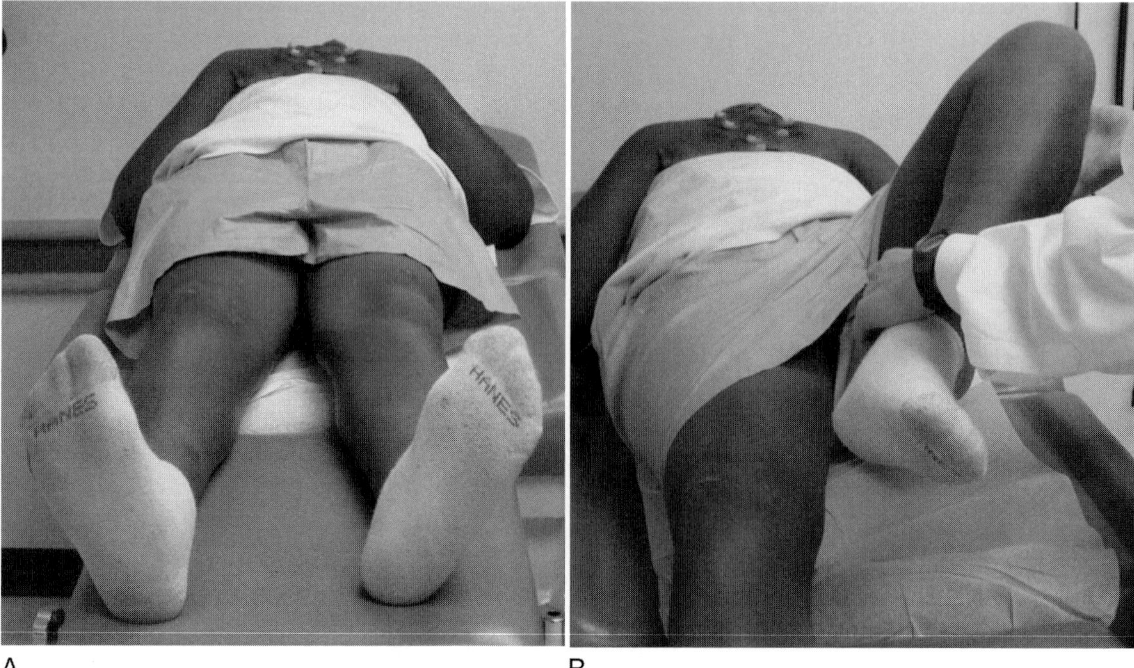

Figure 10–26: Physical examination of a patient with SCFE. A, Note the lateral rotation of the affected limb when the patient is lying supine. B, Passive hip flexion results in obligatory lateral rotation of the hip because of the distorted morphology of the proximal femur in this disorder. From Dormans JP, ed (2004) Pediatric Orthopaedics and Sports Medicine. Philadelphia: Mosby.

epiphysis. As progressive displacement of the epiphysis occurs in SCFE, the amount of Klein's line that intersects the epiphysis decreases, compared with the uninvolved hip, and eventually the line fully misses intersection with the proximal femoral epiphysis (Figures 10–27 and 10–28, *A*).

- A true lateral (cross-table lateral) radiographic view of the hip better defines the extent of posterior displacement of the femoral epiphysis. This view may help to diagnose minimal slips because it better elucidates the posterior displacement.
- The frog-leg lateral view usually demonstrates the posterior displacement and step-off of the epiphysis on the femoral neck (Figure 10–28).
  - This view has several advantages:
    1. It is easily obtained by having the patient flex and abduct the hips.
    2. Soft tissue obscuring of the bony image is minimized.
    3. Both hips can be visualized on one film.
  - The frog-leg lateral view should be avoided in the acute (unstable) presentation because of the potential of increasing the physeal displacement during positioning for the radiography.
- When the slip is acute, little or no remodeling of the femoral neck will be apparent on radiographs.
- When the slip has been present for some time, allowing for some remodeling of the femoral neck, this remodeling will appear as a bending of the femoral neck in the direction of the "slipping" CFE.[1,2]

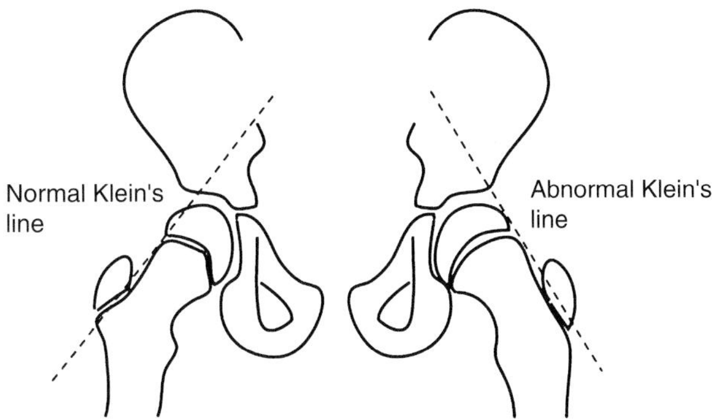

Figure 10–27: Klein's line, drawn along the superior cortex of the femoral neck on the anteroposterior view of the pelvis, normally intersects the lateral capital epiphysis. When typical posterior displacement of the capital epiphysis has occurred, this line will intersect a smaller portion of the epiphysis or will not intersect it.

Computerized Tomography and Technetium-99m Bone Scan

- CT scan can be used to confirm epiphyseal displacement and accurately measure the amount of displacement in patients with symptoms suggestive of a SCFE but without documentation on plain radiographs.
- CT can also be helpful in demonstrating whether penetration of the hip joint by fixation devices has occurred.
- Another indication for CT is to confirm closure of the proximal femoral physis, which can be difficult by plain radiography.

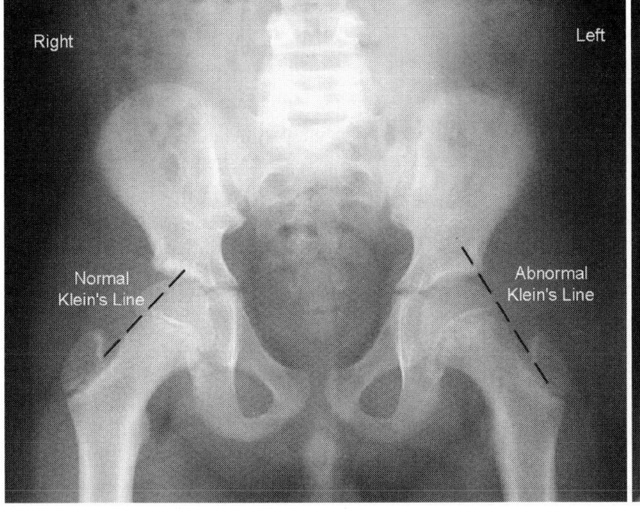

A

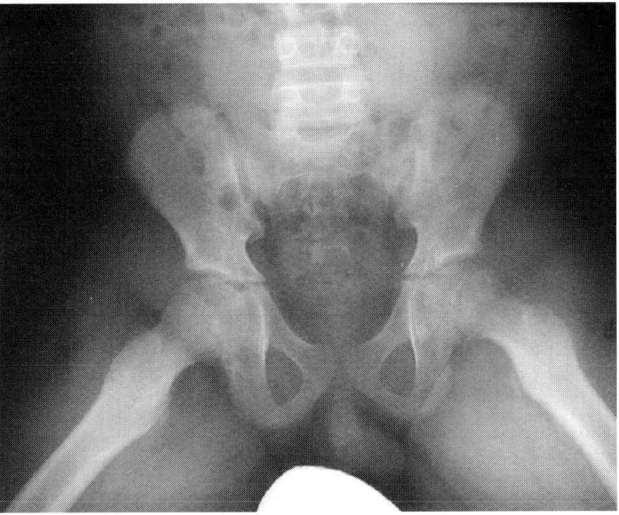

B

Figure 10–28: A, The right hip in this 12-year-old boy is normal, and the Klein's line intersects the lateral capital epiphysis. The left hip has SCFE; the femoral neck has moved proximally and anteriorly relative to the epiphysis, so the Klein's line no longer intersects the epiphysis. B, The "slip" is more easily noted on the frog-leg lateral view. From Dormans JP, ed (2004) Pediatric Orthopaedics and Sports Medicine. Philadelphia: Mosby.

- Three-dimensional reconstructed CT images can be used to assess the severity of residual deformity of the upper femur, especially when reconstructive osteotomy is being considered.
- Bone scanning will show increased uptake in the capital femoral physis of an involved hip, decreased uptake in the presence of osteonecrosis, and increased uptake in the joint space in the presence of chondrolysis.

Ultrasonography

- Ultrasonography recently has been proposed in the diagnosis and evaluation of SCFE.
- It is useful in the detection of early slips by demonstrating joint effusion and a "step" between the femoral neck and the epiphysis created by slipping.
- The severity of slipping could be accurately staged by determining the step at the anterior physeal outline.

Magnetic Resonance Imaging

- MRI can be of assistance in the early diagnosis of SCFE by identifying morphological and signal abnormalities around the affected physeal plate when plain radiographs, and even CT scans, may appear normal.
- MRI is not used as a routine radiological procedure for diagnosis of SCFE but may be rarely indicated in cases of hip pain associated with a high clinical suspicion of SCFE despite negative plain radiographs.

Natural History

- The natural history of SCFE without treatment is difficult to ascertain. The two main concerns are slip progression and the development of degenerative joint disease.
- The incidence of degenerative joint disease of the hip associated with previous SCFE remains unknown.
- The risk of developing osteoarthritis in patients with untreated SCFE depends on the severity of the displacement.[18]
  - Those with mild or moderate slips have positive clinical outcomes because the congruity of the femoral head with the acetabulum is maintained.
  - More severe displacement is associated with early onset degenerative arthritis and may result in injury to the posterosuperior epiphyseal vessels causing osteonecrosis of the femoral head.
- Patients with an untreated, unstable SCFE may develop limitations in hip range of motion because of residual deformity of the proximal femur.
- Long-term studies of the available treatment options have shown that SCFE patients who underwent in situ screw fixation had the best results, regardless of the severity of the slip. In situ screw fixation is associated with the best long-term function, the lowest risk of complications, and the most effective delay of degenerative arthritis.[1]

Treatment

- Treatment can be divided into three categories: treatment to prevent further slippage, treatment to reduce the degree of slippage, and salvage treatment.

Treatment to Prevent Further Slippage

- Prevention of further slippage can be accomplished by spica cast immobilization, in situ metallic pin or screw fixation, and bone graft epiphysiodesis.
- *In situ fixation* of the displaced femoral head, with metallic pins or screws, historically has been and remains the most commonly used method of stabilization in SCFE.
  - The term *in situ* implies that no effort is made to reduce the displacement between the epiphysis and the femoral neck.
  - The goal of in situ pinning is to stabilize the capital epiphysis to the femoral neck to prevent further slippage.
- The combination of improvement in instrumentation, improvement in fluoroscopic visualization of the femoral epiphysis during surgery, and better understanding of the anatomy and pathoanatomy found in SCFE have improved and simplified the performance of the procedure, leading to improved outcomes.
- Advantages of in situ fixation performed percutaneously or through a minimal incision are as follows:
  - Minimal blood loss
  - Avoidance of opening of the hip joint
  - Minimal requirement for postoperative hospitalization and rehabilitation
- The following are disadvantages inherent with the technique:
  - The possibility of persistent penetration of the hip joint by the fixation device
  - Technical difficulty in some severe slips
- In situ fixation remains a surgical technique that depends on biplane fluoroscopy to perform properly.
- A single cannulated screw should enter the anterior aspect of the proximal femur, cross the physis at 90 degrees, and enter the center of the epiphysis with the tip below subchondral bone[2,3] (Figure 10–29).
  - In a typical SCFE, the metaphysis of the femoral neck displaces anteriorly from the femoral head as the femoral head rotates posteriorly around the axis of femoral neck.

1. For the fixation device to enter and stay central in the femoral head, it must be placed perpendicular to the plane of the proximal femoral physis. This can be accomplished if the starting position for the fixation is on the anterior femoral neck.
2. The proper starting point on the femoral neck is determined by the severity of displacement of the femoral head; with increasing severity of the slip, the

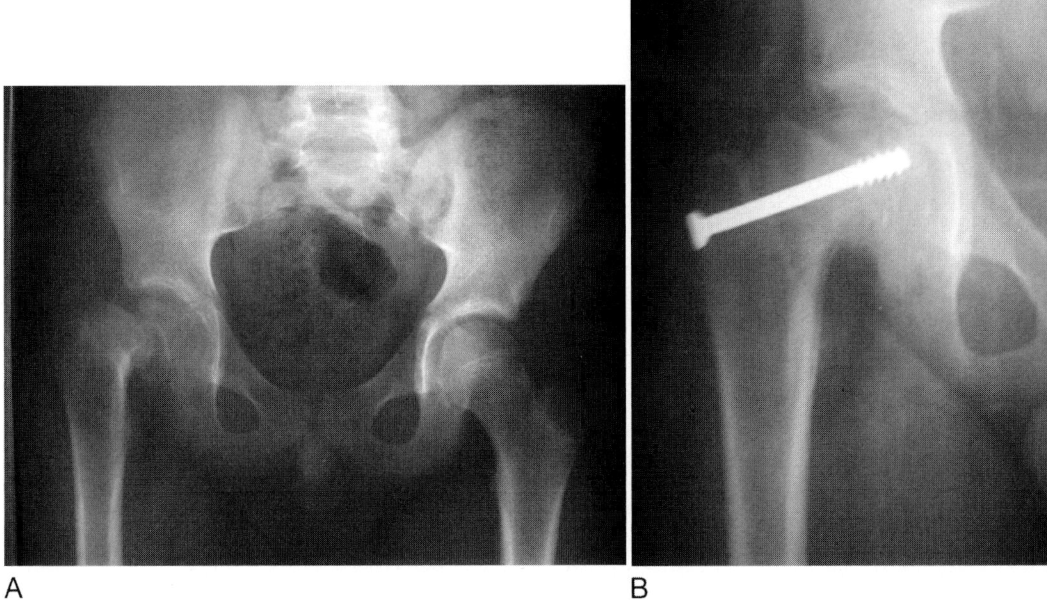

Figure 10–29: This patient underwent in situ screw fixation of the right hip for treatment of SCFE. A, The displacement of the epiphysis was not reduced before placement of the screw. B, A single cannulated screw entered the anterior aspect of the proximal femur, crossed the physis at 90 degrees, and entered the center of the epiphysis with the tip below subchondral bone.

entry point will be found progressively more superior on the femoral neck.

- The central axis of the femoral head remains the safest position for the fixation device. There is only one central axis in the femoral head, so the use of multiple pins or screws must position some of the devices off the central axis and increase the incidence of potential femoral head penetration.

- The internal fixation device should always avoid the superior and anterior quadrant of the femoral head. The terminal branches of the lateral ascending cervical artery are at high risk for injury leading to segmental osteonecrosis of the femoral head if the fixation device is placed in the superior quadrant of the femoral head.
- Following fixation, radiographic confirmation that the fixation device has not penetrated the joint space is mandatory.
- The metallic device used for femoral head stabilization must be of appropriate strength to avoid failure before physeal plate closure. By adhering to the treatment guidelines and principles, almost all SCFEs should be able to be stabilized with percutaneous placement of a single 6.5- to 7.5-mm cannulated screw.
- In situ pin and screw fixation of SCFE accelerates closure of the affected physeal plate.
- In open *bone graft epiphysiodesis,* a portion of the residual physis is removed by drilling and curettage, and a dowel or peg of autologous bone graft (usually harvested from the ipsilateral iliac crest) is inserted across the femoral neck into the epiphysis through a drill hole fashioned to receive the graft.
  - This procedure may be combined with open reduction of the epiphysis and may be used to treat either stable or unstable slips.
  - In unstable slips, supplementary internal fixation, postoperative traction, or spica cast immobilization for 3 to 8 weeks until early stabilization have all been recommended.
  - The disadvantages associated with bone graft epiphysiodesis include extensive surgical approach, greater blood loss, longer hospitalization, problems related with bone graft insufficiency, and potential for continued femoral head displacement before physeal plate closure.

    1. These disadvantages preclude this technique from being recommended for the routine stabilization of the physeal plate in SCFE.
    2. It is probably best indicated for the management of chronic slips of such severity that the treating surgeon is uncomfortable with the feasibility of pinning in situ or for slips that have progressed despite apparently adequate pinning.

- Although treatment with *spica cast immobilization* to prevent further slippage has been considered as an alternative in patients with chronic SCFE, abandoning its use because of the high rate of associated serious, long-term complications (i.e., recurrent slip after cast removal, osteonecrosis of the femoral head, and chondrolysis) is recommended.

Treatment to Reduce the Degree of Slippage

- Treatment methods that reduce the degree of slip, and create a more anatomical relation of the femoral head with the remainder of the femur, should lead to improved function and motion and should delay the onset of degenerative joint disease.
- Techniques to reduce the degree of slip include closed manipulation before physeal plate stabilization and osteotomies of the proximal femur, performed either with physeal stabilization or after physeal closure.
- Closed manipulation can only be considered in patients with acute or acute-on-chronic slips with severe displacement. Closed manipulation can be performed either by slow reduction with skeletal traction over a period of days before stabilization or by a gentle reduction performed at surgical stabilization.
- Osteotomies about the proximal femur in SCFE are designed as realignment procedures through which restoration of a more normal relation among the femoral head, the femoral neck and shaft, and the acetabulum can be achieved.
  - Several osteotomies, performed at various levels along the femoral neck and proximal femur, have been described in SCFE.
  - Intertrochanteric osteotomies remain the most frequently used procedures for realignment in SCFE. Intertrochanteric osteotomies enjoy a low incidence of osteonecrosis of the femoral head compared with femoral neck osteotomies.

Salvage Procedures

- If the femoral head becomes severely deformed and the joint becomes stiff and painful as a result of osteonecrosis or chondrolysis, salvage procedures are indicated to relieve pain and improve function.
- Hip arthrodesis is recommended in adolescents and young adults.[3]
  - This procedure relieves pain and allows the patient a high level of activity and employment at most occupations.
  - The proper position for the hip during arthrodesis is 20 degrees of flexion with neutral rotation and neutral to slight adduction.
  - Hip arthrodesis can be converted to total hip replacement if required.
- Arthroplasty of the affected hip is not recommended for most adolescents and young adults; severe unilateral hip osteoarthritis is associated with SCFE.[2,3] The potential for early component loosening and wear, the need for several revisions over the patient's lifetime, and subsequent risk of chronic infection preclude total hip arthroplasty as the recommended procedure in younger patients.

Prophylactic Pinning of the Contralateral Hip

- The prevalence of contralateral slip, even in an asymptomatic patient, has led many authors to recommend prophylactic pinning.
- On the other hand, the opponents of prophylactic pinning stress that in situ pinning can be associated with severe complications that can be more devastating to hip function than the slip itself.
- Observation of the unaffected hip rather than prophylactic pinning remains the most appropriate treatment in patients with unilateral SCFE.[2,3] The patient and parents must be carefully warned of the potential risk of development of a slip on the contralateral side and instructed to report immediately the development of any lower extremity symptoms on the contralateral limb.
- In patients who have SCFE associated with known metabolic and endocrine disorders, in which the risk of a contralateral slip is extremely high, prophylactic pinning of the contralateral hip may be appropriate.[2]

Complications

- Two major complications, osteonecrosis and chondrolysis, are specifically associated with SCFE.
- *Osteonecrosis* of the femoral head has been reported to occur in 10 to 15% of patients with SCFE. More recent studies report a much lower incidence (0 to 5%) because of improvements in slip stabilization techniques.[1]
  - Osteonecrosis is more frequently associated with acute and unstable slips and is most likely secondary to vascular injury associated with the initial femoral head displacement. Severe slips, which may involve greater insults to the femoral head vascular supply at the time of physeal displacement, are associated with a higher rate of osteonecrosis.
  - Iatrogenic injury to the extraosseous epiphyseal vessels may occur during aggressive manipulation of the femoral head, stabilization of the femoral head if the fixation device violates the posterior cortex of the femoral neck, and realignment of the femoral head through osteotomy of the femoral neck.
  - After the diagnosis has been made, treatment must be directed at maintaining motion and preventing collapse by decreasing the magnitude of the forces at the affected hip through relieved weight-bearing status until healing occurs.

    1. If an implant is encroaching on the joint surface, it should be removed, partially withdrawn, or replaced

so that the residual epiphysis is still stabilized to the femoral neck without further compromise of the articular surface.
2. The use of vascularized bone graft and redirectional intertrochanteric osteotomy, with bone grafting to the femoral head, has been proposed to improve outcome.

- Long-term studies show that hips affected with osteonecrosis have a poorer outcome that continues to deteriorate over time.[3]

- *Chondrolysis* is defined as an acute dissolution of articular cartilage in association with rapid progressive joint stiffness and pain.
  - The diagnosis can be made easily by the characteristic clinical findings and the radiographic confirmation of joint space narrowing (3 mm or less).
  - The etiology for chondrolysis is unknown, but proposed causes include immunological or autoimmune disorders within the hip joint.[1]
  - The incidence has been reported to average 16 to 20% (within a range of 1.8 to 55%).[2,3]
  - Although this complication can occur in the untreated hip, most chondrolysis in SCFE has been reported to follow treatment. Manipulative reduction, prolonged immobilization, realignment osteotomies, and particularly persistent pin penetration of the femoral head are shown to be associated with an increased incidence of chondrolysis.
  - In recent years, improvement in screw placement technique has led to a decline in the rate of chondrolysis.
  - If chondrolysis follows surgical treatment of SCFE, a septic process mimicking chondrolysis must always be ruled out by hip aspiration.
  - The early supportive care for chondrolysis should include modification of activities, use of crutches, gentle range of motion exercises to maintain motion, and anti-inflammatory medications.
  - Patients who do not recover adequate range of motion or who have severe continued pain may require arthrodesis or total joint arthroplasty.

Idiopathic Chondrolysis of the Hip

- Idiopathic chondrolysis of the hip is characterized by acute and rapidly progressive destruction of the articular cartilage of both femoral and acetabular surfaces, resulting in secondary joint space narrowing and stiffness.
- This condition is seen most frequently in adolescents, with isolated involvement of the hip joint and no demonstrable cause.[3]

Etiology

- As the name implies, the cause of idiopathic chondrolysis of the hip remains unknown.
- Previously proposed theories about the cause of idiopathic chondrolysis of the hip include nutritional abnormalities, mechanical injury, ischemia, abnormal capsular pressure, and inherently abnormal chondrocyte metabolism within the articular cartilage.
- Chondrolysis is thought by many to be autoimmune in origin; articular cartilage resorption occurs secondary to an autoimmune response within the hip joint in genetically susceptible individuals.[3]
  - Synovial tissue from involved hip joints has routinely demonstrated an increase in the presence of chronic inflammatory cells, including lymphocytes, plasma cells, and monocytes concentrated in a perivascular pattern.
  - In addition, immunocomplex deposition of immunoglobulin M and the C3 component of complement in the synovium of involved joints have been demonstrated.

Epidemiology

- Idiopathic chondrolysis of the hip is a rare condition, and its true incidence is unclear.
- This condition affects girls five times more frequently than boys.
- The reported age at the onset of symptoms averages 12.5 years for girls (with a range of 9 to18 years) and 14.5 years for boys (with a range of 13 to 20 years).
- The right hip is slightly more likely to be involved. Bilateral involvement has been reported.
- Approximately half of patients with idiopathic chondrolysis of the hip are of African descent.

Clinical Presentation

- The most frequent presenting complaint is the insidious onset of pain in the anterior or medial side of the affected hip in an afebrile patient.
- The pain is associated with progressive joint stiffness and a limp.
- Contractures about the affected hip may lead to pelvic obliquity and an apparent limb length discrepancy.
- Physical examination of the chondrolytic hip demonstrates significant restriction of motion in all planes and associated muscle spasm.
- In the most common presenting pattern of contracture, the hip is fixed in flexion, abduction, and external rotation.
- Complete blood count, urinalysis, rheumatoid factor, antinuclear antibody, human leukocyte antigen-B27 (HLA-B27) marker, blood culture, and tuberculin skin testing are usually within normal limits.

Radiographic Findings

- In most cases with idiopathic chondrolysis of the hip, the diagnosis can be made by the patient's clinical presentation and plain radiographs.

- The radiographic hallmark of idiopathic chondrolysis of the hip is narrowing of the joint space of the involved hip from its normal 3 to 5 mm to a value less than 3 mm.[1] Complete obliteration of the joint space rarely occurs.
- Osteopenia of the periarticular osseous structures, irregular blurring of the subchondral sclerotic lines at the femoral and acetabular joint surfaces, and enlargement of the fovea are common radiographic findings.
- A mild protrusio acetabuli with a buttressing osteophyte at the lateral margin of the acetabulum may develop in about half of the patients.
- Premature closure of the proximal femoral physis and the trochanteric apophysis may be seen.
- Although not routinely used, arthrography of the hip can document articular cartilage loss and secondary joint space narrowing.
- Scintigraphic evaluation of the hip in the early (active) stage of this condition usually demonstrates a generalized increase in uptake, secondary to inflammatory and hyperemic response.
- CT can demonstrate local changes in subchondral bone, cartilage loss, and narrowing of the joint space.
- Local changes in osseous and cartilage tissue can be assessed by MRI.
- The routine use of arthrography, scintigraphy, CT, and MRI is not recommended in idiopathic chondrolysis of the hip. These modalities may be helpful in making the correct diagnosis when idiopathic chondrolysis of the hip is clinically suspected but cannot be confirmed with plain radiographs.

Differential Diagnosis

- The differential diagnosis for idiopathic chondrolysis of the hip includes pyogenic arthritis, tuberculous arthritis, juvenile rheumatoid arthritis, seronegative spondyloarthropathy, and pigmented villonodular synovitis.[3]
- A patient with pyogenic arthritis is usually febrile and systemically ill.
  - Hip pain of acute onset is associated with intense guarding against passive movement of the hip.
  - Laboratory values such as white blood cell count, erythrocyte sedimentation rate, and C-reactive protein are generally elevated in pyogenic arthritis.
- Seronegative spondyloarthropathy is usually seen in patients who are positive for the HLA-B27 marker and has additional joint involvement later in the course of the disease.
- The chondrolysis associated with tuberculous arthritis and juvenile rheumatoid arthritis occurs only after a prolonged period of symptoms, and the limitation of hip motion rarely reaches the degree of restriction seen in idiopathic chondrolysis.
- Pigmented villonodular synovitis of the hip often has a chronic and prolonged clinical course, with radiographs demonstrating cystic erosions in the subchondral bone on both sides of the joint.

Natural History

- The course of idiopathic chondrolysis of the hip appears to have two separate stages: acute and chronic.
  - The acute stage, lasting 6 to 16 months, begins with the onset of symptoms.
    1. An inflammatory state leads to a painful hip with reduced range of motion and loss of articular cartilage.
    2. Over time, the synovial inflammation decreases and the synovium shows an increase in fibrous tissue deposition.
  - The chronic stage, which may last 3 to 5 years, is characterized by one of three possible outcomes:
    1. In some patients, the involved hip may continue to deteriorate to an ultimately painful and malpositioned ankylosis.
    2. In others, the hip may become painlessly ankylosed in a position that causes some limitation of hip function.
    3. In the third group, the involved hip may have resolution of pain, with a partial or complete return of motion and improved joint space width on plain radiographs.
- Further investigation is needed to fully understand the natural history of this condition.

Treatment

- Current recommendations for the management of idiopathic chondrolysis of the hip focus on control of synovial inflammation, maintenance of hip motion, and prolonged relief of the need to bear weight on the involved joint.
  - The administration of nonsteroidal anti-inflammatory medications at therapeutic doses can help to limit the inflammation.
  - Periodic use of skin traction and bed rest can also provide relief during acute exacerbation of joint pain and motion loss.
  - Surgical release of persistent contractures and an aggressive physical therapy program may help to maintain hip motion.
  - The use of crutches to allow the patient to have non–weight-bearing or partial weight-bearing status is also an essential part of the management plan.
- Patients recalcitrant to nonoperative management may require a hip fusion.

Coxa Vara

- Coxa vara is a varus deformity of the proximal femur. The neck–shaft angle drawn between the line of the femoral neck and the line of the femoral shaft viewed on the anteroposterior radiograph is between 130 and 145 degrees in normal children. In coxa vara, the angle is typically less than 110 degrees.
- This varus deformity of the hip can be roughly classified into three types: congenital, developmental, and acquired coxa vara (Table 10–4).[1]

Developmental Coxa Vara

- *Developmental coxa vara,* also known as *infantile* or *cervical coxa vara,* is not present at birth. It develops in early childhood and is typically associated with mild limb shortening and characteristic radiographic features.
- This condition produces progressive deterioration of the proximal femoral neck–shaft angle during growth.
- Developmental coxa vara is different from dysplastic coxa vara, which may be associated with skeletal dysplasias and diseases.

Epidemiology

- Developmental coxa vara is a rare entity with a reported incidence of 1 in 25,000 live births worldwide.[2]

Table 10–4: Classification of Coxa Vara

CLASS	FEATURES
Developmental coxa vara	Physeal involvement with a postnatal onset Unilateral or bilateral, often progressive, and does not remodel Metaphyseal region—Spondylometaphyseal dysplasia, spondyloepiphyseal dysplasia, and cleidocranial dysplasia
Congenital coxa vara (congenital femoral deficiency with coxa vara)	Subtrochanteric area and present at birth Unilateral, not progressive, and does not remodel May be associated with proximal femora focal deficiency, congenital short femur, or congenital bowed femur
Traumatic coxa vara	Physeal involvement but not associated with generalized dysplasia Progressive deformity (no spontaneous remodeling), physeal insufficiency, trochanteric overgrowth, and septic hip (destruction of the femoral head) Vascular injuries to the physis and epiphysis; Legg-Calve-Perthes disease Osteonecrosis (femoral neck fracture, traumatic hip dislocation, and complication after reduction of developmental dysplasia of the hip)
Dysplastic coxa vara	Metaphyseal or subtrochanteric regions Bilateral, often progressive, and does not remodel Associated with generalized dysplasia and diseases Spontaneous remodeling (with a nonprogressive deformity) Fracture or osteotomy of the femur

- There is no racial predilection.
- The disorder appears to be equally common in males and females.
- Bilateral involvement occurs in 30 to 50% of patients.[1]
- There is no predilection for the right or the left hip.

Etiology

- The cause of developmental coxa vara remains unclear.
- The most widely accepted hypothesis postulates a primary ossification defect in the inferior femoral neck.[3] This ossification defect predisposes the local dystrophic bone to fatigue in response to weight-bearing shearing stresses, leading to a progressive varus deformity.
- Histological studies have shown that abnormal chondrocyte development in the growth plate cartilage prevents the formation of a solid connection between the physis and the adjacent metaphyseal bone, leading to progressive varus deformity of the femoral neck.
- Unlike SCFE, there is no slippage between the epiphysis and the metaphysis.

Clinical Presentation

- Most patients with developmental coxa vara show symptoms sometime between initiation of ambulation and 6 years of age.
- The most frequent complaint is a progressive gait abnormality. Pain is rarely reported.
  - Gait abnormality is caused by a combination of true Trendelenburg gait (abductor muscle weakness) and relatively minor limb length inequality in unilateral cases.
  - In patients with bilateral involvement, the complaint is usually of a waddling gait, similar to that seen with bilateral dysplasia of the hips.
- Physical examination usually reveals a somewhat prominent and elevated greater trochanter, often associated with an abductor muscle weakness and a positive Trendelenburg testing.
- Shortening is present in unilateral cases but seldom exceeds 3 cm at skeletal maturity, even in untreated cases.
- The range of motion of the affected hip is usually restricted in all planes of motion, with the most significant limitations occurring in abduction and internal rotation.
- An associated hip flexion contracture is often identified.
- Associated musculoskeletal anomalies are rare.

Radiographic Findings

- The diagnosis of developmental coxa vara, and its differentiation from other forms of coxa vara, depends on the identification of certain classic radiographic findings.

- Anteroposterior and frog-leg lateral views of both hips are required to evaluate cases of suspected coxa vara.
- The radiographic features include a decreased femoral neck–shaft angle; a more vertical position of the physeal plate; a triangular metaphyseal fragment in the inferior femoral neck, surrounded by an inverted radiolucent Y pattern; a decrease in normal anteversion of the proximal femur, which may become true retroversion; coxa breva; and in some patients, a mild acetabular dysplasia[2,3] (Figure 10–30).
  - The neck–shaft angle of the hip is 130 to 145 degrees in normal children. This angle is decreased to less than 110 degrees, and typically is about 90 degrees, in a child with coxa vara (Figure 10–31, *A*).
  - The Hilgenreiner–epiphyseal (H–E) angle—the angle formed between Hilgenreiner's line and a line parallel to the epiphysis—is normally less than 25 degrees. In coxa vara, the H–E angle is greater than 25 degrees, typically progressing to a range between 45 and 70 degrees (Figure 10–31, *B*). The anteroposterior view demonstrates the vertical position of the physis.
  - An inverted Y pattern in the inferior femoral neck is the hallmark of this condition. The lucencies are in the shape of the letter Y and represent the widened physes. The interposed triangular segment is an area of dystrophic bone.

Natural History

- Patients with developmental coxa vara are at risk for stress-fracture–related nonunion of the femoral neck and premature osteoarthritis of the hip.
- Studies demonstrated that the determining factor for progression of the varus deformity was the H–E angle.[3] The patients with a more horizontally oriented physis (less than 45 degrees) more commonly had spontaneous healing of the femoral neck defect and an associated arrest in progression of the varus deformity.
- Patients with a relatively vertically oriented physis (greater than 45 degrees) were found to more commonly manifest the more classic progressive pattern.

Treatment

- The goals of treatment are to stimulate ossification and healing of the defective femoral neck, to correct the femoral head–shaft angle to normal, and to restore normal mechanical muscle function to the hip abductors.

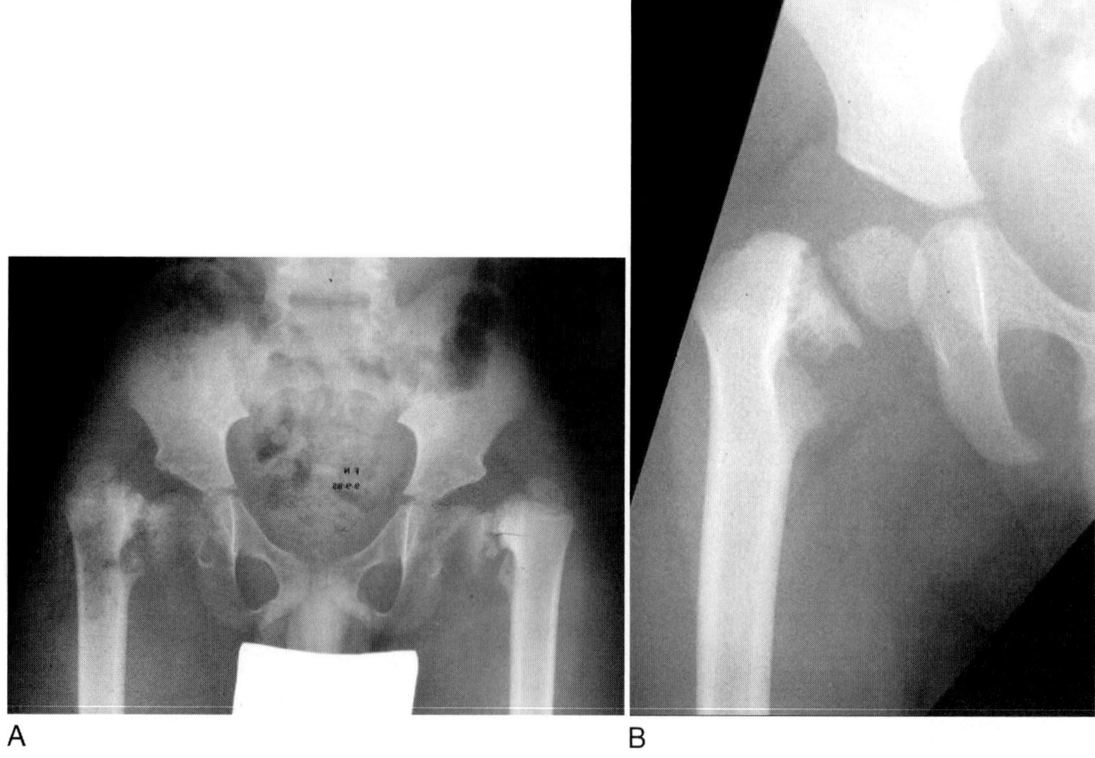

Figure 10–30: Anteroposterior plain radiographs of these bilateral (A) and unilateral (B) cases demonstrate the classic radiographic findings in developmental coxa vara, which include a decreased femoral neck–shaft angle, a more vertical physeal plate, an inferior triangular metaphyseal fragment surrounded by an inverted radiolucent Y, and coxa breva.

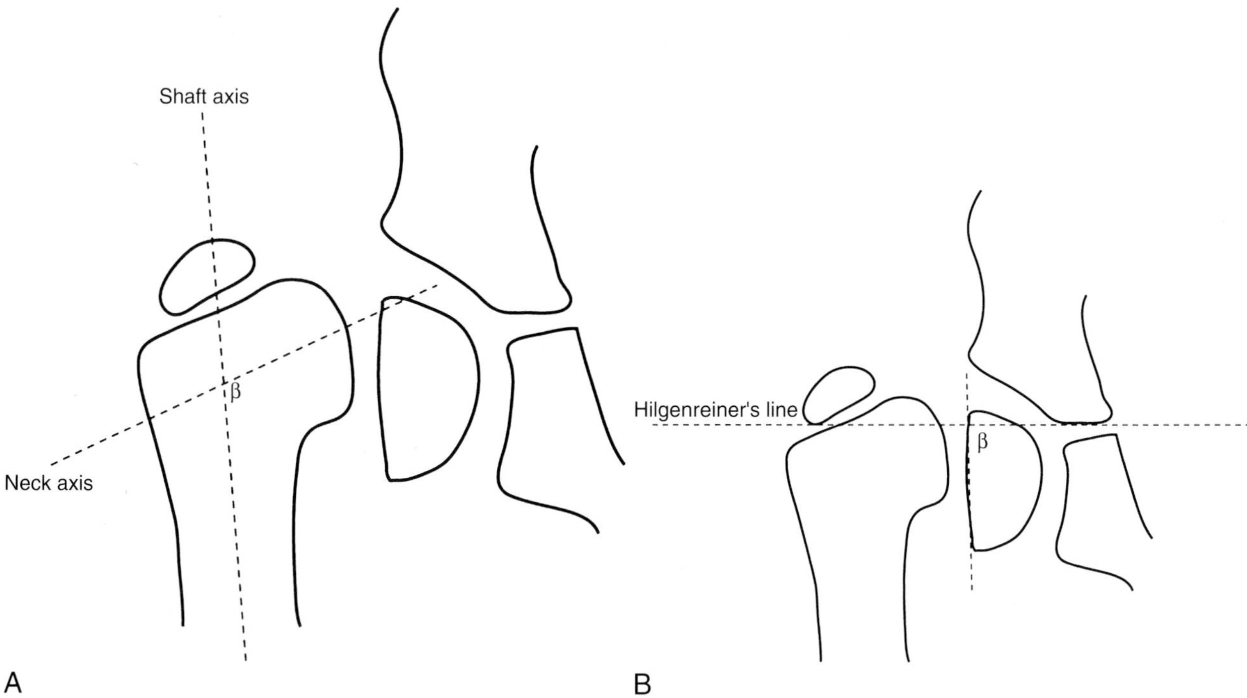

Figure 10–31: Quantification of the extent of radiographic deformity of the proximal femur in developmental coxa vara. A, The neck–shaft angle is the angle between the axis of the femoral shaft and the axis of the femoral neck. B, The H–E angle is the angle between Hilgenreiner's line and a line drawn parallel to the capital femoral physis.

- Nonoperative treatment measures, including abduction splinting, traction, and exercise have not resulted in satisfactory outcomes for developmental coxa vara.
- The presence of symptoms and the extent of proximal femoral deformity as quantified by the H–E angle are the primary determinants of the need for surgical correction of the deformity (Figure 10–32, *A*).
- Valgus osteotomy of the upper femur at the intertrochanteric or subtrochanteric level is the most effective way to correct the varus deformity, to rotate the proximal femoral physis from a vertical to horizontal position (relieving shear stress on it), and to enhance ossification of the defect[2] (Figure 10–32, *B*).
  - Pauwels's Y-shaped osteotomy and Langenskiold's valgus-producing osteotomy are examples of intertrochanteric corrective osteotomies that have produced good results.
  - Subtrochanteric valgus-producing osteotomies also remain well-proven forms of successful therapy in achieving the goals of surgical treatment.
- To prevent loss of the surgical correction achieved before healing of the osteotomy, firm internal fixation, by a tension band technique, blade plate, or nail plate system, is recommended.
  - Violation of the physeal plate by the internal fixation device should be avoided if possible.
  - A spica cast may or may not be applied depending on the stability of the internal fixation and patient compliance.
- To minimize the risk of recurrence, the goal of the operation is to decrease the H–E angle to less than 40 degrees or to increase the neck–shaft angle to greater than 160 degrees.[2]
- Proper treatment of developmental coxa vara can result in a painless and functional hip with a negative Trendelenburg gait. A mild, clinically insignificant length discrepancy may result after surgery.

Congenital Coxa Vara

- *Congenital coxa vara* is more accurately described as *congenital femoral deficiency with coxa vara*.
- Congenital coxa vara is present at birth and is thought to be caused by an embryonic limb bud abnormality.
- The condition is nearly always unilateral.
- Associated congenital musculoskeletal abnormalities and significant limb length inequality, secondary to femoral segment shortening, are common.
- This category includes cases of proximal femoral focal deficiency (PFFD), congenital short femur, and congenital bowed femur.[1]
- The primary etiology of congenital coxa vara, PFFD, will be the focus of this section.

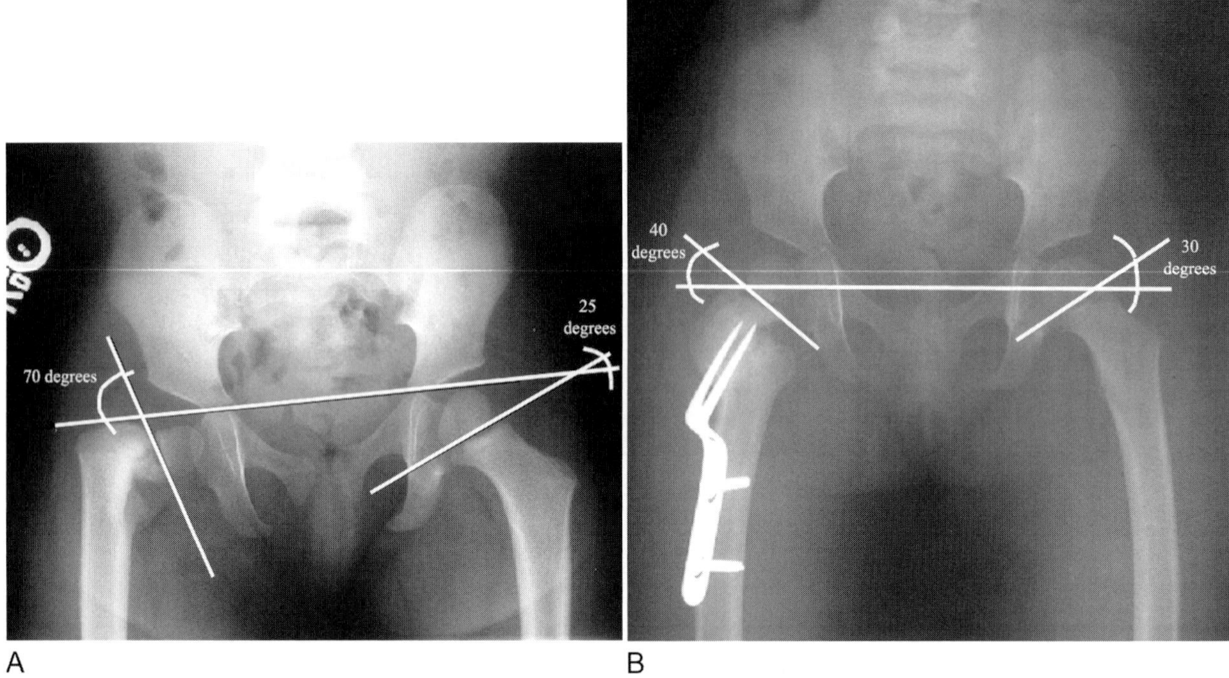

Figure 10–32: A 5-year-old boy with leg length discrepancy was noted to have right hip coxa vara. A, Measurement of the H–E angle was close to 90 degrees. B, A valgus osteotomy of the proximal femur was applied to correct the varus deformity. From Dormans JP, ed (2004) Pediatric Orthopaedics and Sports Medicine. Philadelphia: Mosby.

Classification of Proximal Femoral Focal Deficiency

Aitken Classification

- The *Aitken classification* is the most widely used system for classifying femoral deficiencies. PFFDs are categorized as class A, B, C, or D[19] (Figure 10–33, Table 10–5).

Class A

- The femoral shaft is short but present. The femoral head is also present.
- The acetabulum is normal.
- A bony connection exists between all components of the femur.
- A varus deformity of the subtrochanteric region of the femur (coxa vara), often caused by a pseudarthrosis, is characteristic of this condition.
- The femoral shaft may be positioned near the femoral head.

Class B

- Class B is characterized by a shorter femoral shaft with a bony tuft at the proximal end of the femur.
- The femoral head is present but cannot be visualized initially until the head ossifies.
- The acetabulum is dysplastic.
- Even at maturity, there is no bony continuity between the femoral head and the shaft.
- The proximal end of the femoral shaft is near the acetabulum.

Class C

- In class C, there is a short femoral segment with proximal tapering.
- The femoral head is either absent or represented by an ossicle.
- The acetabulum is severely dysplastic.

Class D

- In class D, the shaft of the femur is extremely short or absent.
- There is no femoral head.
- The acetabulum is either poorly developed or not present.

Gillespie Classification

- Gillespie classification, which categorizes femoral deficiencies into three groups, is useful for planning surgical treatment[20] (Figure 10–34).
- The patient with group A PFFD is considered a candidate for limb lengthening because the length of the affected femur is at least 60% that of the normal femur.

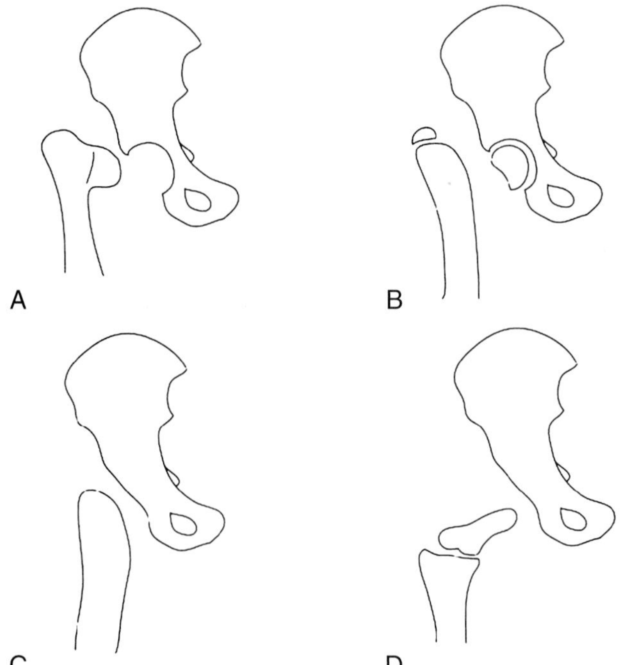

Figure 10–33: Aitken classification for PFFD. **A, In class A, all proximal femoral components eventually ossify with severe subtrochanteric varus, often with pseudarthrosis. B, In class B, the head of the femur is in a competent acetabulum, but there is never bony or cartilaginous continuity between the shaft and the head. C, Class C disease consists of absence of the head, acetabulum, and apophysis at the proximal end of the femur. D, In class D, in addition to absence of the acetabulum and femoral head, the femoral segment is abnormally short and severely flexed with no proximal femoral apophysis. Most bilateral cases of PFFD are class D.**

- The foot of the affected limb is at midtibia level or below compared with the unaffected limb, even with the presence of a flexion contracture in the shorter limb.
- Knee function may be either good or bad.

- In Group B disease, the length of the affected femur is less than 50% of that of the normal side.
  - The foot of the affected limb is at the level between the knee and the midtibia of the unaffected limb.
  - A surgical conversion, such as a knee fusion or a Van Nes rotationplasty, followed by prosthetic fitting would be most suitable in children with this condition.
- Group C PFFD is characterized by virtual absence of the femur with the affected foot positioned at the level of the unaffected knee or above.
  - These patients should be managed with prostheses.
  - Retaining the foot within the socket of the prosthesis may improve suspension and control.

Etiology

- The specific causes of congenital limb deficiencies are unknown in most cases and may be multifactorial.
- Lower limb embryogenesis begins between the fourth and the sixth weeks of gestation; developmental disturbances during this time of limb bud growth and differentiation may lead to femoral defects.
- Environmental and genetic factors may play roles in the development of some limb deficiencies. Thalidomide is one teratogenic drug associated with numerous limb abnormalities.[1]

Clinical Presentation

- Congenital coxa vara is associated with PFFD and congenital shortening of the femur, but the hip deformity generally is not the presenting complaint.
- Patients with PFFD typically have an extremely short and bulky thigh, a flexed and abducted hip, and a laterally rotated limb.
  - The affected foot is usually at the level of the unaffected knee.
  - Because of hip and knee flexion contractures, the limb often appears shorter than it is anatomically.
  - An ipsilateral fibular hemimelia—failure of proper formation of the fibula—may be present.
- Patients with congenital shortening of the femur, a disorder related to PFFD, have a more subtle clinical presentation.

Table 10–5: Aitken Classification of Proximal Focal Femoral Deficiency

CLASS	FEMORAL HEAD	ACETABULUM	FEMORAL SEGMENT	RELATIONSHIP BETWEEN FEMUR AND ACETABULUM
A	Present	Normal	Short	Bony connection between components Femoral head in acetabulum Subtrochanteric varus angulation
B	Present	Moderately dysplastic	Short Proximal bony tuft	No bony connection between head and shaft Femoral head in acetabulum
C	Absent or represented by ossicle	Severely dysplastic	Short Proximal tapering	May be bony connection between shaft and proximal ossicle No articular relationship between femur and acetabulum
D	Absent	Absent	Short Deformed	None

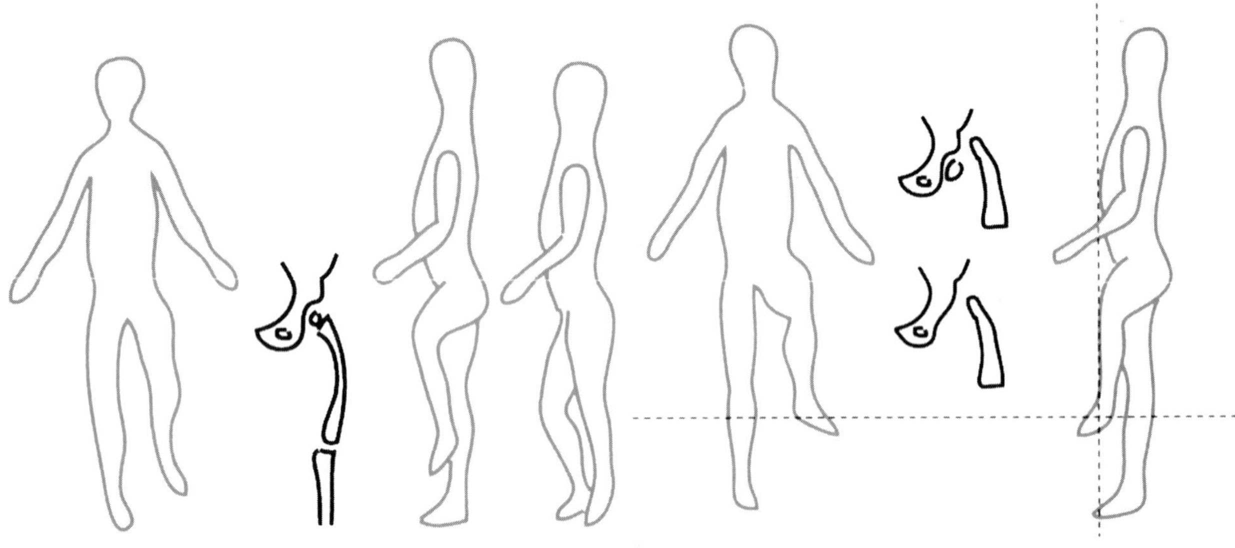

Figure 10–34: Gillespie classification for PFFD. The vertical line in *panels B* and *C* indicates anterior displacement of the weight-bearing axis of the tibia, and the horizontal line indicates the length relationship to the other leg. A, In a congenitally short femur (group A), the child can bear weight on the leg by extending the hip and knee; the child has a sense of proximal stability, and leg length discrepancy is around 20%. B, In group B PFFD (Aitken A, B, and C), the leg length discrepancy is around 40% with characteristic anterior projection of the thigh and flexed knee. C, In group C (Aitken D), the thigh is short and bulbous, and the leg is externally rotated with the foot at or near the level of the other knee.

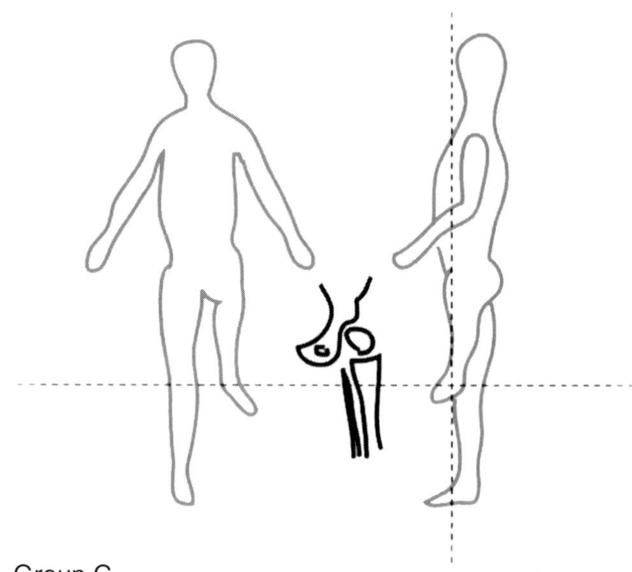

  - The affected thigh is shorter than the contralateral thigh, and the leg may be shorter.
  - The femur may have an anterolateral bow, and the overlying skin may be dimpled.
  - Other features may include femoral retroversion (lateral rotation of the femur), valgus and lateral rotation deformity of the knee, and ipsilateral fibular hemimelia.

Radiographic Findings

- The diagnosis of congenital coxa vara can usually be made with plain radiographs (Figure 10–35).
  - Attention to the acetabulum, the femoral head, and the femoral shaft can help to classify the limb deficiency.
  - Scanograms or orthoroentgenograms, radiographs taken with a ruler, can determine the overall limb length discrepancy. The clinician should be aware that hip or knee flexion contractures may influence the measurement of limb lengths.

Treatment

- Each patient with PFFD must be evaluated carefully to enable development of an appropriate management plan.
- The *abductor lurch* (Trendelenburg gait) associated with congenital coxa vara and PFFD can be addressed with fusion of the femur to the ilium, thus stabilizing the hip.

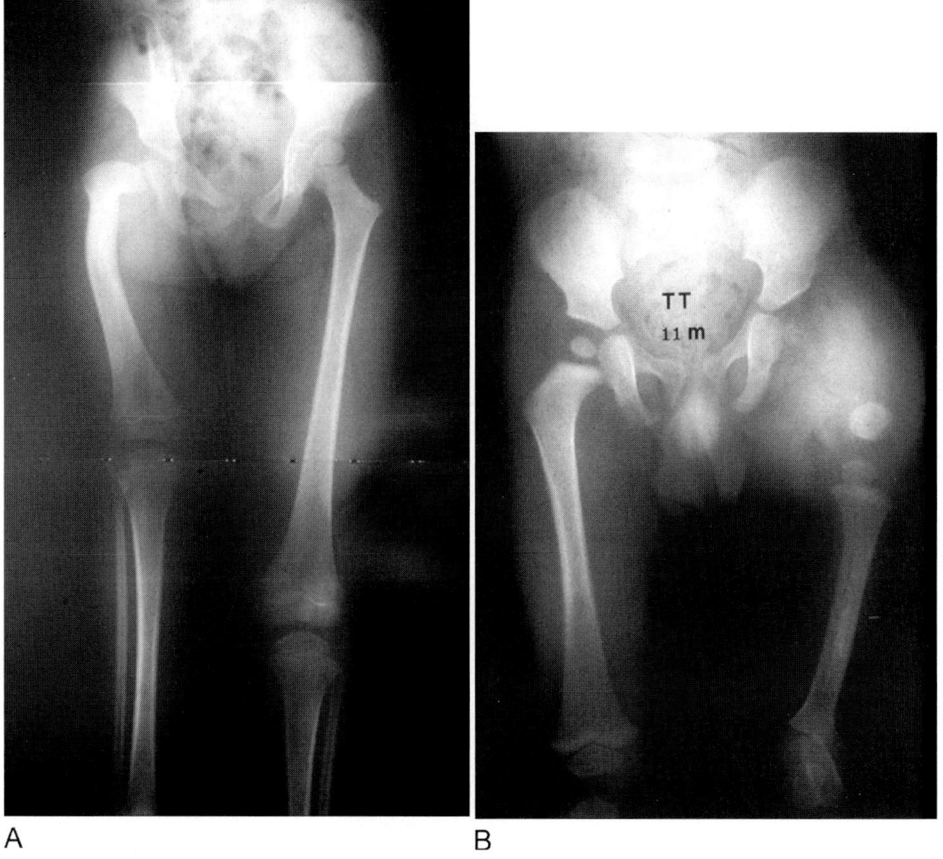

Figure 10–35: Plain radiographs showing two patients with PFFD. A, Note the shortening of the right femur with associated coxa vara of the right hip. B, This patient has more severe involvement with near-complete absence of the left femur.

- Limb length discrepancy in PFFD can be treated either with or without an operation.
  - Many patients, particularly those with Gillespie group C deficiencies, are candidates for prosthetic fitting.
  - Indications for limb lengthening include prediction of the affected femur length to be at least half the length of the normal femur at maturity, with a predicted limb length discrepancy of 17 to 20 cm.[2]
- Correction should be achieved with no more than three separate procedures.
  - Hip abnormalities, such as coxa vara and hip retroversion, should be corrected before lengthening to avoid iatrogenic hip dislocations.
  - In addition to hip stability, knee stability is important. Crossing the knee joint with the external fixator frame (such as the Ilizarov frame) and performing soft tissue lengthening may prevent knee joint subluxation.
- A Syme amputation (at the ankle joint) with a knee arthrodesis can be performed at the same time to create a long bone consisting of a short femur fused to the tibia.
  - This has the advantage of providing an effectively longer femur with an end-bearing limb suitable for prosthetic fitting after a single operation.
  - The drawbacks, however, are that the limb is often too long and that it lacks knee motion or control.
- The Van Nes rotationplasty creates a knee joint by attaching the ankle backward to the distal femur, thus creating a knee joint with a backward ankle joint (the heel is pointing forward) (Figure 10–36).
  - Motor control and sensory feedback are excellent after this technically challenging procedure.
  - Prosthesis fitting and training allow the patient to walk without significant gait disturbances.
  - The disadvantage of this procedure is poor cosmesis and derotation (loss of rotated position) over time.
  - Contraindications for Van Nes rotationplasty include severe foot and ankle deformities and bilateral femoral deficiency.

Acquired Coxa Vara

- *Acquired coxa vara,* or *traumatic coxa vara,* can result from direct injury to the proximal femoral physis and the proximal femur from infections, vascular injuries, and fractures.
- This condition is not associated with any generalized skeletal dysplasias.

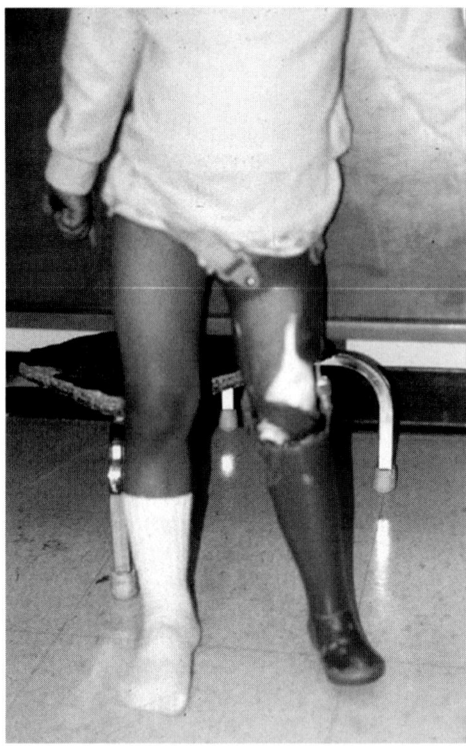

Figure 10–36: A patient with PFFD who underwent a Van Nes rotationplasty.

Etiology and Epidemiology

- Conditions leading to progressive varus hip deformity include hip infection, LCPD, SCFE, osteonecrosis of the femoral epiphysis resulting from several causes, and pathological bone disease.
  - A septic hip, if not treated promptly, can lead to septic necrosis of the hip and complete destruction of the femoral head.
  - Femoral neck fractures or traumatic hip dislocations can cause osteonecrosis of the femoral head by disrupting its vascular supply.
  - In a child with DDH, reduction of a dislocated hip and application of a spica cast in excessive abduction can lead to acquired coxa vara by compromising blood flow to the femoral head.
  - Pathological bone disorders that may lead to acquired coxa vara include osteogenesis imperfecta, fibrous dysplasia, renal osteodystrophy, and osteopetrosis.
  - Coxa vara can occur after a perinatal epiphyseal separation associated with a difficult breech delivery.
  - A varus hip position can result from malunion of a femoral neck or intertrochanteric fracture or from a varus-producing femoral osteotomy.
- The incidence of acquired coxa vara depends on the rate of complications associated with conditions such as septic hip, osteonecrosis of the femoral head, LCPD, perinatal epiphyseal separation, proximal femoral fractures, and varus-producing proximal femoral osteotomies.

Clinical Presentation

- Patients with acquired coxa vara are generally older than those with developmental or congenital coxa vara.
- They are usually ambulatory and are noted to have a limp and an associated limb length discrepancy, both of which may be more severe if the initial insult occurred early in life.
  - Limb length discrepancy may be seen as a result of altered growth through the proximal femoral physis.
- A Trendelenburg sign or gait may be present because of altered hip abductor mechanics.

Radiographic Findings and Natural History

- Plain radiographs usually yield sufficient evidence from which to make the diagnosis of coxa vara.
- Vascular injury to the proximal femoral epiphysis and the physis are suggested by failure of growth of the ossific nucleus, fragmentation and deformity of the femoral head, and failure of growth of the femoral neck.
- Relative overgrowth of the greater trochanter may be noted.
- Comparison with the unaffected hip may be helpful.
- The natural course for patients with acquired coxa vara depends on the natural history of the underlying conditions.

Treatment

- Alteration of hip mechanics because of trochanteric overgrowth can be corrected with epiphysiodesis of the greater trochanter physis once the apophysis becomes visible at age 5.
- In children older than 9 years, the greater trochanter can be transferred distally to increase the length of the hip abductors, improving their mechanics to allow them to keep the pelvis level throughout the gait cycle.
- Osteonecrosis of the hip typically leads to a painful, arthritic hip joint, which may require surgical intervention. Management decisions should be made on an individual basis.
  - Even with marked deformity and advanced degenerative changes, a patient's function may be adequate to forestall an operation.
  - A total hip replacement can provide a pain-free mobile joint. In a young person, such a procedure may have to be revised multiple times during a lifetime because the prosthesis can wear out in active people.
- In a patient with a history of septic necrosis of the hip, the risk of prosthesis infection may make total hip replacement a less attractive treatment strategy.

Femoral Anteversion

- Femoral anteversion, or medial femoral torsion, is a common cause of in-toeing in younger children.
  - The deformity is not in the tibia or the foot but rather in the proximal femur.
  - In the normal child, the femoral head is directed approximately 15 degrees anterior to the shaft of femur and therefore has 15 degrees of femoral anteversion. A larger femoral anteversion forces the entire limb to be medially rotated to maintain the normal relationship between the acetabulum and the femoral head, leading to in-toeing.

Clinical Presentation

- The child is typically brought in by the caregiver with the chief complaint of in-toeing or clumsiness.
- Although these children tend to fall often, they are usually good sprinters.
- Medial rotation of more than 60 degrees and limited lateral rotation of the thigh to less than 20 degrees is highly suggestive of femoral anteversion.[1]
- Femoral anteversion may be confused with internal tibial torsion.
  - Observation of the orientation of the patella helps to distinguish these two conditions.
    1. In internal tibial torsion, the patellae are in typical anatomical alignment, but in femoral anteversion, they are medially rotated.
    2. Alignment of the patellae with the second metatarsals rules out internal tibial torsion.
- A child with femoral anteversion will often be observed sitting in the reverse tailor position (i.e., the W position).

Treatment

- The patient and the caregiver should be encouraged to adopt a different sitting style, such as the "Indian style" position.
- The natural course of femoral anteversion is improvement over time. In addition, as the child's pelvis widens, the medially rotated feet will not collide as much during ambulation.

References

1. Tamai J, Erol B, Dormans JP (2004) Hip disorders. In: Pediatric Orthopaedics and Sports Medicine: The Requisites in Pediatrics (Dormans JP, ed). Philadelphia: Mosby pp 175-212.

2. Herring JA (2002) Tachdjian's Pediatric Orthopaedics, 3rd edition. Philadelphia: WB Saunders.

3. Morrissy RT, Weinstein SL (2001) Lowell and Winter's Pediatric Orthopaedics, 5th edition. Philadelphia: Lippincott Williams & Wilkins.

4. Weinstein SL, Mubarak SJ, Wenger DR (2004) Developmental hip dysplasia and dislocation: Part I. Instr Course Lect 53: 523-530.

   Thorough knowledge of the normal growth and development of the hip, the causes of abnormal development, and the structural and functional changes that result from developmental hip dysplasia and dislocation provide needed information for treatment. Ultrasonography, newborn screening, and radiographic evaluation are important diagnostic tools.

5. Weinstein SL, Mubarak SJ, Wenger DR (2004) Developmental hip dysplasia and dislocation: Part II. Instr Course Lect 53: 531-542.

   Both nonsurgical and surgical options are available for the treatment of developmental hip dysplasia and dislocation. The advantages, pitfalls, and techniques for using the Pavlik harness should be thoroughly examined before treatment. Early diagnosis and treatment lead to the best long-term results.

6. Ramsey P, Lasser S, MacEwen G (1976) Congenital dislocation of the hip. J Bone Joint Surg Am 58(7): 1000-1004.

   From 1968 to 1972, 23 infants under 6 months with 27 dislocated hips were treated with a Pavlik harness. All dislocations except 3 were successfully reduced. In infants, the Pavlik harness successfully uses the principle of reduction in flexion, avoiding forced abduction.

7. Thompson GH, Price CT, Roy D, Meehan PL, Richards BS (2002) Legg-Calve-Perthes disease. Instr Course Lect 51: 367-384.

8. Catterall A (1971) The natural history of Perthes' disease. J Bone Joint Surgery Br 53(1): 37-53.

9. Salter RB, Thompson GH (1984) Legg-Calve-Perthes' disease: The prognostic significance of the subchondral fracture and a two-group classification of the femoral head involvement. J Bone Joint Surgery Am 66(4): 479-489.

   In the early stage of LCPD, the extent of the subchondral fracture is of prognostic significance in predicting the eventual extent of involvement of the femoral head. The authors propose a two-group classification of the extent of involvement of the femoral head: group A (less than half of the head) and group B (more than half of the head).

10. Herring JA, Neustadt JB, Williams JJ, Early JS, Browne RH (1992) The lateral pillar classification of Legg-Calve-Perthes disease. J Pediatr Orthop 12(2): 143-150.

    Hips were classified during LCPD fragmentation based on radiolucency in the femoral head's lateral pillar. Group A had a uniformly good outcome; group B had a good outcome in patients younger than 9 years at onset but a less favorable one in older patients. Most group C femoral heads became aspherical in both age groups. Classification was a stronger predictive determinant than age of onset.

11. Mose K (1980) Methods of measuring in Legg-Calve-Perthes disease with special regard to the prognosis. Clin Orthop 150: 103-109.

A standard classification of the LCPD stage and a precise definition of the evaluation method of the results are necessary. Precise measurements of the sphericity of the head, epiphyseal quotient, joint surface quotient, and radius quotient are recommended. Measurements ought to be made no earlier than age 16, when growth has stopped and quotients no longer change.

12. Stulberg SD, Cooperman DR, Wallansten R (1981) The natural history of Legg-Calve-Perthes disease. J Bone Joint Surg Am 63(7): 1095-1108.
    Each hip in two study groups of LCPD patients could be placed into one of five classes of deformity based on its radiographic appearance at maturity. Three types of congruency between the femoral head and the acetabulum were recognized: spherical congruency (class I and II), aspherical congruency (class III and IV), and aspherical incongruency (class V).

13. McAndrew MP, Weinstein SL (1984) A long-term follow-up of Legg-Calve-Perthes disease. J Bone Joint Surg Am 66(6): 860-869.
    The authors obtained data on 35 patients with 37 hips affected by LCPD (average follow-up of 47.7 years). Statistically significant correlations were found between clinical outcome (as measured by the Iowa hip rating and by the incidence of arthroplasty) and Catterall head-at-risk signs, femoral head/size ratio, and age at onset of the disease.

14. Loder RT, Richards BS, Shapiro PS, Reznick LR, Aronson DD (1993) Acute slipped capital femoral epiphysis: The importance of physeal stability. J Bone Joint Surg Am 75(8): 1134-1140.
    To test the traditional classification system of SCFE, the authors reclassified the slipped epiphyses as unstable or stable rather than acute, chronic, or acute on chronic. Slips were considered unstable when severe pain prevented the patient from bearing weight even with crutches. Slips were stable when the patient could bear weight with or without crutches.

15. Southwick WO (1967) Osteotomy through the lesser trochanter for slipped capital femoral epiphysis. J Bone Joint Surg Am 49(5): 807-835.

16. Loder RT, Aronsson DD, Dobbs MB, Weinstein SL (2001) Slipped capital femoral epiphysis. Instr Course Lect 50: 555-570.

17. Loder RT, Aronson DD, Greenfield ML (1993) The epidemiology of bilateral slipped capital femoral epiphysis: A study of children in Michigan. J Bone Joint Surg Am 75(8): 1141-1147.
    The records of 82 children who had a bilateral SCFE and no underlying metabolic or endocrine disorder were studied. Compared with children whose hips were diagnosed simultaneously, children whose hips were diagnosed sequentially had a shorter duration of symptoms before the first diagnosis, were younger at the first diagnosis, and tended to be more obese.

18. Carney BT, Weinstein SL (1996) Natural history of untreated chronic slipped capital femoral epiphysis. Clin Orthop 322: 43-47.
    From 1915 to 1952, 31 hips in 28 patients with SCFE were observed without interventional treatment. Degenerative arthritis developed in hips with displaced SCFE. Untreated SCFE can progress to a severe degree. The natural history of chronic SCFE is favorable provided that displacement is minimal and remains so.

19. Aitken GT (1972) The child amputee: An overview. Orthop Clin North Am 3(2): 447-472.

20. Gillespie R (1998) Classification of congenital abnormalities of the femur. In: The Child with a Limb Deficiency (Herring JA, Birch JG, eds). Rosemonth, IL: American Academy of Orthopaedic Surgeons pp 63.

CHAPTER

11

Spinal Disorders

Kristan A. Pierz* and John P. Dormans†

*MD, Surgeon, Department of Orthopaedics, Connecticut Children's Medical Center, Hartford, CT; Assistant Professor of Orthopaedics, University of Connecticut School of Medicine, Hartford, CT
†MD, Chief of Orthopaedic Surgery, The Children's Hospital of Philadelphia, Philadelphia, PA; Professor of Orthopaedic Surgery, University of Pennsylvania School of Medicine, Philadelphia, PA

Introduction

- Pediatric spinal disorders include numerous conditions that may be local, diffuse, static, or progressive.
- Detection of spinal disorders may occur *in utero,* during infancy, during childhood, or late in adolescence.
- Pediatric spinal disorders may occur in isolation or may be associated with other manifestations of a particular disease, state, or condition.
- Pain, deformity, and neurological changes may or may not be present depending on the specific condition.
- Orthopaedists, regardless of their subspecialty, may be the first to detect an underlying medical problem in a child because of back complaints or physical findings.

Clinically Relevant Anatomy

Embryology

- Spinal development is a complex process, and errors occurring at any stage of formation may result in spinal anomalies.[1] In addition, other organs that form simultaneously may be affected by the same insults disrupting spinal development. Approximately 60% of individuals with spinal anomalies may have associated malformations. The acronym VATER refers to associations among vertebral defects, anal atresia, tracheoesophageal fistula, and radial and renal dysplasias (Box 11–1).

Box 11–1 Multiple Malformations Associated with Spinal Anomalies

Because of simultaneous organogenesis, the following areas should be examined if any spinal anomaly is detected:

- Vertebral (other levels)—Warrants radiographic imaging of the entire spine
- Lower gastrointestinal tract
- Trachea and esophagus
- Renal tract—Warrants a renal ultrasound or intravenous pyelography
- Lungs
- Heart
- Radius
- Ear
- Lip and palate

- Axial skeleton formation involves movement of embryonic cells and formation of the ectoderm, endoderm, and mesoderm.
- The primitive streak occurs caudally in the ectoderm during the second week of gestation.
- Mesenchymal tissue on either side of the primitive streak becomes mesoderm.
- The notochord elongates from the primitive streak between the ectoderm and the endoderm in a caudal-to-cranial sequence and has been implicated in developing individual somites.

- The notochord induces the neural plate, which curves dorsally and fuses to form a neural tube. Fusion begins centrally and progresses in both caudal and cranial directions, producing the central nervous system (Figure 11–1). Failure of complete closure results in neural tube defects such as spina bifida.
- By the third week of gestation, mesodermal cells begin to condense along the notochord and form paired somites, which further differentiate into the dermatome (future skin and subcutaneous tissue), the myotome (future striated muscle), and the sclerotome (future skeletal tissue).
- A pair of bilateral somites forms one intervertebral disk plus the adjoining vertebrae; the anterior vertebral body and posterior neural (vertebral) arch development are influenced by different factors. Somite segmentation must then occur to separate each vertebra.
- Chondrification begins during the sixth week of gestation.
- Ossification begins in the ninth or tenth week of gestation, except for in C1 and C2, with three primary ossification centers forming in the body (centrum) and each neural (vertebral) arch. The centrum ossification center of the atlas (C1) commonly appears 9 to 12 months after birth, and the axis (C2) develops from five primary and two secondary centers of ossification. Synchondroses between ossification centers may not close until 5 to 7 years and may be mistaken for fractures on radiographs.

Spinal Maturation

- Horizontal growth of vertebral bodies occurs by periosteal ossification. Growth is fastest during the first 7 years and usually ceases by 25 years.
- Vertical growth occurs through superior and inferior growth plates. In the lumbar spine, sagittal lordosis occurs because the vertebral body grows faster than posterior elements; in the thoracic spine, faster posterior growth results in sagittal kyphosis (Box 11–2).

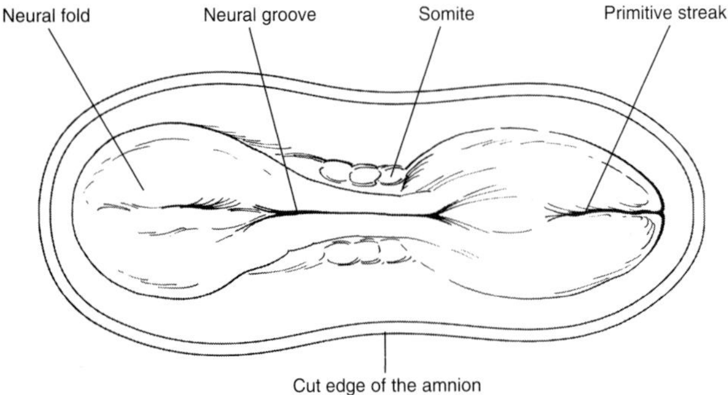

Figure 11–1: During the second and third weeks of gestation, the neural plate begins to curve dorsally to form a neural tube, with somite formation occurring within the adjacent mesoderm.

Box 11–2 Anatomical Definitions

- *Lordosis*—Anterior curvature of the spine in the sagittal plane, as seen in the cervical and lumbar spine
- *Kyphosis*—Posterior curvature of the spine in the sagittal plane, as seen in the thoracic spine
- *Scoliosis*—Lateral curvature of the spine in the coronal plane, frequently associated with rotation

- Ring apophyses form at the upper and lower borders of developing vertebrae and begin to ossify between 11 and 15 years. Irregularities in this ossification may be associated with Scheuermann's disease.
- With growth, the level of the spinal cord termination changes from S1 at six months of gestation to L2 or L3 in the newborn to the inferior border of L1 in adults. The nerves extending from the termination of the spinal cord are referred to as the *cauda equina* (horse's tail).

Bony Structures

- C1 (atlas) is shaped like a ring. Each lateral mass has a concave superior facet, which articulates with the corresponding occipital condyle and allows significant flexion, extension, and some lateral bending. The inferior facets articulate with C2 (axis) and allow rotation. The anterior arch has a dorsal facet, which articulates with the dens of C2.
- Cervical vertebrae have foramen in the transverse processes through which the vertebral artery passes.
- In the cervical vertebrae, superior facet orientation in the sagittal plane increases from 35 degrees to the horizontal in C2 to 55 degrees at C7.
- The 12 thoracic vertebrae articulate with ribs through superior and inferior costal facets (demifacets).
- Superior facet orientation in the sagittal plane ranges from 60 degrees to the horizontal at T1 to approximately 77 degrees at T12, and the facet joints permit mainly lateral bending.
- Superior facet orientation of the five lumbar vertebrae in the sagittal plane decrease from approximately 137 degrees to the horizontal at L1 to approximately 118 degrees at L5, with facet orientation allowing mostly flexion.
- Details regarding pedicle morphology are important, especially when surgically placing pedicle screws.[2]

History and Physical Examination

- Obtaining a complete history, including history of the present illness, medical past, and family, is critical when evaluating any patient with a spinal disorder (Box 11–3).
- The physical examination should include the entire body.
- The patient should be examined in a hospital gown open in the back and worn over underpants or shorts. Long hair should be lifted.

Box 11–3 Key Questions to Ask When Obtaining a History

- What is the chief complaint (pain, deformity, or dysfunction)?
- If painful, where and when does it occur (locally, diffusedly, with activity, or at night)?
- How long has the condition existed? Is it progressing?
- Who first noticed the problem (the patient, a parent, a school nurse, or a pediatrician)?
- Is there a history of trauma (acute versus repetitive microtrauma)?
- Are there associated concerns (fever, chills, weight loss, limb length inequality, limp, weakness, sensory changes, bowel or bladder changes, pulmonary concerns, or cutaneous lesions)?
- If female, have menses started?
- Is there a history of previous surgery (spinal or other major organs)?
- Is there a positive family history?

Box 11–4 General Physical Examination

- Overall state (emotional or developmental maturity, nutritional status, etc.)
- Gait (assistive devices, limp, or weakness)
- Body habitus (Note that Marfan's syndrome is associated with excessive height, increased arm span, cardiovascular and ocular abnormalities, scoliosis, and spondylolisthesis. Dwarfism encompasses a variety of bone dysplasias and may be associated with scoliosis, kyphosis, cervical instability, and lumbar stenosis.)
- Physical maturity (spinal deformities frequently progress during pubertal growth spurt)
- Cutaneous lesions (sacral dimple or hair patch associated with spina bifida or café-au-lait spots associated with neurofibromatosis)
- Ligamentous laxity (knee, elbow, or metacarpal–phalangeal hyperextension and thumb touching volar forearm may indicate connective tissue disorder)

Then, proceed with spine and neurological examination

- Before examining the spine, perform a general examination (Box 11–4).
- Proceed to the spine examination, noting the location and direction of any deformities (Figure 11–2, Box 11–5).
- Perform a neurological examination (Box 11–6, Table 11–1).

Radiological Examination

- When evaluating for spinal deformity, obtain standing, 3-foot, extended, length radiographs from the shoulders to the pelvis in both the coronal (posteroanterior) and the sagittal (lateral) planes (Figure 11–3, A-B). Sitting films may be obtained for individuals unable to stand. Bending films can be obtained to assess curve flexibility, especially when planning surgery. To assess flexibility in the coronal plane, patients may maximally bend to the left or right (Figure 11–3, C-D), or they may be assisted by bending over an object such as an assistant's hand in a lead glove. To assess kyphotic flexibility, patients may lie over a bolster. In addition, traction films may be obtained by having assistants pull on the patient's shoulders and pelvis simultaneously. This is especially helpful with a

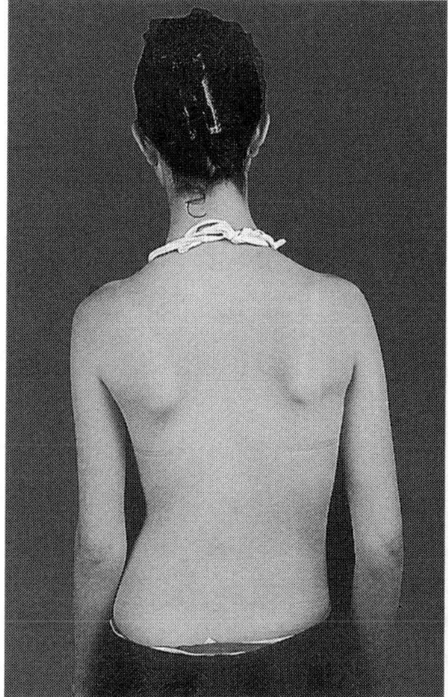

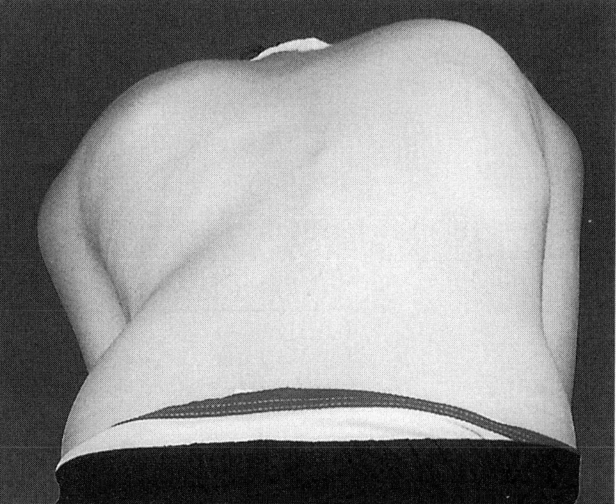

A B

Figure 11–2: A, Clinical photo of a patient with AIS. Note the shoulder and waist asymmetry. B, The rib asymmetry is more noticeable during the Adams forward bend test.

Box 11–5 Physical Examination of the Spine

- Hairline or neck (low hairline, webbed neck, and limited motion suggests Klippel-Feil syndrome)
- Shoulder asymmetry
- Location or direction of curve or deformity
- Waist asymmetry
- Decompensation (plumb line dropped from C7 should pass through gluteal cleft)
- Limb length discrepancy or pelvic obliquity (place block under short limb to level pelvis)
- Evidence of dysraphism (hairy patches, dimples, or lipomas)
- Adams' forward bend test (Feet together, bent forward from waist, and arms hanging freely with palms opposed—assess for rib hump or rotational deformity using a scoliometer)

nonambulatory patient with neuromuscular deformities who cannot stand independently.

- Keeping the tube-to-film distance constant at 72 inches allows uniform comparison among serial films.
- Radiation exposure to the breasts and thyroid can be limited by obtaining posteroanterior views rather than anteroposterior views. Breast, gonadal, or both types of shields may also be used to limit exposure; however, initial films should usually be obtained without shields to avoid obscuring associated anomalies. Bending films should not be reserved for preoperative planning but should not be obtained at every visit.
- Because scoliosis can progress approximately 1 degree per month during rapid growth spurts, serial radiographs are obtained every 4 to 6 months during early adolescence in patients known to have curves. In patients with curves that remain unchanged on serial radiographs, or before or after pubertal growth spurts, the frequency with which radiographs are obtained can be decreased to every 6 to 12 months.
- By convention, posteroanterior radiographs are viewed as if viewing the patient from behind, with the cardiac silhouette and gastric bubble on the left.
- Curves are characterized by location (cervical, thoracic, lumbar, or junctional), direction (convex left, convex right, kyphotic, or lordotic), and magnitude (degree).

Box 11–6 Neurological Examination

- Assess gait or balance.
- Have the patient heel walk, toe walk, and walk in a deep squat to assess strength.
- Trendelenburg test—When standing on one leg, a "normal" patient keeps the pelvis level. A dip from the stance leg suggests hip abductor weakness (L5) of the stance leg.
- Gower test—Difficulty getting up from a seated position without using hands to walk up thighs suggests proximal muscle weakness as seen in Duchenne muscular dystrophy.
- Assess reflexes—Biceps (C5), brachioradialis (C6), triceps (C7), patella (L4), and Achilles (S1).
- Babinski sign—Stroke from the lateral heel to the forefoot and then across the metatarsal heads. In an abnormal (positive) response, the great toe extends and the lesser toes fan out.
- Oppenheim's reflex—Firmly stroke down anterior tibial crest; response is the same as that to a Babinski sign.
- Umbilical—Stroke along all four quadrants adjacent to umbilicus. Normally, the umbilicus deviates (winks) toward each area being stroked.
- Lhermitte's sign—Passive flexion and compression of the neck may result in shock-like pain radiating down arms and legs.
- Hoffman's sign—A pathological reflex is elicited by "flicking" the middle finger of a hand at rest and watching for flexion of the distal thumb and index finger.
- Clonus—Quickly and passively dorsiflex the foot at the ankle; watch for abnormal repetitive planar flexion.
- Straight leg raise—Assesses nerve root tension.
- Assess for lower extremity abnormalities (cavus foot, clubfoot, vertical talus, and clawing of digits).

- The Cobb technique is routinely used to measure curves (Figure 11–4). To perform a Cobb measurement on either a posteroanterior or a lateral radiograph, identify the vertebrae most tilted with respect to the horizontal (the end vertebrae). Draw a line along the upper endplate of the most cranial end vertebra and a line perpendicular to this extending inferiorly. Then, identify the most caudal end vertebra and draw a line along its inferior endplate

Table 11–1: Neurological Levels

ROOT	REFLEX	MUSCLES	SENSATION
C5	Biceps	Deltoid, biceps	Lateral arm (axillary nerve)
C6	Brachioradialis	Wrist extension, biceps	Lateral forearm (musculocutaneous nerve)
C7	Triceps	Wrist flexors, finger extension, triceps	Middle finger
C8		Finger flexion, hand intrinsics	Medial forearm (medial antebrachial cutaneous nerve)
T1		Hand intrinsics	Medial arm (medial brachial cutaneous nerve)
L2		Iliopsoas (+/– quadriceps)	Anterior thigh, groin
L3	Patella	Quadriceps	Anterior and lateral thigh
L4	Patella	Quadriceps, anterior tibialis	Medial leg, malleolus, foot
L5	+/– posterior tibialis	Extensor hallucis longus, hip abductors	Lateral leg and dorsum of foot, first web space
S1	Achilles	Peroneus longus and brevis, gastroc-soleus	Lateral foot, little toe

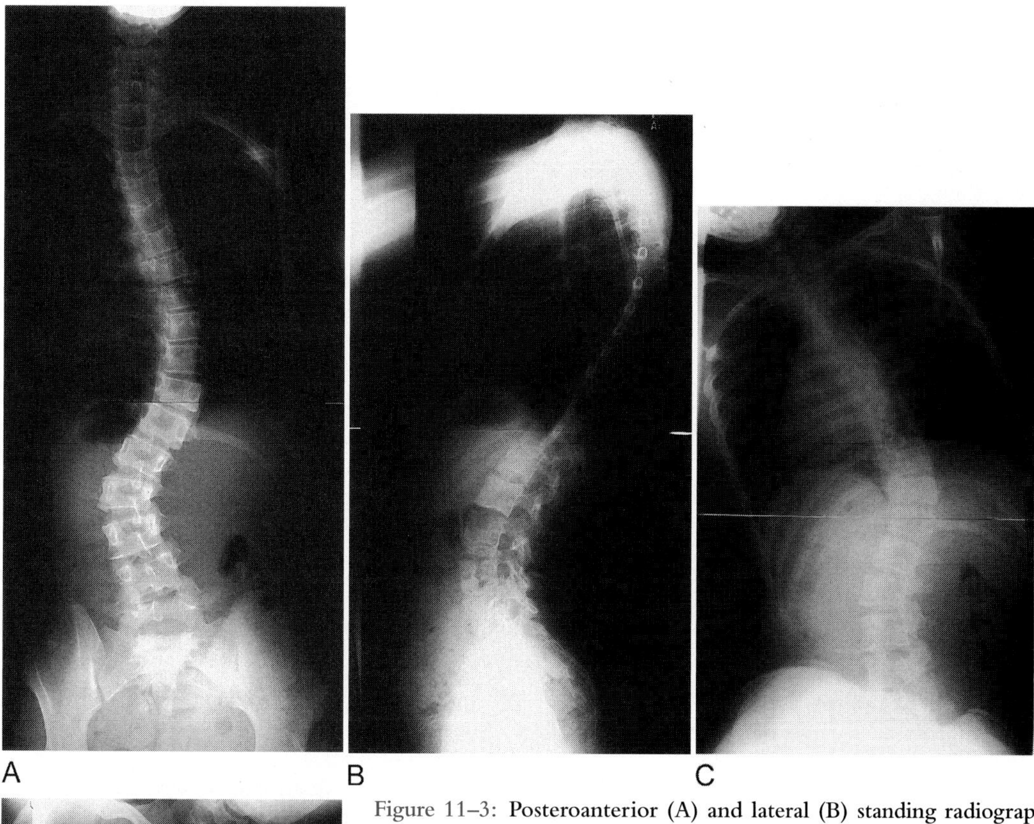

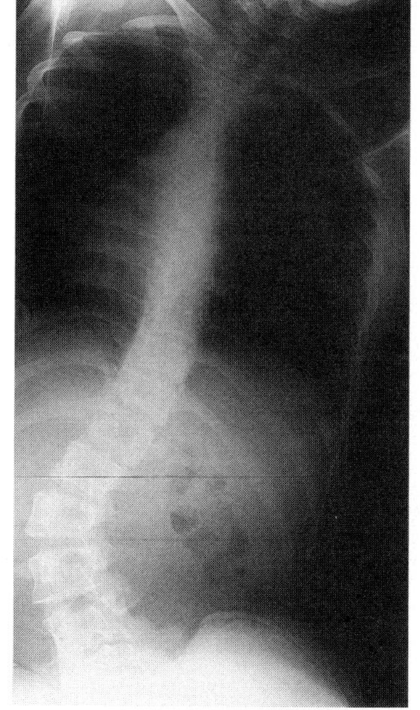

Figure 11–3: Posteroanterior (A) and lateral (B) standing radiographs of a patient with AIS. Curve flexibility can be demonstrated by having the patient bend to the left (C) or right (D).

with a perpendicular line extending proximally. The intersection of the perpendicular lines forms an angle, known as the *Cobb angle,* that represents the degree of scoliosis, kyphosis, or lordosis depending on the plane and directions. If multiple curves exist, the caudal end vertebra of the cranial curve is also the cranial end vertebra of the next caudal curve, referred to as a *transitional vertebra.*

- Scoliosis is frequently associated with rotational deformity that may manifest itself as rib asymmetry on lateral radiographs or pedicle asymmetry on posteroanterior radiographs.
- On a posteroanterior view, a plumb line dropped from C7 should pass through the center sacral line. On a lateral image, a vertical line passing through the body of C7 should intersect the body of S2. The amount by which

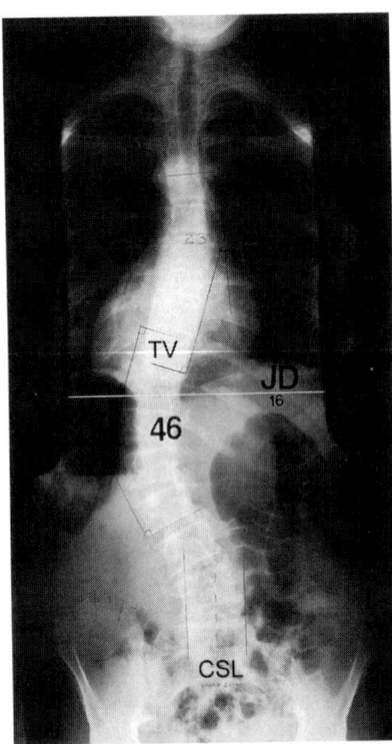

Figure 11–4: Posteroanterior radiograph of a 16-year-old male with AIS. The Cobb technique reveals a 46-degree major curve and a compensatory 23-degree thoracic curve. Based on the iliac crest, this patient is Risser 4. *CSL,* center sacral line that bisects the stable zone of Harrington; *TV,* transitional vertebra.

the vertical axis deviates from the sacral reference point is referred to as decompensation.

- The stable zone of Harrington refers to an imaginary column formed by extending perpendicular lines up from the lumbosacral facets on the posteroanterior radiograph[3] (Figure 11–4).
- The *stable vertebra* refers to the vertebra within a curve that is most closely bisected by the center sacral vertical line.
- The *apical vertebra* is the one most laterally deviated from the center sacral line.
- The Risser sign can be used to assess skeletal maturity and can be seen on posteroanterior radiographs that include the iliac crests (Figure 11–4). Although the iliac crest apophysis ossifies from anterior to posterior, radiographically, it appears to progress from lateral to medial. The apophysis is divided into imaginary quarters. Risser 0 occurs before any ossification; Risser 1 to 4 describe sequential increases in ossification; Risser 5 represents fusion of the apophysis with the iliac crest. Risser 1 corresponds to the most rapid skeletal growth spurt and may be associated with curve progression. (In addition, premenarcheal status and presence of an open triradiate cartilage indicate skeletal immaturity. A more precise skeletal bone age can be determined with a radiograph of the left hand and wrist, which is then compared with normal standards in the Greulich and Pyle *Radiographic Atlas of Skeletal Development of the Hand and Wrist.*)
- Specific areas of concern, such as the lumbosacral junction in patients with suspected spondylolysis or painful areas in patients with trauma or suspected tumors, can be evaluated with cone-down or oblique radiographs focused to highlight the anatomical region.
- In oblique radiographs of the lumbosacral spine, the outline of a Scottie dog can be traced. The ears are the superior articular process, the nose is the transverse process, the eye is the pedicle, the neck is the pars, the back is the lamina, and the front leg is the inferior articular process. Isthmic defects of the pars, as in spondylolysis, appear as a collar on the dog (Figure 11–5).
- Magnetic resonance imaging (MRI) is useful for identifying spinal cord pathology such as syringomyelia, Arnold-Chiari malformations, tethered cords, and tumors. Such imaging is recommended for any atypical curves (Figure 11–6, A-B).
- Computerized tomography (CT) is useful when fine bony detail is desired—for example, when evaluating acute fractures, spondylolysis, and bone tumors such as aneurysmal bone cysts, osteoid osteomas, and osteoblastomas (Figure 11–6, C). Three-dimensional reconstructions can be created to better represent complex deformities.
- Myelography, which involves injecting contrast material into the subarachnoid space followed by imaging with CT or

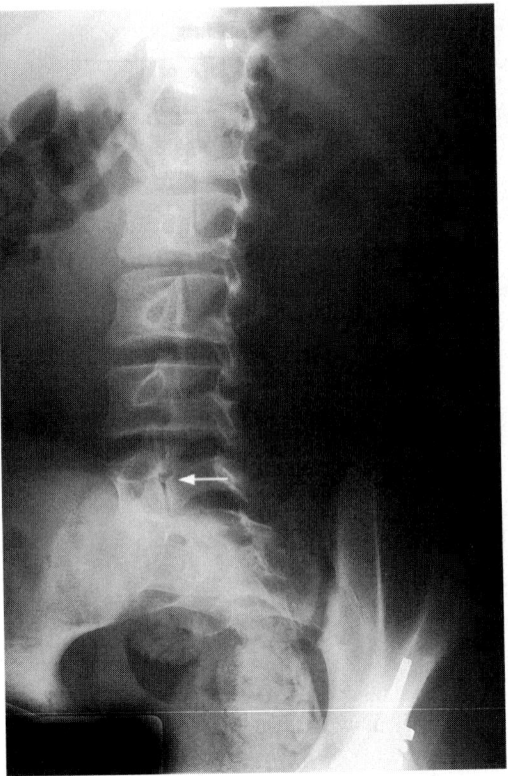

Figure 11–5: Oblique radiograph of the lumbosacral spine with spondylolysis *(arrow).* This pars defect appears as a collar on a Scottie dog (see text for explanation).

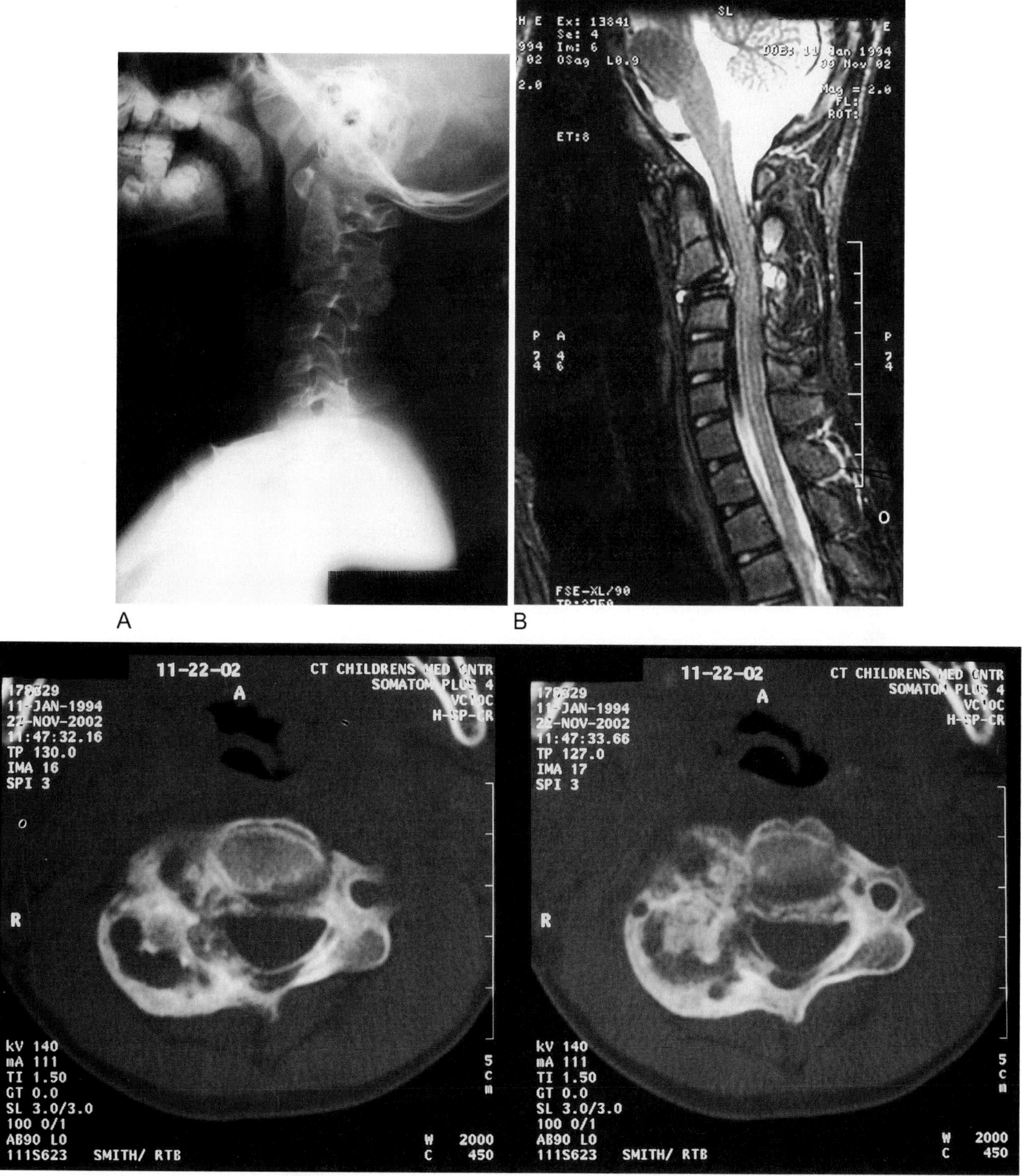

Figure 11–6: A, A lateral radiograph demonstrating kyphosis caused by a spinal tumor. B, An MRI scan demonstrates the loss of anterior vertebral height and mild cord impingement caused by the aneurysmal bone cyst. C, Axial CT images better demonstrate the bony detail.

plain radiographs, can be used to localize areas of spinal cord impingement caused by tumors, dysraphism, or deformity. Since the advent of MRI, myelography is used less frequently and usually reserved for complex deformities.

- Radionuclide bone imaging (also known as scintigraphy or bone scanning) typically involves injecting technetium-99m methylene diphosphonate intravenously to localize areas of increased bone activity. Imaging with single-photon emission computerized tomography (SPECT) provides excellent spatial resolution and is frequently used to evaluate low back pain or suspected spondylolysis (Figure 11–7). Gallium-67 citrate or indium-111–labeled white blood cells can be used to detect the foci of infection.

Laboratory Studies

- Blood tests are not required for all cases of spinal disorders.
- Patients with night pain or constitutional symptoms suggesting infection or neoplasm should be studied with a complete blood count, erythrocyte sedimentation rate, and C-reactive protein evaluation. Blood cultures may be obtained but are frequently inconclusive.
- Patients suspected of having a rheumatological condition should have their rheumatoid factor, antinuclear antibody, and human leukocyte antigen B27 levels tested. Morning stiffness, multiple joint involvement, sacroiliitis, or associated iritis or urethritis warrants a rheumatological evaluation.
- Lyme disease has become endemic in certain geographical regions, and its presenting symptoms may include diffuse aches such as back pain. Although not a typical cause of back complaints, Lyme disease can be tested with a Lyme titer followed by a Western blot analysis.

Adolescent Idiopathic Scoliosis

- *Idiopathic Scoliosis* refers to scoliosis (lateral deviation with associated rotational deformity and a Cobb measurement of more than 10 degrees) that is not associated with any other condition or identifiable cause and that can be subclassified into infantile, juvenile, and adolescent types based on the age of onset. (Each subtype will be addressed in a separate section.)
- Adolescent idiopathic scoliosis (AIS), with age of onset after 10 years, is the most common form of scoliosis, with a prevalence of approximately 25 per 1,000. Smaller curves are more prevalent than larger curves, and females are affected more than males (Table 11–2).
- Patients with AIS have a positive family history approximately 30% of the time. A specific gene or mode of inheritance has not yet been identified; however, multifactorial or autosomal dominance with variable expressivity seem most likely.
- Growth hormone, melatonin, calmodulin, vestibular–ocular–proprioceptive functions, and connective tissue alterations have all been implicated in the etiology, although the cause is still unknown.
- Curves are described by location and direction, with right thoracic curves most common followed by double major (right thoracic, left lumbar), left lumbar, and right lumbar

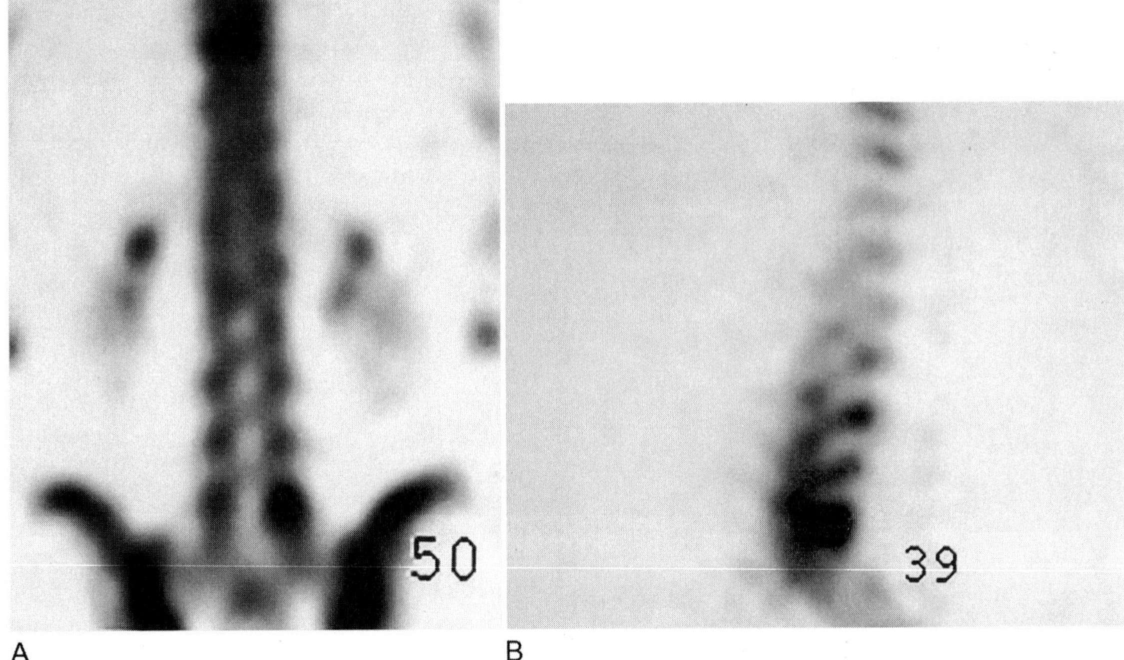

Figure 11–7: Coronal (A) and sagittal (B) SPECT images of the patient in Figure 11–5 with spondylolysis of L5-S1.

Table 11–2: Prevalence of Adolescent Idiopathic Scoliosis

COBB ANGLE (DEGREES)	FEMALE-TO-MALE RATIO	PREVALENCE (%)
>10	1.4-2:1	2-3
>20	5.4:1	0.3-0.5
>30	10:1	0.1-0.3
>40		<0.1

From Weinstein SL (2001) Adolescent idiopathic scoliosis: Natural history. In: The Pediatric Spine: Principles and Practice, 2nd edition (Weinstein SL, ed). Philadelphia: Lippincott Williams & Wilkins.

curves. Left lumbar curves are considered atypical and warrant MRI evaluation.

- School screening has been endorsed by the American Academy of Orthopaedic Surgeons and the Scoliosis Research Society for girls 11 and 13 years and boys 13 or 14 years. The individual is examined while performing an Adam's forward bend test. A scoliometer can be used to detect the degree of rotational deformity, with 7 degrees warranting referral to a physician because of its acceptable referral rate (3%) and positive predictive value[4] (Figure 11–8).
- Patients at greatest risk for curve progression are those with double curve patterns, large curve magnitude, younger age, presentation of curve before menarche, and lower Risser grade at time of detection.[5] For a given magnitude of curve, females are at greater risk of progression than males.
- A careful history and physical examination is performed (as described in the previous sections), and radiographs are obtained to characterize the curve.

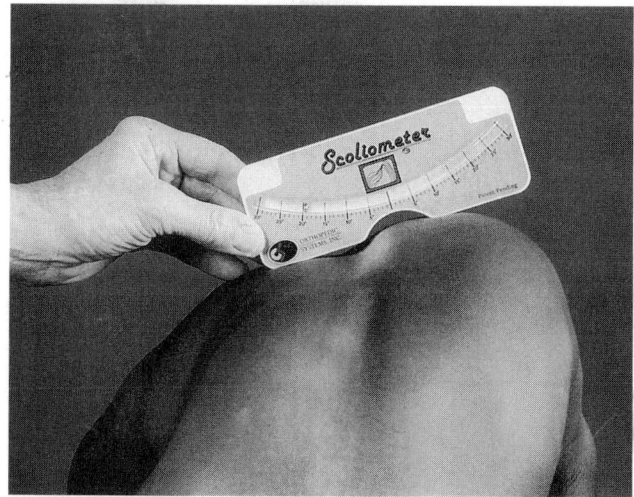

Figure 11–8: Clinical photo of a patient performing an Adams forward bend test demonstrating 20 degrees of rotation with a scoliometer. From Pierz KA, Dormans JP (2004) Spinal disorders: The essentials for the pediatrician. In: Requisites in Pediatrics: Orthopedics and Sports Medicine (Dormans JP, ed). Philadelphia: Mosby.

- Treatment should prevent curve progression so that patients can enter adulthood with curves less than 50 degrees, a balanced spine, and cosmetic acceptability.
- Treatment is based on magnitude of deformity, curve progression, and patient maturity:
  - Curves less than 25 degrees in an immature patient—Observe serially
  - Curves 25 to 30 degrees in an immature patient with 5 to 10 degrees of progression—Brace
  - Curves 30 to 40 degrees in an immature patient—Brace
  - Curves greater than 40 in an immature patient (or greater than 50 degrees in a mature patient)—Surgery

Treatment Options

- Treatment options include observation, bracing, and surgery.

Observation and Bracing

- Observation is recommended for small (less than 30 degrees), nonprogressive curves or for patients approaching skeletal maturity (Risser 4 or 5).
- Bracing is recommended in immature patients with curves greater than 30 degrees (or greater than 25 degrees and evidence of progression). Patients with hypokyphosis or thoracic lordosis may not respond to bracing. To be most effective, bracing is usually prescribed for full-time usage (22 to 23 hours/day) until a patient is 1.5 to 2 years postmenarcheal or at least Risser 4.[6]
  - The Milwaukee brace is a cervical thoracolumbosacral orthosis (CTLSO) consisting of a molded pelvic portion, metallic upright supports, pressure pads along the thoracic apices, a throat mold, and an occipital upper portion (Figure 11–9). Compliance is an issue because of the high profile and visibility of the cervical extension. This brace is still recommended for curves with apices above T7.
  - The Boston brace is a thoracolumbosacral orthosis (TLSO) with prefabricated pelvic and thoracolumbar modules and custom lateral pressure pads (Figure 11–10). Similar braces include the Wilmington brace and the Miami brace. Compliance is improved because of the low profile of the TLSO.
  - The Charleston bending brace and the Providence brace are TLSOs that provide a bending force against the curve and are designed to be worn only at night (Figure 11–11).

Surgery

- Surgery is indicated for patients with large or progressive curves. Posterior spinal fusion (PSF) with instrumentation remains the gold standard for most thoracic or double major curves (Figure 11–12); however, anterior spinal fusion (ASF) with instrumentation has gained acceptance in treating thoracolumbar and lumbar curves (Figure 11–13).

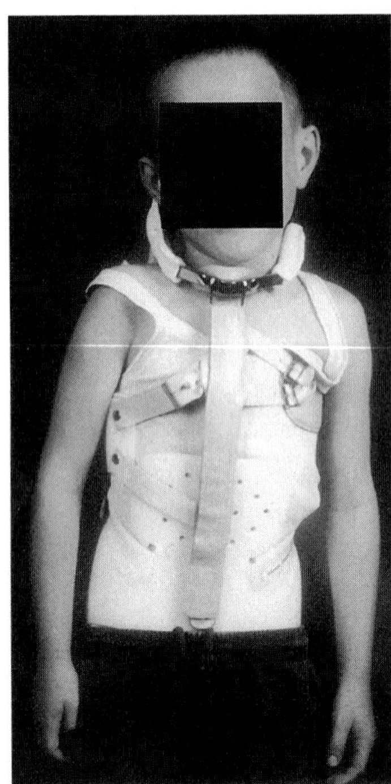

Figure 11–9: Clinical photo of a patient wearing a Milwaukee CTLSO. From Pierz KA, Dormans JP (2004) Spinal disorders: The essentials for the pediatrician. In: Requisites in Pediatrics: Orthopedics and Sports Medicine (Dormans JP, ed). Philadelphia: Mosby.

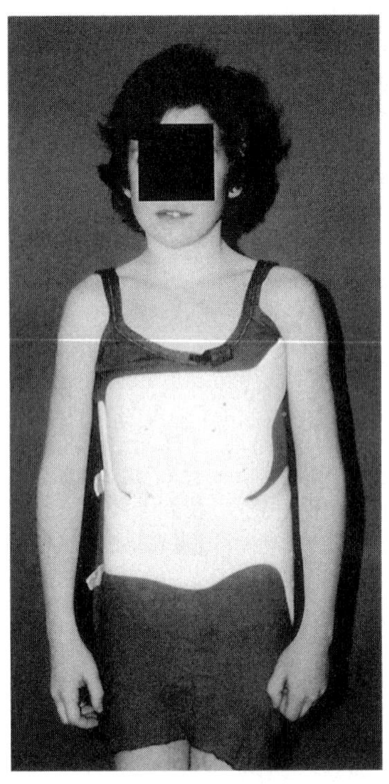

Figure 11–10: Clinical photo of a patient wearing a Boston TLSO. From Pierz KA, Dormans JP (2004) Spinal disorders: The essentials for the pediatrician. In: Requisites in Pediatrics: Orthopedics and Sports Medicine (Dormans JP, ed). Philadelphia: Mosby.

ASF with instrumentation may save lower fusion levels and improve correction by creating increased mobility through anterior disk excision. To prevent the lumbar kyphosis associated with anterior instrumentation, structural autograft or allograft can be placed to create structural interbody support. Combining ASF and PSF is indicated for severe curves (greater than 70 degrees), for stiff curves (those that don't correct less than 50 degrees on bending films), and to prevent crankshaft (in girls younger than 10 years or boys younger than 13 years with open triradiate cartilage). The goals of surgical correction are to achieve (A) a solid *arthrodesis* or fusion to prevent future pain and curve progression, (B) a *balanced* spine with the head centered over the sacrum, and (C) a *correction* of the deformity to produce acceptable cosmetic results.

- Because scoliosis is a three-dimensional deformity, surgical correction should be aimed at correcting the entire deformity. Original posterior techniques with Harrington instrumentation involved placing hooks above and below the curves and distracting along a rod. This allowed correction in the coronal plane but frequently flattened the spine in the sagittal plane. Newer techniques use hooks, sublaminar wires, pedicle screws, or a combination of these to provide multiple points of fixation. Precontouring the rods and derotating can produce harmonious correction of the deformity in all planes[7] (Figure 11–14).
- The King-Moe classification has been used to describe and to plan surgical correction of idiopathic scoliosis[3] (Figure 11–15). Although useful for treating many thoracic or thoracolumbar curves, this system fails to acknowledge the sagittal plane. Care must be taken to avoid overcorrecting types II, III, and IV curves to prevent postoperative decompensation.

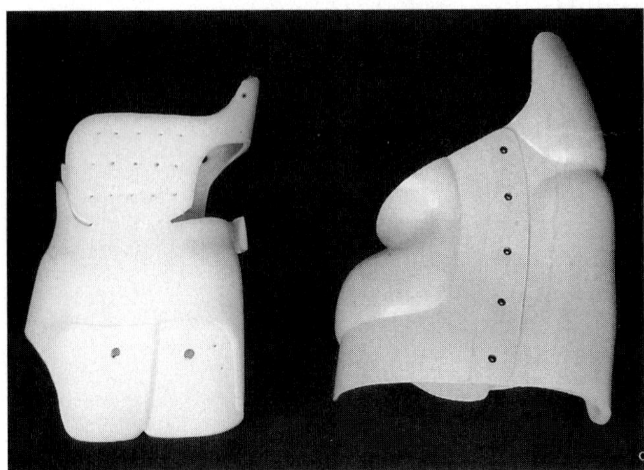

Figure 11–11: A typical Boston TLSO *(left)* next to a night-time bending brace *(right)*. From Pierz KA, Dormans JP (2004) Spinal disorders: The essentials for the pediatrician. In: Requisites in Pediatrics: Orthopedics and Sports Medicine (Dormans JP, ed). Philadelphia: Mosby.

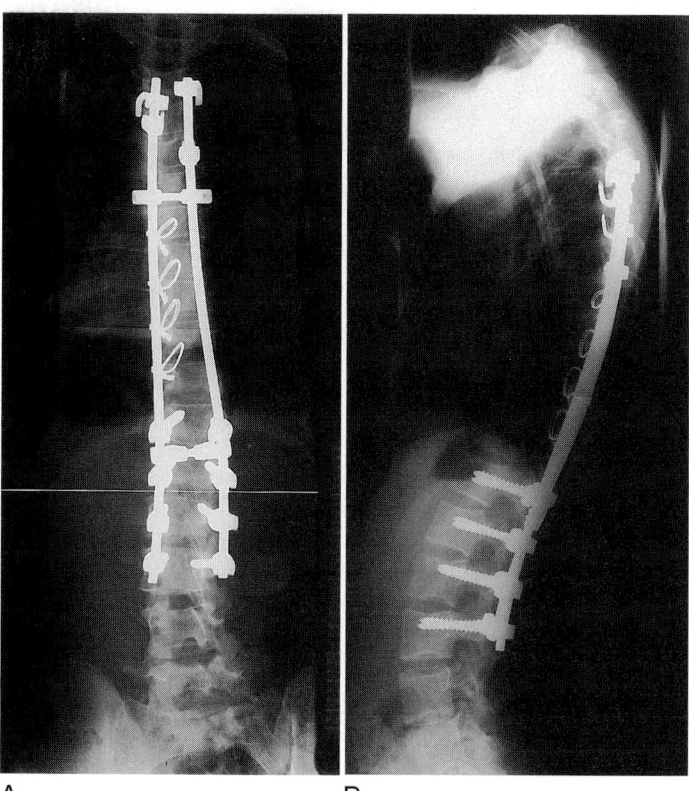

Figure 11–12: Posteroanterior (A) and lateral (B) radiographs of the patient from Figure 11–3 after undergoing PSF and instrumentation.

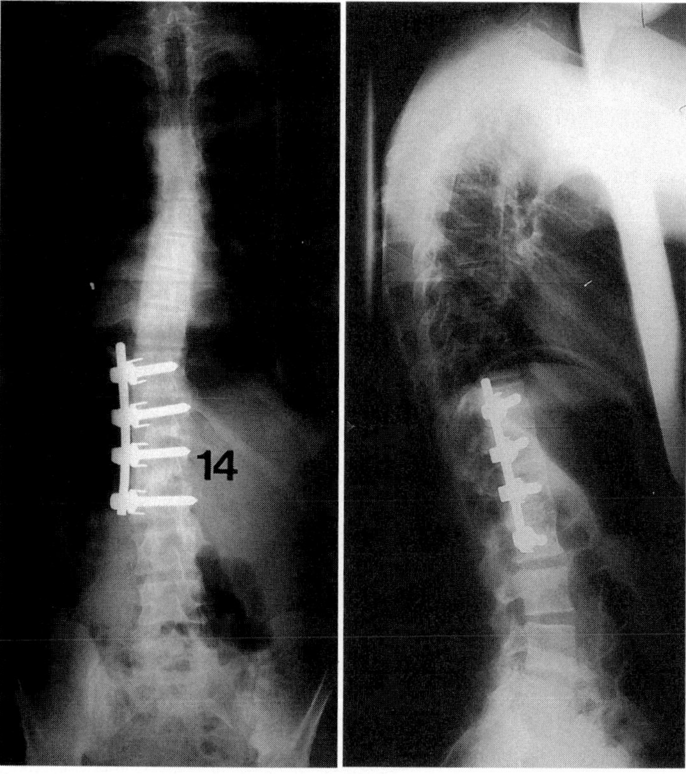

Figure 11–13: Posteroanterior (A) and lateral (B) radiographs of the patient from Figure 11–4 after undergoing ASF and instrumentation.

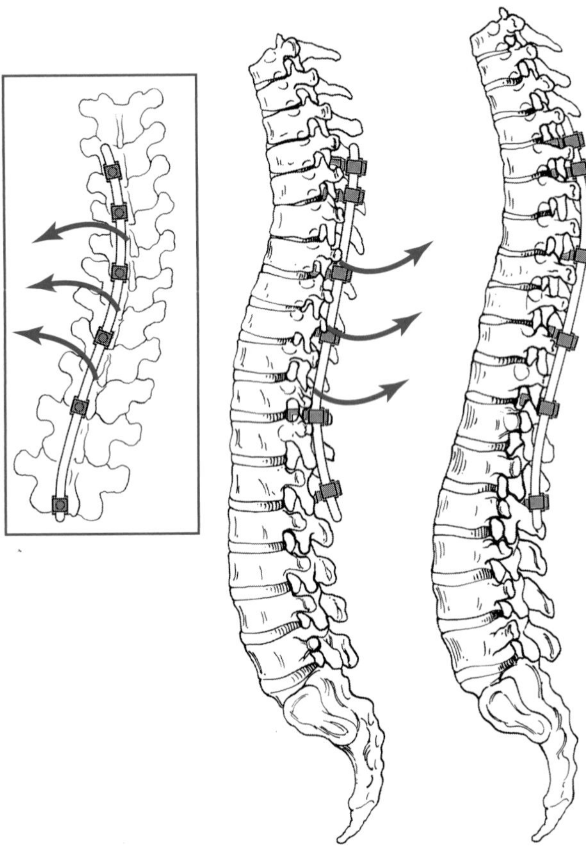

Figure 11–14: Rotating a concave rod applies translational corrective forces to scoliosis, pulls the instrumented segment back to the midline, and restores sagittal balance. **From Zeller RD, Dubousset J (2001) Idiopathic scoliosis treated by a posterior approach. In: Surgical Techniques in Orthopaedics and Traumatology. Paris: Elsevier, pp 1-9.**

- A King-Moe type I curve is a double major curve with the lumbar curve greater and less flexible than the thoracic curve. PSF should include both curves; however, ASF may be considered to treat the lumbar curve alone.
- A King-Moe type II curve is a double major curve with the thoracic curve greater and less flexible than the lumbar curve. If the lumbar curve is greater than 50 degrees, both curves should be included in the PSF.
- A King-Moe type III curve is a thoracic curve in which the lumbar curve is nonexistent or does not cross the midline. Only the thoracic curve needs to be included in the fusion.
- A King-Moe type IV curve is a long thoracic of thoracolumbar curve, with L4 typically tilted into the curve. Pedicle screws may provide better control of these curves posteriorly. ASF has also gained popularity.
- A King-Moe type V curve is a double thoracic curve. Typically, the high left curve should be addressed to avoid further elevation of the left shoulder upon correction of the right thoracic curve. Usually, the fusion does not involve the compensatory lumbar curve.

- To overcome the limitations of the King-Moe classification, the Lenke system has been established and is rapidly gaining popularity[8] (Figure 11–16). This classification method includes six characteristic curve patterns in the coronal plane, lumbar spine modifiers (based on where the center sacral vertical line passes with respect to the apical vertebra), and sagittal thoracic modifiers.
- Surgical intervention can result in complications. The risk of postoperative neurological deficit can be minimized by monitoring intraoperative somatosensory-evoked potentials and making intraoperative adjustments (such as increasing blood pressure or decreasing correction) if changes occur. The Stagnara wake-up test can also detect whether an injury has occurred but cannot detect individual motor units. Spinal decompensation may result from incorrect selection of fusion levels. Partial thoracoplasty (removing portions of the apical ribs) can decrease the risk of persistent rib prominence. Flatback syndrome can be minimized with proper rod contouring. Crankshaft can be prevented by performing anterior diskectomy and fusion in immature patients. Pseudarthroses (1 to 2%), wound infection (1%), and hardware failure or prominence (10 to 15%) are also potential complications.

Juvenile Idiopathic Scoliosis

- Juvenile idiopathic scoliosis (JIS) has an age of onset between 3 and 10 years.
- JIS accounts for 12 to 21% of all idiopathic scolioses.[9]
- Presentation and treatment are similar to that of AIS.
- Curve progression is common, and approximately 70% require treatment (about 50% require bracing; the other 50% require surgery).
- Although it is desirable to delay surgery until after the onset of the pubertal growth spurt, curves greater than 50 degrees may warrant earlier treatment. Spinal instrumentation without fusion may be used to delay definitive surgery. Combining an anterior fusion with a posterior fusion with instrumentation can be performed to decrease the risk of crankshaft phenomenon, as with infantile scoliosis.

Infantile Idiopathic Scoliosis

- Infantile idiopathic scoliosis (IIS) presents symptoms before 3 years of age.
- It is more common in Europe than the United States.
- Supine or semisupine infant positioning may play a role.
- It affects males more than females.
- A higher rate of cardiopulmonary compromise is found in those younger than 5 years and may be caused by inadequate alveoli formation.

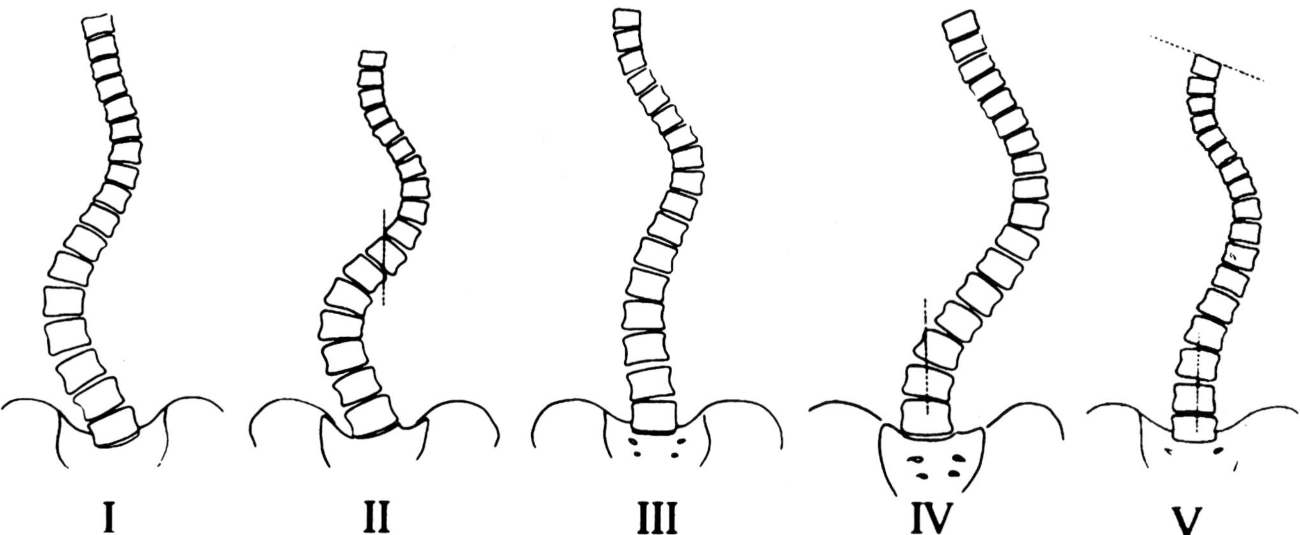

Figure 11–15: Illustration of the five King-Moe patterns of AIS (see text for details). Adapted from King HA, Moe JH, Bradford DS, et al. (1983) The selection of fusion levels in idiopathic scoliosis. J Bone Joint Surg Am 65: 1302-1313.

Curve Type

Type	Proximal Thoracic	Main Thoracic	Thoracolumbar / Lumbar	Curve Type
1	Non-Structural	Structural (Major*)	Non-Structural	Main Thoracic (MT)
2	Structural	Structural (Major*)	Non-Structural	Double Thoracic (DT)
3	Non-Structural	Structural (Major*)	Structural	Double Major (DM)
4	Structural	Structural (Major*)	Structural	Triple Major (TM)
5	Non-Structural	Non-Structural	Structural (Major*)	Thoracolumbar / Lumbar (TL/L)
6	Non-Structural	Structural	Structural (Major*)	Thoracolumbar / Lumbar - Main Thoracic (TL/L - MT)

*Major = Largest Cobb Measurement, always structural
Minor = all other curves with structural criteria applied

STRUCTURAL CRITERIA
(Minor Curves)

Proximal Thoracic: - Side Bending Cobb ≥ 25°
- T2 - T5 Kyphosis ≥ +20°

Main Thoracic: - Side Bending Cobb ≥ 25°
- T10 - L2 Kyphosis ≥ +20°

Thoracolumbar / Lumbar: - Side Bending Cobb ≥ 25°
- T10 - L2 Kyphosis ≥ +20°

LOCATION OF APEX
(SRS definition)

CURVE	APEX
THORACIC	T2 - T11-12 DISC
THORACOLUMBAR	T12 - L1
LUMBAR	L1-2 DISC - L4

Modifiers

Lumbar Spine Modifier	CSVL to Lumbar Apex
A	CSVL Between Pedicles
B	CSVL Touches Apical Body(ies)
C	CSVL Completely Medial

A B C

Thoracic Sagittal Profile T5 - T12	
− (Hypo)	< 10°
N (Normal)	10°- 40°
+ (Hyper)	> 40°

Curve Type (1-6) **+** Lumbar Spine Modifier (A, B, or C) **+** Thoracic Sagittal Modifier (−,*N*, or +)

Classification (e.g.1B+):__________

Figure 11–16: Summary of the Lenke classification system for spinal deformity. Similar to the King-Moe system, the main curve types (I-VI) are based on the location and flexibility of the curves. Location is defined by the apex of the curve, as described by the Scoliosis Research Society. The lumbar modifier (A-C) defines where the center–sacral–vertical line falls with respect to the lumbar vertebrae. The thoracic modifier (positive, normal, or negative) refers to the amount of sagittal kyphosis. From Lenke LG, Betz RR, Harms J, et al. (2001) Adolescent idiopathic scoliosis: A new classification to determine extent of spinal arthrodesis. J Bone Joint Surg Am 83: 1172.

- Plagiocephaly and developmental hip dysplasia may be associated.
- Left thoracic curves are most common followed by thoracolumbar curves.
- IIS is classified according to Mehta.[10] The rib–vertebral angle difference (RVAD) is a predictor or curve progression (Figure 11–17).
  - Measure the angle formed by the rib on the convex side of the curve to a perpendicular to the vertebral endplate *(A)*.
  - Measure the angle formed by the rib on the concave side of the curve to a perpendicular to the vertebral endplate *(B)*.
  - Subtract *A* from *B* to calculate the RVAD. An RVAD >20 degrees is likely to progress.
- Nonprogressive curves (below 25 degrees) frequently resolve spontaneously without treatment.
- Progressive curves are relentless and usually require treatment.
  - For curves between 25 and 30 degrees with an RVAD between 20 and 25 degrees, casting or bracing is indicated, especially if the curve progresses 10 degrees. Casting can be performed to decrease the curve to 25 degrees before implementing a brace.
  - For curves greater than 35 degrees, surgery is indicated. Instrumentation without fusion (subcutaneous "growing rods") may allow continued growth. Anterior and posterior fusion with instrumentation should be combined to decrease the risk of crankshaft phenomenon that can occur with unopposed anterior growth following isolated posterior fusions in skeletally immature patients.

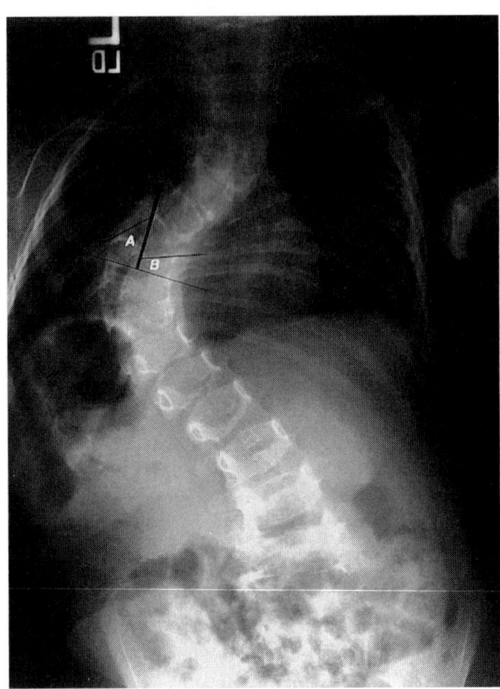

Figure 11–17: Posteroanterior radiograph of a 3-year-old girl with IIS. RVAD = B to A.

Neuromuscular Scoliosis

- Any condition that affects the ability of the central nervous system to control distal motor units can potentially deform the spine.
- Cerebral palsy, myelodysplasia, muscular dystrophies, spinal muscular atrophy, Friedreich ataxia, traumatic paralysis, and neurofibromatosis are some of the conditions that may have associated scoliosis (Table 11–3).
- Neuromuscular curves are frequently long, sweeping curves with pelvic obliquity and other skeletal involvement. Neurofibromatosis, however, is associated with short, severe curves.
- Neuromuscular curves tend to progress more rapidly than idiopathic curves; they continue progressing after skeletal maturity.
- Severe curves and pelvic obliquity may make wheelchair seating difficult.
- Neuromuscular patients are more prone to pulmonary complications, which may be compounded by severe curves.
- Bracing is less effective than with idiopathic scoliosis. It may be used to try to slow curve progression until about 10 to 12 years of age, but corrective surgery is usually the treatment of choice for large curves.
- The goal of surgery should be to achieve a stable spine with the trunk centered over a level pelvis.[11] This facilitates seating and transfers.
- Because of the potential for curves to progress above or below the fusion mass, surgery usually includes T2 to the pelvis for nonambulatory patients. Inclusion of the pelvis in ambulators may potentially limit their ability to walk.
- *Luque-Galveston technique* involves segmental sublaminar wire fixation of the spine to paired rods (Luque) and attachment to the pelvis by bending the caudal ends from the lamina of S1 into the posterosuperior iliac spines extending between the inner and the outer tables of the

Table 11–3: Neuromuscular Disorders and Associated Spinal Deformities

NEUROMUSCULAR DISORDER DEFORMITY (%)	PATIENTS WITH SPINAL
Cerebral palsy	25
Myelodysplasia	60 (higher in thoracic levels)
Spinal muscular atrophy	65
Friedreich ataxia	80
Duchenne muscular dystrophy	90
Traumatic paralysis	Depends on level (>90 for cervical)
Marfan's syndrome	75
Achondroplasia	20 (kyphosis)
Osteogenesis imperfecta	50

ilium (Galveston). The *unit rod* is a single rod precontoured into a U shape with thoracic kyphosis, lumbar lordosis, and pelvic extensions.

- Nutritional status can affect healing and should be optimized preoperatively.

Specific Conditions

- *Cerebral palsy*—This upper motor neuron syndrome causes abnormal control of motor function (usually spasticity) because of insult to the immature brain before 2 years; intelligence may or may not be affected.
  - Quadriplegia affects all four extremities, diplegia affects lower extremities more than upper extremities, and hemiplegia affects one side of body.
  - Spinal deformities may be postural or structural.
  - Scoliosis is most common in patients with quadriplegia; lordosis is common in patients with hip flexion contractures, and kyphosis is common in patients with hamstring contractures or poor sitting balance.
  - Thoracolumbar spinal orthosis or seating modifications may be tried initially.
  - Surgery is indicated for progressive curves greater than 45 to 50 degrees (Usually Luque-Galveston or unit rod techniques unless still ambulatory) (Figure 11–18).
  - Anterior release and fusion may be combined with posterior fusion for patients with skeletal immaturity or severe curves.
  - Complication rates are generally lower in patients with anterior and posterior fusions performed the same day rather than staged over 1 to 2 weeks; however, the patient's medical stability and the surgeon's skill must be considered before attempting a same-day combined procedure.
- *Myelodysplasia* (also known as *spina bifida* or *spinal dysraphism*)—This condition is caused by a defect occurring during the formation of the neural tube.
  - Failed neural tube closure may result in defects of the bony posterior arch alone *(spina bifida occulta),* herniation of the meninges *(meningocele)* or the spinal cord and meninges *(myelomeningocele)* through the posterior spine into a sac protruding from the patient's back, or completely uncovered neural elements *(rachischisis)* with symptoms based on the level and severity of the lesion.
  - Diagnosis can be made *in utero* based on increased α-fetoprotein levels.
  - Rapid curve progression or sudden neurological changes (increased spasticity, bowel or bladder changes, or new deformities) may be caused by a *tethered cord, hydrocephalus,* or *hydromyelia* and may warrant investigation with MRI or myelography.
  - Scoliosis is present in almost all patients with thoracic level function, in approximately 60% of patients with L4 level function, and less commonly in patients with lower level lesions.
  - Nonambulatory patients are at the greatest risk for curve progression, and bracing may be complicated by a lack of protective sensation resulting in pressure sores and rib cage deformity.
  - Curves greater than 40 degrees frequently progress and are usually treated with surgery. Anterior and posterior fusions with Luque-Galveston instrumentation are recommended (Figure 11–19).
  - Kyphosis may be treated with partial or complete vertebral body resection, fusion, and instrumentation.

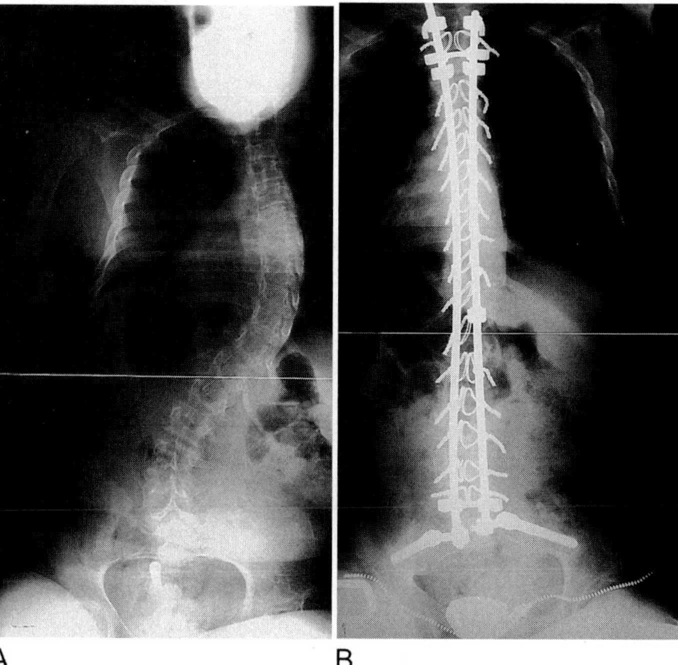

Figure 11–18: Preoperative (A) and postoperative (B) radiographs of a boy with cerebral palsy and neuromuscular scoliosis. **PSF and instrumentation to the pelvis allowed restoration of sitting balance.**

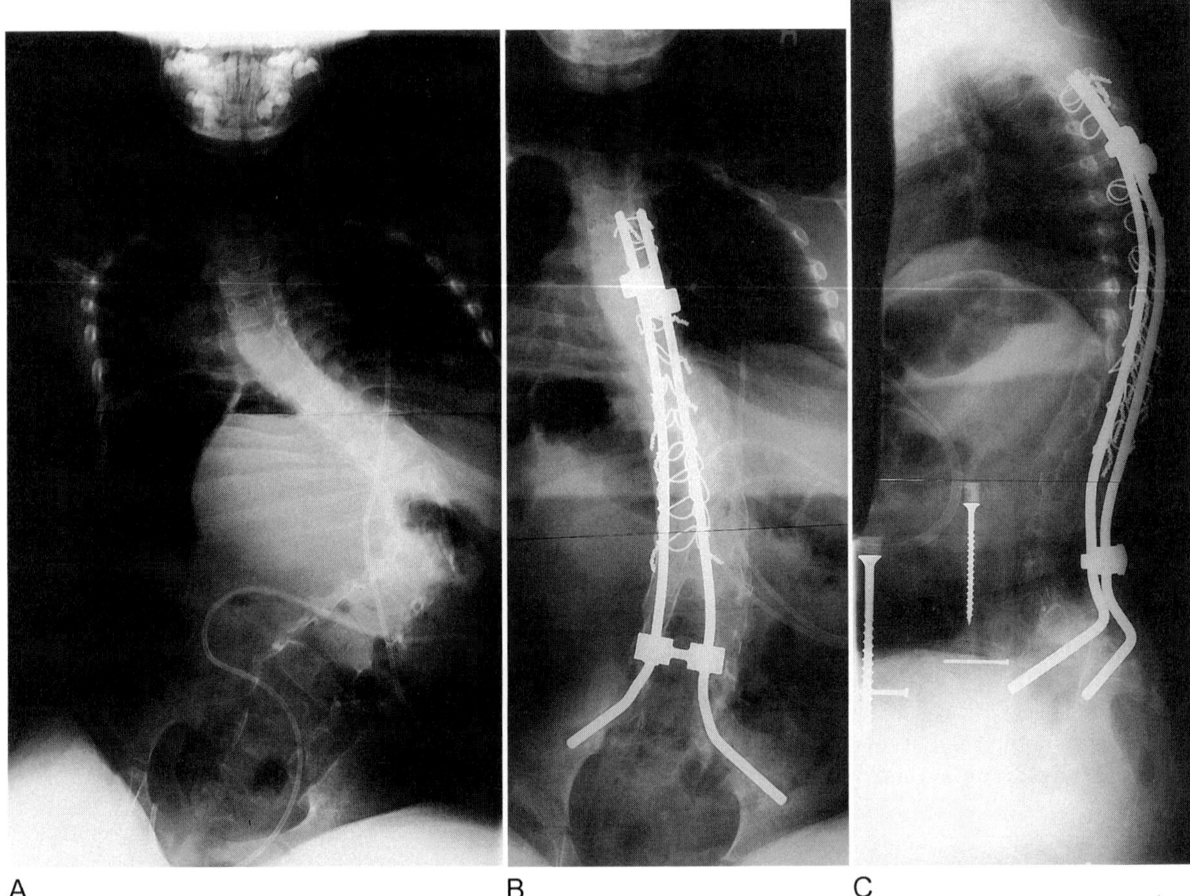

Figure 11–19: Preoperative (A) and postoperative (B and C) radiographs of a patient with severe scoliosis secondary to spina bifida. **Note the ventriculoperitoneal shunt catheter previously placed to decompress hydrocephalus.**

  - Surgical complications caused by infection, skin breakdown, and pseudarthrosis are common.
- *Duchenne muscular dystrophy*—This sex-linked recessive abnormality of boys is characterized by absent dystrophin protein and elevated creatine phosphokinase.
  - It can be diagnosed by muscle biopsy or deoxyribonucleic acid testing.
  - Connective tissue infiltration of muscles results in progressive weakness, decreased motor skills, and calf pseudohypertrophy.
  - Patients typically become wheelchair-bound by 15 years.
  - Scoliosis affects almost all patients and progresses rapidly after patients lose ambulatory status (about 10 degrees/year).
  - Surgery is indicated for patients with curves greater than 20 to 30 degrees to improve seating position, feeding, respiratory function, and self-image.
  - Pulmonary function declines rapidly and is best monitored by the percentage of forced vital capacity (FVC). Spinal surgery should ideally be performed before the FVC falls below 40%.
  - Segmental instrumentation from the upper thorax to L5 may be sufficient in curves less than 25 degrees, but extension to the pelvis (Luque-Galveston technique or unit rod) is recommended for curves greater than 40 degrees or in the presence of any pelvic obliquity.
  - Becker's dystrophy is a milder form seen in patients who live beyond the second decade.
- *Spinal muscular atrophy*—This autosomal recessive disorder is caused by a loss of anterior horn cells from the spinal cord with progressive motor loss.
  - Werdnig-Hoffman disease is present at birth and rapidly progresses, whereas less severe forms may not present symptoms until early childhood and are associated with better motor function.
  - Scoliosis is seen in 50 to 100% of cases depending on the severity of the disease.
  - Treatment is similar to that for muscular dystrophy.

- *Friedreich ataxia*—This spinocerebellar degenerative disease involves motor and sensory defects.
  - Patients frequently have a wide-based gait, cardiomyopathy, nystagmus, cavus feet, and scoliosis.
  - Scoliosis treatment is similar to that for idiopathic scoliosis.
- *Neurofibromatosis*—This is an autosomal dominant disorder of neural crest origin. Multiple types exist; the most common are neurofibromatosis type I, or von Recklinghausen disease, and neurofibromatosis type II, which includes acoustical neuromas and rarely has peripheral manifestations. Neurofibromatosis type I will be described later because of its skeletal manifestations.
  - The diagnosis of neurofibromatosis type I requires two of seven criteria (Box 11–7).
  - Vertebral scalloping and enlarged foramina may produce the appearance of "dumbbell vertebrae" on radiographs.
  - Nondystrophic curves, or idiopathic-like scoliosis, may be managed similarly to idiopathic scoliosis.
  - Dystrophic curves are characterized by short, tight, kyphoscoliotic curves with severe apical rotation. Such curves are relentlessly progressive and do not respond to bracing.
  - Surgery should include anterior and posterior fusion to decrease the rate of pseudarthrosis.
  - Preoperative MRI or myelogram is indicated to rule out intraspinal tumors or dural ectasia (Figure 11–20).
- *Marfan's syndrome*—This autosomal dominant disorder of collagen synthesis is associated with ligamentous laxity, tall height, arachnodactyly (long, thin fingers), cardiac valve problems, superior lens dislocations of the eyes, pectus (sternal) deformities, and spinal disorders, including scoliosis, lordosis, and spondylolisthesis.
  - Approximately 75% of patients develop scoliosis, most before 9 years of age.
  - Curves tend to be rigid and rapidly progressive during adolescence. Pain and respiratory problems may also be associated.
  - Bracing is usually unsuccessful.
  - Surgical treatment is similar to that for idiopathic scoliosis; however, pseudarthrosis rates are more common. Adding an anterior fusion and postoperative bracing may decrease the rate of pseudarthrosis but may increase the rate of superior mesenteric artery syndrome (prolonged ileus secondary to pressure or stretch on the superior mesenteric artery).
- *Osteogenesis imperfecta*—This autosomal dominant or autosomal recessive disorder is characterized by a defect in type I collagen (procollagen to type I collagen sequence defect resulting in abnormal cross-linking).
  - Spinal deformities occur in 20 to 80% of patients depending on disease severity.
  - Bracing is ineffective.
  - Surgery is indicated for progressive curves above 35 degrees. Segmental sublaminar wiring is recommended.
  - Cervical spine deformities may be associated with basilar impressions. Treatment should include anterior decompression and posterior fusion.
- *Achondroplasia*—One of many skeletal dysplasias, this autosomal dominant condition has an 80% spontaneous mutation rate and results in disproportionate, short-limbed dwarfism caused by abnormal enchondral bone formation. Individuals are characterized by a normal trunk and short limbs (rhizomelia), frontal bossing, small nasal bridge, trident hands, radial head subluxation, thoracolumbar kyphosis, lumbar stenosis, and excessive lordosis.
  - Thoracolumbar kyphosis is common before walking age and usually resolves spontaneously.
  - Anterior fusion with strut grafting and PSF are indicated for kyphosis more than 60 degrees in older children and adults.
  - Stenosis may occur because of excessive periosteal bone formation and short pedicles resulting in narrow canals and foramina.
  - Back pain occurs in 50% of cases.
  - Surgical decompression is recommended for those with neurological deficits and progressive symptoms. Fusion can be added to prevent postlaminectomy instability.

Box 11–7 Diagnostic Criteria for Neurofibromatosis Type I

(At least two are required for diagnosis)

- At least six café-au-lait spots (more than 5 mm in children; more than 15 mm in adults)
- At least two neurofibromas or one plexiform neurofibroma
- Axillary or inguinal freckling
- Osseous lesion (such as vertebral scalloping, scoliosis, or congenital pseudarthrosis)
- An optic glioma
- At least two Lisch nodules (hamartoma of the iris detected through slit lamp examination)
- First-degree relative with neurofibromatosis type I

Congenital Scoliosis

- Lateral curvature of the spine is caused by vertebral anomalies that develop in the embryonic period (Figure 11–21).
- Although the anomaly is present at birth, the clinical deformity may not be detected until later in life.
- Because some anomalies produce no deformity and are never detected, the true incidence remains unknown.
- *Failures of formation* occur when bilateral pairs of somites fail to condense their sclerotomal tissue into an intervertebral disk with adjoining vertebral segments during the third and fourth weeks of gestation.[12]
  - Incomplete material is available to form a vertebra.

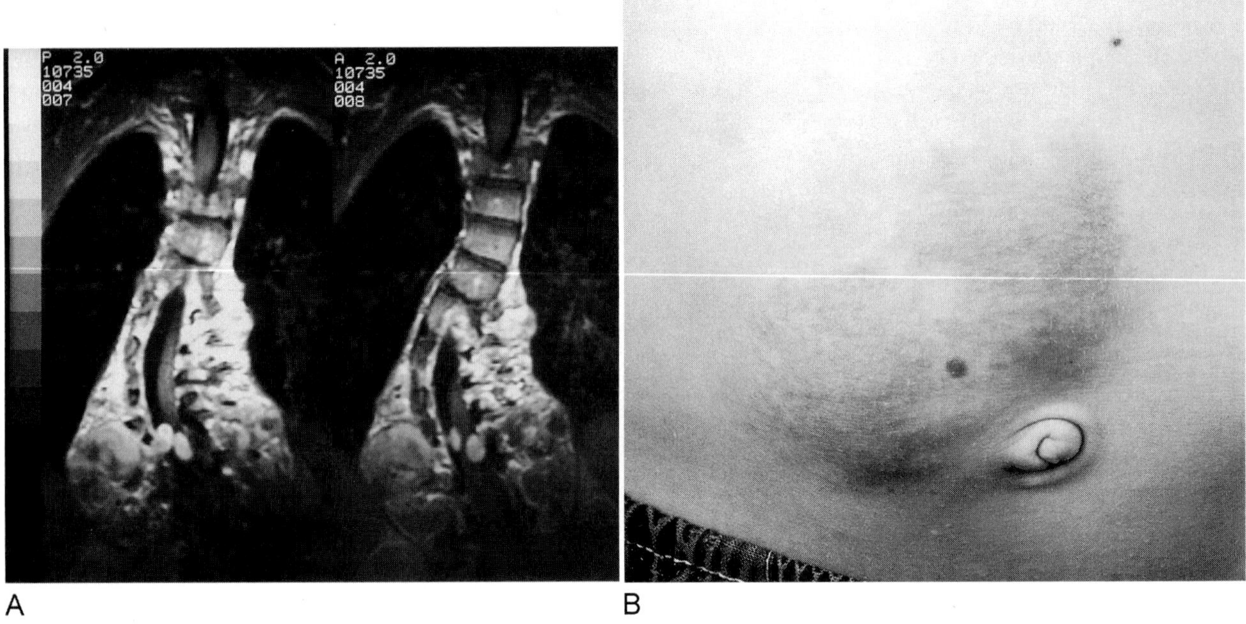

Figure 11–20: A, MRI of a boy with neurofibromatosis demonstrating a larger plexiform neurofibroma affecting the thoracic spine. B, Plexiform neurofibromas also resulted in cutaneous markings adjacent to the umbilicus.

- Unilateral complete failure of the formation of a vertebral structure results in a hemivertebra.
- Continued growth from the cranial, caudal, or both ends of hemivertebrae can cause angular deformity and produce scoliosis.
- Partial failure of formation results in a less severe deformity.

• *Failures of segmentation* occur when the caudal half of one sclerotome fails to merge with the cranial half of the adjacent sclerotome to produce a precartilaginous vertebral body.

- Complete failure of segmentation produces a block vertebra that may be well balanced, such as with *Klippel-Feil syndrome* (congenital fusion of cervical vertebrae).
- Partial failure of segmentation may produce a unilateral bar that tethers adjacent vertebrae and causes a concavity on the unsegmented side, thus producing scoliosis.
- Fully segmented vertebrae have growth potential both cranially and caudally, whereas unsegmented vertebrae lack their disk and growth potential.

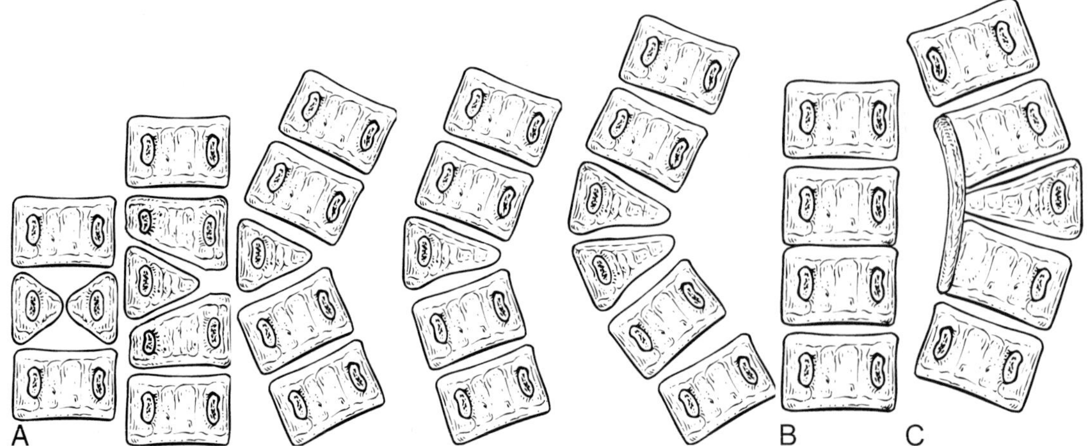

Figure 11–21: The defects of segmentation and formation that can occur during spinal development (see text for a description). From Freeman BL III (2003) Scoliosis and kyphosis. In: Campbell's Operative Orthopaedics, 10th edition (Canale ST ed). Philadelphia: Mosby. A and B redrawn from Bradford DS, Hensinger RM (1985) The Pediatric Spine, New York: Thieme. C redrawn from Lubicky JP (1997) Congenital scoliosis. In: The Textbook of Spinal Surgery, 2nd edition (Bridwell KH, DeWald RL, eds). Philadelphia: Lippincott-Raven.

- The combination of a unilateral bar with a contralateral hemivertebra produces the most severe and progressive scoliosis because one side remains tethered and the other side continues to grow from both ends.

- Semisegmented or nonsegmented hemivertebrae lack growth potential on one or both ends, thus limiting their potential for deformity.
- An incarcerated hemivertebra is smaller than a fully segmented hemivertebra and remains tucked within a niche scalloped out of adjacent vertebrae. Because of poor growth potential above and below the incarcerated vertebrae, associated scoliosis rarely requires treatment.
- Treatment is based on the potential for curve progression.
- Bracing is almost never successful.
- Nonprogressive curves may be observed, but surgery is indicated once progression is established before deterioration of the deformity.
- Because a unilateral unsegmented bar combined with a contralateral hemivertebra has such a bad prognosis, surgery is indicated at the time of diagnosis.
- An MRI is indicated preoperatively to look for associated anomalies such as diastematomyelia (localized split in the spinal cord caused by an osseous or fibrocartilaginous spur projecting posteriorly from a vertebral body), diplomyelia (cord duplication), tethered cord, low-lying conus, teratoma, or syringomyelia (spinal cord cyst).[13] Genitourinary and cardiac anomalies may also be present.
- Surgery should be aimed at preventing deformity rather than correcting it.
  - Prophylactic convex growth arrest involves anterior and posterior convex hemiepiphysiodesis and tries to halt growth of the convexity but allow continued growth on the concave side.
  - Excision of the hemivertebra removes the source of the scoliosis and allows some correction. The procedure involves anterior and posterior vertebral resection and may or may not require instrumentation.
  - Prophylactic early spine arthrodesis in situ should be performed before significant deformity and may be done posteriorly with or without anterior fusion.
  - Correction and posterior spinal arthrodesis and instrumentation are indicated in an older child whose curve remains relatively flexible.
  - Anterior and posterior spinal osteotomy, vertebrectomy, correction, and arthrodesis form a salvage procedure indicated for severe deformity that usually could have been prevented by an earlier, less complicated procedure.

Congenital Kyphosis

- As with congenital scoliosis, failed formation or failed segmentation can produce deformity. In addition, rotatory dislocation of the spine can occur if a kyphotic zone is located between areas of congenital scoliosis.
- Progressive neurological deficit is common, especially in those with a dislocated spinal canal and total failure of vertebral body formation.
- Bracing is ineffective.
- Posterior fusion may be adequate for curves less than 50 degrees; combined anterior and posterior fusions are indicated for greater curves.

Scheuermann's Kyphosis

- Normal sagittal kyphosis is between 20 and 50 degrees.
- Excessive kyphosis may be caused by postural round back or structural abnormalities.
- Postural round back is flexible, corrects with hyperextension, lacks structural changes within the vertebral bodies or intervertebral disks, and may improve with hyperextension exercises.
- Scheuermann's kyphosis is characterized by increased kyphosis in adolescence, vertebral wedging of 5 degrees or more at more than three adjacent levels, and irregularities of the vertebral endplates[14,15] (Figure 11–22).
- Radiographic changes are not seen before 10 years of age.

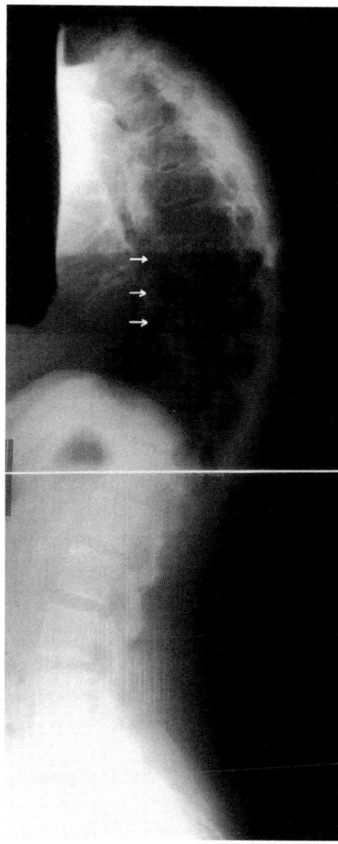

Figure 11–22: Lateral radiograph of a patient with anterior wedging of three thoracic vertebrae *(arrows)* consistent with Scheuermann's kyphosis.

- There is an incidence of 0.4 to 8% and a male predominance.
- The classic thoracic form has an apex between T7 and T9 and may have a mild associated scoliosis.
- A thoracolumbar or lumbar form, with an apex between T10 and T12, also exists. It is associated with chronic backache, irregular vertebral endplates, Schmorl's nodes, and reduction in disk space height without associated vertebral wedging.
- Schmorl's nodes may be seen on radiographs because of protrusion or herniation of disk material into the vertebral body.
- Theories regarding the etiology of Scheuermann's kyphosis include aseptic necrosis of the ring apophysis, mechanical weakening of the cartilaginous vertebral endplates, familial predisposition, elevated growth hormone levels, collagen defects, juvenile osteoporosis, osteochondrosis, tight hamstring muscles, and vitamin deficiencies.
- Clinical presentation includes back pain and cosmetic deformity.
- Radiographic evaluation should include a standing lateral projection of the entire spine, a passive hyperextension view with the patient lying supine over a wedge placed just below the apex of the deformity, and a standing posteroanterior view.
- Treatment is based on the degree of deformity and symptoms.
  - Physical therapy may be useful in relieving pain and improving postural round back, but it cannot correct structural deformity.
  - Bracing is most effective in skeletally immature patients with curves between 50 and 75 degrees that correct at least 40% with hyperextension.
  - The Milwaukee brace is recommended for curves with apices between T6 and T9, but compliance is frequently limited because of the high profile of the occipital chin ring.
  - Full-time bracing is recommended for 12 to 18 months followed by weaning to part-time bracing until skeletal maturity.
  - Casting may be used to improve correction and flexibility before casting or to relieve severe pain.
  - Surgery is indicated for curves that, despite bracing, progress beyond 70 degrees or are associated with unacceptable cosmesis or pain.
  - Long, instrumented, posterior fusions with facetectomies of the kyphotic segment and sequential segmental compression are recommended. Anterior release and fusion are added to those patients with curves greater than 75 degrees and wedging greater than 10 degrees.

Spondylolysis and Spondylolisthesis

- In Greek, *spondylos* means vertebra, *lysis* means break or defect, and *olisthesis* means movement or slipping.
- Spondylolysis refers to a bony defect of the pars interarticularis and may be described by the Wiltse classification[16] (Figure 11–23).
  - Type 1: Congenital or dysplastic—Dysplastic posterior elements result in deficient facet joints that may allow slippage, usually of L5 on S1.
  - Type 2: Isthmic—This defect of the pars interarticularis with normal facets may be (1) a lytic stress fracture, (2) an elongated pars, or (3) an acute pars fracture.
  - Type 3: Degenerative—Degenerative arthritis disrupts facet joints.
  - Type 4: Post-traumatic—Acute fracture, ligamentous injury, or both to posterior elements other than the pars interarticularis results in instability.
  - Type 5: Pathological—Generalized or local bone disease causes destruction of the posterior elements, thus allowing slippage.
  - Type 6: Post-surgical—A loss of posterior elements follows surgery.
- Isthmic spondylolysis is not seen at birth but has an incidence of 5% by 6 years of age. (The incidence is higher in Alaskan Eskimos.)
- Spondylolysis increases during teenage years and is common in athletes exposed to hyperlordosis, such as gymnasts, football linemen, wrestlers, ice hockey players, and butterfly swimmers.
- Spondylolysis may be asymptomatic or associated with pain, tight hamstrings, and a flexed hip gait.
- The pars defect may be detected on a standard lateral radiograph or better seen on oblique views of the LS spine (Figure 11–5). SPECT or CT can be more sensitive (Figure 11–7).
- Spondylolisthesis occurs when the superior vertebra slips forward on the inferior vertebra and is usually described by the Meyerding classification (Figure 11–24):
  - Grade 0—No slippage
  - Grade 1—Slippage of less than 25%
  - Grade 2—Slippage of 25 to 50%
  - Grade 3—Slippage of 51 to 75%
  - Grade 4—Slippage of more than 75%
  - Spondyloptosis—Complete translation greater than 100%
- Progression is predicted based on the slip angle, determined by drawing a line parallel to the posterior cortex of the sacrum and measuring the angle between its perpendicular and a line parallel to the inferior border of L5. Normally, the angle is 0 degrees to −10 degrees; however, angles greater than 55 degrees are associated with progression (Figure 11–25).
- Treatment is based on symptoms and the degree of slippage.[17]
  - Grade 0 (spondylolysis) and grade 1 spondylolisthesis, may respond to a period of rest, bracing, and physical therapy to improve abdominal strength and hamstring flexibility.

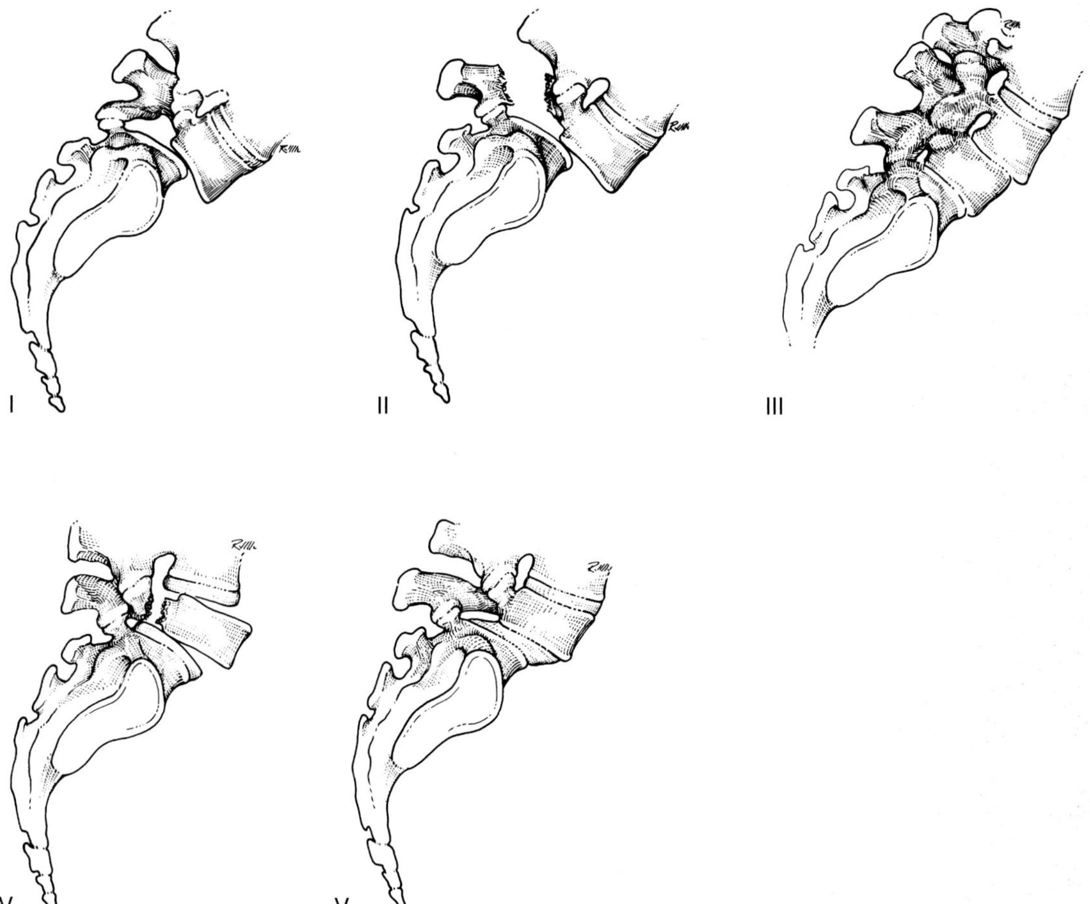

Figure 11–23: Types of defects that can occur in the pars interarticularis, as described by Wiltse. **Type I is dysplastic and has a congenitally deficient facet joint. Type II is isthmic and has a lesion within the pars. Type III results from a degenerative process. Type IV results from acute trauma to an area other than the pars. Type V occurs after generalized or local bone disease, such as osteoporosis or tumors. From Freeman BL III (2003) Scoliosis and kyphosis. In: Campbell's Operative Orthopaedics, 10th edition (Canale ST ed). Philadelphia: Mosby. Redrawn from Hensinger RN (1983) Instr Course Lect 32: 132.**

- Surgery is indicated if pain or neurological symptoms persist despite nonoperative treatment, if slippage progresses beyond 25%, if initial presentation has more than 50% slippage, or if postural deformities and gait abnormalities are worsening.
- Single-level bilateral lateral fusion in situ through a posterolateral (Wiltse) approach is indicated for symptomatic patients with less than 50% slippage. A direct repair of the pars can be performed if slippage is less than 25% through oblique screw or transverse process to spinous process wiring with bone graft.
- Slippage greater than 50% can be treated with a two-level bilateral fusion in situ from L4 to the sacrum.
- If severe radiculopathy exists, decompression can be performed through a midline approach, but fusion is still required to prevent further slippage following laminectomy.
- Postoperative extension casting with thigh extension may improve fusion rates.
- Greater slippage may benefit from a combined posterior and anterior approach to improve stability. In addition, preoperative traction may be tried to reduce slippage. Vertebral body resection with spinal realignment and spinal instrumentation may be performed; however, such procedures are associated with high complication rates and should be performed only by those with extensive subspecialty training.

Back Pain

- Less common than in adults, back pain nevertheless more frequently has an identifiable cause[18] (Box 11–8).
- Prevalence increases with age—from 12% at 11 years to 50% by 15 years.
- History should include the following:
  - Location of pain (focal or diffuse)
  - Any associated deformity
  - Onset (acute trauma or gradual)

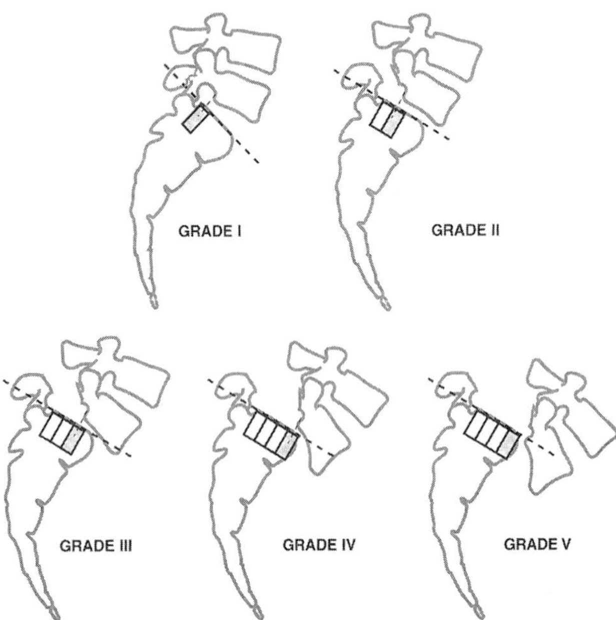

Figure 11–24: Meyerding classification of spondylolisthesis showing normal, Grade I, or 0 to 25% slippage; Grade II, or 26 to 50% slippage; Grade III, or 51 to 75% slippage; Grade IV, or 76 to 100% slippage; and Grade V, or complete slippage. **From Herring JA, ed (2002) Tachdjian's Pediatric Orthopaedics: From the Texas Scottish Rite Hospital for Children, 3rd edition. Philadelphia: Saunders.**

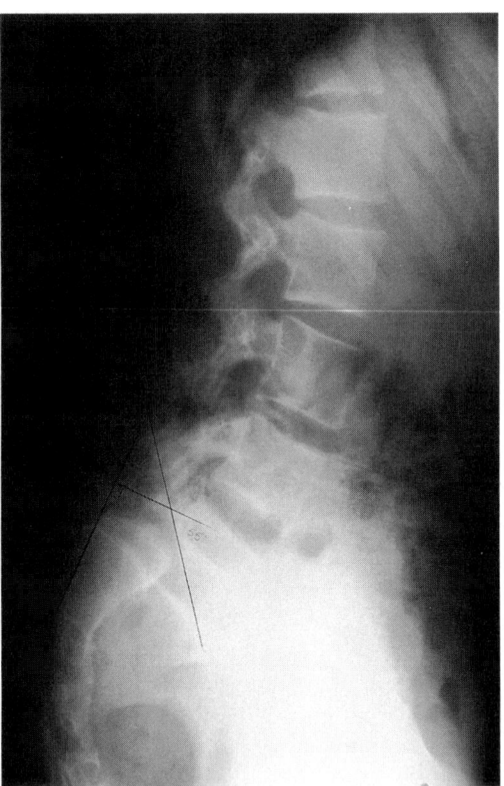

Figure 11–25: Radiograph of an adolescent male with spondylolisthesis demonstrating a slip angle of 55 degrees.

  - Duration
  - Any related activity
  - Waking from sleep
  - Associated neurological changes (numbness or weakness)
  - Constitutional symptoms (fevers or weight loss)
- During traumatic events, the bones and ligaments of the pediatric spine can tolerate more stretch than the spinal cord; therefore, children may sustain neurological injury despite completely normal-appearing radiographs. Such an injury is a spinal cord injury without radiographic abnormality. MRI is recommended to search for such injury.
- Spine infections may involve the disk space (diskitis), the vertebral body (osteomyelitis), or an entire vertebra–disk–vertebra unit (spondylitis).
  - Elevated erythrocyte sedimentation rate and C-reactive protein are more sensitive than the white blood cell count for detecting infection.
  - MRI is best to localize an infection.
  - *Staphylococcus aureus* is the most common pathogen and can usually be treated with antibiotics rather than surgery.
- Tumors frequently present symptoms including pain, often at night. Associated symptoms, such as fever and weight loss, may suggest malignancy.[19]
  - Plain radiographs, a complete blood count, and an erythrocyte sedimentation rate should be obtained. Often bone scans are useful for localizing the site, but MRIs and CT scans are more specific for identifying the type of lesion.
  - Biopsy may be needed to confirm the diagnosis.
  - Benign tumors (approximately 70%), such as aneurysmal bone cysts and osteoid osteomas, may require excision for pain relief. Osteoid osteomas, however, may become asymptomatic with aspirin or nonsteroidal anti-inflammatory treatment. Langerhans cell histiocytosis usually resolves without surgery.
  - Malignant tumors are usually treated with a combination of resection and radiation or chemotherapy.
  - Deformity may be caused by true structural changes of the spinal architecture or caused by muscular spasm.

Cervical Spinal Deformities[20]

Klippel-Feil Syndrome

- Klippel-Feil syndrome is congenital failure of segmentation in the cervical spine.
- The classical triad is short neck, low posterior hairline, and limited neck range of motion (seen in 40 to 50% of patients).
- It may be associated with other conditions—fetal alcohol syndrome, Goldenhar's syndrome (ocular–auricular–vertebral dysplasia), VATER, genitourinary problems,

Box 11–8 Differential Diagnoses of Back Pain in Childhood and Adolescence

Mechanical or Traumatic

- Muscle strain or overuse injuries
- Fracture
- Spondylolysis or spondylolisthesis
- Herniated disk
- Slipped vertebral apophysis

Developmental

- Spondylolysis or spondylolisthesis
- Scheuermann's kyphosis
- Painful scoliosis

Inflammatory

- Diskitis or vertebral osteomyelitis
- Tuberculous spondylitis
- Disk space calcification
- Ankylosing spondylitis
- Juvenile rheumatoid arthritis
- Other rheumatological conditions

Neoplastic

- Benign
  - Anterior
    1. Langerhans cell histiocytosis or eosinophilic granuloma
    2. Giant cell
  - Posterior
    1. Aneurysmal bone cyst
    2. Osteoid osteoma–osteoblastoma
- Malignant
  - Leukemia or lymphoma
  - Ewing's sarcoma
  - Metastatic (neuroblastoma, Wilms tumor, etc.)
  - Spinal cord–meningeal–epidural tumors
  - Rhabdomyosarcoma

Visceral

- Appendicitis
- Pyelonephritis
- Retroperitoneal abscess

Psychological

- Rare—Consider this diagnosis only after a complete workup for other sources.

From Pierz KA, Dormans JP (2004) Spinal disorders: The essentials for the pediatrician. In: Requisites in Pediatrics: Orthopedics and Sports Medicine (Dormans JP, ed). Philadelphia: Mosby.

cardiovascular anomalies, clubfoot, Sprengel's deformity (undescended scapula), developmental dysplasia of the hip, and idiopathic and congenital scoliosis.

- Evaluation should include cervical flexion and extension lateral radiographs to assess instability, a renal ultrasound or intravenous pyelogram, and a thorough cardiac examination.
- Patients should be advised to avoid contact sports.

Torticollis

- Clinically identified by head tilt toward and rotatory deviation from the affected side's sternocleidomastoid (SCM) muscle ("cocked robin deformity"). To simulate the deformity, place your index finger just in front of your ear and your thumb on your ipsilateral medial clavicle. Gently squeeze your fingers together and allow your head to tilt toward and rotate from your hand.
- Torticollis may be caused by congenital occipitocervical anomalies, muscular conditions, or an acquired deformity.
- Congenital muscular torticollis is the most common etiology, usually presenting symptoms in the first few months of life.
  - A palpable mass may be felt in the SCM muscle.
  - Etiology may be caused by intrauterine positioning or compartment syndrome of the SCM muscle.
  - Developmental dysplasia of the hip present symptoms in 20% of cases.
  - Plagiocephaly may develop because of asymmetrical pressure on the young skull.
  - Radiographs can be used to rule out congenital cervical anomalies.
  - Treatment begins with careful stretching, which is successful in 90% of cases.
  - Recalcitrant cases may be treated surgically with release of the attachments of the SCM muscle. Bipolar techniques release both the proximal and the distal (clavicular and sternal heads) attachments, whereas unipolar techniques release only the proximal or the distal attachment.
- Acquired torticollis may have various causes.
  - Sandifer's syndrome—Abnormal head tilt secondary to gastroesophageal reflux
  - Posterior fossa tumors
  - Ocular dysfunction—Superior oblique muscle weakness
  - Inflammation or infection—Grisel syndrome
  - Basilar impression, atlanto-occipital anomalies, or cervical dysplasia
  - Atlantoaxial rotatory subluxation—Best seen on dynamic CT scan with images taken in neutral and with the head rotated maximally to the left and right. Rest, a soft cervical collar, and nonsteroidal anti-inflammatory medication may be successful treatment in the first week. After the first week, halter traction may be added. Posterior cervical fusion may be required in long-standing cases.

Down's (Trisomy 21) Syndrome

- Down's syndrome is a chromosomal abnormality associated with ligamentous laxity, hypotonia, mental retardation, heart disease, and endocrine disorders.
- Occipital-C1 or atlantoaxial instability (evidenced by an atlantodens interval of more than 5 mm on flexion

radiographs) is common, but symptoms are present in only 2 to 3% of patients.
- Asymptomatic children with atlantoaxial instability should avoid contact sports.
- Patients with neurological symptoms or an atlantodens interval greater than 10 mm should undergo surgical stabilization, although the complication rate is high.

Pseudosubluxation

- Subluxation of C2 on C3 (or C3 on C4) of up to 4 mm or 40% is a normal variant in children younger than 8.
- The posterior interspinous distances and the posterior spinolaminar line (Swischuk's line) should remain well aligned.
- Patients should be asymptomatic with no associated soft tissue swelling.

References

1. Ganey TM, Ogden JA (2001) Development and maturation of the axial skeleton. In: The Pediatric Spine: Principles and Practice, 2nd edition (Weinstein SL, ed). Philadelphia: Lippincott Williams & Wilkins.
   This chapter describes the morphogenesis of the axial skeleton and alterations in the process that may result in spinal abnormalities. Embryology, postnatal development, and clinical applications are reviewed.

2. Vaccaro AR, Rizzolo SJ, Balderston RA, Allardyce TJ, Garfin SR, Dolinskas C, An HS (1995) Placement of pedicle screws in the thoracic spine: Part II—An anatomical and radiographic assessment. J Bone Joint Surg Am 77: 1200-1206.
   Using CT scans and subsequent dissections, the authors studied 90 pedicle screws placed into the fourth through twelfth cadaveric thoracic vertebrae. Of the screws, 37 had penetrated the cortex of the pedicle, 21 medially and 16 laterally. Anteriorly, the aorta and esophagus were at risk.

3. King HA, Moe JH, Bradford DS, Winter RB (1983) The selection of fusion levels in idiopathic scoliosis. J Bone Joint Surg Am 65: 1302-1313.
   This article describes the King-Moe classification method of idiopathic scoliosis, including the selection of thoracic fusion levels. The concept of identifying the neutral and stable vertebrae is presented.

4. Bunnell W (1993) Outcome of spinal screening. Spine 18: 1572-1580.
   Spinal screening using a scoliometer was performed on 1000 high school students to determine the prevalence of spinal deformity and the appropriate degree of deformity to be used as a selection criterion. An angle of trunk rotation of 7 degrees resulted in a referral rate of 3% and a reduction in the need for surgical treatment of scoliosis.

5. Weinstein SL, Ponseti IV (1983) Curve progression in idiopathic scoliosis. J Bone Joint Surg Am 65: 447-455.
   This study followed 133 curves in 102 patients for an average of 40.5 years to quantitate curve progression after skeletal maturity and to identify prognostic factors leading to curve progression. Of the curves, 68% progressed after skeletal maturity. In general, curves that were less than 30 degrees at skeletal maturity tended not to progress regardless of curve pattern. Curves that measured between 50 and 75 degrees at skeletal maturity, particularly thoracic curves, progressed the most.

6. Nachemson AL, Peterson LE (1995) Effectiveness of treatment with a brace in girls who have adolescent idiopathic scoliosis: A prospective, controlled study based on data from the brace study of the Scoliosis Research Society. J Bone Joint Surg Am 77: 815-822.
   In a prospective study, 286 girls with AIS were followed to determine the effect of treatment. Brace treatment was associated with a success rate of 74%, whereas observation alone had a success rate of 34%.

7. Zeller RD, Dubousset J (2001) Idiopathic scoliosis treated by a posterior approach. In: Surgical Techniques in Orthopaedics and Traumatology. Paris: Elsevier.
   This chapter provides a strategy for correcting the three-dimensional deformity of scoliosis with posterior fusion and instrumentation. Preoperative planning, surgical techniques, and postoperative care are reviewed.

8. Lenke LG, Betz RR, Harms J, Bridwell KH, Clements DH, Lowe TA, Blanke K (2001) Adolescent idiopathic scoliosis: A new classification to determine extent of spinal arthrodesis. J Bone Joint Surg Am 83: 1169-1181.
   In this article, the authors introduce a new classification method and describe the six coronal curve types, the lumbar spine modifiers, and the sagittal thoracic modifiers. Interobserver and intraobserver κ values were determined and found to be higher than those for the King-Moe system.

9. Koop SE (1988) Infantile and juvenile idiopathic scoliosis. Orthop Clin North Am 19: 331-337.
   This review article focuses on how IIS and JIS differ from AIS. Differences regarding presentations, natural histories, associated anomalies, frequency and rate of deformity progression, and treatments are described.

10. Mehta M (1972) The rib–vertebral angle in the early diagnosis between resolving and progressive infantile scoliosis. J Bone Joint Surg Br 54: 230-243.
    In this article, the author defines the RVAD and applies it to predicting which infantile curves are more likely to progress and require treatment. Curves with an RVAD > 20 degrees are likely to progress.

11. McCarthy RE (1999) Management of neuromuscular scoliosis. Orthop Clin North Am 3: 435-449.
    This review article highlights important features regarding neuromuscular scoliosis. Differences between neuropathic (such as cerebral palsy) and myopathic (such as Duchenne muscular dystrophy) are described. The high failure rate of nonoperative management and the surgical goals of corrective management are reviewed.

12. McMaster MJ, David CV (1986) Hemivertebra as a cause of scoliosis: A study of 104 patients. J Bone Joint Surg Br 68: 588-595.

Based on a review of the natural history of congenital scoliosis, the following risk factors for curve progression were identified: hemivertebral type, site, number, relationship to other vertebrae, and patient age.

13. Bradford DS, Heithoff KB, Cohen M (1991) Intraspinal abnormalities and congenital spine deformities: A radiographic and MRI study. J Pediatr Orthop 11: 36-41.
    In a study of 42 patients with congenital spinal deformities, 16 were noted to have intraspinal anomalies based on MRI. The authors recommend obtaining an MRI study in any patient with a congenital spinal deformity before surgical stabilization and when associated with lumbosacral kyphosis, pain, neurological findings, or a cutaneous hairy patch.

14. Scheuermann HW (1920) Kyphosis dorsalis juvenilis. Ugeskr Laeger 82: 385-393.
    In this manuscript, Scheuermann described the radiographic characteristics of the condition that now bears his name: Increased kyphosis in adolescence, wedging of vertebral bodies, and irregularities of vertebral endplates.

15. Sorensen KH (1964) Scheuermann's Juvenile Kyphosis: Clinical Appearances, Radiography, Aetiology, and Prognosis. Copenhagen: Munksgaard.
    Following Scheuermann's original article, this manuscript added the criteria of vertebral wedging of 5 degrees or more and provided epidemiological information regarding Scheuermann's kyphosis.

16. Wiltse LL, Newman PH, Macnab I (1976) Classification of spondylolysis and spondylolisthesis. Clin Orthop 117: 23-29.
    The etiological and anatomical features of spondylolysis and spondylolisthesis are presented and used to develop a working classification of the disorders.

17. Burkus JK, Lonstein JE, Winter RB, Denis F (1992) Long-term evaluation of adolescents treated operatively for spondylolisthesis: A comparison of in situ arthrodesis only with in situ arthrodesis and reduction followed by immobilization in a cast. J Bone Joint Surg Am 74: 693-704.
    In this study, 42 adolescents with spondylolisthesis were treated with in situ arthrodesis with or without reduction and casting. Casting decreased progressive sagittal translation and lumbosacral kyphosis. Neurological problems were not seen, and persistent low back pain was only seen in 4 patients.

18. Turner P, Green J, Galasko C (1989) Back pain in childhood. Spine 14: 812-814.
    Of 61 children with back pain, 50% had serious spinal disease. Clinical findings can be unreliable, but radiographs, white cell count, and sedimentation rate can be useful in identifying potential problems.

19. Dormans JP, Pill SG (2000) Benign and malignant tumors of the spine in children. In: Strategies in the Pediatric Spine: State of the Art Reviews (Drummond DS, ed). Philadelphia: Hanley and Belfus.
    This review describes benign and malignant tumors of the spine. Clinical presentation, imaging modalities, and management techniques are covered. Attention is given to eosinophilic granuloma, osteochondroma, osteoblastoma–osteoid osteoma, aneurysmal bone cyst, hemangioma, giant-cell tumor, Ewing's sarcoma, osteogenic sarcoma, and leukemia.

20. Herman MJ, Pizzutillo PD (1999) Cervical spine disorders in children. Clin Orthop North Am 30: 457-466.
    This review focuses on anatomical and biological features of the developing pediatric spine that can complicate the evaluation and treatment of children. Congenital and developmental alterations, seen with Down's syndrome, Klippel-Feil syndrome, osteochondrodysplasias, mucopolysaccharidoses, and post-traumatic instability, are described.

CHAPTER 12

Musculoskeletal Tumors in Children

Bülent Erol* and John P. Dormans†

*MD, Attending Surgeon, Department of Orthopaedic Surgery, The Hospital of University of Marmara, Marmara University School of Medicine, Istanbul, Turkey
†MD, Chief of Orthopaedics Surgery, The Children's Hospital of Philadelphia, Philadelphia, PA; Professor of Orthopaedic Surgery, University of Pennsylvania School of Medicine, Philadelphia, PA

- Pediatric musculoskeletal tumors are uncommon; when they occur, they usually are benign.
- Early detection of a malignant musculoskeletal tumor not only may make the difference between life and death but also may allow successful salvage surgery rather than amputation of the limb.
- The primary bone and soft tissue tumors of childhood can be classified based on their tissue origin (Box 12–1).

Evaluation

History

- Children with a musculoskeletal tumor usually have pain, mass, pathological fracture, or incidental findings on radiographs (Box 12–2).
- The characteristics of the pain can help to determine the diagnosis.
  1. Patients who have active benign tumors (e.g., aneurysmal bone cyst or chondroblastoma) usually have a mild, dull, slowly progressive pain that is worse at night and aggravated by activity.
  2. Patients with malignant musculoskeletal tumors complain of a more rapidly progressive symptom complex, not specifically related to activity, that often awakens them at night.
  3. Occasionally, the pain pattern is diagnostic (e.g., osteoid osteoma).

Box 12–1 Classification of Pediatric Musculoskeletal Tumors Based on Tissue of Origin

- Bone tumors
  - Bone origin—Osteoid osteoma, osteoblastoma, and osteosarcoma
  - Cartilaginous origin—Osteochondroma, chondroblastoma, chondromyxoid fibroma, enchondroma, and periosteal chondroma
  - Fibrous origin—Nonossifying fibroma, fibrous dysplasia, osteofibrous dysplasia, and desmoplastic fibroma
  - Miscellaneous—Unicameral bone cyst, aneurysmal bone cyst, giant cell tumor, Langerhans cell histiocytosis, and Ewing sarcoma–PNET
  - Musculoskeletal manifestations of leukemia
  - Bone lymphomas
  - Metastatic tumors—Neuroblastoma, retinoblastoma, and hepatoblastoma
- Soft tissue tumors
  - Vascular tumors—Hemangioma and vascular malformations
  - Nerve origin—Neurolemmoma, neurofibroma, and malignant peripheral nerve sheath tumor
  - Fibrous origin—Fibromatosis and fibrosarcoma
  - Muscular origin—Rhabdomyosarcoma
  - Miscellaneous—Synovial cell sarcoma
  - Ganglion and synovial cyst

Box 12–2 Clinical Presentations of Pediatric Musculoskeletal Tumors

1. Pain
   - Duration
   - Localization
   - Severity
   - Character
   - Relief and how obtained
2. Mass
   - Duration
   - Size
   - Consistency
   - Mobility
3. Pathological fracture spectrum from microfractures to displaced fractures
   - Prior symptoms and signs
   - Mechanism of fracture
   - Characteristics of fracture
4. Incidental radiographic findings
   - Prior symptoms and signs
   - Why radiograph was obtained

- A child with a pathological fracture should be questioned about the specifics of the injury that produced the fracture. A child who has a pathological fracture without prior symptoms most often has a benign lesion of bone that gradually weakened the cortex, resulting in a fatigue fracture.
- Most patients with musculoskeletal tumors do not have systemic symptoms. Even children with large, primary, malignant musculoskeletal tumors usually appear healthy.
- The age of the patient is important in establishing a differential diagnosis, because certain tumors tend to occur in certain age groups (Table 12–1).
- Most musculoskeletal tumors occur more in boys than in girls. The gender of the patient usually does not play a significant role in formulating the differential diagnosis.

Physical Examination

- The physical examination of a patient with a musculoskeletal tumor should include a neurovascular examination of the affected extremity, the range of motion of the adjacent joint, and the gait pattern of the patient.
- The size, consistency, and mobility of a mass should be evaluated (Box 12–2).
  - For soft tissue masses, small (<5 cm), superficial, soft, and movable masses usually are benign.
  - On the other hand, large (>5 cm), deep, firm, fixed, and tender masses raise suspicion of malignancy and are less commonly benign.
  - It is important to measure and record the size of the tumor as accurately as possible for comparison and subsequent examinations.

Table 12–1: Peak Ages of Common Pediatric Musculoskeletal Tumors

AGE (YEARS)	BENIGN	MALIGNANT
0-5	Langerhans cell histiocytosis Osteomyelitis	Fibrosarcoma Metastatic tumors Leukemia Ewing sarcoma Rhabdomyosarcoma
5-10	Unicameral bone cyst Aneurysmal bone cyst Nonossifying fibroma Fibrous dysplasia Osteoid osteoma Langerhans cell histiocytosis	Osteosarcoma Rhabdomyosarcoma
10-20	Fibrous dysplasia Osteoid osteoma Fibroma Aneurysmal bone cyst Chondroblastoma Osteofibrous dysplasia	Osteosarcoma Ewing sarcoma Chondrosarcoma Rhabdomyosarcoma Synovial cell sarcoma

Plain Radiograph Examination

- Plain radiographs give the most detailed information about skeletal lesions.
  1. Plain radiographs, at least in two views (anteroposterior and lateral), showing the entire lesion are necessary.
  2. Before changes can be seen in plain radiographs, 30 to 40% of a bone must be destroyed.
  3. It is often difficult to see soft tissue tumors and soft tissue extension from bony neoplasms with plain radiographs.
- It is useful to ask some questions when evaluating plain radiographs of bony lesions: Where is the lesion located in the bone? What is the lesion doing to the bone? What is the bone doing to the lesion? What is the periosteal response?[1]
  - The anatomical location of a bony lesion is an important diagnostic clue.
    1. The lesions involving long bones should be identified as epiphyseal, metaphyseal, or diaphyseal, and central or eccentric (Table 12–2).
    2. The portion of the skeleton involved is also of diagnostic importance (e.g., lesions involving spine or pelvis).
  - The lesion may be destroying or replacing the existing bone.
    1. Bone destruction can be described as geographic, moth-eaten, and permeative (Figure 12–1). Although none of these features are pathognomonic for any specific neoplasm, the type of destruction may suggest a benign or a malignant process.

Table 12–2: Common Locations of Pediatric Bone Tumors

EPIPHYSIS	METAPHYSIS
Chondroblastoma Brodie's abscess of the epiphyses Giant cell tumor Fibrous dysplasia	Any tumor
DIAPHYSIS (FAHEL)	**MULTIPLE**
Fibrous dysplasia Osteofibrous dysplasia Langerhans cell histiocytosis Ewing sarcoma Leukemia, lymphoma: *Occasional diaphyseal* Osteoid osteoma Unicameral bone cyst	Leukemia (metastasis) Multiple hereditary exostoses Langerhans cell histiocytosis Polyostotic fibrous dysplasia Enchondromatosis
ANTERIOR ELEMENTS OF SPINE	**POSTERIOR ELEMENTS OF SPINE**
Langerhans cell histiocytosis Leukemia Metastatic Giant cell tumor	Aneurysmal bone cyst Osteoblastoma Osteoid osteoma
PELVIS	**RIB**
Ewing sarcoma Osteosarcoma Osteochondroma Metastasis Fibrous dysplasia	Fibrous dysplasia Langerhans cell histiocytosis Ewing sarcoma Metastasis

2. Geographical bone destruction typifies slow-growing, benign lesions, whereas moth-eaten (i.e., characterized by multiple, small, often clustered lytic areas) and permeative (i.e., characterized by ill-defined, tiny, oval radiolucencies or lucent streaks) types of bone destruction mark rapidly growing, infiltrating tumors.[2]

– The response of the bone to the neoplastic process involves the response of the adjacent cortex and periosteum.[3]
1. The lesion may be contained by the cortex or "walled off" by dense sclerotic bone, implying a slow-growing or static lesion, or it may destroy the cortex and form a soft tissue mass, mostly indicating an aggressive neoplastic process.
2. Like the pattern of bone destruction, the pattern of periosteal reaction is an indicator of the biological activity of a lesion. Although no single periosteal response is unique for a given lesion, a continuous periosteal reaction indicates a long-standing (slow-growing) and benign process. An interrupted periosteal reaction, on the other hand, is commonly seen in malignant tumors; in these tumors, the periosteal reaction may appear in a sunburst ("hair-on-end") or onionskin (lamellated) pattern. A reactive periosteal cuff at the periphery of the tumor, a Codman triangle, also may form (Figure 12–2).

• Most bone tumors can be diagnosed correctly after obtaining the history, performing a physical examination,

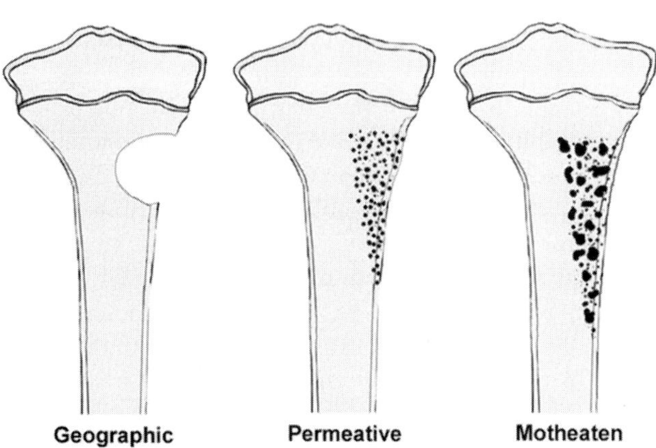

Figure 12–1: Different patterns of bone destruction. Modified from Madewell JE, Ragsdale BD, Sweet DE (1981) Radiologic and pathologic analysis of solitary bone lesions: Part I—Internal margins. Radiol Clin North Am 19(4): 715-748. 22. Glotzbecker M, Carpentieri D, Dormans J (2004) Langerhans cell histiocytosis: a primary infection of bone? Human Herpes virus 6 latent protein detected in lymphocytes from tissue of children. J Pediatr Orthop. Jan–Feb; 24(1): 123–129. The findings reported in this article suggest a role for the HHV-6B in the etiology of LCH.

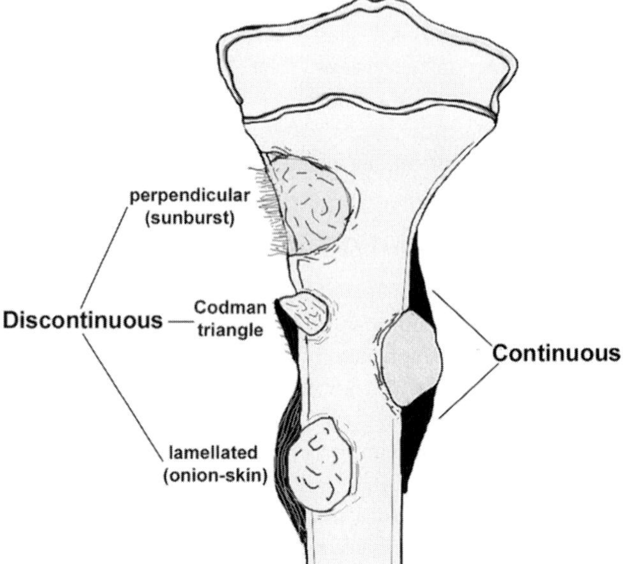

Figure 12–2: Different patterns of periosteal reaction. Modified from Greenspan A, Wolfgang R (1998) Radiologic and pathologic approach to bone tumors. In: Differential Diagnosis of Tumors and Tumor-Like Lesions of Bones and Joints (Greenspan A, Wolfgang R, eds). Philadelphia: Lippincott-Raven, pp 1-24.

and examining the plain radiograph. If the radiographs reveal a lesion that has a potential for malignancy or if they do not confirm a specific diagnosis, further staging studies are indicated.

Additional Diagnostic Studies

Magnetic Resonance Imaging

- Magnetic resonance imaging (MRI) is the single most important diagnostic test after physical examination and plain radiography for evaluating a musculoskeletal lesion.
- The ability of MRI to produce images of the body in three planes (axial, sagittal, and coronal) provides a significant advantage in defining the extent of many tumors.[4]
  1. The coronal and sagittal planes show a long axis view and can determine both the location and extent (intraosseous component and soft tissue extension) of a lesion. This modality also can identify skip lesions in the bone marrow.
  2. The axial plane can best define the anatomical relationships among tumor, bone, soft tissue, nerves, and vessels.
- MRI remains the modality of choice for staging, for evaluating response to preoperative chemotherapy, and for long-term follow-up of most bone and soft tissue sarcomas (Box 12–3).

Computed Tomography

- Computed tomography (CT) is particularly helpful in the evaluation of bone tumors involving axial skeleton (e.g., spine and pelvis).
- CT remains most useful in the evaluation of small lesions in or immediately adjacent to the cortex (e.g., osteoid osteoma) and lesions with fine mineralization or calcifications (e.g., chondroblastoma).[5]
- Percutaneous biopsies of musculoskeletal lesions can be performed with the assistance of localization obtained with CT.
- For all other situations, MRI has replaced CT.

Radionuclide Scans

- Technetium bone scanning is a readily available, safe, and excellent method for evaluating the activity of the primary lesion. In addition, bone scanning is the most practical method of surveying the entire skeleton.
  - A disorder associated with an increase in bone production increases the local concentration of technetium-99 and produces a "hot spot" on the scan (e.g., osteoid osteoma or osteoblastoma).
  - In some cases, the bone scan is normal, or there is decreased activity at the site of the lesion (e.g., Langerhans cell histiocytosis or myeloma).
- Gallium-67 imaging is another radionuclide study that can help to differentiate a musculoskeletal infection from a neoplasia.

Box 12–3 Current Treatment Principles of Osteosarcoma and Ewing Sarcoma

- Staging of primary lesion and search for other lesions
  - MRI of the primary site including the joint above and below
  - Total body radionuclide bone scan to search for bone metastases and skip lesions
  - CT of the chest to search for lung metastases
- Pediatric oncology evaluation
- Incisional biopsy
  - Intraoperative frozen section
  - Bone marrow aspiration for Ewing sarcoma
  - Broviac placement for chemotherapy
- Preoperative neoadjuvant chemotherapy (usually multiagent chemotherapy)
- Repeat MRI after chemotherapy and before definitive surgery
  - Radiographic evaluation of the tumor response to chemotherapy (e.g., change in the size of the tumor, change in the amount of tumor edema, and the involvement of neurovascular structures)
  - Surgical planning
- Surgery to excise the tumor with wide surgical margins
  - Limb salvage surgery to resection the tumor with wide surgical margins and to reconstruct; possible in most patients with extremity sarcoma
  - Amputation
- Histological examination of resection specimen
  - Histological evaluation of the tumor response to chemotherapy (>90% tumor necrosis demonstrates good response)
  - Verification of wide surgical margins
- Continued chemotherapy (adjuvant chemotherapy) after local control surgery
  - Usually the same protocol as with neoadjuvant chemotherapy if tumor response to chemotherapy is good
- Follow-up
  - Every 3 months first year then at 6- to 12-month intervals

Biopsy

- Biopsy should be the last step in the evaluation of a patient with a bone or soft tissue sarcoma and should be performed following completion of the radiographic staging, which includes a total body bone scan, a CT scan of the chest, and an MRI of the primary lesion (Box 12–3).
- The purpose of the biopsy is to confirm the diagnosis suspected by the physician after the evaluation or to determine which diagnosis, among a limited differential diagnosis, is correct.
- A well-planned biopsy provides an accurate diagnosis and facilitates treatment. On the other hand, a poorly performed biopsy may fail to provide a diagnosis and, more importantly, may have a negative effect on treatment options, survival, or both.
- The best biopsy method for a musculoskeletal neoplasm depends on the differential diagnosis, the location of the

neoplasm, and the ability of the pathologist to make a diagnosis on a sample of tissue.

  - Needle aspiration may provide adequate tissue for a histological diagnosis; however, many oncological surgeons prefer an open incisional technique, which also provides sufficient tissue for the multiple studies often needed, including newer molecular diagnostics.
  - Incisional biopsy involves removing only a portion of the tumor without contaminating the surrounding soft tissue structures.
- A biopsy is best accomplished at the institution that would perform the definitive surgery if it becomes necessary.[6]
- Box 12–4 summarizes the basic principles that should be followed in performing an incisional biopsy.

Classification

- Enneking and colleagues proposed a musculoskeletal staging system.[1] This system was designed to be simple, straightforward, and clinically practical.
  - The tumors are separated into only two histological grades (I, low; II, high) and two anatomical extends (A, intracompartmental; B, extracompartmental). Patients with metastatic disease in either a regional lymph node or a distant site are grouped as stage III. There are five stages (IA, IB, IIA, IIB, and III) in this system (Table 12–3).

Treatment

- A precise definition and classification of surgical margins are useful for evaluation, planning, and treatment in the care of musculoskeletal tumors.
- Four types of surgical margins of resection have been defined: intralesional (or intracapsular), marginal, wide, and radical[1] (Figure 12–3, Table 12–4).
  1. An intralesional margin is the surgical margin achieved when a tumor's pseudocapsule is violated and a gross tumor is removed from within the pseudocapsule. Incisional biopsy and curettage are two common examples of intralesional margin.
  2. A marginal surgical margin is achieved when a tumor is removed by dissecting between the normal tissue and the tumor's pseudocapsule. Because the pseudocapsule contains tumor cells, this excision leaves viable tumor in the surrounding local tissues. This excision is inadequate for local removal of a malignancy.
  3. A wide surgical margin is achieved when the tumor is removed with a surrounding cuff of normal, uninvolved tissue.
  4. A radical surgical margin is achieved when the tumor and the entire compartment (or compartments) are removed together.
- As a rule, benign lesions can be managed with an intralesional or marginal surgical margin, but malignant tumors require a wide surgical margin. Radical surgical margins are reserved for recurrent tumors and the most infiltrative malignancies.

Box 12–4 Basic Principles of an Incisional Biopsy

- Longitudinal incisions should be used in the extremities.
- The smallest incision compatible with obtaining an adequate tumor specimen should be used.
- The most direct route from the skin to the tumor should be taken; to prevent tumor spreading, the biopsy should go through muscle rather than through intermuscular planes and should avoid exposure of neurovascular bundle or joint.
- An intraoperative frozen section should be done to confirm the adequacy of the specimen.
- Meticulous hemostasis should be obtained for the prevention of tumor spread by hematoma.
- Drains should be placed close to and in line with the incision.

Table 12–3: Surgical Stages

STAGE	GRADE	SITE	METASTASES
IA	Low	Intracompartmental	None
IB	Low	Extracompartmental	None
IIA	High	Intracompartmental	None
IIB	High	Extracompartmental	None
III	Low or high	Intracompartmental or extracompartmental	Yes

Specific Bone Tumors

Tumors of Bone Origin

Osteoid Osteoma

- Osteoid osteoma is a benign bone tumor characterized by a nidus of osteoid tissue surrounded by dense reactive bone.

Table 12–4: Surgical Margins

SURGICAL MARGINS	LIMB SALVAGE	AMPUTATION	HISTOLOGY
Intralesional	Curettage, piecemeal resection within lesion	Through tumor	Tumor at margin
Marginal	Marginal excision through reactive tissue	Along reactive tissue	Reactive tissue +/– satellites
Wide	Wide excision through normal surrounding tissue	Through normal tissue in compartment	Normal tissue +/– skip lesions
Radical	Radical resection with entire compartment	Extracompartmental amputation or disarticulation	Normal tissue

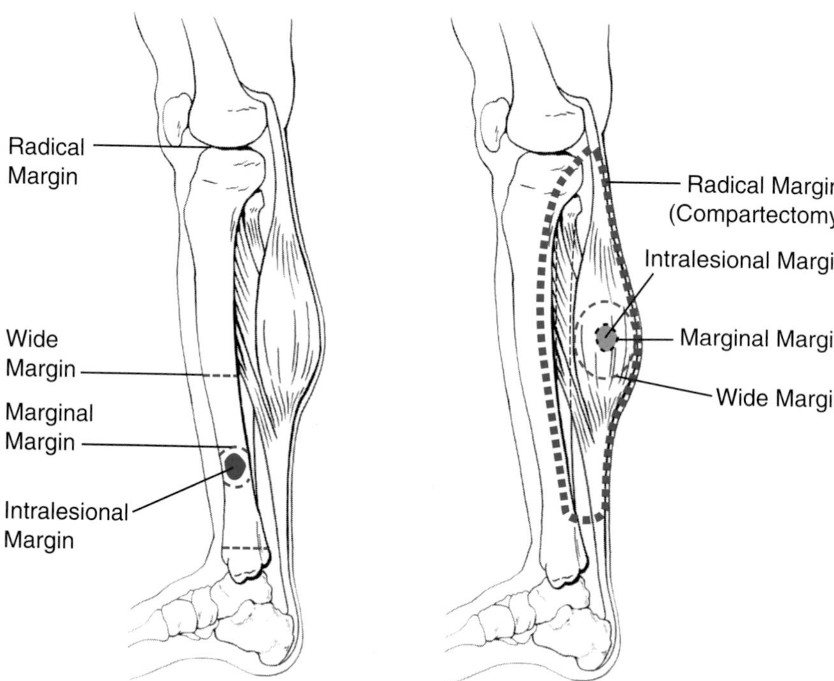

Figure 12–3: Surgical margins for bone (*left*) and soft tissue (*right*) lesions. The intralesional margin is within the lesion, the marginal marginis is through the reactive zone of the lesion, the wide margin is beyond the reactive zone through normal tissue within the compartment, and the radical margin is normal tissue that is extracompartmental. From Himelstein BP, Dormans JP (1996) Malignant bone tumors of childhood. Pediatr Clin North Am 43(4): 967-984.

- It accounts for approximately 10% of benign bone tumors.[7]
- Males are affected more than females at a ratio of 3:1.

Clinical Findings

- The most commonly involved site is the lower extremity, particularly the metaphyseal or diaphyseal regions of the femur and tibia.
- Patients with osteoid osteoma typically have a history of dull, aching pain in the region overlying the affected long bone. The pain tends to be worse at night and is relieved significantly by salicylates and nonsteroidal anti-inflammatory drugs.[4,8,9]
- Limping and atrophy of the involved extremity may be associated.
- Painful scoliosis may develop because of spinal involvement.

Radiographic and Histological Features

- See Table 12–5 for the typical radiographic and histological features of osteoid osteoma (Figure 12–4).

Treatment

- Osteoid osteomas are described as self-limiting lesions that may mature spontaneously over several years.
- Treatment of osteoid osteoma usually involves complete surgical removal of the nidus.[4,5] Complete removal of the nidus relieves the patient's pain.
- There are two surgical methods of removing the nidus: extended curettage and en bloc excision.

Table 12–5: Typical Features of Osteoid Osteoma and Osteoblastoma

	OSTEOID OSTEOMA	OSTEOBLASTOMA
Histological Features		
Gross (macroscopic)	Round or oval, reddish brown, most ≤1 cm in diameter	Similar but larger than osteoid osteoma (most 2-6 cm)
Histological (microscopic)	Distinct demarcation between nidus and surrounding reactive bone Interlacing network of immature bone and bony trabeculae, with focal areas of osteoblastic and osteoclastic activity	Insignificant demarcation Interlacing woven bone lined by osteoblasts within a fibrovascular stroma
Radiographic Features		
Plain radiographs	Spine—Posterior elements Long bone—Metaphysis or diaphysis Small (≤1 cm), round–elliptical, lucent, intracortical (mostly) lesion surrounded by extensive reactive sclerotic bone	Spine—Posterior elements Long bone—Metaphysis or diaphysis 2-6 cm, round–elliptical lytic lesion surrounded by moderate reactive sclerotic bone Expansion of the involved bone with intralesional stippled ossifications
Computed tomography	Thin (1-2 mm) sections Provides exact localization of the nidus	

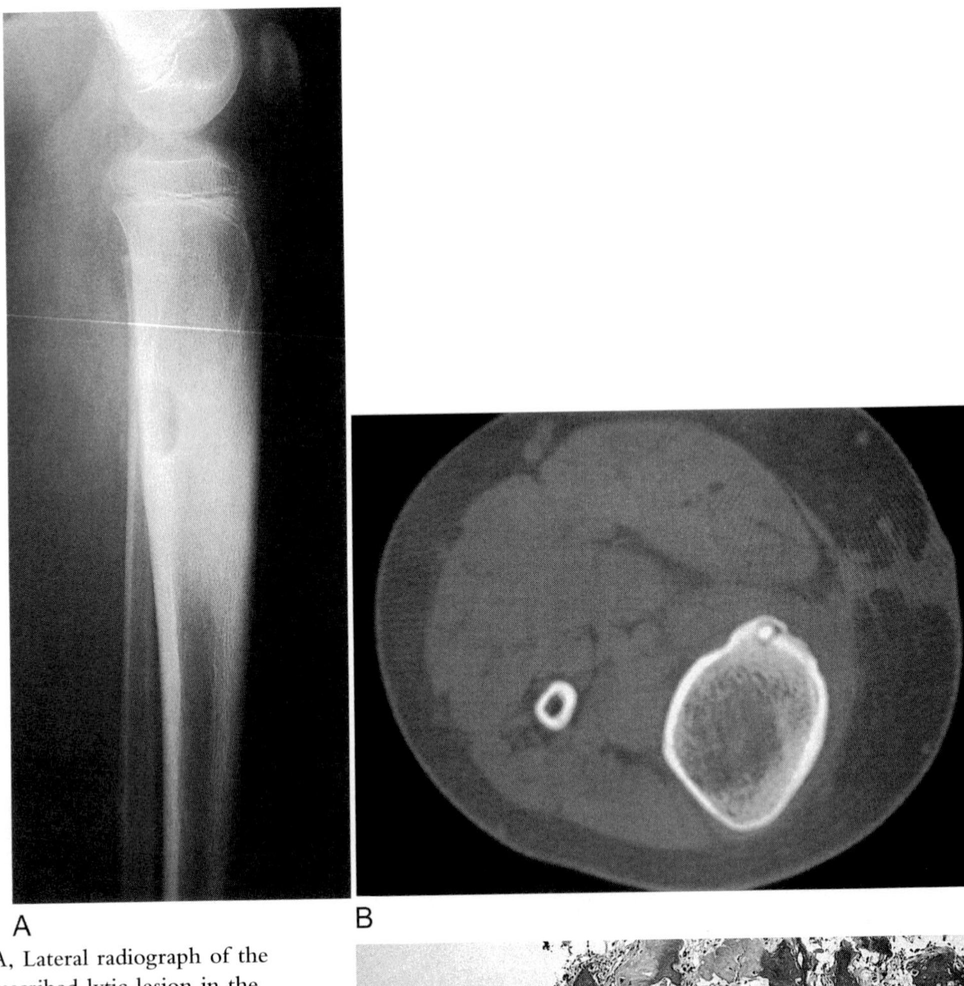

Figure 12–4: Osteoid osteoma. A, Lateral radiograph of the proximal leg shows a well-circumscribed lytic lesion in the posterior cortex of the proximal tibia. There is significant cortical thickening surrounding the lesion. The cortical thickening has caused widening of the tibia. B, Axial CT image demonstrates the cortical location of the lesion. There is a dense, central nidus surrounded by a lucent rim. Note the extensive cortical thickening. C, Photomicrograph of the lesion shows a nidus composed of irregular woven bone trabeculae within a background fibroblastic stroma that is rich in blood vessels.

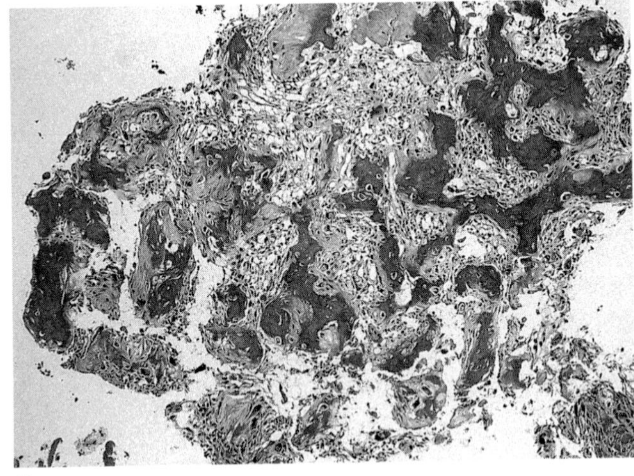

- The most widely used method of treatment is intralesional extended curettage using a high-speed burr, or the *burr-down technique*.
  1. This technique removes the entire nidus but leaves the surrounding reactive bone.
  2. The burr-down technique does not weaken the bone significantly; it is associated with a shorter duration of protected weight-bearing ability and an earlier return to activity.
  3. Bone grafting usually is not required.[4,5]
  4. If curettage is the excision technique used, the nidus must be accurately localized preoperatively and seen intraoperatively. Although some methods—such as CT-guided exploration, intraop-

erative radionuclide scanning, and intraoperative tetracycline–fluorescence demonstration—have been described to find the nidus in the operating room, preoperative planning and careful localization of the nidus makes the use of these methods unnecessary and is usually sufficient to find the nidus intraoperatively.[5]

- When the nidus cannot be localized accurately preoperatively or seen intraoperatively, block excision is preferred.
  1. En bloc resection is performed by placing drill bits around the lesion and confirming their placement with fluoroscopy in the operating room. The lesion is then removed en bloc with the margins of reactive bone.
  2. The advantage of the block resection is the greater assurance that all of the nidus is removed.
  3. This method requires removal of a segment of the cortex, producing a marked reduction in the strength of the bone. The extremity may need to be protected for an extended period.
  4. Bone grafting may be needed to fill the defect.

- CT-guided percutaneous techniques are showing favorable results.[4]
  - These techniques include CT-guided percutaneous excision using a trephine and CT-guided percutaneous radiofrequency coagulation. A radiofrequency probe is placed in the center of the lesion, and a 1-cm area around the bone is heated to destroy the nidus (Figure 12–5).
  - These are outpatient procedures with a low risk of pathological fracture, and the convalescence is rapid.
- Medical management with long-term salicylates occasionally may be considered for lesions that are difficult to remove surgically, such as certain acetabular or spinal lesions. However, long-term use of salicylates may be associated with some complications, such as gastrointestinal bleeding.

Osteoblastoma

- Osteoblastoma is sometimes called *giant osteoid osteoma* because it is histologically identical to osteoid osteoma but is larger.
- Osteoblastoma is less common than osteoid osteoma, accounting for less than 1% of primary bone tumors.[7,8]

Clinical Findings

- Approximately 30 to 40% of osteoblastomas are found in the spine, where they most often affect the posterior elements, including spinous and transverse processes, lamina, and pedicles.[7,9] All areas of the spine may be involved, from the upper cervical region to the sacrum.
- The diaphysis of long bones, particularly the femur and tibia, is also a common site.
- Spinal involvement may appear with myelopathic or radicular symptoms, progressive painful scoliosis, or torticollis if the lesion is in the cervical spine.
- In nonvertebral locations, pain is usually the prominent complaint. The pain is less local than the pain of osteoid osteomas and is much less likely to be relieved by salicylates.
- Osteoblastomas are tender, and direct palpation often localizes a lesion, even when it cannot be seen on a plain radiograph.

Radiographic and Histological Features

- See Table 12–5 for the typical radiographic and histological features of osteoblastoma (Figure 12–6).

Treatment

- Osteoblastoma is a benign but locally aggressive lesion (Box 12–5). The tumor should be excised surgically;

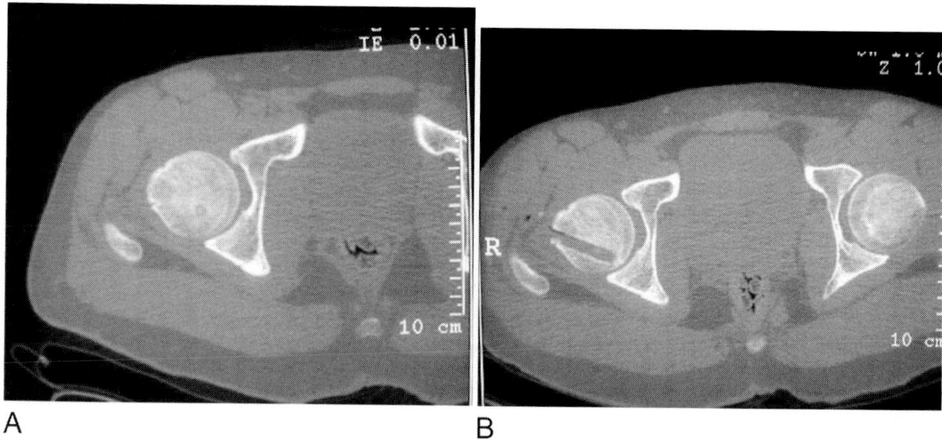

Figure 12–5: Osteoid osteoma. An osteoid osteoma located in the femoral head was treated by CT-guided percutaneous radiofrequency coagulation.

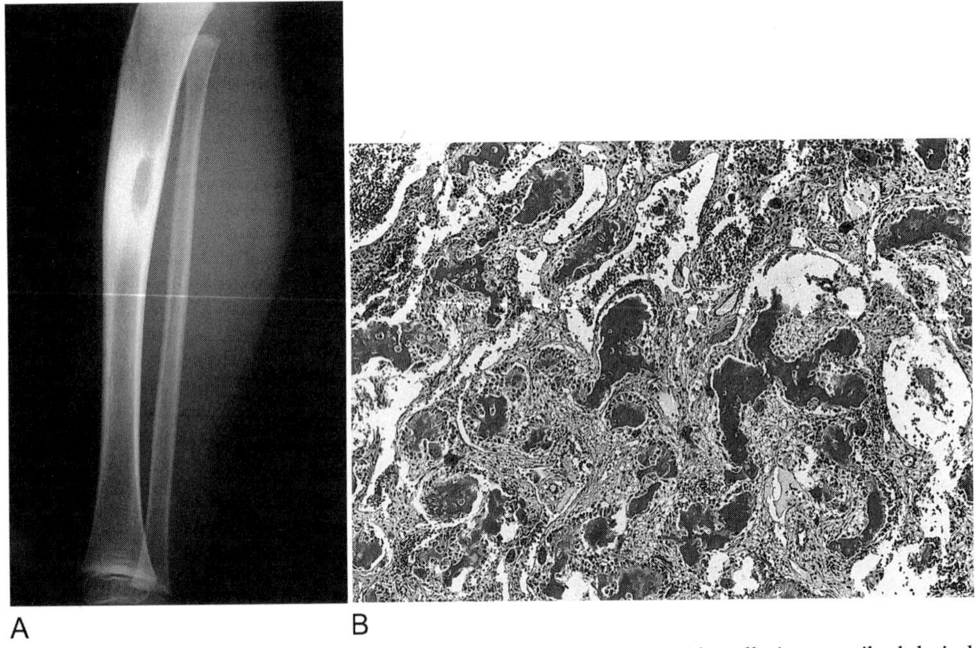

Figure 12–6: Osteoblastoma. A, Lateral radiograph of the leg shows an ovoid, well-circumscribed, lytic lesion in the diaphysis of the tibia with extensive reactive sclerosis and cortical thickening. B, Photomicrograph of the lesion demonstrates haphazard trabeculae of woven immature bone in a fibrovascular stroma, histologically similar to osteoid osteoma.

otherwise, it continues to enlarge and damage the bone and adjacent structures.

- Intralesional extended curettage is the preferred treatment for most lesions. As much of the surrounding bone should be removed as possible. Most osteoblastomas are controlled by extended curettage, but recurrence is not uncommon (approximately 10 to 20%).[4,5,10]
- En bloc excision may be preferred for lesions in expandable bones (e.g., the fibula), aggressive-appearing lesions, and some vertebral lesions.
  1. Reconstruction of the defect formed by excision depends on the site, but most defects require bone grafting.
  2. For extremity lesions, an extended period of protection may be needed.
- Osteoblastomas located in sites inaccessible to surgical excision have been reported to respond to radiation therapy or chemotherapy.

Box 12–5 Benign But Locally Aggressive Bone Tumors

- Osteoblastoma
- Chondroblastoma
- Osteofibrous dysplasia
- Aneurysmal bone cyst (variable)
- Giant cell tumor
- Chondromyxoid fibroma

Osteosarcoma

- Osteosarcoma (osteogenic sarcoma) is the most common malignant bone tumor in children and adolescents.
- There are two major variants that have significantly different clinical presentations and prognoses. The more common osteosarcoma is classic high grade or conventional, and the other is juxtacortical.
- Osteosarcomas generally have complex karyotypic abnormalities without chromosomal translocations. Several nonrandom deletions have been identified, however. The two most obvious gene deletions in osteosarcomas are located on chromosome 13 and 17, the chromosomes containing tumor suppressor genes—retinoblastoma (RB1) and protein 53 (p53) genes, respectively.[4]

Classic High-Grade Osteosarcoma (Conventional Osteosarcoma)

- Classic high-grade osteosarcoma constitutes approximately 85% of all forms of osteosarcoma.
- It is a highly malignant spindle cell sarcoma of bone in which the malignant cells produce osteoid.
- Boys and girls are affected with equal frequency.

Clinical Findings

- High-grade osteosarcoma usually occurs at the metaphyseal ends of the long bones that have the greatest growth potential, but on occasion it may be diaphyseal in location.

- The most common sites, accounting for more than 50% of cases, are the lower end of the femur and the upper end of the tibia.[7,8] The proximal humerus, proximal femur, and pelvis are the next most common sites.
- Pain is the most prevalent presenting symptom in osteosarcoma, occurring in 85% of patients. A palpable or visible mass is noted in about 40% of cases. Less common findings include a limp, weakness, and decreased range of motion in associated joints.
- The patients usually do not have systemic symptoms and usually feel well.
- Approximately 15% of patients with high-grade osteosarcoma have clinically evident metastases, most commonly in the lungs but also in other bone locations and brain.[5,11] Metastases at diagnosis indicates poor prognosis.

Radiographic and Histological Features

Radiographic Features

- Plain radiographs demonstrate a metaphyseal lesion involving the medullary canal with mixed lytic (radiolucent) and blastic (radiodense) activity.
  - The overall appearance of the tumor is one of an aggressive process characterized by the destruction of both cortical and cancellous bone and by a wide (permeative) zone of transition between the tumor and the normal host bone.[9]
  - Extensive periosteal reaction may be seen; the most common periosteal reactions are the sunburst type and the Codman triangle (Figure 12–7, *A*).
  - The presence of a soft tissue mass, which may contain sclerotic foci (tumor bone formation), is also a common finding.
- MRI is the method of choice for evaluating the tumor.
  - MRI can effectively demonstrate the extent of the lesion, including the intraosseous component, the soft tissue extension, and the peritumoral edema (Figure 12–7, *B*).
  - The relation of the tumor to the major neurovascular bundle, the muscles invaded by the soft tissue component, and the involvement of the adjacent joint are all important points that should be evaluated by MRI before definitive surgery.
- Bone scan shows increased uptake in the area of the tumor. It is an excellent screen of the entire skeleton for occult bone lesions.
- Chest radiography and whole-lung CT are performed because of the relatively high incidence of patients with pulmonary metastasis.

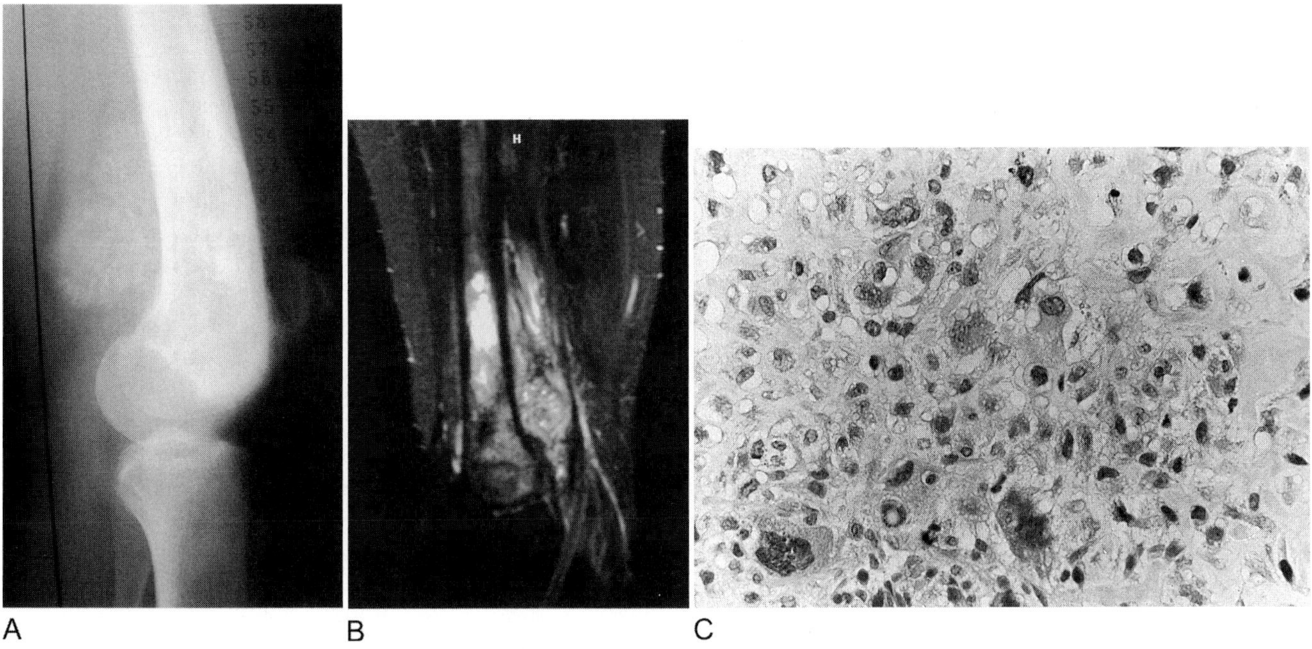

Figure 12–7: High-grade intramedullary osteosarcoma (conventional osteosarcoma). A, Lateral radiograph of the knee shows a lacy, spiculated mass of new bone formation in the metaphysis of the distal femur. Irregular, patchy sclerosis is seen in the metaphysis and epiphysis. B, On a sagittal T2-weighted image, a heterogenous mass is seen in the marrow of the metaphysis and epiphysis with extension into the soft tissues posterior to the femur. C, Photomicrograph (high-power magnification) of the lesion reveals a cellular neoplasm with scattered pleomorphic and bizarre nuclei. Focal osteoid production is evident.

Histological Features

- Gross examination of an osteosarcoma specimen most often reveals a soft tissue mass originating in the medullary canal and extending beyond the cortex. The inner part of the mass is usually more heavily mineralized than the periphery.
- High-grade osteosarcoma has been divided into several histological subtypes based on the predominant cell type of the tumor: osteoblastic, chondroblastic, fibroblastic, mixed, and telangiectatic.
  - Although initially it was thought that the different types had distinct prognoses, it is now recognized that, if matched for size and histological grade, all types have the same prognosis.[5]
  - These tumors are graded on a scale of either 1 to 3 or 1 to 4; the higher the histological grade, the worse the prognosis. Most osteosarcomas are grade 3 or 4 and are of the mixed type.
- Histological examination will reveal frankly malignant cells producing osteoid (Figure 12–7, *C*). These cells are pleomorphic and exhibit mitotic activity. There are often areas of spontaneous tumor necrosis. In addition, the background stroma may be predominantly fibrous or chondroid.

Treatment

- Surgery alone was the treatment for patients with classic high-grade osteosarcoma before 1970, and 80% of the patients died with metastatic disease. Over the next 2 decades, great strides were made in the treatment of classic high-grade osteosarcoma so that, currently, approximately 70% of patients with the disease survive and limb-sparing surgery is possible in about 90% of patients.
- Modern therapy for osteosarcoma begins with accurate staging, the final step of which is biopsy (Box 12–3). The current standard of treatment is multiagent preoperative (neoadjuvant) chemotherapy with wide resection or amputation followed by postoperative (adjuvant) chemotherapy[4,5,11] (Box 12–3). The entire treatment takes approximately 1 year. Osteosarcoma responds poorly to radiation therapy.
  - Neoadjuvant chemotherapy is given for osteosarcoma to treat the micrometastatic disease, to cause necrosis of the primary tumor, and to decrease the primary tumor size, facilitating limb salvage procedures. Most current protocols incorporate doxorubicin, cisplatin, and high-dose methotrexate. The combination of bleomycin, cyclophosphamide, and actinomycin D is also used.[5,11]
  - Following surgical resection, adjuvant chemotherapy is continued to eliminate any micrometastases still present.
  - A good response to chemotherapy, usually defined as greater than 90% necrosis of the tumor (detected in the resection specimen), is associated with higher survival rates than a poorer response.[12]
  - Surgery is the mainstay of local control of osteosarcoma. Excision of the tumor with wide surgical margins, which can be achieved through limb salvage or amputation, is the goal of the surgery. Currently, limb salvage is possible for most patients with an extremity osteosarcoma.[4,5,11]
    1. Limb salvage surgery is indicated for patients in whom wide margins can be obtained without sacrificing so much tissue that the remaining limb is nonfunctional. Usually, the determining factor is the ability to spare major nerves. Major vessels need to be preserved or reconstructed.
    2. There must be adequate soft tissue coverage either locally or in the form of flaps to ensure survival of the reconstruction.
    3. The overall reconstruction should function as well as or better than an appropriate prosthesis after an amputation.
    4. The options for reconstructing the skeletal defect include osteoarticular allograft, intercalary allograft, a metal endoprosthesis (Figure 12–8, *A* and *B*), an allograft–prosthesis composite, arthrodesis, rotationplasty (Figure 12– 8, *C-F*), and free vascularized fibular transfer. In some locations, such as the fibula and clavicle, no bony reconstruction is necessary.
    5. The indications for an amputation are an inability to achieve wide surgical margins, a grossly displaced pathological fracture, a tumor that enlarges during preoperative chemotherapy, and a neurovascular bundle involvement that cannot be appropriately addressed with reconstructive techniques.
- Patients who have clinically apparent metastases at presentation fare considerably worse, with 5-year survival rates of between 10% and 20%.
- When pulmonary metastases develop after the completion of therapy and the metastases can be resected, a 5-year survival rate of 20% to 40% can be expected.

Surface or Juxtacortical Osteosarcoma

- The term *juxtacortical* is a general designation for a group of osteosarcomas that arise on the surface of a bone. Three subtypes are recognized: parosteal, periosteal, and high grade.
- Most juxtacortical osteosarcomas are low-grade tumors (parosteal osteosarcoma), although there are moderately (periosteal osteosarcoma) and highly malignant (high-grade surface osteosarcoma) variants.

Parosteal Osteosarcoma

- Parosteal osteosarcoma, which accounts for about 5% of all osteosarcomas, is seen in patients in their third and fourth decades.

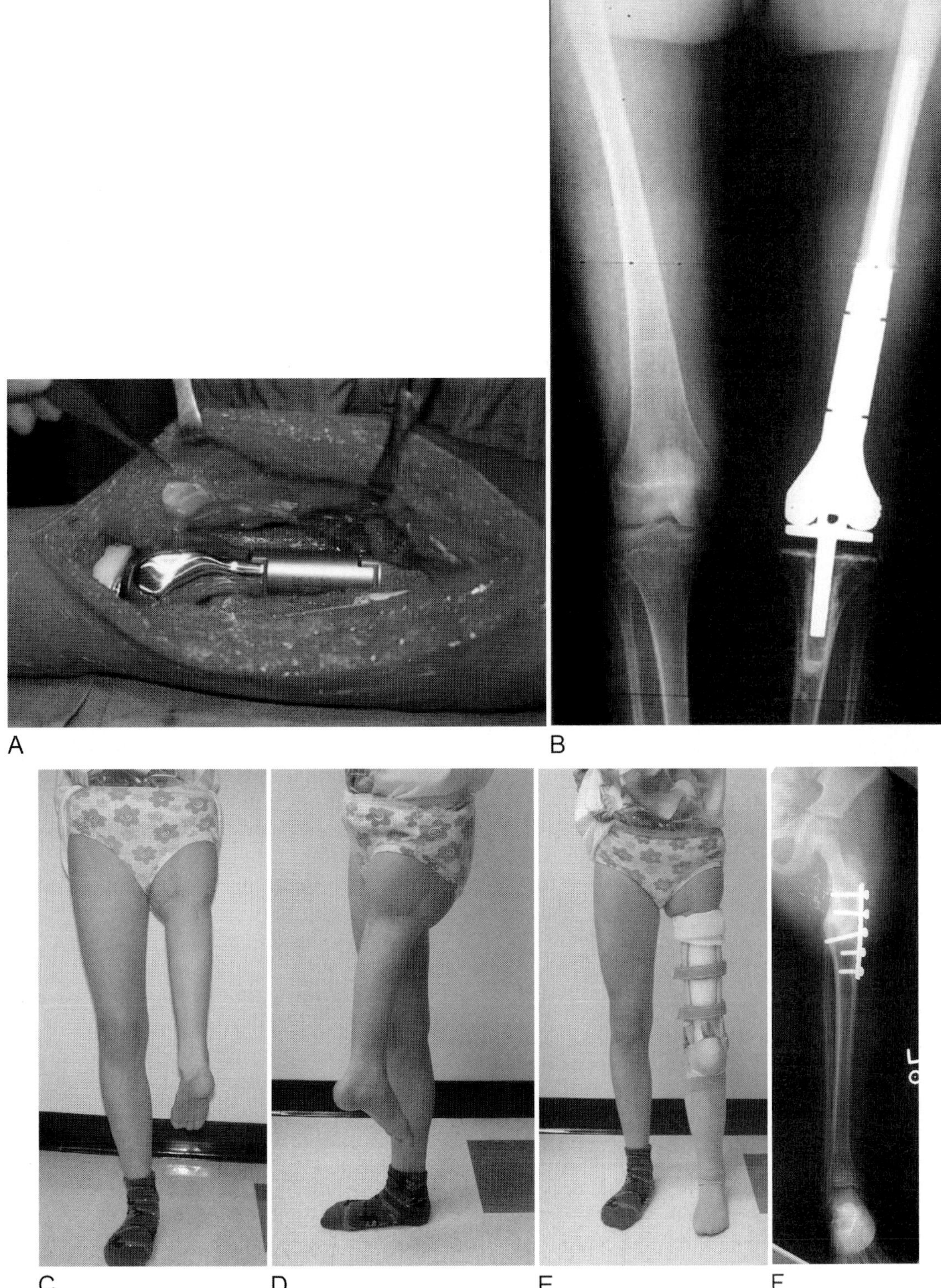

Figure 12–8: Reconstruction of skeletal defects following limb salvage surgery, with metal endoprosthesis (A and B) and rotationplasty (C-F).

- The tumor characteristically affects the posterior aspect of the distal femur. Other sites include the humerus, tibia, and proximal femur.
- Parosteal osteosarcoma often presents symptoms including a painless or vaguely aching, slow-growing mass.
- Radiographically, parosteal osteosarcoma appears as a large, ossified mass with a broad base, which may be confused with an osteochondroma. The medullary cavity is usually spared unless the lesion has long been present.[9]
- Although these features can be adequately demonstrated by conventional radiography, MRI is often necessary to determine the extent of cortical penetration and intramedullary invasion by the tumor.
- Histologically, the tumor demonstrates the features of a low-grade malignancy. There is a fibroblastic stroma with multiple parallel trabecular bone in different stages of maturation, ranging from woven to more organized lamellar bone. The trabeculae are lined with spindle cells that may demonstrate varying degrees of atypia.

Periosteal Osteosarcoma

- This rare type of osteosarcoma, which accounts for 1 to 2% of all osteosarcomas, is most commonly seen in adolescence.
- Periosteal osteosarcoma is usually located in the diaphysis of long bones, most commonly the tibia and femur.
- Radiographically, periosteal osteosarcoma is characterized by its surface origin, bony spicule formation perpendicular to the shaft of the underlying bone, and chondroblastic matrix.
- Histologically, it is a low- or medium-grade malignancy and is composed mainly of lobulated chondroid tissue with moderate cellularity. The tumor characteristically exhibits large amounts of cartilage matrix undergoing calcification or endochondral ossification and small amounts of fine, lace-like osteoid surrounding malignant cells.

High-Grade Surface Osteosarcoma

- A small percentage of juxtacortical osteosarcomas consists of high-grade tumors; these carry the same prognosis as conventional osteosarcoma.
- High-grade tumors account for less than 1% of all osteosarcomas.
- They are most common in the second and third decades, and the femur is the most common site.
- Radiographically, high-grade tumors have an appearance similar to that of parosteal osteosarcomas, but histologically they are high-grade lesions.

Treatment

- Low-grade juxtacortical osteosarcomas (parosteal and periosteal) should be treated with wide excision. Although the metastatic potential of these low-grade surface lesions is much lower than conventional osteosarcoma, these are locally aggressive, malignant tumors and inadequate resection will result in recurrence. Local recurrence also may progress the tumor to a more aggressive, high-grade lesion.[4]
- High-grade surface osteosarcomas require aggressive treatment similar to that of conventional osteosarcoma.

Tumors of Cartilaginous Origin

Osteochondroma

- Osteochondroma, also known as *exostosis,* is the most common skeletal tumor; it accounts for 20 to 50% of benign bone tumors and 10 to 15% of all bone tumors.[5,9]
- There appears to be a slight predominance in male patients.
- Osteochondroma is characterized by a cartilage-capped osseous projection protruding from the surface of the affected bone.
- The exostosis is produced by progressive endochondral ossification of the hyaline cartilaginous cap, which essentially functions as a growth plate.
- Unlike the more extensive hereditary (autosomal dominant) multiple exostosis, solitary osteochondromas do not appear to be genetically transmitted.

Clinical Findings

- Osteochondroma most commonly involves the metaphysis of long bones, particularly around the knee (40% of lesions) and the proximal humerus.[7,8] Other areas in which solitary osteochondromas may be found include the distal radius, distal tibia, proximal and distal fibula, and occasionally flat bones such as the scapulae, ilium, or ribs.
- The most common finding is a firm mass, usually of long duration, adjacent to a joint.
- Pain may result from irritation of overlying soft tissues by the lesion.
- On physical examination, the mass is nontender, hard, and fixed to the bone.

Radiographic and Histological Features

Radiographic Features

- The characteristic radiographic appearance of osteochondroma is a bony projection composed of a cortex continuous with that of the underlying bone and a similarly continuous spongiosa.
  - The lesion protrudes from the host bone on either a sessile (broad-based) or pedunculated bony stalk (Figure 12–9).
  - Osteochondroma occurs either in the metaphysis or, as the main epiphyseal plate grows away from the lesion, in the diaphysis. It is never found in the epiphysis.
  - The lesion usually points from the joint.
  - Irregular zones of calcification, especially in the cartilaginous cap, may be present.

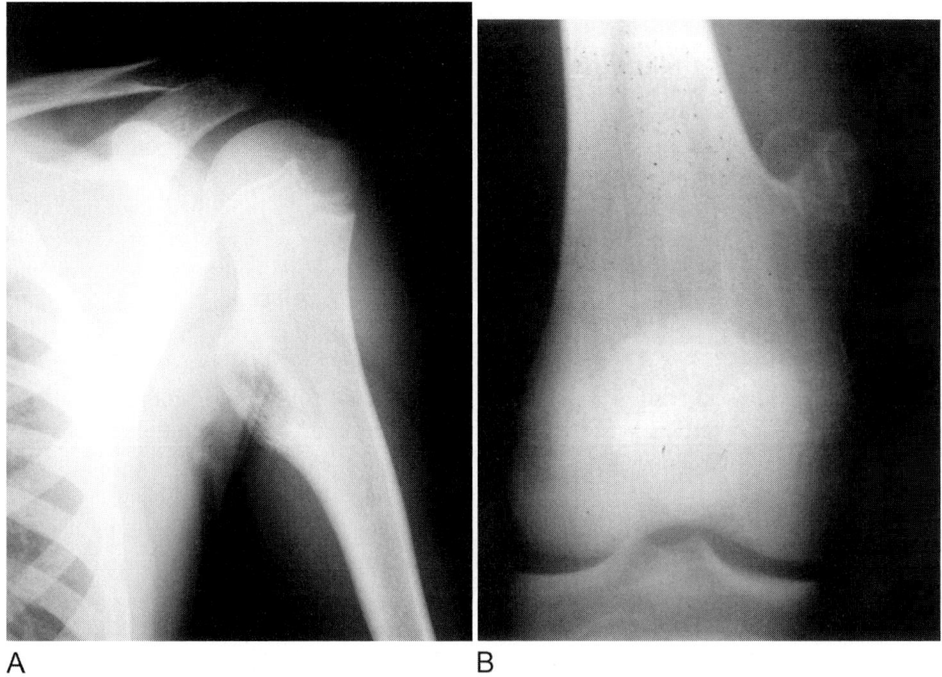

Figure 12–9: Osteochondroma. A, Anteroposterior radiograph of the proximal humerus shows a broad-based lesion arising from the cortex. Note the presence of trabecula within the bony mass. The cartilaginous cap is not visible. B, A different patient with a pedunculated osteochondroma. Note the narrow pedicle. *B* from Erol B, States L, Pawel BR, Tamai J, Dormans JP (2004) Musculoskeletal tumors in children. In: Pediatric Orthopaedics and Sports Medicine (Dormans JP, ed). Philadelphia: Mosby.

- CT can demonstrate the continuity of cancellous portions of the lesion and host bone and the thickness of the noncalcified cap (usually <3 mm in children). CT may be useful in differentiating atypical osteochondromas from malignant lesions such as chondrosarcoma and juxtacortical osteosarcoma.[9]

Histological Features

- Grossly, an osteochondroma looks like a cauliflower.
- Histologically, the lesion is composed of a cartilaginous cap with a pedunculated or sessile base of bone. The cartilaginous cap is usually 1 to 3 cm thick, but in the younger patient it may be noticeably thicker. The thickness of the cartilaginous cap may be much greater if the tumor has undergone sarcomatous change.[7] Deep to the cartilaginous cap there is a variable amount of calcification, an enchondral ossification, and a normal bone with a cortex and cancellous marrow cavity (Figure 12–10).

Treatment

- Osteochondromas may continue to grow until skeletal maturity. This is not a sign of malignancy. Malignant transformation is extremely rare in children and uncommon in adults. In a skeletally mature patient, a growing lesion with a thick cartilaginous cap, particularly in an axial location (i.e., the pelvis or scapula), is highly suspicious for this complication.[5,10]
- Asymptomatic osteochondromas do not require treatment.

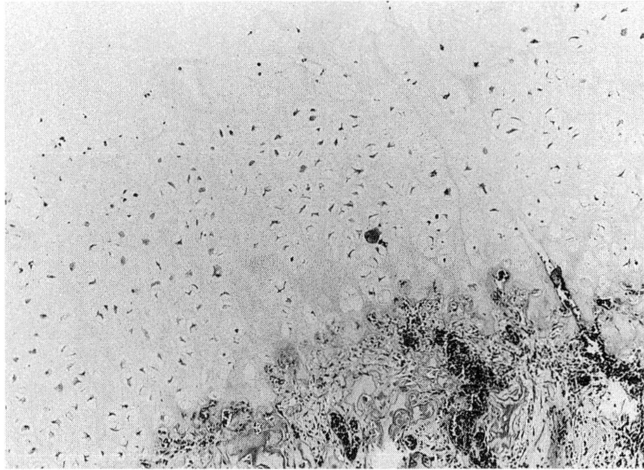

Figure 12–10: Photomicrograph of osteochondroma, demonstrating a thick cartilaginous cap overlying cancellous bone.

- Excision usually is reserved for lesions that cause pain, cause symptomatic impingement on neurovascular structures, or interfere with joint function.
  - Sometimes the osteochondroma is considered cosmetically unacceptable and the adolescent will ask to have it removed, preferring a scar to a bump.
  - Removal in a young child may damage the growth plate and cause a recurrence of the lesion. Excision of osteochondromas should be postponed, if possible, until there is intervening bone between the osteochondroma and the physis so that the risk of physeal damage is decreased.
  - The incidence of local recurrence after surgical excision is low (<2%). The entire cartilaginous cap should be removed to prevent recurrence.

Hereditary Multiple Exostosis

- See Chapter 14.

Dysplasia Epiphysealis Hemimelica

- Dysplasia epiphysealis hemimelica, also known as *Trevor disease,* is a condition that manifests as an intra-articular osteochondroma (Figure 12–11).[9]
- This disorder is characterized by asymmetrical cartilaginous overgrowth of one or more epiphyses in the lower and, occasionally, upper extremities.

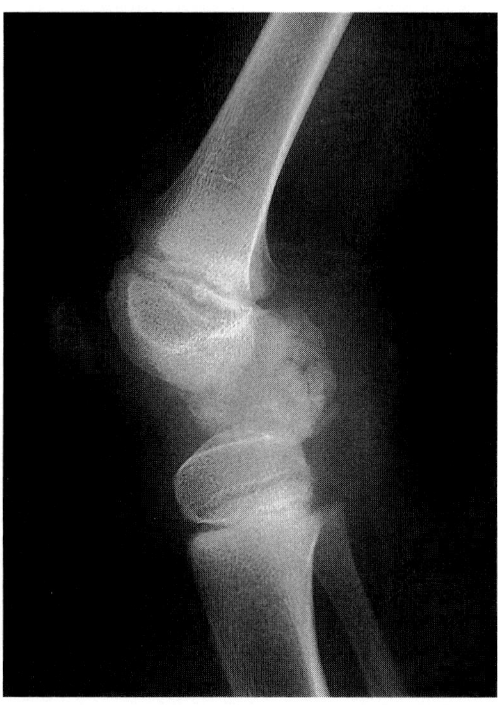

Figure 12–11: Dysplasia epiphysealis hemimelica (Trevor disease). **Lateral radiograph of the knee shows marked enlargement of posterior aspect of the medial femoral condyle. Multiple, rounded, ossific densities representing osteochondromas blend with the trabeculae. Note the loss of the cortex.**

- Dysplasia epiphysealis hemimelica presents symptoms of pain, deformity, and restricted motion in the affected joint.
- Histological examination of the lesion is almost identical to that for osteochondroma.
- Dysplasia epiphysealis hemimelica usually stops growing once maturity is reached. Incongruity that occurs in the joint will lead to subsequent osteoarthritis.
- This condition remains benign; malignant transformation has not been reported in dysplasia epiphysealis hemimelica.
- Observation is warranted if the condition is asymptomatic and has not led to angular deformity or significantly limited joint range of motion.
- Surgical excision should be undertaken if the lesion is painful, the deformity is occurring, or the joint function is limited. Recurrence is common, and repeated local excision is often required.

Chondroblastoma

- Chondroblastoma is a rare neoplasm accounting for 1% of all benign bone tumors.
- Males are affected almost twice as frequently as females.
- Abnormalities in chromosomes 5 and 8 have been reported in chondroblastomas; however, specific locations have not been clearly identified.

Clinical Findings

- Chondroblastoma occurs primarily in the epiphysis of the growing skeleton. In children, it is the most common neoplastic lesion of the secondary ossification center.[7,10]
- The most common sites of involvement are the proximal humerus, the proximal and distal femur, and the proximal tibia.
- Patients with chondroblastoma usually have joint complaints; pain is the initial symptom, followed by effusion and diminished motion in the adjacent joint.
- Frequently the patient is believed to have chronic synovitis because there are no other symptoms or abnormal physical findings.

Radiographic and Histological Features

Radiographic Features

- Chondroblastomas usually have an eccentric location, involving less than one half of the entire epiphysis.
- Plain radiographs show a well-marginated, radiolucent lesion, usually with a sclerotic rim of bone (Figure 12–12, *A*). Small punctuate calcifications may be present within the tumor.
- CT scan is superior to radiography when observing intralesional calcifications and demonstrating the extent of the lesion within the epiphysis.
- The edema associated with chondroblastoma can be appreciated on MRI.

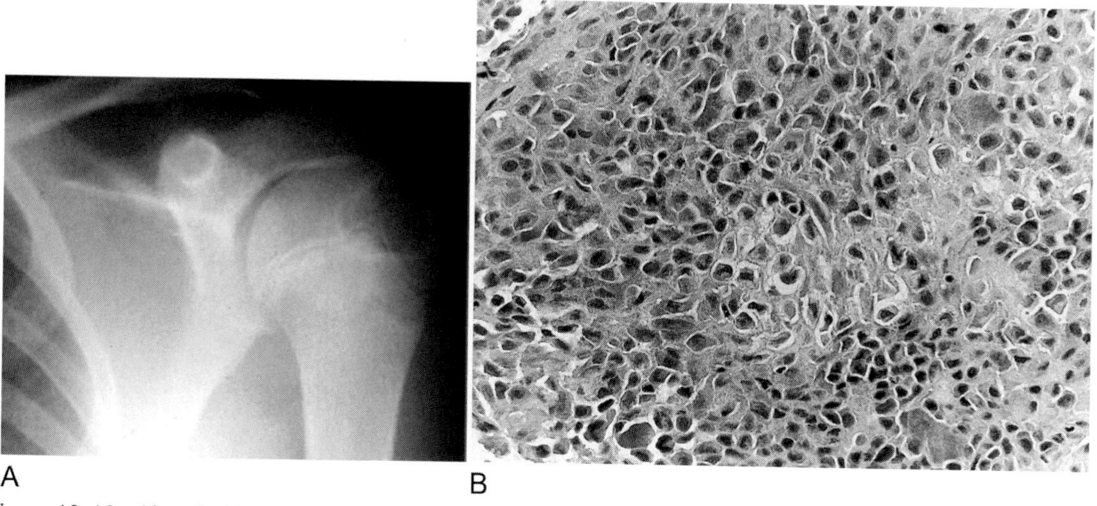

Figure 12–12: Chondroblastoma. A, Anteroposterior radiograph of the shoulder shows a well-circumscribed, lytic lesion in the lateral epiphysis of the humerus. The lesion does not cross the physis. B, Photomicrograph of the lesion demonstrates tumor cells that are uniform, closely packed, and polyhedral and that are focally enveloped by a lace-like, lightly calcified chondroid matrix.

- Chest radiography or CT should be performed, because chondroblastoma is one of the benign tumors that can have lung metastasis.

Histological Features

- Gross specimens are often characterized by pieces of gray pink or hemorrhagic tissues intermixed with calcified, cholesterol-laden tissues.
- Histologically, the lesion consists of small, closely packed cuboidal cells (chondroblasts) that give the appearance of a cobblestone street (Figure 12–12, *B*). There are areas with varying amounts of amorphous matrix, which often contains streaks of calcification ("chicken-wire" calcification), and there are numerous multinucleated giant cells.[9,10]

Treatment

- Chondroblastomas may progress and invade the joint (Box 12–5). They should be treated when detected.[10]
- Extended curettage is the initial treatment of choice.
  - The lesion should be exposed and visualized adequately at the time of curettage, and the curettage should be extended beyond the reactive rim.[4,5,10]
  - Intra-articular surgical exposure is sometimes needed if this facilitates visualization.
  - The cavity is filled with bone graft.
  - Recurrence rates of approximately 10 to 30% have been reported after intralesional excision. Most recurrences are adequately addressed with a second curettage, but a rare lesion can be locally aggressive and requires a wide en bloc resection.
  - Reconstruction after wide resection may require a partial or full osteoarticular allograft or an endoprosthetic reconstruction.[5]
- Most patients with chondroblastoma are close to skeletal maturity when the diagnosis is made, and the risk of growth disturbance from the tumor or its treatment is minimal.

Chondromyxoid Fibroma

- Chondromyxoid fibroma is a rare bone tumor.
- Males are more frequently affected than females at a ratio of 2:1.
- Although most of the lesions are found in the tibia, other sites of predilection include the femur, fibula, metatarsals, and calcaneus.
- Patients with chondromyxoid fibroma complain of a dull, steady pain, usually worse at night.
- Plain radiographs show a well-localized, eccentric, oval, radiolucent lesion located primarily in the metaphysis of a long bone. Expansion and bubbling of the cortex may occur. The radiographic differential diagnosis includes nonossifying fibroma, aneurysmal bone cyst, and chondroblastoma.
- Histologically, the lesion often is lobular with areas of distinct fibromyxoid cartilage.
- The natural history is not fully understood because of infrequency and because surgical treatment is usually performed early. Chondromyxoid fibromas are accepted as benign but locally aggressive lesions, and extended curettage and bone grafting are recommended.

Enchondroma

- Enchondroma is a relatively common tumor of mature hyaline cartilage, accounting for approximately 10% of benign bone tumors.

- Enchondroma may result from epiphyseal growth cartilage that does not remodel and persists in the metaphysis, or it may result from persistence of the original cartilaginous anlage of the bone.

Clinical Findings

- Enchondromas usually appears as solitary lesions; the short tubular bones of the hand (50%) and foot are common sites, followed in frequency by the distal femur and proximal humerus.[7,8]
- Most patients have a pathological fracture through a lesion in the phalanx or as an incidental finding on a radiograph taken for another reason. An enchondroma should not produce symptoms unless there is a pathological fracture.

Radiographic and Histological Features

Radiographic Features

- Plain radiographs show a sharply circumscribed radiolucent lesion located centrally in the medullary canal (Figure 12–13, *A*). The lesions usually are metaphyseal in location.
  - The bone may be wider than normal, but this is believed to be caused by the lack of remodeling in the metaphysis rather than by expansion of the bone by the tumor.
  - Calcification is usually within the lesion in older patients and appears as fine punctate stippling.
  - In the pediatric patient, unicameral bone cysts may have a similar radiographic appearance, but they are most common in the proximal femur and proximal humerus.

Histological Features

- Grossly, enchondromas are lobular lesions with a bluish color.
- Histologically, lobules of hyaline cartilage with varying cellularity are seen and are recognized by their blue matrix (Figure 12–13, *B*). The chondrocytes are located in rounded spaces called *lacunae*. Foci of calcification are present.

Treatment

- Malignant transformation of enchondromas occurs infrequently (<1%) and is rare before skeletal maturity.[7,9]
  - Patients experiencing pain in a previously asymptomatic lesion without evidence of a pathological fracture should be evaluated for this possibility.
  - In a solitary enchondroma, this more likely occurs in the axial skeleton or a proximal portion of a long bone and rarely occurs in a short tubular bone.
- Asymptomatic solitary enchondromas usually do not require treatment other than a periodic follow-up evaluation; a repeat plain radiography and physical examination should be performed in approximately 6 weeks then every 3 to 6 months for 2 years.[5]

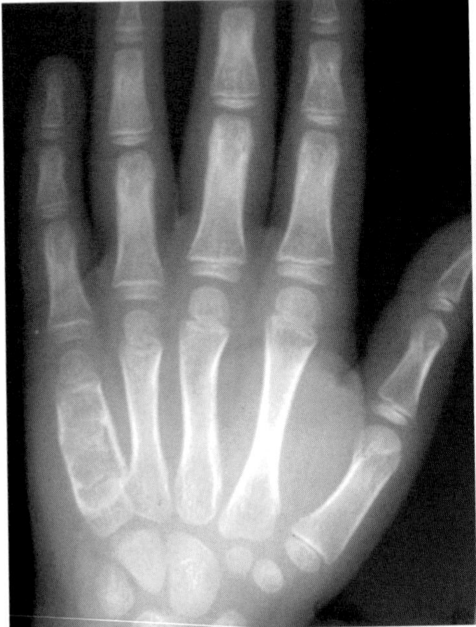

A

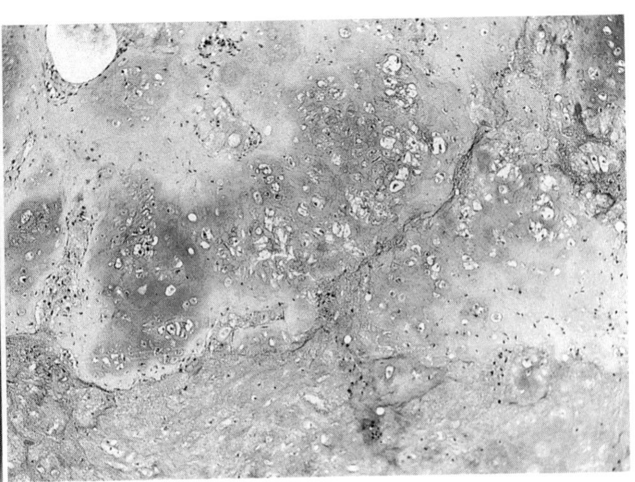

B

Figure 12–13: Enchondroma. A, Anteroposterior radiograph of the hand shows an expansile, lytic lesion involving the diaphysis of the fifth metacarpal with extension into the distal metaphysis. There is saucerization (scalloping) of the inner cortex. B, Photomicrograph demonstrates a lobular lesion composed of mature cartilaginous tissue.

- Incisional biopsy usually is not necessary for asymptomatic lesions. If surgery is indicated, biopsy for histological confirmation should be done.
  - An incisional biopsy alters the histological and radiographic status of the lesion and may make subsequent evaluation difficult. Pathologists may have difficulty distinguishing active enchondroma (most pediatric patients have active lesions) and low-grade chondrosarcoma.
  - If the patient or the patient's parents insist on biopsy, it is best to remove the entire lesion.[5]
- Symptomatic or large lesions in the short tubular bones of the hand without a pathological fracture can be managed with curettage and bone grafting.
- If a pathological fracture occurs through an enchondroma, the fracture should be allowed to heal before curettage and bone grafting (Figure 12–14).
- Recurrence after curettage and bone grafting is rare.

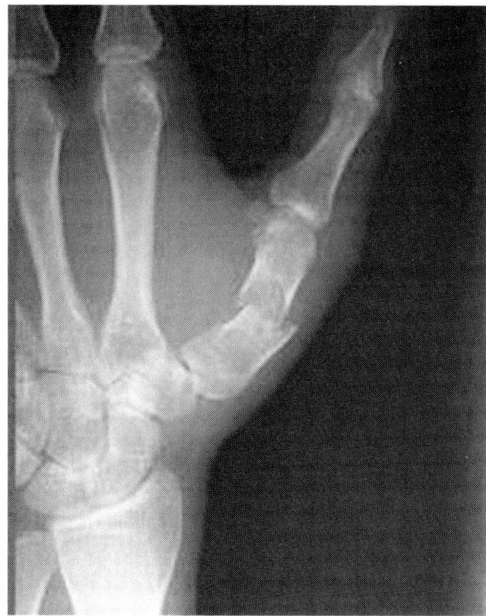

Figure 12–14: Enchondroma. Anteroposterior radiograph of the radial three digits of the hand shows a pathological facture in the first metacarpal through an enchondroma.

Multiple Enchondromatosis

- Multiple enchondromatosis, also known as *Ollier disease,* is an inherited condition with widespread enchondromas.
- It is much less common than solitary enchondroma.
- Most patients have bilateral involvement but have unilateral predominance.
- Unlike solitary enchondroma, Ollier disease can result in symptoms at an early age; shortening of the involved bone, angular deformity, and pathological fracture are commonly seen (Figure 12–15).
- Patients with Ollier disease have an increased risk of later developing secondary chondrosarcoma.[8,9,10] The pelvis and shoulder girdle (axial skeleton) are the most common locations of secondary chondrosarcoma.
- Multiple enchondromatosis with vascular anomalies of soft tissues is known as *Maffucci's syndrome* (see the section on

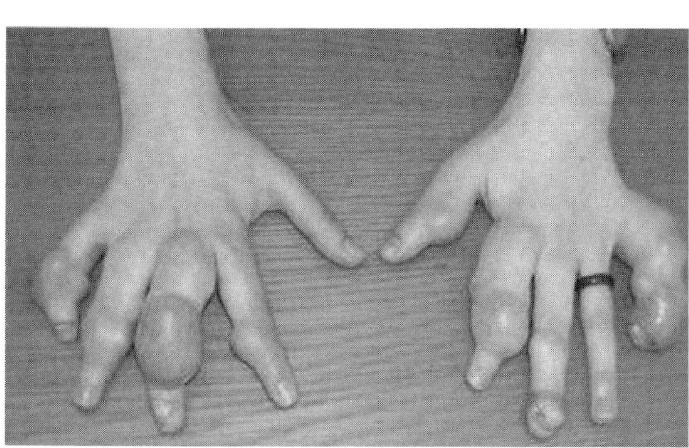

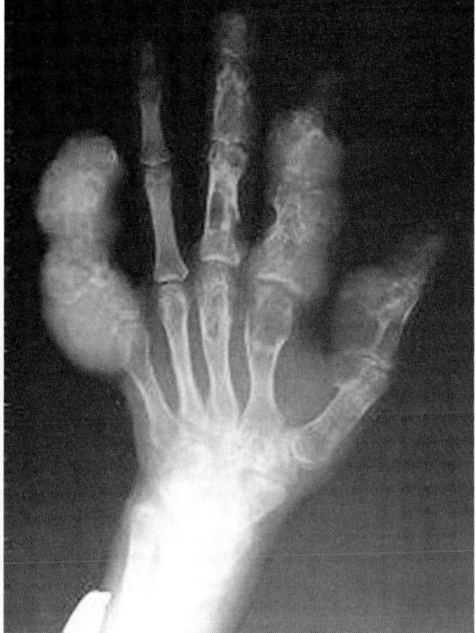

A B

Figure 12–15: Multiple enchondromatosis (Ollier disease). This young female patient with multiple enchondromatosis has multiple lesions involving the digits of both hands.

vascular tumors). Patients with this disorder have an even greater risk of developing malignant cartilage tumors than patients with Ollier disease; importantly, they also have a greater risk of developing carcinoma of an internal organ.

Periosteal Chondroma

- Periosteal chondromas, also known as *juxtacortical chondromas,* are extremely rare benign cartilaginous tumors forming beneath the periosteum and outside the cortex of bone.[7,9]
- The proximal humerus is the classical location, followed by small bones of the hands or feet.
- Patients usually complain of pain at the side of the lesion.
- Radiographs show a cup-shaped or saucer-shaped erosion of the cortex with surrounding sclerotic bone (Figure 12–16, *A*).
- Histologically, periosteal chondroma is benign cartilage, but it appears more active than enchondroma (Figure 12–16, *B*).
- Malignant transformation of periosteal chondromas has not been reported.
- Treatment of periosteal chondroma is surgical.
  - Extended curettage with an intact narrow rim of normal bone is the treatment of choice.
  - Curettage has a relatively high risk of recurrence. Spilling the cartilage into the soft tissues by curettage increases the risk of local recurrence.
  - Bone grafting may be indicated depending on the size of the lesion.

Tumors of Fibrous Origin

Nonossifying Fibroma

- *Nonossifying fibroma, fibrous cortical defect, metaphyseal fibrous defect,* and *fibroma* all refer to the same histopathological process in bone. These lesions differ in size and in radiographic appearance, which reflects the varying phases of the development of the same lesion.
- These lesions are not true neoplasms but rather are a developmental defect in which areas that normally ossify are occupied by fibrous connective tissue.

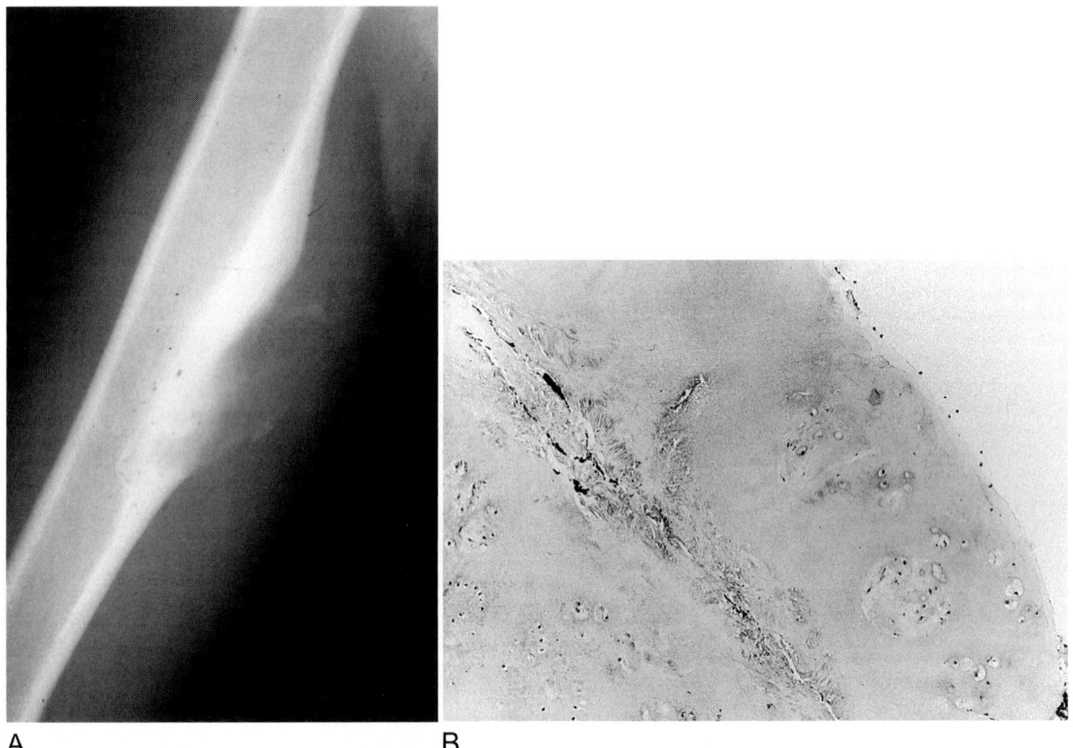

Figure 12–16: Periosteal chondroma. A, Anteroposterior radiograph of the humerus shows spicules of bone formation within a lucent mass. Note the fusiform area of cortical thickening with a central pattern of erosion, referred to as saucerization. The axis of the mass is parallel with the bone, and the cortex at each end of the lesion has a triangle configuration, keys to the origin of the lesion. B, Photomicrograph shows a thin periosteal covering and underlying cartilage of normal cellularity. *A* from Erol B, States L, Pawel BR, Tamai J, Dormans JP (2004) Musculoskeletal tumors in children. In: Pediatric Orthopaedics and Sports Medicine (Dormans JP, ed). Philadelphia: Mosby.

- Nonossifying fibroma is one of the most common benign bone lesions. Because of its harmless course and its classic radiographic appearance, few are biopsied. Consequently, it accounts for only 2% of all benign bone biopsies reported in large series.[5]

Clinical Findings

- The term *fibrous cortical defect* refers to the small, asymptomatic fibrous lesions that occur in young children. These developmental defects usually regress spontaneously, becoming smaller and less distinct then eventually disappearing. Occasionally, these lesions proliferate and grow, extending into the medullary cavity and involving a greater portion of the width of the bone. At this stage, the diagnosis of nonossifying fibroma is made.
- Approximately 90% of fibrous cortical defects and nonossifying fibromas occur in the distal femur.[7,9]
- These are asymptomatic lesions found only if a radiograph is taken for another reason or when the patient has a pathological fracture.

Radiographic and Histological Features

Radiographic Features

- Both lesions are sharply delineated, radiolucent, multiloculated, eccentric, and outlined by a sclerotic border. They are usually metaphyseal in location and the long axes of the lesions are aligned with the long axes of the affected bone.
- Fibrous cortical defect is a small (<0.5 cm) lesion within the cortex, whereas nonossifying fibroma is larger (0.5 to 7 cm) and involves the medullary canal (Figure 12–17, *A* and *B*).

Histological Features

- Surgical curettage usually reveals soft, friable, yellow or brown tissue. Hemosiderin pigment contributes to the brownish color.
- Both lesions consist of benign, spindle, fibroblastic cells arranged in a storiform pattern (Figure 12–17, *C*). Multinucleated giant cells are common, and foam cells containing lipid often can be seen. Hemosiderin within the spindle cells and multinucleated giant cells is usual. Typically, the lesions do not contain bone.

Treatment

- Fibrous cortical defects need no treatment but should be observed. Repeat radiographs at 3- to 6-month intervals for 1 to 2 years are suggested. These lesions should heal spontaneously.
- Large nonossifying fibromas may need surgery.
  - Asymptomatic lesions that are less than 50% of the diameter of the bone can be merely observed.

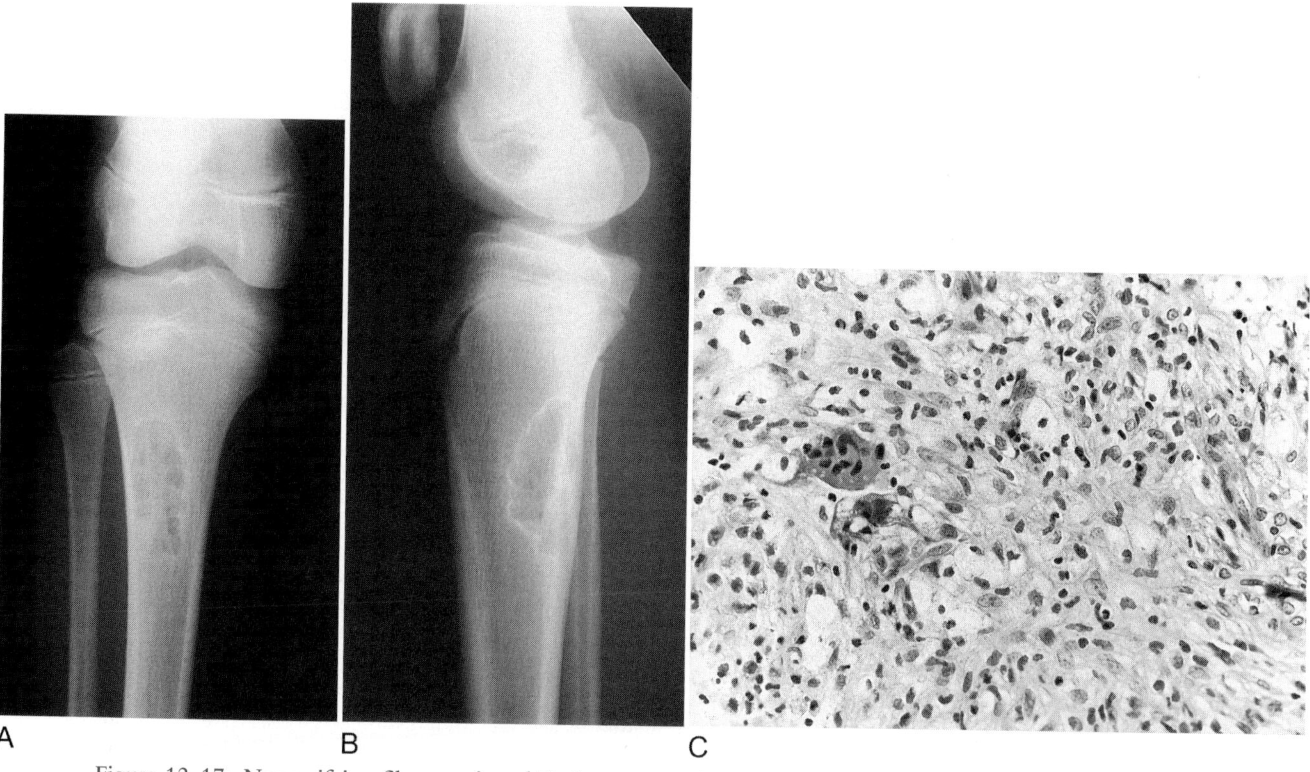

Figure 12–17: Nonossifying fibroma. A and B, Anteroposterior and lateral radiographs of the knee show a large, cortically based, lobulated, lytic lesion with a sclerotic border in the metadiaphysis of the tibia. C, Photomicrograph (high-power magnification) of the lesion demonstrates foamy histiocytic cells, and giant cells are discerned within the fibroinflammatory spindle cell stroma.

They may undergo spontaneous healing by the remodeling process of the tubular bone. If the lesion enlarges, curettage and bone grafting should be considered.

– Large nonossifying fibromas, occupying more than 50% of the diameter of the bone, have an increased risk of developing a pathological fracture. These lesions should be considered for surgical treatment consisting of curettage and bone grafting. Prophylactic internal fixation may be required in high-stress locations, such as the proximal femur[13,14] (Figure 12–18).

- Minimally invasive surgical techniques for treating nonossifying fibromas are becoming more widely accepted.
- Patients who have pathological fractures should have the fractures treated nonoperatively if possible.[13]
  – There is little evidence to suggest that the healing of the fracture increases the chances of spontaneous healing of a nonossifying fibroma or of most other benign lesions.[5]
  – Patients with pathological fractures must be followed until the callus has remodeled sufficiently so that a final

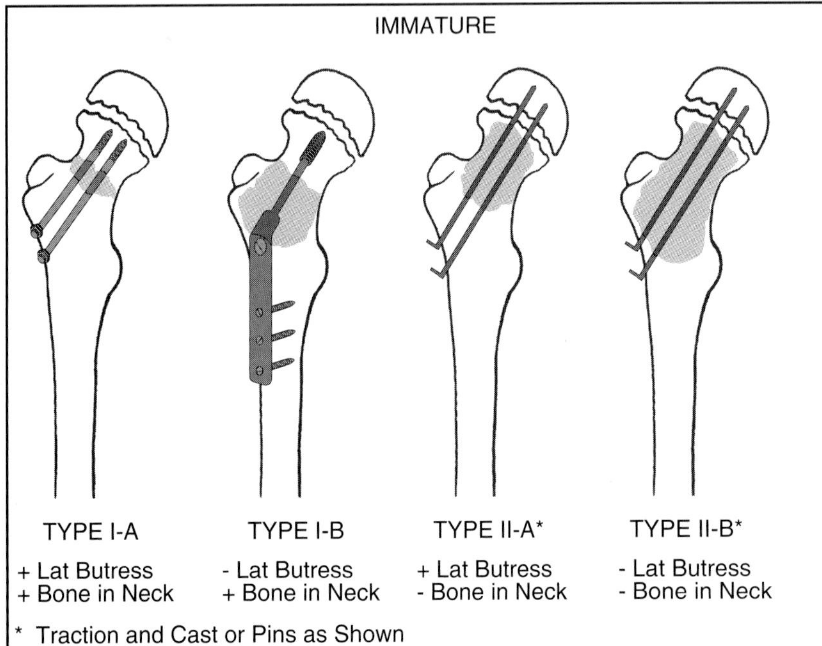

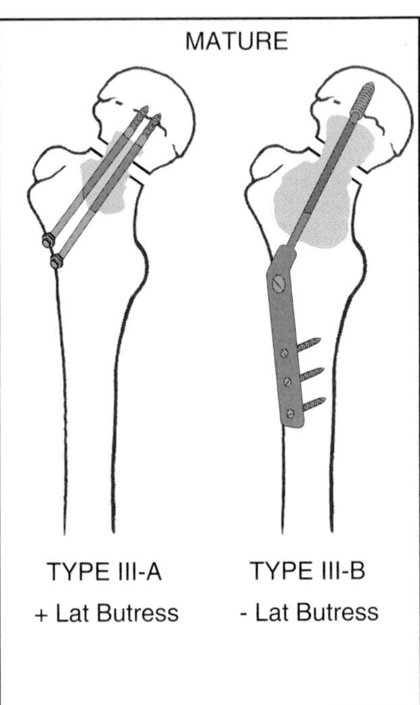

Figure 12–18: The authors' classification system for the treatment of pathological fractures of the proximal femur in children. All small lesions (<50% cortical involvement of femoral neck or trochanteric region) are included in type I. The authors recommend observation for asymptomatic lesions or lesions with transient symptoms. For type I lesions with persistent symptoms, open or percutaneous curettage and bone grafting (bone graft substitutes for percutaneous procedures) can be performed regardless of the skeletal maturity and localization of the lesion. Moderate or large lesions (>50% cortical involvement of femoral neck or trochanteric region) formed type II, III, and IV lesions. In type IIA, a moderately sized lesion is present in the middle of the femoral neck. There is enough bone in the femoral neck and lateral proximal femur (lateral buttress) to allow fixation with cannulated screws after curettage and bone grafting. A pediatric hip screw and side plate can also be used. In type IIB, a large lesion is present at the base of the femoral neck. Although there is enough bone in the femoral neck, there is loss of lateral buttress, so a pediatric hip screw and a side plate should be considered rather than cannulated screws after curettage and bone grafting. In type IIIA-B, a large lesion is present in the femoral neck, so there is not enough bone beneath the physis to accept screws. There are three options for treatment of these bone lesions: (1) After curettage and bone grafting, internal fixation with parallel pins across the physis can be applied; (2) the patient can be treated in skeletal traction until the fracture heals (with subsequent spica cast) followed by open curettage and bone grafting; and (3) the patient can be treated by open curettage and bone grafting at the initial presentation. In type IVA-B, the physis is closing or closed. The lateral buttress is present in type IVA lesions, so cannulated screws (or compression screw and side plate) can be used to stabilize the fracture after curettage and bone grafting. In type IVB hips, the loss of lateral buttress makes it necessary to use a pediatric hip screw and a side plate following curettage and bone grafting. In all types, the authors recommend a representative biopsy specimen for frozen section. Spica cast (or "walking hip spica cast" in selected cases) immobilization following procedures done for moderate or large lesions is also required.

determination can be made about the status of the underlying lesion. If the lesion persists after the fracture has healed, curettage and bone grafting are recommended.

Fibrous Dysplasia

- Fibrous dysplasia is a fibro-osseous lesion characterized by the replacement of a normal lamellar cancellous bone with an abnormal fibrous tissue.
- It is a common disorder that produces a variety of complaints and physical findings.
- Fibrous dysplasia occurs more frequently in females than in males.
- Although most lesions are probably present in early childhood, they usually do not become evident before late childhood or adolescence.
- Most patients (approximately 85%), have a single skeletal lesion (monostotic fibrous dysplasia); the remainder have numerous lesions (polyostotic fibrous dysplasia).[9,10]

Clinical Findings

- The most common locations for monostotic fibrous dysplasia are the ribs, proximal femur, tibia, and base of the skull.[7]
- Monostotic fibrous dysplasia is usually asymptomatic and is discovered incidentally on radiographs obtained for unrelated reasons. Occasionally, the child has a pathological fracture or deformity.
- The skeletal changes are usually more severe in the polyostotic form and may result in pain, swelling, deformity, and limb length discrepancies.
- Repetitive microfractures in the proximal femur can lead to a *shepherd's crook* deformity, with pain, significant varus at the femoral neck, shortening of the femur, an obvious Trendelenburg gait, and limited mobility. Deformity can occur in all of the long bones but usually not to the degree seen in the femur.

Radiographic and Histological Features

- Fibrous dysplasia usually involves the diaphysis of the long bones. It is a medullary process that typically involves the full width of the bone (Table 12–6).

Table 12–6: Differences Between Osteofibrous and Fibrous Dysplasia

OSTEOFIBROUS DYSPLASIA	FIBROUS DYSPLASIA
Has a predilection for tibia	Can occur in any or many locations
Associated with bowing of the tibia in later stages	Associated with bowing of the femur in later stages
Arises from cortex	Arises from medulla
Has trabeculae of woven bone in a fibrous background with osteoblast lining	Has trabeculae of woven in a fibrous background without osteoblast lining
Has cytokeratin-positive cells (+)	Has cytokeratin-negative cells (–)

- Plain radiographs show a radiolucent lesion with slight expansion and thinning of the cortex and a partial loss of the trabecular pattern in the cancellous bone, which gives the characteristic "ground glass" appearance[7,9] (Figure 12–19, *A*).
- There may be an angular deformity or bowing in the bone, especially when the lesion is large. Deformities most commonly occur in the proximal femur (a shepherd's crook deformity) (Figure 12–19, *A*) followed by the proximal humerus.
- The differential diagnosis of fibrous dysplasia may include other common diaphyseal lesions of bone.
- On the bone scan, uptake within the lesion is usually intense.
- Histologically, fibrous dysplasia (both the monostotic and polyostotic variants) is composed of trabeculae of immature, woven bone within a background stroma of collagen-rich tissue (Figure 12–19, *B;* Table 12–6). The osteoid and bone appear to arise in a haphazard fashion from the fibrous stroma. The trabeculae often obtain a variety of shapes (Cs and Os) and are sometimes referred to as alphabet soup or Chinese letters.[7]

Treatment

- Monostotic fibrous dysplasia usually does not require treatment other than observation.
- Surgical treatment may be required for lesions that are large or enlarging, are in a high-stress location (e.g., the proximal femur), or have become symptomatic.
  - Intralesional extended curettage is performed to eradicate the lesion; curettage often results in healing with dysplastic, mechanically deficient bone similar to the pattern of fracture healing in fibrous dysplasia. Therefore, the goals of surgical treatment, when indicated, are clearly different from those of other benign active or aggressive lesions. Rather than resect the lesional tissue, the goals are to stabilize the bone, prevent or correct deformity, and relieve pain.[4,10]
  - Prophylactic internal fixation may be required depending on the size and location of the lesion (Figure 12–18).
  - Small lesions can be packed with cortical cancellous bone graft (autogenous or allogenic), whereas large lesions in long bones, especially the proximal femur, are probably better treated with cortical bone grafts, such as fibular strut. Cortical bone, especially allograft, is useful because of its limited ability to incorporate, which parallels its lower rate of resorption.
  - If the lesion is complicated by a pathological fracture, internal fixation may be required with the curettage and grafting.[13]
  - Resorption of the bone graft with recurrence of fibrous dysplasia can occur, and the patient should be followed for up to 5 years.

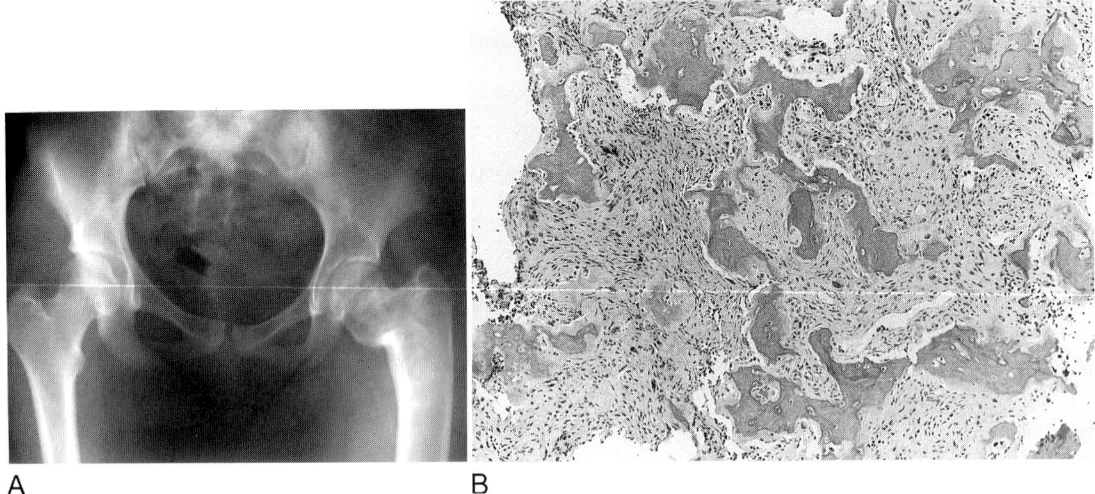

Figure 12–19: Monostotic fibrous dysplasia. A, Anteroposterior radiograph of the pelvis shows widening of the left femoral neck and proximal diaphysis with a diffuse, ground-glass density and scattered lucencies. Note the shepherd's crook deformity of the femoral neck. B, Photomicrograph of the lesion demonstrates irregular woven bone trabeculae (so-called Chinese letters) in a background of bland fibroblastic stroma. Note absence of osteoblastic rimming.

- With polyostotic disease, problem areas usually require straightening and strengthening procedures. Extensive involvement of long bones may be successfully treated with long-term intramedullary stabilization and corrective osteotomies.

Albright's Syndrome

- Polyostotic fibrous dysplasia may occur as part of a condition known as *McCune-Albright's syndrome,* characterized by a classical triad of polyostotic fibrous dysplasia, café-au-lait skin lesions, and precocious puberty (Figure 12–20).
- Activating missense mutations of the guanine nucleotide-binding protein gene encoding the α subunit of the stimulatory G protein (GNAS) have been identified in patients with this syndrome. Recently, the occurrence of GNAS mutations has been shown in individual cases of fibrous dysplasia.

Osteofibrous Dysplasia

- Osteofibrous dysplasia, or *Kempson-Campanacci* lesion (formerly called *ossifying fibroma*), is a rare disorder of childhood.
- The lesion is slightly more common in males.
- Osteofibrous dysplasia has been described as a variant of fibrous dysplasia; however, it differs from fibrous dysplasia in site of involvement, radiographic and histological features, and clinical course (Table 12–6).
- Osteofibrous dysplasia may have a histogenetic relationship to adamantinoma; cytokeratin-positive cells

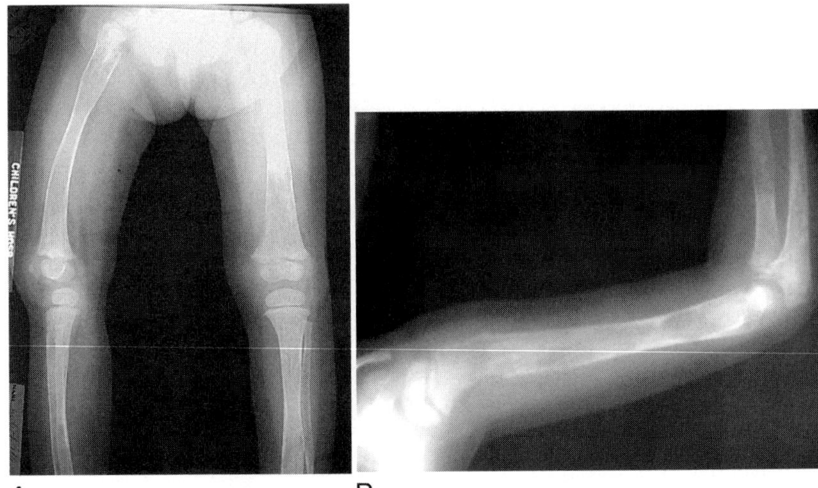

Figure 12–20: Polyostotic fibrous dysplasia (McCune-Albright's syndrome). A and B, Anteroposterior radiographs of the lower and upper extremities reveal expansion of the diaphyses of all the bones with ground-glass opacity.

are found in the stroma of both osteofibrous dysplasia and adamantinoma but not in fibrous dysplasia. Most recent literature has demonstrated the transmission from osteofibrous dysplasia to adamantinoma.[15]

Clinical Findings

- Osteofibrous dysplasia is almost always located within the anterior cortex of the tibia. Ipsilateral fibula may also be affected.
- Osteofibrous dysplasia is usually asymptomatic. Occasionally, its presenting symptoms may include a firm swelling over the tibia with associated mild to moderate anterior tibial bowing.

Radiographic and Histological Features

Radiographic Features

- Plain radiographs show a diaphyseal, intracortical radiolucent lesion associated with expansion and thinning of the cortex and lobulated sclerotic margins (Figure 12–21). In the tibia, the lesion rarely involves the entire circumference of the shaft, but in the fibula, this may occur.

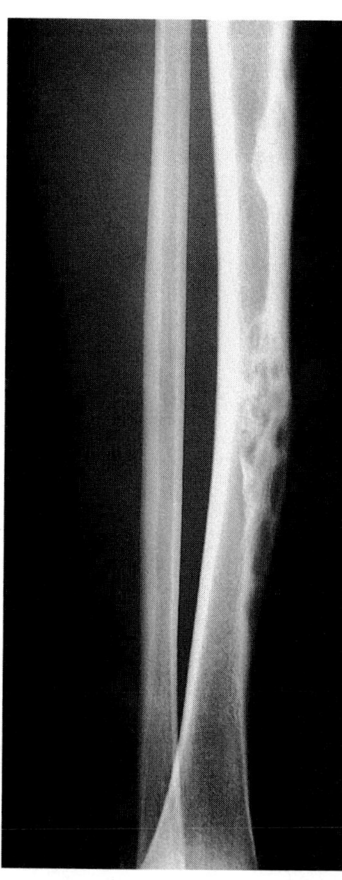

Figure 12–21: Osteofibrous dysplasia. **Lateral radiograph of the tibia shows a cortically based lesion with both sclerotic and multilocular components. Multiple, well-defined, lytic lesions expand the cortex.**

- On bone scan, there is increased uptake in the area of the lesion.

Histological Features

- The tissue is similar to fibrous dysplasia with irregular spicules of trabecular bone and fibrous or collagenous stroma. In contrast to fibrous dysplasia, the spicules are usually lined with osteoblasts. The finding of woven bone with juxtaposed lamellar bone (from osteoblasts) is thought to be characteristic of osteofibrous dysplasia.[7,9]
- Recent immunohistochemical studies have demonstrated isolated cytokeratin-positive cells in the stroma of osteofibrous dysplasia. These cells are not seen in fibrous dysplasia but are found in adamantinomas.

Treatment

- The natural history of osteofibrous dysplasia varies: the lesion may grow slowly, it may expand rapidly into the entire diaphysis (Box 12–5), or occasionally it may regress. The most common clinical course is one of steady growth and expansion during the first 5 to 10 years. Growth then slows, and after maturity the lesion stops expanding.
- Treatment of osteofibrous dysplasia depends on the course of the specific lesion, the age of the child, the radiological characteristics of the lesion, the presence or absence of progression of the lesion, and biopsy information, if available.[5]
- Observation is recommended when the child is younger than 10 years and the lesion is asymptomatic and nonprogressive.
- Incisional biopsy is not necessary in most patients because the clinical presentation is often diagnostic and the biopsy often does not change the initial treatment.
- Bracing may be tried if the child has progressive bowing of the tibia, but it usually cannot prevent progression of the bowing.
- If the lesion progresses (before the closure of the growth plate), biopsy and resection are suggested.
- If the patient presents symptoms after the age of 10 (or after the closure of the growth plate), especially if the lesion is large (more than 3 or 4 cm in diameter) or has aggressive features on the plain radiographs, a biopsy is suggested to rule out an adamantinoma.[5]
    1. Adamantinoma has a similar clinical presentation with osteofibrous dysplasia; however, usually the patient is older (in the third decade of life) and the lesion appears more aggressive on the radiographs (i.e., it has a soft tissue extension, an acute periosteal reaction, a large size, and the involvement of the medullary canal).
    2. An adamantinoma requires a wider resection than an enlarging osteofibrous dysplasia. En bloc resection with wide surgical margins and reconstruction is the treatment of choice. Local recurrence rates are 20 to 30% with intralesional excision compared with 5 to 10% with en bloc excision.

- If the biopsy reveals osteofibrous dysplasia, excision of the entire lesion is recommended for complete histological examination to rule out the possibility of a focus of adamantinoma.
- If the lesion is small (less than 3 cm) and the patient is asymptomatic, continued observation is suggested.

Miscellaneous Lesions

Unicameral Bone Cyst (Simple Bone Cyst)

- Unicameral bone cysts are benign tumors of childhood and adolescence. They represent approximately 3% of all biopsied primary bone tumors.
- There is a male predominance with a 2:1 male/female ratio.
- The pathogenesis of unicameral bone cysts remains unclear, but favored theories include hemodynamic alterations, trauma-related defects in endochondral bone formation, and the presence of local factors causing bone resorption such as prostaglandins.
- The term *unicameral bone cyst* implies that one chamber exists. Although one large cavity is usually found, a cyst may become multiloculated following a fracture because of the formation of multiple bony septations, thus making the term *unicameral* technically incorrect.
- Unicameral bone cysts are often categorized as *active* or *latent* based on their proximity to the growth plate.
  - A cyst that is juxtaphyseal (less than 0.5 cm from the physis) is considered active and possesses greater potential for growth.
  - A cyst that has grown from the plate is considered latent and, theoretically, no longer has the capacity for growth.

Clinical Findings

- Unicameral bone cyst arises on the metaphyseal side of the growth plate and is displaced from the physis with skeletal growth.
- The most common locations are the proximal humerus and femur, accounting 90% of lesions, followed by calcaneus.[4,7]
- Unicameral bone cysts can be asymptomatic and may be discovered incidentally when radiographs (e.g., chest film) are obtained for other reasons.
- A mild pain reflecting a microscopic pathological fracture or a more abrupt discomfort because of a displaced pathological fracture may be presenting symptoms.

Radiographic and Histological Features

- See Table 12–7 for the typical radiographic and histological features of unicameral bone cysts (Figure 12–22, *A* and *B*).

Table 12–7: Typical Features of Aneurysmal and Unicameral Bone Cysts

	ANEURYSMAL BONE CYST	UNICAMERAL BONE CYST
Histological Features		
Gross (macroscopic)	Blood-filled sponge with thin periosteal membrane	Cystic cavity usually filled with yellowish fluid
Histological (microscopic)	Cavernous blood-filled spaces lacking endothelial cell lining Fibrous septa forming the walls contain woven bone trabeculae, giant cells, hemosiderin-laden macrophages	Cyst lining consisting of a single layer of mesothelial cells with underlying connective tissue or bone
Radiographic Features		
Plain radiographs	Metaphysis of long bones Eccentric or involving the entire width of the bone Expansile, lytic lesion circumscribed with a thinned but intact bony cortex Internal septations within the lesion	Metaphysis of long bones Centrally located Well-circumscribed, lucent lesion with sclerotic margins
Magnetic resonance imaging	Internal septations and multiple fluid–fluid levels Marked bony expansion	Fluid–fluid levels only if hemorrhage has occurred Minimal bony expansion

Treatment

- A unicameral bone cyst tends to enlarge with skeletal growth in young children and, consequently, may become symptomatic (pain secondary to a microfracture) or may be associated with a pathological fracture. After skeletal maturity, the lesion enters a latent phase, ceases growing, is resorbed, and is replaced by normal bone.
- The goal of treatment of unicameral bone cysts is to prevent a pathological fracture.
  - Some unicameral bone cysts remain small and do not present a significant risk of pathological fracture. Observation and activity restriction may be all that are necessary for these lesions.
  - Other lesions are large (e.g., proximal humeral lesions), are in high-stress anatomical sites (e.g., the femoral neck), or persist after the patient has become a young adult. Treatment should be directed to these lesions, which are at risk for pathological fracture.[13]

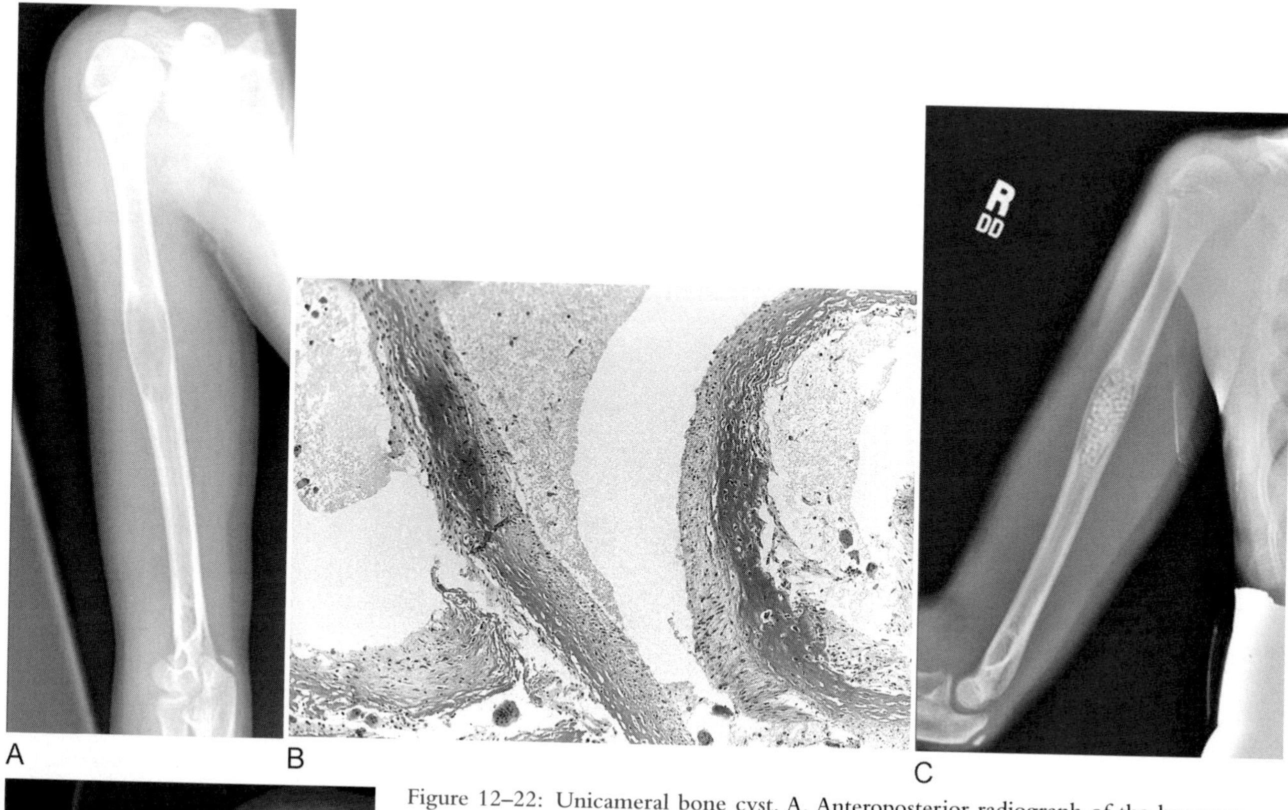

D

Figure 12–22: Unicameral bone cyst. A, Anteroposterior radiograph of the humerus shows a lytic lesion with sclerotic borders filling the entire medullary canal. B, Photomicrograph of the lesion demonstrates cyst membranes lined by loose connective tissue with underlying bands of osteoid. Amorphous debris partially fills the cyst cavities. C, This lesion was treated by percutaneous intramedullary decompression, biopsy, curettage, and grafting with calcium sulfate pellets. C, Postoperative 1-year follow-up radiograph shows complete healing of the lesion.

- Traditional surgical treatment options include fluoroscopically guided percutaneous corticosteroid injection, open curettage, and bone grafting.
  - Intracystic injection of corticosteroids (most commonly methylprednisolone acetate) has been used extensively and is an established method of treatment of a unicameral bone cyst.
    1. This procedure should be performed with anesthesia (usually general anesthesia) and with the aid of fluoroscopic visualization.
    2. Intracystic corticosteroid injection has induced at least a partial response in 50 to 80% of cases; however, it has been limited by the need for repeated injections and a significant rate of incomplete healing.[16]
    3. In addition, growth arrest and limb length discrepancies have been reported in 5 to 15% of cases treated with steroid injections.
  - Open curettage and bone grafting have been associated with a recurrence risk as high as 45% and with complications such as prolonged immobilization, donor site morbidity, and postoperative pathological fracture.[4] However, there are some cysts for which curettage followed by bone grafting remains necessary. Patients with displaced pathological fractures of the hip may need open reduction and internal fixation. At the time of internal fixation, curettage of the cyst and bone grafting are performed.
- Newer techniques in the treatment of unicameral bone cysts include injection with autologous bone marrow or demineralized bone matrix and percutaneous intramedullary decompression, curettage, and grafting using bone graft substitutes (calcium sulfate pellets) (Figure 12–22, *C*). The short-term results of these techniques are promising, with high healing and low complication and recurrence rates (Figure 12–22, *D*).[5]
- Microfractures associated with unicameral bone cysts in the upper and lower extremities (excluding the hip) are common; more extensive fractures occur but are less common, and displacement is usually minimal.
  - Large unicameral bone cysts associated with pathological microfractures (excluding the hip) can be managed by simple immobilization, if the fracture is stable and nondisplaced, to allow fracture stabilization and healing.
  - In addition to fracture healing, cyst healing can occur, although this is infrequent.
  - Once the fracture has healed, the unicameral bone cyst can be treated when necessary and appropriate (e.g., when there is a risk of refracture).
- Displaced pathological fractures of the proximal femur can be challenging to treat. If there is a significant loss of bone, coxa vara is likely to occur without internal fixation. Both the location of the cyst and the amount of bone loss dictate whether fixation can stabilize the fracture after grafting and what type of fixation would be most ideal (see Figure 12–18).[14]

Aneurysmal Bone Cyst

- Aneurysmal bone cysts are vascular lesions consisting of widely dilated vascular channels that are not lined by identifiable endothelium.
- They account for 1 to 2% of all benign bone lesions.
- The etiology of aneurysmal bone cysts is not certain. In most instances, they are primary lesions; occasionally they are secondary to or associated with other lesions, such as unicameral bone cyst, nonossifying fibroma, fibrous dysplasia, or osteogenic sarcoma.

Clinical Findings

- Aneurysmal bone cysts involve the long bones in 75% of patients. In order of decreasing frequency, the most commonly involved long bones are the distal femur, proximal tibia, proximal humerus, and distal radius.[7,8,16] Vertebral involvement is seen in 12 to 27% of patients; the lumbar vertebrae are most commonly affected.
- The patients usually complain of a mild, dull pain lasting several weeks or months, and only rarely is there a clinically apparent pathological fracture.
- When the cyst involves the spine, progressive enlargement may compress the spinal cord or nerve roots, resulting in neurological deficits such as motor weakness, sensory disturbance, and loss of bowel and bladder control.

Radiographic and Histological Features

- See Table 12–7 for the typical radiographic and histological features of aneurysmal bone cysts (Figure 12–23, *A* and *B*).

Treatment

- Although aneurysmal bone cysts have a well-differentiated benign histology, most are aggressive and they grow and invade rapidly (see Box 12–5). Treatment should be prompt once the diagnosis is made.
- The first step in the effective treatment of a patient with an aneurysmal bone cyst is to confirm the diagnosis with open biopsy and frozen section (Box 12–6). The biopsy is usually done in the same surgical setting as the definitive surgical procedure.
- A four-step approach is recommended in the surgical treatment of aneurysmal bone cysts: (1) curettage, (2) exploration of the cyst wall with a cautery, (3) use of a high-speed burr, and occasionally (4) use of adjuvants (e.g., hydrogen peroxide or phenol) for aggressive or recurrent aneurysmal bone cysts[14,17] (Figure 12–23, *C;* Box 12–6).
  - Making a large cortical window to adequately remove all portions of the tumor followed by burring the entire cavity are key aspects of the procedure.

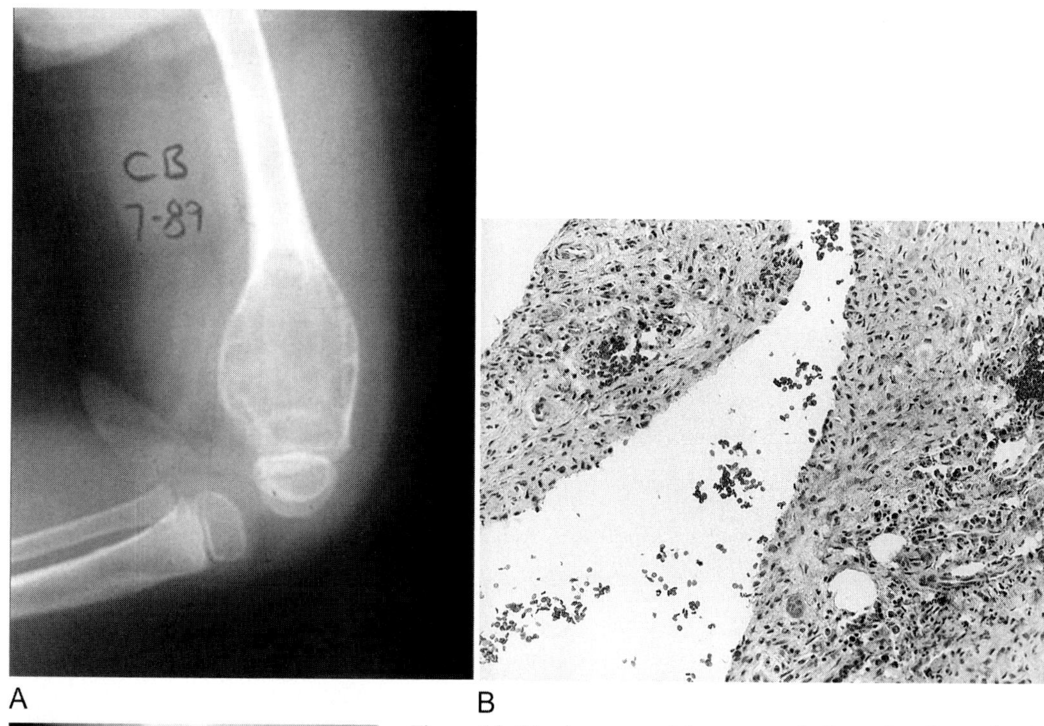

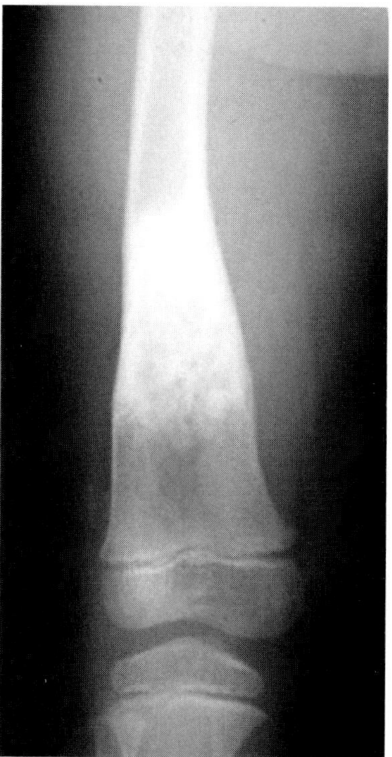

Figure 12–23: Aneurysmal bone cyst. A, Lateral radiograph of the knee shows a large lytic lesion expanding the distal femoral metaphysis. Note the trabeculated, nonossified matrix. B, Photomicrograph of this lesion demonstrates salient features including scattered erythrocytes within the cyst cavity, a lack of an endothelial lining, and an occasional giant cell in the underlying stroma. C, This lesion was treated by a four-step approach.

- Bone grafting can consist of autograft, allograft, bone substitutes, or a combination of these.
- The persistence–recurrence rate after curettage and use of a high-speed burr has been reported at 10%. The first recurrence can be recuretted and grafted.
- Large lesions located in high-stress locations (e.g., the proximal femur), associated with unstable pathological fractures, or both may require internal stabilization (Figures 12–18 and 12–24).

- Aneurysmal bone cysts in expendable bones, such as the fibula, ribs, distal ulna, metacarpal, and metatarsal bones, may be treated by en bloc resection.[4] Resection is also appropriate for recurrent aggressive lesions.

Box 12–6 Surgical Steps in the Management of Aneurysmal Bone Cysts

- Frozen section
- Curettage through a large cortical window
- Electrocautery
- High-speed burring
- Adjuvants (e.g., hydrogen peroxide or phenol) for aggressive or recurrent lesions
- Grafting (autograft, allograft, bone substitutes, or a combination of these)
- Internal fixation if indicated

- Irradiation should be avoided because it has been associated with later development of sarcoma. It also may damage reproductive organs and the active growth areas of long bones and may cause other complications.
- Selective arterial embolization can be used as definitive treatment or preoperatively with other procedures. It is used most commonly in the spine, the pelvis, and the proximal portion of the extremities when surgical exposure is more difficult and invasive and when blood loss with standard surgery can be significant.
- An aneurysmal bone cyst of the spine can present a challenging problem.
  - The lesion most commonly involves the elements of the posterior column, but it may extend anteriorly into the vertebral body.
  - Surgery is recommended for all patients as the initial means of treatment.[5] Most cases are controlled with simple curettage; the posterior elements are resected, and involvement of the pedicles or the body is curetted. If a complete laminectomy is performed, a short posterior fusion is advised.
  - Radiotherapy can be used in the postoperative period, but usually this is reserved for the rare case of rapid recurrence with soft tissue infiltration.

Langerhans Cell Histiocytosis

- Langerhans cell histiocytosis is a spectrum of diseases that primarily affects the skeleton but can involve the reticuloendothelial system and viscera.

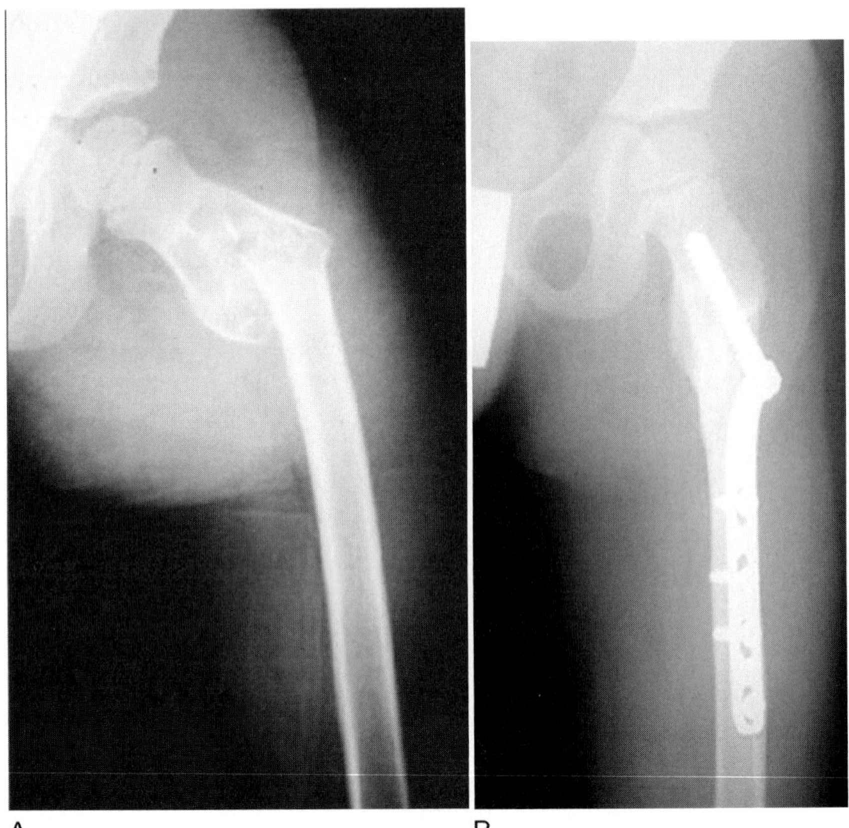

Figure 12–24: Aneurysmal bone cyst. A, Anteroposterior radiograph of the femur shows a pathological fracture through an aneurysmal bone cyst. B, This lesion was treated with extended curettage and grafting followed by internal fixation.

 - Langerhans cell histiocytosis in its simplest form, *eosinophilic granuloma,* involves the skeleton as either a single lesion or in multiple sites.
 - In another form, Hand-Schüller-Christian disease, it is a combination of multiple osseous lesions, exophthalmos, and diabetes insipidus.
 - The most extreme form of Langerhans cell histiocytosis is Letterer-Siwe disease, which occurs in infants as a combination of polyostotic lesions and multiple organ involvement.
- Although etiology and pathogenesis remain unsettled, Langerhans cell histiocytosis is now considered a disorder of immune regulation, possibly with a primary viral infection of bone, rather than a neoplastic process.[9,18]

Clinical Findings

- The skull is the most commonly involved site. Many of the skull lesions probably are not diagnosed because the only abnormality is a painless, small, spontaneously resolving lump in the scalp.
- The long bones (particularly femur), pelvis, ribs, and vertebral bodies are the next most common sites of involvement.
- Those lesions in long bones may weaken the bone sufficiently that the patient has activity-related pain suggestive of a fatigue fracture or has a pathological fracture.
- Patients with Langerhans cell histiocytosis may also have systemic symptoms such as fever and malaise.

Radiographic and Histological Features

- The radiographic appearance of Langerhans cell histiocytosis is highly variable. Depending on the stage of the process at which the radiographs are taken, the lesion may appear similar to numerous benign and malignant processes and is appropriately referred to as the "great mimicker."[9,10]
 - Its radiographic appearance ranges from a focal, well-marginated radiolucency to a permeative appearance with expansion of the overlying cortex, periosteal new bone formation, surrounding sclerosis, and associated soft tissue mass (Figure 12–25, *A*).
 - Spinal involvement usually results in variable compression of the vertebral body, known as *vertebra plana* when there is complete collapse (Figure 12–26, *A*).
- On bone scan, most of the lesions show increased uptake, but up to 25% of lesions will not be associated with abnormal bone scan. Therefore, some recommend a skeletal survey to look for other isolated bone lesions.
- Histologically, the lesion is characterized by a proliferation of lipid-laden histiocytes–Langerhans cells in an inflammatory background (Figure 12–25, *B*). These cells frequently have ill-defined cytoplasmic boundaries and characteristically contain an oval or intended nucleus. Birbeck granules, tennis racket-shaped cytoplasmic structures identified only by electron microscopy, are found within the histiocytes and are pathognomonic. Immunohistochemical phenotype shows that Langerhans cells react positively for S100, CD1a, CD11, and CD14[7,9] (Figure 12–25, *C*).

Treatment

- Patients with eosinophilic granuloma do not progress to Hand-Schüller-Christian or Letterer-Siwe diseases but should be evaluated on presentation to exclude the presence of these syndromes. A skeletal survey and some urine and blood tests (e.g., liver enzymes) should be performed for all patients, then the patient should be referred to a pediatric hematologist.
- Patients with solitary eosinophilic granulomas generally have a benign clinical course. They have a good chance of spontaneous remission and a favorable outcome over a period of months to years. The single bony lesion usually does not require treatment other than a biopsy to confirm the diagnosis.[4]
- In the spine, no treatment is generally needed or recommended unless deformity or neurological deficit is present. Variable rates of vertebral body restoration are seen with time (Figure 12–26, *B*).
- Patients with Hand-Schüller-Christian disease are usually treated with systemic corticosteroids and chemotherapy. An aggressive chemotherapy protocol is also required for Letterer-Siwe disease.

Ewing Sarcoma and Peripheral Neuroectodermal Tumor

- Ewing sarcoma is a malignant, small, round-cell tumor.
- It is the second most common primary malignant bone tumor in children and accounts for approximately 10% of all primary malignant bone tumors.
- Recent genetic, biochemical, and electron microscopic studies suggest that Ewing sarcoma is a spectrum of tumors.
 - Ewing sarcoma is closely related with peripheral (or primitive) neuroectodermal tumor (PNET); both of these tumors have the same chromosomal translocation between chromosomes 11 and 22, similar presentations, identical treatments, and almost identical histological characteristics (Table 12–8).[4]
 - Ewing sarcoma and PNETs are thought to arise from the neural crest.

Clinical Findings

- The femur is the most common site of origin (20%); the pelvis and the humerus are also common sites.
- In the long tubular bones, the lesion is more often situated in the diaphysis than in the metaphysis.
- Pain and local swelling, representing an associated soft tissue mass, are the most common clinical findings in patients with Ewing sarcoma–PNET. The mass is warm, firm, and tender.

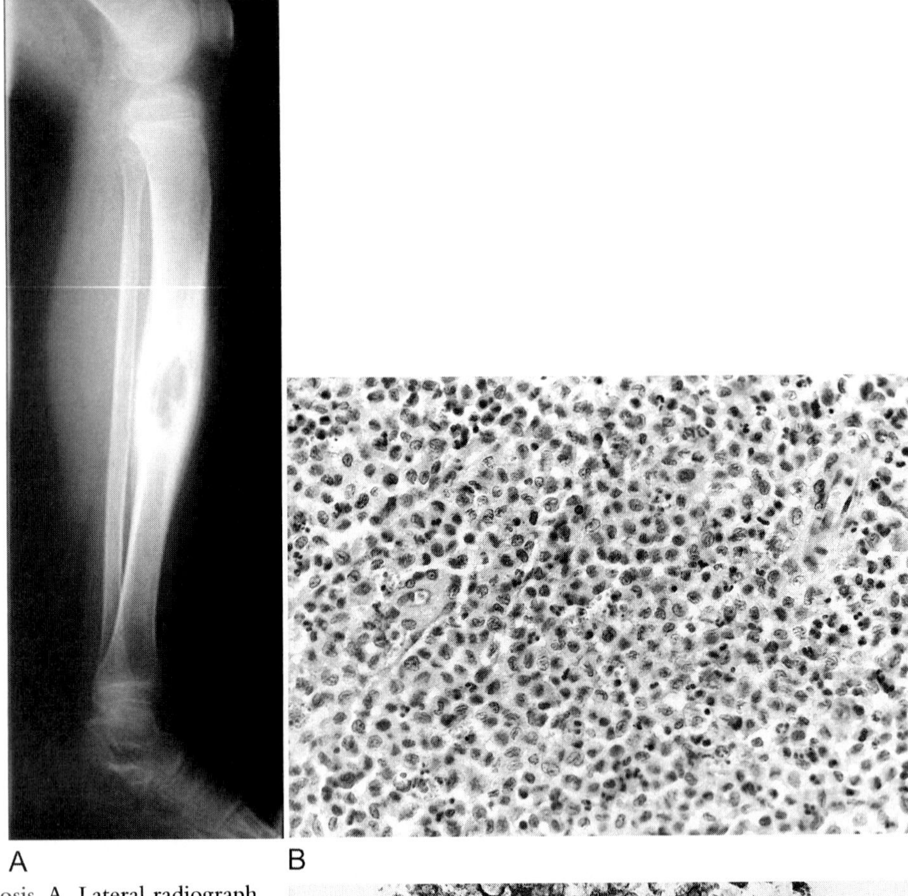

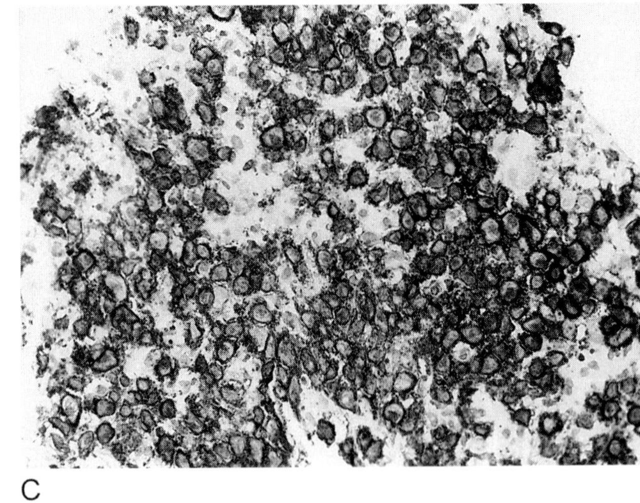

Figure 12–25: Langerhans cell histiocytosis. A, Lateral radiograph of the leg shows a cluster of lytic lesions in the diaphysis of the tibia associated with extensive sclerosis. The lesions have sharply defined borders. There is, however, destruction of the cortex seen both anteriorly and posteriorly. Thick periosteal new-bone formation bridges the areas of destruction and extends along the diaphysis. B, Photomicrograph of the lesion shows sheets of Langerhans cells, many with characteristic deep nuclear clefts and nuclear grooves. Smaller, darkly staining cells are eosinophils. C, Photomicrograph of CD1a immunohistochemical preparation demonstrates crisp cell membrane positivity.

- Constitutional symptoms, such as fever and malaise, may be present in patients with Ewing sarcoma–PNET, especially those patients with metastatic disease. These symptoms, with common laboratory findings of high white cell counts and elevated sedimentation rates, may suggest osteomyelitis as a differential diagnosis.[11]
- Approximately 25% of patients with Ewing sarcoma–PNET have overt metastases, typically in the lungs, bone marrow, or bone. Metastasis at diagnosis is a poor prognostic finding for these tumors.

Radiographic and Histological Features

Radiographic Features

- Any portion of any bone may be involved by Ewing sarcoma–PNET.

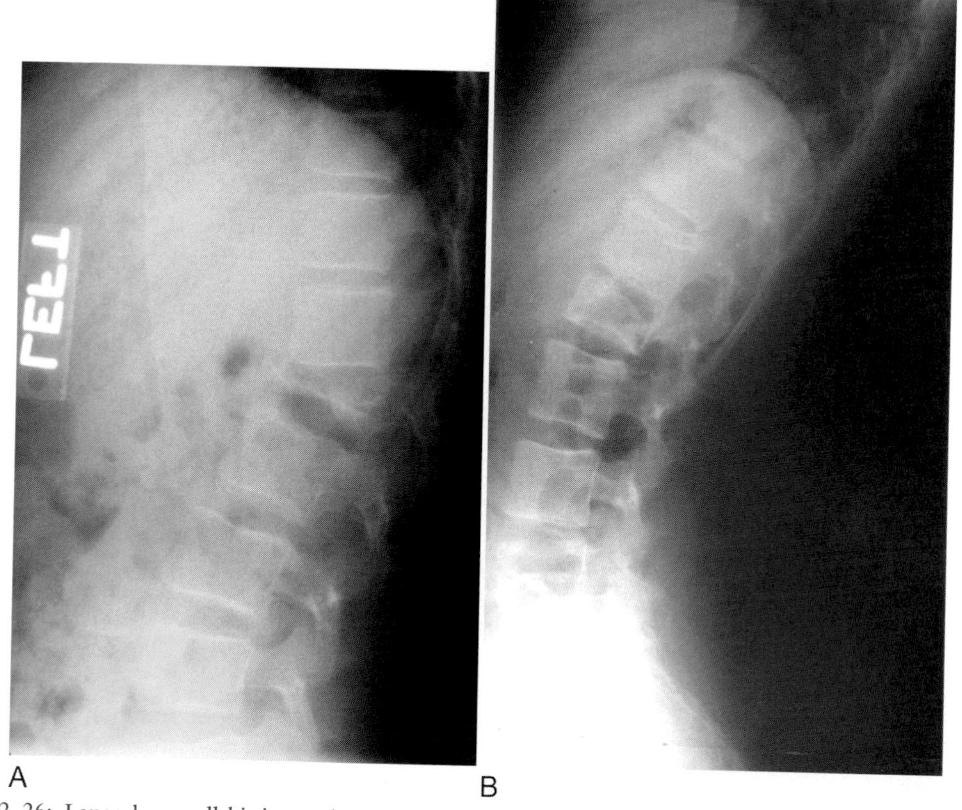

Figure 12–26: Langerhans cell histiocytosis. A, Lateral radiograph of the spine shows complete collapse of the first lumbar vertebral body that results in kyphosis. This "vertebra plana" appearance is a classic feature of Langerhans cell histiocytosis. Note the preservation of the disk spaces. B, A follow-up radiograph taken 4 years after the initial diagnosis demonstrates the significant improvement in the restoration of the vertebral body.

- The typical plain radiograph of Ewing sarcoma–PNET reveals diffuse destruction of the bone, extension of the tumor through the cortex, a soft tissue component, and a periosteal reaction[9,11] (Figure 12–27, *A*). The periosteal reaction may produce a Codman triangle, an onionskin appearance, or a sunburst appearance.
- The extraosseous soft tissue mass and medullary canal involvement can be best seen on MRI scans, which are usually more extensive than what was expected from the plain radiographs (Figure 12–27, *B and C*).

Table 12–8: Pediatric Musculoskeletal Tumors with Nonrandom or Specific Translocations

TUMOR	TRANSLOCATION
Ewing sarcoma–PNET*	t(11;22), t(21;22)
Alveolar rhabdomyosarcoma	t(2;13), t(1;13)
Synovial sarcoma	t(X;18)
Myxoid liposarcoma	t(12;16)

PNET, peripheral neuroectodermal tumor.

  - The MRI scan is repeated after several cycles of chemotherapy to assess the response of the tumor to the neoadjuvant regimen and to help to plan definitive treatment of the primary lesion.
  - There has been recent interest in the use of dynamic MRI scans to assess more accurately the viability of the tumor before definitive local control is undertaken.
- The presence and extent of metastatic disease is evaluated with a radiograph and CT scan of the chest, a whole-body bone scan, and a bone marrow aspirate.
- The bone scan is important because 10% of patients have involvement of multiple bones at presentation.

Histological Features

- Grossly, Ewing sarcoma–PNET is a gray white tumor with a variable amount of necrosis, hemorrhage, or cyst formation. At times, the tumor tissue may be almost liquid, mimicking purulence.
- Histologically, the tumor is composed of numerous small, round cells with a diffuse homogeneous growth pattern and sparse intercellular stroma. The cells have ill-defined borders and a finely dispersed chromatin

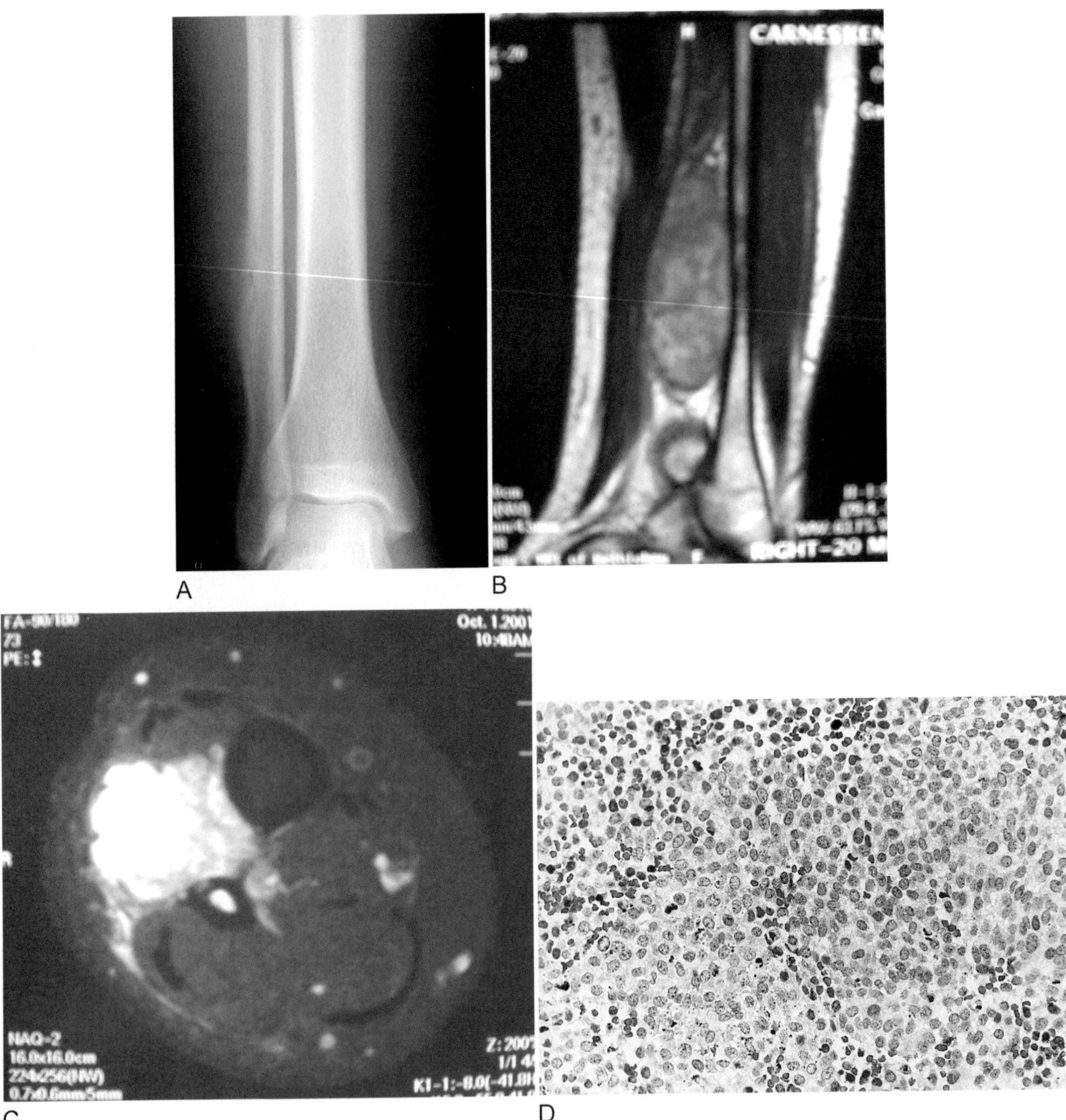

Figure 12–27: Ewing sarcoma. A, Anteroposterior radiograph of the lower leg shows a moth-eaten pattern of bone destruction within a fusiform area of cortical thickening in the distal fibular diaphysis. An ill-defined layer of new bone formation is present. B, On a coronal T1-weighted MRI, a heterogenous signal is seen within the marrow of the distal fibula. The extraosseous component of the lesion has well-circumscribed borders. C, Axial T2-weighted image shows a high-signal intensity mass in the anterior compartment of the leg. Extension of the tumor is seen across the interosseous membrane into the posterior compartment and laterally along the fascia. Note the high signal in the medullary cavity of the fibula and the cortex. D, Photomicrograph of the lesion demonstrates monotonous sheets of small, round cells with scattered mitoses and ill-defined cytoplasm.

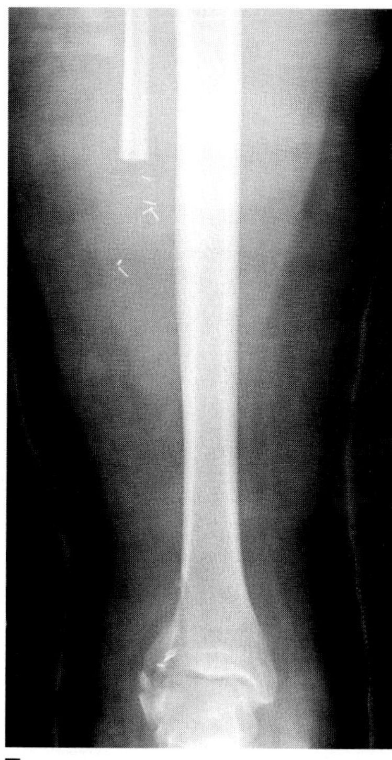

Figure 12–27, cont'd: **E, The treatment of this patient consisted of administration of multiagent chemotherapy followed by resection of the lesion with wide surgical margins.**

pattern (Figure 12–27, *D*). Mitotic activity is seldom high, and the cells are quite uniform. There are glycogen granules in the cytoplasm, and these produce the positive periodic acid-Schiff stain on routine histology.

- Advances in cytogenetics and immunohistochemistry allow more precise diagnostic evaluations.
  - Ewing sarcoma–PNET cells strongly express the p30/32 MIC2 antigen, which is a cell-surface glycoprotein encoded by the MIC2 gene. The MIC2 analysis has a sensitivity of up to 95% in the diagnosis of Ewing sarcoma–PNET.
  - Cytogenetic studies have revealed that 85% of Ewing sarcoma–PNET contain a translocation either of chromosomes 11 and 22 [t(11;22)] or of chromosomes 21 and 22 [t(21;22)] (Table 12–8). The resultant fusion gene is composed of part of the EWS gene from chromosome 22 and the FLY1 gene of chromosome 11 or the ERG gene from chromosome 21. The t(11;22) translocation is the most common translocation, and t(21;22) is the next most common.

Treatment

- Modern chemotherapy has made a significant difference in the prognosis for patients with Ewing sarcoma–PNET, improving the long-term survival rate from between 5 and 10% to more than 70%.
- The treatment of patients with nonmetastatic Ewing sarcoma–PNET consists of administration of multiagent chemotherapy and efforts to achieve local control.[4,5,11]
  - The treatment principles of Ewing sarcoma–PNET are summarized in Box 12–3.
  - The chemotherapeutic agents most widely used for Ewing sarcoma–PNET are vincristine, cyclophosphamide, doxorubicin, ifosfamide, and etoposide. Actinomycin D, a drug used previously, is currently used less often. Chemotherapy dramatically reduces the soft tissue component of the lesion in most cases.
  - Resection of the primary lesion with wide surgical margins is recommended for local control of Ewing sarcoma–PNET if the functional consequences of the resection are acceptable. Limb salvage surgery is possible for most patients (Figure 12–27, *E*).
  - Amputation may be required if the limb salvage surgery is contraindicated.
  - Postoperative irradiation is recommended when the surgical margins are close and a significant viable tumor is present in the resected specimen.
- If the primary tumor cannot be resected without undue morbidity, irradiation alone can be used. The total dosage should be kept as low as possible—usually around 50 gray (Gy) and certainly less than 60 Gy, because dosages of more than 60 Gy are associated with an unacceptable incidence of later irradiation-associated sarcomas.[5]

Musculoskeletal Manifestations of Leukemia

- Acute leukemia is the most common cancer in childhood, and acute lymphoblastic leukemia represents 80% of cases.
- Leukemic involvement of bones and joints occurs frequently in patients with acute lymphoblastic leukemia; leukemic involvement of bone should be suspected in a child with bone pain who also has cytopenia, fever, bleeding manifestations, hepatosplenomegaly, or lymphadenopathy.
- Box 12–7 summarizes the musculoskeletal manifestations (clinical and radiographic) of leukemia.[7] (Figure 12–28, *A*).
- The diagnosis should be made if typical leukemic blasts are seen in an aspiration specimen of the bone marrow (Figure 12–28, *B*).
- Treatment involves prolonged multiagent chemotherapy, with overall survival rates approaching 70% for children with acute lymphoblastic leukemia.

Specific Soft Tissue Tumors

- Most soft tissue tumors in children are benign.
- Soft tissue sarcomas represent only 7% of all malignancies in children younger than 15 years.

Box 12–7 Musculoskeletal Manifestations of Leukemia

Clinical

- Musculoskeletal pain
  - Bone pain—Intermittent, local, sharp, severe, and sudden in onset
  - Joint pain—Migratory

Radiographic

- Diffuse osteopenia—Alterations in protein and mineral metabolism
- Radiolucent metaphyseal bands (generally is the first roentgenographic abnormality)—Diminished osteogenesis of the epiphyseal growth plate
- Periosteal bone formation—Leukemic infiltration that lifts the periosteum from the cortex of the bone
- Osteolytic lesions—Leukemic infiltration of the bone marrow, local hemorrhage, and osteonecrosis of adjacent trabecular bone
- Osteosclerosis—Late manifestation
- Mixed lesions—Simultaneous production of bone by osteoblasts at one site and increased osteoclastic activity at a separate site
- Permeative pattern—Indicator of an aggressive lesion with rapid growth
- Pathological fracture—Most commonly associated with osteoporosis of the spine; occurs at other locations following minor trauma

- Rhabdomyosarcoma accounts for 45 to 50% of all soft tissue sarcomas in children.
- The physician must be aware of the possibility of a malignant soft tissue tumor in the child and evaluate any lump carefully.

Vascular Tumors

- Vascular anomalies have been divided into two groups, hemangiomas and vascular malformations, by a biological classification proposed by Mulliken and Glowacki.[19]

Hemangiomas

- Hemangiomas are true neoplastic lesions with endothelial hyperplasia.
- They are the most common benign soft tissue tumors of childhood, occurring in 4 to 10% of all children.

Clinical Findings

- Hemangiomas infrequently are present at birth but grow rapidly during the first 2 to 3 weeks.[20,21]
- Hemangiomas may be located in the superficial or deep dermis, subcutaneous tissue, musculature, bone, or viscera.
- Head and neck are the most commonly involved sites.
- Hemangioma of bone may be solitary or diffuse.

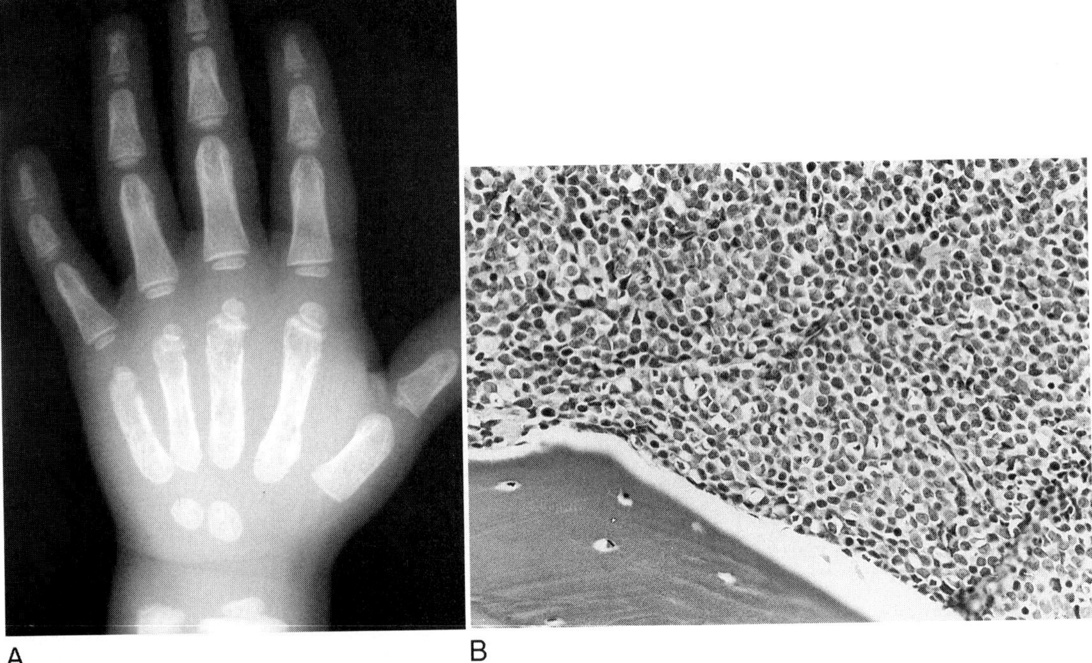

Figure 12–28: Musculoskeletal manifestations of leukemia. A, Anteroposterior radiograph of the hand shows a moth-eaten pattern of bone destruction and a single layer of periosteal new-bone formation in all metacarpals except the first. Also note the lucent metaphyseal bands in the distal radius and ulna. B, Photomicrograph demonstrates features of high cellularity and inconspicuous cytoplasmic borders.

- Solitary lesions may occur in any bone, but the vertebral bodies are the most common sites. These lesions usually do not produce symptoms and are found when a radiograph is taken for another reason.
- Multiple lesions usually involve the long bones of the extremities and the short bones of the hands and feet, leading to weakening of the involved bones.

Radiographic and Histological Features

- Ultrasound or color Doppler may also be used.
- Table 12–9 summarizes the clinical presentation or natural history and the typical radiographic (MRI findings) and histological features of hemangiomas and different types of vascular malformations (Figures 12–29 and 12–30).

Treatment

- In the absence of intervention, partial or complete involution of hemangiomas usually occurs, and correction of cosmetic defects typically follows. Capillary hemangiomas, the largest group of benign vascular tumors, enlarge for the first 6 months of life, then regress and become 75 to 90% involuted by the age of 7 years.[5,20,21]

Table 12–9: Presentation, History, and Features of Hemangiomas and Vascular Malformations

ANOMALY TYPE	CLINICAL PRESENTATION OR NATURAL HISTORY	HISTOLOGICAL FEATURES	MRI FEATURES
Venous malformation	Growth proportionate with child Possible presenting symptoms of thrombosis, thrombophlebitis, or low-grade disseminated intravascular coagulation	Dilated, thin-walled channels with smooth muscle fibers in clumps Flattened endothelial cells	T1—Low intensity T2—High intensity Possible variable intensity because of hemorrhage or thrombosis
Arteriovenous malformation	Noticeable at birth because of cutaneous blushing and localized warmth Four stages (some never pass first stage)—Quiescence, expansion, destruction, decompensation	Heterogeneous lesion with large vessels Intimal thickening of veins Tortuosity of vessels Increased fibrin deposition (stage III)	T1—Low intensity T2—High intensity Flow voids caused by rapid, turbulent blood flow
Lymphatic malformation	Mild to massive lymphedema or Multicystic masses with viral–bacterial infection Localized multicystic lesions with vesicle rupture, weeping of lymphatic fluid Frequent with capillary, venous, or arteriovenous malformation Most commonly hypoplastic but can be hyperplastic or multicystic	Hypoplastic—Small lymphatic channels and fibrotic lymph nodes Hyperplastic—Enlarged lymphatic channels lacking valves, small and space lymph nodes Multicystic—Numerous lymphatic sacs with normal lymph channels	T1—Low intensity (occasionally variable) T2—High intensity Slow flow lesion Possibly enhanced septa following gadolinium
Capillary malformation	Noticeable at birth Growth proportionate with child with some dilation and darkening with age Macular at birth and raised in adulthood Intermittent breakdown and bleeding Possible mixed type containing venous, arteriovenous, or lymphatic components	Dilated capillary network of variable density located in the dermis Paucity of intradermal nerve fibers in the area of capillary dilation	Not applicable
Mixed-type malformation	Possible overlapping characteristics depending upon composition No improvement to vascular malformations with time	Possible overlapping characteristics depending upon composition	Variable Consistent with findings of individual components
Hemangioma	Rare bone or muscle hypertrophy Most cases noticeable during the first month Initially cutaneous blanching, telangiectasia, or small red papule Three phases—Proliferative (1-8 months), involution (8 months-2 years), involuted (75-95% resolve by 7 years)	Plump, rapidly dividing endothelial cell Increased number of mast cells Multilaminated basement membrane	T1—Intermediate intensity T2—High intensity Lobulated soft tissue mass with well-defined borders Possible flow voids Equatorially located feeding the draining vessels

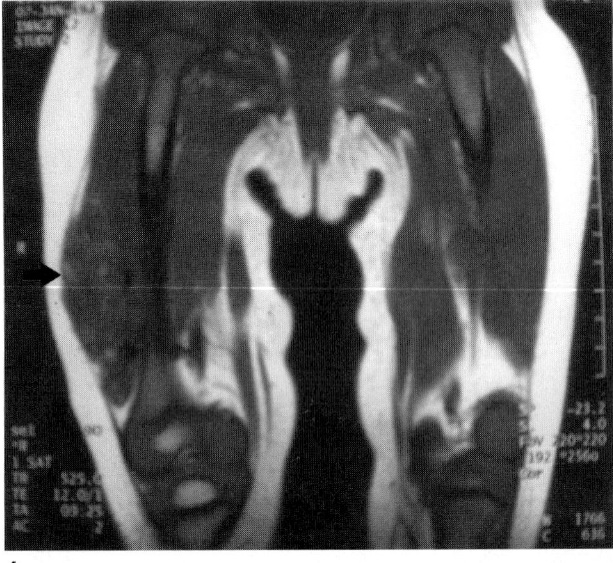

A

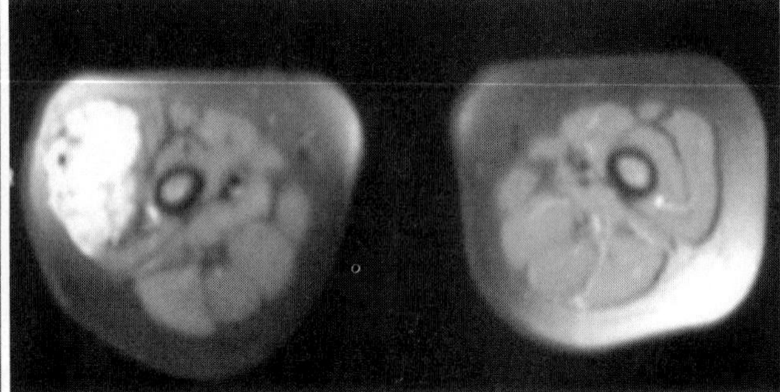

B

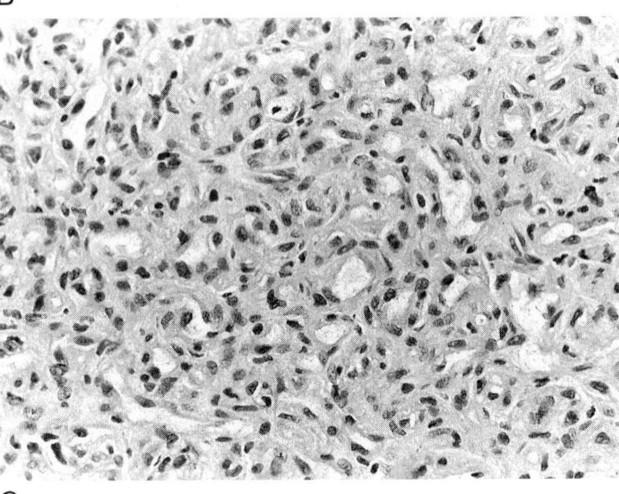

C

Figure 12–29: Hemangioma. A, On a coronal T1-weighted MRI of the thighs, a mass is seen in the lateral soft tissues of the right thigh *(arrow)*. It is the same signal intensity as muscle. The slight heterogeneity and bulging of the muscle planes are the only clues to the presence of the mass. B, Axial T2-weighted image shows the large, lobulated, high-signal soft tissue mass in the vastus lateralis muscle. Low-signal septations are scattered throughout the mass. C, Histopathology of hemangioma. Photomicrograph of this juvenile capillary hemangioma shows small capillary channels scattered throughout a background of compressed, plump endothelial cells. *A and B* from Erol B, States L, Pawel BR, Tamai J, Dormans JP (2004) Musculoskeletal tumors in children. In: Pediatric Orthopaedics and Sports Medicine (Dormans JP, ed). Philadelphia: Mosby.

- When intervention for a rapidly expanding hemangioma is necessary, the first line of treatment is intralesional or systemic corticosteroids.
- Occasionally, when surgical resection is indicated for larger, deeper lesions that threaten normal function, staged excisions may be considered.
- Irradiation has been used for persistent hemangiomas with various results.
- Embolization also has been used for patients who have severe pain.
- Solitary bone hemangiomas usually do not require any treatment. Treatment of diffuse bone hemangiomas should be symptomatic, with curettage and bone grafting for lesions that weaken the bone.

Vascular Malformations

- The second category of vascular anomalies is vascular malformations, which are congenital lesions with normal endothelial turnover.
- They are subclassified by the predominant vessel found in the lesion (i.e., venous, arterial, capillary, lymphatic, or mixed) and by the blood flow within the lesion (high versus low flow).
- Vascular malformations are not as common as hemangiomas.

Clinical Findings

- Many of the common vascular malformations present symptoms at birth; however, some may manifest in adolescence or adulthood.

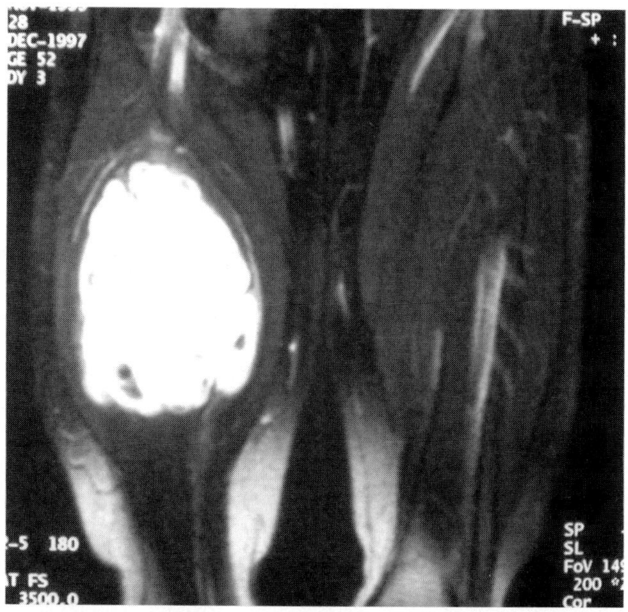

A

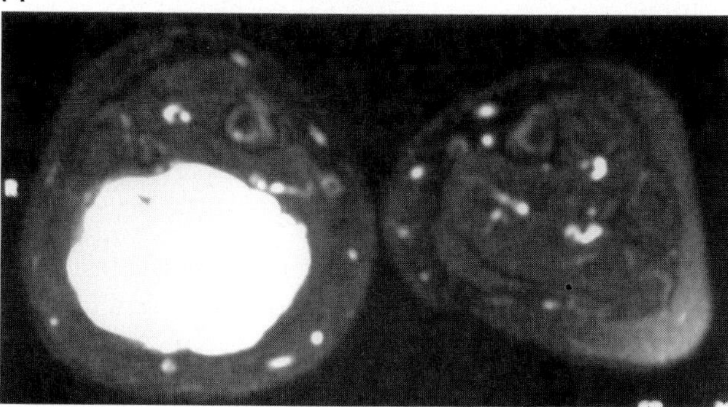

B

Figure 12–30: Vascular malformation (venous malformation). A, Sagittal T2-weighted MRI of the lower legs shows a large, lobulated, high-signal mass in the right calf. The low-signal intensity areas represent blood products caused by hemorrhage in the mass. B, Axial T2-weighted image demonstrates the displacement of the muscles of the posterior compartment by this large soft tissue mass. From Erol B, States L, Pawel BR, Tamai J, Dormans JP (2004) Musculoskeletal tumors in children. In: Pediatric Orthopaedics and Sports Medicine (Dormans JP, ed). Philadelphia: Mosby.

- Most of these lesions involve the skin and subcutaneous tissue, but deep or extensive involvement of structures such as muscle, joint, bone, abdominal viscera, and the central nervous system is not uncommon.
- The most commonly affected sites are the head and neck.

Radiographic and Histological Features

- MRI is an excellent imaging modality for confirming the nature of vascular anomalies and defining their relationship to adjacent structures.[19,20]
- Ultrasound or color Doppler may also be used.
- Table 12–9 summarizes the clinical presentation or natural history and the typical radiographic (MRI findings) and histological features of hemangiomas and different types of vascular malformations (Figures 12–29 and 12–30).

Treatment

Venous Malformations

- Compression stockings to prevent progressive venous dilation, pain, ulceration, and bleeding are the mainstay of treatment. Low-dose aspirin may also be used to minimize thrombophlebitis.
- When the patient does not adequately benefit from compression stockings, laser surgery, sclerotherapy (i.e., 100% ethanol), and surgical resection are all widely accepted treatment methods.
- Surgical intervention may be required for deep venous malformations involving muscle or bone that have led to pain, functional impairment, or pathological fracture.
- Epiphysiodesis may be applied for patients with extensive venous malformations that have resulted in skeletal overgrowth.

Arteriovenous Malformations

- Arteriovenous malformations can prove deceptively problematic and even dangerous to treat.
- Most authors agree that conservative treatment is preferred in the absence of significant symptoms.[19,20]
- Deep arteriovenous malformations may cause significant muscle or bone changes and may necessitate surgical debulking or epiphysiodesis.
- When surgery is required, angiographic studies followed by selective embolization are usually done 24 or 72 hours before resection. Embolization or ligation of feeding arteries without surgical resection is contraindicated because occlusion of the major feeding arteries usually results in rapid recruitment and dilation of previously microscopic collateral blood flow.[19]

Lymphatic Malformations

- Compression garments are the mainstay of treatment and can be used to diminish the accompanying chronic lymphedema, skin breakdown, and skeletal and soft tissue overgrowth.
- When compression garments fail, surgical debulking procedures or epiphysiodesis may be required. Because of the diffuse nature of these lesions, surgery is most often aimed at palliative debulking of soft tissues.
- Sclerotherapy with 100% ethanol can also be used.

Capillary Malformations

- In the absence of venous, arteriovenous, or lymphatic involvement, capillary malformations are best treated with pulsed yellow-dye laser therapy under the care of a plastic surgeon or dermatologist.

Associated Syndromes

- Vascular malformations may be part of several rare syndromes.

Maffucci's Syndrome

- Maffucci's syndrome is a premalignant condition with venous vascular malformations and enchondromas.
- The vascular lesions often are present at birth, and enchondromas develop at a later age.
- This syndrome often occurs in the subcutaneous tissue and bones of the limbs.
- The cartilage tumors have a high risk of malignant transformation to chondrosarcomas.

Angiomatosis

- Angiomatosis is a vascular syndrome that usually involves multiple tissue types (e.g., subcutis, muscle, and bone).
- Generally, angiomatomas grow commensurately with the child.
- The characteristics of angiomatosis are haphazard proliferations of small or medium blood vessels that diffusely infiltrate the skin, muscle, or bone.
- Treatment options include compression stockings, laser ablation, embolization, electrocautery, irradiation, local or systemic steroids, antiangiogenic therapies, and surgery.

Tumors of Nerve Origin

Benign Tumors of Nerve Origin

- Neurolemmoma and neurofibroma are the most common benign tumors of peripheral nerves.
- Both tumors arise from benign proliferation of periaxonal Schwann cells that embryologically arise from the neural crest.
- Although, neurolemmoma and neurofibroma share a common cell of origin, the clinical and morphological findings separate the two into distinct entities.[20]

Clinical Findings

Neurolemmoma

- Neurolemmomas, also known as *schwannomas,* can be seen in patients of all ages, but they are most often seen during early childhood.
- They have a predilection for the head, neck, and flexor surfaces of the extremities (e.g., peroneal and ulnar nerves).
- The patients with neurolemmoma usually have a painless, slow-growing, solitary mass in the subcutaneous tissue.
- The mass may be from any nerve, but it often arises from a small, superficial sensory nerve.
- A positive Tinel sign with percussion over the mass is not uncommon.
- Although neurolemmomas arise from the nerve sheath, nerve dysfunction is uncommon and is seen only when the nerve is compressed between the tumor and an adjacent rigid structure.[5]
- Patients with superficial nerve lesions usually present symptoms early with small tumors, but deep-seated lesions may be large before they are discovered.
- Neurolemmomas rarely are associated with neurofibromatosis.[20,21]

Neurofibroma

- Neurofibromas, like neurolemmomas, usually occur in early childhood.
- Neurofibromas may arise as a solitary lesion or multiple lesions. The solitary lesions account about 90% of neurofibromas and are not associated with neurofibromatosis.
- The clinical presentation of neurofibromas is similar to that of neurolemmomas; the lesions grow slowly as a painless mass in the skin, subcutaneous tissue, or distribution of a peripheral nerve.
- A positive Tinel sign is present in most cases.
- Neurofibromas, unlike neurolemmomas, tend to be intimately associated with the nerve fibers.[20,21]

Radiographic and Histological Features

- See Table 12–10 for typical radiographic and histological features of neurolemmoma and neurofibroma (Figure 12–31).

Treatment

- The risk of malignant transformation of neurolemmomas or solitary neurofibromas is exceedingly rare. In contrast, malignant transformation of neurofibromas in the face of neurofibromatosis is well documented; this risk has been reported in about 2% of patients.[20]
  - Patients and parents should be aware of the clinical symptoms leading to suspicion of malignant transformation, such as enlargement of a neurofibroma and pain.
  - If sarcomatous degeneration occurs, the prognosis for long-term survival is poor.
- Treatment of neurolemmomas consists of marginal surgical excision. Overlying nerve fibers can usually be mobilized easily and preserved as the lesion is marginally shelled out.
- Neurolemmoma usually does not recur following marginal excision.
- For symptomatic solitary neurofibromas that involve a peripheral nerve, marginal surgical excision is recommended (Figure 12–32).
- Lesions arising from a major nerve can be resected, but the nerve fascicles must be split and the neurofibroma must be removed from between them.

Table 12–10: Typical Features of Neurolemmoma and Neurofibroma

	NEUROLEMMOMA	NEUROFIBROMA
Histological Features		
Gross (macroscopic)	Truly encapsulated by the epineurium overlying the lesion and nerve fibers Typically fusiform and eccentric from the underlying nerve	Nonencapsulated Invading the nerve fibers Centrally located fusiform mass within a peripheral nerve
Histological (microscopic)	Pattern of alternating Antoni type A (compact spindle-shaped cells and Verocay bodies) and B areas Ultrastructurally a single cell type—Schwann cells	Interlacing bundles of elongated cells with wavy, dark-staining nuclei Usually neurites within the lesion
Radiographic Features		
Magnetic resonance imaging	Well-circumscribed round or ovoid masses Low to intermediate signal on T1-weighted images High signal on T2-weighted images Rare target sign* on T2-weighted images	Well-circumscribed round or ovoid masses Low to intermediate signal on T1-weighed images High signal on T2-weighted images Frequent target sign* on T2-weighted images

*Target sign—Peripheral high-signal intensity area surrounding a central low-signal intensity core on T2-weighted images.

Malignant Peripheral Nerve Sheath Tumors

- Malignant peripheral nerve sheath tumors or *neurofibrosarcomas* are uncommon in children and adolescents. They account for about 5% of pediatric soft tissue sarcomas.

Clinical Findings

- Most occur after the age of 10 with an equal sex distribution.
- Neurofibrosarcomas may arise in a preexisting neurofibroma or *de novo* in the subcutaneous or deep soft tissues of the extremities or trunk.[4,21]
- An enlarging soft tissue mass with pain or dysesthesia is the most common presentation in children.

Radiographic and Histological Features

- Although, MRI findings of malignant and benign peripheral nerve sheath tumors are usually similar, neurofibrosarcomas may show variable intensities on both T1- and T2-weighted images depending on the degree of intratumoral necrosis.[20] The extent and aggressiveness of the tumor can be evaluated well with MRI (Figure 12–33, *A* and *B*).
- CT scans demonstrate a bulky soft tissue mass that may have areas of necrosis or calcification.
- Histologically, a nerve of origin and an associated neurofibroma can be identified in most cases. The tumor displays interlacing fascicles of spindle cells, with pale, indistinct cytoplasm and elongated nuclei. Focal hemorrhage, necrosis, and cystic changes are usually seen (Figure 12–33, *C*).

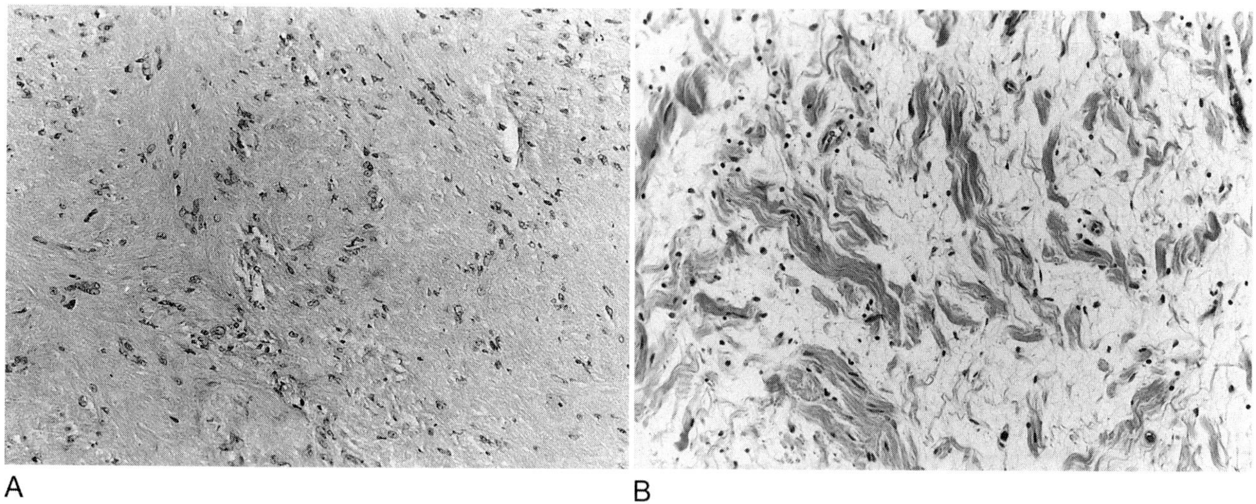

Figure 12–31: Histopathology of benign peripheral nerve sheath tumors. A, Neurolemmoma. This tumor demonstrates a classic palisading of Schwann cells (Verocay bodies) within a spindle cell background. B, Neurofibroma. The lesion is composed of fascicles of Schwann cells and fibroblasts within an edematous and mildly inflamed background stroma, imparting a histological appearance that has been compared with shredded carrots.

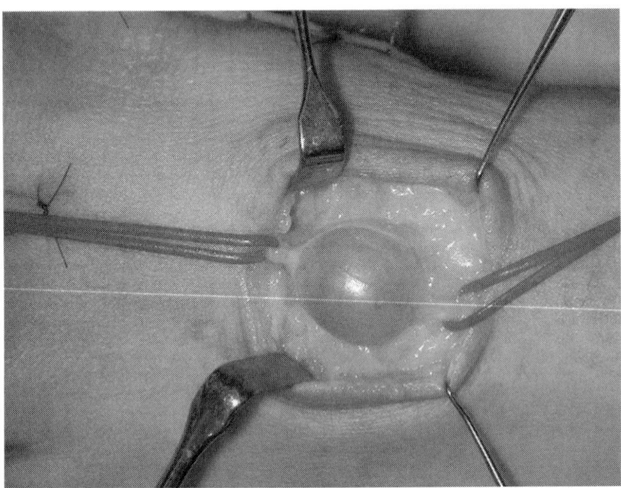

Figure 12–32: Benign peripheral nerve sheath tumors. **This symptomatic neurofibroma was treated surgically by marginal excision.**

Treatment

- Wide excision with resection of the entire tumor bed is the mainstay of the treatment for neurofibrosarcomas.[4,21] Adjuvant radiation therapy is recommended for many after surgery and appears to improve survival. The efficacy of adjuvant chemotherapy remains unproven.

Tumors of Fibrous Tissue Origin

Fibromatosis

- The term *fibromatosis* refers a variety of benign fibrous lesions with different manifestations.
- Benign fibrous lesions are relatively common in children and are divided into two groups.
  - The first group includes aggressive fibromatosis or extra-abdominal desmoid, which affects children.
  - The second, less common group is that of fibrous lesions (e.g., fibrous hamartoma of infancy and infantile myofibromatosis) peculiar to infancy and childhood.[20,21] The more common lesions will be described in this section.

Aggressive Fibromatosis

Clinical Findings

- Aggressive fibromatosis is the most common benign fibrous tumor in patients older than 10 years.[5]
- It typically arises from the connective tissue of muscle or its overlying fascia.

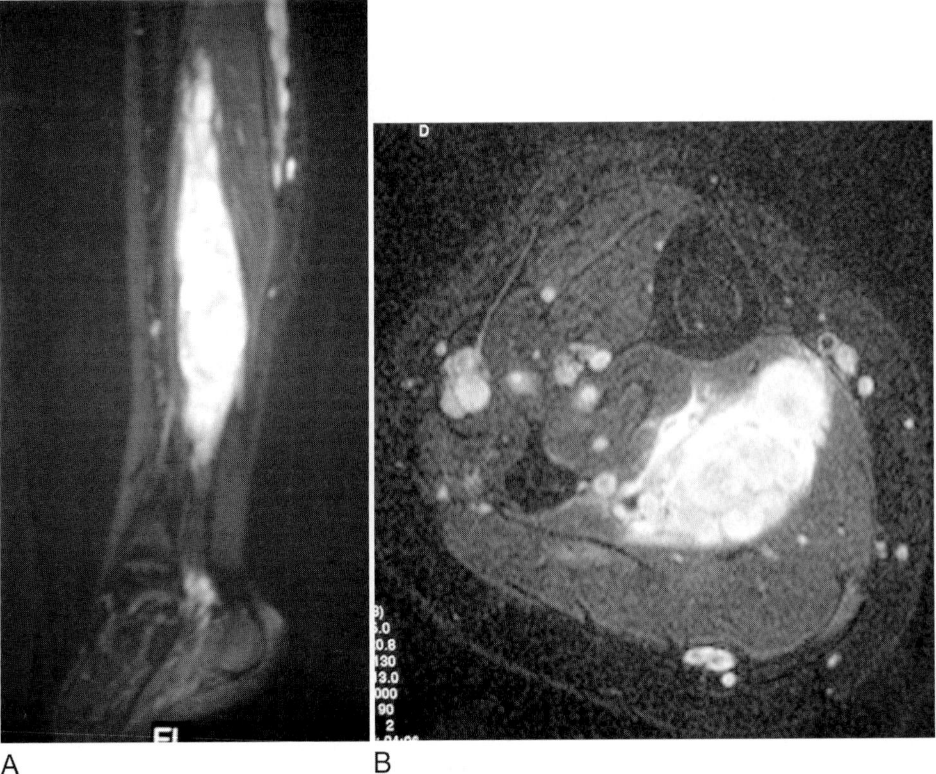

Figure 12–33: Malignant peripheral nerve sheath tumor (neurofibrosarcoma). **A, Sagittal T2-weighted MRI of the leg shows fusiform, lobulated, elongated masses of high signal following the neurovascular bundle. B, Axial T2-weighted image demonstrates a cluster of nodular, high-signal intensity masses. Only the rapid increase in size can help distinguish benignity from malignancy.**

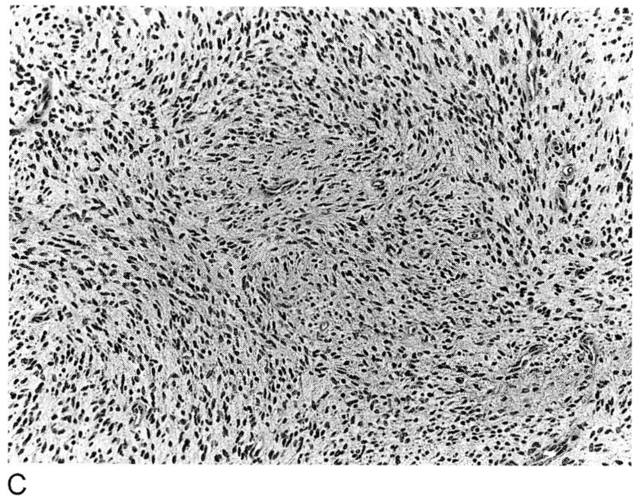

Figure 12–33, cont'd: **C, Photomicrograph demonstrates a lesion composed of interlacing cellular spindle cell fascicles.**

- The biological activity is, in general, between that of other benign fibrous lesions and fibrosarcoma (e.g., locally aggressive), but it does not have the ability to metastasize.
- The principal location of the tumor is the musculature of shoulder followed by the chest wall, back, thigh, and mesentery.
- Patients with aggressive fibromatosis usually have a slowly enlarging mass that typically causes little or no pain. The mass usually is deep seated, firm, and slightly tender.

Radiographic and Histological Features

- Plain radiographs may reveal a soft tissue mass if the lesion is large but there are no distinguishing features.
- MRI shows a lesion of low-signal intensity on both T1- and T2-weighted images. However, because the cellularity varies, fibromatosis may have an appearance on MRI similar to any soft tissue neoplasia (Figure 12–34, *A*).
- On bone scan, aggressive fibromatosis usually shows an increased uptake.
- Histologically, aggressive fibromatosis appears similar to scar tissue. The tumor is poorly circumscribed and infiltrates the surrounding normal tissue. It consists of elongated spindle-shaped cells of uniform appearance, within dense bundles of collagen. The nuclei are small, pale staining, and sharply defined (Figure 12–34, *B*). The cell of origin is believed to be the myofibroblast.

Treatment

- Malignant transformation of aggressive fibromatosis is extremely rare, but the tumor may behave in a locally aggressive manner.[22]

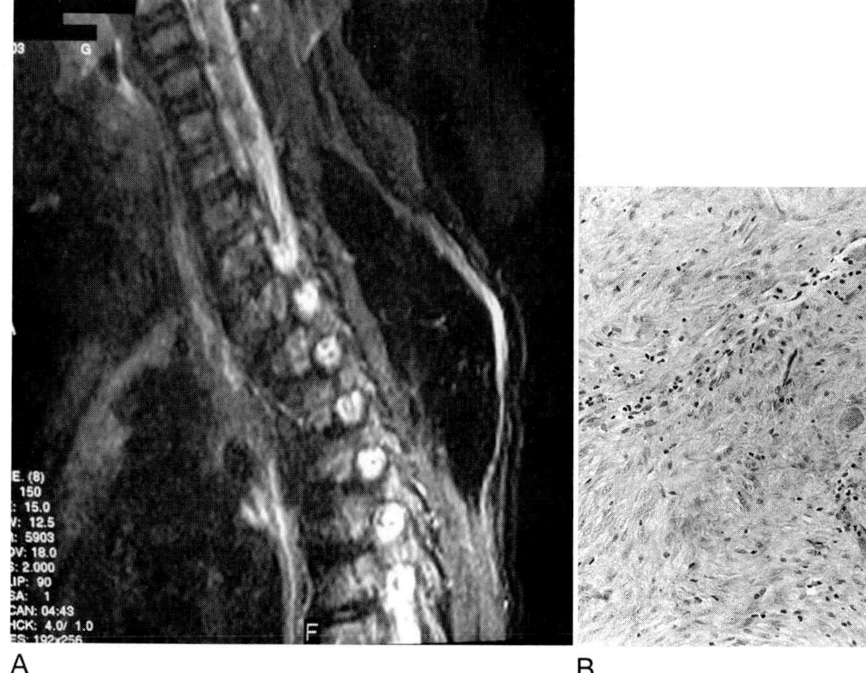

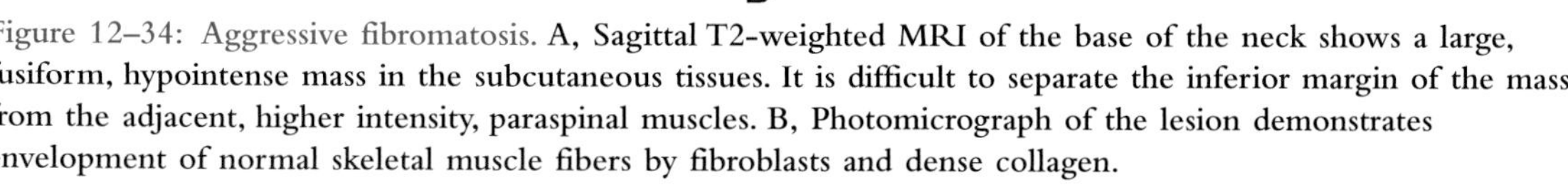

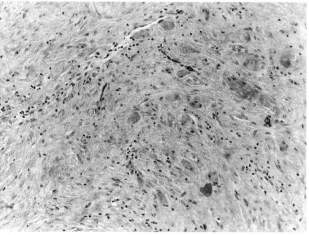

Figure 12–34: Aggressive fibromatosis. **A, Sagittal T2-weighted MRI of the base of the neck shows a large, fusiform, hypointense mass in the subcutaneous tissues. It is difficult to separate the inferior margin of the mass from the adjacent, higher intensity, paraspinal muscles. B, Photomicrograph of the lesion demonstrates envelopment of normal skeletal muscle fibers by fibroblasts and dense collagen.**

- The preferred treatment for aggressive fibromatosis is wide excision; however, because of the tumor's infiltrative nature, this may not be possible or appropriate without debilitating surgery.[5,22] The presence of a positive margin at the initial resection does not always lead to a local recurrence, and it is recommended to observe the patient for a local recurrence.
- Approximately half of patients with aggressive fibromatosis will develop recurrent disease regardless of the histological margin. Patients younger than 10 years have a greater risk of developing a local recurrence than older patients. If the lesion recurs, a repeat wide surgical resection with the excision of the recurrence should be attempted; this usually provides local control of the tumor.
- When the second surgical margin is microscopically positive, irradiation (a dose averaging 55 Gy) is recommended. This combination, surgery and irradiation, will achieve local control of the tumor in most the patients.[5]
- Irradiation has also been successful for surgically inaccessible lesions.
- Chemotherapy appears to be effective in children with aggressive fibromatosis. Low-dose methotrexate and vinblastin have been used in some patients with initial good results, but the effect of this treatment is unpredictable.

Tumors of Muscular Origin

Rhabdomyosarcoma

- Rhabdomyosarcoma is the most common malignant soft tissue tumor in children, accounting for approximately 5% of all pediatric cancers.
- This highly malignant tumor accounts for well over half the soft tissue sarcomas in childhood.

Clinical Findings

- Rhabdomyosarcoma may occur at any time in childhood or even in adulthood; however, the peak incidence is in the 1- to 5-year age group.[21]
- Boys are affected slightly more often than girls.
- Rhabdomyosarcoma is a malignancy that arises from the embryonal mesenchyme destined to produce striated skeletal muscle.
- There are four histological patterns: embryonal, botryoid-type, alveolar, and pleomorphic. Embryonal and alveolar types are common. Embryonal tumors are most often found in the head and neck or the genitourinary tract, whereas alveolar rhabdomyosarcomas are more commonly found in the extremities and trunk.[5,20,21]
- Patients with alveolar rhabdomyosarcoma usually have a rapidly growing, painless mass deep within the muscle. This occurs with equal frequency in the upper and lower extremities.
- Paravertebral tumors may cause back pain.
- There are usually no generalized or systemic signs. Laboratory findings are normal.
- The regional lymph nodes should be carefully assessed clinically in patients with rhabdomyosarcoma. Unlike in bone sarcomas, regional lymph nodes are involved with a tumor in approximately 15% of the cases, and this worsens the prognosis.
- Characteristic chromosomal abnormalities have been identified in the alveolar rhabdomyosarcoma (Table 12–8). Approximately 70% of the tumors will have a translocation between chromosome 13 and chromosome 2 [t(2;13) (q35:q14)], whereas another 30% will have the translocation between chromosome 13 and chromosome 1 [t(1;13) (p36:q14)].[21] Other mutations in oncogenes or tumor suppressor genes such as *p53* and overproduction of insulin-like growth factor 2 have been identified and may be of importance in the pathogenesis of rhabdomyosarcoma.

Radiographic and Histological Features

Radiographic Features

- MRI shows a heterogeneous mass, indicating the presence of blood or necrosis. Tumor invasion and extent are variable; they can be well circumscribed or poorly defined and infiltrative (Figure 12–35, *A* and *B*). MRI provides important information about tumor extent, particularly the relationship of the tumor to bone and neurovascular structures, which is needed for treatment planning.
- Besides clinical examination, the regional lymph nodes should be carefully assessed by MRI.
- Chest CT should be performed to assess for the presence of lung metastases.
- A bone scan is obtained to exclude bony metastases.

Histological Features

- Embryonal rhabdomyosarcoma consists of poorly differentiated rhabdomyoblasts with a limited collagen matrix. The rhabdomyoblasts are small, round to oval cells with dark-staining nuclei and limited amounts of eosinophilic cytoplasm (Figure 12–35, *C*).[20]
- Alveolar rhabdomyosarcoma is composed of poorly differentiated, small, round to oval tumor cells that show central loss of cellular cohesion and formation of irregular alveolar spaces. The individual cellular aggregates are separated and surrounded by irregularly shaped fibrous trabeculae.

Treatment

- Prognostic variables for rhabdomyosarcomas include the histological subtype, the size of the tumor, the site of the tumor, and the age of the patient.

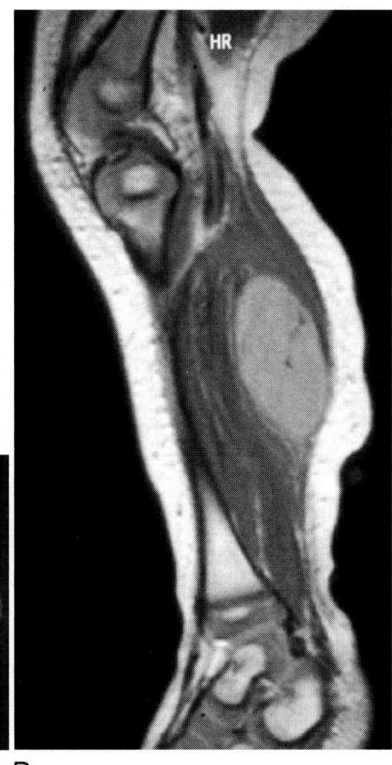

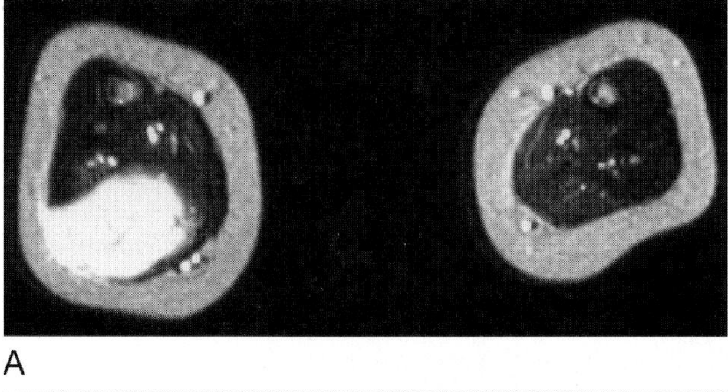

A B

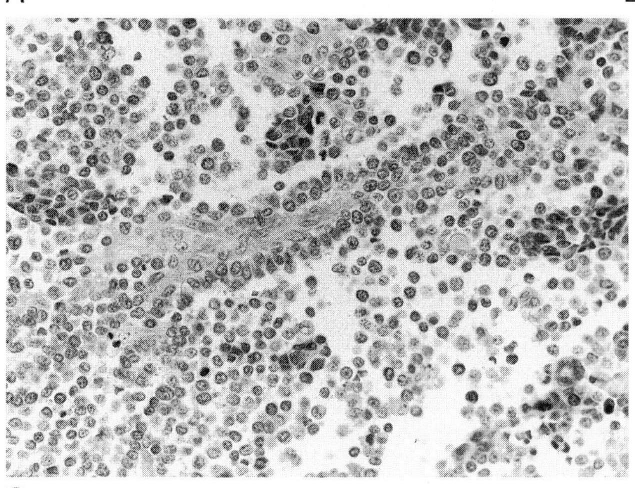

C

Figure 12–35: Alveolar rhabdomyosarcoma. A, Axial T2-weighted MRI of the calf shows a high-signal mass replacing the lateral gastrocnemius muscle. The neurovascular bundles are well visualized separate from the mass. From Erol B, States L, Pawel BR, Tamai J, Dormans JP (2004) Musculoskeletal tumors in children. In: Pediatric Orthopaedics and Sports Medicine (Dormans JP, ed). Philadelphia: Mosby. B, After the administration of intravenous contrast, the enhancement of the mass is seen on the sagittal view. C, Photomicrograph of the lesion demonstrates undifferentiated, small, round cells with inconspicuous cytoplasm, which are discohesive and line fibrous septae.

  - An alveolar subtype, larger tumors, an extremity location, and patients older than 10 years are more often associated with a poorer prognosis.[5,20]
  - Children with nonmetastatic, extremity rhabdomyosarcoma have an estimated 5-year survival rate of 74%, which is worse than survival from disease at other sites, such as orbital or genitourinary sites.
- Alveolar rhabdomyosarcoma, like the other subtypes, is treated with a combination of chemotherapy and surgery.
  - Total resection of the tumor with wide surgical margins is recommended, and preoperative chemotherapy often makes total resection of an extremity lesion possible.[20,21]
  - Irradiation can be used if total surgical resection cannot be achieved without excessive morbidity.
- Lymph node biopsy should be considered if the patient has any suggestion of lymph node involvement (i.e., palpable lymph node enlargement).
- Postoperative irradiation may be used when the surgical margins are positive for tumor or there is poor necrosis of the excised tumor from chemotherapy.
- About 20% of patients with rhabdomyosarcoma have metastatic disease at diagnosis; their prognosis is much poorer. Five-year survival rates are about 20 to 30% overall. These patients are treated with more intensive chemotherapy and radiation therapy delivered to the primary tumor.

- Patients with local relapse should be restaged. If the recurrence is local, surgical resection is used if possible. This is often combined with chemotherapy and radiation therapy.
- Patients with local relapse and distant metastases or with distant metastases alone are most often treated with chemotherapy and palliative radiation therapy.

Synovial Cell Sarcoma

- Synovial cell sarcoma is a well-known adult soft tissue sarcoma that occurs in teenagers and, occasionally, in younger children.
- Synovial cell sarcoma accounts for 10% of all soft tissue sarcomas.
- Most patients are between 15 and 35 years, and males predominate slightly.
- Synovial cell sarcoma arises from primitive synovial cells but rarely occurs within a joint.[20]
- The tumor occurs primarily in the para-articular regions, usually associated with tendon sheaths, bursae, and joint capsules.

Clinical Findings

- Synovial cell sarcoma may manifest in all parts of the body. The upper and lower extremities account for more than 50% of the lesions; the trunk accounts for 15% of them. Almost 10% of the lesions arise in the hands and feet, which is not a characteristic of other soft tissue sarcomas.[21]
- The most common presenting symptom is a deep-seated swelling or a mass that may be accompanied by pain or tenderness.
- The lymph nodes should be examined carefully because up to 25% of the patients have metastasis to regional lymph nodes.[5,20]
- At least 90% of synovial sarcomas display the translocation t(X;18)(p11;q11), and many of the remainder have variant translocations involving either chromosome X or chromosome 18 and a different partner[21] (Table 12–8).

Radiographic and Histological Features

Radiographic Features

- Plain radiographs show calcifications or ossifications within the tumor.
- CT scan demonstrates a soft tissue mass, with calcified densities deep within the tumor.
- MRI, although it does not show the small foci of calcified densities as well as CT, is the preferred test for evaluation and staging of the tumor.

Histological Features

- Grossly, the tumor appears to be well encapsulated with white areas of calcification on the cut surface.
- Histologically, the classical pattern is biphasic consisting of epithelial cells and spindle cells. Usually the spindle cell component predominates (Figure 12–36). The epithelioid foci contain glands with a central lumen lined by cuboidal or tall columnar cells in a spindle cell background. Some synovial cell sarcomas have a monophasic pattern consisting of only a spindle cell component. There seems to be no clinically significant differences between the biphasic and the monophasic types.[5]

Treatment

- The preferred treatment for synovial cell sarcoma is wide excision with limb salvage if possible; adjuvant chemotherapy or irradiation may be required for some patients.
- In adults and older children with synovial cell sarcoma, as in those with other soft tissue sarcomas, preoperative radiotherapy may be used with nonradical surgery in an attempt to avoid amputation and achieve local control.[21]
  - Adjuvant irradiation and marginal resection can be performed in most synovial cell sarcomas of the feet and hands with preservation of a functioning extremity.*
  - Preoperative irradiation and surgery are recommended for most soft tissue sarcomas of the feet. Although, this is successful in saving extremities and controlling the disease locally, the incidence of metastatic disease remains high, at slightly more than 50%.[5]

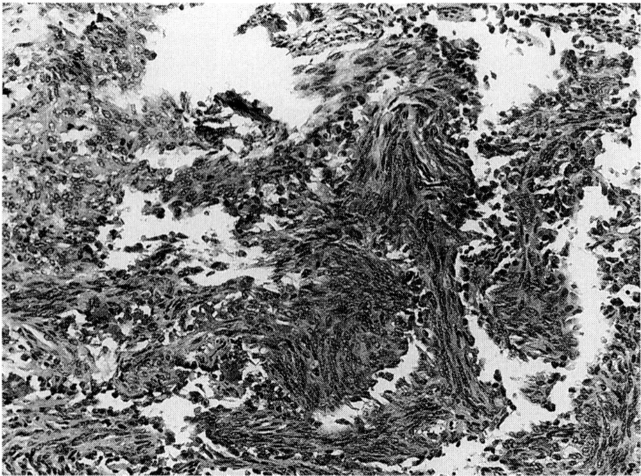

Figure 12–36: Histopathology of synovial cell sarcoma. **Dense fascicles of atypical spindle cells occupy this field. A glandular component could not be demonstrated in this tumor, although immunohistochemistry revealed the presence of epithelial differentiation.**

References

1. Enneking WF (1983) Musculoskeletal Tumor Surgery. New York: Churchill Livingstone.

2. Madewell JE, Ragsdale BD, Sweet DE (1981) Radiologic and pathologic analysis of solitary bone lesions: Part I—Internal margins. Radiol Clin North Am 19(4): 715-748.
   The authors provide a review of the radiographic appearance of solitary bone lesions in this classic reference.

3. Ragsdale BD, Madewell JE, Sweet DE (1981) Radiologic and pathologic analysis of solitary bone lesions: Part II—Periosteal reactions. Radiol Clin North Am 19(4): 749-783.
   The authors describe histological changes associated with solitary bone lesions in this classic reference.

4. Heinrich SD, Scarborough MT, eds, Pediatric Orthopaedic Oncology. Orthop Clin North Am, July, 1996.

5. Springfield DS, Gebhardt MC (2001) Bone and soft tissue tumors. In: Lovell and Winter's Pediatric Orthopaedics, 5th edition (Morrissy RT, Weinstein SL, eds). Philadelphia: Lippincott Williams & Wilkins, pp 507-562.

6. Simon MA, Biermann JS (1993) Biopsy of bone and soft tissue lesions. J Bone Joint Surg Am 75(4): 616-621.

7. Unni K (1996) Dahlin's Bone Tumors: General Aspects and Data on 11,087 Cases, 5th edition. Philadelphia: Lippincott-Raven.

8. Huvos AG (1991) Bone Tumors: Diagnosis, Treatment, and Prognosis, 2nd edition. Philadelphia: WB Saunders.

9. Greenspan A, Remagen W (1998) Differential Diagnosis of Tumors and Tumor-Like Lesions of Bones and Joints. Philadelphia: Lippincott-Raven.

10. Copley L, Dormans JP (1996) Benign pediatric bone tumors: Evaluation and treatment. Pediatr Clin North Am 43(4): 949-966.
    The authors describe advanced and new techniques in the diagnosis and treatment of children with benign bone lesions.

11. Himelstein BP, Dormans JP (1996) Malignant bone tumors of childhood. Pediatr Clin North Am 43(4): 967-984.
    The authors discuss improvements in diagnosis and treatment of children with malignant bone tumors. New molecular genetic discoveries, and the potential for novel therapeutic modalities using hybrid transcripts interfere with aberrant transcriptional activation.

12. Picci PL, Sangiorgi L, Rougraff B, Neff J, Casadei R, Campanacci M (1994) Relationship of chemotherapy-induced necrosis and surgical margins to local recurrence in osteosarcoma. J Clin Oncol 12(12): 2699-2705.
    OBJECTIVE: The authors reviewed 59 cases of high-grade osteosarcoma with follow-up of 65 months in surviving patients. There were 28 local recurrences in this study (7%): 4 patients (81%) who had wide amputations, 1 intralesional amputation, and 23(10%) who had limb salvage surgery. There were no recurrences in patients treated with radical amputation or rotationplasty.
    CONCLUSION: Chemotherapy response, age, and surgical margins were predictive for recurrent disease.

13. Dormans JP, Flynn JM (2001) Pathologic fractures associated with tumors and unique conditions of the musculoskeletal system. In: Rockwood and Wilkins' Fractures in Children, 5th edition (Beaty JH, Kasser JR, eds). Philadelphia: Lippincott Williams & Wilkins.

14. Dormans JP, Pill SG (2002) Fractures through bone cysts: Unicameral bone cysts, aneurysmal bone cysts, fibrous cortical defects, and nonossifying fibromas. Instr Course Lect 51: 457-467.

15. Springfield DS, Rosenberg AE, Mankin HJ, Mindell ER (1994) Relationship between osteofibrous dysplasia and adamantinoma. Clin Orthop 309: 234-244.
    The authors reviewed 32 patients with ossifying fibroma, fibrous dysplasia, osteofibrous dysplasia-like adamantinoma, or adamantinoma of the tibia and found that 19 patients had their diagnosis changed because of a recurrence or through a review of their histology. The authors propose: (1) many patients with a diagnosis of fibrous dysplasia or osteofibrous dysplasia of the tibia actually have an adamantinoma, (2) osteofibrous dysplasia is often a locally aggressive lesion, and (3) osteofibrous dysplasia may be a precursor of adamantinoma.

16. Campanacci M, Capanna R, Picci P (1986) Unicameral and aneurysmal bone cysts. Clin Orthop 204: 25-36.
    The authors compared 178 cases of unicameral bone cysts treated with curettage and bone grafting with 141 cases treated with cortisone injections. The results were comparable in the two groups. The authors present new radiographic classification of aneurysmal bone cyst based on 198 cases. The authors recommend surgical treatment based on radiographic aspect and the rate of growth of the cyst.

17. Dormans JP, Hanna BG, Johnston DR, Khurana JS (2004) Surgical treatment and recurrence rate of aneurysmal bone cysts in children. Clin Orthop 421: 205-211.

18. Glotzbecker M, Carpentieri D, Dormans J (2004) Langerhans cell histiocytosis: a primary infection of bone? Human Herpes virus 6 latent protein detected in lymphocytes from tissue of children. J Pediatr Orthop. Jan–Feb; 24(1): 123-129.
    The findings reported in this article suggest a role for the HHV-6B in the etiology of LCH.

19. Mulliken JB, Glowacki J (1982) Hemangiomas and vascular malformations in infants and children: A classification based on endothelial characteristics. Plast Reconstr Surg 69(3): 412-422.
    The authors analyzed 49 specimens from a variety of vascular lesions for cellular characteristics and described two major categories of lesions. The authors propose cell-oriented analysis as the basis for the classification of vascular lesions of infancy and childhood and to guide diagnosis and management.

20. Enzinger FM, Weiss SW (1995) Soft Tissue Tumors, 3rd edition. St. Louis: Mosby.

21. Coffin CM, Dehner LP, O'Shea PA (1997) Pediatric Soft Tissue Tumors: A Clinical, Pathological, and Therapeutic Approach. Baltimore: Williams & Wilkins.

22. Spiegel DA, Dormans JP, Meyer JS, et al. (1999) Aggressive fibromatosis from infancy to adolescence. J Pediatr Orthop 19(6): 776-784.

Eighteen patients with extra-abdominal fibromatosis are described. The authors suggest that conservative surgery with wide margins and adjuvant therapies may result in adequate control of disease from infancy to adolescence.

Musculoskeletal Infections

Lawson A.B. Copley* and John P. Dormans†

*MD, Assistant Professor of Orthopaedic Surgery, University of Texas Southwestern, Dallas, TX; Staff Orthopaedic Surgeon, Texas Scottish Rite Hospital for Children, Children's Medical Center of Dallas, Dallas, TX
†MD, Chief of Orthopaedic Surgery, The Children's Hospital of Philadelphia, Philadelphia, PA; Professor of Orthopaedic Surgery, University of Pennsylvania School of Medicine, Philadelphia, PA

Introduction

- Infections of the musculoskeletal system in children comprise a range of disorders that vary in severity and complexity.
- Diversity of the clinical picture ranges from obvious and acute to insidious and chronic.
- Septic arthritis, which most commonly occurs during the first 5 years, is about twice as common as osteomyelitis, which typically occurs between 5 and 10 years.[1]
- Simultaneous infection of bone and its adjacent joint has been reported in 20 to 33% of cases.[1,2]
- Appropriate and timely workup may yield an accurate diagnosis and enable prompt treatment to improve outcomes, even in sequela-prone children.[3,4]
- A thorough history and physical examination with appropriately selected radiological and laboratory studies should result in a timely and correct diagnosis in most cases.
- Every effort should be made to properly identify the causative organism by obtaining blood cultures and aspirating the involved bone and joint.
- *Staphylococcus aureus* is the most commonly isolated organism in all age categories.[5,6]
- Extra vigilance is necessary in neonates and in those children with vague complaints in reference to the spine, pelvis, or foot.[7-9]

Clinically Relevant Anatomy

- In infants younger than 18 months, the metaphyseal circulation is in continuity with the epiphyseal circulation, which may be a predisposing factor to simultaneous bone and joint infection in this age group.
- The metaphyseal circulation is derived from two sources—the nutrient artery, which supplies the central region, and the perichondral vessels, which supply the peripheral regions (Figure 13–1).
- The terminal portions of the metaphyseal circulation form a series of loops that penetrate between the trabeculae to reach the margin of the physis.
- The venular side of the metaphyseal loop enlarges to form a sinusoid, which creates turbulent blood flow that may play a causative role in the aggregation of infection in this region.
- Certain joints are predisposed to simultaneous infection of the adjacent bone because of the intracapsular or intra-articular location of the metaphysis. The most common sites of dual involvement of bone and joint are the knee (31%), hip (23%), ankle (18%), and shoulder (14%).[1-4]
- The circulatory anatomy of the spine is relevant to the likely cause of hematogenous dissemination of diskitis and osteomyelitis. Retrograde flow occurs from the pelvic venous plexus to the perivertebral venous plexus through valveless menignorrhachidian veins. An end-arteriolar

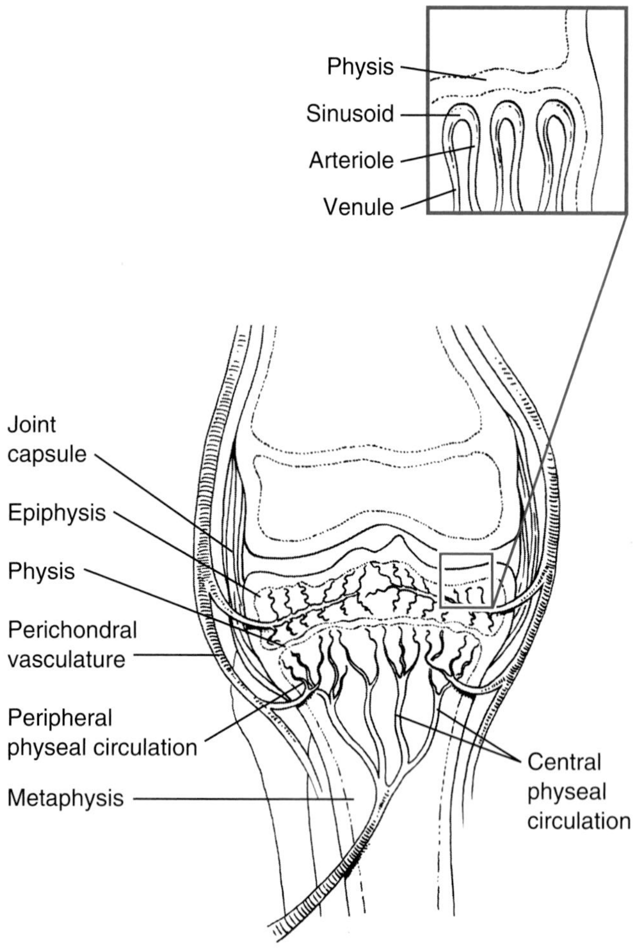

Figure 13–1: Blood supply of the epiphysis, physis, and metaphysis of long bones. **Also shown is the anatomy of the venous sinusoid, which results in turbulent blood flow near the physis.**

network near the vertebral endplate may also contribute to the cause of infection.[9]

Physical Examination

- Although difficult to perform with small or frightened children, the physical examination is important in the diagnostic process.
- Children should be examined in a comfortable environment in the presence of their parents and away from loud noises and bright lights.
- Proceed with physical examination only after all relevant historical information has been obtained and a positive rapport has been established with the parents and child.
- Begin the examination away from the suspected area of involvement and leave the most tender area to be examined last.
- It is sometimes necessary to leave extremely anxious children alone with their parents after demonstrating to them how to elicit the focal points of tenderness or the limitation of joint motion. The parents may then be better able to establish the most likely region of involvement toward which to direct subsequent radiographic studies.
- Relevant physical findings include fever higher than 38° C, focal tenderness, warmth, erythema, swelling, limited range of motion, pseudoparalysis, limp, refusal to walk, loss of normal spinal rhythm on forward bending, rash, synovitis, and joint effusion.
- Even in the absence of discrete physical findings, infection must be maintained in the differential diagnosis when children have musculoskeletal pain because this may be the only symptom in subacute cases (Boxes 13–1 and 13–2).[10]

Radiological Examination

- High-quality plain radiographs are essential in all cases of suspected musculoskeletal infection.
- Comparison views of the uninvolved extremity are often useful in distinguishing subtle abnormalities such as lytic or blastic skeletal lesions, periosteal elevation, fracture, tumor, osteopenia, or deep soft tissue swelling.
- Deep soft tissue swelling is the first radiographic manifestation of musculoskeletal infection.[11]
- Classic radiographic signs of bone resorption and periosteal new bone formation may not occur for 1 or 2 weeks after the onset of infection.[11]
- Ultrasound is a low-cost, noninvasive means of detecting musculoskeletal infection in certain regions without exposure to radiation. It is most useful in detecting fluid in the hip joint or abscesses of the psoas muscle (Figure 13–2).
- Ultrasonic features of osteomyelitis include deep soft tissue swelling, periosteal thickening, subperiosteal fluid collections, and cortical breach or destruction.[12]
- Bone scintigraphy has value in localizing a specific area of skeletal involvement when history and physical examination have suggested infection but not identified a location.

Box 13–1 Relevant Historical Features in the Evaluation of Pediatric Musculoskeletal Infection

- Timing of onset
- Recent systemic illness or upper respiratory infection
- Recent travel to area with known endemic pathogens
- Constitutional symptoms (fever, chills, night sweats, or malaise)
- Pain not responding to conservative treatment
- Progressive worsening of symptoms and limitation of motion or activity

Box 13–2 Relevant Physical Findings in the Evaluation of Pediatric Musculoskeletal Infection

- Temperature >38.5° C
- Refusal to walk
- Limp
- Loss of normal spinal rhythm on forward bending
- Rash
- Pseudoparalysis
- Erythema, warmth, swelling, and tenderness near the ends of long bones
- Joint effusion or synovitis
- Limited range of motion of joints

- Three phases of technetium-99m diphosphonate scanning are commonly used: blood flow (performed immediately following injection), blood pool (performed after a brief period to evaluate soft tissue pooling), and delayed (performed after 2 to 3 hours to evaluate radionuclide deposition in bone) (Figure 13–3).
- Osteomyelitis is identified as focally increased radioactivity in all three phases, whereas cellulitis will cause uptake on only the first two phases.
- Photopenic or cold bone scans may occur in 8 to 20% of cases of osteomyelitis and are thought to be caused by compression of the microcirculation of the medullary canal. This finding may be associated with more aggressive infection because of the obscurity of the regional blood flow caused by the infection.
- Special techniques are useful in pediatric bone scintigraphy to differentiate the areas of increased activity in the metaphysis in cases of early osteomyelitis from the normally occurring increased activity of the growth plate. These include pinhole or converging collimation.[11]
- Bone scans may be difficult to interpret in neonates and in certain anatomical areas, such as the spine and pelvis.[8,9]
- Gallium-67 imaging may be useful when a technetium bone scan is normal but the clinical suspicion of osteomyelitis remains high. The combination of gallium and technetium scans may help to differentiate infarct from infection in children with sickle cell disease.[11,13]
- Septic arthritis is more difficult to evaluate with nuclear imaging with frequent false-positive (32%) and false-negative (30%) results.[11]
- Magnetic resonance imaging (MRI) has been found to have a sensitivity of 97% and a specificity of 92% in evaluating musculoskeletal infection. Unfortunately the cost and requirement for monitored sedation limit the usefulness of MRI.[11,14]
- Characteristics of infection seen on MRI include dark marrow on T1-weighted images and increased marrow signal on T2-weighted images (Figure 13–4).
- Abscess formation in bone and subperiosteal fluid collections may also be identified.
- Caution should be used in interpreting an abnormal marrow signal adjacent to joint effusions, which may be seen in up to 60% of uncomplicated septic arthritis.[14]
- MRI is greatly useful in the evaluation of the spine, pelvis, or foot because it provides high resolution and

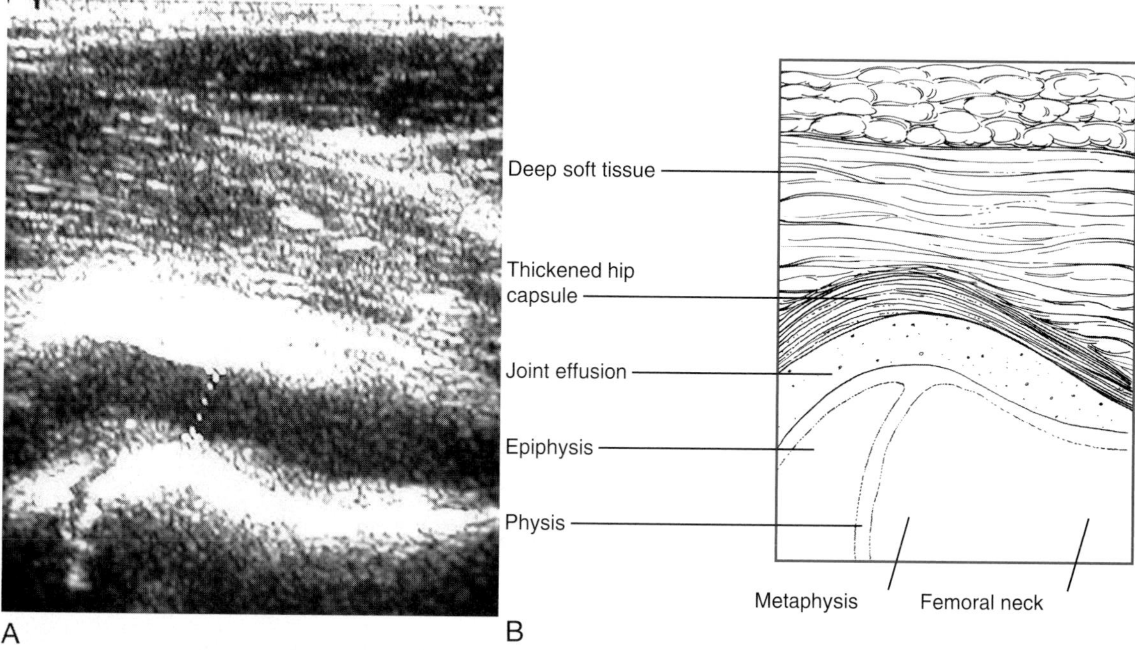

Figure 13–2: A, Ultrasound findings of septic arthritis with deep soft tissue swelling, capsular thickening, and elevation by joint fluid. B, Details of the ultrasound.

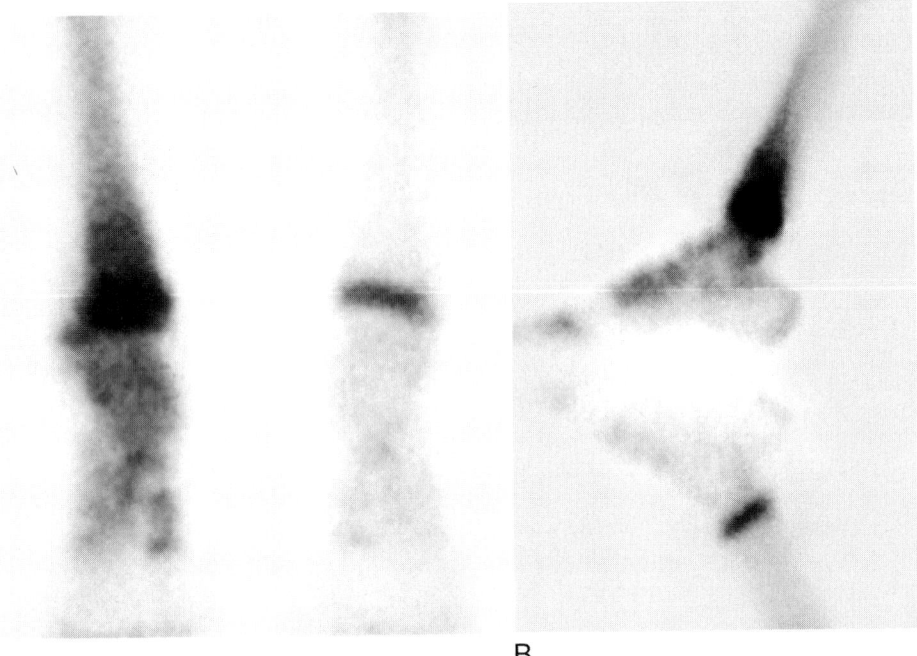

Figure 13–3: Technetium-99m diphosphonate bone scan demonstrating increased uptake in the distal tibial metaphysis on anteroposterior (A) and lateral (B) images.

multiplane imaging in these areas that are otherwise difficult to visualize.[14]

- Table 13–1 list the rationale for the selection of specific studies in the evaluation of infection in children.

Laboratory Tests

- Initial studies that should be obtained include complete blood count with differential leukocyte count, erythrocyte sedimentation rate (ESR), C-reactive protein (CRP) and blood cultures from two separate sites.[3,4] See Table 13–2 for additional laboratory studies and their indications in the work-up of infection.
- The white blood cell (WBC) count is elevated in only 25 to 35% of children with acute hematogenous osteomyelitis (AHO) but may be useful in excluding other disorders from the differential (Box 13–3).[4]

Figure 13–4: MRI scan of fibular osteomyelitis with findings of reduced marrow signal in the distal fibular metaphysis on the T1-weighted image (A) and increased uptake from marrow edema on the T2-weighted image (B).

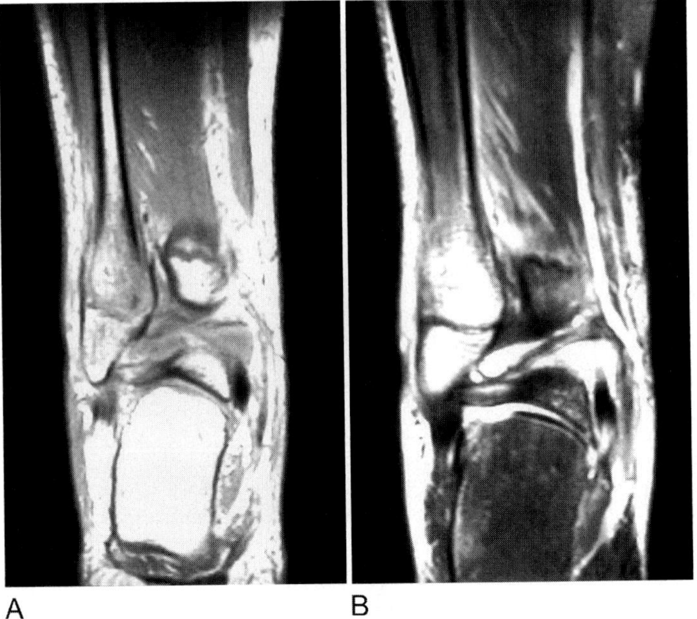

Table 13–1: Indications for Selected Additional Studies in Workup for Infection

STUDY	ADVANTAGES	DISADVANTAGES	INDICATIONS	FINDINGS
X-ray film	Low cost Noninvasive Low radiation exposure	Technique dependent in early stages of infection	Should be obtained in all cases of suspected infection May need to be repeated	Early—Deep soft tissue swelling Late—Cortical erosion or osseous destruction
Ultrasound	Low cost Noninvasive No radiation	Technique dependent	Most useful to evaluate septic arthritis of hip or psoas abscess	Joint fluid collections Deep soft tissue swelling, subperiosteal fluid collections
Bone scan	Lower cost than MRI Identifies site or sites of infection	Difficult to interpret in spine or pelvic infections or in neonates Significant radiation exposure with gallium scanning False positives (32%) and false negatives (30%) in septic arthritis Requires special techniques of pinhole collimation to avoid obscurity caused by physeal activity	Useful when infection is suggested but location is not clear from history, physical examination, and laboratory tests	Increased activity in the area of involvement in all three phases of technetium scan Cold scans (photopenic, 8 to 20%) may suggest more aggressive infections
MRI	Clear visualization of regional anatomy No radiation Helpful for infections of spine, pelvis, or foot	Expensive Requires sedation in small children False positives (60%) of suggested osteomyelitis in cases of uncomplicated septic arthritis	Useful for suspected infections of pelvis, spine, or foot	Dark marrow on T1 Increased marrow signal on T2 Intraosseous abscess identified by loculated fluid Joint fluid collections visualized Deep soft tissue collections (abscess) visualized

Table 13–2: Supplemental Studies and Their Indications When Evaluating Infection

ADDITIONAL STUDIES	INDICATIONS
Anti-streptolysin O, anti-DNAse B, streptozyme, or throat swab for Group A streptococcus	History of recurrent or untreated streptococcus infections, migratory arthritis, arthralgias, myalgias, or scarlatiniform rash
ELISA for Lyme antibody titer, and Western blot (IgG; IgM)	History of ECM rash larger than 5 cm, tick bite, cardiac, neurological or orthopedic manifestations, or travel or residence in the northeastern United States (outdoor activity)
ANA, BUN/creatine, and urinalysis	Morning stiffness, rash, or oligoarticular arthritis. Referral to ophthalmologist if ANA is positive
HLA-B27	Spine stiffness and pain, sacroiliac inflammation, or enthesopathy
Purified protein derivative skin test	Exposure to tuberculosis or constitutional symptoms (night sweats, weight loss, or fever), chest x-ray film
Coags, LFTs, electrolytes, BUN/creatinine, fibrin split products, and fibrinogen	Shock, sepsis, or evidence of multiple organ system involvement
Inspection of the peripheral smear and bone marrow biopsy	Pancytopenia, leukocytosis, or constitutional symptoms
Albumin, total protein, fibrinogen, total lymphocyte count, and HIV test	Chronic osteomyelitis, unusual opportunistic infections, or tuberculosis

ANA, antinuclear antibody; *BUN*, blood urea nitrogen; *Coags*, blood coagulation studies; *ECM*, erythema chronicum migrans; *ELISA*, enzyme-linked immunosorbent assay; *HIV*, human immunodeficiency virus; *HLA*, human leukocyte antigen; *IgG and IgM*, immunoglobulin G and M; *LFT*, liver function test.

- The ESR rises to a peak within 3 to 5 days of the onset of infection, with mean values of 58 mm/hr. It slowly returns to normal over approximately 3 weeks.[4]
- The ESR should not be significantly elevated in response to trauma or stress fracture.
- The CRP is an acute-phase reactive protein synthesized by the liver in response to bacterial infection.
- CRP begins to rise within 6 hours of the triggering response, reaching a peak within 36 to 50 hours with mean values of 71 mg/L.[3,4]

Box 13–3 Laboratory Findings in Pediatric Musculoskeletal Infection

- WBC count is elevated in only 25 to 35% of children with AHO.
- ESR reaches a peak 3 to 5 days after the onset of infection, with a mean of 58 mm/hr, and normalizes in 3 weeks following effective treatment.
- CRP reaches a peak 36 to 50 hours after the onset of infection, with a mean of 71 mg/L, and normalizes within 7 days following effective treatment. The likelihood of sequelae is suggested if the CRP doubles in 24 hours or remains significantly elevated 4 to 6 days following the initiation of treatment.
- Blood cultures are positive in only 30 to 50% of cases of septic arthritis or AHO but should always be obtained because this might be the only positive identification of causative organism in some cases.

- Resolution of the CRP to normal following appropriate treatment of the infection commonly occurs within 7 days in uncomplicated cases.[3,4]
- Adverse sequelae of infection have been shown to occur more commonly in those children who have a CRP that remains significantly above the mean of those children without sequelae during the first 4 to 6 days of treatment.[3]
- Because CRP is an easy study for laboratories to perform with results available in less than 1 hour, consideration should be given to daily CRP levels during the early course of treatment to monitor improvement.
- Blood cultures yield positive results in only 30 to 50% of children with either septic arthritis or AHO but should be obtained in all cases because they render the only isolate of the causative organism that may guide treatment.[9]
- Joint aspiration is essential in cases of suspected septic arthritis. The fluid should be sent for WBC count with a differential percentage of polymorphonuclear (PMN) cells, gram stain, culture, and sensitivity.
- A cell count greater than 80,000/mL with greater than 75% PMN cells suggests infection, whereas a cell count less than 15,000/mL with less than 25% PMN cells suggests inflammation.
- Bone or periosteal fluid aspiration may prove useful in cases of osteomyelitis to isolate the causative organism. Attempted aspiration does not appear to alter the results of subsequent nuclear imaging or MRI.[11]

Classification Methods

- Musculoskeletal infections are typically classified by definitions and the relationship of the suspected time of onset to the time of diagnosis.
- Presenting symptoms of AHO include a rapid development of focal bone pain, fever, and malaise, which occur within the first several days of onset.
- Subacute osteomyelitis results in pain that is present for at least 2 weeks but possibly for months. The onset is insidious, and the progression is gradual. Rarely are there signs of systemic illness.
- Subacute osteomyelitis creates diverse radiographic findings classified according to location (epiphysis, metaphysis, or diaphysis) and appearance (aggressive or benign).[15]
- Chronic osteomyelitis, although rare in the United States, usually occurs from delayed or inadequate treatment of AHO.
- Classic features of chronic osteomyelitis include the presence of dead bone (sequestrum) surrounded by gross purulence and reactive new bone (involucrum).
- Chronic recurrent multifocal osteomyelitis (CRMO) is a condition of insidious onset involving multiple bone locations associated with pain and malaise.
- Blood and bone cultures are negative in CRMO, and antibiotics have been ineffective in treatment. Overall, CRMO is considered a benign and self-limited condition.
- Infections may also be classified by patient age (neonate, child, or adult), route of infection (hematogenous or direct inoculation), or causative organism (pyogenic or granulomatous).

Causative Organisms

Staphylococcus Aureus

- *S. aureus* remains the most common causative organism for bone or joint infection in all age categories.
- Empirical antibiotic therapy includes nafcillin and gentamicin for neonates and nafcillin, oxacillin, clindamycin, or cefazolin for all other age categories (Table 13–3).

Streptococcus Pyogenes

- Group A streptococcus is responsible for a spectrum of musculoskeletal infection in children.
- A toxic shock-like syndrome, which causes musculoskeletal complaints in up to 87% of cases, may cause severe local tissue destruction and life-threatening multisystem disease.[16]
- Aggressive resuscitation is necessary with the timely surgical decompression of foci of infection in the musculoskeletal system.[16]
- Group A streptococcal pharyngitis may be followed by acute rheumatic fever (ARF) or poststreptococcal reactive arthritis (PSRA).[17]
- Orthopaedic manifestations typically include migratory polyarthritis, usually affecting the lower extremities first.
- The modified Jones criteria are helpful in establishing a diagnosis. Two major criteria (carditis, polyarthritis, subcutaneous nodules, erythema marginatum, and chorea) or one major and two minor criteria (fever, arthralgia, elevated ESR or CRP, and prolonged PR interval on electrocardiogram) with evidence of a preceding streptococcal infection are necessary for diagnosis.
- Salicylates and antibiotic treatment appear to have a significant role in the management and prevention of long-term sequelae of ARF or PSRA.[17]

Table 13-3: Causative Organism and Empiric Antibiotic by Age Group

AGE	ORGANISM	EMPIRIC ANTIBIOTIC (IV)
Neonate (up to 8 weeks)	*Staphylococcus aureus* Group B streptococcus *Staphylococcus epidermidis* Enterococcus, *Escherichia coli, Salmonella sp.* *Neisseria gonorrhoeae*	Nafcillin and gentamicin or cefotaxime
Infant and child (≤3 years)	*Staphylococcus aureus* *Kingella kingae* *Streptococcus pneumoniae* Group A streptococcus	Nafcillin, oxacillin, clindamycin, or cefazolin Non-Hib-immunized: Cefuroxime
Child (>3 years)	*Staphylococcus aureus* Group A streptococcus *Pseudomonas aeruginosa* (foot puncture)	Nafcillin, oxacillin, clindamycin, or cefazolin Ceftazidime Cefuroxime
Adolescent	*Salmonella sp.* (SSD) *Staphylococcus aureus* *Neisseria gonorrhoeae*	 Nafcillin, oxacillin, clindamycin, or cefazolin Ceftriaxone or cefotaxime

Hib, Haemophilus influenzae type B; *sp*, Species nova (new species); SSD, Sickle Cell Disease

Kingella Kingae

- There has been a rising incidence of bone and joint infections caused by *Kingella kingae* within the past 3 decades.
- Up to 17% of infections in children up to 3 years of age involve *K. kingae,* replacing *Haemophilus influenzae* as the most common gram-negative organism in this age group.[5]
- The decreased incidence of *H. influenzae* has likely resulted from an improved vaccine.[5]
- Specific acquisition methods and culture conditions are needed to identify this organism and should be requested when sending specimens for culture in children younger than 3 years.

Neisseria Meningitidis

- *Neisseria meningitidis* is significant as a causal organism in purpura fulminans, characterized by progressive dermal vascular thrombosis, disseminated intravascular coagulation, and shock.
- Peripheral cutaneous lesions caused by the avascular infarction are initially sterile but may become superinfected and gangrenous.
- Affected extremities gradually heal with demarcation of the necrotic tissues followed by scarring and autoamputation.
- Treatment involves initial resuscitation efforts with appropriate antibiotics, usually a third-generation cephalosporin, aggressive fluid management with invasive monitoring of volume status, correction of coagulopathy with fresh frozen plasma and vitamin K, and appropriate use of cardiac inotropic agents.
- Successful surgical reconstruction is often delayed until a clear demarcation of nonviable tissues is apparent.

A multidisciplinary approach with an intensivist, an infectious disease specialist, an orthopaedic surgeon, and a plastic surgeon is helpful.

Streptococcus Pneumoniae

- Pneumococcus has been reported in osteomyelitis and septic arthritis in children between the ages of 3 and 24 months.
- Pneumococcal infection has been identified as another cause of purpura fulminans in children that is thought to be mediated by the pneumococcal autolysin.

Neisseria Gonorrhoeae

- Pediatric patients are affected by gonococcal arthritis in three situations: (1) transmission to neonates who pass through the birth canal in infected mothers, (2) transmission through sexual abuse of children or adolescents, and (3) transmission through sexual activity in adolescents.
- Disseminated disease, which occurs from days to months following the initial infection, is identified by polyarthralgias involving the knee, ankle, or wrist associated with fever, chills, rash, and tenosynovitis of the dorsum of the hand.
- When gonococcal infection is suspected, cultures should be obtained from the joint fluid, the cervix of postpubertal girls, the urethral or prostatic discharge of males, and the vagina, pharynx and rectum of children suspected to be victims of sexual abuse.
- Special handling instructions are necessary for laboratory specimens to increase the potential of positively identifying the organism.
- Treatment involves local aspiration and intravenous administration of a third-generation cephalosporin.

- The decision for surgical arthrotomy and drainage of a joint should be made on a case-by-case basis.

Mycobacterium Tuberculosis

- Tuberculosis infections have been increasing in incidence in the United States since 1985.
- Extrapulmonary tuberculosis is more common in children younger than 5 years, occurring in 5 to 10% of infected children.
- Osteomyelitis, dactylitis, or septic arthritis may take 1 to 3 years to manifest after the initial infection.
- More than half of all cases of tubercular osteomyelitis involve the spine, followed in incidence by infections around the hip and knee.[10]
- Spinal involvement usually occurs in the anterior one third of the vertebral body with destructive bone lesions that create collapse and kyphosis.
- Paravertebral abscess and calcification are almost pathognomonic for spinal tuberculosis.
- Diagnosis requires a high index of suspicion. Skin testing should be performed using purified protein derivative, and culture material should be obtained because positive cultures can be obtained in 80% of children with extrapulmonary disease.[10]
- Treatment recommendations for skeletal tuberculosis include four-drug therapy (isoniazid, rifampin, pyrazinamide, and streptomycin) for 2 months followed by isoniazid and rifampin for 10 months.[10]
- Surgical decompression of the foci of infection is rarely necessary. Indications for spinal surgery include neurological involvement, spinal instability, and failure of medical treatment.

Borrelia Burgdorferi

- Lyme disease most commonly occurs in the northeast, mid-Atlantic, and north–central regions of the United States after inoculation with the spirochete *Borrelia burgdorferi* by the deer tick *(Ixodes dammini)*. The delay before systemic manifestations is 2 to 30 days.
- Multisystem infection may be mistaken for juvenile arthritis or septic arthritis. In one series, 7 of 10 children with Lyme arthritis underwent emergent joint irrigation and debridement for presumed septic arthritis based on a fever of 38° C or higher and elevated ESR and CRP.[18]
- The Centers for Disease Control (CDC) diagnostic criteria are an erythema chronicum migrans (ECM) rash 5 cm in diameter and one cardiac, neurological (aseptic meningitis or Bell's palsy), or musculoskeletal manifestation of the disease.
- Immunoglobulin M (IgM) enzyme-linked immunosorbent assay (ELISA) may not be positive for the first 3 to 6 weeks. Positive or equivocal results need to be confirmed by a Western blot test that should include both the IgM and IgG procedures during the first 4 weeks of suspected infection.
- The availability of a rapid (<1 hour) Lyme enzyme immunoassay may help to differentiate Lyme arthritis from septic arthritis before a commitment to surgical management is made. This should be considered in endemic areas.[18]
- Treatment consists of 10 to 30 days of oral antibiotic (amoxicillin or doxycycline). Intravenous ceftriaxone may be necessary for 2 to 4 weeks in cases of severe neurological or cardiac manifestations.
- Post-Lyme disease syndrome with recurrent arthralgias, myalgias, headache, neck pain, and fatigue should be expected to resolve spontaneously within 6 months. Antibiotic use in these cases is controversial.

Challenging Locations

Spine

- The classic presentation of diskitis and vertebral osteomyelitis with refusal to walk and back pain is found in fewer than 50% of children or adolescents.[9]
- Insidious onset with minimal signs or symptoms is typical. Vague symptoms of abdominal pain or poor appetite with equivocal laboratory and radiology studies may be misleading and may delay diagnosis.
- Supplemental studies of the spine such as single-photon emission computerized tomography (SPECT) scanning or MRI should be obtained whenever infection is suspected.[11]
- MRI has a sensitivity of 96% and a specificity of 93% in detecting infections of the spine.[11]
- MRI findings of bone marrow edema located in adjacent vertebrae and altered signal of the disk space suggests infection.
- Extensive destruction of adjacent vertebrae is suggestive of tuberculosis, whereas vertebral collapse with disk space preservation is consistent with eosinophilic granuloma or leukemia.[10]
- Antibiotic treatment has been controversial with some evidence suggesting a similar outcome whether or not antibiotics are administered. One study showed a more rapid resolution of symptoms and a low likelihood of recurrence with at least 6 days of intravenous antibiotics.
- Because *S. aureus* is the most common causative organism, empirical antibiotic therapy consists of a semisynthetic penicillin or first-generation cephalosporin for 4 weeks.[9]
- If a trial of antibiotics is initiated without favorable response, then antibiotics should be suspended for 3 to 4 days before a computerized tomography (CT)-guided biopsy is performed. This will ensure greater accuracy from the cultures.
- CT-guided biopsy has been shown to yield positive results in 60 to 70% of cases.[9]
- Bracing is recommended to reduce pain by immobilizing the spine. Bracing is considered necessary with destructive lesions to prevent vertebral collapse and kyphosis until some reconstitution of the vertebral height occurs.

- The long-term effect on the disk space is persistent narrowing or fusion rather than restitution. This finding may be associated with persistent complaints of backache.

Pelvis

- The variety of symptoms, equivocal nature of physical findings, negative routine radiographs, and equivocal laboratory studies often lead to uncertainty and delay in diagnosis.
- Pelvic osteomyelitis and sacroiliac septic arthritis should be in the differential diagnosis for children or adolescents who have vague hip, lumbosacral, buttock, or abdominal complaints.[8]
- Physical examination should include palpation of the pelvic crests, spines, tuberosities, and rami; range of motion of both hips; and rectal examination to elicit tenderness along the inner margins of the pelvis or sacrum.
- CT, SPECT, or MRI are useful supplemental studies to adequately locate and visualize the infection.[11]
- Treatment may be facilitated by CT- or ultrasound-guided needle aspiration and drain placement for pelvic abscesses located on the inner margin of the pelvis (Figure 13–5).

Foot

- Two clinically important foot infection problems are hematogenous calcaneal osteomyelitis and sequelae of puncture wounds.
- Puncture wounds are extremely common in children, but less than 1% result in deep infections (osteomyelitis, septic arthritis, or abscess).
- A reasonable protocol for management of puncture wounds includes superficial cleansing, tetanus prophylaxis, radiographs to ensure no retained foreign body, and close outpatient follow-up after counseling the family about the signs and symptoms of infection (Box 13–4).
- If deep infection develops, then *Pseudomonas aeruginosa* is the most likely causative organism.
- Exploration with irrigation and debridement and administration of an intravenous antipseudomonal antibiotic is necessary in suspected deep infection. Conversion to an oral fluoroquinolone antibiotic may be considered after clinical and laboratory improvement.
- Hematogenous calcaneal osteomyelitis is responsible for up to 8% of bone infections in children.[7]
- Because calcaneal infection can mimic a variety of common childhood conditions (apophysitis, enthesopathy, contusion, or stress fracture), a high index of suspicion should be maintained and an MRI should be considered to aid in the diagnosis (Figure 13–6).
- The universal site of involvement is the metaphyseal equivalent of the portion of the posterior tuberosity. The alteration of the physis in this area may produce a growth arrest with loss of calcaneal length and secondary deformity.[7]
- Those presenting symptoms more than 5 days after the onset of symptoms have required surgical decompression in up to 75% of cases.[7]

Neonatal Infections

- Neonatal infections occur because of the immaturity of the immune system during the first 8 weeks.
- Neonatal infections are classified as two varieties: nosocomial (polyarticular) and community acquired (monoarticular).

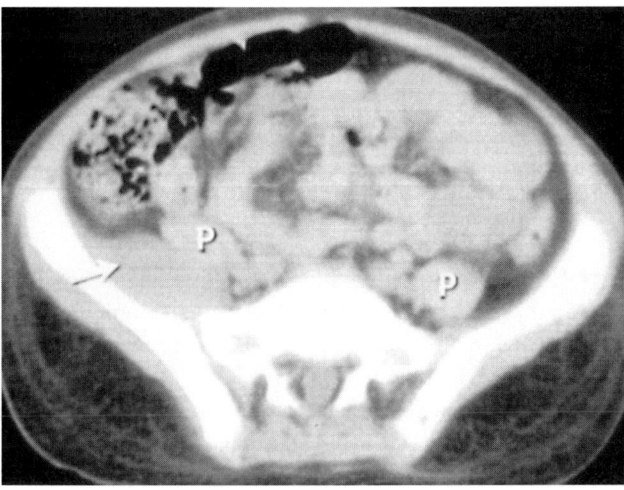

A

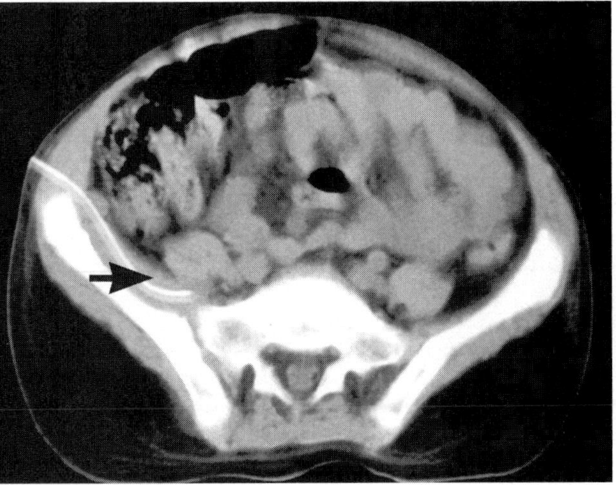

B

Figure 13–5: CT-guided aspiration and placement of drain for treatment of a psoas abscess before (A) and after (B) drain placement. Herring JA, ed (2002) Chapter 34: Bone and joint infections. In: Tachdjian's Pediatric Orthopaedics, 3rd edition, Volume 3. Philadelphia: WB Saunders.

Box 13–4 Protocol for Management of Foot Puncture Wounds

- Cleanse and dress wound
- Verify or administer tetanus prophylaxis
- Obtain radiographs to ensure no retained foreign body
- Counsel family regarding signs and symptoms of infection
- Maintain close outpatient follow-up
- Avoid antibiotic use initially because deep infection occurs in less than 1% of cases
- Surgically debride deep infections and administer an anti-pseudomonal antibiotic

- Premature infants who spend substantial time in the intensive care unit and undergo frequent invasive procedures acquire nosocomial infections in multiple sites.
- Consideration should be given routinely to bilateral hip aspirations in cases of suspected neonatal infections.
- Term infants discharged from the hospital without evidence of infection may subsequently develop a monoarticular infection, which usually occurs between 2 and 4 weeks.
- Transphyseal vessels persist until 12 to 18 months. In older children, the physis serves as a mechanical barrier to infection.
- Neonates are unable to mount a significant inflammatory response to infection and frequently demonstrate normal temperature and WBC count in the presence of infection.
- A high index of suspicion must be maintained in the presence of any musculoskeletal swelling or joint stiffness because these findings may be less impressive than would be seen in an older child.
- Aspiration should be performed on any suspicious bone or joint.

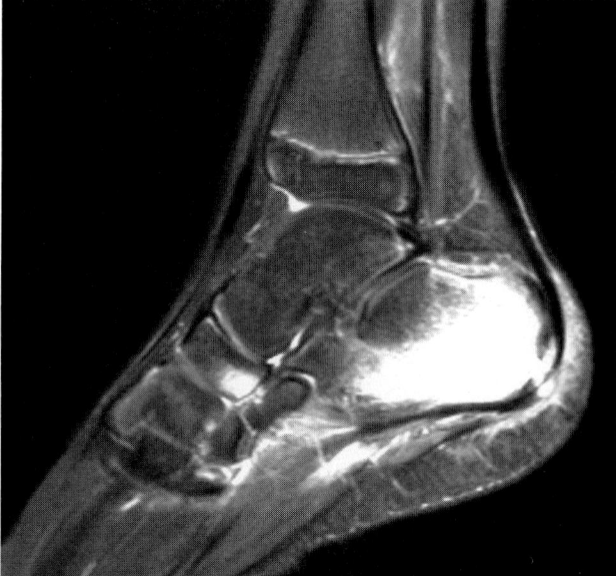

Figure 13–6: MRI showing increased uptake in the posterior tuberosity and body of the calcaneus on a T2-weighted image consistent with hematogenous calcaneal osteomyelitis.

Differential Diagnosis

Eosinophilic Granuloma

- Eosinophilic granuloma commonly presents symptoms including localized pain, tenderness, and swelling, which may be suggestive of infection.
- Plain radiographic lesions may mimic osteomyelitis, Brodie's abscess, Ewing sarcoma, osteolytic osteogenic sarcoma, or neuroblastoma.
- Bone scans are often unpredictable.
- Common sites of involvement are the skull, femur, pelvis, ribs, humerus, spine, clavicle, mandible, tibia, scapula, and fibula.
- Biopsy of lesions is necessary to rule out more serious conditions.
- Treatment options include observation, curettage and bone graft, irradiation, and steroid injections.

Malignant Bone Tumors

- Malignant bone tumors include neuroblastoma (in children younger than 5 years), osteogenic sarcoma (10 to 15 years), and Ewing's sarcoma (approximately 15 years).
- Such tumors may present symptoms including pain, localized tenderness, and swelling at the site of tumor involvement.
- Radiographic findings may include subcortical erosions, permeative diaphyseal destructive lesions, stippled metaphyseal osteolysis, and periosteal elevation with an onionskin layering or sunburst appearance (Figure 13–7).
- Referral to an orthopaedic oncologist for biopsy and definitive treatment may be necessary for aggressive-appearing lesions.

Leukemia

- Leukemia commonly presents symptoms including bone pain, fever, and anemia.
- Presenting symptoms may include migratory arthritis.
- Leukocytosis or leukopenia may be seen.
- Manual inspection of the peripheral blood smear should reveal the presence of leukoblasts.
- X-ray appearance demonstrates diffuse demineralization with widening of the medullary canal, thinning of the cortex, and a characteristic radiolucent metaphyseal band.
- Bone marrow biopsy is diagnostic.

Gaucher's Disease

- Gaucher's disease may present symptoms including crises of bone or joint pain for 1 to 2 days with associated focal musculoskeletal warmth, redness, and tenderness.

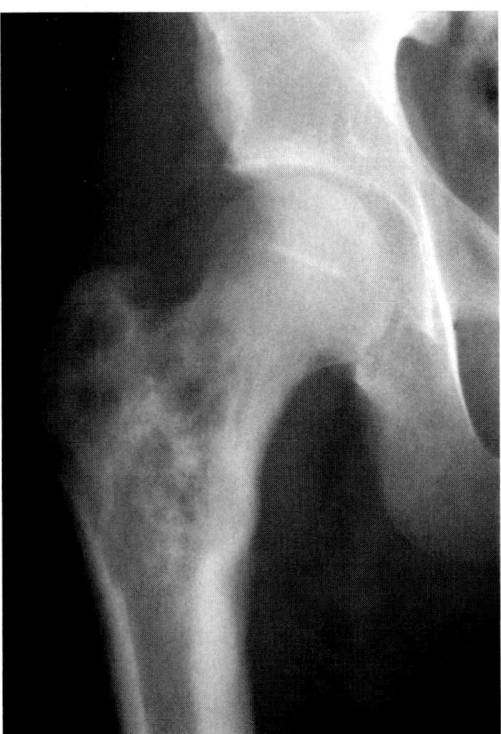

Figure 13–7: Plain x-ray film of the proximal femur of a patient with a 2-month history of pain and an elevated ESR. **Biopsy established the diagnosis of Ewing's sarcoma.**

- This disease is difficult to distinguish from osteomyelitis because of leukocytosis and elevated ESR.
- Aspiration of the affected bone is sometimes necessary to establish the diagnosis because up to 10% of children with Gaucher's disease acquire AHO.
- Combined technetium and gallium scans may be useful in the diagnosis.

Sickle Cell Disease

- Acute bone infarct causing crisis in patients with sickle cell disease may be difficult to distinguish from osteomyelitis.
- Common presenting features of bone infarction include pain, swelling, tenderness, warmth, and erythema of the affected extremity, which may be associated with a low-grade fever.
- Bone infarction is about 50 times more common than infection in patients with sickle cell disease.
- Osteomyelitis is typically accompanied by a high fever in sickle cell patients.
- A three-phase technetium bone scan with subsequent gallium scanning or aspiration of the suspected site of infection may be helpful in situations of diagnostic uncertainty.

Myelodysplasia with Fracture

- Children with myelodysplasia are at risk for occult pathological fracture from low-energy mechanisms because of osteopenia caused by disuse and a lack of bearing weight.
- Lack of sensation in the lower extremities and failure to recognize the occurrence of injury commonly result in these fractures presenting symptoms including the appearance of warmth, erythema, and swelling that may mimic infection.
- Children with higher levels of involvement, particularly thoracic level spina bifida, have a higher risk for this occurrence.
- Immobilization with care to protect the skin frequently resolves rapidly the warmth, erythema, and swelling associated with these injuries.

Treatment

- Delivery of the appropriate concentration of the most specific antibiotic to the site of infection for an adequate duration to completely eradicate infection is the goal of treatment.
- Cost, compliance, and convenience to the patient's family and the treating physician are important but remain secondary in the decision for a treatment regimen.
- In an effort to avoid confusion in large hospital settings, consideration should be given to forming a multidisciplinary team involving pediatrics, infectious disease, orthopaedic surgery and pharmacy to establish evidence-based protocols for the treatment of musculoskeletal infections.

Antibiotic

- A diligent initial effort should be made in all cases to obtain culture material to positively identify the causative organism and its sensitivity to antibiotics.
- In the absence of a positive culture, empirical antibiotic selection is based on the most likely causative organism for each age category. This should be correct in most cases.
- If an organism is identified, then sensitivity data is used to determine a selection of antibiotics to which the organism is susceptible. An organism is considered susceptible if serial dilutions of the antibiotic in a ratio of 1:8 still demonstrate bactericidal properties.
- The antibiotic with the narrowest spectrum of coverage, but capable of destroying the organism, should be selected.

Route

- During the initial treatment, when close monitoring of the clinical and laboratory response is necessary, intravenous antibiotic delivery is essential.

- Oral antibiotic administration is less expensive, more convenient, and capable of achieving adequate serum, bone, and joint bactericidal concentrations.
- It is reasonable to consider converting from the parenteral to the oral route after an appropriate response to treatment has been demonstrated.
- Contraindications to oral therapy include minimal clinical and laboratory improvement with intravenous antibiotic, uncertainty about compliance of the family, gastrointestinal disturbances that may affect absorption, and virulent or resistant organisms that necessitate a greater degree of confidence during treatment.
- With current methods of peripherally inserted central catheter (PICC) or central venous line (CVL) placement, long-term home antibiotic therapy is possible at a fraction of the cost of hospitalization during treatment.[19]
- A home health team can directly monitor the course of treatment and the status of the intravenous site.
- Outpatient parenteral antimicrobial therapy has been found to be safe and effective in children with resolution of the osteoarticular infection in 98% of 179 individuals treated with this method in one study.[19]
- With oral antibiotic therapy, some have recommended monitoring serum peak (at least 1:8) and trough (at least 1:2) bactericidal titers, but others have found this to be unnecessary.[20]

Duration

- In general, bone infections require a longer treatment course than joint infections because of the possibility of chronic infection of bone.
- The typical duration of antibiotic therapy for uncomplicated osteomyelitis is approximately 6 weeks, and that for uncomplicated septic arthritis is approximately 4 weeks.
- Close clinical and laboratory monitoring near the end of the treatment course is helpful in identifying patients that may benefit from longer treatment or another alteration of the regimen.
- It is important to have clear communication between the various treating physicians who continue to follow the patient to determine who will make the final decision regarding the end of treatment and the discontinuation of intravenous access.

Surgical Decision Making

- Most cases of septic arthritis should be addressed surgically to reduce the leukocytosis and the release of destructive enzymes within the joint space.
- An alternate form of treatment for septic arthritis involves serial bedside aspirations during the initial intravenous antibiotic administration. Problems with this form of treatment include poor tolerance in small children and failure to adequately debride thickened exudates within the joint.
- Arthroscopy provides a minimally invasive alternative to open joint debridement and is feasible for knee, shoulder, elbow, wrist, and ankle infections. However, hip infections are more difficult to treat without open arthrotomy.
- In cases of osteomyelitis, most children respond well to nonsurgical treatment.
- An ultrasound study demonstrated resolution of as much as 3 mm of subperiosteal fluid by the use of antibiotics alone.[12]
- In cases with radiographically demonstrable deep soft tissue or intraosseous abscess formation, surgical decompression is necessary to allow eventual resolution of the musculoskeletal infection.
- If significant clinical and laboratory improvement has not resulted within 48 to 72 hours, regardless of radiographic appearance, then surgical treatment should be considered.
- Children older than 1 year who present symptoms within 48 hours of the onset of illness do well with antibiotic treatment alone.[3,4]
- Children younger than 1 year and older children presenting symptoms 5 or more days after the onset of illness have a high likelihood of requiring surgical drainage.[1,3,4]
- Surgical decisions should be made on a case-by-case basis that takes into account all clinical, laboratory, and radiological information and maintains close communication with the primary treating physician, infectious disease consultant, and radiologist (Box 13–5).
- Chronic osteomyelitis is treated surgically with surgical debridement of all necrotic tissue and identification of the causal organism to ensure that the most appropriate antibiotic is selected for long-term treatment.
- Serial surgical debridements may be necessary and consideration may be given to temporarily placing antibiotic-impregnated cement beads to increase the

Box 13–5 Surgical Principles in Treatment of Chronic Osteomyelitis

- Obtain adequate cultures to isolate the causal organism and determine the most specific antibiotic for long-term treatment.
- Surgically debride all necrotic tissue regardless of the degree to which this destabilizes the limb.
- Apply supportive external support as needed to establish limb stability between and after debridements.
- Delay attempts at soft tissue or bone reconstruction until after the infection has resolved.
- Establish multidisciplinary teams with ongoing communication, including the orthopaedic surgeon, the plastic surgeon, the infectious disease specialist, the primary treating physician, and the pharmacy.

antibiotic concentration in the immediate area of infection.

- Only after the infection has resolved should the attempt be made to reconstruct any bone or soft tissue deficiencies.
- Several methods have been described for filling bone defects, including open bone grafting, fibular transposition, and vascularized bone grafting.
- Large segmental bone defects, which may follow radical debridement of the necrotic bone, can be addressed using a bone transport method with an Ilizarov frame (Figure 13–8).
- Surgical treatment, including reconstruction, should involve multidisciplinary communication that includes orthopaedic surgery, plastic surgery, infectious disease, and the physician primarily responsible for the patient.

Follow-up

- Outpatient surveillance is necessary for all children with septic arthritis or osteomyelitis to ensure complete resolution of the infection and restoration of full function.
- Musculoskeletal infection may produce joint stiffness because of the direct involvement of the joint in septic arthritis or because of the proximity of infection in cases of metaphyseal osteomyelitis.
- Surgical treatment of septic arthritis or osteomyelitis and brief periods of postoperative disuse and immobilization may further lead to joint stiffness and muscle atrophy.
- Most children will spontaneously recover their range of motion and function within 4 to 6 weeks following discharge from the hospital.
- Physical or occupational therapy may be necessary for children who had extensive surgical treatment or who demonstrate minimal improvement in function after 2 to 4 weeks of observation.
- Radiographic and laboratory data should be considered 6 to 8 weeks after the onset of illness to ensure resolution. This should include routine radiographs of the involved area, ESR, and CRP.
- The ESR may remain slightly elevated for several months, especially in postsurgical patients, but it should be trending toward normal. The CRP should be normal.
- Metaphyseal osteomyelitis can arrest central growth by dissolving the physis. This may result in physeal tenting caused by continued peripheral growth.
- Plain radiographic follow-up is indicated when potential for physeal arrest exists. Most growth disturbances will be identifiable 6 to 12 months following the insult.

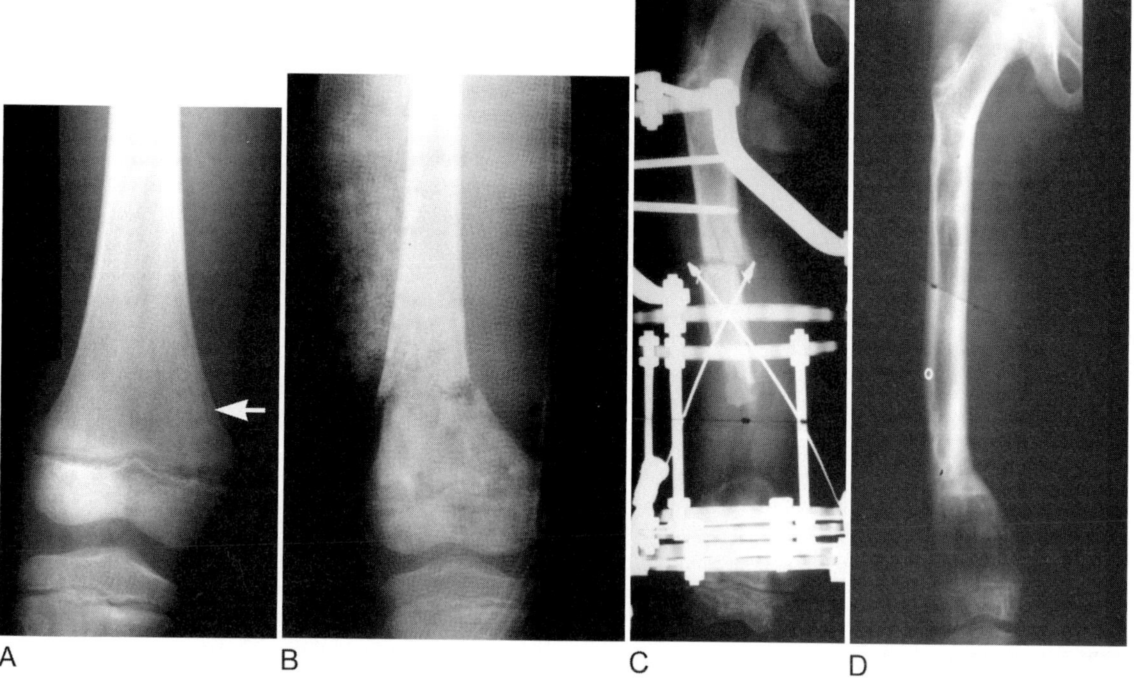

Figure 13–8: A, Chronic osteomyelitis involving the distal metaphysis of the femur. Initial radiographs demonstrate acute osteomyelitis. B, Pathological fracture through the area of chronic osteomyelitis. C, Oblique wire transport of bone to fill the segmental defect. D, Result after maturation of the regenerate and consolidation of the docking site. From Herring JA, ed (2002) Chapter 34: Bone and joint infections. In: Tachdjian's Pediatric Orthopaedics, 3rd edition, Volume 3. Philadelphia: WB Saunders.

- Oral administration of indomethacin after incision and drainage may help to prevent bony bridging following physeal-penetrating lesions.
- If a central physeal arrest occurs, then treatment should be considered based on years of remaining growth, presence of deformity or limb length inequality, and percentage of growth plate involvement.
- Treatment principles for partial physeal arrest include mapping the physeal involvement with plain radiographs, tomography, MRI, or CT; determining limb length discrepancy and the presence of angular deformity; and deciding whether surgical intervention or observation is necessary.
- Surgical goals are to reestablish normal anatomical relationships and proportions and to prevent further deformity.
- Surgical options will include completion of the growth arrest, resection of physeal bar with placement of interposition materials to prevent recurrent bar formation, corrective osteotomy for angular deformity, elongation through chondrodiastasis or distraction osteosynthesis to correct limb length inequality, or a combination of these options.

Concerns

- As physicians have learned in the past several decades, the epidemiology of musculoskeletal infection is constantly changing in light of new diagnostic imaging techniques, new treatment methods, the rise of resistant organisms, cost-saving measures to deliver treatment, and an increase in the number of neonatal patients at risk for acquiring nosocomial infections.[21]
- Vigilance is necessary to identify unusual manifestations of subacute and chronic infections of the musculoskeletal system that might otherwise go unnoticed because they lack the presenting clinical and radiographic features of AHO.
- Continued effort must identify new treatment modalities that reliably eradicate infection as soon as it is identified to prevent sequelae.

References

1. Jackson MA, Burry VF, Olson LC (1992) Pyogenic arthritis associated with adjacent osteomyelitis: Identification of the sequela-prone child. Pediatr Infect Dis J 11: 9-13.

   Of 96 children with septic arthritis, 17% were found to have concurrent osteomyelitis in the adjacent bone. These were thought to be indistinguishable by presenting symptoms. Patients with adjacent osteomyelitis tended to be younger, symptomatic more than 7 days, and likely to have received prior antibiotics.

2. Perlman MH, Patzakis MJ, Kumar PJ, Holtom P (2000) The incidence of joint involvement with adjacent osteomyelitis in pediatric patients. J Pediatr Orthop 20: 40-43.

   This study found that the incidence of simultaneous bone and joint infection was 33%, with the knee as the most common site for dual involvement. There was no difference in incidence between the infant (18 months and younger) and childhood groups, which disputes the general literature on this subject.

3. Roine I, Arguedas A, Faingezicht I, Rodriguez F (1997) Early detection of sequela-prone osteomyelitis in children with use of simple clinical and laboratory criteria. Clin Infect Dis 24: 849-853.

   Accurate predication of sequelae was possible with serial CRP measurement and a daily clinical scoring system. Those children with sequelae had a higher CRP during the first 6 days of treatment and were found to have at least one of the following: temperature above 37.4° C for more than 7 days, local swelling or warmth for more than 10 days, limited motion for more than 10 days, repeated surgical drainage, multiple foci of osteomyelitis, or septic shock.

4. Unkila-Kallio L, Kallio MJT, Peltola H (1994) The usefulness of C-reactive protein levels in the identification of concurrent septic arthritis in children who have acute hematogenous osteomyelitis. J Bone Joint Surg 76A(6): 848-853.

   CRP was found to be the most useful indicator of concurrent osteomyelitis and septic arthritis. In positive cases, the CRP level increased almost twofold within 24 hours and failed to decrease rapidly from that point forward. Changes in the ESR gave the same information but did not become evident until 5 to 14 days after admission.

5. Bowerman SG, Green NE, Mencio GA (1997) Decline of bone and joint infections attributable to Haemophilus influenzae type B. Clin Orthop 341: 128-133.

   In October 1990, licensing was approved for vaccination of infants beginning at 2 months of age with the conjugate vaccine for H. influenzae type B. This has effectively reduced the incidence of bone and joint infection from this organism to nearly zero in children 3 years and younger. Because of this change in epidemiology, K. kingae has significantly risen in incidence in the same patient population.

6. Marshall GS, Mudido P, Rabalais GP, Adams G (1996) Organism isolation and serum bactericidal titers in oral antibiotic therapy for pediatric osteomyelitis. South Med J 89(1): 68-70.

   Sequential parenteral–oral therapy was demonstrated to be effective for pediatric patients with hematogenous osteomyelitis regardless of the monitoring of serum bactericidal titers or identification of a specific organism. Older children, in particular, may be changed to oral therapy without monitoring if they have responded well to the initial course of empirical parenteral antistaphylococcal antibiotic.

7. Jaakkola J, Kehl D (1999) Hematogenous calcaneal osteomyelitis in children. J Pediatr Orthop 19: 699-704.

   Hematogenous calcaneal osteomyelitis usually has less dramatic signs and symptoms than long-bone infections, which may result in diagnostic delay. If the patient is diagnosed within 4 to 5 days of symptom onset, antibiotics alone will cure most cases. Growth disturbance may result from inadequate treatment because the infection most commonly occurs in the metaphyseal-equivalent portion of the calcaneus adjacent to the apophysis.

8. Mustafa MM, Saez-Llorens X, McCracken GH, Nelson JD (1990) Acute hematogenous pelvic osteomyelitis in infants and children. Pediatr Infect Dis J 9: 416-421.
   In a 27-year retrospective review at a large, children's medical center, only 6.3% of 365 bone infections involved the pelvis. Delay in diagnosis was common and, in some cases, resulted in long-term morbidity.

9. Song KS, Ogden JA, Ganey T, Guidera KJ (1997) Contiguous diskitis and osteomyelitis in children. J Pediatr Orthop 17: 470-477.
   MRI proved to be the most useful diagnostic tool in these challenging cases by defining the anatomical location and the extent of vertebral and soft tissue involvement. The authors noted that disk-space height decreased by 43% in affected segments and that there was no restitution of the disk space at long-term follow-up.

10. Vohra R, Kang H, Dogra S, Saggar R, Sharma R (1997) Tuberculous osteomyelitis. J Bone Joint Surg 79B(4): 562-566.
   This study documents the spectrum of findings in tuberculous osteomyelitis in an endemic population. Delay in diagnosis ranged up to 39 months, often initially treated with nonsteroidal anti-inflammatory medication that failed to provide relief. Advanced skeletal lesions were difficult to distinguish from chronic pyogenic osteomyelitis, Brodie's abscess, neoplasms or granulomatous lesions. Biopsy is considered mandatory to confirm the diagnosis.

11. Kothari NA, Pelchovitz DJ, Meyer JS (2001) Imaging of musculoskeletal infections. Radiol Clin North Am 39(4): 653-671.
   This is a thorough review of the modern methods of musculoskeletal imaging often used in the evaluation of infection. The sensitivity and specificity of each imaging modality are reviewed. Recommendations are given regarding useful studies for conditions that often lead to diagnostic uncertainty.

12. Mah ET, LeQuesne GW, Gent RJ, Paterson DC (1994) Ultrasonic features of acute osteomyelitis in children. J Bone Joint Surg 76B(6): 969-974.
   Ultrasound was used to categorize four time-related groups of osteomyelitis based on the interval between the onset of symptoms and the ultrasound examination. Deep soft tissue swelling is followed by periosteal fluid elevation with a thin layer of fluid. Subperiosteal abscess is the third stage, which eventually produces cortical erosion and breach. The final stage of cortical involvement is commonly found in children who have had symptoms for more than 1 week.

13. Chambers JB, Forsythe DA, Bertrand SL, Iwinski HJ, Steflik DE (2000) Retrospective review of osteoarticular infections in a pediatric sickle cell age group. J Pediatr Orthop 20: 682-685.
   A 22-year retrospective review in a single institution of osteoarticular infections in children with sickle cell disease found that the rare infections may be differentiated from the frequent crises by carefully considering clinical, laboratory, and radiographic data. Positive studies combined with high fever, chills, and "toxicity" increase the suspicion for infection. Sickle cell patients are much more prone to Salmonella osteomyelitis than unaffected children.

14. Mazur JM, Ross G, Cummings RJ, Hahn GA, McCluskey WP (1995) Usefulness of magnetic resonance imaging for the diagnosis of acute musculoskeletal infections in children. J Pediatr Orthop 15: 144-147.
   MRI was found to have a sensitivity of 0.97 and a specificity of 0.92 with significantly fewer false-positive and false-negative studies than bone scanning. MRI was found to be particularly useful in identifying musculoskeletal infection in difficult cases and in cases with spinal or pelvic involvement.

15. Hamdy RC, Lawton L, Carey T, Wiley J, Marton D (1996) Subacute hematogenous osteomyelitis: are biopsy and surgery always indicated? J Pediatr Orthop 16: 220-223.
   Careful assessment of the radiographic features of lesions suspected of subacute osteomyelitis may help to differentiate benign-appearing lesions from those with more aggressive features. Open biopsy and surgical debridement should be reserved for cases that do not respond to antibiotics or that lack a benign radiographic appearance.

16. Jackson MA, Burry VF, Olson LC (1991) Multisystem group A b-hemolytic streptococcal disease in children. Rev Infect Dis 13: 783-788.
   A toxic shock syndrome is associated with streptococcal infection characterized by severe local tissue destruction and life-threatening systemic manifestations. Musculoskeletal involvement was noted in seven of eight children in this review. Surgical debridement of the foci of infection was necessary in most cases.

17. Moon RY, Greene MG, Rehe GT, Katona IM (1995) Poststreptococcal reactive arthritis in children: A potential predecessor of rheumatic heart disease. J Rheumatol 22(3): 529-532.
   This large retrospective study from a tertiary pediatric rheumatology clinic evaluated the epidemiology and treatment of PSRA. PSRA should be considered in any pediatric patient with the acute onset of arthritis. Throat culture and serological testing for streptococcal infection should be performed. If confirmed, cardiac evaluation is warranted.

18. Willis AA, Widmann RF, Flynn JM, Green DW, Onel KB (2003) Lyme arthritis presenting as acute septic arthritis in children. J Pediatr Orthop 23: 114-118.
   Because of the considerable overlap of clinical and laboratory findings in cases of Lyme arthritis and septic arthritis, the authors suggest that children who have possible septic arthritis in endemic regions should also be evaluated for Lyme disease according to CDC guidelines. A rapid Lyme enzyme immunoassay with results available within 1 hour helped to differentiate Lyme arthritis from septic arthritis and prevented unnecessary surgery.

19. Maraqa NF, Gomez MM, Rathore MH (2002) Outpatient parenteral antimicrobial therapy in osteoarticular infections in children. J Pediatr Orthop 22: 506-510.
Osteoarticular infections in children can be safely managed on an outpatient basis with CVLs and PICCs. Catheter-related complications occurred in 30% of cases. The PICC mechanical complication rate was higher than that related to CVL (10.6 versus 4.2 per 1,000 catheter days).

20. Kim HKW, Alman B, Cole WG (2000) A shortened course of parenteral antibiotic therapy in the management of acute septic arthritis of the hip. J Pediatr Orthop 20: 44-47.
The authors found that it was possible to switch from parenteral to oral antibiotics within 7 to 10 days of the onset of treatment as long as the child demonstrated a good response before making the change. Those children who failed to respond favorably to parenteral antibiotics were treated with repeated arthrotomy and longer parenteral and oral antibiotic therapies.

21. Dormans JP, Drummond DS (1994) Pediatric hematogenous osteomyelitis: New trends in presentation, diagnosis, and treatment. J Am Acad Orthop Surgeons 2(6): 333-341.
This review demonstrates the changing epidemiology of AHO in the past several decades. Current treatment methods have resulted in more frequent subacute osteomyelitis, and the rise of neonatal intensive care treatment has led to a higher incidence of neonatal osteomyelitis.

CHAPTER 14

Skeletal Dysplasias

Bülent Erol*, Leslie A. Moroz[†], and John P. Dormans[‡]

*MD, Attending Surgeon, Department of Orthopaedic Surgery, The Hospital of University of Marmara, Marmara University School of Medicine, Istanbul, Turkey
[†]BA, Clinical Research Coordinator, Division of Orthopaedic Surgery, The Children's Hospital of Philadelphia, Philadelphia, PA
[‡]MD, Chief of Orthopaedic Surgery, The Children's Hospital of Philadelphia, Philadelphia, PA; Professor of Orthopaedic Surgery, University of Pennsylvania School of Medicine, Philadelphia, PA

- The skeletal dysplasias, also known as *osteochondrodysplasias*, are a heterogeneous group of conditions characterized by generalized disorders of growth and development of bone and cartilage.
- There are more than 200 described bone dysplasias; most of are extremely rare.
- Generalized disturbances in the development of the skeleton affect the skull, spine, and extremities in varying degrees.
  - There are often abnormalities in the facial structures.
  - The resulting alterations in the size and shape of the limbs and trunk frequently are associated with disproportionate short stature (dwarfism).
  - Disproportionate short stature is characteristic of the skeletal dysplasias, which differentiates these conditions from endocrine (i.e., absent growth hormone) and metabolic (i.e., rickets) disorders that cause proportionate short stature.
- Dwarfing conditions frequently are referred to as short-limb or short-trunk dysplasias according to whether limbs or trunk are more extensively involved (Box 14–1).
  - In short-limb dysplasias, the extremities are disproportionately short compared with the trunk.
  - In contrast, short-trunk dysplasias produce greater shortening of the spine relative to the limbs.
  - Disproportionate involvement of the trunk is known as *microcormia*.
  - Disproportionate involvement of the limbs is known as *micromelia*. Micromelia divides into subtypes: *rhizomelic* (proximal), *mesomelic* (middle), and *acromelic* (distal) are used to describe the segment of the limb with the greatest involvement. These terms refer to the arm, forearm, and hand or to the thigh, leg, and foot, respectively.
- Some skeletal dysplasias are genetically transmitted; others are not inherited.
  - Recent research has focused on molecular genetics: the chromosomes on which the dysplasias are transmitted, the genes that have mutations, the specific products (e.g., proteins) encoded by these genes, and the roles of these gene products in skeletal development are all being investigated.
  - Although specific gene therapy is not yet possible, much new information is rapidly becoming available, advancing our understanding of the mechanism of bone dysplasias.
- The diversity of the skeletal dysplasias and the heterogeneity that may exist within a specific disorder has made classification difficult. They have been classified according to the pattern of bone involvement, as in the International Classification of Osteochondrodysplasias (Box 14–2).[1] The newer trend, however, is to group them according to the specific causative protein, enzyme, or gene defect when such information is known (Box 14–3).
- Management of the skeletal dysplasias includes accurate genetic counseling and the recognition and treatment of musculoskeletal abnormalities and associated intrinsic medical problems. Detailed chromosomal studies are available for some of the skeletal dysplasias. With the

Box 14–1 Dwarfing (Disproportionate Short Stature) Conditions in Skeletal Dysplasias

- Micromelia—Short-limb dwarfism
  - Rhizomelia—Proximal segment (arm or thigh)
  - Mesomelia—Middle segment (forearm or leg)
  - Acromelia—Distal segment (hand or foot)
- Microcormia—Short-trunk dwarfism

increasing availability of prenatal screening, more patients with skeletal dysplasia are being diagnosed before birth.

Achondroplasia

- Achondroplasia is the most frequent form of short-limb dwarfism, with an estimated prevalence of approximately 1 in 30,000 to 50,000.[2]
- Affected individuals exhibit short stature caused by rhizomelic shortening of the limbs, characteristic facies with frontal bossing and midface hypoplasia, limitation of elbow extension, genu varum, and trident hand.
- Achondroplasia is an autosomal dominant condition, although two thirds of cases arise by spontaneous new mutations. The mutation of achondroplasia is an activating missense mutation in the gene encoding fibroblast growth factor receptor-3 (FGFR-3). The mutation has been mapped to chromosome 4.[3] Normally, the FGFR-3 gene is expressed in articular chondrocytes, and the gene product restrains cell division in the proliferative cells of the growth plate. The activating mutations in the FGFR-3 gene lead to further retardation of cell division in the proliferative zone of the growth plates, resulting in phenotypical features of achondroplasia. The primary defect is abnormal endochondral bone formation. Periosteal and intramembranous ossification processes are normal.
- The risk of having a child with achondroplasia increases with paternal age.

Clinical Features

- Achondroplasia is recognizable at birth as a disproportionate short-limbed rhizomelic dysplasia. The proximal segments of the limbs—the humeri and femora—are the most foreshortened. Trunk height tends to be normal, but arm span and standing height are diminished (Figure 14–1).
- The predicted adult height is 132 cm for men and 122 cm for women.
- Developmental motor milestones are frequently delayed, although normal motor coordination is achieved in later childhood, with independent ambulation typically occurring from 18 to 24 months.[4,5]

Box 14–2 1992 International Classification of Skeletal Dysplasias*

Defects of the Tubular Bones, Flat Bones, and Axial Skeleton

Achondroplasias
- Achondroplasia
- Hypochondroplasia
- Thanatophoric dysplasia

Metatropic dysplasias
Atelosteogenesis–diastrophic dysplasias
Osteogenesis imperfecta
Kniest-Stickler dysplasias
SED congenitas
Other SED–metaphyseal dysplasias
- X-linked SED tarda
- Pseudoachondroplasia

Dysostosis multiplexes
- MPSs
- Mucolipidoses

Epiphyseal dysplasias
- MED

Chondrodysplasia punctata
Metaphyseal dysplasias
Mesomelic dysplasias
- Dyschondrosteosis

Dysplasias with significant (but not exclusive) membranous bone involvement
- Cleidocranial dysplasia

Multiple dislocations with dysplasias
- Larsen syndrome

Dysplasias with decreased bone density
- Osteogenesis imperfecta (several types)
- Idiopathic juvenile osteoporosis

Dysplasias with defective mineralization
- Hypophosphatasia
- Hypophosphatemic rickets

Dysplasias with increased bone density

Disorganized Development of Cartilaginous and Fibrous Components of the Skeleton

Dysplasia epiphysealis hemimelica
Multiple hereditary exostoses
Enchondromatosis
Fibrous dysplasia

Idiopathic Osteolyses

*A partial list.

- Patients with achondroplasia have a typical facial appearance characterized by frontal bossing and midface hypoplasia (Figure 14–1).[6]
- The digits of the hand have extra space between the third and fourth rays so that the digits, including the thumb, are separated into three groups—the *trident hand.*
- There is usually a flexion contracture of the elbow, and the radial heads may be subluxated (Figure 14–1).

Box 14–3 Classification of Skeletal Dysplasias Based on Etiology

FGFR-3 group (local regulator of cartilage growth)
- Achondroplasia
- Hypochondroplasia
- Thanatophoric dysplasia

Sulfate transporter protein group (sulfate transportation)
- Diastrophic dysplasia

COL2A1 group (type II collagen and structural cartilage protein)
- Kniest dysplasia
- SED congenita

COMP group (structural cartilage protein)
- Pseudoachondroplasia
- MED

Storage disorders
- MPSs
- Mucolipidoses

COL1A1 group (structural osseous protein)
- Osteogenesis imperfecta

- Kyphosis at the thoracolumbar junction may be seen in infancy, but this deformity usually improves spontaneously by independent ambulation.
- Ligamentous laxity is present in most patients, leading to external rotation of the lower limbs and genu recurvatum in infancy. The knees are most commonly in varus alignment but may be in excessive valgus.

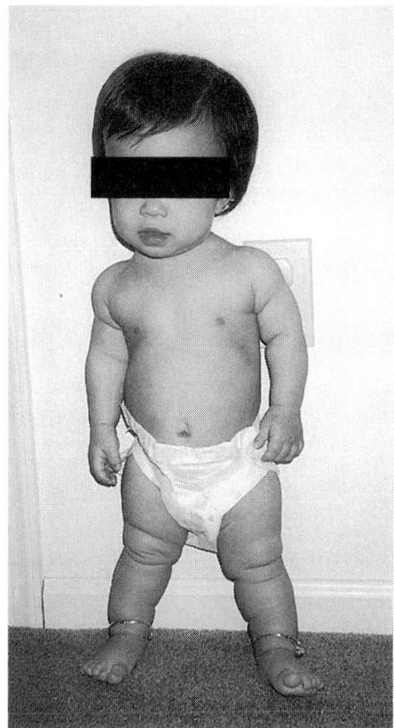

Figure 14–1: An 18-month-old girl with achondroplasia. The trunk length is normal, and the proximal segments of the limbs are short (rhizomelic pattern). The elbows have a mild flexion contracture. Note typical facial features: frontal bossing, flattening of the nasal bridge, and midface hypoplasia.

- Intelligence is normal unless hydrocephalus or other central nervous system complications arise.

Radiographic Findings

- The facial bones, skull base, and foramen magnum are underdeveloped, whereas the cranial bones are normal in size and shape.[5]
- Foramen magnum stenosis is common because of disproportionate growth of the chondrocranium and neurocranium and is measured most accurately by computerized tomography (CT) or magnetic resonance imaging (MRI) (Figure 14–2).
- The spine displays central and foraminal stenosis, which is most common in the lumbar spine. The spinal canal, as measured by the interpedicular distance, normally widens proceeding distally in the lumbar spine from L1 to L5. However, in patients with achondroplasia, the spinal canal narrows and the interpedicular distance decreases.
- The vertebral bodies have a scalloped appearance in patients with achondroplasia. Before walking age, a kyphosis at the thoracolumbar junction may be seen (Table 14–1). Significant scoliosis is rare.
- In achondroplasia the pelvis characteristically appears broad and flat with squared iliac wings. The sciatic notches are small. The acetabular roof is horizontal, and the femoral heads are well covered.
- The proximal femoral metaphyses are widened and the femoral necks are short as a result of the abnormalities in longitudinal growth.
- The long bones are short and thick with metaphyseal flaring.

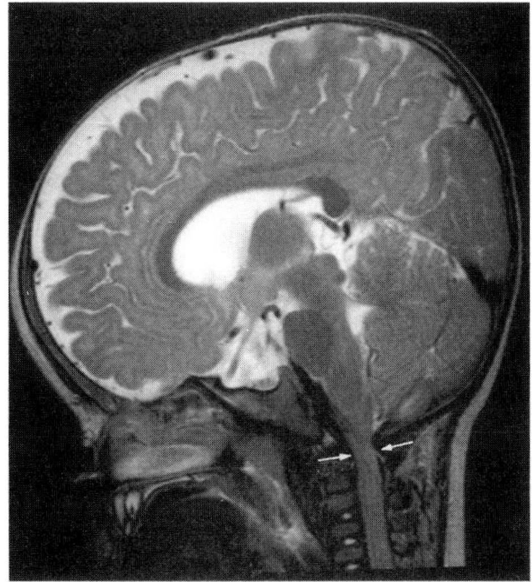

Figure 14–2: MRI of a 6-month-old infant with achondroplasia shows the characteristic narrow foramen magnum *(arrows)*. From Erol B, Dormans JP, States L, Kaplan FS (2004) Skeletal dysplasias and metabolic disorders of bone: Musculoskeletal tumors in children. In: Pediatric Orthopaedics and Sports Medicine (Dormans JP, ed). Philadelphia: Mosby.

Table 14–1: Spinal Abnormalities Seen in Various Skeletal Dysplasias

	CERVICAL SPINE	THORACOLUMBAR SPINE
Achondroplasia	Foramen magnum stenosis	Stenosis and kyphosis at the thoracolumbar junction
Metatropic dysplasia	Atlantoaxial instability	Kyphosis and scoliosis
Diastrophic dysplasia	Cervical kyphosis	Kyphosis and scoliosis
Kniest dysplasia	Atlantoaxial instability	Kyphosis and scoliosis
Spondyloepiphyseal dysplasia (congenita and tarda)	Atlantoaxial instability	Kyphosis and scoliosis
Pseudoachondroplasia	Atlantoaxial instability	Kyphosis and scoliosis
Mucopolysaccharidoses	Cervical instability	Kyphosis and scoliosis
Chondrodysplasia punctate	Atlantoaxial instability	Kyphosis and scoliosis
Metaphyseal chondrodysplasia (McKusick type)	Atlantoaxial instability	
Cleidocranial dysplasia		Scoliosis (with syringomyelia in some)
Larsen syndrome	Cervical kyphosis and midcervical instability	Scoliosis

- Angulation at both the distal femoral and the proximal tibial metaphyses contributes to abnormal knee alignment (Figure 14–3).

Medical Problems

- People with achondroplasia have a continuous challenge in identifying and maintaining ideal body weight. Obesity is more common than in the general population. It typically begins in early childhood and is a lifelong problem.[4]

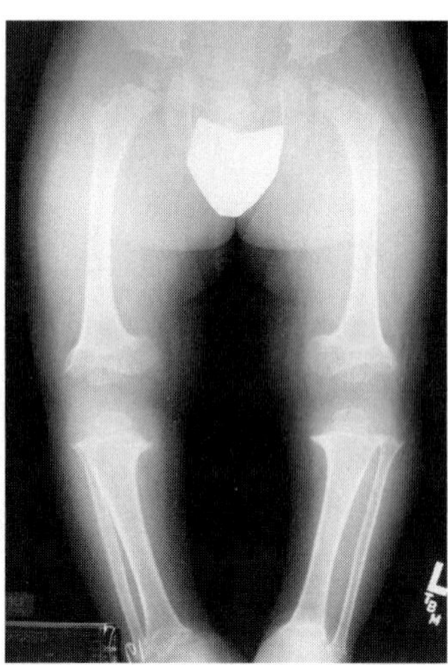

Figure 14–3: The lower extremities in a young walking child with achondroplasia show abnormal metaphyseal flaring and broadening throughout all the long bones. **Medial tibial spurs are related to mild genu varum. Also note the deep acetabula.**

- In achondroplasia patients several ear, nose, and throat problems occur as a result of underdevelopment of the midfacial skeleton. Recurrent ear infections may lead to hearing loss. Obstructive sleep apnea is found in three fourths of these children when studied in the sleep laboratory.
- The chest wall diameter is narrowed; as a consequence, pulmonary function, particularly vital capacity, is reduced.
- Narrowing of the foramen magnum is a typical problem in first several years of life and may result in a variety of neurological signs, including developmental delay, hypotonia, sleep apnea, and feeding difficulties. Decompression of the brain stem often provides improvement of neurological symptoms.[5]
- Enlargement of head circumference (megacephaly) is common but does not necessarily indicate hydrocephalus that needs to be shunted.
- Although patients with achondroplasia are among the most stable and healthy of those with skeletal dysplasias, mortality rates are nevertheless elevated in all age groups. An increased incidence of sudden death is seen among young infants. Central nervous system events or respiratory problems occur more frequently in older children and young adults, and cardiovascular problems in older adults with achondroplasia.

Orthopaedic Considerations

- Lumbar spinal stenosis is the most common and disabling problem in the adult with achondroplasia (Table 14–1).
  - Onset of symptoms is typical in the third decade, but earlier presentation may be seen.
  - Patients with spinal stenosis complain of *neurogenic claudication*, or pain in the lower back or legs exacerbated by activity. As the stenosis continues, walking endurance decreases and neurological signs such as clonus, hyperreflexia, lower extremity weakness, and myelopathy may develop. Paresthesias are quite common.
  - MRI is useful in identifying the extent of the stenosis. CT myelography documents the stenosis well.[4]
  - Spinal decompression is indicated as soon as the diagnosis has been confirmed. A wide decompression must be performed with foraminotomies of the lateral recesses. This decompression should extend from several levels above the myelographic block down to the second sacral vertebra.
  - Because instability rarely develops, even after wide decompression, primary fusion is generally not indicated. When fusion is performed, instrumentation within the canal is contraindicated because of the risk of paraplegia.
- Kyphosis at the thoracolumbar junction is seen in almost all young babies with achondroplasia, presumably because of low muscle tone, ligamentous laxity, and a large cranium.

- As the child learns to walk, muscle tone and trunk control improve and the kyphosis usually resolves without treatment. However, between 10 and 15% of patients retain kyphosis, which can increase the risk of symptomatic stenosis through pressure on the conus (Figure 14–4).
- Prevention of unsupported sitting has been recommended in achondroplastic infants, and kyphosis is present. Bracing (thoracolumbosacral orthosis) is indicated if the deformity is accompanied by significant and progressive structural changes in the anterior vertebral bodies (e.g., anterior beaking and wedging).
- For children who fail bracing, posterior spinal fusion without instrumentation (fusion in situ) is performed. Halo body cast is applied following fusion in situ.

- Genu varum affects at least 50% of people who have achondroplasia. This deformity is usually progressive and requires treatment.
  - There is no evidence that bracing children with achondroplasia is effective.
  - The treatment of genu varum usually involves surgical correction by proximal tibiofibular realignment osteotomy. Stabilization of osteotomy has been achieved with crossed pins, internal fixation, and external fixation.
  - Despite angular deformity, degenerative arthritic changes in the knees are rare.
- Significant controversy still exists regarding the lengthening of short extremities in patients with achondroplasia to achieve a taller stature. In contrast to most other skeletal dysplasias, conditions are favorable for extensive lengthening in that the joints are normal and the musculotendinous units and nerves have excellent tolerance for stretch.[5] Gradual distraction of the bone using special external fixators has substantially elongated overall height between femur and tibia—up to 30 cm. Care must be taken to minimize the complications of angular deformity and joint stiffness.
- Growth hormone is used to augment the height of patients with achondroplasia. Early results indicate that some children with achondroplasia experience increased longitudinal growth while receiving growth hormone. The greatest acceleration in growth velocity has been seen during the first year of treatment. Administration of growth hormone continues on an investigational basis, and final judgment of its efficacy should be reserved until the patients involved in these studies reach their final adult height.

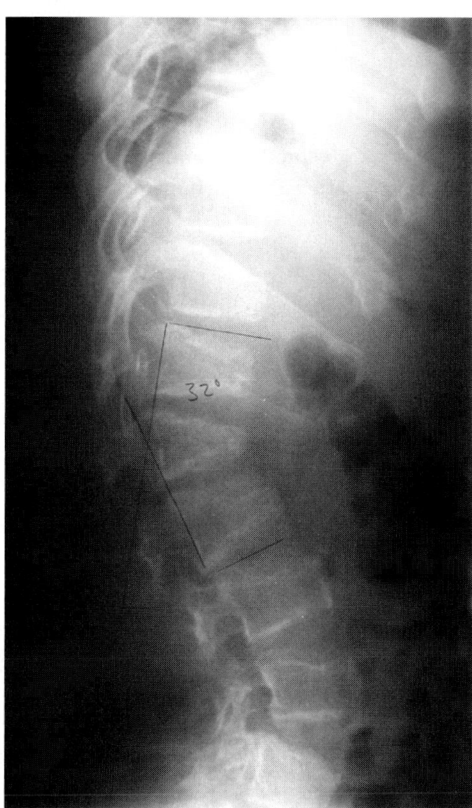

Figure 14–4: A 4-year-old boy with achondroplasia. The lateral radiograph of the spine shows a kyphosis with a sharp apex centered at a wedge-shaped first lumbar vertebra. Diffuse irregularity of the vertebral body endplates and rib ends is seen. The spinal deformity of this patient required bracing.

Hypochondroplasia

- Hypochondroplasia is a rare form of short-limb dwarfism that resembles achondroplasia but is less severe. The estimated incidence of hypochondroplasia is 3 to 4 per 1 million live births.
- Hypochondroplasia also is transmitted as an autosomal dominant trait, and its gene defect encodes for FGFR-3. However, the mutation occurs in a different region of the gene from that occurring in achondroplasia (the tyrosine kinase domain in hypochondroplasia in contrast to the transmembrane domain in achondroplasia).[3]
- There does not appear to be an increased paternal age in fathers of children with hypochondroplasia.

Clinical Features

- Hypochondroplasia is one of the most subtle of the skeletal dysplasias. Clinically, patients with hypochondroplasia are short but less so than those with achondroplasia.
- The spectrum of severity is wide, ranging from severe short-limbed (mesomelic) dwarfism to short, apparently normal prepubertal children who manifest disproportion only after failure to achieve a pubertal growth spurt.[5]
- The eventual height ranges from 118 to 160 cm.
- Except for mild frontal bossing, the facial appearance is normal.
- Spinal deformities are rarely seen, although mild ligamentous laxity persists.

- Mild spinal stenosis has been reported in one third of patients.
- Varus angulation of the knees is mild and may resolve with growth. Significant genu varum occurs in less than 10% of these patients.

Radiographic Findings

- Radiographic findings, as with clinical findings, are generally subtle in hypochondroplasia.
- Primary and secondary criteria have been proposed.
  - The primary criteria are narrowing of the lumbar interpedicular distances; short, square iliac crests; short, broad femoral necks; mild metaphyseal flaring; and shortening of the long tubular bones (Figure 14–5).
  - Secondary criteria are shortening of the lumbar pedicles, concavity of the posterior vertebral bodies, elongation of the distal fibula, and shortening of the distal ulna.[7]

Differential Diagnosis

- Hypochondroplasia has more phenotypical variation than achondroplasia in its severity.
  - In its severe from, it may resemble achondroplasia.
  - Conversely, its mild form may be mistaken for constitutionally short stature.
  - In its classical presentation with mild short stature and mild genu varum deformity, it may resemble Schmid metaphyseal chondrodysplasia.

Orthopaedic Considerations

- The skeletal abnormalities seen in hypochondroplasia usually are mild and rarely require surgical intervention.
- Mild interpedicular narrowing can predispose some patients to symptomatic spinal stenosis, but it is usually mild and does not require surgical treatment.
- Occasionally, significant genu varum requiring realignment osteotomy may develop.
- Limb lengthening is usually as successful as it is in achondroplasia and can result in enough gain in length to place the child in the low–normal range.
- Growth hormone therapy remains investigational.

Metatropic Dysplasia

- Metatropic dysplasia is a rare skeletal dysplasia characterized by a change in body proportions with growth.
- It is a rare condition, which may be transmitted in an autosomal dominant or recessive manner.
- The cause of metatropic dysplasia has not been elucidated, but it is thought to result from a defect in endochondral ossification. Some histological abnormalities of the growth plate, causing developmental arrest, have been studied and appear to be characteristic. In a study published by Boden et al., the major histological findings were the absence of formation of normal primary spongiosa in the metaphysis, the presence of a thin seal of bone at the chondro-osseous junction with abnormal metaphyseal vascular invasion and arrest of endochondral growth, and normal-appearing perichondral ring structures with persistence of circumferential growth.[8] These findings suggested an uncoupling of endochondral and perichondral growth and offered an explanation for the dumbbell-shaped morphological structure of the osseous metaphysis seen in patients with metatropic dysplasia.

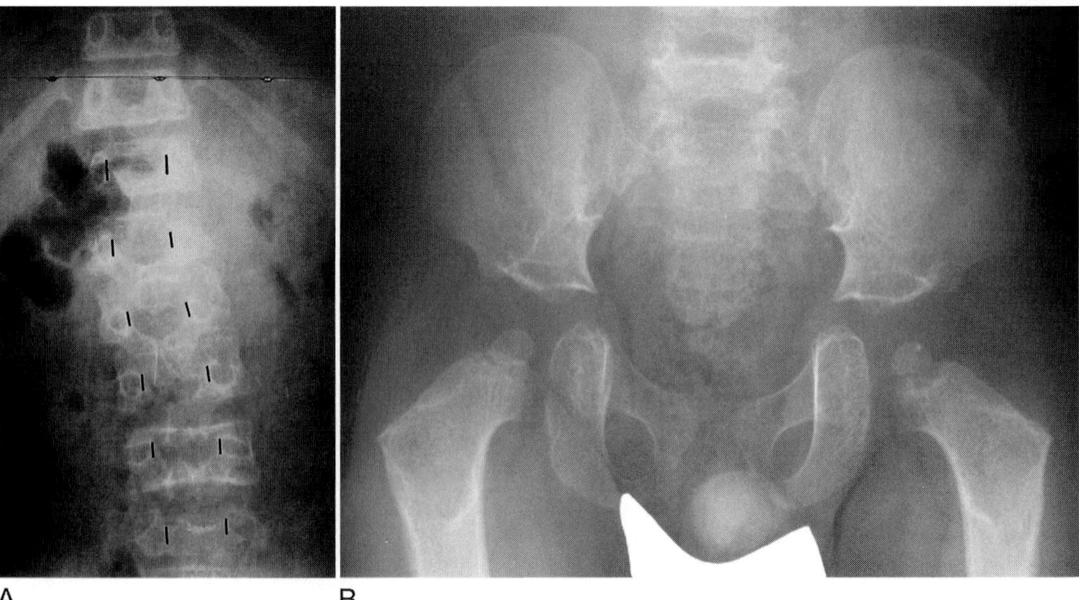

Figure 14–5: A 7-year-old boy with hypochondroplasia. A, A primary criterion for hypochondroplasia is a decrease in the interpedicular distance in the lower lumbar spine. B, The pelvis in this patient shows square iliac wings; short, broad femoral necks; and deep acetabula.

Clinical Features

- During infancy, short limbs and a relatively long trunk are characteristic. With growth, a severe kyphoscoliosis typically develops, apparently shortening the trunk and reversing body proportions.[4]
- Many patients with metatropic dysplasia have a small, tail-like appendage overlying the lower sacrum. It is usually a few centimeters long and arises from the gluteal fold.
- The head and face are usually normal.
- Upper cervical spine instability develops in some patients.
- The limbs are significantly short, with bulbous enlargement of the metaphyses of the long bones and severe joint contractures (i.e., flexion contractures up to 40 degrees).
- These patients usually have difficulty in achieving an upright posture because of joint contractures. More importantly, their ambulation may then deteriorate because of progression of these contractures.
- Adult height varies from 110 to 120 cm.

Radiographic Findings

- Prenatal ultrasonographic diagnosis may be possible in the first or second trimester with finding of significant dwarfism, narrow thorax, and enlarged metaphyses.[5]
- Odontoid hypoplasia with upper cervical spine instability (atlantoaxial instability) frequently exists in patients with metatropic dysplasia (Table 14–1).
- Spinal involvement is characterized with severe platyspondyly (flatness of the vertebral bodies) and delayed ossification of the vertebral bodies. Progressive deformities of the thoracolumbar spine, kyphosis and scoliosis, are almost always seen in infancy (Figure 14–6, *A*).
- The ribs are short and flared with cupping at the costochondral junction.
- Flaring of the metaphyseal regions of the long bones gives them a dumbbell-shaped appearance (Figure 14–6, *B*).
- Joint incongruity may be seen as a result of delayed and irregular epiphyseal ossification. Degenerative changes of major joints often occur in adulthood.

Medical Problems

- Patients with metatropic dysplasia frequently have severe restrictive pulmonary disease that is life threatening. These children have a small, stiff thorax, which may be further compromised by the development of spinal deformities. Death can occur in infancy from pulmonary insufficiency.
- A high incidence of upper cervical spine (C1-C2) abnormalities occurs in metatropic dysplasia, which may lead to myelopathic changes.

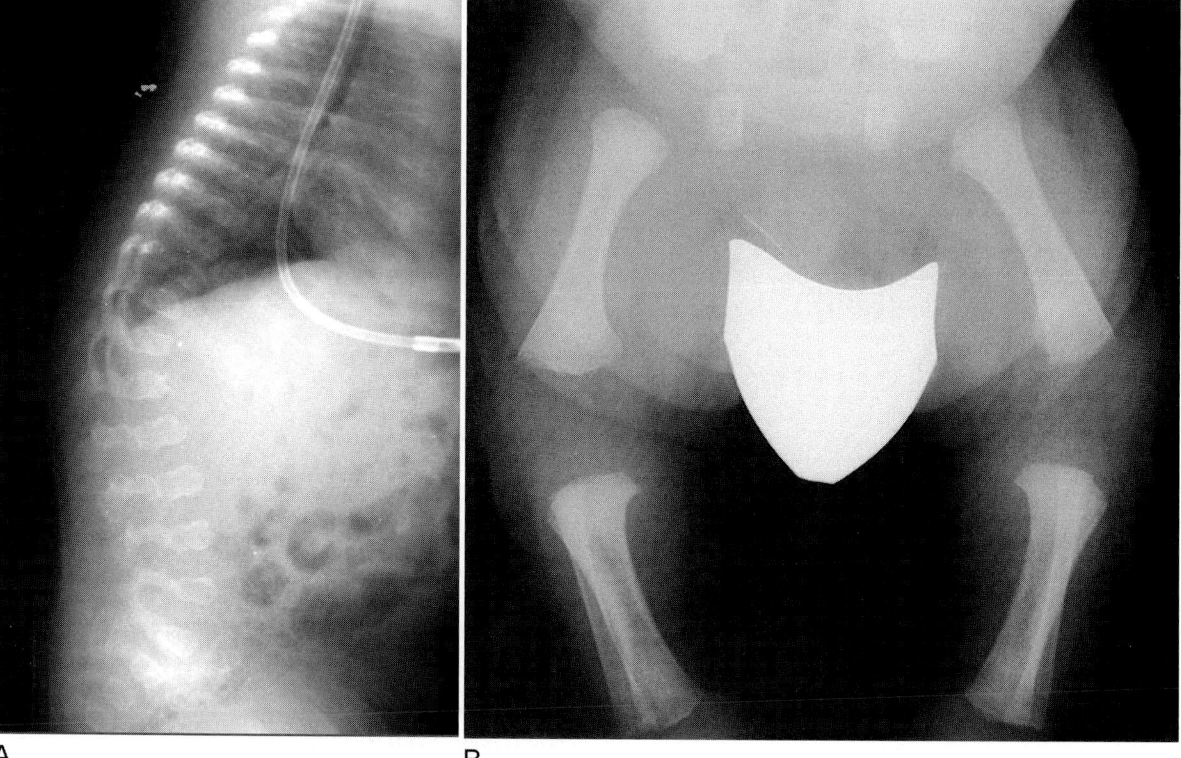

Figure 14–6: A 5-month-old patient with metatropic dysplasia. A, A thoracolumbar kyphosis is centered at a hypoplastic first lumbar vertebra. The lower thoracic vertebrae and lumbar vertebrae are abnormally shaped. B, All the long bones are short and broad with flaring of the metaphyses, creating the characteristic dumbbell-shaped appearance in this patient. Note the deep acetabula.

- Ventriculomegaly or hydrocephalus has been reported in up to 25% of patients.[4]

Orthopaedic Considerations

- Stability of the upper cervical spine should be evaluated periodically (in a growing child at 1 year intervals) with lateral flexion–extension radiographs.
  - An atlantodens interval (ADI) greater than 4 to 5 mm indicates instability, although many of these patients are asymptomatic.
  - For asymptomatic patients with radiographic evidence of instability, a flexion–extension MRI should be obtained to evaluate cord compression.
  - ADI greater than 5 mm may require posterior spinal fusion (occipitocervical fusion) with or without decompression if there are neurological signs and symptoms or evidence of cord compression demonstrated by MRI.[4,5] Halo vest immobilization is used for 8 to 12 weeks postoperatively.
- Kyphoscoliosis may progress rapidly during the first few years of life, typically with rigid deformities. Because of the rigidity of the spine, any pelvic obliquity caused by asymmetrical lower extremity deformities will exacerbate the labored posture and gait.
  - There is no documentation of the efficacy of brace treatment for this condition. It may be tried in small curves (<45 degrees) in young patients or those who need support to sit, but for large curves, orthotic treatment is not recommended.
  - Spinal fusion is advisable for more severe, progressive curves. Anterior as well as posterior fusion is usually recommended because of the high rate of pseudarthrosis in this condition. Presence of spinal stenosis, diminutive spinal elements, and osteoporosis makes instrumentation difficult, so fusion in situ usually is preferred. Halo body cast may be applied following spinal fusion.
- The hip and knee flexion contractures frequently require surgical intervention, including soft tissue releases and rarely osteotomies.
- Premature osteoarthritis of the hips and knees is a common problem. Total joint arthroplasty is successful for severely symptomatic adult patients.

Chondroectodermal Dysplasia

- Chondroectodermal dysplasia, also known as *Ellis-van Creveld syndrome*, is an extremely rare form of skeletal dysplasias with a prevalence of 0.1 per 1 million.
- As its name implies, this syndrome affects both mesodermal and ectodermal tissues and is characterized by short-limb disproportionate dwarfism; postaxial polydactyly; abnormalities of the nails, hair, and teeth; and congenital heart failure.[6]
- Chondroectodermal dysplasia is transmitted as an autosomal recessive condition and is more common in closely knit populations, most notably in the Pennsylvania Amish community.
- A novel gene, the Ellis-van Creveld syndrome gene (EVC), on the short arm of chromosome 4 was identified in individuals with chondroectodermal dysplasia.[3] In bone, EVC was expressed in the developing vertebral bodies, ribs, and both upper and lower limbs. The EVC gene encodes a 992-aminoacid protein that has no homology to known proteins other than in a short region that may be a leucine zipper.

Clinical Features

- The patients with chondroectodermal dysplasia are characterized by acromelic shortness of the limbs with a normal spine. The shortening is most prominent in the most distal aspects of the limbs (e.g., the phalanges).
- The short stature is primarily because of the shortness of the lower legs; the tibia and fibula are also short. This distal shortening is the opposite of that seen in achondroplasia.
- Postaxial (small finger-sided) polydactyly of the hands is typical and occasionally involves the feet.
- Syndactyly (webbed digits) and dysplastic nails of the fingers and toes may also occur.
- The ligaments are lax, and there is often significant genu valgum. Rotational abnormalities often accompany this, such as external rotation of the femur and internal rotation of the tibia.

Radiographic Findings

- Patients with chondroectodermal dysplasia have a long, narrow chest with short ribs.
- The bones of the forearm are disproportionately short with hypoplasia of the proximal radius and distal ulna. The fingers are very short (Figure 14–7, *A*).
- Ossification centers of the distal phalanges may be absent.
- The wrists display fusions of the carpal bones, most commonly the capitate and hamate. Tarsal coalitions may also be present.[4,5]
- The spine is normal.
- The pelvis has a distinctive appearance with small iliac crests and sciatic notches.
- The hip joints are congruous, but femoral necks are generally in valgus position (Figure 14–7, *B*).
- Bilateral valgus deformity of the knees usually is relatively symmetrical. It is partially because of uneven growth of the proximal tibial epiphysis in which the lateral side is underdeveloped.

Medical Problems

- One third of infants with chondroectodermal dysplasia are stillborn or die of cardiorespiratory complications in the neonatal period.

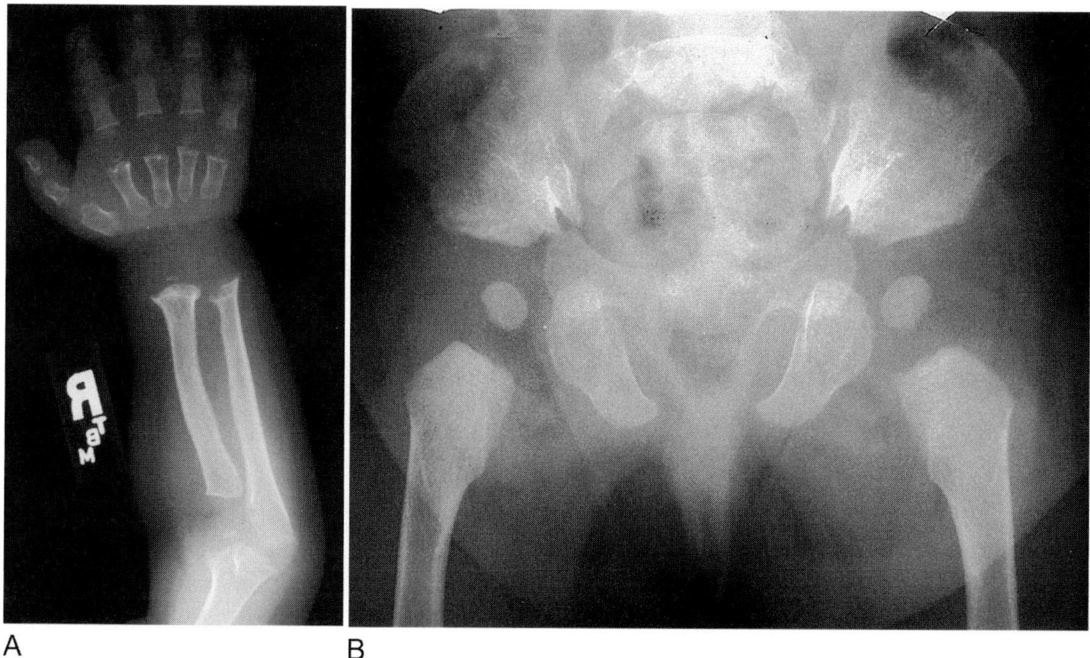

Figure 14–7: A 9-month-old patient with chondroectodermal dysplasia. A, The bones of the forearm are disproportionately short with hypoplasia of the proximal radius and distal ulna. Note the shortening of the small bones of the hand. B, The pelvis has small iliac bones and narrow sciatic notches. This child also has bilateral coxa valga (increased femoral neck angle).

- Congenital cardiac defects are present in about one half of patients and most commonly consist of atrial septal defects or single atrium.
- The children with chondroectodermal dysplasia frequently display abnormalities of the nails, hair, and teeth. The nails are small, hypoplastic, and dystrophic. The teeth are conical with wide spaces and are lost early.
- Genitourinary system abnormalities include hypospadias, epispadias, and undescended testes.
- Mental retardation has been reported in some patients.[6]

Orthopaedic Considerations

- The cardiac status of the patients should be evaluated carefully before any surgical intervention.
- Excision of polydactyly of the hands and feet and release of syndactylies are usually required.
- Genu valgum deformity should be addressed when it becomes clinically significant or rapidly progressing, usually about 20 degrees.
  - Bracing seems to have little or no effect, and surgery remains the mainstay of treatment.[4,5]
  - Surgical intervention usually consists of proximal tibial realignment osteotomy. Usually external fixation is the most expeditious way of handling the correction. If the deformity is one of simple valgus, simple medial hemiepiphyseal stapling may be adequate.
  - In severe cases of genu valgum, medial femoral condylar overgrowth contributes to the deformity. In such cases, distal femoral osteotomy should be performed with the proximal tibial osteotomy.
  - Genu valgum may recur after osteotomy because of the continued growth disturbance of the lateral proximal tibial epiphysis, so continued follow-up until skeletal maturity is required.
- Patellar dislocation can occur because of the genu valgum. Surgical realignment of the quadriceps mechanism and of the bony anatomy is the treatment of choice.

Diastrophic Dysplasia

- Diastrophic dysplasia is an extremely rare skeletal dysplasia characterized by severe short-limb dwarfism with extensive spinal deformities and specific hand, foot, and ear abnormalities.
- The disease occurs in most populations, but it is particularly prevalent in Finland, where between 1 and 2% of the population are carriers because of an apparent founder effect.
- Diastrophic dysplasia is inherited as an autosomal recessive trait. The responsible gene is located on the distal part of the long arm of chromosome 5 and encodes a unique sulfate transporter protein (diastrophic dysplasia sulfate transporter).[3] Impaired function of this protein leads to undersulfation of proteoglycans in cartilage matrix, which impairs the growth response of these cells to FGF, thus stunting enchondral growth.

- Histopathology reveals atypical chondrocytes with extreme variation in size and shape and with premature cytoplasmic degeneration. The chondrocytes are larger and clearer than normal with more rounded nuclei. Prominent, densely staining fibrotic foci are present throughout the cartilage, and the collagen in these foci is remarkably abnormal.[4]

Clinical Features

- Diastrophic dysplasia is easily recognizable at birth. The affected newborn is severely dwarfed, with micromelic shortening of the limbs and marked bilateral clubfeet.
- The median adult height is 136 cm for male patients and 129 cm for females.
- The head is normocephalic, and the facial appearance is characteristic with a narrow nasal bridge, broadened midnose, and flared nostrils.
- The ears are normal at birth, but in a few weeks, swelling of the external ears develops that subsequently calcifies and ossifies, forming the *cauliflower ear* deformity.
- Specific hand and foot malformations are universal in patients with diastrophic dysplasia.[6]
  - The hands are short, broad, and ulnarly deviated.
  - The *hitchhiker's thumb*, a distinctive feature of the dysplasia, is caused by excessive shortening of the first metacarpal, leading to radial subluxation of the metacarpophalangeal joint of the thumb.
  - Symphalangism (stiffness of the interphalangeal joints) of the fingers is frequently observed.
  - Bilateral rigid equinovarus is another distinctive feature of diastrophic dysplasia.
  - The great toe may be in additional varus beyond the degree commonly seen in idiopathic clubfoot. This is analogous to the hitchhiker's thumb.
- Flexion contractures of the elbow, hip, and knee joints are commonly seen in patients with diastrophic dysplasia, and marked limitation of motion occurs in the involved joints.
  - The functional length of the limbs is further compromised by these contractures.
  - Persistent hip flexion contractures may lead to progressive deformation of the proximal femoral epiphyses. Arthritic changes develop by early to middle adulthood.
  - Knee flexion contractures are frequently associated with epiphyseal deformation, excessive valgus, and dislocation of the patella.
- The spine appears normal at birth, but as the child becomes ambulatory, scoliosis and kyphosis develop.
  - Two types of scoliosis have been described: idiopathic-like or sharply angular.[9] The sharply angular type is usually characterized by kyphosis at the same level as the scoliosis.
  - Spinal deformity is progressive in nearly all cases.
- Lumbar lordosis may develop secondary to hip flexion contractures.
- Cervical kyphosis is seen in one third to one half of patients. Its course is variable, from spontaneous resolution to severe involvement with quadriparesis.

Radiographic Findings

- Prenatal diagnosis may be made by ultrasonography in the second trimester with the demonstration of short limbs, clubfeet, and hitchhiker's thumb.[5]
- On spinal radiographs, the vertebral bodies may show some irregularities or wedging.
- The lower cervical spine may demonstrate kyphosis with hypoplasia of the vertebral bodies. Spina bifida of the cervical spine is common.
- Kyphosis or scoliosis of the thoracolumbar spine occurs in more than 80% of patients and frequently develops into a severe, progressive structural curve (Table 14–1). Exaggerated lumbar lordosis may also be detected (Figure 14–8).
- The first metacarpal and first metatarsal are triangular, leading to the hitchhiker's thumb in the upper extremity.

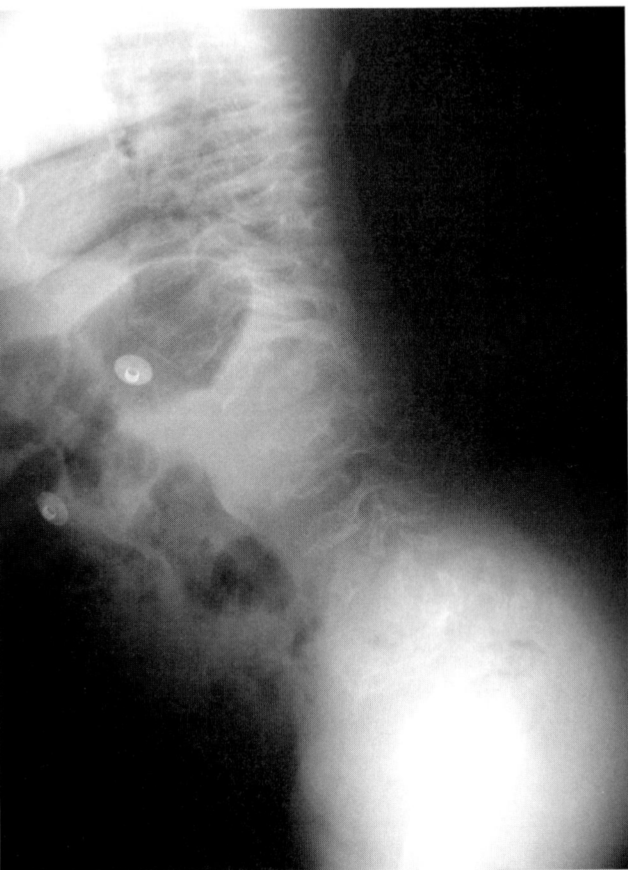

Figure 14–8: A thoracolumbar kyphosis with an exaggerated lumbar lordosis is seen in this young child with diastrophic dysplasia. **There is generalized platyspondyly with anterior beaking of the lumbar vertebrae. A hypoplastic first lumbar vertebra is seen at the apex of the kyphosis. Note the flared ribs with irregular rib ends.**

- Long bones are usually short and broad with metaphyseal flaring.
- The epiphyses of both the proximal and the distal femur are delayed in appearance.
- Coxa vara is common, and hip dislocation is present in about 25% of patients.
- The feet usually demonstrate a severe equinovarus deformity.

Medical Problems

- Early comprehensive medical attention is required for respiratory difficulties. Some patients die in infancy of respiratory failure, but most have a normal life span unless there are cardiopulmonary sequelae from severe scoliosis or quadriplegia secondary to cervical kyphosis.
- Cleft palate may contribute to respiratory difficulties, because aspiration with feeding may occur. Surgical repair is required in most patients.
- Hearing impairment secondary to stenosis of the external auditory canal may develop.

Orthopaedic Considerations

- If cervical kyphosis is noted, the patient should be followed with clinical and radiographic examinations every 6 months. Lateral flexion–extension radiographs and sometimes flexion–extension MRI of the cervical spine should be obtained.
  - If the cervical kyphosis is not progressive and there is no instability or neurological signs, it can be observed and may improve spontaneously.
  - Progressive deformities with instability should be treated surgically by posterior cervical fusion. Deficiencies of the posterior elements of the cervical spine make posterior spinal fusion difficult.[5] Immobilization by a halo and vest is needed for 2 to 3 months postoperatively.
  - If there is severe anterior cord compression, corpectomy and strut graft should be considered with posterior fusion.
- Scoliosis often begins early in childhood in diastrophic dysplasia.
  - For the idiopathic-like curves smaller than 45 degrees, bracing is recommended. Sharply angular curves with kyphosis usually do not respond to brace treatment.[5]
  - Surgical intervention is required to prevent progression for curves over about 50 degrees. Posterior spinal fusion is the mainstay of the treatment. In the presence of associated kyphosis over 50 degrees, anterior spinal fusion may be added.
- Lumbar hyperlordosis usually is not progressive, and surgical correction is not indicated.
- Hip and knee flexion contractures should be assessed together.
  - Physical therapy and splinting may be instituted early for the management of these contractures.
  - Joint deformity and motion should be carefully assessed before any surgical procedure to the joints.
    1. If there is a significant (>40 degrees) hip flexion contracture, soft tissue release may be considered if an arthrogram shows no epiphyseal flattening and good potential for gaining range of motion. If there is epiphyseal flattening, it is probably better to avoid releases because recurrence is likely.[4,5]
    2. Proximal femoral valgus-extension osteotomy is performed for residual contractures, improving function.
- Femoral head deformity and joint contractures make reduction of dislocated hip challenging in patients with diastrophic dysplasia. The dislocations are teratological and therefore do not respond to closed forms of treatment. The surgeon should use individual judgment as to whether to perform an open reduction associated with acetabular augmentation and femoral osteotomy or to leave the hip dislocated.
- Because the irregularity of the femoral head is inherent to the dysplasia, surgical treatment in early childhood does not prevent degenerative changes. Total joint arthroplasty is successful for the severely symptomatic adult patients. Custom-made prostheses are usually needed.
- Knee flexion contractures require soft tissue releases, which should be combined with simultaneous release of the hip flexion contractures. Although, soft tissue releases may improve soft tissue contractures, skeletal malalignment and intra-articular pathology can prevent achieving full correction. Residual contracture at maturity may be diminished by distal femoral osteotomy.
- Genu valgum is common in patients with diastrophic dysplasia but does not require corrective osteotomy in most cases. Patellar subluxation–dislocation should be treated surgically to improve extensor power.
- In diastrophic dysplasia, equinovarus foot deformity is common.
  - The feet are usually rigid and resistant to conservative treatment by serial casting.
  - Surgical treatment is required in most patients to achieve a plantigrade foot. Operation should be deferred until the feet are large enough to work on, which usually is at or slightly older than 1 year. Soft tissue release should be as extensive as needed to correct the deformity. Postoperative bracing with ankle–foot orthoses is recommended to delay recurrence.
  - Partial recurrence of deformity is common and requires repeat surgery, which is even less likely to achieve a plantigrade foot. Salvage procedures including talectomy, talocalcaneal decancellation, and arthrodesis (in the older child) may be necessary.[5]

Kniest Dysplasia

- Kniest syndrome is a severe skeletal dysplasia characterized by disproportionate short-trunk dwarfism, kyphoscoliosis, typical facial features, large stiff joints with contractures, and hearing and visual impairment.[6]

- It has been likened to metatropic dysplasia, because of the enlarged stiff joints, and to spondyloepiphyseal dysplasia (SED), because of the generalized disorder of both spinal and epiphyseal growth.
- Kniest dysplasia is an autosomal dominant disorder. Mutations in the gene that encodes type II collagen, the predominant protein of cartilage, have been identified in several individuals with Kniest dysplasia.[3] Most mutations are between exons 12 and 24 of the COL2A1 gene and result in alternate splicing and interruption of the triple helix of α-1 chains of type II collagen.
- Histopathological findings include a disorganized physeal growth plate, soft crumbly cartilage with a "Swiss cheese" appearance, and diastase resistant intracytoplasmic inclusions in the resting chondrocytes. Scanning electron microscopy demonstrates striking fragmentation and disintegration of collagen fibrils, resulting in large, open, cyst-like spaces, and deficiency and disorganization of the collagen fibrils.[10]

Clinical Features

- Kniest dysplasia can be recognized at birth in most patients, but in mild involvement recognition may be delayed.
- By 1 year, contractures of the elbows, fingers, hips, and knees are evident. Affected children cannot fully close the hand into a fist because of contractures. Contractures and joint stiffness cause delayed motor development.
- By 3 years, all of the usual manifestations of Kniest dysplasia are evident. There is significant disproportionate short-trunk dwarfism and rhizomelic involvement of the limbs. The trunk is short and broad.
- The face is flat with widely spaced, prominent eyes and a flat nasal bridge.
- Kyphoscoliosis and marked lumbar lordosis with hip flexion contractures further contribute to the short stature.
- The elbows, wrists, knees, and ankles are enlarged and prominent.
- Adult height ranges from 106 to 145 cm.

Radiographic Findings

- Osteoporosis of the spine and limbs is evident from birth.
- Hand involvement is significant with generalized osteoporosis and narrowing of the intercarpal and interphalangeal joints.
- All regions of the spine are affected.
  - Abnormalities of the odontoid with atlantoaxial instability and hypoplasia of the cervical vertebrae may occur (Table 14–1).
  - Generalized platyspondyly and vertical clefting in the vertebral bodies are common findings.
  - There is kyphosis, and often mild scoliosis, in the thoracolumbar spine (Figure 14–9, *A*).
- The pelvis is characteristic with short, broad iliac crests and small, insufficient acetabula (Figure 14–9, *B*).
- The appearance of the epiphyses, in particular the femoral heads, is delayed. There are irregular calcifications in the epiphyseal and metaphyseal regions.

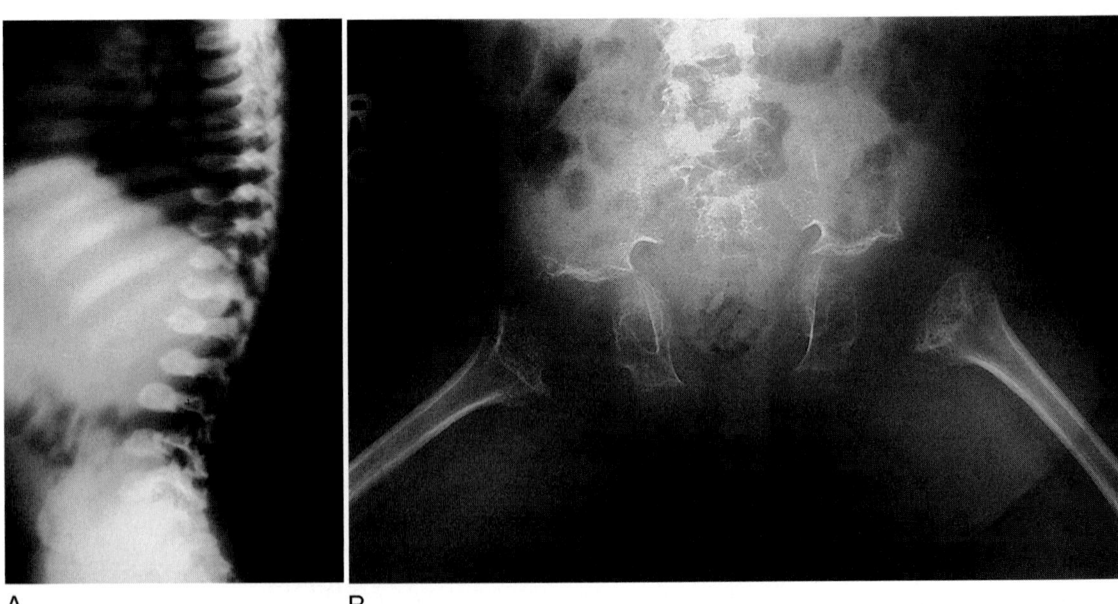

Figure 14–9: A 6-month-old patient with Kniest dysplasia. **A, A lateral view of the spine shows anterior beaking of the vertebrae throughout the spine. B, The pelvis is characteristic with short, broad iliac crests and small, insufficient acetabula. The appearance of the proximal femoral epiphyses is delayed with irregular calcifications in the metaphyseal regions.**

- The epiphyses are irregular in shape and therefore lead to angular deformities of the lower extremities.
- The dumbbell-shaped long bones have short, broad metaphyses leading to the appearance of joint enlargement.

Medical Problems

- Severe respiratory distress and recurrent pulmonary infections, requiring appropriate treatment, may occur frequently during infancy.
- Cleft palate is found in at least 50% of patients with Kniest dysplasia and usually requires surgical treatment.
- Hearing losses are frequent and appear to be related to chronic otitis media.
- The frequency of severe myopia and retinal detachment makes ophthalmological examination essential.

Orthopaedic Considerations

- Evaluation of upper cervical spine instability is essential by lateral flexion–extension radiographs and may be required by flexion–extension MRI. If significant instability or neurological signs exists, posterior cervical fusion with halo immobilization should be performed.
- Thoracic kyphoscoliosis is usually not severe, and surgical treatment is not required.
- Joint stiffness and contractures require early physical and occupational therapy to gain and maintain motion, especially in the small joints of the hands, hips, knees, and ankles.
- Angular deformities of the lower extremities are best treated by osteotomy in the ambulatory patient, although recurrence of deformity is common.
- Osteoarthritis of the hip is common in the second or third decade, and total hip arthroplasty is the only reasonable alternative for symptomatic hips.

Spondyloepiphyseal Dysplasia Congenita

- SED is descriptive for a group of rare disorders characterized by disproportionate short-trunk dwarfism with primary involvement of the vertebrae and epiphyseal centers.
- SED congenita is the most common type with an estimated prevalence of 3 to 4 per 1 million.
- SED congenita is transmitted in an autosomal dominant manner, but most patients acquire the disease because of a new mutation. The gene defect has been linked to a deletion at the type II collagen gene locus, COL2A1, on chromosome 12.[3] This is the predominant protein of cartilage, and mutations have been observed in the α-1 chain, altering length. Electron microscopy has demonstrated intracellular inclusions, which are probably caused by intracellular retention of procollagen.

Clinical Features

- SED congenita can be diagnosed in infancy. There is disproportionate short-trunk dwarfism and rhizomelic involvement of the limbs (Figure 14–10, *A* and *B*).
- Head circumference is normal with flattened facies and wide-set eyes.
- The neck is short, and the chest is barrel-shaped with pectus carinatum deformity (Figure 14–11, *A*).[6]
- Scoliosis and kyphosis usually develop in adolescence. Lumbar lordosis may be accentuated and is usually caused by hip flexion contractures.
- Angular deformities of the lower extremities including coxa vara; more commonly, genu valgum may be seen. A waddling gate is produced by the coxa vara.
- The most common foot deformity is equinovarus.
- The estimated adult height of patients with SED congenita varies from 90 to 125 cm.

Radiographic Findings

- The development of ossification centers is delayed in SED congenita patients.
- Spinal abnormalities are commonly detected.
  - There are various degrees of platyspondyly. The vertebral bodies are initially biconvex but become progressively flattened with age, and the endplates become irregular.
  - The odontoid may be hypoplastic or absent leading to atlantoaxial instability that may cause neurological compromise, even in early childhood (Figure 14–11, *B* and *C*) (Table 14–1).
  - Progressive kyphoscoliosis may develop in late childhood (Figure 14–10, *C* and *D*).
- Iliac crests are short and small with horizontal acetabular roofs.
- The proximal femora are in varus with short necks, but the degree of this involvement varies (Figure 14–10, *E*). The proximal femur may not ossify for up to 9 years.[11]
- The ossification centers of the distal femur and proximal tibia are also delayed, with flattening and irregularity of the articular surfaces (Figure 14–10, *F*). Genu valgum is more common than genu varum.
- Early osteoarthritis is likely in the hips, more so than in the knee.
- The carpals are delayed in ossification, but the tubular bones of the hands are nearly normal.

Medical Problems

- Restrictive lung disease may develop in infancy because of the small thorax, but most of these children survive.
- Retinal detachment or severe myopia is common in patients with SED congenita, so periodic ophthalmological surveillance is indicated.
- Cleft palate may occur and usually requires surgical treatment.

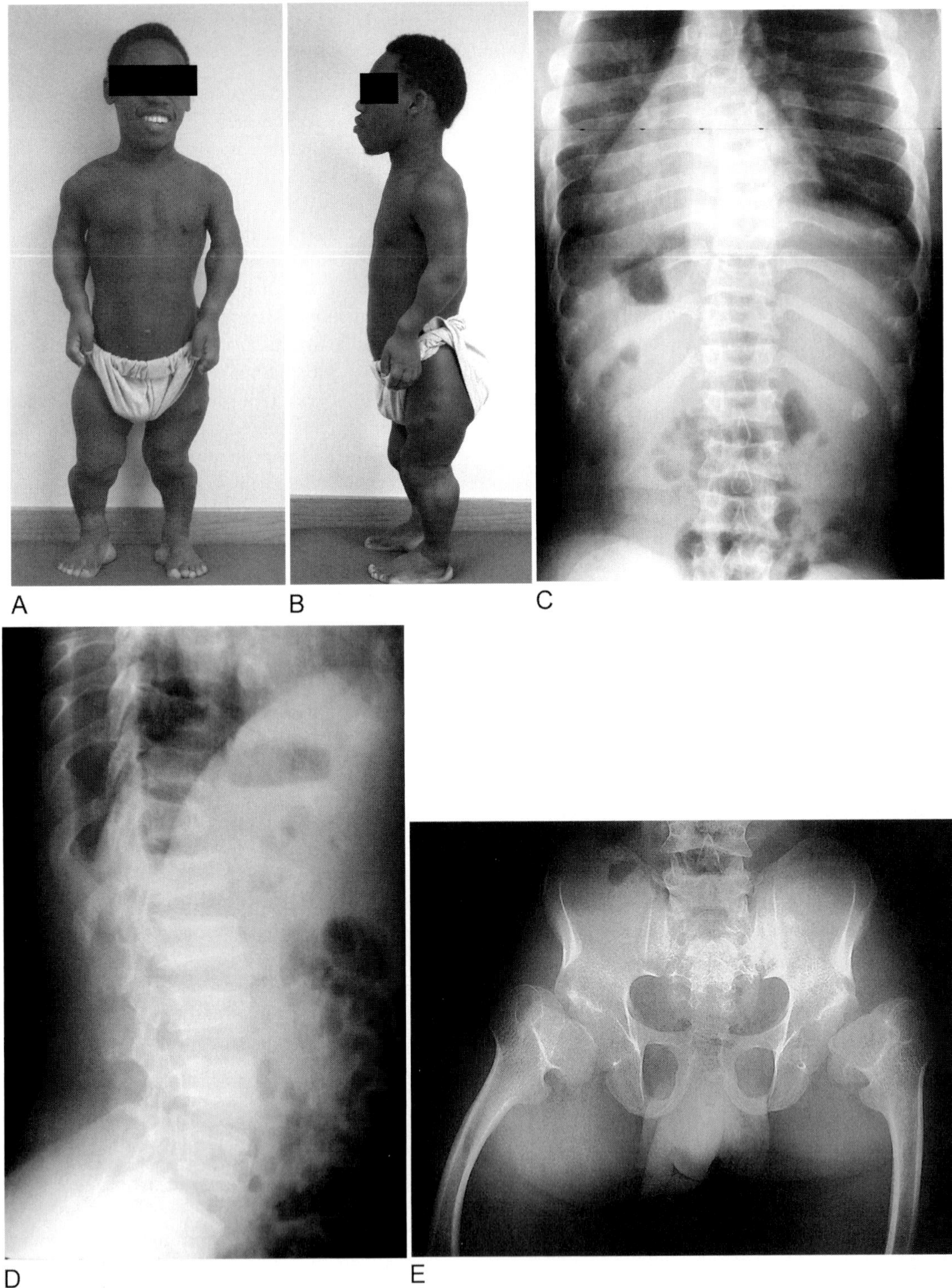

Figure 14–10: A 19-year-old patient with SED congenita. A and B, Note the markedly short stature with a short trunk and rhizomelic involvement of the limbs. There are angular deformities of the lower limbs, including bilateral genu valgum and bowing of the femur and tibia. The elbows have a flexion contracture. C, On the posterior–anterior radiograph of the spine, a thoracic scoliosis is seen. The ribs are broad and short, resulting in a small thorax. D, A lateral radiograph of the spine shows diffuse platyspondyly and mild kyphosis centered at a hypoplastic T11. E, This patient has marked coxa vara associated with hip flexion contractures. The femoral necks are short, the heads are broad, and there is overgrowth of the greater trochanters. These abnormalities lead to the shallow, dysplastic acetabula seen here. Note the small, vertical iliac wings.

Continued

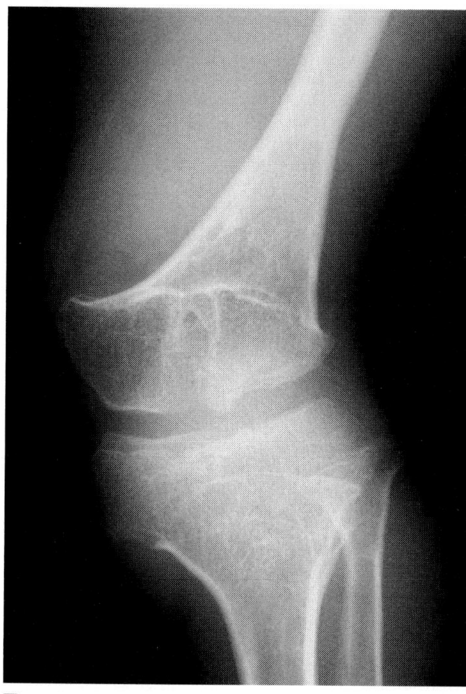

F

Figure 14–10, cont'd: **F, At the knee, a valgus deformity results from a hypoplastic lateral femoral condyle. Both the femoral and the tibial epiphyses are abnormally flattened and broad.**

Orthopaedic Considerations

- Upper cervical spine instability or spinal stenosis may be associated with cord compression and myelopathic changes in children with SED congenita.[4,5]
  - Periodic evaluation of cervical instability by lateral flexion–extension radiographs and flexion–extension MRI is essential. MRI is also helpful in evaluating spinal stenosis.
  - If instability or cord compression exists, posterior cervical fusion with halo vest immobilization should be performed (Figure 14–11, *D*). Decompression may be considered if there is significant stenosis.
- Scoliosis is present in more than one half of patients with SED congenita. Scoliosis may be associated with severe kyphosis.
  - Scoliotic curves smaller than 45 degrees may require bracing, although the response to bracing in patients with SED is somewhat unpredictable.
  - Progressive curves that are more than 50 degrees frequently require posterior spinal fusion and instrumentation with additional anterior fusion for large or rigid curves. The canal size typically is adequate for instrumentation, but preoperative MRI should be done for assessment.
- Hip osteotomies are indicated if the neck–shaft angle is less than 100 degrees.
  - Insufficient correction makes recurrence more likely.
  - Coxa vara may be associated with hip flexion contracture. It is helpful to correct any flexion contracture at the same time if enough flexion will remain. The procedure of choice is the proximal femoral valgus-extension osteotomy.
- Severe angular deformities around the knee are treated by realignment osteotomies.
  - Genu valgum is quite common, and distal femoral varus osteotomy is performed to surgically correct this condition.
  - Recurrence is a frequent complication.
- Total joint replacement may be considered for selected adult patients with symptomatic osteoarthritis of the hips and knees.
- Equinovarus deformity usually is resistant to conservative treatment, so surgical correction with soft tissue releases is required in most patients.

Spondyloepiphyseal Dysplasia Tarda

- SED tarda is a disorder of endochondral bone formation characterized by disproportionate short stature with short neck and trunk. It occurs in approximately 2 of every 1 million people.
- SED tarda is distinguished from SED congenita by the later age at diagnosis and the milder involvement.
- Several genetic patterns of transmission have been reported. The most common is X-linked in which male patients are more commonly and more severely affected. Obligate female carriers are commonly clinically and radiographically indistinguishable from the general population, although some cases have phenotypical changes consistent with expression of the gene defect. A recessive form has also been reported. X-linked SED tarda can be caused by mutations in sedlin (SEDL) gene localized to the X chromosome.[3] SEDL is widely expressed in tissues including fibroblasts, lymphoblasts, and fetal cartilage and encodes a protein (sedlin) with a putative role in endoplasmic reticulum-to-Golgi vesicular transport.

Clinical Features

- SED tarda is not recognized at birth but becomes apparent as the growth rate of the child slows in midchildhood or adolescence. Stature is mildly shortened.
- SED tarda affects primarily the spine and the large joints; the changes become evident between 10 and 14 years.
- Thoracic kyphoscoliosis associated with back pain may be seen.
- Patients usually develop hip pain, and they may be diagnosed as having bilateral Perthes disease initially.[12]
- Progressive osteoarthritis of the hips and knees may be seen by early adolescence.
- Angular deformities of the lower extremities are rare.

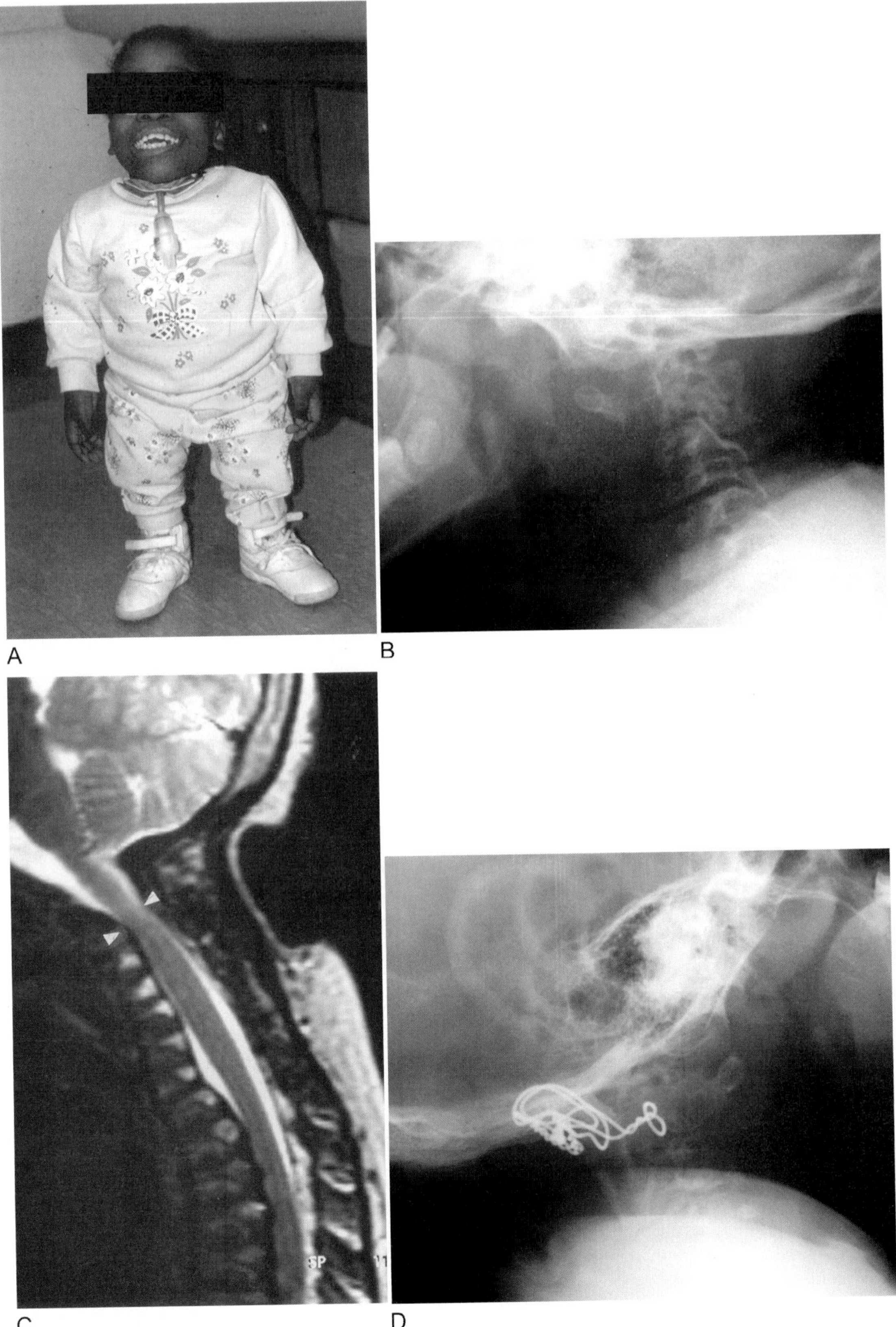

Figure 14–11: A 10-year-old girl with SED congenita. A, Note the markedly short stature with a short neck. B, A lateral cervical spine radiograph depicts a hypoplastic, barely visible odontoid and a significantly widened ADI characteristic of cervical instability. C, MRI of the cervical spine shows narrowing of the spinal canal at the level of the atlas (C1) *(arrows)*. The spinal cord appears thinned at and just above this level. D, This patient had posterior cervical fusion (occiput to the first, second, and third cervical vertebra) and decompression. Wires and a bone graft are seen. *A* and *C* from Erol B, Dormans JP, States L, Kaplan FS (2004) Skeletal dysplasias and metabolic disorders of bone: Musculoskeletal tumors in children. In: Pediatric Orthopaedics and Sports Medicine. (Dormans JP, ed). Philadelphia: Mosby.

Radiographic Findings

- Involvement of the shoulders, hips, and knees predominates.
- Radiographic changes in the hip are typical, including abnormal femoral heads (with coxa magna, flattening, and subluxation), acetabular insufficiency, and premature osteoarthritis (Figure 14–12, *A*). These features may mimic bilateral Perthes disease. However, in SED involvement is symmetrical, and in bilateral Perthes disease involvement is discordant, with one hip more radiographically affected than the other.[12]
- Mild genu varum or valgum may be seen with flattening of the femoral condyles and deformation of the tibial articular surfaces (Figure 14–12, *B*).

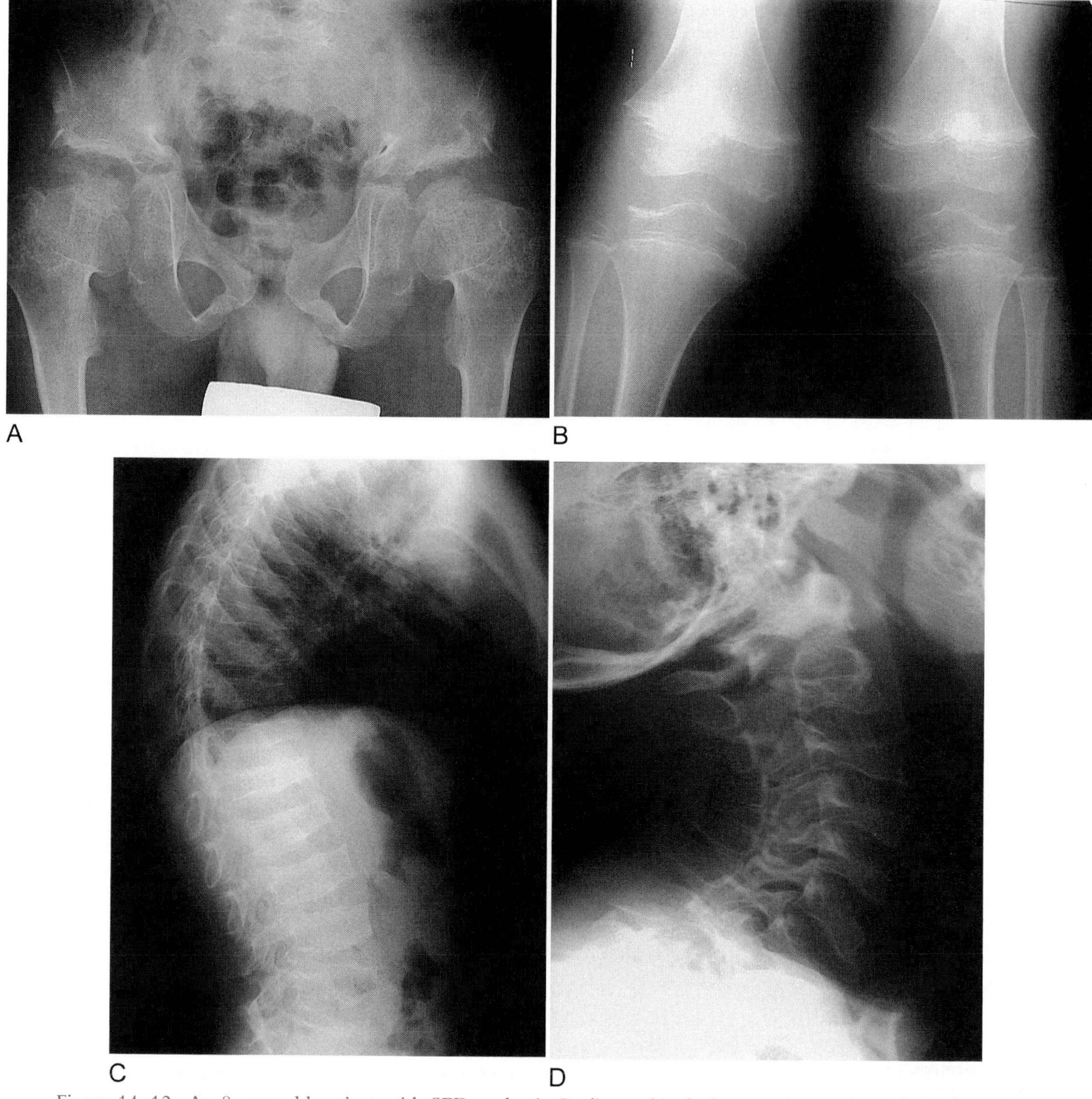

Figure 14–12: An 8-year-old patient with SED tarda. A, Radiographic findings in the proximal femur include a small femoral head with delayed ossification and enlargement of the metaphyses and coxa magna. Note the deep acetabula with a horizontal acetabular roof. B, At the knees, the long bones have irregular, flattened epiphyses and enlarged metaphyses. Mild genu valgum is seen. C, The thoracolumbar spine has significantly flattened and elongated vertebra throughout characteristic of diffuse platyspondyly. A moderate thoracolumbar kyphosis is also present. D, A lateral view of the cervical spine shows a hypoplastic odontoid and platyspondyly.

- Spinal involvement including platyspondyly or anterior wedging of the vertebral bodies usually affects the thoracic spine and may result in kyphoscoliosis (Figure 14–12, *C*). Odontoid hypoplasia may cause atlantoaxial instability (Figure 14–12, *D*) (Table 14–1).

Orthopaedic Considerations

- All patients with SED tarda should be evaluated for atlantoaxial instability, and cervical fusion should be considered if significant instability is detected.
- Scoliotic curves are usually mild to moderate in severity and are managed by observation or bracing. Surgery is indicated for the rare patient in whom the scoliotic curve exceeds 50 degrees.
- Hip problems frequently require surgical intervention. A valgus or valgus-extension osteotomy may help to provide joint congruity or to decrease hinge abduction.
- Angular deformities of the knees usually do not require treatment.
- Degenerative arthritis in adulthood is treated by total joint arthroplasty. Custom components may be necessary because of the anatomy and length of the femur.

Pseudoachondroplasia

- Pseudoachondroplasia is one of the most frequent skeletal dysplasias with a prevalence of 4 per 1 million. It was first described as a form of SED; however, it is a distinct dwarfing condition readily differentiated from SED, because of late-onset physical findings and milder spinal involvement.
- Pseudoachondroplasia is characterized by rhizomelic short-limb dwarfism in which both the epiphyses and the metaphyses are involved.
- Affected individuals have significantly short stature and a predisposition to premature osteoarthritis.
- Pseudoachondroplasia is usually transmitted as an autosomal dominant trait. A gene for this disorder has recently been localized to the pericentromeric region of chromosome 19. This region encodes for cartilage oligomeric matrix protein (COMP), a glycoprotein that plays a role in calcium binding within cartilage.[3] The disruption of calcium-dependent proteoglycan binding by COMP may result in an accumulation of proteoglycan in chondrocytes. COMP is also expressed in tendon and ligament, and abnormal COMP in these tissues is plausibly responsible for the loose joints that are a consistent feature of this disorder.
- Histological studies of cartilage from patients with pseudoachondroplasia reveal noncollagenous protein accumulated in the rough endoplasmic reticulum of chondrocytes.
- Pseudoachondroplasia resembles achondroplasia because of its rhizomelic pattern but otherwise has little in common with it.

Clinical Features

- The patients with pseudoachondroplasia appear normal at birth, and growth retardation is seldom recognized until the second year of life or later, at which time body proportions resemble those of persons with achondroplasia.[4]
- Adult height ranges from 106 to 130 cm.
- Unlike in achondroplasia, the head and face are normal in pseudoachondroplasia.
- Cervical instability is present in a minority of cases. Patients may have mild thoracolumbar kyphosis, and a few patients develop scoliosis (Table 14–1).
- In almost all cases, the hips are dysplastic and the patient exhibits a waddling gait.
- Varus, valgus, and recurvatum deformities of the knees are common and result from osseous changes and marked ligamentous laxity. Some children develop "windswept" deformities of the knees in which genu valgum is present on one side and genu varum is present on the other.
- The fingers and toes of patients with pseudoachondroplasia are short and thick.
- No changes outside the skeletal system have been noted as part of the disorder. Patients have normal intelligence and a normal life expectancy.

Radiographic Findings

- All regions of the spine are affected in patients with pseudoachondroplasia.
  - The radiographs of the spine usually show a mild platyspondyly, with anterior tongue-like projections and irregular endplates.
  - The interpedicular distance in the lumbar spine is normal in pseudoachondroplasia, unlike achondroplasia.
  - Almost one half of the patients have odontoid hypoplasia or aplasia.
  - Scoliosis may be present in teenage patients.
- The long bones are short and broad, with flaring of the metaphyses (Figure 14–13).
- The epiphyses have delayed and fragmented ossification; in the proximal femur, this may be mistaken for SEDs and even bilateral Perthes disease. Pseudoachondroplasia can be distinguished from bilateral Perthes disease by its synchronous symmetrical involvement.[12]
- Epiphyseal involvement leads to flattening and enlargement of the femoral heads with subluxation of the hip. The epiphyseal irregularity may lead to degenerative joint disease.

Orthopaedic Considerations

- Periodic evaluation of upper cervical spine instability is essential for patients with pseudoachondroplasia. Lateral flexion–extension radiographs and, when required, flexion–extension MRI should be obtained and

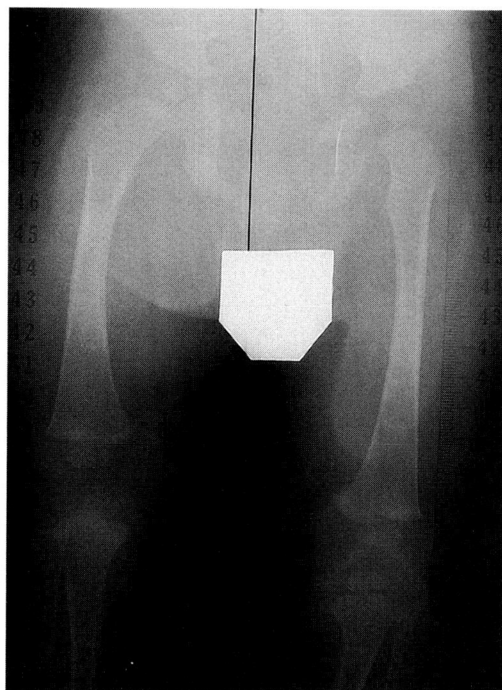

Figure 14–13: A young child with pseudoachondroplasia has asymmetrical widening of the metaphyses, greater on the right than on the left, and shortening of the right femur.

cervical fusion should be considered if significant instability is detected.

- Scoliotic curves are usually mild (<25 degrees) and are followed periodically without any treatment. Occasionally, larger curves requiring bracing (between 25 and 45 degrees) or even surgery (>50 degrees) may be seen.
- Surgical treatment of hip subluxation–dislocation is difficult because of the incongruity of the femoral head with the acetabulum.
  - Proximal femoral valgus osteotomy may improve joint congruity and enhances abductor function by moving the greater trochanter distally and laterally.
  - A Chiari osteotomy or shelf acetabular augmentation may be required to achieve coverage.
  - Rotational iliac osteotomies of the pelvis (e.g., Salter osteotomy and triple osteotomy) are usually not helpful in pseudoachondroplasia because a prerequisite for these osteotomies is concentric congruity of the joint.
- Angular deformities of the knee usually do not respond to conservative treatment modalities and usually require surgical correction. The objective of the procedure is to obtain a horizontal joint surface with a well-aligned knee. Both tibial and femoral procedures may be necessary. Recurrence is common, and repeat surgery may be needed.
- Total joint arthroplasty is the treatment of choice for premature osteoarthritis of the knee and hip joints.

Mucopolysaccharidoses

- The mucopolysaccharidoses (MPSs) are a group of inherited metabolic disorders caused by deficiency of specific lysosomal enzymes, which results in intracellular accumulation of partially degraded glycosaminoglycans.
- The overall incidence of the MPSs is 1 in 25,000 live births.
- The MPSs are subdivided based on their enzyme deficiency and the type of substance that accumulates (Table 14–2).
- Although there is phenotypic variability, these disorders share some common clinical features, such as facial dysmorphism, short stature, organomegaly, cardiac problems, and joint contractures.[6] Mental retardation may be associated with some types.
- Most of the MPSs show similar changes in the cartilage; resting cartilage consists of uniformly stained matrix with chondrocytes that are larger than normal and stain positively for glycosaminoglycans.[3]
- The most common of the MPSs are Morquio and Hurler syndrome.
- The MPSs can be diagnosed by some laboratory studies after birth.

Table 14–2: Mucopolysaccharidoses and Specific Enzyme Deficiencies

MUCOPOLYSACCHARIDOSES	ENZYME DEFICIENCY	GENE LOCUS
MPS I (Hurler syndrome)	α-L-iduronidase	Chromosome 4
MPS II (Hunter's disease)	Iduronate-2-sulfatase	X chromosome
MPS III (Sanfilippo syndrome)		
A	Heparan sulfate sulfatase	
B	α-N-acetylglucosaminidase	
C	Acetyl CoA—α-glucosaminide-N-acetyltransferase	
D	N-acetyl-glucosaminide-6-sulphatase	Chromosome 12
MPS IV (Morquio syndrome)		
A	Galactosamine-6-sulphate-sulphatase	
B	β-galactosidase	
MPS VI (polydystrophic dysplasia)	Arylsulfatase B	Chromosome 5

MPS, mucopolysaccharidoses.

- The mucopolysaccharides, including heparan sulfate, dermatan sulfate, and keratin sulfate, are accumulated and excreted by the urine. Biochemical analysis of the urine can lead to the diagnosis of the specific MPS.
- Identification of the MPSs is also possible through skin fibroblast culture. The fibroblasts are assayed for specific enzyme activity known to be abnormal in the different MPSs.
- Molecular genetic research determines the specific mutations that result in MPSs.[5] Specific mutations are described individually for each type of MPS (Table 14–2).

Clinical Features

- The clinical diagnosis of MPSs is usually made between 6 months and 10 years depending on the type.
- A flat nasal bridge, hypertelorism, and corneal clouding are typical facial features seen in children with MPSs (Figure 14–14, *A*).
- Short stature, short neck, and joint contractures occur almost in all types (Figure 14–14, *B* and *C*).
- Cervical instability and thoracolumbar kyphoscoliosis are common spinal problems (Table 14–1).
- Dysplasia of the pelvis and broadening and shortening of the long bones may be seen.
- Generalized joint laxity is a feature of Morquio syndrome, making it distinctly different from the other MPS in which joint stiffness is the rule (Figure 14–14, *D*).
- The patients with MPS I (Hurler syndrome) and MPS IV (Morquio syndrome) are usually more severely affected than those with the other types.

Radiographic Findings

- The MPSs may share some common radiographic findings.
  - Radiographic changes are commonly seen in the skull; the skull is enlarged with a thick calvarium.
  - The clavicles are broad, especially medially. The ribs are oar shaped and broader anteriorly than posteriorly.
  - The vertebral bodies are ovoid when immature. Scoliosis and kyphosis are frequently present.
  - The iliac wings are flared, and the acetabula are dysplastic. Coxa valga is common, and the long bones often have thickened cortices (Figure 14–15).
  - There is delay in the ossification of the carpal bones.

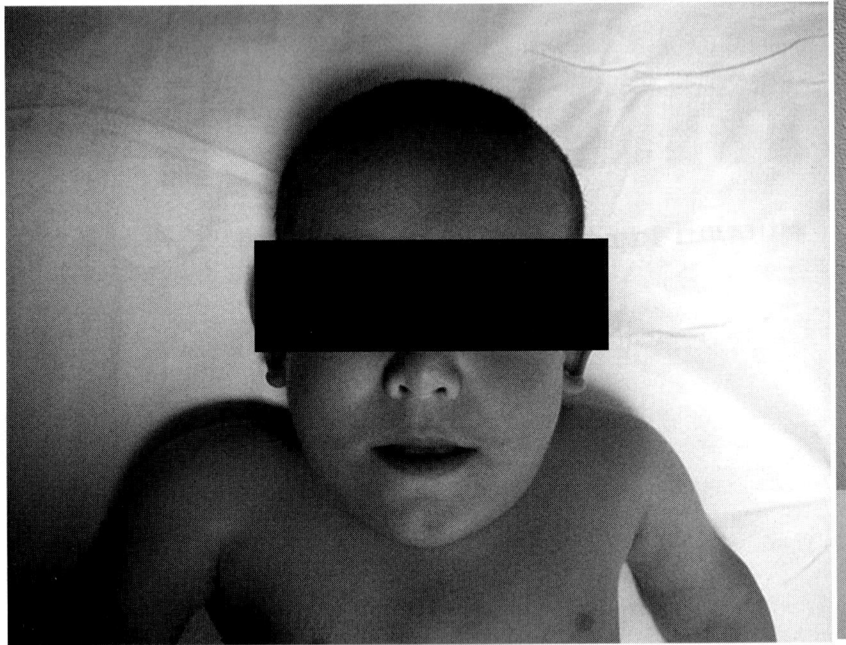
A

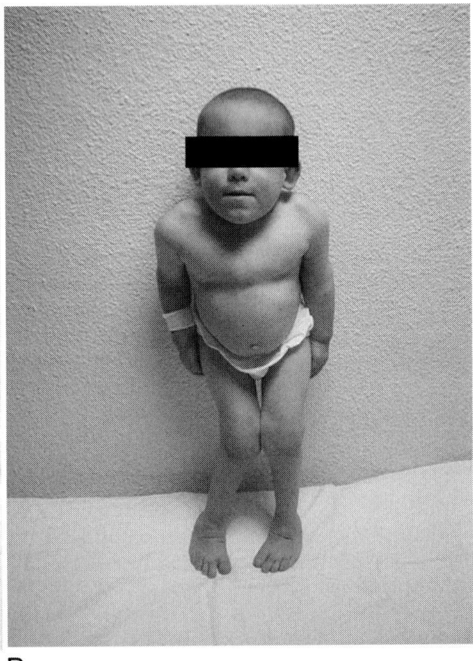
B

Figure 14–14: A 5-year-old boy with MPS IV (Morquio syndrome). A, Note the typical facial features, including a depressed nasal bridge, hypertelorism, and a prominent forehead. B and C, Dwarfing is primarily because of shortness of the trunk rather than shortness of the limbs. The neck is short. The child stands with his knees and hips flexed in a crouched position and his head thrust forward and sunk between his high shoulders. Also note the thoracolumbar kyphoscoliosis and protrusion of his abdomen. D, There is generalized joint laxity, a feature of the Morquio syndrome differentiating it from the other MPSs.

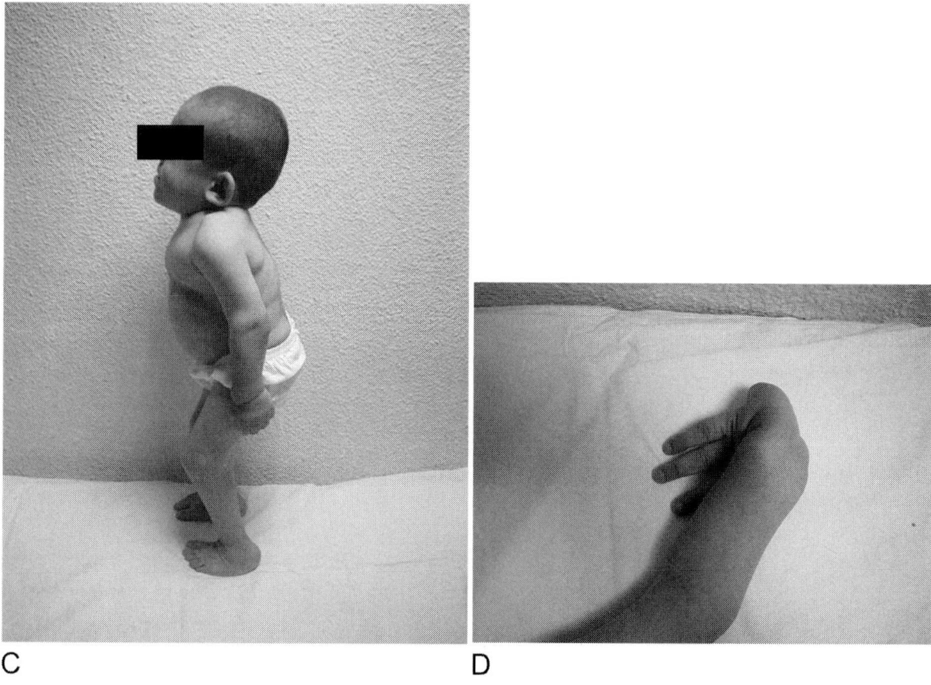

Figure 14–14, cont'd.

- It is difficult to differentiate the various types of MPSs on the basis radiographic findings alone.

Orthopaedic Considerations

- Genetic counseling is essential for all children diagnosed as having MPSs.
- Medical problems require appropriate treatment.
- Orthopaedic treatment usually consists of symptomatic corrective measures: fusion of cervical spine instability and conservative or surgical treatment of spinal curvatures and joint contractures.

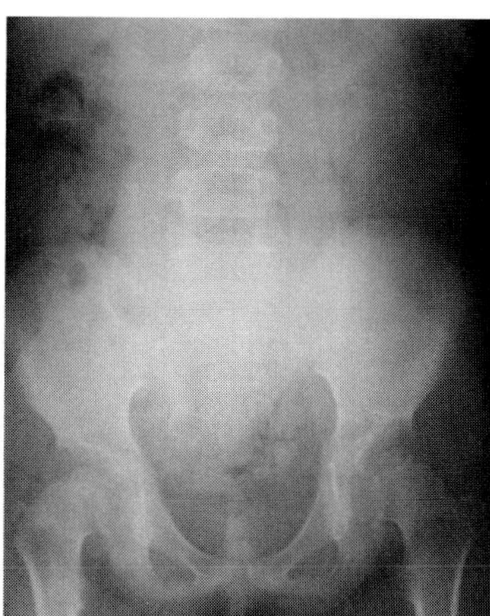
Figure 14–15: The pelvis of an 8-year-old girl with mucopolysaccharidosis type I (Hurler syndrome) has small iliac bones and dysplastic acetabula. The patient also has bilateral coxa valga.

Multiple Epiphyseal Dysplasia

- Multiple epiphyseal dysplasia (MED) is one of the most common skeletal dysplasias characterized by delayed epiphyseal ossification, mild short stature, limb deformities, and early-onset osteoarthritis.
- It affects many epiphyses, produces symptoms mainly in those with significant load-bearing capability, and has few changes in the physes or metaphyses.
- MED is broadly categorized into the more severe Fairbank type (type I) and the milder Ribbing type (type II). In most patients, the dysplasia is inherited by autosomal dominant transmission. A rare autosomal recessive form also exists. There is genetic variability between families, which is expected because there are variable forms of the disease.
  - Fairbank type I MED has been mapped to chromosome 19, and its gene product is COMP, the same gene that is abnormal in pseudoachondroplasia.
  - In Ribbing type II MED, abnormalities have been found on chromosome 1 in the gene encoding for the α-2 fibers of type IX collagen (COL9A2).[3] Type IX collagen is a cartilage-specific fibril-associated collagen and is located on the fibril surfaces. It may form a macromolecular bridge between type II collagen fibrils and other matrix components. It thus may be important for the adhesive properties of cartilage.
- Histologically, intracytoplasmic inclusions within chondrocytes are seen. These inclusions, which are dilations

of the rough endoplasmic reticulum, are similar to but not so severe as those seen in pseudoachondroplasia. Growth plate organization is noticeably abnormal despite the minimal changes seen in the metaphyses.

Clinical Features

- MED is not recognizable at birth. Often the diagnosis is not made until early adolescence.
- The head and face are normal.
- The spine is minimally involved and usually asymptomatic.
- These children are usually referred to orthopaedic surgeons, later in childhood, for joint pain in the lower limbs, decreased range of motion of the hips and knees, or gait disturbance.
- Angular deformities of the lower limbs including coxa vara, genu varum, and genu valgum are common.
- There may be flexion contractures of knees and elbows.
- Shortening of the digits of the hands and feet is the only typical clinical feature of patients with MED.
- These patients have minimal short stature, ranging from 145 to 170 cm.
- There is no visceral involvement, and the intelligence is not affected.

Radiographic Findings

- The principal finding on radiographs is a delay in the appearance of the ossification centers.
  - In the growing patient, the epiphyses are fragmented, mottled, and small.
  - After maturity, there is some degree of flattening of the major load-bearing epiphyses: flattened femoral condyles, an ovoid femoral head, decreased sphericity of the humeral head, and squared talus.
  - In adulthood, major joints develop premature osteoarthritis. This is most common and most severe in the hips.
- The findings on hip radiographs may be easily confused with those of bilateral Perthes disease. Several radiographic clues may be helpful.[12]
  - The radiographic changes are symmetrical and fairly synchronous in MED in contrast to asymmetrical and metachronous involvement in Perthes disease.
  - In Perthes disease, usually one hip is involved before the other, so each hip is in a different stage of the disease.
  - In addition, acetabular changes are more pronounced and seen more frequently in MED.
  - Presence of epiphyseal irregularities in other joints will support the diagnosis of MED.
- Avascular necrosis occurs frequently in the hips of patients with MED.[4,13]
  - Radiographic changes include subchondral fractures, resorption of ossified cartilage, reossification, and sometimes metaphyseal cysts.
  - MRI may show loss of signal in a portion of the femoral head.
  - Superimposed avascular necrosis of the femoral head may further hamper the differential diagnosis of MED and Perthes disease because the imaging studies, bone scan or MRI, will demonstrate avascularity and subsequent changes for both diseases.
- Angular deformities of the lower limbs may occur because of asymmetrical physeal growth.
  - Coxa vara may occur but is not necessarily bilateral. The femoral necks appear short.
  - Radiographs of the knee may show valgus deformity with flattened femoral condyles and shallow intercondylar notch.
  - The ankles in MED usually are in valgus; changes occur more in the talus than in the distal tibia.
- Upper extremity involvement is less severe; there may be irregularities in the proximal and distal humerus and radius (Figure 14–16). The tubular bones of the hands often are shortened, with maximal involvement of the middle and distal phalanges.
- MEDs are distinguished from SEDs by the absence of severe vertebral changes. Mild endplate irregularities may be present.

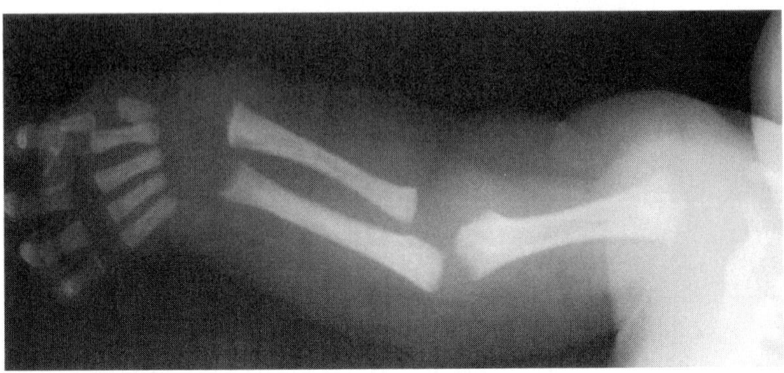

Figure 14–16: Ossification centers are delayed in this 6-month-old patient with MED. The long bones are broad and have flared ends, especially the humerus and ulna. Both ends of the bones are abnormal.

Orthopaedic Considerations

- Orthopaedic treatment is rarely necessary in early childhood. Once the diagnosis is established, maintenance of range of motion is initiated.
- Realignment osteotomies may be performed with little benefit in the early, deforming period of the hip if there is progressive subluxation and pain. Pain is more likely to occur in cases complicated by avascular necrosis. Proximal femoral varus osteotomy is contraindicated because of preexisting coxa vara. Acetabular shelf augmentation is recommended in these instances to improve coverage of the misshapen femoral head.[4]
- Osteotomies may be helpful in realigning the lower extremity deformities.
  - Valgus osteotomy of the proximal femur is the treatment for coxa vara, but recurrence is quite common.
  - Valgus alignment of the knees and ankles usually require surgical correction by varus osteotomies. These deformities may reoccur after surgical correction because of asymmetrical physeal and epiphyseal growth.
  - Realignment osteotomies are usually performed closer to skeletal maturity because of a high recurrence risk.
- Degenerative arthritis usually occurs in the second or third decade. It usually develops in hips that are incongruent with large, flat heads and poor acetabular coverage. If the femoral head is well formed at maturity, the onset of arthritis is delayed. For late cases, total joint arthroplasty may be the only reasonable treatment option.

Chondrodysplasia Punctata

- Chondrodysplasia punctata is a rare skeletal dysplasia characterized by short-limb dwarfism and multiple punctate epiphyseal calcifications, which are present at birth and resolve over the first year.[14]
- It has been subclassified into three groups: the most common X-linked dominant type, also known as *Conradi-Hünermann syndrome;* an autosomal recessive rhizomelic type, which is usually lethal in infancy; and a rare X-linked recessive type.[3] Other forms of the disease exist and are becoming better understood as the molecular genetics of the subtypes are discovered. Although the appearance of neonatal epiphyseal calcification is striking, it is not specific. Some other conditions, such as Zellweger (cerebrohepatorenal) syndrome, gangliosidosis, rubella, trisomy 18 or 21 vitamin K deficiency, hypothyroidism, or fetal alcohol or hydantoin syndromes, may present with the same phenomenon.[4]
  - *Conradi-Hünermann* syndrome is inherited as an autosomal dominant trait with variable expression. The mutations in the gene encoding emopamil-binding protein (EBP), which catalyses an intermediate step in the cholesterol biosynthesis, are thought to be responsible for this syndrome. EBP mutations that produce truncated proteins result in typical *Conradi-Hünermann* syndrome, whereas phenotypes resulting from missense mutations are not always typical for this disorder.[3]
  - Rhizomelic chondrodysplasia punctata type I is caused by mutations in the peroxin 7 gene, which encodes receptors required for import of matrix proteins into peroxisomes. Rhizomelic chondrodysplasia punctata type II shows deficiency of the enzyme acyl-CoA:dihydroxyacetone phosphate acyltransferase; it is often fatal in the first year of life.
  - The X-linked recessive chondrodysplasia punctata (CDPX) is caused by mutations in the arylsulfatase E gene (ARSE), resulting in a sulfatase deficiency. The nature of the CDPX phenotype bone development. The importance of several lysosomal sulfatases in cartilage and bone development is evident from their involvement in the catabolic pathway of sulfated glycosaminoglycans, which are essential components of the extracellular matrix of cartilage.
- Specimens obtained from patients with rhizomelic chondrodysplasia punctata exhibit marked irregularity of vascularization of the epiphyses, disturbance of chondroblastic maturation, and mucoid degeneration of cartilage. In other forms of the dysplasia, there are irregular areas of calcification and cyst formation within the epiphyseal cartilage.

Clinical Features

- Patients with Conradi-Hünermann syndrome are characterized by typical facial features including hypertelorism, a depressed nasal bridge, and a bifid nasal tip. A dysmorphic face with a depressed nasal bridge is also a characteristic of rhizomelic type.
- Patients with Conradi-Hünermann syndrome or rhizomelic type of chondrodysplasia punctata may share some common musculoskeletal abnormalities.
  - These patients frequently have symmetrical shortening of the proximal limbs, contractures of the joints, subluxation–dislocation of the hips, limb length inequality, and coxa vara.[4,6]
  - Spinal findings include atlantoaxial instability, congenital scoliosis, and kyphosis.
  - Equinovarus or other foot deformities may be seen.

Radiographic Findings

- The prenatal diagnosis of chondrodysplasia punctata has been made with ultrasound. The punctuate calcifications can be seen in late pregnancy in the rhizomelic form; limb shortening is apparent earlier.
- The characteristic multiple punctate opacities are observed radiographically at birth and usually

disappear by 1 year (Figure 14–17). These involve the epiphyses of the long bones, the carpal and tarsal bones, the pelvis, and the vertebrae. Stippling may also occur in the trachea and the larynx and can result in upper airway obstruction.

- Other radiographic findings include upper cervical spine abnormalities such as odontoid hypoplasia or os odontoideum. Congenital vertebral anomalies (e.g., hemivertebra, unilateral unsegmented bar, and block vertebra) causing congenital spinal deformities are commonly detected (Table 14–1).
- The appearance of the secondary centers of ossification is often delayed.
- Unilateral or bilateral coxa vara deformity may develop and is frequently associated with asymmetrical shortening of the femur (Figure 14–18).

Medical Problems

- The patients with the rhizomelic type of chondrodysplasia punctata usually die of respiratory complications or seizure-related disorders during the first year of life. In patients who survive, there is a high rate of associated spasticity, psychomotor retardation, growth failure, seizures, thermoregulatory instability, feeding difficulty, and pneumonia.
- Patients with Conradi-Hünermann syndrome have a normal life span.
- The frequency of bilateral congenital cataract and optic atrophy makes ophthalmological consultation essential for patients with chondrodysplasia punctata.
- The possibility of renal abnormalities and congenital heart disease requires careful evaluation.

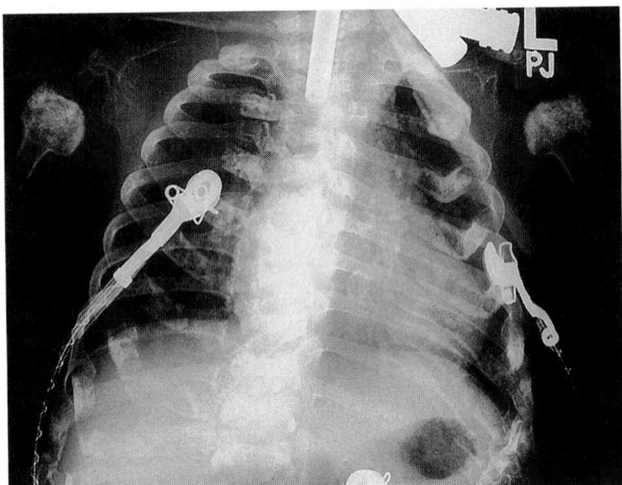

Figure 14–17: A 3-month-old patient with chondrodysplasia punctata has dense, punctate calcifications in the humeral heads and anterior rib ends characteristic of this disorder. A small thorax resulted in restrictive lung disease.

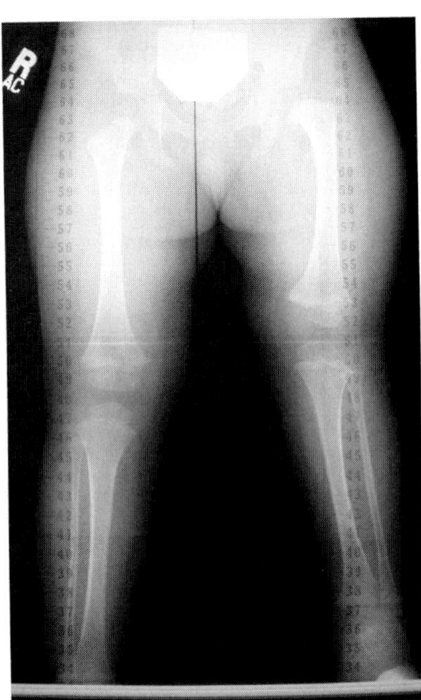

Figure 14–18: During development, the epiphyses develop a more normal appearance, as seen in this 18-month-old patient with chondrodysplasia punctata. The long bones are broad. There is a delay in ossification of the left femoral head and significant shortening of the left femur, resulting in a limb length inequality, a frequent finding in these children. Coxa vara, seen in the left proximal femur, may develop from flexion contractures.

Orthopaedic Considerations

- Orthopaedic treatment consists primarily of managing the congenital spinal deformities, particularly of scoliosis.
  - In most patients, congenital scoliosis and kyphosis progress rapidly during the first 1 or 2 years.
  - Bracing is rarely useful, and most patients require surgical intervention.
  - Surgical treatment consists of early anterior and posterior spinal fusion.
- Atlantoaxial instability must be assessed by lateral flexion–extension radiographs and, if required, flexion–extension MRI. Occasionally, significant cervical instability requiring posterior cervical fusion may develop.
- Coxa vara, when severe (neck–shaft angle < 100 degrees), is treated by valgus osteotomy of the proximal femur.
- Limb length inequalities more than 3 to 4 cm may occur, and limb lengthening may be considered in some patients. Discrepancies are not treated by epiphysiodesis because these patients are already below the 3rd percentile.
- Most flexion contractures are not severe enough to require surgical intervention and are well maintained by physical therapy.

Metaphyseal Chondrodysplasia

- Metaphyseal chondrodysplasias are a group of disorders characterized by metaphyseal deformity and irregularity adjacent to the physes with little or no epiphyseal involvement.
- The defect is in the growth plate; the metaphyseal changes are the results. Histological studies of the growth plate show abnormalities in columniation with nests and clusters of chondrocytes instead of orderly rows.
- Because the longitudinal growth of the bone is diminished, affected patients are short and angular deformities may occur.
- In all types of this dysplasia the epiphyses are spared, and thus arthritis rarely develops.
- Schmid, McKusick, and Jansen dysplasias are the most common types of metaphyseal chondrodysplasia.
- Metaphyseal chondrodysplasia must be differentiated from vitamin D metabolism disorders.
  - The radiographic changes in the metaphyseal regions of the long bones and angular deformities of the lower limbs may resemble various types of rickets.
  - Epiphyseal and physeal involvement is not as severe in metaphyseal chondrodysplasia as it is in rickets.
  - Apart from the radiographic differences, biochemical abnormalities are not found in metaphyseal chondrodysplasia.

Schmid Metaphyseal Chondrodysplasia

- The Schmid type is the most common form of metaphyseal chondrodysplasia.
- It is an autosomal dominant disorder with a mutation in the gene for the α-1 chain of type X collagen (COL10A1).[3] Type X collagen is synthesized specifically and transiently by hypertrophic chondrocytes at sites of endochondral ossification, such as growth plates. However, the precise function of type X collagen is unknown.
- On histological examination, cartilage islands that extend into the metaphyses can be seen.

Clinical Features

- Patients with Schmid metaphyseal chondrodysplasia are normal at birth. They are diagnosed between 2 and 3 years.
- These patients show rather minimal clinical abnormalities, and the adult height is minimally shortened. The head and face are not affected, and the upper extremity involvement is mild. The thorax and the spine have a normal appearance except for increased lumbar lordosis in some patients.
- The patients usually came to the orthopaedic surgeon because of leg pain, a waddling gait, varus angulation of the knee, or short stature.

Radiographic Findings

- Spinal changes occur infrequently in patients with Schmid metaphyseal chondrodysplasia.
- The epiphyses are usually normal. Radiographic changes characteristically occur at the metaphyseal regions of the long bones; the metaphyses are widened and scalloped, and they may have cysts.
- The proximal femoral metaphysis is particularly irregular and splayed, and there is medial beaking. Some widening of the physis occurs but not to the extent observed in rickets. Coxa vara is present to varying degrees.
- Shortening and bowing of the long bones and genu varum may be seen.

Orthopaedic Considerations

- Lower extremity deformities may require orthopaedic treatment.
  - Valgus osteotomy of the proximal femur may be indicated for children with significant coxa vara.
  - Usually the entire femur has a varus bow, with the clinical appearance of genu varum. The varus alignment may improve spontaneously during childhood. If surgical realignment of genu varum is performed, distal femoral and proximal tibial osteotomies are usually required.
  - Following osteotomies, recurrence of deformity with growth is common.

McKusick Metaphyseal Chondrodysplasia

- McKusick metaphyseal chondrodysplasia, also known as *cartilage–hair hypoplasia*, is particularly prevalent in the Amish community of Lancaster county of Pennsylvania and in Finland.
- It is an autosomal recessive disorder, and the gene defect is located on chromosome 9. Recently, it was shown that mutations in the RMRP gene, which encodes the ribonucleic acid (RNA) component of mitochondrial RNA-processing endoribonuclease (RNAase MRP), are responsible for this disorder.[3] The RNAase MRP consists of an RNA molecule bound to several proteins. It has at least two functions, namely, cleavage of RNA in mitochondrial deoxyribonucleic acid synthesis and nucleolar cleaving of pre-rRNA. The mutations in the RMRP gene cause McKusick metaphyseal chondrodysplasia by disrupting a function of this enzyme that affects multiple organ systems.

Clinical Features

- McKusick metaphyseal chondrodysplasia is diagnosed between 2 and 3 years.
- Patients with this disorder have light-colored, sparse hair. Microscopically, the hair is smaller in diameter than normal hair and often lacks pigmentation.

- Progressive dwarfing results in markedly short adult stature. The adult height is 106 to 147 cm.
- These patients have generalized ligamentous laxity, but the elbow extension may be limited.
- Scoliosis may be present in up to one fourth of patients. Pectus excavatum or carinatum may be observed.
- Mild genu varum is common.

Radiographic Findings

- Atlantoaxial instability and some minimal changes in the thoracolumbar spine, which are not of much clinical importance, may be seen in McKusick metaphyseal chondrodysplasia (Table 14–1).
- The metaphyseal involvement is more evenly distributed, and there is more shortening and less varus angulation of the long bones than seen in the Schmid type.
- Radiographic changes in the thorax—including changes at the costochondral junctions—Harrison grooves, and a prominent sternum, occur in two thirds of the patients.

Medical Problems

- Immunological abnormalities are found more than half of the patients with McKusick metaphyseal chondrodysplasia.[4]
  - An alteration in T-cell immunity makes these patients susceptible to viral infections in childhood with a predisposition to severe varicella-zoster infections.
  - Continued antibiotic prophylaxis in the first 6 months is recommended.[15]
- These patients have an increased tendency to hematological problems, including lymphopenia, neutropenia, and anemia.
- There is an increased risk of malignancy, such as lymphoma, sarcoma, and skin cancer.
- Hirschsprung disease, intestinal malabsorption, and megacolon may also develop.

Orthopaedic Considerations

- Patients with McKusick metaphyseal chondrodysplasia should be evaluated for atlantoaxial instability, and if significant instability exists, posterior cervical fusion should be performed.
- Genu varum usually improves with growth during the first decade. Rarely, it does not improve but progresses to a severe deformity that requires surgical correction by proximal tibiofibular osteotomy.

Jansen Metaphyseal Chondrodysplasia

- Jansen metaphyseal chondrodysplasia is a rare autosomal dominant disorder characterized by abnormal growth plate maturation and laboratory findings indistinguishable from hyperparathyroidism.
- This disorder is caused by activating mutations in the receptor for parathyroid hormone (PTH) and PTH-related peptide (PTHrP).[3] By somatic cell hybrid analysis, the mutations in the PTH receptor gene have been mapped to chromosome 3 in humans.
- Jansen metaphyseal chondrodysplasia is usually apparent at birth because of severe short stature, severe shortening of the limbs, frontal bossing, widely spaced eyes, and exophthalmos. The angular deformities of the lower limbs and flexion contractures of the major joints may develop.
- Radiographs show bulbous expansion of the metaphyses.
- Abnormal laboratory findings are typical in this disorder and include hypercalcemia, hypophosphatemia, increased renal excretion of phosphate, cAMP, and hydroxyproline, despite normal or undetectable levels of PTH and PTHrP.

Dyschondrosteosis (Leri-Weill Syndrome)

- Dyschondrosteosis is a rare skeletal dysplasia characterized by disproportionate short stature with predominantly mesomelic limb shortening.
- Expression is variable and consistently more severe in females, who frequently display the Madelung deformity of the forearm.
- Dyschondrosteosis is inherited in an autosomal dominant fashion. It is caused by a mutation in the short stature homeobox-containing gene (SHOX) or the SHOX Y-linked gene (SHOXY) located on the X and Y chromosomes.[3] SHOX gene has previously been described as the short stature gene implicated in Turner syndrome. It functions as a repressor for growth plate fusion and skeletal maturation in the distal limbs and, thus, counteracts the skeletal maturing effects of estrogens.

Clinical Features

- The diagnosis is usually made in late childhood or adolescence with short stature or wrist pain and deformity.[16]
- The growth disturbance of the middle segments of the extremities is most notable in the distal radius, causing a Madelung deformity. This deformity results in bowed forearms with wrist pain and limited wrist, forearm, and elbow motion.
- Lower limb changes are usually less severe; only a mild genu varum or ankle valgus exists.
- Short stature is usually a feature; adult height ranges from 135 to 170 cm.

Radiographic Findings

- Radiographic changes are found in the ulna, radius, tibia, and fibula in patients with dyschondrosteosis.

- Madelung deformity is a failure of development of the volar–ulnar part of the distal radial epiphysis. The distal radial epiphysis develops a triangular appearance and a tilt of joint surface. There is shortening, bowing, and broadening of the radius (Figure 14–19, *A*).
- The ulna is also shortened but not to the extent that the radius is shortened. The dorsal subluxation of the distal ulna is also detected (Figure 14–19, *B*).
- The tibia and fibula are short with the fibula longer than the tibia in most patients. Mild genu varum or valgus angulation of the ankle may be seen.

Differential Diagnosis

- The differential diagnosis of dyschondrosteosis includes other disorders associated with bilateral Madelung deformity, such as Turner syndrome, multiple hereditary exostoses, or Ollier disease.
- Trauma (i.e., epiphyseal fractures) may cause premature closure of the ulnar–volar portion of the distal radial epiphysis, producing a similar deformity—although most cases are unilateral.

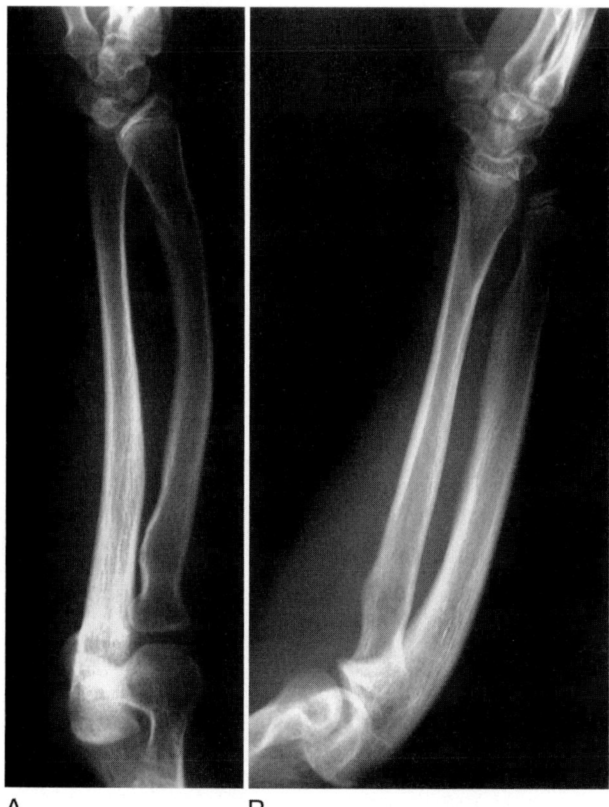

Figure 14–19: Madelung deformity in the forearm of a patient with dyschondrosteosis. A, There is shortening, bowing, and broadening of the radius. B, The ulna is also shortened. Note the dorsal subluxation of the distal ulna. From Erol B, Dormans JP, States L, Kaplan FS (2004) Skeletal dysplasias and metabolic disorders of bone: Musculoskeletal tumors in children. In: Pediatric Orthopaedics and Sports Medicine. (Dormans JP, ed). Philadelphia: Mosby.

Orthopaedic Considerations

- Patients concerned about short stature may be referred to an endocrinologist for discussion of human growth hormone treatment.
- Patients with wrist pain may be treated initially by a wrist splint and nonsteroidal anti-inflammatory agents. If the pain persists, surgical treatment may be considered. Surgical treatment of the Madelung deformity includes realignment osteotomy of the distal radius with shortening of the distal ulna. This procedure improves symptoms and clinical appearance.
- Genu varum and ankle valgus usually do not require surgical correction.

Cleidocranial Dysplasia

- Although its name highlights the two most prominent features of this disorder, this autosomal dominant dysplasia involves multiple skeletal abnormalities, especially in bones of intramembranous origin.
- Classic features of cleidocranial dysplasia include a widening of the cranium and dysplasia of the clavicle and pelvis.
- The prevalence is estimated at 1:200,000.
- Cleidocranial dysplasia is inherited as an autosomal dominant trait. The disease gene has been mapped to chromosome 6 within a region containing core-binding factor α-1 (CBFA1), a member of the runt family of transcription factors.[3] CBFA1 controls differentiation of precursor cells into osteoblasts and is thus essential for intramembranous and endochondral bone formation.

Clinical Features

- Typically, the disease is identified within the first 2 years. The patients have mildly to moderately diminished stature with most female and some male patients below the 5th percentile for age.
- Large, broad, and short cranium; frontal bossing; hypertelorism; a depressed nasal bridge; and midface hypoplasia are typical facial findings. Fontanelles and open sutures persist for years or for life. Cleft palate and dental abnormalities are common.
- The shoulders look droopy, and the upper thorax is narrow. Sternal abnormalities result from the abnormal intramembranous ossification, and pectus excavatum is common.
- The clavicles are partially or completely absent. The most common defect is loss of the lateral end of the clavicle; the second most frequent is failure of development of the middle third of the clavicle.[5]

- Hypermobility of the shoulders is typical; many patients are able to completely appose the shoulders anteriorly (Figure 14–20, *A*).[4,6]
- Coxa vara is a frequent problem and may limit abduction and cause a Trendelenburg gait.
- Kyphoscoliosis occurs in minority of the patients, and it has been reported with syringomyelia in several patients (Figure 14–20, *B*).
- Hand abnormalities include short, tapered fingers and thumb.

Radiographic Findings

- Hypoplasia or absence of the clavicles is obvious on radiographs (Figure 14–20, *C*). Absence of the clavicles has even been seen on prenatal ultrasound.
- Skull radiographs show multiple wormian bones and poor mineralization of the cranium. Closure of the sutures is markedly delayed, and the anterior fontanelle is enlarged.
- The pelvis is narrow with widening of the triradiate cartilage and delay in the ossification of pubic symphysis.
- Hip abnormalities, such as unilateral or bilateral coxa vara, and shortening and broadening of the femoral head and neck are commonly detected.
- Spinal deformities including scoliosis may occur because of abnormal development of ossification centers (Table 14–1). Spina bifida occulta may be present in the thoracic and lumbar spine. Lumbar spondylolysis has also been reported in one fourth of patients.
- Ossification of the carpal and tarsal bones is delayed. There may be underdevelopment of the distal phalanges of fingers.

Orthopaedic Considerations

- Clavicular defects found in patients with cleidocranial dysplasia do not require surgical intervention. These defects are asymptomatic, and attempts to reconstruct the clavicles are not recommended.[4,5]
- The coxa vara is usually progressive and treated by proximal femoral valgus osteotomy if the neck shaft angle is less than 100 degrees.
- If there is acetabular dysplasia, a pelvic osteotomy is recommended to improve the containment of the hip.
- Scoliosis should be treated according to the usual guidelines.

Larsen Syndrome

- Larsen syndrome is characterized by multiple congenital dislocations of large joints, facial dysmorphism, ligamentous laxity, and foot deformities.
- Autosomal dominant and recessive forms have been described. By linkage analysis, the gene for autosomal dominant Larsen syndrome (LAR1) has been mapped to chromosome 3 near (but distinct from) the *COL7A1* locus, but the biochemical defect is unknown.[3]
- Hyperelasticity syndromes, including Marfan syndrome or Ehlers-Danlos syndrome, and arthrogryposis multiplex

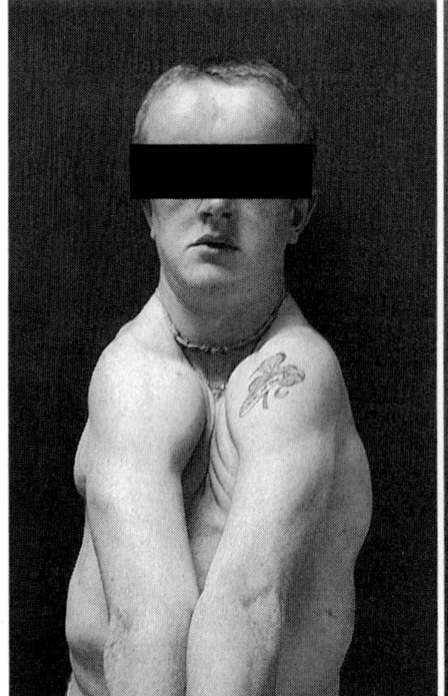
A

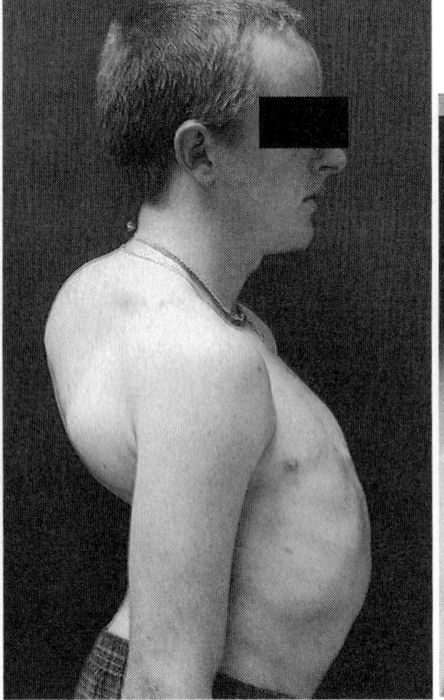
B

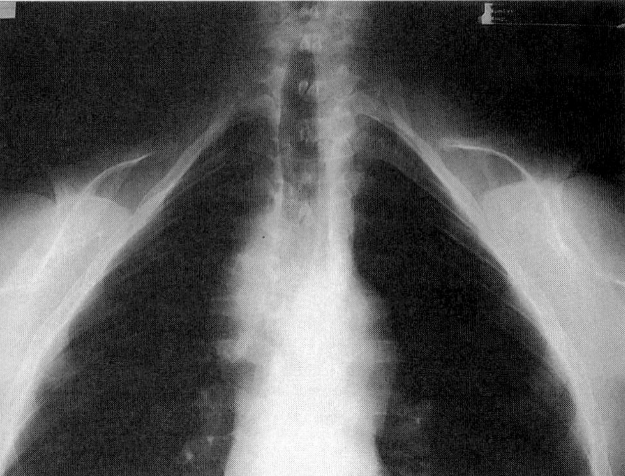
C

Figure 14–20: A, A 20-year-old patient with cleidocranial dysplasia has excessive shoulder mobility. B, The patient has thoracal kyphoscoliosis and increased lumbar lordosis. C, Complete absence of both clavicles contributes to the abnormal appearance of the bell-shaped thorax.

congenita should be kept in the differential diagnosis of Larsen syndrome.

Clinical Features

- Larsen syndrome is recognizable at birth. A broad face with hypertelorism, depressed nasal bridge, and prominent forehead is typical.
- Congenital spinal deformities are frequently seen.[17,18]
  - The cervical spine is the most commonly and severely affected; severe cervical kyphosis or cervical instability may be associated with significant neurological alterations.
  - Scoliosis may affect the thoracic and lumbar spine.
- Ligamentous laxity and congenital joint dislocations, especially of the hips, knees, and elbows, are common.
  - The knee deformity spans a range from simple congenital hyperextension deformity to complete anterior dislocation of the tibia on the femur. The more severe dislocation is common.
  - The hips are often teratologically dislocated with obvious foreshortening of the thighs.
  - The elbows frequently demonstrate radiohumeral dislocation with lateral prominence of the radial heads even in the infant, and there may be more extensive dislocation with a total disruption of the radiocapitellar and the humeroulnar joints.
- The thumb has a wide distal phalanx, and the fingers are cylindrical with broad ends and short nails.
- Characteristic foot deformities include equinovarus and equinovalgus.

Radiographic Findings

- Congenital defects of the cervical, thoracic, and lumbar spine occur frequently in patients with Larsen syndrome (Table 14–1).
  - Cervical spinal defects, including vertebral body hypoplasia (especially C4 and C5), posterior element dysraphism, and segmentation abnormalities may result in severe cervical kyphosis and midcervical instability.
  - Thoracolumbar scoliosis secondary to congenital vertebral anomalies may be seen.
  - In the lumbar spine, spondylolysis and back pain may occur.
  - Sacral spina bifida is common, but no neurological compromise is reported.
- Congenital dislocations of the hips, knees, and elbows are frequently detected.
- One of the characteristic findings in Larsen syndrome is accessory calcaneal or carpal ossification centers. Shortened metacarpals and terminal phalanges are also noted (Figure 14–21).

Orthopaedic Considerations

- Cervical spine problems should be evaluated carefully in patients with Larsen syndrome.[17,18]

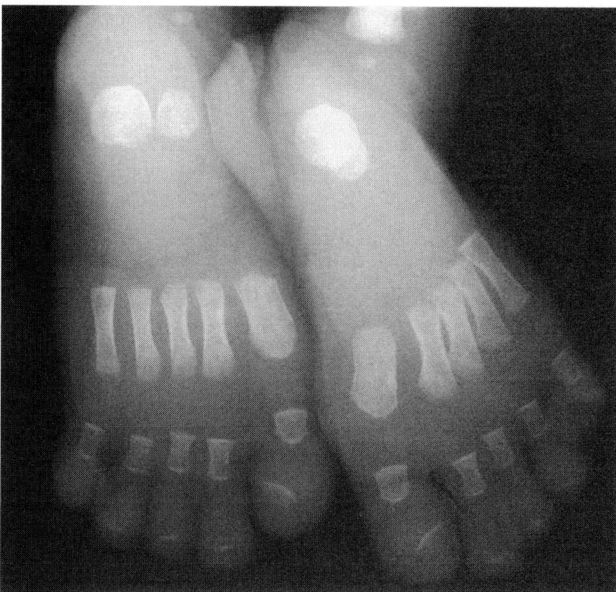

Figure 14–21: Both feet in this infant with Larsen syndrome have short terminal phalanges. The middle phalanges are not ossified. Equinovarus is seen on the right foot, and equinovalgus is seen on the left foot.

  - Cervical kyphosis is usually progressive and requires surgical intervention.
  - The treatment of cervical kyphosis may not be required early in the absence of objective signs of spinal cord compression. Early MRI evaluation is crucial to determine the urgency of stabilization.
  - In infants younger than 12 months, posterior spinal fusion is associated with a definite risk of pseudarthrosis. Therefore delaying the posterior cervical fusion until around 18 months is usually recommended to obtain a higher rate of fusion and subsequent correction of the deformity by continued anterior growth.
  - Posterior fusion alone over the involved segments is usually successful; however, in some severe cases (if the kyphosis progresses to the point of myelopathy) anterior fusion may be required in addition to posterior fusion. After surgery, the patient should be in a brace, halo ring and vest, for 4 to 6 months.
- Approximately half of the patients with Larsen syndrome and scoliosis undergo surgical stabilization.
  - Because of the earlier onset of the deformity, early spinal fusion should be considered to obtain the best results.
  - Most patients will require anterior and posterior fusion to eliminate the crankshaft phenomenon.
- The lower extremity problems in patients with Larsen syndrome are usually treated in a sequence: the feet, the knees, then the hips. These problems usually are resistant to conservative treatment modalities.

- Treatment for clubfeet may be started early, inasmuch as some respond to manipulation and cast treatment with tenotomy. Recurrence is common and should be treated with complete subtalar release and shortening osteotomy or decancellation as necessary.
- Knees that are hyperextended or subluxatable may be treated with casts, but this is unlikely to succeed in cases of complete dislocation.
  1. Open reduction of congenital dislocation of the knee is probably the second most important operative procedure performed, after cervical spine stabilization, if the patient is to have good functional outcome and ambulatory ability as an adult.
  2. The best results are obtained when the knees are reduced by the age of 2.
  3. The traditional treatment consists of open reduction with V-Y quadricepsplasty, anterior capsulotomy, and release of the anterior portions of the collateral ligaments.
  4. If cruciate deficiency leads to persistent anterior instability, reconstruction using parapatellar fascia is usually successful.
- Congenital dislocation of the hip may seem teratological in patients with Larsen syndrome, but closed reduction and stabilization have been successfully performed.
  1. Knee hyperextension and congenital dislocation of the hip can be treated simultaneously in the neonate by a Pavlik harness.[5] If hip stability is not achieved with the harness, maintaining the knees in flexion is still beneficial for subsequent closed or open reduction of the hips, which will then be immobilized in a spica cast.
  2. Attempts to reduce the hip with close methods may fail frequently, and open reduction is required. Anterior open reduction and capsulorrhaphy of the hip is best performed around the age of 1. If the ipsilateral hip and knee are both dislocated, surgical treatment of both joints in the same extremity should be combined.

Multiple Hereditary Exostoses

- Multiple hereditary exostoses are among the most common skeletal dysplasias seen by orthopaedic surgeons with an estimated prevalence of approximately 1 in 18,000.
- It is characterized by cartilage-capped prominences that develop from the epiphyses of the long bones.
- The disorder is of autosomal dominant inheritance with penetrance approaching 96%.[5] Numerous genetic studies have found anomalies on at least three genes, termed *exostosin* (EXT) genes, making this a genetically heterogeneous disorder. The three described EXT loci have been recently mapped: EXT1 on chromosome 8, EXT2 on chromosome 11, and EXT3 on chromosome 19.[3] According to linkage analysis, the EXT1 and EXT2 loci appear to be altered in most families and EXT3, which has not been fully isolated and characterized, is probably less frequently affected. EXT1 and EXT2 function as tumor-suppressor genes and encode two homologous glycoproteins expressed throughout the musculoskeletal system. Both glycoproteins are glycosyltransferases that are located in the membrane of the endoplasmic reticulum and that have a role in modifying and enhancing the synthesis and expression of heparan sulfate. Heparan sulfate is a complex polysaccharide implicated in a variety of cellular processes, including cell adhesion, growth factor signaling, and cell proliferation.
- The gross pathological and microscopical features of multiple hereditary exostoses are similar to those described for solitary osteochondromas.

Clinical Features

- The exostoses usually appear after 3 to 4 years. On presentation, five or six exostoses typically may be found involving both the upper and the lower limbs.
- Over time, the upper and lower extremities may appear short in relation to the trunk. Shortening of the limbs is usually disproportionate.
- Affected persons are at the low end of normal for stature.
- Distal femur, proximal tibia, proximal humerus, scapula and ribs, proximal fibula, and distal radius and ulna are the most commonly involved sites.[20]
- Problems from this condition may be divided into four categories: (1) local prominence and impingement by the exostoses; (2) asymmetrical growth of two-bone segments, such as the forearm and the leg; (3) limb length inequality; and (4) late degeneration into chondrosarcoma.
  - Local prominence may cause pressure on muscles, tendons, or nerves, resulting in pain, limited motion (e.g., forearm motion), or nerve palsy (i.e., peroneal palsy from a proximal fibular lesion).
  - Asymmetrical growth often results in angular deformities of the upper and lower limbs (Figure 14–22). Valgus may develop at the wrist, knee, and ankle. The natural history of these deformities has been described as progressive with variable weakness, functional impairment, and worsening cosmetic deformity of the extremity.
  - Limb length inequality is common because one limb is more involved than the other.
  - Malignant transformation in the pediatric age group is rare and is difficult to monitor. The most practical way is educating patients and parents about signs of malignant transformation, such as increased growth of an exostosis or pain over an exostosis.

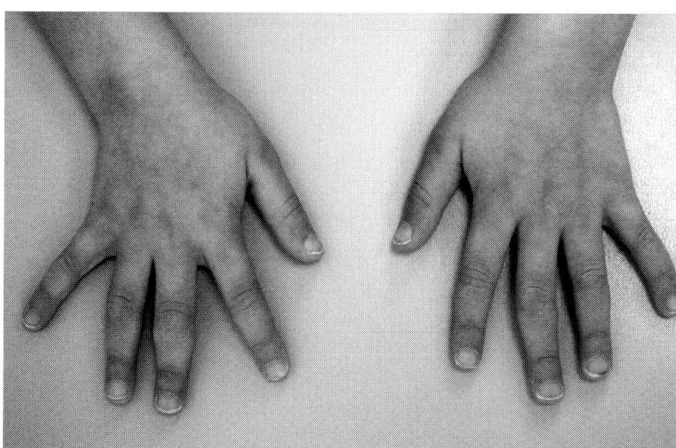

Figure 14–22: A 7-year-old boy with multiple hereditary exostoses. Note the angular deformities of the fingers.

Radiographic Findings

- Unlike solitary osteochondromas, multiple hereditary exostoses involve a significantly greater portion of the metaphysis or diaphysis and are generally more irregular in shape. Over time, lesions that begin in the metaphyseal region migrate into the diaphysis of the long bones.
- The exostoses vary in number, size, and configuration.
- Like solitary osteochondromas, they may grow perpendicular to the bone in a sessile or pedunculated fashion (Figure 14–23). They nearly always point away from the physis.
- The cortex of the exostosis is contiguous with that of the bone.
- Exostoses on the undersurface of the scapula may be identified on plain films but are best evaluated by CT.
- The ulna is shorter than the radius, and the radius is bowed laterally with its concavity toward the short ulna. Often the distal end of the ulna is more severely affected than the distal end of the radius, leading to this discrepancy in length (Figure 14–24). Subluxation–dislocation of the radial head occurs and is usually associated with a negative ulnar variance.
- The femoral necks are usually wide and in valgus (Figure 14–25). Genu valgum and ankle valgus may be seen.

Orthopaedic Considerations

- Because the lesions are numerous and multiple bones are affected, a careful evaluation of the upper and lower limbs, including range of motion of the joints, neurological examination, and measurement of the angular deformities, should be performed.[19]

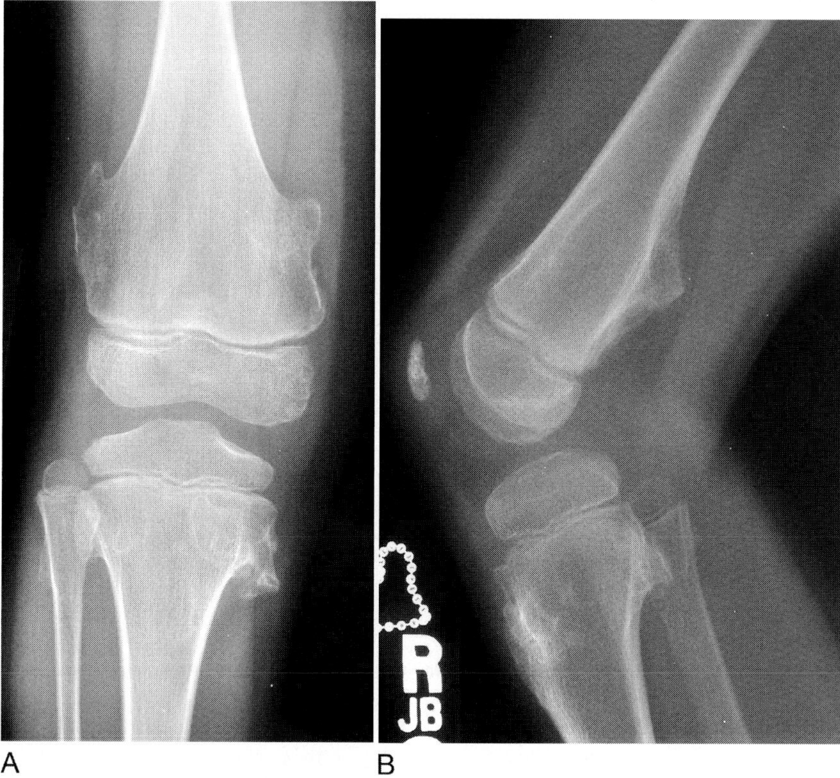

Figure 14–23: A and B, Wide based, bony protuberances are seen in the distal femur, proximal tibia, and proximal fibula. The cortex is continuous with the bone. A normal trabecular pattern is seen.

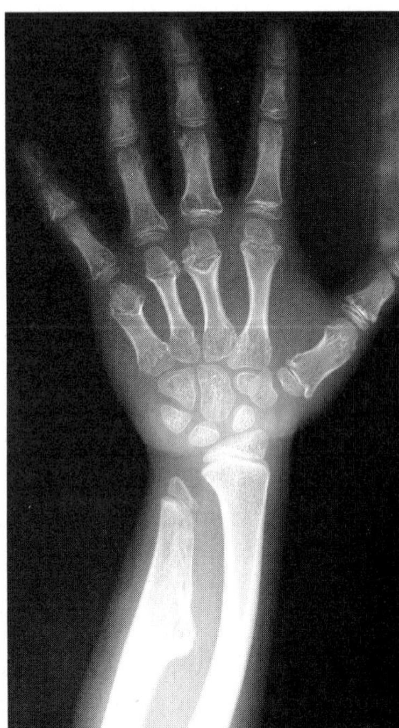

Figure 14–24: An 8-year-old girl with multiple hereditary exostoses. The ulna is shorter than the radius, and the radius is bowed laterally with its concavity toward the short ulna. The distal end of ulna is more severely affected than the distal end of the radius, leading to discrepancy in length.

- Any exostoses causing significant symptoms should be excised. Reasonable indications include pain, growth disturbance leading to angular deformity or limb length discrepancy, joint motion compromised by juxta-articular lesions, soft tissue impingement or tethering, false aneurysm produced by an osteochondroma, painful bursa formation, obvious cosmetic deformity, and rapid growth of a lesion.
- Osteochondromas involving the forearm frequently lead to surgical intervention.
  - Early excision of the lesions on the radius and ulna does not alter or correct an existing deformity, but it may delay progression of the deformity.
  - If ulnar shortening has occurred with bowing of the radius, lengthening of the ulna with distal radial osteotomy or hemiepiphysiodesis has been found to effectively correct the deformity.
  - Painful radial head dislocations can be safely excised following skeletal maturity.
- Significant valgus deformities of the knee and ankle are treated by osteotomy or hemiepiphysiodesis when young or corrective varus osteotomy when older (near maturity).
- Epiphysiodesis is the most appropriate treatment for significant limb length inequality in growing patients.

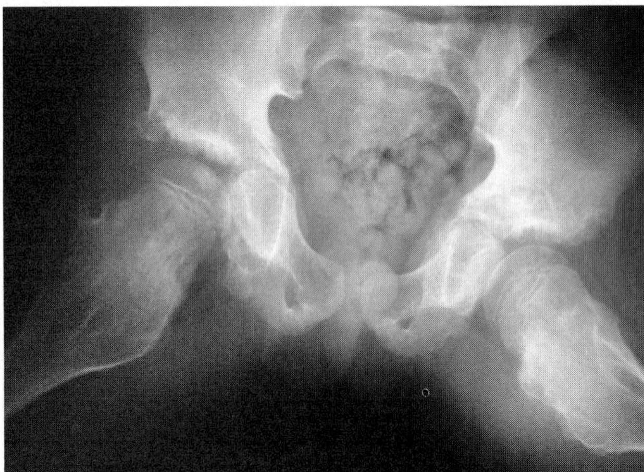

Figure 14–25: In both proximal femora, multiple exostoses cause widening of the femoral necks. Bilateral coxa valga is seen. Irregularity of the bones of the pelvis is caused by small exostoses.

References

1. Beighton P, Giedion ZA, Gorlin R, Hall J, Horton B, Kozlowski K, Lachman R, Langer LO, Maroteaux P, Poznanski A (1992) International classification of osteochondrodysplasias. Am J Med Genet 44: 223.

   The authors report histological findings that suggest an uncoupling of endochondral and perichondral growth that explains the dumbbell-shaped morphological structure of the osseous metaphysis seen in patients who have metatropic dysplasia.

2. Dietz FR, Matthews KD (1996) Current concepts review: Update on the genetic bases of disorders with orthopaedic manifestations. J Bone Joint Surg 78A: 1583.

3. McKusick VA, ed (2000) Online Mendelian Inheritance in Man. Baltimore: McKusick-Nathans Institute for Genetic Medicine, John Hopkins University. Bethesda, MD: National Center for Biotechnology Information, National Library of Medicine. http://www.ncbi.nlm.nih.gov/entrez/query.fcgi?db=OMIM.

4. Sponseller PD (2001) The skeletal dysplasias. In: Lovell and Winter's Pediatric Orthopaedics, 5th edition (Morrisy RT, Weinstein SL, eds). Philadelphia: Lippincott Williams & Wilkins.

5. Herring JA (2002) Tachdjian's Pediatric Orthopaedics, 3rd edition. Philadelphia: WB Saunders.

6. Jones KL (1997) Smith's Recognizable Patterns of Human Malformations, 5th edition. Philadelphia: WB Saunders.

7. Fasanelli S (1999) Hypochondroplasia: Radiological diagnosis and differential diagnosis. In: Achondroplasia: Human Achondroplasia, a Multidisciplinary Approach (Nicoletti B, ed). New York: Plenum.

8. Boden SD, Kaplan FS, Fallon MD, Ruddy R, Belik J, Anday E, Zackai E, Ellis J (1987) Metatropic dwarfism: Uncoupling of endochondral and perichondral growth. J Bone Joint Surg 69A: 174.

Review of spinal deformities associated with Larsen syndrome consisting of vertebral anomalies, spondylolysis, and scoliosis.

9. Tolo VT, Kopits SE (1983) Spinal deformity in diastrophic dysplasia. Orthop Trans 7.

10. Gilbert-Barnes E, Langer LO (1996) Kniest dysplasia: Radiologic, histopathologic, and scanning EM findings. Am J Med Genet 63: 34.
    Radiographic and histologic features of severe neonatal Kniest dysplasia. Radiologically, bone are short, bowed, and tubular with an exaggerated metaphyseal flare; vertebral bodies exhibit moderate platyspondyly with vertical clefts. Pathological findings showed a disorganized physeal growth plate; soft, crumbly cartilage with a "Swiss cheese" appearance; and diastase-resistant intracytoplasmic inclusions in the resting chondrocytes.

11. Wynne-Davies R, Hall C (1982) Two clinical variants of spondyloepiphyseal dysplasia congenita. J Bone Joint Surg 64B: 435.
    The authors report 17 cases of congenital SED including two variants. The authors conclude that both groups can be diagnosed at birth, but the two cannot be differentiated on clinical and radiological grounds until after 3 years, when the developing severe coxa vara and difference in stature become apparent.

12. Crossan JF, Wynne-Davis R, Fulford GE (1986) Bilateral failure of the capital femoral epiphysis: Bilateral Perthes disease, multiple epiphyseal dysplasia, pseudoachondroplasia, and spondyloepiphyseal dysplasia. Pediatr Orthop 8: 197.
    The authors compare a series of 25 patients with bilateral Perthes disease to cases of inherited skeletal dysplasias also affecting the hip joints.

13. MacKenzie WG, Bassett GS, Mandell GA, Scott CI Jr (1989) Avascular necrosis of the hip in multiple epiphyseal dysplasia. J Pediatr Orthop 9: 666.
    The authors observed radiographic changes of avascular necrosis of the capital femoral epiphysis in nine hips of 11 patients with MED, with plain roentgenography, bone scintigraphy, and MRI studies.

14. Sheffield LJ, Halliday JL, Danks DM, et al. (1989) Clinical, radiologic, and biochemical classification of chondrodysplasia punctata. Am J Med Gen 45 (suppl. A): A64.

15. Makitie O, Kaitila I (1993) Cartilage–hair hypoplasia: Clinical manifestations in 108 Finnish patients. Eur J Pediatr 152: 211.
    Review of the clinical characteristics of 108 patients with cartilage-hair hypoplasia.

16. Cook PA, Yu JS, Wiand W, Lubbers L, Coleman CR, Cook AJ 2nd, Kean JR, Cook AJ (1996) Madelung deformity in skeletally immature patients: Morphologic assessment using radiography, CT and MRI. J Comput Assist Tomogr 20: 505.
    Radiographic features of skeletally immature patients with the Madelung deformity.

17. Laville JM, Lakermore P, Limouzy F (1994) Larsen's syndrome: Review of the literature and analysis of thirty-eight cases. J Pediatr Orthop 14: 63.
    The authors report 38 cases of Larsen syndrome with an average follow-up of 13 years.

18. Bowen JR, Ortega K, Ray S, MacEwen GD (1985) Spinal deformities in Larsen's syndrome. Clin Orthop 197: 159.

19. Erol B, Dormans JP, States L, Kaplan FS (2004) Skeletal dysplasias and metabolic disorders of bone. In: Pediatric Orthopaedics and Sports Medicine: The Requisites in Pediatrics (Dormans JP, ed), Philadelphia: Mosby.

20. Steiber JR, Dormans JP (In Press) Manifestations of hereditary multiple exostoses. J Am Acad Orthop Surg.

CHAPTER 15

Metabolic Disorders of Bone

Bülent Erol* and John P. Dormans†

*MD, Attending Surgeon, Department of Orthopaedic Surgery, The Hospital of University of Marmara, Marmara University School of Medicine, Istanbul, Turkey
†MD, Chief of Orthopaedic Surgery, The Children's Hospital of Philadelphia, Philadelphia, PA; Professor of Orthopaedic Surgery, University of Pennsylvania School of Medicine, Philadelphia, PA

- Metabolic bone disease can be defined as impairment of the shape, strength, and composition of bone because of altered bone mineral homeostasis.
- The major factors affecting this homeostasis are the ions, hormones, and signal transduction pathways. Intracellular and extracellular levels of three ions (calcium, phosphorus, and magnesium), which are regulated by three hormones (parathyroid hormone, or PTH; calcitonin; and 1,25-dihydroxyvitamin D), act upon three tissues (bone, intestine, and kidney) to provide this homeostasis. Other minerals, hormones, and target tissues are involved, making these diseases a complex interaction of many exogenous and endogenous factors.
- Frequent clinical features include electrolyte disturbances, fractures, bone deformities, abnormal gait, and short stature.
- The most common forms of metabolic bone disease in children are the various types of rickets and renal osteodystrophy.

Mineral Metabolism

Calcium and Phosphorus Homeostasis

- Three principles govern calcium and phosphate shifts in the body.[1]
  - First, if the concentrations of Ca_2^+ and HPO_4^- exceed the critical solubility product, ectopic calcification will occur. The solubility of the $CaHPO_4$ salt is increased (consequently, the tendency for ectopic calcification is decreased) by mild to moderate acidosis.
  - Second, the irritability and conductivity of nervous tissue and muscle tissue (smooth and skeletal muscle) are inversely proportional, and the irritability and conductivity of cardiac muscle is directly proportional, to the concentrations of Ca_2^+. The margin of safety is small. With hypocalcemia, there is hypertonia, hyperreflexia, convulsions, and death in diastole. With hypercalcemia, there is hypotonicity, hyperreflexia, obtundation and death in systole.
  - Third, calcium can not cross cell membranes without a transport system. The cell barrier-transport system for calcium includes 1,25-dihydroxyvitamin D (activated vitamin D), cytosolic phosphate, and to a lesser extent PTH. The 1,25-dihydroxyvitamin D increases the synthesis of calcium-binding proteins such as calbindin or cholecalcin, the phosphate acts at the membrane transport level, and the PTH acts through adenyl cyclase–adenosine 3′,5′-cyclic monophosphate (cAMP) to increase calcium entry to the intracellular space and to activate the release of calcium from the mitochondria. The major controller is 1,25-dihydroxyvitamin D; phosphate acts only by turning off the entry of calcium at a critical level (and therefore protecting against ectopic calcification). The role of PTH is primarily to balance the action of vitamin D through its differential effects on calcium and phosphorus metabolism.

Biology of Vitamin D

- The provitamins D consist of ergosterol ingested in the form of animal fats and 7-dehydrocholesterol synthesized in the liver.
  - Both of these metabolically inactive sterols are stored in the skin and, in the presence of ultraviolet light, are converted to ergocalciferol (vitamin D2) and cholecalciferol (vitamin D3).
  - After transportation to the liver, they are converted to 25-hydroxyvitamin D.
  - The final and most critical conversion occurs in the kidney, where 25-hydroxyvitamin D is converted to either the less active 24,25-dihydroxyvitamin D or the highly active 1,25-dihydroxy form (Figure 15–1).
  - A low serum calcium level, a low serum phosphate level, and a high PTH level favor conversion to the 1,25 analog. On the other hand, a high serum calcium level, a high serum phosphate level, and a low PTH level favor formation of the less potent 24,25-dihydroxyvitamin D.
- The 1,25-dihydroxyvitamin D controls calcium metabolism in the gut, proximal tubule, and bone.
  - The major function is to increase the efficiency of the small intestine to absorb dietary calcium and transfer it into the circulation.
  - It also increases calcium absorption from the proximal tubules.
  - In bone, vitamin D enhances the mobilization of calcium stores when dietary calcium is inadequate to maintain serum blood calcium levels within the normal range.

Biology of Parathyroid Hormone

- PTH is synthesized in the parathyroid glands from a biosynthetic precursor pro-PTH.
- Serum calcium levels carefully regulate release of the hormone: the lower the serum calcium level, the more PTH is synthesized and elaborated.
- Maintenance of extracellular calcium homeostasis is the primary role of PTH. Its action is synergistic with 1,25-dihydroxyvitamin D, which is to increase calcium transport from the gut and renal tubules and to promote calcium release from the bone (lysis of hydroxyapatite crystals).
- PTH acts independent of vitamin D to activate the osteoclast population to resorb bone. Another action of PTH (also independent of vitamin D) is to diminish the tubular reabsorption of phosphate.

Maintenance of Serum Calcium

- Multicellular organisms require a highly regulated concentration of calcium in the extracellular fluid. The absorption of calcium from the gastrointestinal tract, the reabsorption of calcium from the renal tubule, and the bone–blood exchange are the three major components of the calcium control system.
  - All these components are under the control of the 1,25-dihydroxyvitamin D and PTH synergistic transport system. The lowered serum calcium

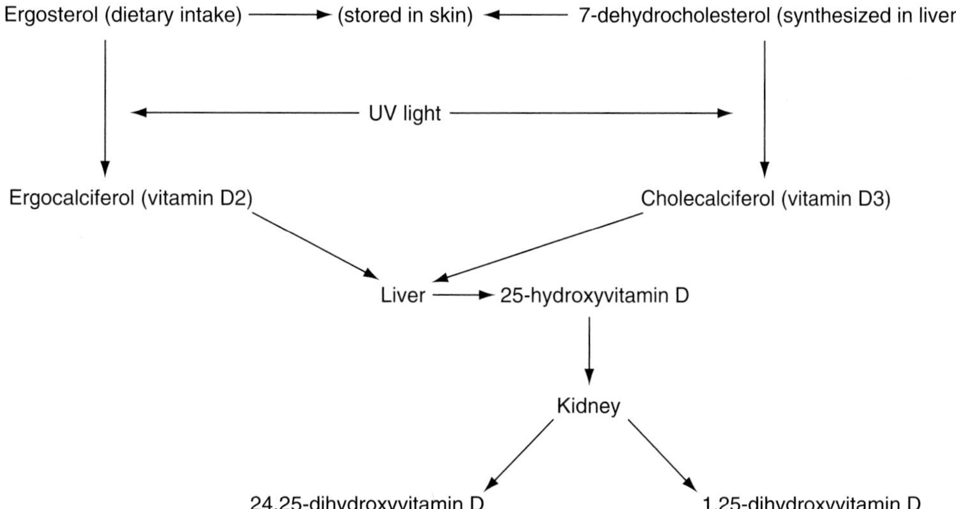

Figure 15–1: Biology of vitamin D. The provitamins D (ergosterol and 7-dehydrocholesterol) are stored in the skin and, in the presence of ultraviolet light, are converted to ergocalciferol (vitamin D2) and cholecalciferol (vitamin D3). In the liver, vitamin D2 and vitamin D3 are converted to 25-hydroxyvitamin D. The final step is in the kidney, where 25-hydroxyvitamin D is converted to less active 24, 25-dihydroxyvitamin D or highly active 1,25-dihydroxyvitamin D. From Erol B, Dormans JP, States L, Kaplan FS (2004) Skeletal dysplasias and metabolic disorders of bone. Musculoskeletal Tumors in Children. In Dormans JP (ed) Pediatric Orthopaedics and Sports Medicine. Philadelphia: Mosby.

level stimulates the production and release of PTH, which activates the synthesis of 1,25-dihydroxyvitamin D. Together, the two agents increase calcium absorption from the gut, tubular reabsorption of filtered calcium in the kidney, and resorption of bone (Figure 15–2).
  - Bone resorption occurs by lysis of the crystalline apatite through osteoclastic resorption.
  - Any excess phosphate that appears as a result of the breakdown of bone, under the influence of PTH, is rapidly excreted by the kidney by a marked decrease in the tubular reabsorption of phosphate.
  - In this manner, short-term calcium deficits, even if profound, may be rapidly corrected by a highly effective balance system.[2]

Rickets

- Rickets is a syndrome rather than a specific disease entity.
- Despite the numerous etiological pathways, the main cause of the disorder is the lack of available extracellular calcium, phosphorus, or both, which interferes with physeal growth and mineralization of the skeleton and results in clinical deformities in the growing child.
- The lack of calcium and phosphorus may be caused by inadequate intake of calcium and vitamin D, impaired absorption of phosphorus or vitamin D, decreased conversion of vitamin D to its active form, organ insensitivity to vitamin D, impaired release of calcium from bone, and phosphate wasting (Box 15–1).
- The clinical presentation, histological abnormalities, and radiographic changes are similar in many of the etiologies of rickets with the exception of renal osteodystrophy.
- In rickets, the primary disturbance in bone is failed calcification of cartilage and osteoid tissue.
  - There is failed deposition of calcium along the mature cartilage cell columns followed by disorderly invasion of cartilage by blood vessels, lack of reabsorption at the zone of provisional calcification, and increased thickness of the growth plate.
  - The chondrocytes multiply normally, but the normal process of maturation of cartilage columns fails to take place.
  - There is also failed mineralization of newly formed bone. Osteoid formation proceeds normally; however, osteoclastic resorption of the uncalcified osteoid does not take place. Mineralized segments are surrounded by a layer of unmineralized bone–osteoid seam, which helps to establish the diagnosis.[3]

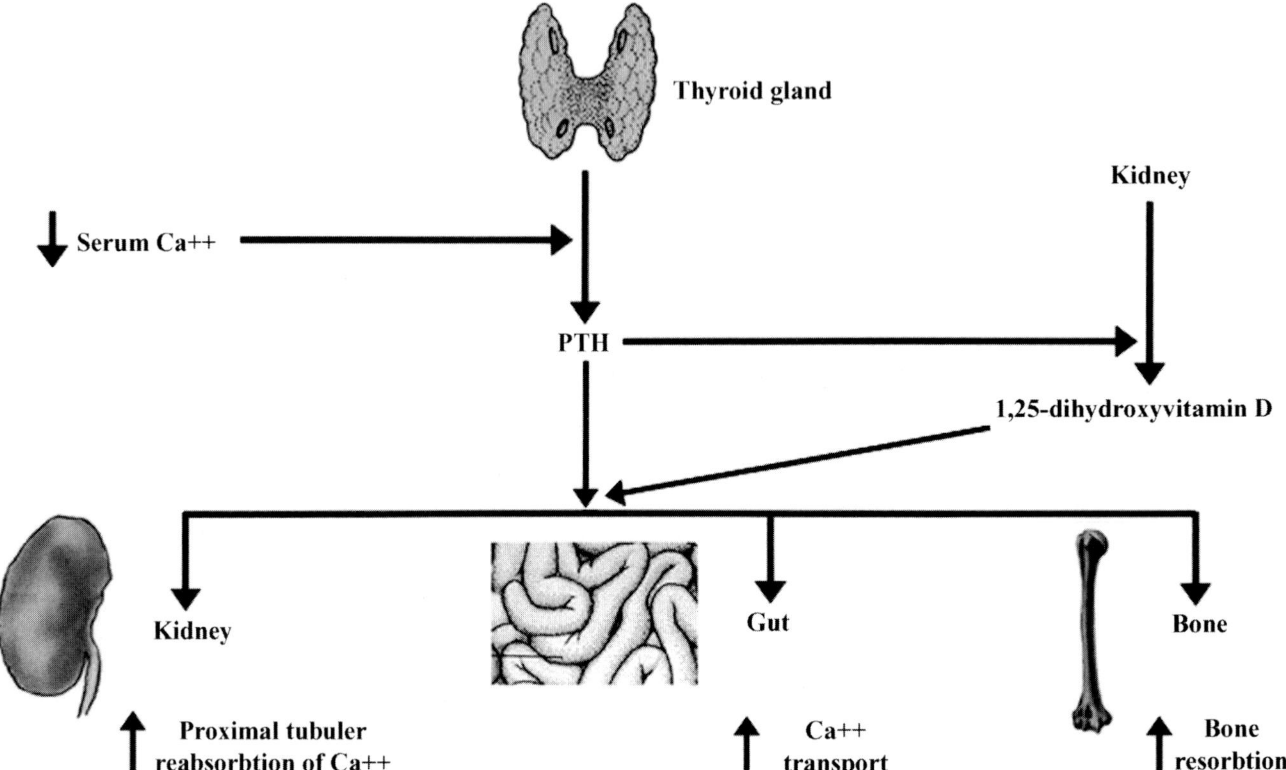

Figure 15–2: Maintenance of serum calcium. The lowered serum calcium level stimulates the production and release of PTH from parathyroid glands. PTH activates the synthesis of 1,25-dihydroxyvitamin D in the kidney. These agents act together to increase tubular reabsorption of filtered calcium in the kidney, calcium transport in the gut, and bone resorption.

Box 15–1 Causes of Rickets

- Deficiency diseases
  - Vitamin D-deficient rickets (inadequate intake of vitamin D with or without sunlight)
  - Chelators in the diet (e.g., phytates and oxalates)
  - Phosphorus deficiency
- Gastrointestinal disorders
  - Gastric rickets
  - Hepatobiliary rickets (free fatty acids in gut bind calcium)
  - Enteric rickets (e.g., inflammatory bowel disease)
- Vitamin D-resistant rickets
  - Hypophosphatemic rickets (decreased tubular reabsorption of phosphate)
  - Decrease in 1,25-dihydroxyvitamin D production
  - Organ insensitivity to autogenous 1,25-dihydroxyvitamin D
  - Renal tubular acidosis
- Unusual forms of rickets
  - Rickets with soft tissue and bone tumors
  - Rickets with fibrous dysplasia
  - Rickets with neurofibromatosis
  - Rickets with anticonvulsant medications
- Renal osteodystrophy

Vitamin D-Resistant Rickets

- Vitamin D-resistant rickets is frequently seen by pediatric orthopaedic surgeons.
- Hypophosphatemic rickets, also known as *phosphate diabetes*, is the common form of vitamin D-resistant rickets and is characterized by a renal tubular defect in phosphate transport.
  - Hypophosphatemic rickets is commonly transmitted as an X-linked dominant disorder. The gene responsible for this disorder was identified by positional cloning and designated PHEX (formerly PEX) to depict a phosphate-regulating gene with homology to endopeptidases on the X chromosome. It appears that this enzyme plays an important role in cleaving endogenous fibroblast growth factor-23, a potent phosphaturic hormone.[4] X-linked, dominant hypophosphatemic rickets is fully expressed in hemizygous male patients. Isolated hypophosphatemia may signify the trait in heterozygous females. With full expression, the condition consists of hypophosphatemia, lower limb deformities, and stunted growth.

Laboratory Findings

- The main diagnostic laboratory tests in rickets include serum calcium, phosphate, alkaline phosphatase, and PTH levels. Other laboratory tests, including serum vitamin D, urine calcium, and urine phosphate levels, may also be helpful.
- In infancy, abnormal laboratory values may be the only findings in a child with rickets.
- In classic or vitamin D-deficient rickets, vitamin D deficiency results in inability to absorb calcium and phosphorus. PTH is released in response to hypocalcemia, which corrects the serum calcium deficit, but hypophosphatemia persists. Serum calcium levels are normal to mildly decreased, phosphate levels are low, and vitamin D levels are decreased, but PTH and alkaline phosphatase levels are high.

Clinical Features

- Children with rickets usually have generalized muscular weakness, lethargy, and irritability. Sitting, standing, and walking are delayed.
- The affected children usually have short stature, often under the 3rd percentile.
- Frontal bossing and enlargement of the suture lines (i.e., caput quadratum) are common. Delayed dentition, enamel defects, and extensive caries are common dental abnormalities.
- Examination of the chest is likely to show enlargement of the costal cartilages (i.e., rachitic rosary), indentation of the lower ribs where the diaphragm inserts (i.e., Harrison groove), and occasionally pectus carinatum.
- The spine is commonly affected, most characteristically with a long thoracic kyphosis.
- Ligamentous laxity is a common finding in children with rickets.
- The long bones are deformed and shortened, usually with bowing abnormalities in the lower limbs. General guidelines are that a disease that manifests during the stage of physiological bowing (age 1-2) results in varus and that an active disease during the stage of physiological genu valgum (age 2-4) produces valgus deformity.[2]
- Upper limbs usually do not have significant deformities.
- Apparent enlargement of the elbows, wrists, knees, and ankles may be detected in physical examination and are caused by metaphyseal enlargement.
- Fractures are common.

Radiographic Findings

- General radiographic findings include osteopenia, thin cortices, and small trabecula with overall decreased bone mass.
  - The osteopenia is more marked in the metaphyses, giving a "washed out" appearance.
  - The cortices, vertebral endplates, and trabeculae often appear fuzzy and indistinct.
- The appearance of the growth plates, including irregular widening or cupping, forms the most classical finding (Figure 15–3).[2,3]
- Looser's lines are ribbon-like linear radiolucencies extending transversely from one cortex across the medullary canal, and represent areas of weakening or

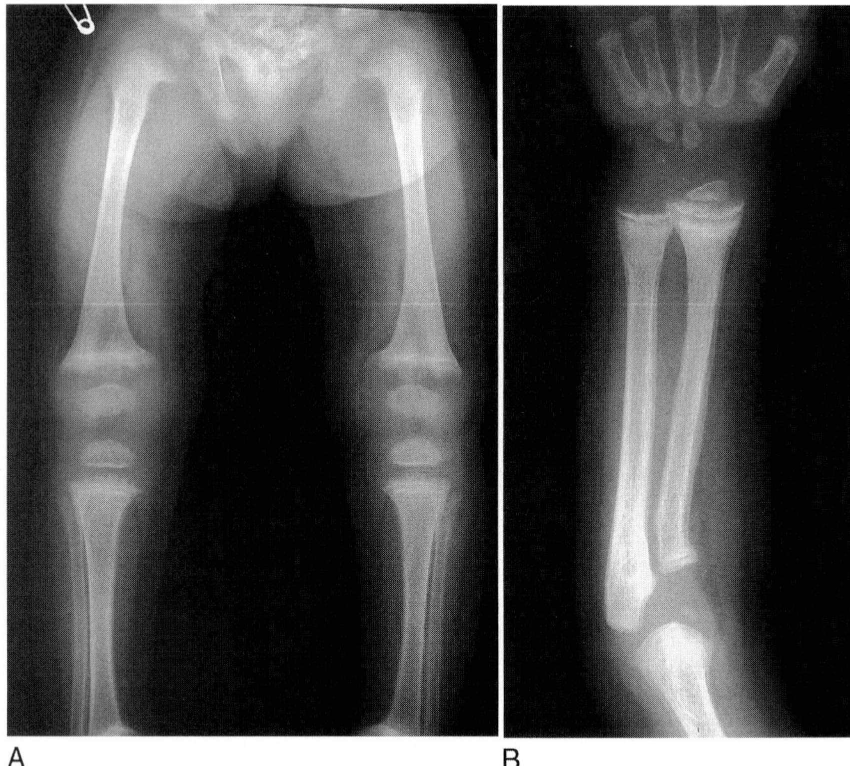

Figure 15–3: The radiographic findings of rickets are most easily seen at the sites of most active growth, the knees and wrists. A, In a 3-year-old boy with active rickets, all the long bones at the knee have widened growth plates with washed-out, irregular metaphyses. Some of the metaphyses have a feathery "paintbrush" appearance. Note the characteristic cupping of the metaphyses and generalized osteopenia. B, The forearm and wrist of a different child depicts dense metaphyseal bands indicating a period of healing. Subcortical tunneling is seen along the radius, ulna, and metacarpals. Generalized osteopenia is seen.

incomplete fractures. They may become complete transverse fractures, sometimes with only minor trauma.

- Bowing of the femur and tibia, and angular deformities of the lower extremities including coxa vara, genu varum, or genu valgum are common radiographic findings (Figure 15–4).

Differential Diagnosis

- Osteomalacia, the adult counterpart of rickets, is also characterized by excessive amounts of unmineralized osteoid, resulting in skeletal deformity. However, it occurs only after the physes have closed and lacks the growth disturbances seen in patients with rickets.
- Physiological genu varum or valgum, Blount's disease, and some skeletal dysplasias with angular deformities of the knee should be considered in the differential diagnosis of rickets.
  - In physiological genu varum or valgum and Blount's disease, the child has no other findings; the stature and development are within normal range.[2,3]
  - Metaphyseal, epiphyseal, or other skeletal dysplasias such as achondroplasia and hypochondroplasia may be associated with short stature and multiple skeletal abnormalities, including angular deformities of the knee.[5]

Renal Osteodystrophy

- Renal osteodystrophy includes bone diseases that occur as a result of renal failure. Improved management of renal bone disease has decreased the incidence of renal osteodystrophy.[1,2]
- In renal osteodystrophy, glomerular damage leads to phosphate retention, and tubular injury causes decreased production of 1,25-dihydroxyvitamin D, the active form of vitamin D. These two factors severely inhibit the gut's ability to absorb calcium. The resultant hypocalcemia triggers severe secondary hyperparathyroidism, which remains ineffective in increasing intestinal absorption of calcium. Therefore, the body's only means of increasing serum calcium levels is by bone resorption.
- Patients with chronic renal disease are hyperphosphatemic, and even when there is reduced pH, which shifts the solubility product, they depend on decreased serum calcium to avoid precipitation of the relatively insoluble $CaHPO_4$. If for any reason (e.g., dietary indiscretion, spontaneous improvement, or dialysis) calcium increases to near-normal levels, calcium salts may be precipitated at a variety of ectopic sites.[2]

Clinical Findings

- Patients with renal osteodystrophy may have all the features of rickets.
- The bones are fragile, and fractures occur frequently with minor trauma.
- Calcification in the conjunctivae and skin can produce significant irritation and itching.
- The periarticular calcification and ossification can cause severe limitation and pain in one or more joints.

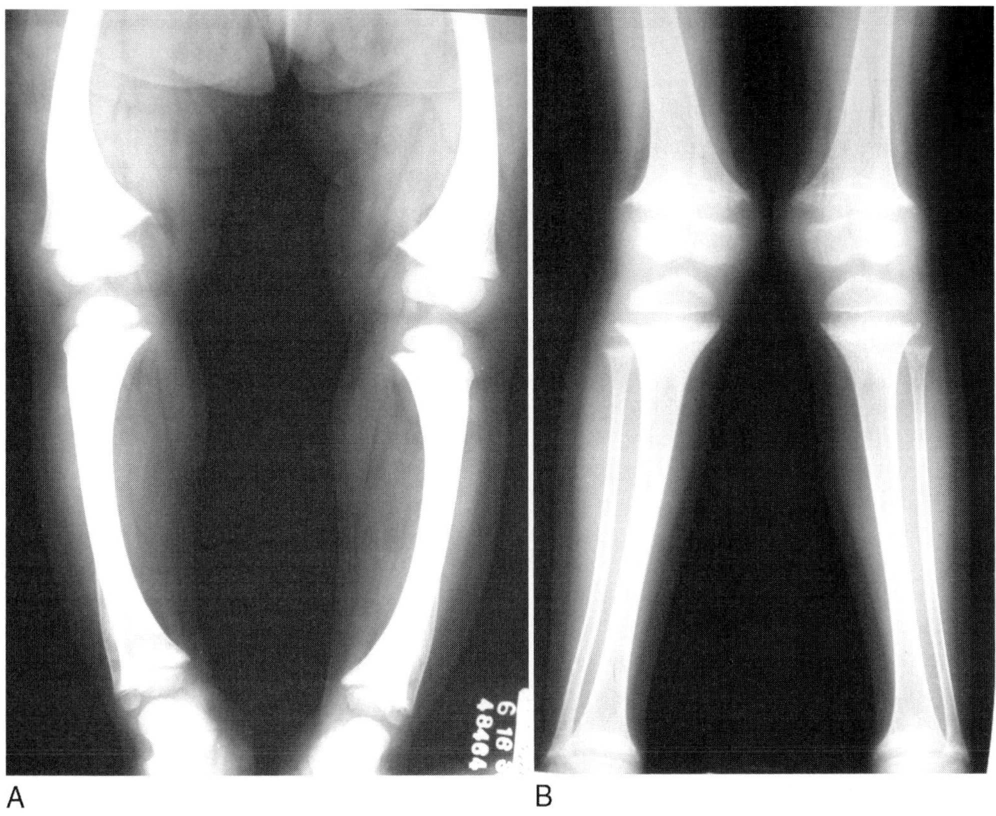

Figure 15–4: A, Genu varum in a 2-year-old patient with rickets. Both femurs, tibias, and fibulas are bowed. B, Genu valgum in a 4-year-old patient with active rickets. The physes are widened, and the metaphyses are cupped and irregular.

- Ligamentous laxity and muscle weakness may be seen.
- Slipped epiphyses, especially in the proximal femur (slipped capital femoral epiphysis, or SCFE), occur frequently.
- Genu valgum is the most commonly seen deformity in the lower extremities, but genu varum may occur in some patients.

Radiographic Features

- Radiographic changes seen in renal osteodystrophy are unique and include a "salt and pepper" skull, the absence of a cortical outline of the outer centimeter of the clavicles, and subperiosteal resorption of the ulnas, terminal tufts of the distal phalanges, and medial proximal tibias.
- Slipped epiphyses and valgus alignment of the knees are also frequently seen in patients with renal osteodystrophy.
- Brown tumors appear as expanded destructive bone lesions and are usually round or ovoid with indistinct margins.
  - These lesions are caused by secondary hyperparathyroidism and are most common in cases of severe and long-standing renal osteodystrophy.
  - Brown tumors may be present in the long bones or pelvis and, when associated with thinning of the cortex, may be the site of pathological fractures.

Treatment of Rickets and Renal Osteodystrophy

- The role of the orthopaedic surgeon has shifted considerably with the understanding of the basic science of disorders associated with rickets and renal osteodystrophy.
- Medical treatment of the underlying metabolic disturbance, coordinated by a pediatrician or a pediatric endocrinologist, is the necessary first step in the management of rachitic disease. Because it alone may be curative, the general health of the individual depends on it and orthopaedic intervention without it will disappoint.
  - In rickets, medical treatment aims to correct the altered physiology with agents such as vitamin D, 1, 25-dihydroxyvitamin D, calcium infusions, neutral phosphate solutions, and other dietary and pharmacological interventions.
  - The extent of remodeling likely to occur depends on the growth remaining after correction of the abnormal physiology. It is usually possible to achieve a cure in many rickets patients with expectations of normal growth and lifestyle.
- In the presence of a fracture or when the deformity exceeds the physiological range and predisposes the

individual to progressive deformity or altered mechanical alignment, orthopaedic treatment is indicated.
  - Fractures require appropriate treatment by closed methods (e.g., casting) or surgical intervention.
  - Lower limb deformities can be managed by bracing or surgery.
    1. Progressive deformities of more than 15 to 20 degrees and failed brace treatment are the indications for surgical intervention.[3]
    2. Realignment of lower limb deformities is the goal of surgical treatment. Multilevel osteotomies usually are required, and these osteotomies are fixed by intramedullary rods; the deformed segment of the bone is divided into multiple straight, smaller segments, and these segments are realigned over the rod.
    3. Healing time can be prolonged. Recurrence risk is about 20 to 25%.
- Management of renal osteodystrophy is more complicated and involves management of the primary disorder by dialysis or renal transplantation and control of the calcium and phosphate levels by appropriate drug treatment and infusions.
- Occasionally, parathyroidectomy is necessary to control the hyperparathyroidism, particularly in patients with tertiary hyperparathyroidism.
- The orthopaedic problems include angular deformities of the lower extremities, fractures, growth disturbances, SCFE, and brown tumors. Only some of these resolve with improvement in metabolic status.
  - Lower extremity deformities seen in patients with renal osteodystrophy usually do not respond well to bracing. If the patient is symptomatic and has had optimal medical management of the osteodystrophy without resolution of deformity, surgical treatment is indicated.
    1. Valgus occurring through the distal femur is common and may be treated with stapling of the medial aspect of the growth plate toward the end of growth. If this option cannot be enacted because insufficient growth remains, metaphyseal osteotomies (mostly distal femoral but sometimes proximal tibial) may be required using internal or external fixation.[2,3]
    2. Recurrence is common in patients with continuing metabolic disease, so medical treatment should be optimized before osteotomy whenever possible.
  - The goal of routine treatment of SCFE is to stop proximal femoral physeal growth and thus to heal the slip. However, this may not be a desirable goal in a very young child with renal osteodystrophy. In additional, physeal healing may be difficult to achieve in the presence of metabolic imbalance.
    1. In many patients with renal SCFE, medical treatment provides good symptomatic relief and narrowing of the proximal femoral physis, making surgical treatment unnecessary for these children.
    2. Surgical treatment is considered if the slip is displaced or if symptoms persist despite good medical control of the disease. In a young child, fixation with partially threaded screws is recommended to achieve stability and to cross (but not close) the physis. In adolescence, after correction of metabolism, fixation to promote growth plate closure can be performed.

Hypophosphatasia

- Hypophosphatasia is a rare metabolic disorder of bone in which there is a deficiency of alkaline phosphatase in the plasma and tissues, leading to abnormal mineralization of bone.
- In most classification systems, hypophosphatasia is included as a cause of rickets. Although there are some clinical and radiographic similarities, hypophosphatasia has a different pathophysiology and should be differentiated from rickets.[2]
- There is a wide variation in the severity of the disease with the prognosis related to the age at onset.
- Several forms of hypophosphatasia exist—perinatal, infantile, childhood, and adult.
  - Severe perinatal, infantile, and childhood types of hypophosphatasia are transmitted in an autosomal recessive manner, whereas the mild adult type may be transmitted as a dominant or recessive trait.
  - The gene for hypophosphatasia is the tissue-nonspecific alkaline phosphatase (TNSALP) gene. Many mutations have been described within the TNSALP gene leading to deficient synthesis of alkaline phosphatase in liver, bone, or kidney.[4] This enzyme is necessary for the maturation of the primary spongiosa in the physes, and its deficiency results in normal production of bone (osteoid) but inadequate mineralization with skeletal deformities that mimic rickets.
  - The physis widens with persistence of the provisional zone of calcification (which cannot calcify) and islands of cartilage continuing down into the metaphysis. The normal columnar arrangement of the chondrocytes of the growth plate is disturbed.

Clinical Features and Radiographic Findings

- The clinical features vary with the age at which the disease manifests.
  - In the severe perinatal form, the babies may be stillborn. If they survive, they frequently have severe respiratory infections that are life threatening.
  - The onset of symptoms in the infantile form is later in infancy, usually around 6 months. These children are usually hypotonic, experiencing anorexia, vomiting, dehydration, and fever.

- The characteristic changes occur early in life in patients with hypophosphatasia.
  1. Absent calcification of the calvaria (craniotabes), late closure of the fontanelles and sutures, and craniosynostosis are common findings. Dentition may be markedly delayed.
  2. Bowing of the long bones and knock-knee deformities are frequently seen.
  3. Fractures following minor trauma may occur.
- Children who survive early infancy tend to improve clinically with time.
- Stature is normal in the infant, but as the child matures, dwarfism caused by a lack of normal endochondral bone growth becomes noticeable.

• Hypophosphatasia can be diagnosed in fetuses; ultrasound may show deficient ossification of the fetal skull.

• Radiographic changes seen with hypophosphatasia are similar to those with rickets.
  - Generalized osteopenia, most marked in the calvarium and metaphyseal regions of the long bones, is seen.
  - The cranial sutures are initially wide but close prematurely, leading to increased intracranial pressure.
  - Broad metaphyses and central cup- or wedge-shaped ossification defects of the central physes are typical radiographic findings (Figure 15–5).
  - Bowing of the long bones and angular deformities of the lower extremities may be seen.

Treatment

• There is no definitive therapy for hypophosphatasia.

• Pathological fractures may be difficult because of the poor quality of the bone.
  - Closed treatment methods are usually employed.
  - If closed treatment fails, surgical intervention is required. Intramedullary fixation can be undertaken in an attempt to avoid growth plate injury.

• Bowing of the long bones and angular deformities of the lower extremities may require treatment if they are progressive and exceed the physiological range. They are managed by bracing or, if indicated, surgical treatment.

Osteogenesis Imperfecta

• Osteogenesis imperfecta (OI) is a genetically transmitted disease resulting in fragility of the entire skeleton. It is seen with varying degrees of severity, from an infant with multiple fractures to a child who has only a few fractures before maturity.

• The clinical variation is caused by differences in the causative mutation. It is now known that at least 90% of individuals with OI have an identifiable genetically determined quantitative, qualitative, or both types of defect in type I collagen formation.[3] Type I collagen is the major structural protein found in bone, skin, tendon, ligament, cornea, sclera, and dentin. It is a triple helix composed of two α-1 chains and one α-2 chain. The mutations in OI involve one of the two genes that encode the chains of type I collagen. The COL1A1 gene on chromosome 17 encodes the α-1 chain, and the COL1A2 gene on chromosome 7 encodes the α-2 chain.[4] Mild forms of OI often result from a reduced amount of type I collagen of normal composition, and severe forms often result from structural abnormalities in type I collagen.

• Numerous classifications have been proposed for OI.

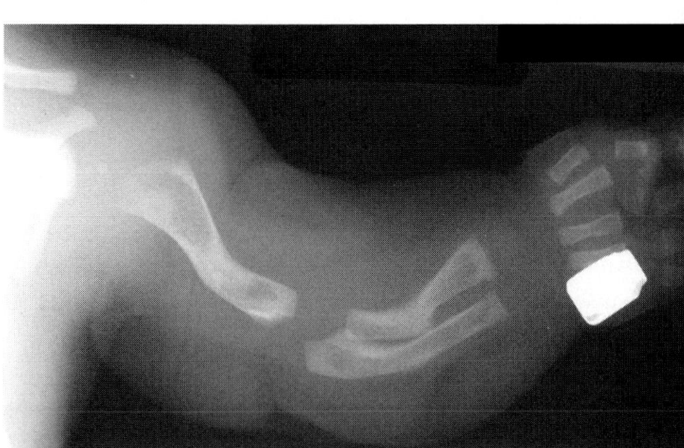

A

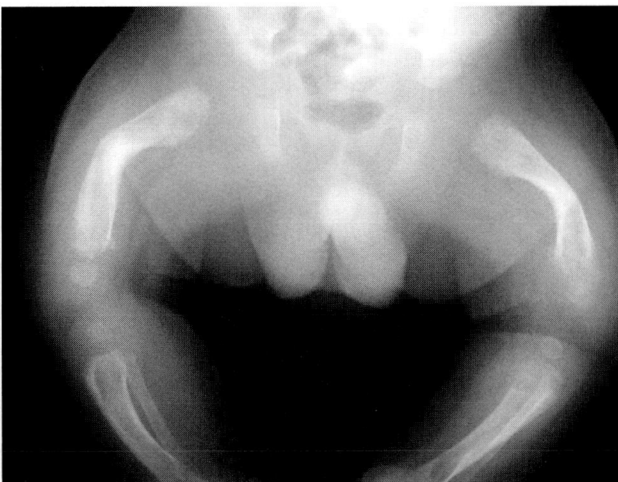

B

Figure 15–5: A 3-month-old patient with hypophosphatasia. A and B, There is generalized osteopenia with bowing of the long bones in both the upper and the lower extremities. Focal round- or wedge-shaped lucencies, representing islands of cartilage, are seen in the metaphyses, a finding unique to hypophosphatasia.

- The Sillence classification is the most commonly used system (Box 15–2).[6] It includes four types: types I and IV are transmitted in an autosomal dominant manner, and types II and III are transmitted in an autosomal recessive manner. Dental findings are used to further subtype OI (i.e., A without and B with dentinogenesis imperfecta).
- Although Sillence remains the most helpful classification for the geneticist ordering the many features of this entity, it may be less helpful for the pediatric orthopaedic surgeon consulted in the perinatal period to estimate the musculoskeletal prognosis. To address this issue, Shapiro advanced a congenita–tarda classification (Box 15–3).[7]

Clinical Features

- The clinical picture varies according to the variety of the disease.
  - In severe congenital form (Sillence II or Shapiro congenita A), multiple fractures from minimal trauma during delivery or *in utero* cause the limbs to be deformed and short. The skull is soft and membranous. This type is usually fatal with death secondary to intracranial hemorrhage or respiratory insufficiency; the infant is stillborn or lives only a short time.
  - In the nonlethal forms of the disease (Sillence I, III, and IV), fragility of the bones is the most prominent feature.
    1. In general, the earlier the fractures occur, the more severe the disease.
    2. Lower limbs are more frequently affected because they are more prone to trauma.
    3. Fractures heal at a normal rate; nonunion is relatively rare.
    4. Growth may be arrested by multiple microfractures at the epiphyseal ends.
    5. The frequency of fractures declines sharply after adolescence.
    6. Deformities of the long bones because of fractures or microfractures usually develop.
- Many patients with OI have small, triangular faces (Figure 15–6, *A*).
  - The sclera may be blue in many cases.

Box 15–2 Sillence Classification of Osteogenesis Imperfecta[6]

Type IA-B—Most common, mild type; mild to moderate bone fragility with little or no deformity
Type II—Perinatal, lethal type; rarely survives infancy and produces extremely fragile bones and severe deformity
Type III—Severe, progressively deforming type; moderate to severe deformity at birth with progressive, neonatal fractures
Type IVA-B—Moderately severe type; mild to moderate bone fragility and long bone–spine deformity

Box 15–3 Shapiro Classification of Osteogenesis Imperfecta[7]

Congenita—Implies that fractures occurred *in utero* or at birth and are diagnosed at birth
  A. Crimpled femurs or ribs
  B. Normal bone contours with fractures
Tarda—Diagnosed later
  A. Fractures before walking
  B. Fractures after walking

  - The defective dentinogenesis of deciduous or permanent teeth or both may be seen (Figure 15–6, *A*).
  - Hearing may be impaired because of defects in the bones of the middle ear.
- The laxity of the ligaments results in hypermobile joints and an increased incidence of joint dislocation.
- Severe spinal deformities may develop because of the combination of marked osteoporosis, compression fractures of the vertebrae, and ligamentous laxity.
- Short stature is common because of deformities of the limbs caused by angulation and overriding of fractures, growth disturbance at the physes, and marked kyphoscoliosis (Figure 15–6).
- Patients with OI frequently have joint contractures, including those of the hips, knees, and elbows.

Radiographic Findings

- Prenatal diagnosis of OI has been accomplished by ultrasound. The ultrasonographic features of type II OI include long bone deformity (implying fracture), severely reduced femoral length, and decreased echogenicity of the skull.[3]
- Some degree of generalized osteopenia is detected in almost all patients with OI. This is evident from visual inspection in most patients, but in even the mildest cases, bone densitometry shows at least a 25% decrease in mineralization.
- The osteopenic vertebrae may fracture easily, resulting in a flattened or biconcave shape. Thoracic or thoracolumbar scoliosis frequently is detected.
- The pelvis may show acetabular protrusion.
- The long bones may be thin and bowed with thin cortices and a poorly developed trabecular pattern. Deformities may result from multiple fractures (Figure 15–7).

Differential Diagnosis

- The differential diagnosis of OI includes child abuse, idiopathic juvenile osteoporosis, and rarely, fibrous dysplasia.
  - History is extremely helpful in differentiating OI from child abuse. Fractures occurring with relatively mild injury; a positive family history; abnormalities of the

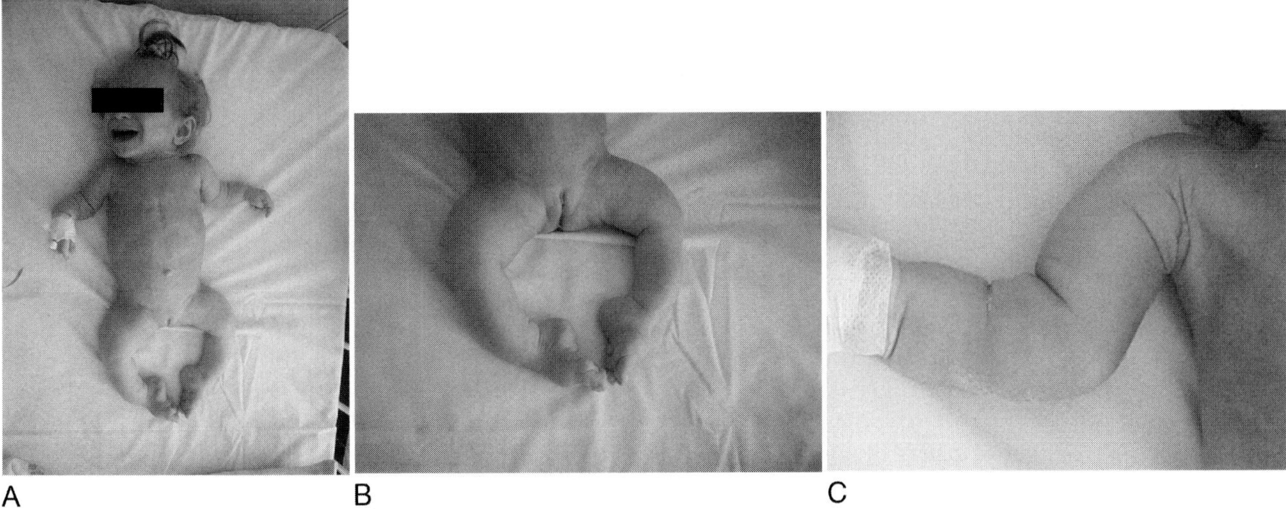

Figure 15–6: A 4-year-old girl with OI. A through C, The patient has a small, triangular face with defective dentinogenesis. The short stature is because of deformities of the limbs caused by angulation and overriding of fractures. Also note the multiple joint contractures including the hips, knees, and elbows.

teeth, sclera, or hearing; or a systemic osteopenia revealed by radiography may suggest OI.
- Idiopathic juvenile osteoporosis may appear with spontaneous or pathological fractures but is usually a transient, self-limited disorder.
- Fibrous dysplasia may exhibit bone deformities and fractures, but the bones are not as tapered and thin as in OI and many of the bones in an affected patient are free of the disease.

Treatment

- There is no specific treatment to correct the basic mutant gene defect in OI.

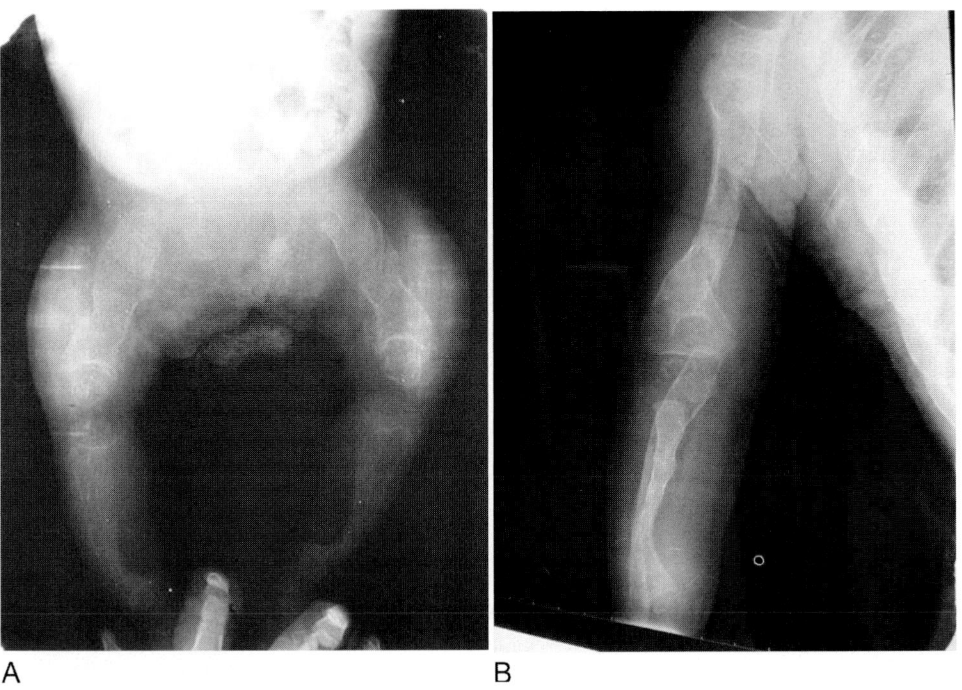

Figure 15–7: A and B, The radiographs of the upper and lower extremities of this young child with OI demonstrate diffusely decreased mineralization, bowing of the long bones, and multiple healing fractures. Also note the thin cortices and the poorly developed trabecular pattern.

- Until recently, efforts to improve bone strength by medical means were largely unsuccessful. The administration of calcium, vitamin C, vitamin D, fluoride, calcitonin, and magnesium were all attempted, usually with no or mixed results.
- Promising studies regarding the use of a bisphosphonate, aminohydroxypropylidene (pamidronate), have been published.[8]
  - This compound inhibits osteoclastic resorption of bone, an activity that appears to be increased in patients with OI.
  - Administration of pamidronate subjectively improved complaints of generalized bone pain and fracture frequency.
  - In addition, increased bone mineral density, as determined from dual-energy x-ray absorptiometry, has been noted.
- Allogenic bone marrow transplant is another treatment being tried for the most severe cases in young infants.[9]
- The goals of orthopaedic treatment are to maximize the affected patient's function, to prevent deformity and disability resulting from fractures, to correct deformities that have developed, and to monitor potential complicating conditions associated with OI.
  - Infants with birth fractures usually need only careful, supportive handling to prevent further injury. If long bone fractures are unstable, minimal external splinting may be used to stabilize the affected limb; such fractures will usually heal within 1 or 2 weeks. Excessive duration of immobilization should be avoided.[3]
  - Protective bracing to prevent fractures and aid ambulation is a mainstay in the conservative management of patients with OI.
    1. Typically, lightweight hip–knee–ankle–foot orthoses (HKAFOs) are required for effective lower extremity bracing in the most severely affected patients.
    2. The braces may allow patients to stand or walk, usually with the upper extremity aids of crutches or a walker.
    3. In addition, HKAFOs can reduce the incidence of lower extremity fractures compared with the incidence in unbraced patients.
  - Treatment of fractures is a major problem in patients with OI (Figure 15–8). Callus formed in response to the fracture is identical in structure with the rest of the skeleton; it is plastic and easily deformed by mechanical forces.
    1. Closed treatment methods usually are employed.
    2. If management by closed means proves difficult, treatment with internal fixation may be considered (Figure 15–9). Intramedullary rods (load-sharing devices) are preferable to plates and screws, which tend to dislodge from the weakened bone.[10]

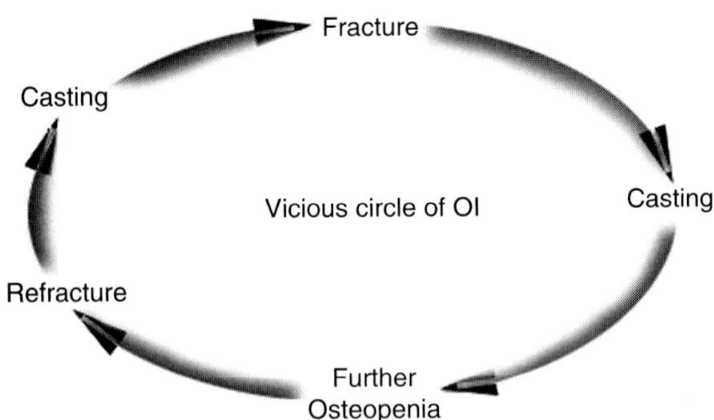

Figure 15–8: Vicious cycle of OI. From Erol B, Dormans JP, States L, Kaplan FS (2004) Skeletal dysplasias and metabolic disorders of bone. Musculoskeletal Tumors in Children. In Dormans JP (ed) Pediatric Orthopaedics and Sports Medicine. Philadelphia: Mosby.

  - Deformities of the long bones may require surgical treatment.
    1. The indications are severe diaphyseal bowing (usually anterolateral bowing of the femur and anterior bowing of the tibia) that prevents standing, recurrent fractures in a given region, and occasionally cosmesis.
    2. Realignment of the deformed bone is provided by multiple osteotomies and intramedullary fixation with expansile rods.
    3. Pseudarthrosis develops in up to 20% of patients.
  - Scoliosis is a difficult problem to treat in OI as in other disorders with osteopenia.

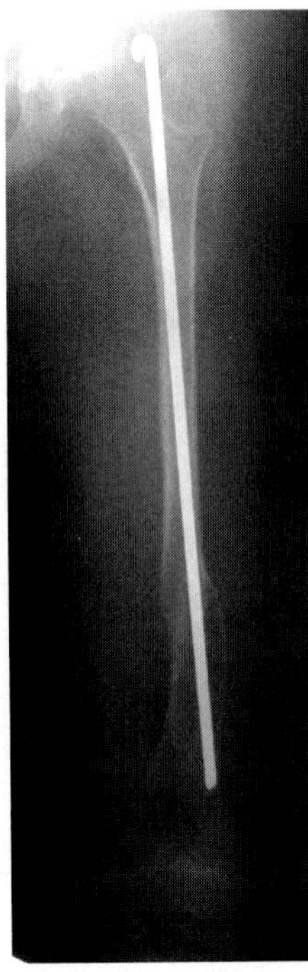

Figure 15–9: An intramedullary rod transfixes a healing fracture in a child with OI.

1. The curves tend to progress relentlessly, and bracing is usually ineffective in controlling the progression of the deformity.
2. Segmental instrumentation is performed because of the poor quality of bone. Spinal curves may be fused early (40 degrees or more) to halt the relentless progression.

– Basilar invagination is present radiographically in up to one quarter of the patients. The deformable bones of OI are unable to stand the increasing weight of the head.

1. Symptoms may include cranial nerve palsies, headaches, respiratory depression, spasticity, nystagmus, or weakness and may lead to early mortality.
2. There is no satisfactory treatment for this complication. Conservative treatment with full-time use of a brace may provide partial symptomatic relief. Surgical therapy also is an option.

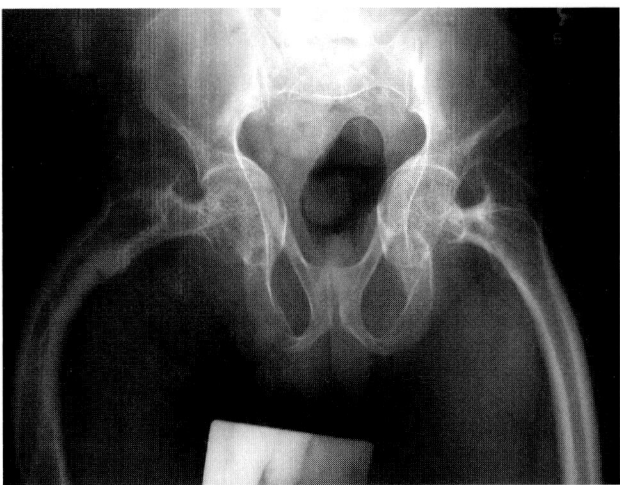

Figure 15–10: A teenager with idiopathic juvenile osteoporosis has diffuse osteopenia and resultant deformity of the pelvis and femurs. **Protrusio acetabuli is severe.**

Idiopathic Juvenile Osteoporosis

- Idiopathic juvenile osteoporosis is a rare, self-limited disorder of unknown etiology that affects previously healthy children. It is characterized by a profound reduction in bone mass.
- The age of onset is usually between 8 and 14 years, and resolution usually occurs spontaneously within 2 to 4 years after onset or after puberty.[11]
- Idiopathic juvenile osteoporosis is not genetically transmitted. The basic mechanism of disease is an imbalance between bone formation and bone resorption.
  - Bone histology usually shows an excess of osteocytes associated with woven bone.
  - Recent studies have shown some abnormalities in collagen metabolism in patients with idiopathic juvenile osteoporosis.[3]

Clinical Features and Radiographic Findings

- Idiopathic juvenile osteoporosis always manifests before puberty. The initial complaints are back pain and leg pain. Patients usually have a slow gait or limp.
- Generalized osteopenia of varying degrees is seen; osteopenia is more marked at the metaphyseal regions of the long bones leading to metaphyseal fractures.
- Spinal deformities (e.g., kyphosis) occur frequently.
- Diffuse generalized osteoporosis is seen on radiographs of the spine and limbs (Figure 15–10). The normal trabecular pattern is markedly decreased and the cortices of the bones are thinned.
- Thoracolumbar kyphosis with anterior wedging of the vertebrae and vertebral compression fractures are common findings.
- Metaphyseal fractures of the long bones tend to occur in the areas of highest stress, such as femoral neck.

Differential Diagnosis

- Idiopathic juvenile osteoporosis must be differentiated from other conditions resulting in osteopenia and bone fragility during childhood, such as OI, hematological malignancies, thyroid disorders, Cushing's disease, steroid-induced osteopenia, and disuse osteopenia. The diagnosis is usually made by demonstrating the features of this disease and by ruling out other conditions with similar manifestations.
  - The most difficult distinction to make is between idiopathic juvenile osteoporosis and mild OI.[2] Rapid progression after many years of normality may help in differentiating idiopathic juvenile osteoporosis from OI. In addition, OI has some distinguishing features unassociated with idiopathic juvenile osteoporosis, such as a positive family history, blue sclera, dentinogenesis imperfecta, and ligamentous laxity.
  - Another important distinction to make clinically is between leukemia and idiopathic juvenile osteoporosis. Children with leukemia may have symptoms of osteopenia and compression fractures. Usually a bone marrow aspirate will be required to rule out leukemia.

Treatment

- Idiopathic juvenile osteoporosis is usually a self-limited disorder that tends to resolve spontaneously.[2] It has been difficult to demonstrate the efficacy of any treatment regimen in altering the natural history of the disease.
- For kyphosis, antikyphotic bracing has been recommended.[5] Surgical intervention is rarely required.
- Metaphyseal fractures require appropriate orthopaedic management. Prolonged disuse or immobilization can worsen the osteoporosis and clinical symptoms.

Osteopetrosis

- Osteopetrosis is a rare metabolic bone disease characterized by a diffuse increase in skeletal density and obliteration of marrow spaces. There is failure of bone resorption because of functional deficiency of the osteoclasts.
- Histologically, the skeleton shows cores of calcified cartilage surrounded by areas of new bone; this new bone formation is normal, but there is a deficiency of bone and cartilage resorption resulting in exceedingly dense bones. The bone contains an increased number of osteoclasts; however, the osteoclasts do not have the ability of resorbing bone, as evidenced by the absence of ruffled borders and clear zones. Calcified chondroid and primitive bone persist, leading to osteosclerosis and increased brittleness of the bones.[12]
- There are three forms of osteopetrosis: infantile malignant, intermediate, and adult tarda.[13] Infantile osteopetrosis is transmitted as an autosomal recessive trait and maps to chromosome 11q13. The intermediate form is also transmitted as an autosomal recessive type. Adult form is inherited in an autosomal dominant pattern, and its gene locus is suspected to be on chromosome 1p21.

Clinical Features and Radiographic Findings

- In infantile osteopetrosis, clinical manifestations appear at birth or in early infancy.
  - This malignant form of osteopetrosis is characterized by pancytopenia, which develops because of the inability of bone marrow to participate in hematopoiesis.
  - Pancytopenia has presenting symptoms of severe anemia, abnormal bleeding, easy bruising, and failure to thrive.
  - Bony overgrowth of the cranial foramina causes cranial nerve palsies, which result in blindness and deafness.
  - Pathological fractures occur frequently in the fragile, brittle bones.
  - The clinical course is rapidly progressive, and death may occur at a young age from anemia or sepsis.
- The intermediate form of osteopetrosis usually is diagnosed in later childhood after a fracture. It may have some features of the infantile form, but presentation is milder.
- The patients with adult form have a normal life expectancy but many orthopaedic problems. Clinical findings include mild anemia, pathological fractures, and premature osteoarthritis. In rare cases, osteomyelitis may characterize the clinical picture.
- Prenatal diagnosis of osteopetrosis has been accomplished in the twenty-fifth week of pregnancy with the use of fetal radiography, which reveals sclerosis of osteopetrotic bone.[3]
- Ultrasound has also been used to identify affected fetuses.
- Generalized increased density of the bones is the main radiographic feature in osteopetrosis (Figure 15–11, *A*).
  - There is no distinction between cortical and cancellous bone, because the intramedullary canal is filled with bone.
  - There may be transverse bands in the metaphyseal regions and longitudinal striations in the shafts.
  - Flaring of the metaphyses of the long bones (best seen in the distal femur), the bone-within-a-bone appearance of the pelvis, and the rugger jersey appearance of the spine are typical radiographic findings (Figure 15–11, *B* and *C*).
  - Deformities may be seen secondary to fractures.

Treatment

- Treatment for infantile osteopetrosis is bone marrow transplantation at a young age with marrow from an appropriately human leukocyte antigen-matched donor.[2] A successful transplant may resolve the hematological abnormalities and can gradually restore patent marrow cavities.
- High-dose 1,25-dihydroxyvitamin D therapy with a low calcium diet has been employed because of its ability to stimulate osteoclasts and bone resorption.[13]
- Fractures in the intermediate and adult forms are common and require appropriate treatment. Healing occurs but may be delayed.
- Deformities caused by fractures may require corrective osteotomies. Intramedullary fixation is desirable, but it may be difficult to apply because of the abnormal structure of the bone.
- Osteomyelitis is common because of the diminished vascularity and defective immune response.

Parathyroid Disorders

Hyperparathyroidism

- Primary hyperparathyroidism results from hyperplasia of the parathyroid glands, which leads to increased secretion of PTH. It should be differentiated from secondary or tertiary hyperparathyroidism, mainly compensatory conditions seen in chronic renal failure.
- The increased PTH stimulates osteoclastic resorption of bone, which produces hypercalcemia.
- The presenting symptoms of hyperparathyroidism are lethargy, bone pain, and abdominal complaints.
  - Bone pain is caused by induced osteoclastic resorption of bone.
  - Abdominal pain and constipation result from the decreased abdominal motility; smooth muscle action in the gut is inhibited by hypercalcemia.
  - The irritability and conductivity of nervous tissue are decreased by hypercalcemia.

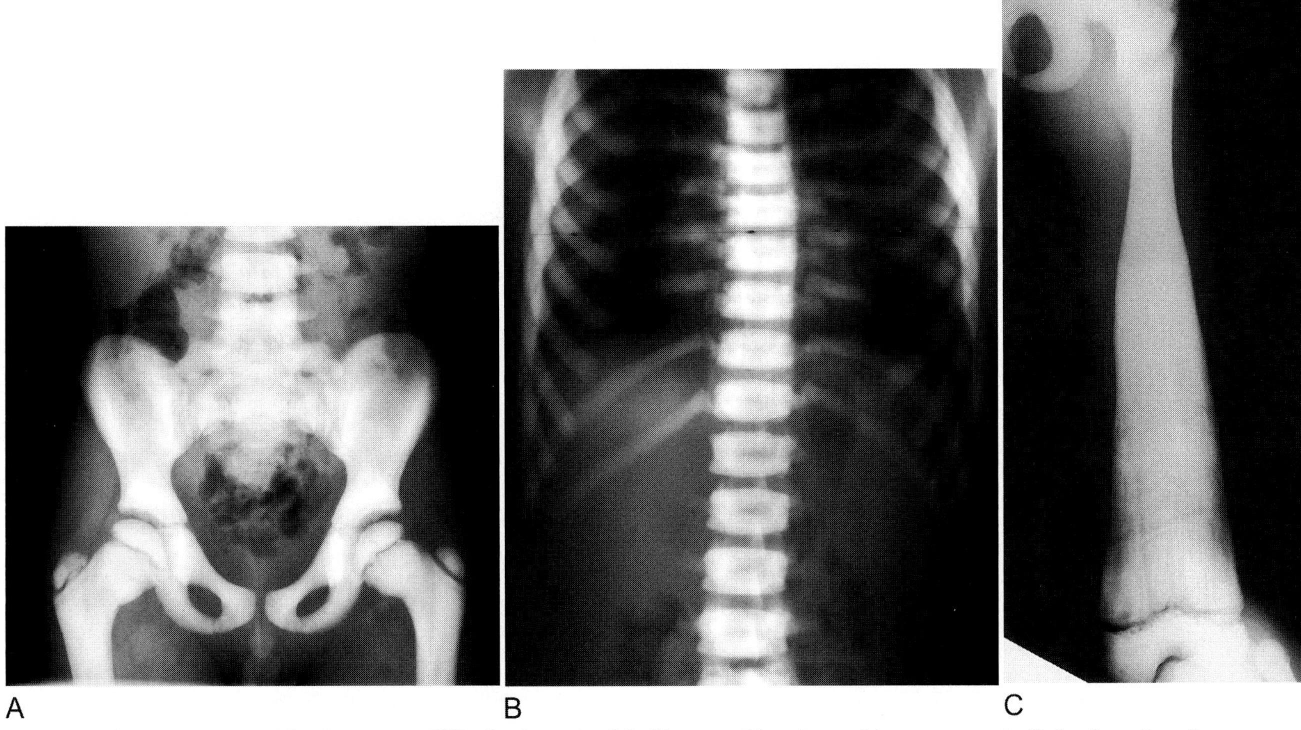

Figure 15–11: **A, The bones are diffusely dense in this 10-year-old patient with osteopetrosis. B, In the spine, the centers of the vertebral bodies are relatively lucent, creating a "rugger jersey" appearance. C, Also note the metaphyseal flaring in the distal femur and a healing fracture in the proximal femur.**

- Prolonged hypercalcemia leads to ectopic calcification and renal calculi formation; the critical solubility product of calcium and phosphorus is exceeded.
- Hypertension is commonly present.

- The radiographic findings resemble those of secondary hyperparathyroidism (renal osteodystrophy); there is generalized osteopenia, cortical thickening, and bony resorption at the terminal tufts of the distal phalanges and the distal clavicles.
- The classic laboratory findings in patients with hyperparathyroidism are elevated serum calcium, decreased serum phosphorus, and elevated alkaline phosphatase. Rarely, the calcium and phosphate concentrations are normal. Further testing, including urinary cAMP measurements and direct assays for serum PTH, may be required.
- Treatment is directed toward correcting the underlying cause of hyperparathyroidism.
  - In cases of adenoma and hyperplasia, treatment is usually surgical. Preliminary metabolic management may be required.
  - Fractures can occur and need to be managed by customary principles.
  - Hypercalcemic crisis is treated by hydration and replacement of sodium losses.

Hypoparathyroidism

- Hypoparathyroidism (idiopathic hypoparathyroidism) is caused by failure of the parathyroid glands to produce PTH. This condition should be distinguished from pseudohypoparathyroidism, in which production of PTH is increased but the organs cannot respond to the hormone.
- Inherited forms of hypoparathyroidism exist.[4]
  - An autosomal dominant type is the result of mutations on chromosome 3q13 in the gene encoding for the G protein-coupled Ca_2^+-sensing receptor, which regulates PTH secretion.
  - Hypoparathyroidism is also associated with deletions in chromosome 22q11, the gene responsible for DiGeorge syndrome and cardiac defects.
  - Other autosomal recessive types associated with growth retardation, seizures, severe mental retardation, and an X-linked recessive type have been described.
- Irritability of nervous and muscle tissue is high because the serum calcium is low; tetany, paresthesias, and alteration in mental status may be seen. The skin is dry; the hair is brittle and scanty. If hypocalcemia occurs early in development, mental retardation may result.

- Radiographic findings include increased density of the long bones and skull. Soft tissue calcifications can occur, including the basal ganglia.
- The classic laboratory findings in patients with hypoparathyroidism are decreased total and serum-ionized calcium and elevated serum phosphorus.
- Treatment of hypoparathyroidism is endocrine related. There is no orthopaedic treatment specific to this disease.
  - Treatment is vitamin D and PTH administration; these two agents work synergistically to transport calcium across the gut, by the renal tubule, and from the bone. Considerably higher than physiological (i.e., pharmacological) doses of vitamin D are required. Management must be carried out carefully to avoid vitamin D toxicity.[2,3]
  - Nephrocalcinosis is a known complication of vitamin D therapy.
  - Infants with hypoparathyroidism complicated by tetany may need calcium infusions.

Hypervitaminosis A

- Vitamin A is a necessary constituent in the synthesis of visual pigments, but it is also required in appropriate amounts for skeletal growth and for maintenance and regeneration of epithelial tissues.
- Hypervitaminosis A is rarely seen. It can be acute or chronic.
  - Acute hypervitaminosis A intoxication causes increased intracranial pressure, vomiting, and lethargy.
  - Chronic hypervitaminosis A usually results from inappropriate use of vitamin supplements.[14]
    1. Several weeks or months of chronic overingestion (if the child survives) leads to a syndrome characterized by pruritus, skin lesions, failure to thrive, and muscle and bone tenderness.
    2. The soft tissues overlying the hyperostotic bones are swollen and tender.
- The development of bony changes is slow, so radiographs are normal initially. In the later phase, periosteal reaction (hyperostosis) and cortical thickening are seen in many of the long bones. Epiphyseal and metaphyseal ossification abnormalities occur with central physeal arrest.
- Bone scintigraphy shows increased uptake.
- The diagnosis is made by determining the plasma level of vitamin A, which will be elevated 5 to 15 times the normal value. Hypercalcemia can be present.
- Histological examination of the bones demonstrates an increase in resorptive surfaces, suggesting that the combination of resorption and formation has been accelerated to a hypermetabolic state.
- Treatment of hypervitaminosis A includes total cessation of administration of vitamin A and eliminating all foods containing vitamin A from the diet. Systemic symptoms resolve quickly; however, hyperostosis will disappear only after a long period because of great body reserves of vitamin A.

Hypervitaminosis D

- Hypervitaminosis D is the result of the ingestion of excessive doses of vitamin D. Patients who take vitamin D and potent 1-hydroxyvitamin D and 1,25-dihydroxyvitamin D for the treatment of their metabolic bone diseases (e.g., rickets, osteomalacia, and hypoparathyroidism) are at risk to have this condition.
- The elevated vitamin D promotes intestinal absorption of calcium, leading to hypercalcemia. Life-threatening hypercalcemia is rarely seen.
- Histologically, wide osteoid seams are found around the trabeculae resembling what is seen in rickets. The physis, however, is well calcified and normal in width and length.[3]
- Metastatic calcifications may be found in the kidneys, arteries, thyroid, pancreas, lungs, stomach, and brain.
- The early manifestations of hypervitaminosis D are anorexia, constipation, nausea, vomiting, polyuria, and thirst. With progression of the intoxication, mental depression and stupor may develop.
- Radiographic findings include dense metaphyseal bands, osteopenia in the diaphyses of the long bones, and metastatic calcifications in soft tissues.
- Hypercalcemia may be severe. The serum phosphate concentration is normal, and the alkaline phosphatase concentration is diminished.
- Treatment consists of decreasing the serum calcium.
  - Vitamin D administration should be stopped immediately.
  - The patient should be promptly treated by diuresis, usually accomplished by administration of large volumes of saline and furosemide. Replacement of urinary losses of water, sodium, and potassium is often necessary; these should be carefully monitored.[2,3]
  - Steroids may be helpful in correcting the calcium level by inhibiting calcium absorption in the kidney and gut.
  - Biphosphonates inhibit bone resorption and have been helpful in treating vitamin D intoxication.
  - Sodium phosphate, advocated in the past, should not be given because its administration leads to ectopic calcification.

Scurvy

- Scurvy is caused by a nutritional deficiency of vitamin C (ascorbic acid).
- All the clinical and pathological manifestations of scurvy are based on the role of vitamin C in the synthesis of collagen.

  - Vitamin C is necessary for the hydroxylation of lysine and proline to hydroxylysine and hydroxyproline, two amino acids crucial to the proper cross-linking of the triple helix of collagen.[15]
  - The deficiency of this vitamin forms primitive collagen seen throughout the body. Blood vessels become excessively permeable and rupture readily, normal bone formation is reduced, and bone that forms lacks tensile strength and is defective in structural arrangement.
- Osteoclasts are normal, but osteoblasts become flattened, resembling connective tissue fibroblasts. The bone trabeculae and the cortices of the long bones are thin and fragile.
- Scurvy develops after 6 to 12 months of dietary deprivation of vitamin C. It is not seen in neonates.[3]
  - Children with scurvy appear undernourished, apathetic, and irritable.
  - Subperiosteal hemorrhage is a distinctive sign, occurring most commonly in the distal femur and tibia and the proximal humerus. The limbs become exquisitely tender, leading to pseudoparalysis.[2,3]
  - Hemorrhages may also develop in the soft tissues, including the joints, the kidneys, and the gut, and petechiae may be seen.
  - Hemorrhage of the gums is a common finding leading to swollen, bluish gums.
  - Anemia and impaired wound healing are common.
- Radiographic findings may be seen in any of the long bones but are most prominent around the knees.[2]
  - Osteopenia is the first sign followed by thinning of the cortices.
  - The zone of provisional calcification increases in width and opacity (i.e., the white line of Fraenkel) because of failed resorption of the calcified cartilaginous matrix and stands out compared with the severely osteopenic metaphyses.
  - Brittleness of the zone of provisional calcification may lead to fractures and marginal spurs (i.e., Pelken sign).
  - The epiphyseal nucleus is markedly radiolucent with relatively sclerotic margins, producing an appearance of ringed epiphyses (i.e., Wimberger sign).
  - The areas of subperiosteal hemorrhage calcify with treatment and have the appearance of periosteal new bone.
- Scurvy may be mistaken for osteomyelitis because of clinical presentation. However, laboratory studies including sedimentation rate, C-reactive protein level, and white blood cell count are normal in scurvy.
- Serum levels of vitamin C may be difficult to interpret in scurvy. A more reliable test is the absence of vitamin C in the buffy coat of centrifuged blood.
- Treatment is replacement of the deficient vitamin C. Rapid recovery is usual with pain and tenderness resolving. Minimal daily requirements are 30 mg for infants and 50 mg for adults. Therapeutic dosages may be 200 mg or higher.[2,3]

References

1. Mankin HJ (1990) Rickets, osteomalacia, and renal osteodystrophy: An update (review article). Orthop Clin North Am 21: 81.
   Review of rickets, osteomalacia, and renal osteodystrophy.

2. Zaleske DJ (2001) Metabolic and endocrine abnormalities. In: Lovell and Winter's Pediatric Orthopaedics, 5th edition (Morrisy RT, Weinstein SL, eds). Philadelphia: Lippincott Williams & Wilkins.

3. Herring JA (2002) Tachdjian's Pediatric Orthopaedics, 3rd edition. Philadelphia: WB Saunders.

4. McKusick VA, ed (2000) Online Mendelian Inheritance in Man. Baltimore: McKusick-Nathans Institute for Genetic Medicine, John Hopkins University. Bethesda, MD: National Center for Biotechnology Information, National Library of Medicine. http://www.ncbi.nlm.nih.gov/entrez/query.fcgi?db=OMIM.

5. Sponseller PD (2001) The skeletal dysplasias. In: Lovell and Winter's Pediatric Orthopaedics, 5th edition (Morrisy RT, Weinstein SL, eds). Philadelphia: Lippincott Williams & Wilkins.

6. Sillence DO (1981) Osteogenesis imperfecta: An expanding panorama of variance. Clin Orthop 159: 11.
   Clinical characteristics and pathogenesis of four variants of OI.

7. Shapiro F (1985) Consequences of an osteogenesis imperfecta diagnosis for survival and ambulation. J Pediatr Orthop 5: 456.
   Review of radiographic findings in patients with OI. Discussion of time of initial fracture and the radiographic appearance of long bones and ribs at the time of initial fracture as prognostic indicators of survival and ambulation.

8. Glorieux FH, Bishop NJ, Plotkin H, Chabot G, Lanoue G, Travers R (1998) Cyclic administration of pamidronate in children with severe osteogenesis imperfecta. N Engl J Med 339: 947.
   The authors assessed the effects of treatment with a bisphosphonate on bone resorption in an observational study of 30 children with severe OI. The authors reported that cyclic administration of intravenous pamidronate improved clinical outcomes, reduced bone resorption, and increased bone density.

9. Marini JC (1998) Osteogenesis imperfecta: Managing brittle bones (editorial). N Engl J Med 339: 947.

10. Dormans JP, Flynn JM (2001) Pathologic fractures associated with tumors and unique conditions of the musculoskeletal system. In: Rockwood and Wilkins' Fractures in Children, 5th edition (Beaty JH, Kasser JR, eds). Philadelphia: Lippincott Williams & Wilkins.

11. Smith R (1995) Idiopathic juvenile osteoporosis: Experience of twenty-one patients. Br J Rheumatol 34: 68.
   The authors review the features and outcome of 21 children with idiopathic juvenile osteoporosis followed for up to 23 years.

12. Shapiro F, Glimcher MJ, Holtrop ME, Tashjian AH Jr, Brickley-Parsons D, Kenzora JE (1980) Human osteopetrosis: A histological, ultrastructural, and biochemical study. J Bone Joint Surg 62A: 384.
    The authors describe histological, ultrastructural, and biochemical studies of the tissues of a patient with osteopetrosis.

13. Shapiro F (1993) Osteopetrosis: Current clinical considerations. Clin Orthop 294: 34.
    The author describes three clinical groups of osteoporosis: infantile-malignant autosomal recessive, fatal within the first few years of life (in the absence of effective therapy); intermediate autosomal recessive, appearing during the first decade of life but not following a malignant course; and autosomal dominant with full-life expectancy but many orthopaedic problems. Clinical and radiographic characteristics, sequelae, and treatment are discussed.

14. Bendich A, Langseth L (1989) Safety of vitamin A. Am J Clin Nutr 49: 358.
    The authors describe Vitamin A deficiency and toxicity.

15. Peterkofsky B (1991) Ascorbate requirement for hydroxylation and secretion of procollagen: Relationship to inhibition of collagen synthesis in scurvy. Am J Clin Nutr 54: 1135.
    The authors describe the association of Vitamin C deficiency with defective connective tissue, particularly in wound healing.

CHAPTER 16

Synovial Disorders

Randy Q. Cron* **and James J. McCarthy†**

*MD, PhD, Attending Physician, Division of Rheumatology, The Children's Hospital of Philadelphia, Philadelphia, PA; Assistant Professor of Pediatrics, University of Pennsylvania, Philadelphia, PA
†MD, Assistant Professor, Temple University, Philadelphia, PA; Assistant Chief of Staff, Shriners Hospital for Children, Philadelphia, PA

Introduction

- Synovial disorders encompass a variety of disease processes common to the orthopaedic surgeon. Within this spectrum, there is a variation from benign pains of childhood to life-threatening malignancies, and the acuity varies from disorders that need immediate treatment to those that are chronic. Unfortunately, many of the topics that fall under the heading of synovial disorders are often not covered within typical orthopaedic training. The complexity of and infrequency in which these disorders are encountered in a typical orthopaedic practice demands that the practicing orthopaedic surgeon become familiar with this information, know how and where to access additional information, and realize when further referral is needed.
- Pain is an extremely common complaint in childhood. As much as 1% of children have pains severe enough to seek medical evaluation, and 15% of children have episodes of skeletal pain when questioned. The differential diagnosis for skeletal pain is enormous, and establishing the correct diagnosis is often difficult. Only a small percentage of children with skeletal pain have significant pathology. Unfortunately, the clinical symptoms may vary little between a benign disorder and a more threatening disorder, such as leukemia. It is therefore critical that working knowledge and an algorithm for skeletal pain is established to determine the diagnosis and subsequent treatment in an efficient and timely manor.
- In this chapter, we introduce the range of synovial disorders and focus on the clinically relevant information as it applies to orthopaedic residents and surgeons. We focus on the physical examination and needed laboratory and radiographic examinations. We also present a differential diagnosis and descriptions and treatments of specific disorders. At the end, a reference list is provided that will direct you toward more detailed information.

Clinically Relevant Anatomy

Joint Anatomy

- There are two types of joints.
  - Synarthroses (solid joints) may be either fibrous or collagenous.
  - Diarthroses (cavitated joints) are synovial joints. Synovial joints are formed at the ends of endochondral bones (with the exceptions of the temporomandibular and clavicular joints).

Joint Development

- The limbs develop between 4 and 6 weeks of gestation and quickly form the upper extremities. A few days later they form the lower extremities.
- Endochondral ossification—Long-bone formation begins as an aggregation of mesenchymal tissue, which subsequently forms a cartilaginous anlage (chondrification). This cartilaginous model is then replaced by endochondral ossification to form bone.
- Intramembranous ossification—Flat bones, such as the scapula and calvarium, are formed directly without a cartilaginous model, and this is termed *intermembranous ossification*.

- The joint is formed during chondrification while the mesenchymal skeleton is gradually replaced by a continuous cartilage. Concomitant changes occur in the regions of the future joints to create the interzones. Cavitation appears initially in this interzone. This is an enzymatic process, independent of joint motion. Interruption of this process will lead to abnormally shaped joints or even absence of a joint.
- The diarthrodial (synovial) joint is made up of the following basic components: (1) articular cartilage, (2) synovial lining, (3) a fibrous capsule, and (4) other nonarticular joint surfaces (Figure 16–1).
- Articular cartilage is formed by a special variety of hyaline cartilage (Box 16–1). It has a wear-resistant, low-friction, lubricated surface that is elastic and compressible. Thickness usually ranges between 1 and 2 mm in small bones and may reach 5 to 7 mm in larger joints. Under direct visualization, it is typically smooth, white, and compressible. With aging, the cartilage becomes thinner, firmer, more brittle, and yellowish.
- Articular cartilage is divided into several layers (Figure 16–1, *inset*).
  - The superficial layer of the articular cartilage is termed the *tangential zone* because of the orientation of the collagen fibers parallel or tangential to the joint surface. The primary functions are to provide smooth articulation and to prevent shearing.
  - The middle zone lies underneath the tangential layer and is called the *transitional zone*.
  - The deep layer is called the *radial zone* because of the vertical or radial orientation of the collagen fibers.

Box 16–1 Articular Cartilage Components

Articular cartilage consists of the following:
- Water (65 to 80% of the wet weight)
- Collagen (10 to 15% of the wet weight)
  - Type II collagen is the predominate type of collagen, but there are also small amounts of types V, VI, IX, X, and XI collagen.
- Proteoglycans (10 to 15% of the wet weight)
  - Proteoglycans are produced by the chondrocytes and secreted into the extracellular matrix. They are composed of subunits known as glycosaminoglycans. These glycosaminoglycans include two subtypes, chondroitin sulfate and keratin sulfate. With aging, the concentration of chondroitin sulfate decreases and that of keratin sulfate increases.
- Chondrocytes (5% of the wet weight).
  - Chondrocytes are active in protein synthesis and produce collagen, proteoglycans, and some enzymes for cartilage metabolism.

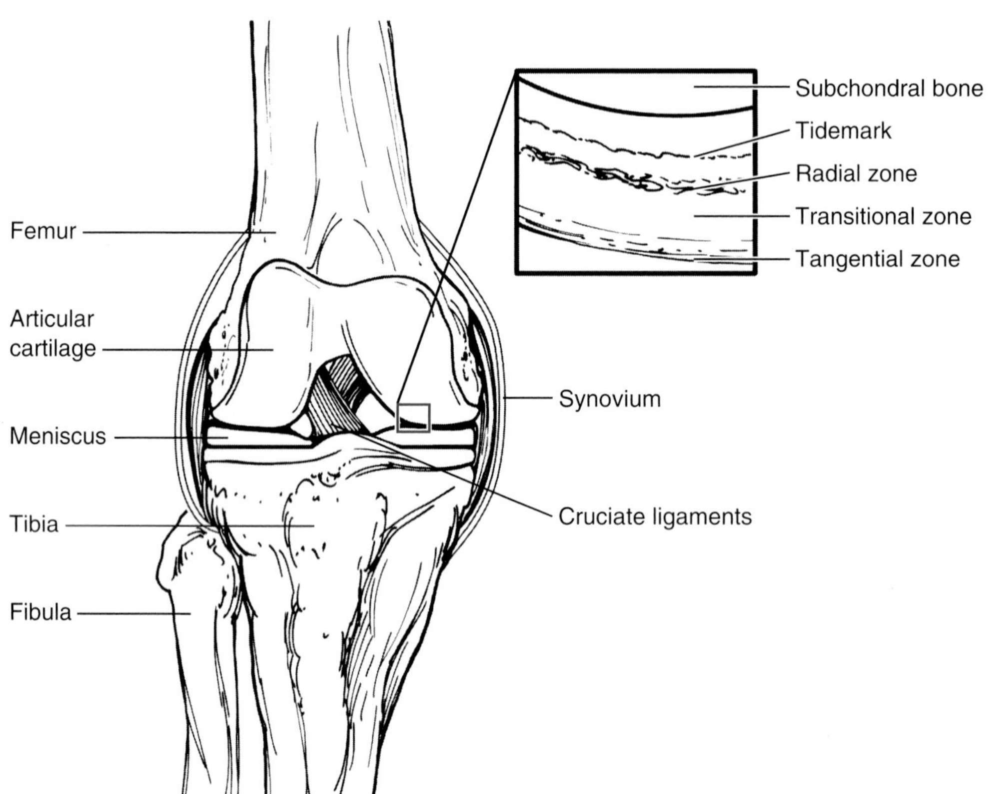

Figure 16–1: Anatomy of a diarthrodial (synovial) joint. The inset portrays the many layers of the articular cartilage.

Both the middle and the deep zones resist compression.
  - Deeper than this is the *tidemark,* an undulating border between the radial zone and the deeper calcifying zone.
  - The *calcifying zone* anchors the articular cartilage to the underlying (subchondral) bone.
- Synovium is the inner lining of the diarthrodial joint. It lines the nonarticular areas of synovial joints, bursa, and tendon sheaths.
  - Joint surfaces are subsequently lubricated by a fluid secreted and absorbed by this membrane. In diarthrodial joints, synovium lines the fibrous capsules and covers most exposed osseous surfaces. It is absent from intra-articular disks, or *menisci,* and from the margins of the articular cartilage.
  - Grossly, healthy synovium is pink, smooth, and shiny, with folds (plica) and fringes. The synovial membrane consists of a cellular intima. Synoviocytes are found in this layer.
- There are two types of synoviocytes.
  - Type A synoviocytes are derived from a macrophage-type cell responsible for phagocytosis and the removal of debris.
  - Type B synoviocytes are primarily responsible for the synthesis of the components of synovial fluid.
  - Deeper than the intimal layer is the subintimal lamina. These two layers are not separated by a basement membrane. Between these two layers are fibroblasts, macrophages, mast cells, and fat cells.
- The fibrous capsule of the joint has condensed, parallel bundles of white type I collagen fibers, often with local thickenings of parallel fibers, which are joint capsular ligaments. These are often named by their attachments. In general, ligaments are firm enough to limit excessive motion yet pliable enough to allow normal range of motion.
- Noncongruent joints, such as the knee, have intra-articular disks, menisci, and labra. These are fibrocartilaginous structures and allow stress transmission across the noncongruent joint surfaces.

Joint Pathoanatomy

- General joint pathology can be divided into four groups.
  - *Noninflammatory arthrosis*—This primarily describes osteoarthrosis but includes joint destruction associated with osteonecrosis and trauma.
  - *Inflammatory arthritides*—This includes a variety of disorders, which will be covered in greater detail later in this chapter. In children, juvenile rheumatoid arthritis (JRA) is the most common of these, but it can be associated with many other systemic disorders.
  - *Infectious arthritides*—This includes septic arthritis, which will be covered in other chapters.
  - *Hemorrhagic arthritides*—This includes hemophilic arthropathy, sickle cell joint destruction, and pigmented villonodular synovitis.
- Pathoanatomy of a joint can occur at the joint surface, synovium, fibrous capsule, or other intra-articular structures.
  - *Articular surface*—In children, osteoarthrosis does not occur unless there is an underlying injury or defect in the quality of the joint surface. In some skeletal dysplasias—such as pseudoachondroplasia; multiple epiphyseal dysplasia, coma, and spondyloepiphyseal dysplasia —there is a primary defect in the quality of the articular surface.
  - *Synovial lining*—Inflammation of the synovial lining can be a result of primary pathology such as occurs with JRA. The synovial membrane will become edematous and infiltrated with mononuclear cells, primarily lymphocytes and plasma cells. The synovium will proliferate; the articular cartilage and subchondral bone are then secondarily affected.
  - *Fibrous capsule*—The fibrous capsule can be primarily affected by trauma or with underlying disorders of type I collagen. This may cause ligamentous laxity and ultimately generalized joint laxity and even subluxation and dislocation of less constrained joints, such as the patellofemoral joint or shoulder.
  - *Other nonarticular joint surfaces*—There can also be injuries to the intra-articular disks, menisci, or labrum. These are common in the knee. The blood supply to the meniscus is in the peripheral 25% of the meniscus. If there is a tear to the meniscus, peripheral tears have a much higher chance of healing and should be repaired. Children may lack complete development of the meniscus, termed *discoid meniscus.* This may lead to pain and locking symptoms. Labral tears in the hip are more becoming frequently recognized and treated with newer techniques, such as hip arthroscopy.

Clinical Features

- Synovial disorders often have specific definitions or criteria for their diagnoses (described later in this chapter). There are often several key characteristics that need to be elicited from the history. Of primary importance are the location of pain; its intensity, duration, and timing; the response to treatment; age; sex; family history; and associated symptoms.
  - *Location–intensity of pain*—The location of pain is important. Various disorders often affect one or more particular joints. Typically, the muscles are not affected, and rarely is there pain over the diaphyseal regions of the long bones. The intensity of pain is crucial. With underlying synovial disorders, the intensity of the pain tends to be moderate. When a child reports severe pain, it typically occurs over a gradual period. This is extremely important because severe pain, especially with new onset, should make you immediately

consider more emergent disorders, such as septic arthritis or trauma. These may need to be treated emergently.

- *Duration and timing of pain*—The duration and timing of the pain are important. Children with synovial disorders frequently will have pain and stiffness, especially in the morning or after resting or sitting for long periods. This is often called *gelling*. This tends to improve shortly after activity is renewed.
- *Treatment response, age, and sex*—Assessing the response to treatment, the effects of activity restriction, or both can be helpful in the differential diagnosis. Synovial disorders typically improve with moderate activity. This contrasts with a traumatic injury, which improves dramatically with immobilization and, as injury heals, is accompanied by a reinstitution of activities without pain. Lack of response to nonsteroidal anti-inflammatory drugs (NSAIDs) argues against an inflammatory etiology. The age of the child can be helpful. The onset of synovial disorders in children typically occurs before 6 years. Although trauma occurs in children of this age, usually the history can easily differentiate between the two disorders. Nonaccidental trauma (child abuse) normally occurs in much younger children and typically consists of multiple bone injuries in multiple stages of healing. Inflammatory disorders are typically more common in girls, as are pain amplification syndromes.
- *Family history and associated symptoms*—A family history should be elicited. Human leukocyte antigen (HLA) B27-associated disorders, for example, tend to affect more than one family member. Associated symptoms can also be helpful in guiding a diagnosis. Fever could be associated with septic arthritis but can also be seen in some forms of JRA. You should also be aware that certain forms of childhood chronic arthritis, including JRA, are associated with uveitis and it is crucial that children who ultimately have the diagnosis of JRA are seen and evaluated by an ophthalmologist.

Physical Examination and Approach to Evaluation

- Secondary to the history, the physical examination is crucial to the evaluation of a child with synovial disorders. General evaluation of the joint should include observation, palpation for the location of tenderness, presence and direction of joint instability, and examination for joint effusion or synovial swelling. Multiple versus single joint inflammation will help with the differential diagnosis. Range of motion of the joint should also be determined. Signs of trauma and areas of point tenderness should be identified and documented. It is important to examine the child walking and playing to determine whether there is a limp. A child who is in excruciating pain, who will not allow you to internally rotate the hip, and who will not bear weight has septic arthritis unless proven otherwise. This is covered more thoroughly in Chapter 13.

Laboratory Evaluation

- The evaluation will be covered more specifically for each disorder. Unfortunately, there are no single tests or multitest panels appropriate for all children with suspected synovial disorders. Therefore, the history and physical examination should guide you toward determining the appropriate laboratory evaluation. That being said, for most children, a complete blood count (CBC) with a differential and platelet count, evaluation of C-reactive protein level, erythrocyte sedimentation rate (ESR), or a combination of these are often indicated.
- The ESR is a nonspecific measurement of underlying inflammation. The ESR in children with synovial disorders is often elevated but typically to less than 100 mm/hr, although there are exceptions. It is nonspecific and more helpful in ruling out synovial and inflammatory disorders. The ESR may be elevated because of a marked anemia or a low serum concentration of albumin. This must be taken into account when evaluating the ESR. The C-reactive protein and, to some degree, platelets from the CBC are evaluations of acute phase reactants. C-reactive protein responds to treatment more quickly and should fall within days of effective treatment; therefore it is helpful in monitoring the response to treatment.
- The antinuclear antibody (ANA) is a measure of serum antibodies that bind to antigens in the nucleus of the cells. Although this is often used as a screening test for synovial disorders, ANAs may be elevated in up to 20% of normal children, typically lower titers. If a child is diagnosed with JRA and the ANA is positive, then that child is at increased risk of developing silent uveitis. All children diagnosed with JRA should receive prompt referral to an ophthalmologist for a slit lamp examination for the presence of uveitis.
- Rheumatoid factor (RF) is an autoreactive antibody that identifies immunoglobulin G as bound to antigen. In children, this is infrequently positive, especially in children younger than 7 years. If this is positive in a child with JRA, however, it is associated with a poor prognosis. RF is likely to be present in children with other diseases; therefore the role of this test for diagnosis in children is limited.

- HLA-B27 is associated with transient reactive arthritis and other enthesitis-related arthritis. Although this is positive in a significant portion (approximately 10%) of the white population, this may be helpful in making a correct diagnosis.
- Synovial fluid analysis in inflammatory arthritis includes white blood cell counts, which are generally between 5000 and 20,000 cells/mm^3. This is in contrast to septic arthritis, which often has cell counts greater than 50,000. However, noninfectious forms of inflammatory arthritis can have blood cell counts this high or higher.

Radiographic Examination and other Diagnostic Imaging

- Radiographs—Radiographic studies of a specific joint should be directed by history and physical examination. The primary role of radiographic examination is to rule out other disorders. It is especially crucial in children who complain primarily of knee, anterior thigh, or groin pain. Anterior thigh or groin pain is commonly misdiagnosed as a groin pull or knee disorder when the true pathology may be a hip disorder, such as a slipped capital femoral epiphysis or Legg-Calve-Perthes disease. If the physical examination demonstrates abnormalities of a specific joint, then radiographic evaluation is indicated. Typically, orthogonal views of each joint, in a weight-bearing position, are indicated, although there are multiple special views for different joints. Radiographic changes consistent with synovial disorders are typically long standing, and bony changes will not be obvious from radiographs taken early in the disease process, although soft tissue swelling may be evident. Over several months, bony resorption may be evident, and the bone may appear more radiolucent. If the disease continues, then evidence of cartilaginous destruction may be evident.
- Other imaging studies—Other imaging studies may be useful. The pathology may be related not only to bony disorders but also to underlying soft tissue disorders.
  - Magnetic resonance imaging (MRI)—MRI is an especially well-recognized tool for the examination of nonbony intra-articular pathology such as meniscal tears and osteochondral lesions.
  - Computerized tomography (CT) is useful for viewing bony abnormalities more accurately and is particularly useful in trauma, such as intra-articular fractures.
  - Bone scans can be helpful for identifying the location (or locations if there are multiple sites) of the disorder. Although nonspecific, an absence of changes on a bone scan can be helpful in ruling out diagnoses or locating different sites of the underlying disorder.

Classifications of Chronic Arthritis in Childhood

- Approximately 1 in 1000 children will develop some form of chronic arthritis (>6 weeks). The most common form of chronic arthritis in childhood is JRA.
- JRA is subdivided into three forms: pauciarticular onset (no more than four joints), polyarticular (more than four joints), and systemic onset (associated with high fevers and an evanescent, salmon-colored rash) (Table 16–1).
- The other major group of chronic arthritides in childhood consists of the HLA-B27–associated spondyloarthropathies. A new classification system for childhood chronic arthritis (the International League of Associations for Rheumatology criteria), which encompasses both JRA and spondyloarthropathies, has been proposed (Table 16–1).
- The childhood spondyloarthropathies are the seronegative enthesopathy and arthropathy (SEA) syndrome, juvenile ankylosing spondylitis (JAS) (similar to the adult form with onset before 18 years), juvenile psoriatic arthritis (chronic arthritis associated with psoriasis), and arthritis associated with inflammatory bowel disease (Crohn's disease and ulcerative colitis) (Table 16–1).
- Other forms of HLA-B27–associated arthritis are reactive arthritis and Reiter syndrome (conjunctivitis, arthritis, and urethritis). These usually occur after infectious gastroenteritis or chlamydial infections. Although they may be recurrent, they are usually not chronic (>6 weeks).
- Acute rheumatic fever is another infection-associated reactive-type arthritis, which is triggered by group A streptococci. It is much less common in the United States these days but is still present. The diagnosis is made using the modified Jones criteria, which also outline the potential manifestations of the illness, including carditis (Table 16–2).

Table 16–1: Subtypes of Childhood Chronic Arthritis and Classification Criteria

JRA	JCA	JIA
Systemic	Systemic	Systemic
Polyarticular	Polyarticular JCA	Polyarticular RF–
	JRA	Polyarticular RF+
Pauciarticular	Pauciarticular	Oligoarticular
		Persistent
		Extended
	Juvenile psoriatic arthritis	Psoriatic arthritis
	Juvenile ankylosing spondylitis	Enthesitis-related arthritis
		Other arthritis

JCA, juvenile chronic arthritis; *JIA*, juvenile idiopathic arthritis; *JRA*, juvenile rheumatoid arthritis; *RF*, rheumatoid factor.

Table 16–2: Modified Jones Criteria for the Diagnosis of Rheumatic Fever*

MAJOR MANIFESTATIONS	MINOR MANIFESTATIONS
Carditis	Prolonged P-R interval
Polyarthritis	Arthralgia
Sydenham's chorea	Fever
Erythema marginatum	Elevated acute phase reactants (ESR or CRP)
Subcutaneous nodules	

CRP, C-reactive protein; *ESR*, erythrocyte sedimentation rate.
* Requires evidence of recent streptococcal infection (positive throat culture, rapid streptococcal antigen test, or elevated or rising streptococcal antibody titer or titers) plus two major or one major and two minor criteria.

- Lyme disease (LD), caused by the spirochete, *Borrelia burgdorferi,* is an antibiotic treatable form of childhood arthritis, which often mimics pauciarticular JRA (pauciJRA) in the New England states and other endemic regions of the United States.
- Other less common forms of chronic arthritis in childhood are associated with rheumatic diseases in which arthritis may be a component. These include the following: systemic lupus erythematosus (SLE), juvenile dermatomyositis (JDMS), sarcoidosis, and systemic vasculitides, such as polyarteritis nodosa.

Differential Diagnosis

- *Benign pains in childhood*—Children often complain of pain. It can be difficult to sort through the multitude of benign disorders and discover the complaints of concern. Complaints often are significant enough that children will show symptoms to their primary care provider or pediatric orthopaedic surgeon. Many children with pain have been diagnosed as having growing pains. It is important to remember that growing pains are a diagnosis of exclusion and that other disorders need to be ruled out. It is not clear that growing pains are related to the growth of children. Growing pains, also called *benign nocturnal limb pains of childhood,* occur in children between the ages of 2 and 12 who have episodes of pain, particularly occurring in the evening, with days of full and normal activity. The pains appear to be improved with rubbing or massage. They typically affect both lower extremities, are not focused at the joints, and involve multiple and different locations. Physical examination and laboratory studies are always normal, and the pain is usually absent during the day. This is episodic. It does not worsen over time and, typically, does not involve a limp. If symptoms are not consistent with the preceding picture or if the pains persist, then further evaluation is warranted. Treatment is typically symptomatic with the use of acetaminophen, ibuprofen, massage, or a combination of these.
- Reflex sympathetic dystrophy (complex regional pain syndrome) can occur in children and young adults, typically secondary to fairly minor trauma, its treatment, or both. Pain even to light touch, swelling, and temperature and skin color changes are associated with this disorder. Regional osteoporosis can be seen several weeks after the onset on radiographs. Bone scans may show a slight increase or decrease in uptake of the involved region, and treatment includes vigorous physical therapy and psychological counseling. Timely diagnoses are crucial because children do better with early diagnosis and treatment.
- *Transient synovitis versus septic arthritis*—Transient synovitis occurs in children, and the primary differential diagnosis is between that and septic arthritis of the hip. In both cases, young children may have significant pain, which can cause crying and limit motion of the hip fairly dramatically. The child may be carried in or limping and may tend to sit or lie with the leg flexed and in external rotation. The differential diagnosis between these two disorders is extremely important and can be difficult. Treatment varies dramatically from open arthrotomy for septic arthritis to simple observation and NSAIDs for transient synovitis. To help make this diagnosis more accurately, Kocher et al. developed four clinical criteria to aid the assessment of the child with a painful hip (Box 16–2). In their study, if all four of the criteria were met, then there was a 99% chance that these children would have septic arthritis. There was a 93% chance of septic arthritis if three of the four criteria were present, a 40% chance if half the criteria were present, and 3% for one criterion. When the study was taken in different populations, however, the correlation was much less dramatic. Despite this, these are excellent clinical factors to help guide your differential diagnosis and subsequent treatment. If the diagnosis is still in question, ultrasound will help to determine whether there is an effusion but will not differentiate between septic arthritis and toxic synovitis. Aspiration of the hip joint and evaluation of the fluid is crucial and can be performed with radiographic (fluoroscopic) or ultrasound guidance. A positive gram stain or a white blood cell count greater than 50,000 indicate septic arthritis, and this would require open or arthroscopic hip decompression. It is important to realize that the evaluation *must rule out* the possibility of septic

Box 16–2 Septic Arthritis versus Toxic Synovitis

Criteria to differentiate septic arthritis from toxic synovitis include the following:

- Inability to ambulate
- White blood cell count greater than 12,000 cells/cc
- ESR of at least 40 mm/hr
- Fever

arthritis of the hip and that if it is suspected it must be treated emergently. Also included in this differential diagnosis are children with congenital coagulopathies, such as hemophilia, and with hemoglobinopathies, including sickle cell disease. These diagnoses should be well established, and in a child with this history, local swelling, and local pain, this diagnosis must be considered in the differential diagnosis with septic arthritis and acute osteomyelitis.

- *Tumors*—Benign bony tumors may be found incidentally or as a cause of pain in the lower extremity. It is not uncommon in a routine workup for joint pain to identify a benign lesion such as a fibrous cortical defect or nonossified fibroma. Typically, these are not painful nor the cause of the pain, but they should be thoroughly evaluated to ensure that they are benign. Other benign lesions, such as osteoid osteoma, which appears as a well-defined sclerotic lesion surrounding a radiolucent center, can cause pain. The patient's response to NSAIDs may help to make this diagnosis. CT evaluation may also be beneficial.
- Pigmented villonodular synovitis is a benign synovial tumor. This is rare in childhood but swells joints. The diagnosis usually can be made from MRI findings or by joint aspiration (high red blood cell count).
- Of greatest concern in differential diagnoses are malignant tumors. Leukemia can present with skeletal pain and must always be kept in the differential diagnosis. Typically, pain is localized not to the joint but to the diaphysis of the long bones. Pain that wakes the child at night who is not completely well during the day is of great concern. Often the ESR is dramatically elevated and the CBC is abnormal in leukemia, although the cells may need to be examined microscopically to identify immature cell lines. Plain radiographs early in the disorder may be deceptively benign. Typically, they display a poorly defined lesion with a periosteal reaction. Other features suggestive of malignancy include nonarticular pain, back pain, bone tenderness, and constitutional symptoms. Night sweats, ecchymosis, abnormal neurological signs, and masses are associated with underlying malignancies. Children with leukemia may also have the unusual combination of an increased ESR with a low platelet count.

Specific Disorders

Juvenile Rheumatoid Arthritis

Systemic Onset

- Systemic onset JRA (SoJRA) can occur at any age during childhood. There is no gender preference, and this form of JRA accounts for about 10 to 20% of all children diagnosed with JRA.
- Children with SoJRA usually appear ill at diagnosis. They experience a daily or twice daily high-spiking fever (a quotidian pattern—see Figure 16–2) that usually returns to below baseline (<37° C). Children with SoJRA may feel relatively well when afebrile.
- The classical quotidian fever pattern often helps to distinguish SoJRA from most infectious illnesses, but

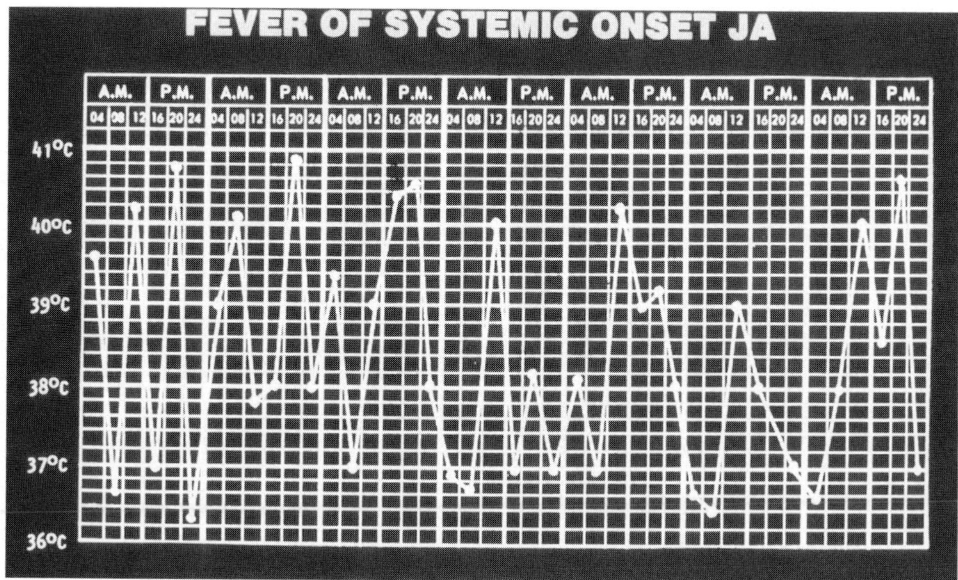

Figure 16–2: Quotidian fever. The classical high-spiking fever of SoJRA usually peaks once daily in the late afternoon. The body temperature usually dips below 37° C after the spike. Graph of patient data courtesy Dr. David Sherry.

SoJRA must always be considered a diagnosis of exclusion. It is particularly important to rule out infectious and neoplastic (including leukemia–lymphoma) disorders before the initiation of immunosuppressive therapy.

- In addition to the fever, children with SoJRA typically experience an evanescent salmon-colored, usually truncal, rash that comes and goes with the fever (Figure 16–3).
- The arthritis of SoJRA may range from monoarticular to polyarticular. In some children, it may be aggressive, leading to erosive disease similar to that seen in RF+ polyarticular JRA (polyJRA). In other children, the arthritis may be mild or even absent (making the diagnosis of SoJRA difficult) but the systemic features may be prominent.
- Besides the rash and fever, other common systemic features of SoJRA include anemia of chronic disease, lymphadenopathy, hepatosplenomegaly, pericarditis, and macrophage activation syndrome (MAS).
- MAS, or hemophagocytic syndrome, is often associated with SoJRA disease flares. It may also be triggered by viral infections. It can be relatively mild but also may range to severe manifestations. At its worst, MAS may lead to disseminated intravascular coagulopathy, which can be fatal.
- Laboratory values associated with MAS include transaminitis, anemia, elevated D-dimer levels, a falling ESR (usually elevated with active disease), a falling white blood cell count (usually high with mostly neutrophils in active SoJRA), and a falling platelet count (usually elevated in SoJRA). A definitive diagnosis of MAS can sometimes be made by observing hemophagocytosis in a bone marrow aspirate specimen (Figure 16–4).
- The ultimate course of SoJRA varies from child to child. Some may "burn out" their illness within months of disease onset, others may have relapsing courses, and still others may have a long-lasting chronically active form (with primarily systemic features, primarily arthritic features, or both).
- Treatment of SoJRA depends on the severity of the illness but often includes systemic (oral and pulse intravenous) and intra-articular administration of corticosteroids, NSAIDs (particularly indomethacin), methotrexate, and tumor necrosis factor (TNF) inhibitors. For severe forms, cyclophosphamide, thalidomide, or autologous stem cell transplantation have been used.

Polyarticular

- Children with polyJRA are typically white females who develop the disease at an early age (<5 years), but a subset will have the disease onset later in childhood, particularly in their teenage years. Some of these older girls may have a form of spondyloarthropathy, but it is often difficult to distinguish these two forms of chronic childhood arthritis.
- Children with polyJRA usually make up about 30 to 40% of all cases of JRA. A small subset (10%, or

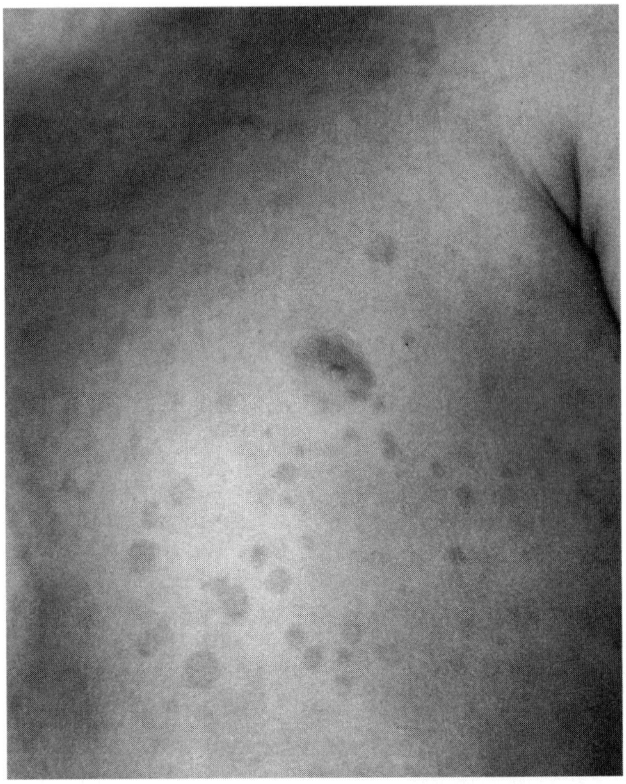

Figure 16–3: The salmon-colored, evanescent rash of SoJRA. **The rash of SoJRA is commonly present on the trunk but may appear elsewhere, including the face. The rash will come and go with the fever and returns in different locations, unlike a vasculitic rash. Photo courtesy Dr. David Sherry.**

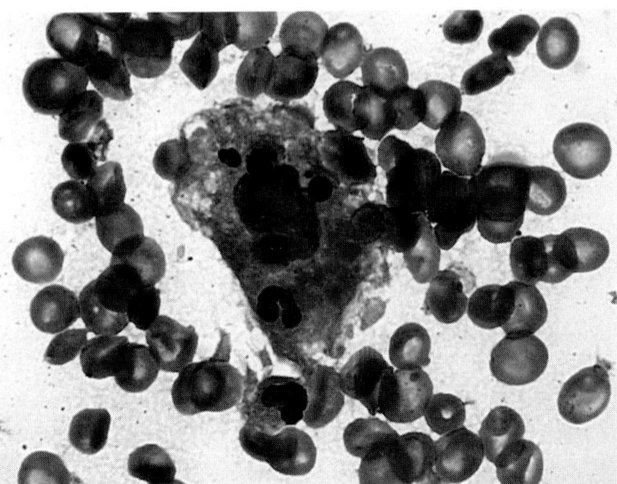

Figure 16–4: MAS. **A hematoxylin and eosin stain from a bone marrow aspirate from Still's disease demonstrating macrophage engulfment of multiple cells, including polymorphonuclear cells. Photo courtesy Dr. Lisabeth Scalzi.**

approximately 4% of all cases of JRA) is associated with RF+. In general, these girls have a more severe–erosive form of arthritis (Figure 16–5).

- By definition, children with polyJRA have five or more involved joints. Certain joints are commonly involved, including the small joints of the hands and feet, and the arthritis tends to be in a symmetrical distribution.
- Nonarticular features of polyJRA include low-grade fevers, hepatosplenomegaly, anemia of chronic disease, subcutaneous nodules (usually in those with RF+ disease), and silent uveitis (particularly in those with a positive ANA).
- The disease course of polyJRA can be variable. Those with RF+ disease most resemble the adult form of rheumatoid arthritis and may have an aggressive form of arthritis.
- Treatment for polyJRA includes intra-articular corticosteroid injections, NSAIDs, methotrexate, TNF inhibitors, and occasionally low-dose oral corticosteroids.

Pauciarticular

- PauciJRA usually affects 1- to 3-year-old white females. By definition, these girls have no more than four joints involved, the most commonly involved joints being the knee and ankle. The distribution of arthritis is often asymmetrical. A subset of children with pauciJRA will progress to a polyarticular variety, which can be difficult to treat.
- Children with pauciJRA appear well but often have a limp and a swollen knee. Up to one third of these girls will have painless arthritis.
- Leg length discrepancies caused by bony overgrowth, usually around an involved knee joint, may develop if the arthritis is not rapidly treated. For this reason and others, intra-articular corticosteroid injections are commonly used to treat children with JRA.
- Because children with pauciJRA have a high incidence of ANAs, they are at high risk of developing silent uveitis. This necessitates frequent slit lamp screening by a pediatric ophthalmologist to help avoid decreased visual acuity and blindness (Table 16–3).

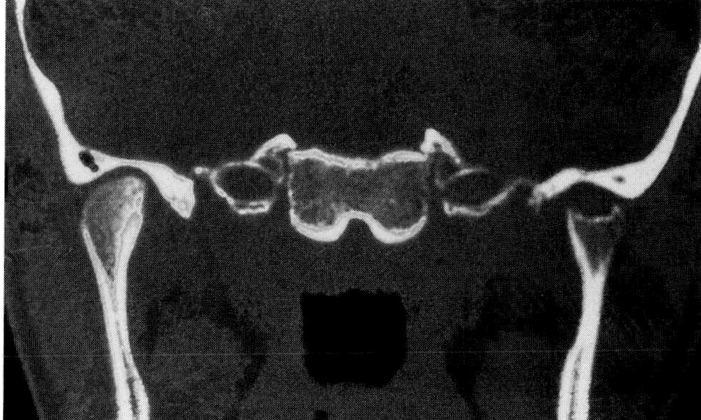

Figure 16–5: Erosive arthritis. This CT scan reveals erosion of the right mandibular condylar head in a child with polyJRA. Photo courtesy Dr. David Sherry.

Spondyloarthropathies

SEA Syndrome

- SEA stands for seronegative (ANA and RF are negative but not mandatory), enthesopathy (pain where ligaments and tendons insert into bone—generally around the knees and feet), and arthropathy (usually of the lower extremities).
- Boys with SEA syndrome outnumber girls 7:1. Greater than 70% of individuals with SEA syndrome are HLA-B27+ compared with less than 10% of the general white population in the United States.
- Children with SEA syndrome may go on to develop inflammatory bowel disease, psoriatic arthritis, or ankylosing spondylitis. Other children may never progress beyond SEA syndrome.

Juvenile Psoriatic Arthritis

- Juvenile psoriatic arthritis is simply chronic arthritis associated with psoriasis onset before age 16. If psoriasis is absent, the diagnosis can still be made in the presence of three of the four following conditions: dactylitis (sausage-shaped digit), nail pitting or onycholysis, a psoriasis-like rash, or a first- or second-degree relative with psoriasis.
- Psoriatic arthritis is the one form of spondyloarthropathy that is slightly more common in girls. Also, the association with HLA-B27 is thought to be less than 50%. Only about 5% of individuals with psoriasis develop arthritis.

Table 16–3: Recommendations for Uveitis Screening in Children with Juvenile Rheumatoid Arthritis*

JRA TYPE	AGE AT ONSET: YOUNGER THAN 7 YEARS	AGE AT ONSET: 7 YEARS OR OLDER
Pauciarticular or polyarticular		
ANA+	Every 3 to 4 months for 4 years, then every 6 months for 3 years, then yearly	Every 6 months or 4 years, then yearly
ANA–	Every 6 months for 7 years, then yearly	As above
Systemic	Yearly	Yearly

ANA, antinuclear antibody; *JRA*, juvenile rheumatoid arthritis.
* Based on a joint statement of ophthalmologists and pediatricians published in Pediatrics (1993) 92:295.

Arthropathy Associated with Inflammatory Bowel Disease

- It is estimated that 10 to 30% of individuals with Crohn's disease and ulcerative colitis will develop chronic arthritis. The arthritis can precede, coincide with, or manifest subsequent to the bowel disease.
- The arthritis usually begins peripherally, primarily in the lower extremities. However, a subset of children may develop a more severe form of arthritis involving the sacroiliac joints and axial skeleton, even after the gastrointestinal disease has resolved.
- Skin manifestations of inflammatory bowel disease include erythema nodosum and pyoderma gangrenosum. When present, these skin findings may help to establish a diagnosis of inflammatory bowel disease. The presence of antisaccharomyces cerevisiae antibodies is also associated with inflammatory bowel disease.

Reactive Arthritis and Reiter Syndrome

- Reactive arthritis and Reiter syndrome occur in response to a prior infection, usually within a few weeks. In addition to the arthritis seen in reactive arthritis, Reiter syndrome includes urethritis and conjunctivitis. In addition, mucocutaneous findings may be present, including the unusual rash keratoderma blennorrhagicum.
- In young children, the arthritis is typically triggered by organisms that lead to gastroenteritis. The most common enteric pathogens implicated are *Salmonella, Shigella, Campylobacter,* and *Yersinia*. However, *Clostridium* and even parasites, such as *Giardia* and *Cryptosporidium,* can trigger disease.
- Older boys will often develop Reiter syndrome from sexually transmitted chlamydial infections.
- Reactive arthritis and Reiter syndrome are usually self-limited but rarely develop a chronic course, which can last more than 1 year.

Juvenile Ankylosing Spondylitis

- JAS is uncommon in childhood partly because of the stringent criteria required to make the diagnosis. JAS is seen in some late adolescent, HLA-B27+ boys. SEA syndrome can be a precursor for JAS as well.
- Like the adult form, JAS involves the peripheral and axial skeleton and can be debilitating. Enthesitis is usually present in JAS.
- Other features of the disease include a red, painful, photophobic iritis (in distinction to the silent uveitis of JRA) and rarely an aortic insufficiency, or central nervous system disease, such as cauda equina syndrome.

Rheumatic Fever and Poststreptococcal Reactive Arthritis

- Rheumatic fever is caused by Group A β-hemolytic streptococci. Rheumatic fever typically occurs in children of both sexes between the ages of 5 and 15 years. Symptoms of rheumatic fever generally appear about 2 weeks after pharyngitis.
- The diagnosis of rheumatic fever is made using the modified Jones criteria (see Table 16–2). There must be evidence of a recent streptococcal infection (positive throat culture or elevated streptococcal serum titers) plus two major or one major and two minor criteria. The major criteria are carditis, polyarthritis, chorea, subcutaneous nodules, and erythema marginatum (Figure 16–6). The minor criteria are a prolonged P-R interval, fever, arthralgia, and elevated ESR or C-reactive protein.
- The arthritis of rheumatic fever is migratory and often involves six large joints or more. The onset of arthritis is acute, painful, and responds well to aspirin. The arthritis typically resolves within 3 weeks without residual deformity.
- Treatment of rheumatic fever includes antibiotic eradication of the streptococcal pharyngitis and early high-dose aspirin followed by low-dose aspirin. Corticosteroids are used for carditis.
- Poststreptococcal reactive arthritis differs from rheumatic fever in that the arthritis often includes both small and large joints and that the arthritis can persist for months. The arthritis is usually more difficult to treat. Fortunately, few individuals with poststreptococcal reactive arthritis go on to develop carditis.

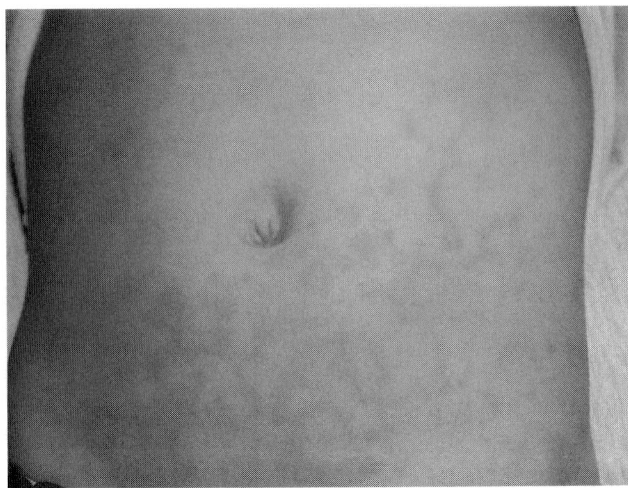

Figure 16–6: Erythema marginatum. **The rash of rheumatic fever on the abdomen of a child. Photo courtesy Dr. Jon Burnham.**

Lyme Disease

- LD is the most common tick-borne disease in the United States. In the United States, LD is usually caused by the spirochete, *B. burgdorferi,* which is commonly transmitted by deer ticks of the genus, *Ixodes*.
- An enzyme-linked immunosorbent assay (ELISA) is used to screen for LD, but Western blot assays are used to confirm the diagnosis when the ELISA is only mildly positive. Many borderline-positive Lyme ELISA results are false positives.
- LD begins with a flu-like illness, usually occurring in the summer. The classic rash of erythema chronicum migrans may or may not be present in infected children. HLA-DR4 and HLA-DR2 are known risk factors for developing arthritis associated with LD.
- The manifestations of LD can be divided into early (days to weeks following infection) and late (months to years) manifestations.
- Early disease manifestations include malaise, fatigue, migratory arthralgias–myalgias, myopericarditis, atrioventricular block, meningitis, Bell's palsy, mononeuritis multiplex, conjunctivitis, and uveitis.
- Late disease manifestations of untreated disease include chronic fatigue, morphea-like skin lesions, chronic episodic oligoarticular large joint (usually a knee or knees) arthritis, Reiter syndrome, heart block, chronic encephalomyelitis, ataxia, and keratitis.
- Treatment for LD varies depending on the chronicity and severity of symptoms and on organ system involvement. Early disease is usually treated with a 14- to 28-day course of penicillin, amoxicillin, or erythromycin (for those allergic to penicillin) for children younger than 8 years. Tetracycline, doxycycline, or amoxicillin is used for those 8 and older.
- Treatment of late disease is as described previously with a 30-day course. If carditis is severe, arthritis is persistent (after 30 to 60 days of treatment), or meningoencephalitis is present treatment with intravenous ceftriaxone for 14 to 21 days is recommended.

Viral Arthritis

Rubella

- Arthritis can occur 2 to 4 weeks following rubella immunization or 1 week after the rash of Rubella infection. The arthritis typically involves the fingers and knee joints and usually lasts less than 1 month.

Parvovirus

- Parvovirus leads to erythema infectiosum (fifth disease, or slapped-cheek syndrome). Arthritis associated with parvovirus is more common in those with HLA-DR4. When present, the arthritis is usually symmetrical and often involves the knees and wrists.

Varicella

- Arthritis is rarely associated with varicella infection, but occasionally chickenpox is associated with psoriatic arthritis.

Epstein-Barr Virus

- Arthritis is rarely associated with infectious mononucleosis (Epstein-Barr virus), but Epstein-Barr virus may play a role in the pathogenesis of systemic lupus.

Hepatitis B

- Hepatitis B may lead to a lower extremity rash and arthritis, which resembles serum sickness. The arthritis is symmetrical, involving the hands, knees, and ankles, and lasts 4 weeks on average.

Connective Tissue Diseases with Associated Chronic Arthritis

Systemic Lupus Erythematosus

- SLE is a multiorgan system autoimmune disease characterized by the presence of antinuclear antibodies. It typically affects females of reproductive age and is more common in blacks.
- Of 11 criteria, 4 are required to make the diagnosis (Box 16–3). The criteria include many of the common disease manifestations: malar rash, photosensitivity rash, palatal ulcers, discoid rash, nephritis, central nervous system disease, serositis, hematopenias, arthritis, ANA+ and dsDNA+ antibodies, evidence of antiphospholipid antibodies, or a combination of these.
- Arthritis is relatively common in SLE. The arthritis is typically painful but nonerosive.

Box 16–3 Criteria for Diagnosing Systemic Lupus Erythematosus

Requires 4 of the following 11 criteria for diagnosis:

1. Malar rash
2. Discoid rash
3. Photosensitivity rash
4. Oral or nasal ulcers
5. Arthritis
6. Pleuritis or pericarditis
7. Nephorosis or nephritis
8. Psychosis
9. Hemolytic anemia, thrombocytopenia, or leukopenia
10. Anti-nuclear antibody
11. Anti–double-stranded DNA antibody, anti-Smith antibody, or evidence of antiphospholipid antibodies

Juvenile Dermatomyositis and Childhood Polymyositis

- Inflammatory myositis involving the proximal flexor muscle groups symmetrically is uncommon in childhood. When the classic heliotrope rash (upper eyelids) and Gottron's papules (knuckles) are present, however, the diagnosis of JDMS is straightforward.
- Serum muscles enzymes, including aldolase, creatine kinase, and lactate dehydrogenase, are often elevated in autoimmune myositis. Muscle inflammation can usually be seen by a T2-weighted MRI of the thighs. This may also be useful for guiding needle muscle biopsies, which are sometimes used for diagnosis.
- Arthritis is present in 7 to 38% of children with JDMS and polymyositis, but the diagnosis of mixed connective tissue disease should be considered if the arthritis is a prominent finding.

Sarcoidosis

- Sarcoidosis may present in late childhood with elevated angiotensin converting enzyme levels and classic pulmonary findings, including noncaseating granulomas and hilar adenopathy.
- An early age of onset (younger than 4 years) for a form of sarcoidosis is also seen in childhood and is characterized by boggy arthritis, uveitis, and a follicular rash. These children are sometimes misdiagnosed as having JRA. A rare familial variety of sarcoidosis is known as Blau syndrome.

Vasculitis-Associated Arthritis

- Arthritis is often a disease manifestation of systemic vasculitides, including Kawasaki disease, polyarteritis nodosa, Henoch-Schönlein purpura, Wegener granulomatosis, and Takayasu arteritis.

Treatment

Medical

- Advances in the medical therapy of childhood arthritis have progressed rapidly in the last 2 decades. The use of methotrexate, in particular, has revolutionized the care of chronic childhood arthritis.
  - NSAIDs, such as naproxen and ibuprofen, are still the most commonly used drugs to treat arthritis in childhood. The most common side effect of NSAID use is gastrointestinal distress, but chronic use requires periodic laboratory screening for renal, hepatic, and hematological toxicities. The recent development of selective cyclo-oxygenase-2 inhibitors, such as celecoxib and rofecoxib, may help to prevent gastritis. Lastly, sun exposure for fair-skinned children can lead to pseudoporphyria and facial scarring in children taking NSAIDs. Proper sun protection is, thus, imperative for these children.
  - For the treatment of childhood chronic arthritis, disease-modifying antirheumatic drugs (DMARDs) are being used earlier in the course of disease. The most commonly used DMARD is methotrexate, given once weekly at doses ranging from 0.3 to 1.0 mg/kg/wk (40 mg maximum). Subcutaneous dosing of methotrexate is preferential to oral dosing because of decreased gastrointestinal and hepatotoxicity (avoiding the first-pass effect on the liver), better absorption, and more consistent dosing. Methotrexate is used for all forms of childhood chronic arthritis, including JRA, the spondyloarthropathies, SLE, JDMS, sarcoidosis, the vasculitides, and other rheumatic disorders. Monthly to bimonthly screening of liver enzymes and CBCs are recommended for those on chronic methotrexate.
  - Sulfasalazine and hydroxychloroquine are other DMARDs used to treat chronic arthritis in childhood, but gold and penicillamine are essentially no longer in use for this indication.
  - Another common therapy for childhood chronic arthritis is intra-articular corticosteroid injections. With long-acting corticosteroids, such as triamcinolone hexacetonide, this form of treatment can keep individual joints quiescent for 6 to 18 months or longer. Use of intra-articular corticosteroid joint injections can also help to prevent leg length discrepancies from bony overgrowth surrounding inflamed joints and to decrease the use of systemic anti-inflammatory drugs. Common side effects include subcutaneous atrophy and hypopigmentation at sites of injection, but, fortunately, infection is extremely rare.
  - Because of the myriad of side effects associated with systemic corticosteroids, they usually are reserved for short-term use of very active arthritis or for DMARD-resistant arthritis. Side effects of systemic corticosteroid use are cushingoid habitus, hyperglycemia, cataracts, glaucoma, osteopenia, aseptic necrosis, and increased risk of infection, to list a few.
  - In the last few years, biological agents have been approved for difficult-to-treat polyarticular childhood arthritis. TNF inhibitors have gained widespread use, but newer agents, such as interleukin-1 inhibitors, are being studied.

Physical Therapy

- Children with underlying synovial disorders sometimes need to be evaluated by an occupational therapist, a physical therapist, or both. Therapy modalities can be employed to help not only with the activities of daily living but also with the maintenance of range of motion and strength.

- Splinting may be employed to maintain alignment and range of motion of an involved joint. Range of motion exercises should begin early in an effort to prevent joint contractures. If joint contractures form, treatment can be much more involved and possibly require surgery. Dynamic splinting may be helpful in preventing or treating relatively mild joint contractures. Serial casting can also be employed in an attempt to improve range of motion.
- Therapy is typically focused on only moderate strengthening gains, avoiding an aggressive high-resistance weight program. Occupational therapy has numerous modalities to help with activities of daily living, including use and training of assistive devices.

Surgical Treatment

- Generally, the use of surgical treatment for children with synovial disorders is limited and is specific to the individual disorder. Surgery is typically reserved until other modalities have failed. The sections that follow describe the general goals for surgery in children with synovial disorders.

Prevention of Worsening Deformity

- Synovectomies can be performed, although there are certain disorders in which this is more effective. Synovectomy for pigmented villonodular synovitis can also be helpful. Synovectomy is more controversial in children with underlying inflammatory disorders because the arthritis may return. Typically, synovectomy will provide a short-term benefit in joint swelling and pain, but long-term improvement is less clear. In young adults with synovial chondromatosis, removal of the multiple loose bodies is helpful. This could be performed either openly or arthroscopically. It is typically a difficult, demanding procedure but provides great benefit.

Improve Overall Function

- Surgical treatment has also been focused on improving range of motion. Soft tissue releases for improvement in motion are typically difficult in that the contractures involve the joint themselves and therefore tendon lengthening, as performed in a child with cerebral palsy, is much less effective. Because the joint capsule is often involved, it needs to be released to improve range of motion. The subsequent chance of scarring and recurrence of contractures is high. Occasionally, osteotomies above or below the joint can be performed with acceptance of the deformity at the joint. The osteotomy then creates a new deformity to compensate for the contracture. This can make future arthroplasty difficult and can be disfiguring. External fixation devices have been used to distract across joints in an attempt to improve motion. This has met mixed results. Typically, range is initially improved, but a recurrence of (on average) 50% of the gained range is not uncommon.
- Progressive leg length inequality is not uncommon; therefore children should be closely monitored for this. Scanograms or long-legged films with a ruler are helpful in determining overall leg length. From these radiographs, the estimated leg length and the timing of an appropriate epiphysiodesis (growth plate ablation) can be determined. In children with synovial disorders, estimations of leg length inequality at maturity can be difficult because the rate of growth of the involved leg may not be constant, as is true for children with congenital leg length inequalities. Involved joints may develop early bony overgrowth, but later their effected growth plates may shut down sooner during the pubertal growth spurt.
- In long-standing synovial disorders in which total joint destruction has occurred, other options must be considered. Arthrodesis can be considered in selective cases, such as the foot or wrist, in children with inflammatory arthrosis. This is much less beneficial in children with systemic disorders of the hip or knee because the remaining joints are often also affected, such as a contralateral hip or ipsilateral knee required for satisfactory function.
- One of the few indications for joint arthroplasty in children with synovial disorders is aseptic necrosis. In children with pain, severe functional limitations, and severe destruction of their joint space, this can be an effective and a relatively long-standing solution. Typically, the most commonly replaced joints are the hip and knee. A surgeon with expertise in this surgery should be consulted. Often, children need special components for their joint replacement, and sizing can be difficult. Long-term follow-up in children with synovial disorders undergoing total joint replacement has been encouraging.

Summary

- Joint complaints in childhood may be detected by an orthopaedic surgeon. The task of the physician is to determine the correct diagnosis from an extensive differential diagnostic list. The history and physical examination are most useful in determining the underlying cause of joint complaints in childhood, but joint fluid analysis can also help to establish a diagnosis of inflammatory arthritis of either infectious or rheumatic origin.
- Septic arthritis must be ruled out in acute forms of childhood arthritis. In addition to bacterial causes, viruses may be associated with childhood arthritis.
- Approximately 1 in 1000 children develops chronic arthritis (>6 weeks). The two most common disorders leading to chronic arthritis in childhood are JRA and the spondyloarthropathies. However, other less common

causes of chronic arthritis in childhood are seen as part of systemic rheumatic diseases, such as SLE.

- There has been and continues to be significant progress in the medical management of chronic childhood arthritis. The use of methotrexate and intra-articular corticosteroid injections has dramatically improved the quality of life in children with chronic arthritis. Newer biological agents, such as TNF inhibitors, have also had a substantial effect on childhood arthritis. Newer therapies are being studied, and the future of medical management for childhood arthritis looks promising.

Bibliography

Bauman C, Cron RQ, Sherry DD, Francis JS (1996) Reiter syndrome initially misdiagnosed as Kawasaki disease. J Pediatr 128: 366.

A comparison of the features that are similar and that distinguish Reiter syndrome and Kawasaki disease is presented. Because of the similarities, Reiter syndrome is commonly misdiagnosed as Kawasaki disease.

Cron RQ (2002) Current treatment for chronic arthritis in childhood. Curr Opin Pediatr 14: 684.

An up-to-date summary of treatment options, including new biological agents and aggressive therapies, for children with chronic arthritis.

Cron RQ, Sharma S, Sherry DD (1999) Current treatment by United States and Canadian pediatric rheumatologists. J Rheumatol 26: 2036.

A recent survey of North American pediatric rheumatologists assessing the frequency of use of various therapies to treat a variety of pediatric rheumatic diseases, including chronic arthritis.

Goodman JE, McGraft PJ (1991) The epidemiology of pain in children and adolescents: A review. Pain 46: 247.

An excellent overview of the (high) incidence of pain in children.

Kocher MS, Zurakowski D, Kasser JR (1999) Differentiation between septic arthritis and transient synovitis of the hip in children: An evidence-based clinical prediction algorithm. J Bone Joint Surg 81A: 1662.

This article provides a set of criteria that allows the clinician to quickly evaluate the probability of septic arthritis in children. This does not apply as well to other populations and is not a definitive diagnostic test. It is, however, an excellent tool to guide your diagnostic evaluation.

Jacobson ST, Levinson JE, Crawford AH (1985) Late results of synovectomy and no synovectomy in patients with juvenile rheumatoid arthritis. J Bone Joint Surg 67A: 8.

An early study showing little long-term benefit of synovectomy in patients with JRA.

Lehman TJ, Edelheit BS (2001) Clinical trials for poststreptococcal reactive arthritis. Curr Rheumatol Rep 3: 363.

A review of poststreptococcal reactive arthritis and its relationship to rheumatic fever.

Lovell DA, Giannini EH, Reiff A, Cawkwell GD, Silverman ED, Nocton JJ, Stein LD, Gedalia A, Ilowite NT, Wallace CA, Whitmore J, Finck BK (2000) Etanercept in children with polyarticular juvenile rheumatoid arthritis (Pediatric Rheumatology Collaborative Study Group). N Engl J Med 342: 763.

The first use of a biological agent, a TNF-α inhibitor, to successfully treat childhood chronic arthritis refractory to methotrexate.

Ostrov BE, Goldsmith DP, Athreya BH (1993) Differentiation of systemic juvenile rheumatoid arthritis from acute leukemia near the onset of disease. J Pediatr 122: 595.

An excellent article comparing disease features that help to distinguish SoJRA from leukemia.

Rosenberg AM, Petty RE (1982) A syndrome of seronegative enthesopathy and arthropathy in children. Arthritis Rheum 25: 1041.

The original description of SEA syndrome in children with HLA-B27–associated chronic arthritis distinct from JRA. SEA syndrome is relatively common, particularly among boys and some older girls with chronic arthritis, but it is often underdiagnosed and is sometimes misdiagnosed as JRA.

Sarokhan AJ, Scott RD, Thomas WH, Sledge CB, Ewald FC, Cloos DW (1983) Total knee arthroplasty in juvenile rheumatoid arthritis. J Bone Joint Surg 65: 1071.

An early review demonstrating good results in patients with JRA undergoing a total knee replacement.

Sherry DD (1999) Pain syndromes. In: Adolescent Rheumatology (Isenberg DA, Miller JJ, eds). London: Martin Dunita.

A framework to organize pain syndromes in children and adolescents.

Sherry DD, Bohnsack J, Salmonson K, Wallace CA, Mellins E (1990) Painless juvenile rheumatoid arthritis. J Pediatr 116: 921.

This study reports that up to one third of children with JRA have painless arthritis, debunking the notion that you do not have arthritis if you do not have pain.

Sherry DD, Stein LD, Reed AM, Schanberg LE, Kredich DW (1999) Prevention of leg length discrepancy in young children with pauciarticular juvenile rheumatoid arthritis by treatment with intra-articular steroids. Arthritis Rheum 42: 2330.

This study demonstrates the benefit of intra-articular corticosteroid injections in preventing leg length discrepancies associated with chronic arthritis of the knee.

Shetty AK, Gedalia A (1998) Sarcoidosis: A pediatric perspective. Clin Pediatr (Phila) 37: 107.

A review of childhood sarcoidosis, including good descriptions of the two forms in childhood. The use of methotrexate as a steroid-sparing agent is also described.

Steere AC (2001) Lyme disease. N Engl J Med 345: 115.

An excellent review of LD from a leader in the field.

Cassidy JT, Petty RE, eds (2001) Textbook of Pediatric Rheumatology, 4th edition. Philadelphia: WB Saunders, pp 214-391.

This is the latest edition of the definitive textbook on pediatric rheumatology. The text is thorough, timely, well written, and well edited. This is a necessity for anyone who cares for children with rheumatic diseases.

Wallace CA (1998) The use of methotrexate in childhood rheumatic diseases. Arthritis Rheum 41: 381.

An excellent summary of the use of methotrexate to treat childhood rheumatic diseases, including the chronic arthritides. Methotrexate use has revolutionized the care of children with chronic arthritis.

Wright DA (2001) Juvenile idiopathic arthritis. In: Lovell and Winter's Pediatric Orthopaedics (Morrissy RT, Weinstein SL, eds), 5th edition. Philadelphia: Lippincott Williams & Wilkins, pp 427-457.

An excellent review of pediatric arthritic disorders.

CHAPTER 17

Neuromuscular Disorders

Cerebral Palsy

David A. Spiegel* and John P. Dormans†

*MD, Associate Professor of Orthopaedic Surgery, University of Pennsylvania, Philadelphia, PA; Staff Surgeon, The Children's Hospital of Philadelphia, Philadelphia, PA
†MD, Chief of Orthopaedic Surgery, The Children's Hospital of Philadelphia, Philadelphia, PA; Professor of Orthopaedic Surgery, University of Pennsylvania School of Medicine, Philadelphia, PA

Definition, Etiology, Epidemiology, and Pathology

Definition and Diagnosis

- Cerebral palsy is a disorder of movement and posture that results from damage to the immature central nervous system (Box 17–1). The central nervous system lesion is not progressive; however, secondary effects on the growth of musculoskeletal tissues may progress until skeletal maturity. Functional capabilities and needs evolve as each child matures into adulthood. Priorities include *communication skills, activities of daily living,* and *mobility.*[1-3] The goals of treatment are to facilitate integration into society and maximize function in later life.
- The diagnosis establishes a disorder of movement and posture, correlates this disorder with damage to the immature brain, and rules out progressive disorders that may have similar clinical findings. The differential diagnosis includes progressive neurodegenerative disorders, genetic syndromes (familial spastic paraparesis and congenital ataxia), and metabolic diseases such as arginase deficiency, Lesch-Nyhan syndrome, Pelizaeus-Merzbacher disease, metachromatic leukodystrophy, and congenital hypothyroidism.

Etiology and Epidemiology

- The prevalence of cerebral palsy has not changed considerably over the past few decades (1-3 per 1000 live births in the United States), and in most cases the etiology remains unknown. Birth asphyxia has become an uncommon cause of cerebral palsy, and prenatal events are thought to be most common (50% have a history of prematurity). In addition, 50% of patients have a history of low birth weight, often less than 1500 grams. Postnatal causes are identified in approximately 5%.[1-3]

Risk Factors

- *Prenatal* factors occur from conception until the onset of labor and include exposure to toxins; infections (toxoplasmosis, rubella, cytomegalovirus, herpes, and syphilis) and chorioamnionitis; genetic syndromes; chromosomal abnormalities; maternal drug use (marijuana, tobacco, or cocaine), alcohol use, or both; and Rhesus incompatibility.
- *Perinatal* factors occur from the onset of labor to the first few days postpartum and include a tight nuchal cord, placental abruption, and birth trauma (rarely intracerebral hemorrhage).
- *Postnatal* risk factors occur from the first few days postpartum to approximately 2 years following birth and include infections (meningitis or encephalitis), hypoxia

Box 17–1 Key Points

- Cerebral palsy is a nonprogressive disorder of movement and posture resulting from damage to the immature brain. The central nervous system lesion is not progressive; however, secondary changes in the musculoskeletal system may progress throughout growth.
- Needs and functional capabilities evolve as each child matures into adulthood. Priorities include communication skills, activities of daily living, and mobility.
- The diagnosis is made by documenting a delay in neurological maturation, identifying upper motor neuron dysfunction, and ruling out progressive neurological conditions.
- Patients may be broadly categorized as to whether they have *pyramidal* (cortical) or *extrapyramidal* (cerebellum and basal ganglia) involvement. Both orthopaedic and neurosurgical interventions are directed toward spasticity (pyramidal) and the musculoskeletal sequelae of spasticity. More specific classification methods include the *physiological* (principle type of movement disorder) and the *geographical* (anatomical distribution of involvement).
- *Spasticity* results from damage to the pyramidal tracts and is a velocity-dependent increase in muscle tone. Patients with spasticity develop muscle contractures with growth; these in turn tether bony growth, resulting in secondary angular and rotational bony deformities.
- Options for the treatment of spasticity include *oral agents* (baclofen, benzodiazepines, and dantrolene), *intramuscular injections* (botox, phenol), *dorsal rhizotomy,* and *intrathecal baclofen.* Each of these methods has specific indications.
- Ambulators commonly require surgical intervention for progressive contractures, deformities associated with muscle imbalance, and rotational deformities of the extremities. Common procedures include muscle lengthening, transfer, or both and osteotomies.
- Treatment goals for the nonambulatory population include setting a comfortable and stable sitting posture, preventing pain, and promoting the ease of care. Nonambulators often benefit from surgical treatment of progressive hip subluxation or dislocation, lower extremity contractures, and scoliosis.
- Realistic goals are essential. Despite successful treatment of both spasticity and musculoskeletal deformities, other components of the patient's motor disorder will persist. These include abnormal patterns of movement such as athetosis, problems with selective motor control, deficiencies in balance and proprioception, muscle weakness, altered cognition, and visual disturbance.

from cardiac arrest, respiratory failure, near drowning, and trauma (accidental or nonaccidental).

Patterns of Injury to the Central Nervous System

- *Hypoxia* creates a diffuse pattern of injury with scattered areas of necrosis in the cerebral cortex, the cerebellum, and the subcortical nuclei.
- *Ischemia* affects "watershed" zones (collateral flow is not well established), most commonly in the deep, periventricular gray matter. This results in periventricular leukomalacia, a common finding on magnetic resonance imaging (MRI) in children with spastic diplegia. Ischemic injury may be associated with intraventricular hemorrhage in approximately 50% of cases.
- *Intracerebral hemorrhage* is usually atraumatic. *Intraventricular* hemorrhage may be associated with either hypoxia or ischemia and is observed in approximately 50% of preterm infants with a birth weight less than 1500 grams. Risk factors include asphyxia, low Apgar scores, respiratory distress, and mechanical ventilation. Grade I hemorrhage involves the germinal matrix, and extension into ventricles occurs in grade II. The ventricles become dilated in grade III, and the hemorrhage extends into the parenchyma in grade IV. Less commonly, traumatic intracerebral hemorrhage may occur (subdural, subarachnoid, or intracerebral).[1]

Coexisting Medical Problems

- A knowledge of coexisting medical problems helps to stratify preoperative risk. Complications following orthopaedic surgery are more frequent in the presence of these comorbidities. For example, the risk of a complication following surgery for neuromuscular hip dysplasia may be 50% in quadriplegic patients who require a gastrostomy tube for nutritional support.
  - Central nervous system problems include mental retardation, seizures, visual problems (strabismus or cortical blindness), behavioral disturbance, and emotional problems.
  - Respiratory problems include recurrent aspiration, with or without pneumonia, and reactive airway disease.
  - Gastrointestinal abnormalities include dysphagia (bulbar involvement), abnormal hypopharyngeal tone (feeding difficulties and aspiration) malnutrition (possibly requiring gastrostomy), abnormal motility (gastroesophageal reflux and possibly needing Nissen fundoplication), delayed gastric emptying, and constipation. In addition, many patients are at an increased risk for fractures (decreased bone mineral density secondary to poor nutrition and decreased mechanical loading).

Classification

- The goal of any classification method (Figure 17–1) is to facilitate treatment decisions. A variety of movement disorders may be seen in children with cerebral palsy, and orthopaedic interventions treat the sequelae of spasticity. In a global sense, patients can be classified as to whether they have pyramidal or extrapyramidal involvement.[1-3] *Pyramidal* involvement includes injury to cortical centers, resulting in spasticity. *Extrapyramidal* involvement results

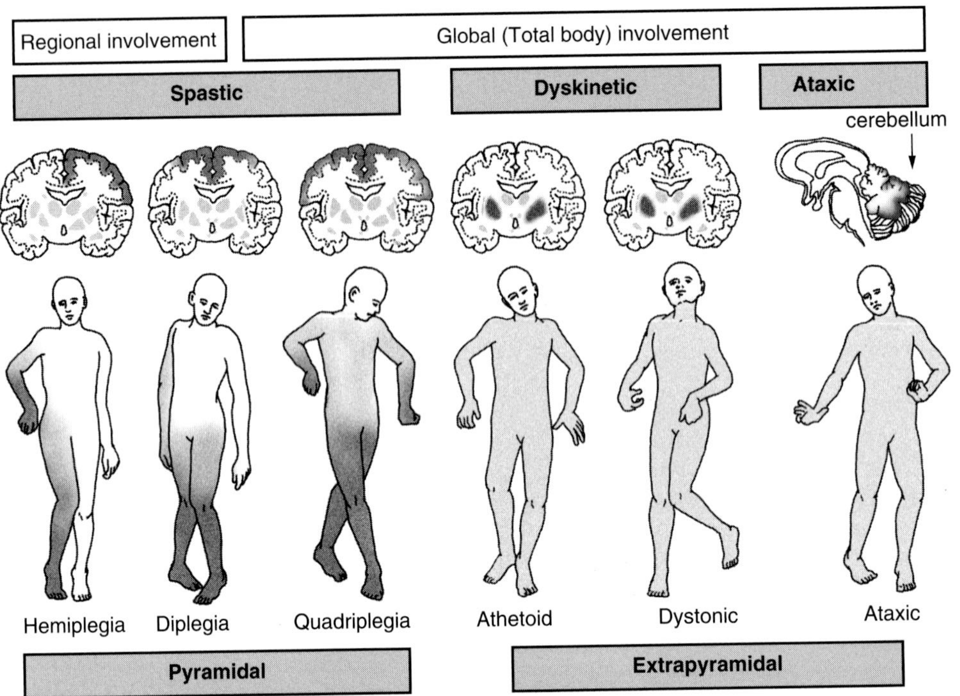

Figure 17–1: Classification of cerebral palsy. **This diagram demonstrates the three major classification systems for cerebral palsy, including the geographical (anatomical distribution of involvement), physiological (type of movement disorder), or presumed neurological substrate (pyramidal versus extrapyramidal). From Pellegrino L, Dormans JP (1998) Definitions, etiology, and epidemiology in making the diagnosis of cerebral palsy. In: Dormans JP, Pellegrino L, eds (1998) Caring for Children with Cerebral Palsy: A Teambased Approach Baltimore: Brookes Publishing, p 33.**

from injury to the cerebellum (ataxia, hypotonia, and tremor) and the basal ganglia (loss of selective motor control, athetosis, chorea, choreoathetosis, and ballismus). Extrapyramidal cerebral palsy is not amenable to orthopaedic intervention. The *physiological* approach defines the type of movement disorder. A subset of patients will demonstrate more than one physiological pattern, although usually only a single type will predominate. The *geographical* classification is based upon regional involvement and is perhaps most practical for orthopaedic surgeons because each major subtype has common orthopaedic problems.

Physiological Classification

- *Spasticity* is seen in approximately 80% of cases of cerebral palsy and represents an increase in muscle tone that is "velocity dependent" (i.e., that varies with the rate of stretching).

Dyskinetic

- *Athetosis* involves slow, writhing, involuntary movements of the hands and fingers, the mouth, and occasionally the toes. Patients with athetosis do not develop contractures unless there is coexisting spasticity.
- *Dystonia* describes involuntary, sustained muscle contractions that result in abnormal postures (head, trunk, and extremities). These result from simultaneous contraction of agonists and antagonists. Physical examination reveals that the muscle tone fluctuates and does not vary with the rate of stretch. Tone often increases with effort and emotion. Primitive reflexes are preserved, and the abnormal tone may cause pain.
- *Chorea* represents involuntary, random movements of the extremities that increase when the muscles are resting. These may improve with voluntary movement.
- *Ballismus* represents spontaneous movements of the proximal joints (especially the shoulders).

Ataxic

- *Ataxia* involves damage to the cerebellum, and problems are seen with balance and coordination.

Geographical Classification

- *Hemiplegia* involves one side of the body, and the upper extremity is often more involved than the lower extremity.
- *Diplegia* predominantly involves both lower extremities, and the upper extremities are involved to a mild degree. This form is commonly associated with prematurity.

- *Triplegia* is similar to diplegia but includes significant involvement in one upper extremity.
- *Quadriplegia* significantly involves both the upper and the lower extremities.

Clinical Evaluation

- The medical history focuses on identifying risk factors for cerebral palsy and documenting a delay in neurological maturation. Although most patients will be referred to an orthopaedic surgeon after a diagnosis has been made, the orthopaedist should have a working knowledge of risk factors, normal developmental milestones, and a focused neurological examination. Important components of the neurological examination are listed in the sections that follow, including the testing of primitive reflexes and postural reactions and the functional assessment of the cerebral cortex, cerebellum, and basal ganglia.[1-3]

History

- Prenatal, perinatal, and postnatal events
- Normal developmental milestones (motor)
  - Controlling the head by 3 to 6 months
  - Sitting by 6 to 9 months
  - Crawling by 8 months
  - Pulling up to stand by 8 to 12 months
  - Ambulating independently by 12 to 18 months
  - Jumping by 2 years
  - Hopping on one foot by 6 years

Neurological Examination

- The focus of an "orthopaedic" neurological examination is to document a delay in neurological development, demonstrate upper motor neuron dysfunction, and describe abnormal patterns of movement. A working knowledge of the infantile reflexes and the protective (postural) reflexes, in addition to the history, helps to identify a delay in neurological maturation. The motor examination will reveal abnormalities in muscle tone (most often spasticity and less often hypotonia), and an attempt should be made to quantify the degree of spasticity. The geographical pattern of involvement should be noted, and close observation should reveal any abnormal patterns of motion, such as athetosis.

Infantile Reflexes

- Infantile reflexes (infantile automatisms) are complex patterns of movement that originate in the brain stem and spinal cord and that are elicited in response to sensory stimulation. These patterns disappear with neurological maturation (inhibitory influences from higher cortical centers), and persistence beyond certain ages suggests a delay in neurological maturation.
  - *Cutaneous* (palmar and plantar grasp reflex and Gallant reflex)
  - *Labyrinthine* (prone and supine tonic labyrinthine reflexes)
  - *Proprioceptive* (tonic and asymmetrical tonic neck reflex)
  - *Multimodal* (Moro reflex)
- The *grasp reflex* is tested by tactile stimulation across the palm, and the normal response is flexion of the fingers. This should disappear by 2 to 4 months of age.
- The *Gallant reflex* is tested by stroking the patient's back on one side, and the normal response is for the back to arch toward the side being stroked.
- The *tonic labyrinthine reflex* is tested in either the prone or supine position. With the patient prone, the neck is flexed. The normal response is flexion of the arms, legs, and trunk with inward movement of the shoulders. Then with the patient supine, the neck is extended. The normal response is extension of the trunk and legs with outward movement of the shoulders.
- In the *asymmetrical tonic neck reflex,* the patient is supine, and the head is turned to one side. A positive test includes extension of the extremities on the side to which the head is turned with flexion on the contralateral side.
- In the *symmetrical tonic neck reflex,* the neck is flexed while the patient is in a sitting position. Normally, there is flexion of the arms and extension of the legs. The opposite should occur if the neck is extended.
- The *Moro reflex* is tested by extending the head and neck while the patient is in the supine position. Alternatively, a loud noise can be made. Normally, there is abduction and extension of all four limbs with extension of the spine and spreading of the digits.

Postural and Protective Reactions

- Postural (head and neck) and protective (extremities) reactions emerge during infancy and facilitate balance and positioning of body segments. Their absence suggests a delay in neurological maturation.

Postural Reactions

- *Segmental rolling* is tested with the patient supine and the head slowly turning to one side. The normal response is sequential rolling of the shoulders, trunk, and pelvis toward the side to which the head is turned.
- *Head and trunk righting* is tested with the patient supine and the upper body tilting to one side. Normally, the head will tilt to maintain a vertical position.
- The *Landau reaction* is tested by lifting the patient from a prone position. The normal response is extension of the arms, trunk, and neck and flexion of the lower extremities.

Protective Reactions

- The *parachute response* is tested by suspending the patient upside down and tilting the patient. Normally, both the arms and legs will extend.
- The *lateral prop reaction* is tested in the sitting position with the patient passively tilted to one side. A normal response is extension of the ipsilateral arm for balance or support.
- In the *foot placement reaction,* the patient is suspended upright and the legs are gently swung forward so that the dorsum of the feet come into contact with the underside of the examining table. Normally, the limbs should flex in an effort to step up onto the table.
- *Extensor thrust* is tested with the patient suspended upright and the plantar surface of the feet touching onto a hard surface. Normally, the limbs should flex; an abnormal response is a gradual and progressive extension of both lower extremities.

Pyramidal Dysfunction (Cerebral Cortex)

- Spasticity is defined by a velocity-dependent increase in muscle tone associated with hyperreflexia and clonus. Grading is most commonly by the *Ashworth scale:* No increase in tone (I), slight increase in tone with a palpable "catch" when stretching the muscle (II), more marked increase in tone (III), considerable increase in tone (IV), and rigidity (V). The grade may vary between examinations.
- Manual muscle testing may be difficult to perform in younger children, and the grade may vary between examinations. Spasticity often masks underlying weakness. Grading is as follows: No muscle activity detected (0), trace of muscle contraction (1), active movement with gravity eliminated (2), active movement against gravity (3), active movement against gravity and some resistance (4), and active movement against full resistance (5).

Cerebellar Dysfunction (Balance and Coordination)

- Ataxia (wide-based gait)
- Abnormal equilibrium reactions may be tested with the patient sitting or standing, and the center of gravity can be manually displaced by a gentle push in any direction. Normally, the seated patient will alter the position of the head and neck and will extend the arm on the lower side. If tested in the standing position, the patient will change foot placement or hop.
- Romberg test, finger to nose, etc.

Basal Ganglia

- Observation of limbs for abnormal movements (chorea, athetosis, etc.)
  - Selective motor control may be tested by asking the patient to isolate the function of one muscle group and observing which muscles contract. Normal individuals should be able to isolate the function of an individual muscle group (or groups with a similar function). Patients with cerebral palsy often exhibit a spread of motor activity to other motor groups within the extremity (e.g., flexion of the hip and knee with attempts to dorsiflex the foot). Grading for each muscle is as follows: patterned movement (0), partially isolated movement (1), and completely isolated movement (2).

Musculoskeletal Assessment

- The musculoskeletal evaluation focuses on the presence of any deformities of the spine or extremities.[1-3] Evaluating joint range of motion allows the examiner to quantify the degree of contracture. *Dynamic contractures* result from spasticity alone, and *myostatic contractures* result from shortening of the muscle–tendon unit. Most patients will have components of both, and an examination under anesthesia may be required to accurately quantify the myostatic component. A rotational profile should be performed to quantify femoral and tibial alignment.
- The spine should be evaluated in both the frontal (scoliosis) plane and the sagittal (kyphosis or lordosis) plane.
  - The *frontal plane* is assessed with the patient either sitting or standing. Any asymmetry or rotational prominence should be investigated further with radiographs. Although the typical criterion for diagnosing scoliosis in the nonneuromuscular population is a curvature greater than 10 degrees, many believe that a minimum value of 20 degrees is more practical in patients with neuromuscular disease. Mild, positional deformities are more common in patients with trunk weakness, impaired balance, or both. Flexibility should be assessed for established deformities. Ambulatory patients may be asked to bend to the side. In nonambulators, the examiner may gently grasp the patient under each axilla and lift upward. Alternatively, the patient may be placed on his or her side, with the apex of the curvature over the examiner's thigh. Although scoliosis is most often the primary problem, the curvature may compensate for an infrapelvic contracture. For example, an abduction contracture of the hip causes pelvic obliquity, and a compensatory lumbar scoliosis may develop to maintain balance.
  - The *sagittal profile* may also be evaluated either sitting or standing. The thoracic spine is normally kyphotic, and the lumbar spine is normally lordotic. Sagittal spinal alignment is influenced by lower extremity alignment, and vice versa, to maintain standing or

sitting balance. Sagittal deformities are rarely a primary deformity; most often these compensate for infrapelvic contractures. For example, lumbar hyperlordosis may compensate for hip flexion contracture in ambulatory patients with spastic diplegia. Excessive thoracic kyphosis may compensate for excessive lumbar lordosis. A loss of lumbar lordosis (or lumbar kyphosis) may compensate for an extension contracture at the hip. Tight hamstrings will tilt the pelvis posteriorly, and the trunk will compensate by leaning forward.

Upper Extremity

Range of Motion

- The examiner needs to differentiate static from dynamic deformities and to assess the degree of spasticity and the passive range of motion.
- The most common deformities are internal rotation of the shoulder; flexion at the elbow, wrist, and fingers; ulnar deviation at the wrist; the thumb in the palm; and a swan neck.

Sensory Function

- Deficiencies in both motor and sensory function are common. The following tests are performed:
  - Rough or smooth
  - Two-point discrimination
  - Proprioception
  - Stereognosis
- Stereognosis is tested by having the patient identify an object placed in the hand without visual information.
  - Gross discrimination—Key, pencil, marble, and others
  - Fine discrimination—Paper clip, coin, rubber band, and others
- Other components of the evaluation may include dynamic electromyogram (EMG, videotaping, and instrumented motion analysis.

Hip Examination

Flexion Contracture (Iliopsoas)

Thomas Test

- The patient is placed supine, and the contralateral hip flexed to flatten out the lumbar spine (Figure 17–2, *A*). The hip is then extended, and the angle between the tabletop and the femur is the degree of flexion contracture.

Staheli Test

- The patient is placed prone with the pelvis at the edge of the table, and the contralateral hip and knee are flexed[4] (Figure 17–2, *B*). The thigh is then extended, and the angle between the thigh and the surface of the examining table is the degree of flexion contracture.

Adduction Contracture

- The patient is supine, and the degree of abduction should be measured with the hip in extension (Figure 17–3).

Femoral Rotational Examination

- *Version* is the normal rotation about an axis, and *torsion* is a pathological deviation in rotational alignment. *Anteversion* is the normal inward rotation of the femoral head and neck relative to an axis through the distal femoral condyles. In normal individuals, anteversion is approximately 40 degrees at birth and decreases to approximately 15 degrees at skeletal maturity. Spasticity or muscle imbalance interferes with normal femoral derotation during growth, resulting in a *persistence of fetal anteversion* (excessive femoral anteversion or femoral torsion).
- The degree of anteversion may be estimated by assessing the degree of medial rotation of the hip. The patient may be tested either prone or supine. In the prone examination, the knee is flexed to 90 degrees, and both medial and lateral rotation are assessed (Figure 17–4). The pelvis should be stabilized, and gravity should be used to identify the endpoint. The angle between the vertical and the lower leg is the degree of medial or lateral rotation, and the combined arc of motion should be approximately 90 degrees. The degree of medial rotation (the leg is rotated from the midline) provides an estimate of anteversion and is graded as mild (60-70 degrees), moderate (70-90 degrees), and severe (>90 degrees).
- Alternatively, the degree of femoral anteversion can be measured clinically. The patient is prone with the knee flexed 90 degrees. The limb is rotated medially until the greater trochanter is palpated to be at its greatest lateral prominence. The angle between the vertical and the lower leg is the degree of femoral anteversion (less than the degree of medial rotation).

Knee and Tibia

Flexion Contracture

- The *popliteal–femoral angle* (Figure 17–5) is tested with the patient supine and the hip flexed 90 degrees. The contralateral hip is extended. The knee is then extended, and the angle between the vertical and the lower limb segment is the popliteal angle (normal is less than 20 degrees). This angle can also be recorded as the angle between the thigh and the lower leg segments. Flexion of the contralateral limb will decrease the popliteal angle when the pelvis is tilted posteriorly and the hamstrings are relaxed. The difference between the measurements with the contralateral hip extended and those with the hip flexed is the *hamstring shift*. The *straight leg raise* is

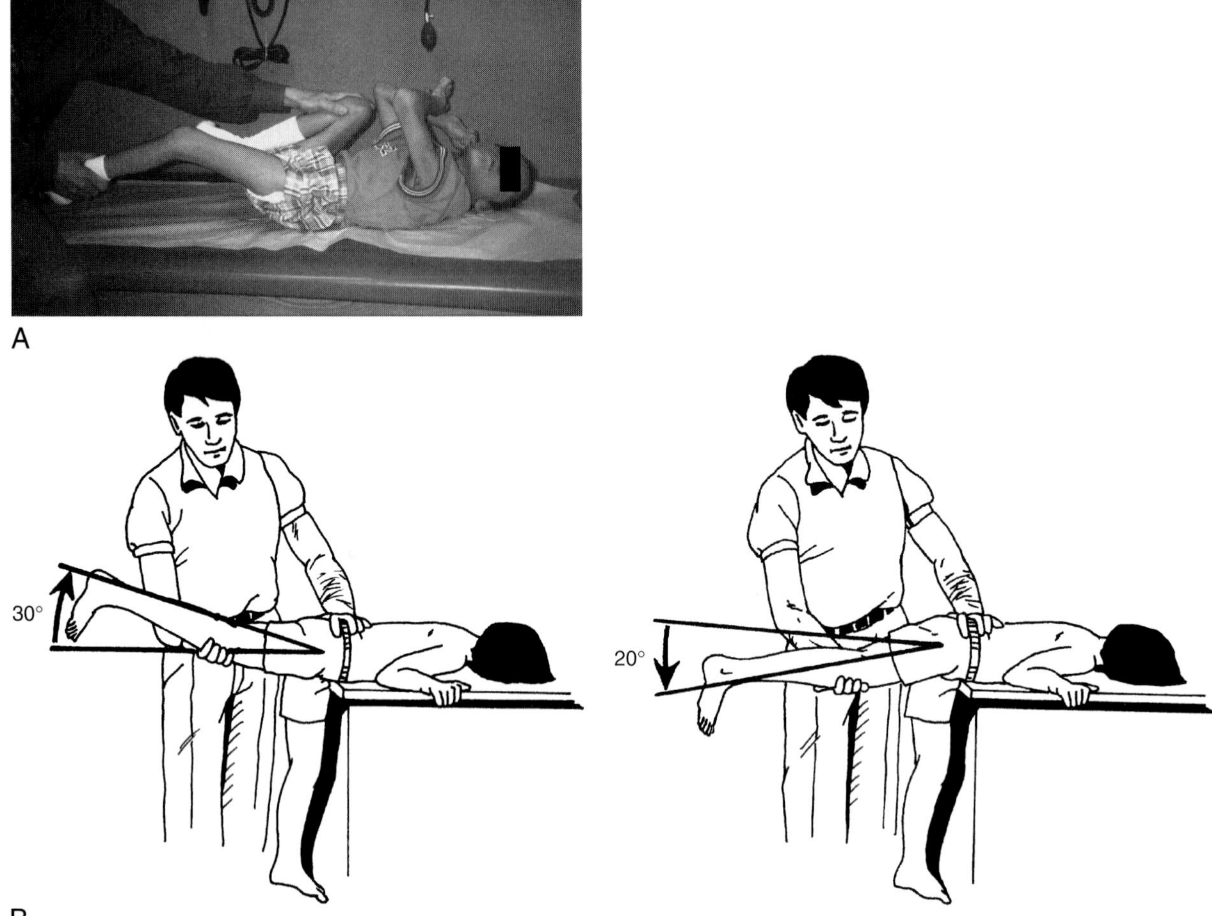

Figure 17–2: Tests for hip flexion contracture. The Thomas test (A) is performed supine, and the lumbar spine is flattened by fully flexing the contralateral hip. The angle between the thigh and the table is the degree of flexion deformity. The Staheli test (B) is performed in the prone position with the contralateral hip flexed and the pelvis at the edge of the table. The angle between the thigh and the horizontal is the degree of hip flexion deformity (loss of extension). A, From Spiegel DA (2004) Cerebral palsy. In: Pediatric Orthopaedics and Sports Medicine (Dormans JP, ed). Philadelphia: Mosby. B, From Herring JA, ed (2001) Tachdjian's Pediatric Orthopaedics, 3rd edition, volume 2. Philadelphia: WB Saunders, p 1179.

another way to assess the degree of contracture; the extremity is extended, and the knee is maintained in a maximally extended position. The angle between the extremity and the table is measured.

- The popliteal–femoral angle reflects contracture of both the hamstring muscles and the posterior capsular structures of the knee. By measuring the degree of knee extension with the hip extended (which relaxes the hamstrings), the examiner can assess the magnitude of posterior capsular contracture.

Rectus Femoris Contracture

- The *prone rectus stretch test* (Duncan-Ely test, Figure 17–6) assesses the degree of rectus femoris spasticity, which may contribute to a stiff knee gait. The patient is placed prone, and the knee is gradually flexed. The examiner feels the degree of spasticity and observes elevation of the contralateral hemipelvis. The test may also be positive in the setting of a significant hip flexion contracture.

Rotational Examination

- The *thigh–foot axis* (Figure 17–7) is tested with the patient in the prone position and the knees flexed 90 degrees. The foot must be in neutral plantar flexion–dorsiflexion because plantar flexion will introduce internal rotation and dorsiflexion will introduce external rotation (through the subtalar joint). The angle between the thigh and a line along the central axis of the foot is the thigh–foot axis. This composite includes both the rotation of the lower limb and the rotation of the hindfoot.

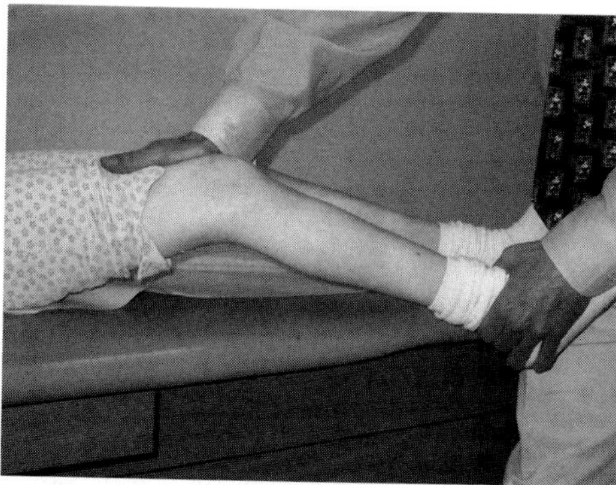

Figure 17–3: Assessment of hip abduction. The degree of abduction is measured with the patient supine and the hips extended. Patients with a combined arc of less than 90 degrees, or with less than 45 degrees on one side, are clinically at risk for progressive hip subluxation and dislocation. From Spiegel DA (2004) Cerebral palsy. In: Pediatric Orthopaedics and Sports Medicine (Dormans JP, ed). Philadelphia: Mosby.

- The *transmalleolar axis* is tested with the patient sitting and the leg hanging over the edge of the examining table. The knee–joint axis placed parallel with the edge of the table, and the angle between the edge of the table (knee axis) and a line through the medial and lateral malleoli is measured. This measurement is not affected by hindfoot alignment.

Ankle

Equinus Deformity

- Dorsiflexion tests should always be completed with the foot inverted to lock the subtalar joint. Otherwise, some dorsiflexion may occur through the midfoot, which will underestimate the degree of dorsiflexion. Equinus contracture may occur in the gastrocnemius (most common in cerebral palsy) or in both the gastrocnemius and the soleus. The *Silverskiöld test* assesses each of these components (Figure 17–8). Ankle dorsiflexion is tested with the knee both flexed (which relaxes the gastrocnemius and tests the soleus) and extended (which tests both the gastrocnemius and the soleus).

Foot

- The foot examination should evaluate the relationships among the forefoot, midfoot, and hindfoot. Range of motion and the degree of spasticity of muscles crossing the ankle should be tested. Common deformities (Figure 17–9) include equinovarus, equinovalgus, and calcaneus.

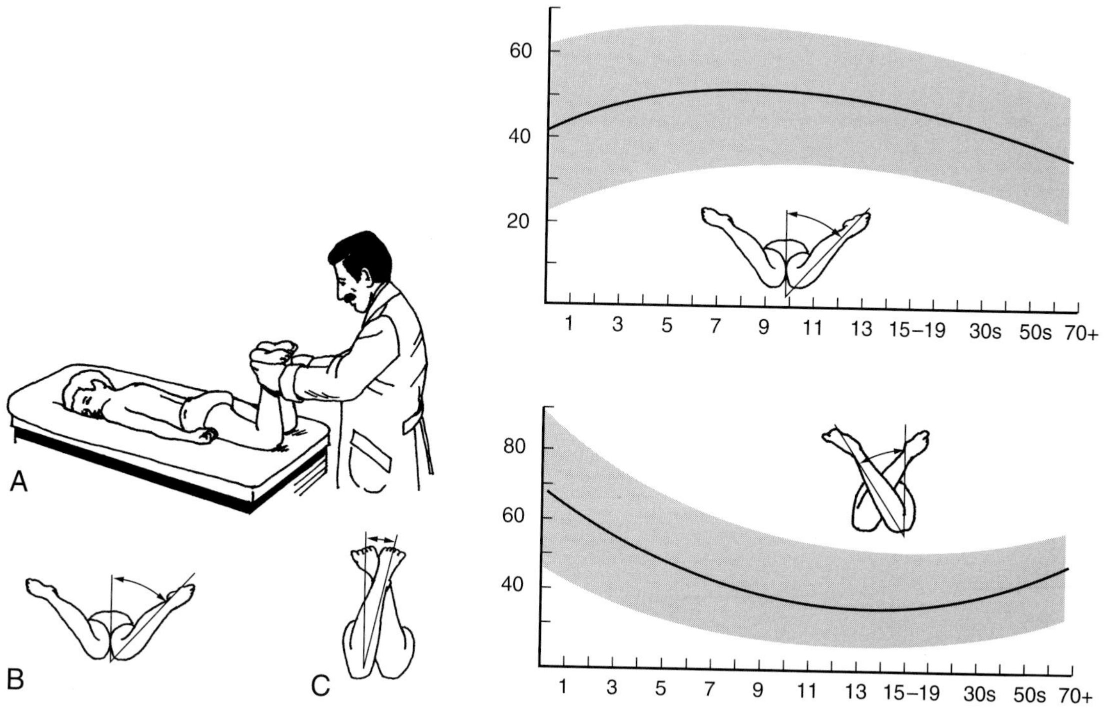

Figure 17–4: Rotational profile at the hip. A, Hip rotation may be tested prone with the hip in an extended position and the knee flexed 90 degrees. B, Medial rotation is tested by allowing each leg to rotate outward. The angle between the vertical and the lower limb segment is the degree of medial rotation. C, Lateral rotation is tested in a similar fashion, but the leg is rotated inward. The range of normal values is shown to the right. From Staheli LT (1998) Lower limb/torsion. In: Fundamentals of Pediatric Orthopaedics. Philadelphia: Lippincott-Raven Publishers, p 32.

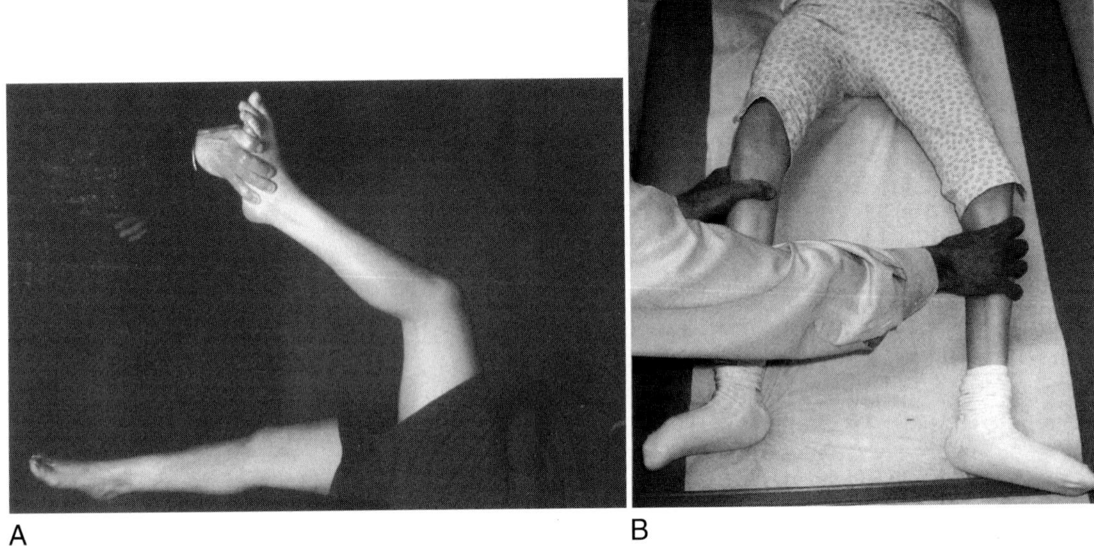

Figure 17–5: Assessment of knee flexion contracture. The popliteal angle (A) is tested with the hip flexed; it evaluates contracture of the hamstring muscles. The degree of knee extension with the hip extended (B) demonstrates the contribution from the posterior capsule of the knee (hamstrings are relaxed by extending the hip). From Spiegel DA (2004) Cerebral palsy. In: Pediatric Orthopaedics and Sports Medicine (Dormans JP, ed). Philadelphia: Mosby.

Management of Spasticity (Tone Reduction)

- Spasticity results from damage to upper motor neurons within the pyramidal system (motor cortex, periventricular white matter, internal capsule, midbrain or pons, and corticospinal tracts). A loss of supraspinal inhibition hyperexcites the stretch reflex. Spasticity impedes function and ease of care and results in secondary musculoskeletal deformities.
- Muscle growth occurs by the addition of sarcomeres at the musculotendinous junction in response to repetitive tensile loading (stretching during normal ambulation). Children with cerebral palsy, particularly with greater degrees of involvement, are less active than age-matched controls. This decreases the volume of stretching and impairs muscle growth, leading to shortening of the muscle tendon unit (myostatic contracture). Myostatic contractures may alter the muscular forces acting upon the skeleton, resulting in tethered growth and angular or rotational deformities.

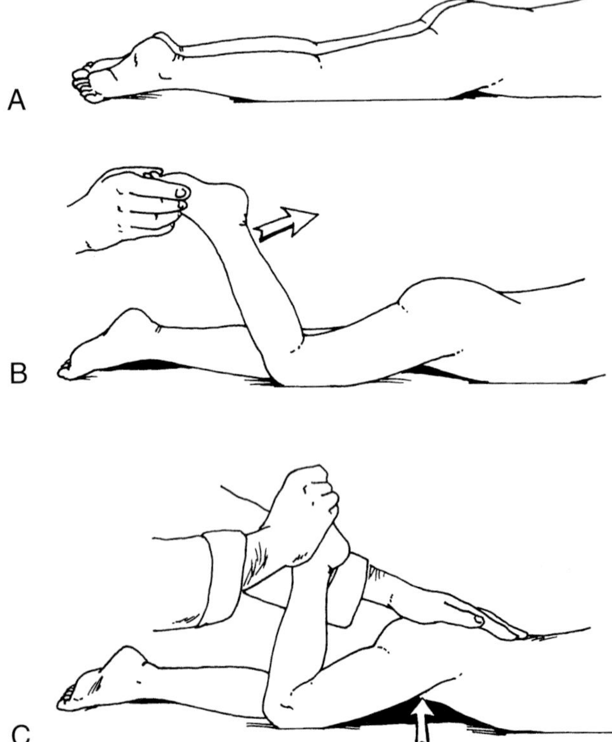

Figure 17–6: The Duncan-Ely test for spasticity of the rectus femoris. With the patient prone, the knee is flexed. Rectus spasticity will raise the ipsilateral pelvis. From Herring JA, ed (2001) Tachdjian's Pediatric Orthopaedics, 3rd edition, volume 2. Philadelphia: WB Saunders, p 1172.

Treatment of Spasticity

Oral Medications

- Although a subset of patients may achieve adequate tone reduction with oral agents, more often than not the effectiveness is limited by side effects, most commonly

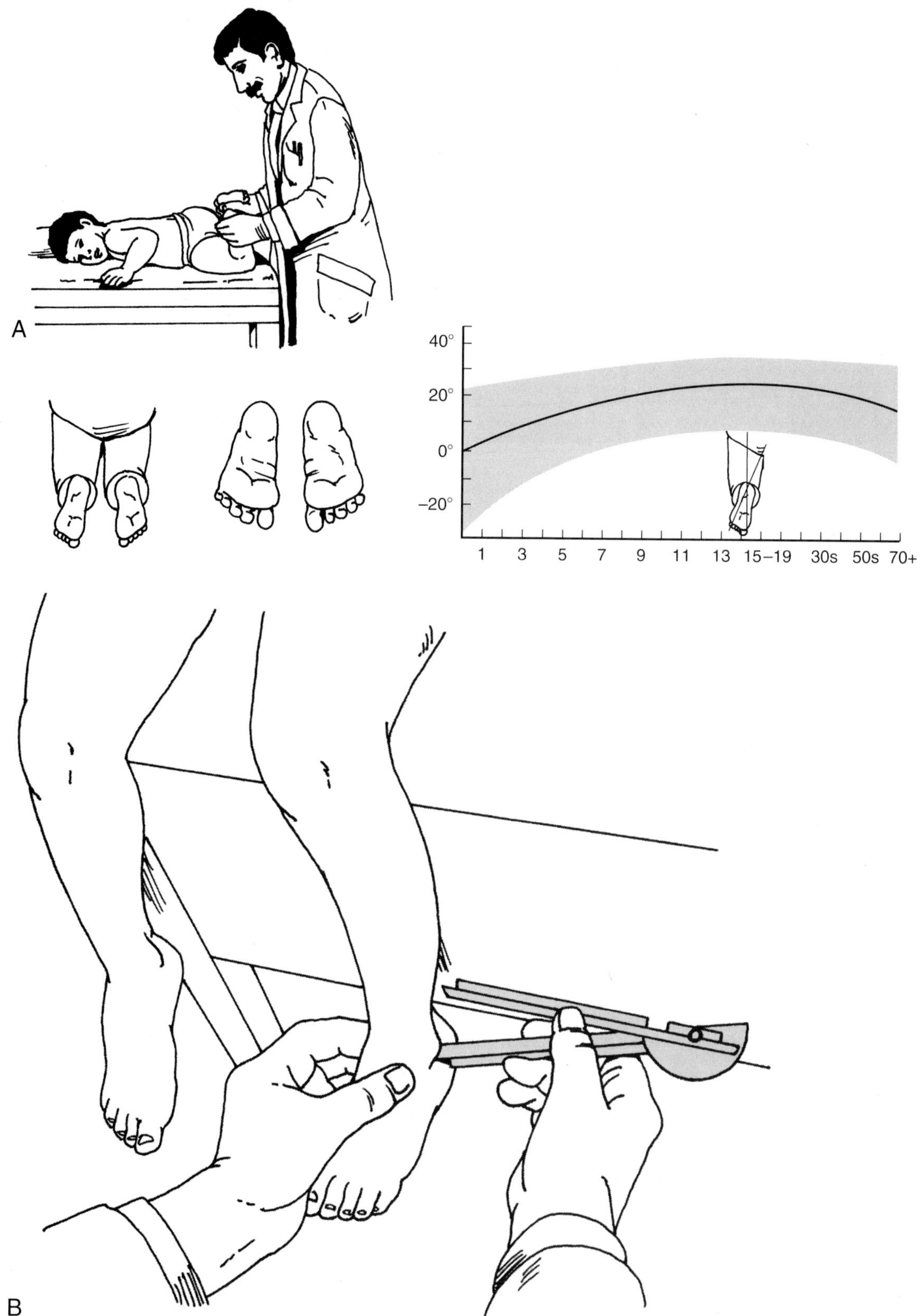

Figure 17–7: Rotational profile of the lower leg. The thigh–foot axis and the transmalleolar axis test rotation below the knee. A, In the former, the patient is prone and the knee is flexed 90 degrees. The angle of the foot (held in neutral dorsiflexion–plantar flexion) relative to the thigh is measured. The normal range of values is shown at the right. This index includes the degree of rotation of both the tibia–fibula and the hindfoot. B, The latter is tested with the patient sitting at the edge of the examining table and the distal femoral condyles aligned with the side of the table. The angle between a line through the medial and lateral malleoli and the edge of the table should be approximately 30 degrees external. A, From Staheli LT (1998) Lower limb/torsion. In: Fundamentals of Pediatric Orthopaedics. Philadelphia: Lippincott-Raven Publishers, p 32. B, From Bleck EE (1987) Orthopaedic Management in Cerebral Palsy. London: Mac Keith Press, p 55.

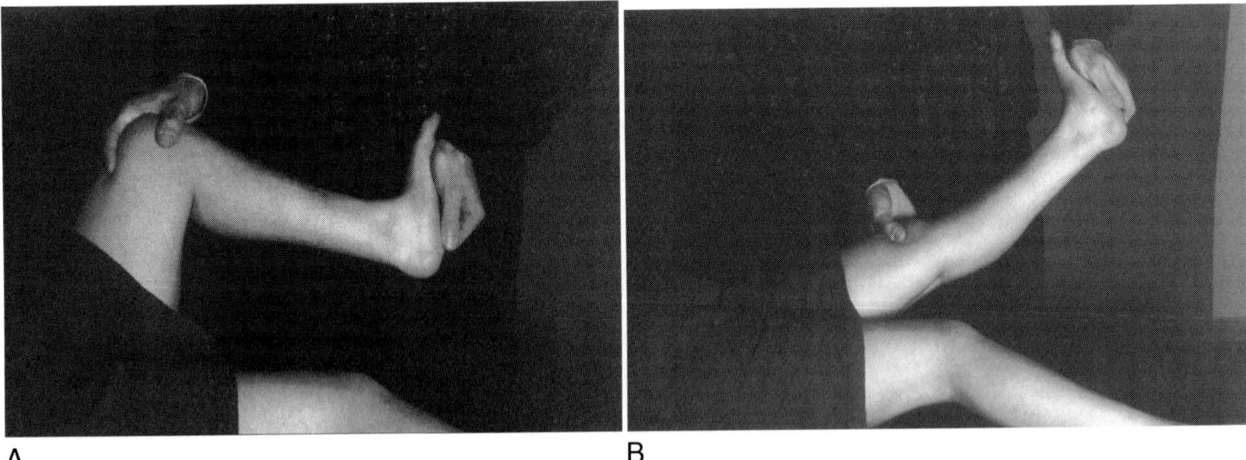

Figure 17–8: The Silverskiöld test for equinus (flexion) contracture at the ankle. The degree of ankle dorsiflexion is tested with the knee both flexed (A) and extended (B). The foot should be inverted to avoid any spurious dorsiflexion through the midfoot. If dorsiflexion is only limited with the knee extended, then an isolated contracture of the gastrocnemius muscle is present. If dorsiflexion is also limited with the knee flexed, this signifies an associated contracture of the soleus. From Spiegel DA (2004) Cerebral palsy. In: Pediatric Orthopaedics and Sports Medicine (Dormans JP, ed). Philadelphia: Mosby.

sedation. Other side effects may include weakness or hypotonia.

Baclofen

- Baclofen (Lioresal) binds to the inhibitory neurotransmitter γ-aminobutyric acid (GABA), resulting in hyperpolarization. Side effects include sedation, confusion, memory loss, dizziness, weakness, ataxia, and attention deficits. Withdrawal may occur, increasing spasticity. Baclofen is most commonly used in children who are too young or too small for a more definitive approach to tone reduction.

Benzodiazepines

- The benzodiazepines (Valium, Ativan, and others) bind to GABA at both spinal and supraspinal levels. Side effects include somnolence and drooling, and patients may develop tolerance. Short-term use of these agents is helpful in controlling postoperative muscle spasm.

Dantrolene Sodium

- Dantrolene sodium acts directly at the level of skeletal muscle to inhibit the release of calcium at sarcoplasmic reticulum, which decreases or inhibits the response to excitatory stimuli. Side effects include weakness and hepatotoxicity.

Tizanidine

- Tizanidine (Zanaflex) acts at central α-2 adrenergic receptor sites (spinal and supraspinal) to prevent the release of excitatory neurotransmitters (glutamate and aspartate). Side effects include somnolence, dizziness, hallucinations, possible hypotension, and hepatotoxicity. There is limited published material on its use in cerebral palsy, although the drug has been effective in spasticity associated with multiple sclerosis and spinal cord injury.

Intramuscular Injections

Botulinum Toxin A[5]

- Botulinum toxin A (botox) is an exotoxin produced by *Clostridium botulinum* that blocks the release of acetylcholine at the neuromuscular junction, resulting in a reversible chemical denervation. The decrease in spasticity usually lasts 4 to 6 months in the upper extremity and 6 to 8 months in the lower extremity. Reinnervation occurs by sprouting at the neuromuscular junction. The goals for this treatment are to delay surgical intervention and to facilitate stretching to regain muscle length. The intramuscular injections are performed under topical anesthesia with or without sedation; general anesthesia is required when multiple sites will be injected or when an EMG is required (especially with small muscle groups in the upper extremities). Side effects are generally minimal and include pain at the injection site and excessive weakening of the muscle group.
- The indications are evolving and include patients with dynamic muscle contracture with a limited number of muscles involved (less than four). Typical injected lower extremity groups include the gastrocnemius, hamstrings,

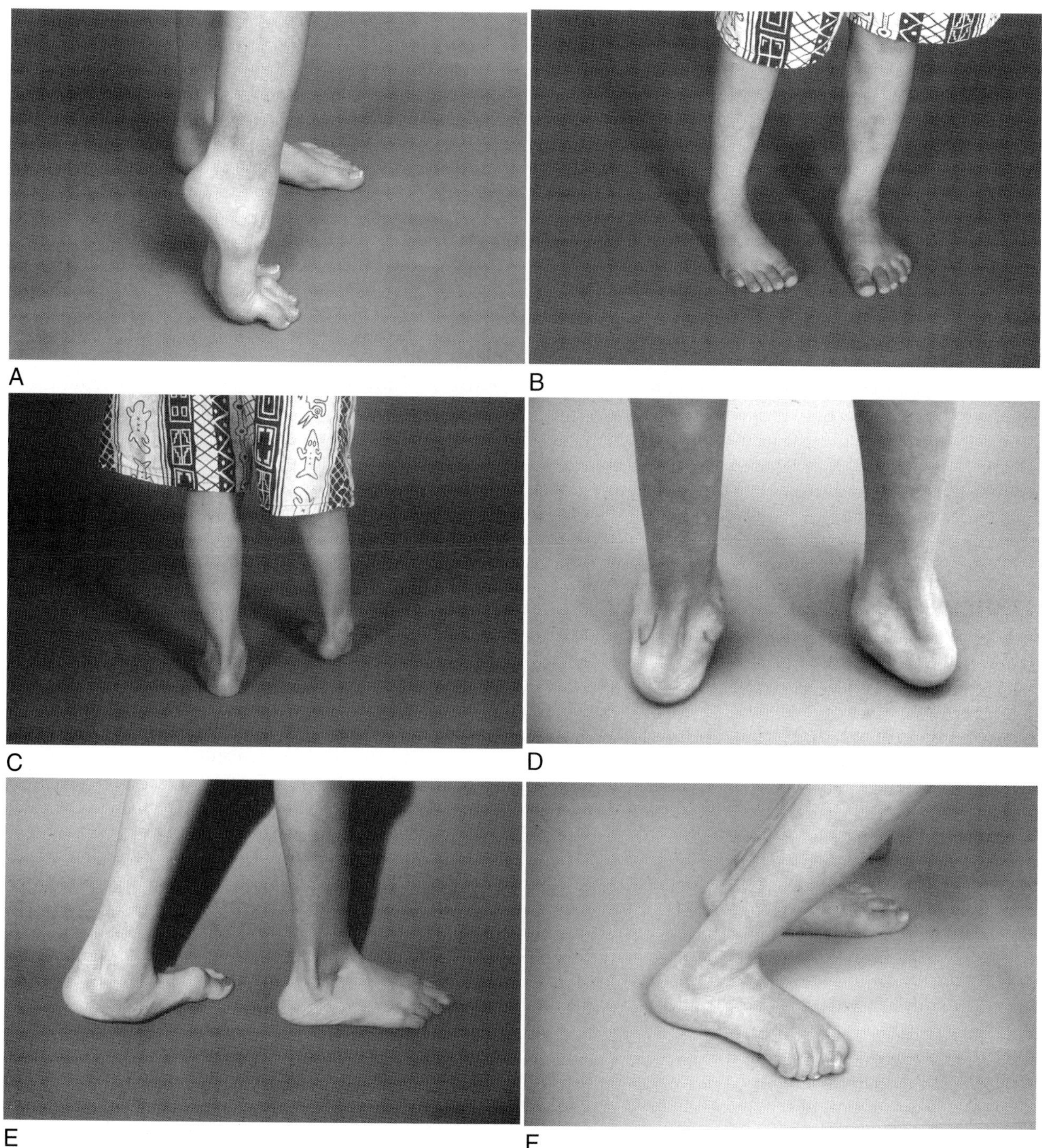

Figure 17–9: Equinus, equinovarus, equinovalgus, and calcaneus deformities. A, An equinus deformity restricts dorsiflexion at the ankle with the heel in neutral alignment. B and C, Equinovarus deformities involve hindfoot equinus and varus. D and E, Equinovalgus deformities have hindfoot equinus valgus. F, Calcaneus deformity involves excessive ankle dorsiflexion (and may have restricted ankle plantar flexion). From Spiegel DA (2004) Cerebral palsy. In: Pediatric Orthopaedics and Sports Medicine (Dormans JP, ed). Philadelphia: Mosby.

adductors, and tibialis posterior. Upper extremity groups include the biceps, flexor carpi ulnaris, pronator teres, and thumb adductor.
- The maximum dosage is 12 U/kg or 400 U. The typical dose for large muscles is 3 to 6 U/kg and for small muscles is 1 to 2 U/kg. The maximum at a single injection site is 50 U. Reinjection can be considered after a minimum of 3 months.

Phenol

- Phenol blocks are performed less commonly and require general anesthesia (electrical stimulation is used to localize the motor end plates). Risks include dysesthesias (15%) and paresthesias. Therapeutic effects last 9 to 12 months.

Dorsal Rhizotomy

- Dorsal rhizotomy (selective or nonselective) is a neurosurgical procedure in which a subset of sensory rootlets is sectioned.[6] Spasticity is decreased, and there is no effect on extrapyramidal dysfunction. Patient selection is critical to success, and the ideal candidate has pure spasticity, has no fixed contractures, ambulates independently, is 4 to 8 years of age, has good selective motor control, and has adequate cognition to cooperate with the extensive postoperative rehabilitation required to optimize the outcome. Some centers perform this procedure in nonambulatory patients to promote ease of care and relieve spasticity-related pain.
- The procedure involves a laminectomy (L1 or L2 to S1) or laminaplasty (preserves the posterior elements). The dorsal rootlets are dissected (L1 or L2 to S1 or S2), and a subset is sectioned. In selective dorsal rhizotomy, each rootlet is stimulated electrically and the response is gauged both by EMG and by physical examination. Only those rootlets with an abnormal response are sectioned, typically between 25% and 50%. An abnormal response may be defined by EMG criteria, often corroborated by the physical findings of contraction of multiple muscle groups with stimulation of a single rootlet (spread). An extensive postoperative rehabilitation program is essential because decreasing spasticity may unmask underlying weakness. Some centers practice nonselective sectioning.
- Acute complications are uncommon and include temporary dysesthesias in the early postoperative period, neurogenic bladder, and sensory loss.
- Benefits include a permanent reduction in spasticity. Supraspinal effects are also seen in a significant number of patients, including improvements in upper extremity function, bladder function, speech, and swallowing. A subset of patients develops the late onset of increased muscle tone, which is thought to represent the development of dystonia rather than the recurrence of spasticity.
- The effects on the musculoskeletal system are variable. Rhizotomy does not appear to alter the need for subsequent orthopaedic surgery because established contractures, rotational deformities, or both will be unaffected. It remains to be determined whether early tone reduction will prevent or minimize the development of musculoskeletal deformities. Possible untoward effects include weakness, a rapidly progressive unilateral hip subluxation, spondylolysis or spondylolisthesis, and scoliosis. Scoliosis is more common in nonambulatory patients undergoing rhizotomy, whereas spondylolysis or spondylolisthesis is more common in the ambulatory patient. Heterotopic ossification may be more common following hip surgery in patients who have previously had a rhizotomy.

Intrathecal Baclofen

- Baclofen may be delivered locally to the superficial layers of the spinal cord. The therapeutic dose is approximately 1% of the oral dose, and the effects are not limited by sedation.[7]
- Indications include spasticity (Ashworth grades III-V), which decreases function, creates difficulties with care, and results in progressive contractures. Patients with dystonia and rigidity may also benefit. The goals are to improve function, facilitate care, and prevent the progression of contractures. Intrathecal baclofen may be indicated for tone reduction in ambulatory patients with poor underlying muscle strength in whom a rhizotomy would be expected to result in excessive postoperative weakness. The indications in nonambulators include impaired upper extremity function, activities of daily living, comfort, or ease of care.
- Patients must weigh 30 to 40 lb to be a candidate for implantation of the device.
- A test dose is delivered through lumbar puncture. If spasticity is deceased significantly (grades I-II on the Ashworth scale), then an intrathecal catheter and a subcutaneous pump are implanted under general anesthesia. The intrathecal catheter is inserted in the lumbar region and advanced to the desired location. The intrathecal concentration varies in different regions of the spinal canal. For example, the lumbar/cervical concentration is 4:1 if the catheter is placed in the lumbar region. The tip of the catheter is positioned from T1 to T4 for spastic quadriparesis, and in the midthoracic to lower thoracic spine for spastic diplegia. A programmable pump (reservoir) is implanted, and the dosage of baclofen can be titrated based on the clinical response. The pump must be refilled (percutaneously) every 3 weeks to 5 months, and both battery changes and ongoing maintenance are required. The procedure is expensive and labor intensive, and side effects include constipation and decreased head–trunk control. Complications are becoming less frequent with more

experience and more advanced pump design. Infection is seen in 10 to 20%, and requires removal of the device and antibiotics. Reimplantation can be considered. Catheter-related problems are seen in approximately 25% of patients, including disconnection, migration, and cerebrospinal fluid leak. Overdose is uncommon and may be treated by stopping the infusion, draining the cerebrospinal fluid to decrease the drug concentration, and supporting respiratory function if necessary. Withdrawal from intrathecal baclofen may occur, and common symptoms include itching, sweating, and hypertonicity. Less common symptoms include dyskinesias, fever, disorientation, psychosis, and hallucinations. The long-term effects on the musculoskeletal system remain to be determined, and the development or progression of scoliosis remains a concern.

Physical and Occupational Therapy

- The goals for physical and occupational therapy include promoting a normal neurodevelopmental sequence, improving functional mobility and activities of daily living, providing adaptive equipment, and improving range of motion and strength postoperatively and during growth and development.
- Therapeutic interventions change throughout the course of growth and development. In infancy and early childhood, these include facilitating sensorineural development, improving alignment and posture, teaching or supervising a home program for stretching and strengthening, and educating patients and caretakers. As the child grows, emphasis is placed upon maximizing ambulatory skills or promoting mobility through the use of a wheelchair. In adolescence, the focus shifts to function in adult life.

Assistive Devices

- *Standers* maintain the patient in an upright position, which facilitates social interaction and provides some mechanical loading (theoretically, it should help to maintain or improve bone mineral density). Standers may also facilitate therapeutic efforts to improve neuromuscular control and range of motion. Prone standers support the anterior surface of the body, and supine standers support the posterior surface of the body.
- A *wheelchair* is required for mobility in many patients. The standard features include the basic frame, the seating system, and positional components. A manual wheelchair requires adequate upper extremity strength and endurance, and a motorized wheelchair requires adequate cognitive skills to operate. The seating system provides comfort and relief of pressure; materials used for cushioning include foam, gel, air, or thermoplastic urethane. Positional components are used to support the head, the trunk, and the lower extremities. These include the headrest, the trunk support system (straps), a waist belt, and an abduction pummel.
- A *walker* is required for *balance* and not for weakness. A posterior (rear) walker is recommended most often and promotes extension of the lower extremities and trunk (Figure 17–10). Anterior walkers permit forward flexion at the hip and are less desirable in patients predisposed to flexion at the hip and knee.
- *Crutches* are also used to improve balance. Options include standard crutches, forearm (Lofstrand) crutches, or a quad cane (Figure 17–11).

Orthoses

- *Lower extremity* orthoses are used to prevent deformity, support weakness, reduce the effects of muscle imbalance, restrict motion in certain planes, and maintain joint alignment.
- *Foot orthoses* (Figure 17–12) are produced from a variety of materials. These may be soft (shock absorptive), semirigid, or rigid (correct malalignment in flexible deformities).
  - The University of California Biomechanics Laboratory (UCBL) orthosis controls the subtalar joint and the midfoot and supports the longitudinal arch. The hindfoot must be flexible, and the most common indication is a planovalgus foot deformity.
  - A *supramalleolar orthosis* extends above the malleoli and provides greater medial–lateral stability than the UCBL. This device allows dorsiflexion and plantar flexion.

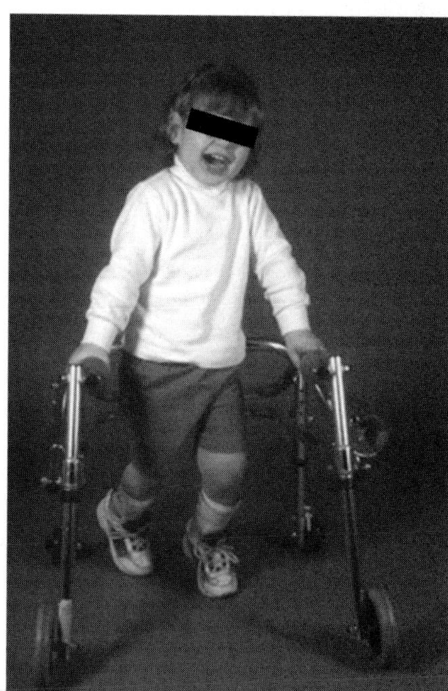

Figure 17–10: A posterior walker promotes extension of the trunk and lower extremities, and either two or four wheels may be added to increase speed in patients with adequate stability. **From Spiegel DA (2004) Cerebral palsy. In: Pediatric Orthopaedics and Sports Medicine (Dormans JP, ed). Philadelphia: Mosby.**

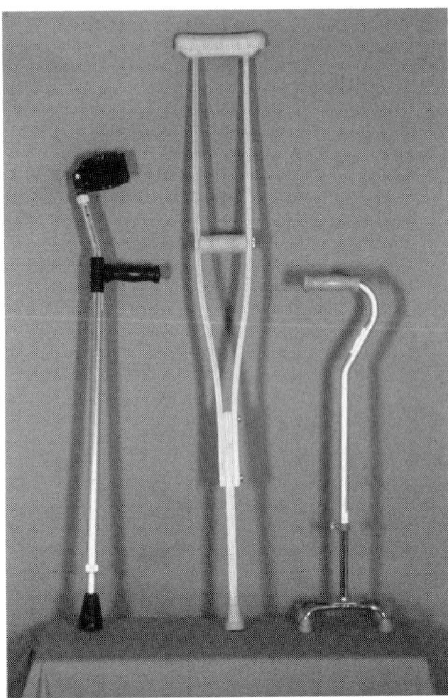

Figure 17–11: Assistive devices. **Many patients will benefit from the support afforded by a cane or crutches. A quad cane *(right)* is held in one hand and offers more stability than a regular cane because of the four points of contact with the ground. Standard or axillary crutches provide the greatest stability *(center)*. Lofstrand crutches transmit forces to the forearm instead of the axilla and require better overall balance than axillary crutches *(left)*. For those who require greater support, a walker may be required.**

Ankle–Foot Orthoses

- A *dynamic* AFO uses a total contact design and is made of more flexible material. This brace controls the midtarsal joint, and styles include solid, articulating, and posterior leaf spring.
  - The *solid* ankle–foot orthosis (AFO) is the most stable and immobilizes the foot and ankle in all three planes. This device helps to facilitate clearance during swing and to preposition the foot for initial contact. Dorsiflexion is blocked, which promotes knee extension.
  - An *articulated* AFO is hinged to allow varying degrees of plantar flexion and dorsiflexion. Dorsiflexion facilitates tibial advancement during the stance phase, and patients should have at least 5 degrees of passive dorsiflexion on examination to benefit from this design. The amount of excursion at the hinge may be adjusted, and designs include unrestricted dorsiflexion and plantar flexion, dorsiflexion assist, and dorsiflexion or plantar flexion stop. The plantar flexion stop is typically set at neutral, which improves clearance during the swing phase (and prevents toe drag by patients with a foot drop). The dorsiflexion stop restricts the degree of dorsiflexion and may be used to prevent excessive dorsiflexion during stance in patients with calcaneus deformity.
  - A *posterior leaf spring* AFO employs a solid design, but the material is thinned over the region of the tendo Achillis, which allows more sagittal ankle motion than a solid AFO.
- A *ground reaction* (floor reaction) AFO employs a solid design, and the foot is placed in neutral to several degrees of plantar flexion to augment the plantar flexion–knee extension couple. An anterior shell is placed over the proximal tibia. This design promotes knee extension in patients with a crouched gait. A prerequisite is less than 10 degrees of fixed flexion contracture at the knee.

Upper Extremity Orthoses

- *Upper extremity* orthoses are used to prevent or correct deformity and to facilitate function (Figure 17–13).
  - A *dynamic finger splint* prevents flexion contracture and provides a constant extension force at the proximal interphalangeal joint while allowing voluntary flexion.
  - A *neoprene splint* is often used during the day to promote functional use of the hand. This design prevents wrist flexion and thumb adduction.
  - *Rigid splints* are often used at night to prevent flexion deformity.
  - A *turnbuckle elbow splint* may be used to treat an established elbow flexion contracture. This dynamic splint is hinged and can be adjusted to gradually stretch out the soft tissues.

Spinal Orthoses

- A *thoracolumbosacral orthosis* (TLSO) may be recommended for scoliosis, and the more rigid materials are often poorly tolerated in this population. The *soft spinal orthosis* is made of more flexible materials to improve tolerance. These orthoses improve sitting balance and may potentially *delay* the progression of spinal deformity.

Orthopaedic Principles Based on Geographical Classification

- One way to conceptualize the relationship between neurological and musculoskeletal problems is to view the central nervous system lesion as primary and the changes in the musculoskeletal system as secondary.
  - *Primary* problems result from injury to the central nervous system and include a loss of selective motor control, abnormal balance, pyramidal dysfunction (spasticity), and extrapyramidal dysfunction (chorea, ataxia, and dystonia). Neurosurgical and

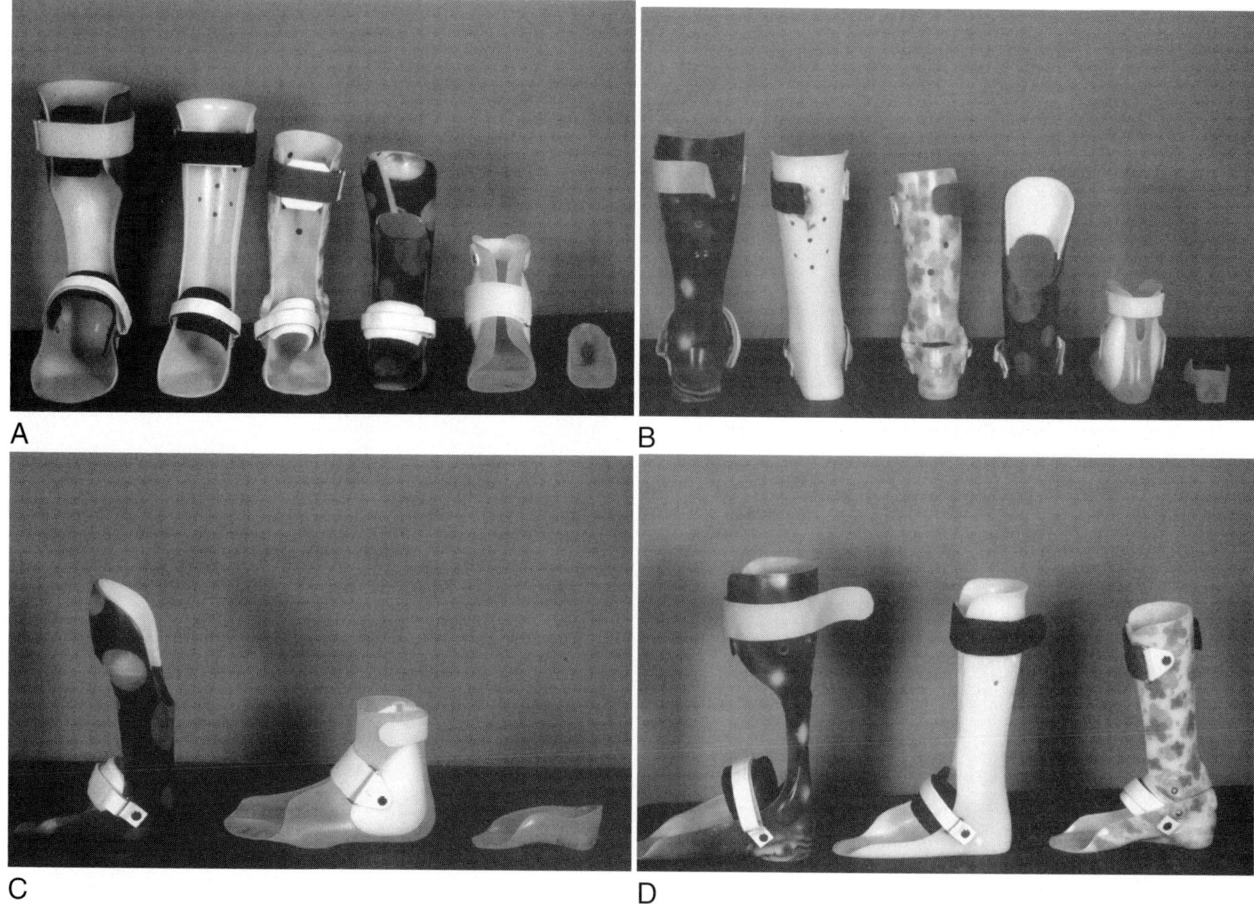

Figure 17–12: Common foot and ankle orthoses viewed from the front (A), the back (B), and the side (C and D). From left to right, these include a floor reaction AFO, a supramalleolar-type orthosis, a UCBL orthosis, a leaf spring AFO, a solid AFO, and an articulating AFO.

pharmacological interventions are directed toward spasticity.

- *Secondary* problems include deformities resulting from growth. These include muscle contractures and bony deformities (hip subluxation–dislocation; femoral, tibial or both types of torsion; and foot deformities). Treatment options include stretching, orthotics, casting or splinting, and orthopaedic surgery.

• Nearly all patients with hemiplegia will ambulate (usually by 18 months) without an assistive device. The goal for treatment of the lower extremities is to improve the efficiency of ambulation. The upper extremity is often more involved than the lower extremity, and a subset of patients will benefit from surgery to improve function, cosmesis, or both.

- Upper extremity problems requiring surgical intervention are seen most frequently in hemiplegics. An extensive evaluation is required to determine which patients are candidates for surgical intervention. A significant percentage of patients will have deficits in sensibility and motor function (selective control, etc.). Limitations in activities of daily living have been correlated with the level of discriminatory sensibility, the level of motor function, the contracture of the forearm (pronation) or the first web space, and the level of motivation.
- Lower extremity involvement varies from isolated contracture of the gastrocnemius to both soft tissue contracture and bony deformity at multiple levels. Patterns of involvement have been classified by Winters and Gage[8] as follows:
  1. *Type I* deformities have a drop foot in the swing phase. An AFO improves clearance during swing phase.
  2. *Type II* deformities include a drop foot with contracture of the gastroc–soleus complex. The most common treatment involves gastroc–soleus lengthening (Strayer +/– soleus fascial release) and an AFO.
  3. *Type III* deformities are similar to type II deformities but also have spasticity or contracture in the hamstrings, rectus femoris, or both with or without

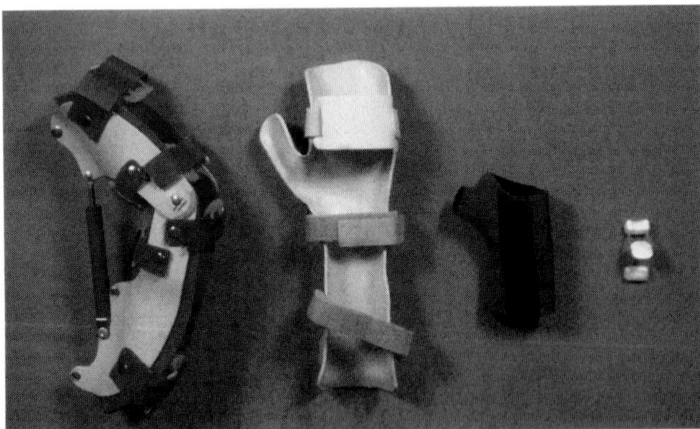

Figure 17–13: Upper extremity orthotics. **A dynamic finger splint *(far right)* allows active flexion of the finger but provides a constant extension force across the proximal interphalangeal joint to help to improve or prevent flexion deformity. A soft, neoprene hand and wrist splint is comfortable and is ideal for use during the day. The thumb is maintained in abduction, and the wrist in minimal dorsiflexion *(center right)*. A more rigid resting splint, which also promotes wrist extension and thumb abduction, is better suited for use at night *(center left)*. A dynamic elbow extension orthosis *(far left)* may be employed as a night splint to promote elbow extension.**

femoral anteversion. The typical treatment lengthens the gastroc–soleus with or without hamstring lengthening (medial), rectus femoris transfer, and femoral derotational osteotomy and involves an AFO.

4. *Type IV* deformities have spasticity or contracture of the iliopsoas in addition to the findings in a type III deformity. The treatment is the same as for the type III deformity with a lengthening of the iliopsoas (over the brim).

 - Leg length discrepancy is common, and shortening occurs on the involved side. The magnitude of discrepancy relates to the degree of neuromuscular involvement, and some patients will require contralateral epiphysiodesis.

- Most patients with spastic diplegia will ambulate (usually by 4 years) with or without an assistive device. Treatment is directed toward improving the efficiency of ambulation. Many patients will benefit from tone reduction, and orthopaedic intervention usually involves multiple lower extremity procedures for contractures, muscle imbalance, and rotational deformities. The trend has been to address all deformities under a single anesthetic, and many centers employ instrumented gait analysis preoperatively. Although the upper extremities are commonly involved, these problems are less likely to require surgical treatment.
- Patients with spastic quadriplegia have the greatest severity of involvement, and only about 20% will ambulate. Treatment goals include stabilizing the sitting posture (straight spine and level pelvis), maximizing the ease of care, preventing or treating deformities, and preventing pain.

Neuromuscular Hip Dysplasia

- Neuromuscular dysplasia is common in patients with greater levels of involvement, and progressive subluxation may culminate in hip dislocation (Figure 17–14).[9,10] The highest risk is in nonambulators with severe spasticity.

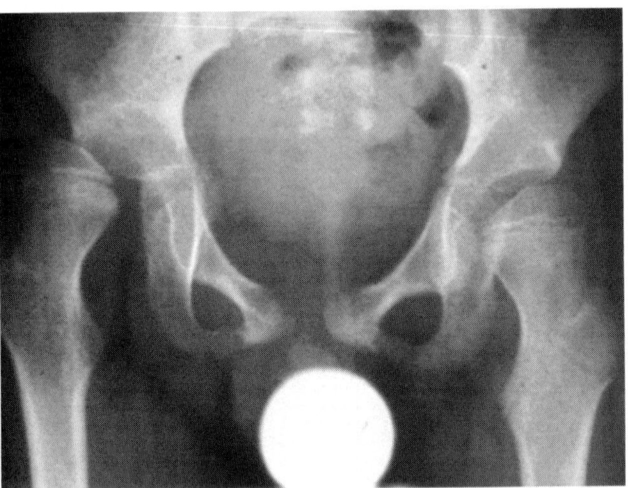

A

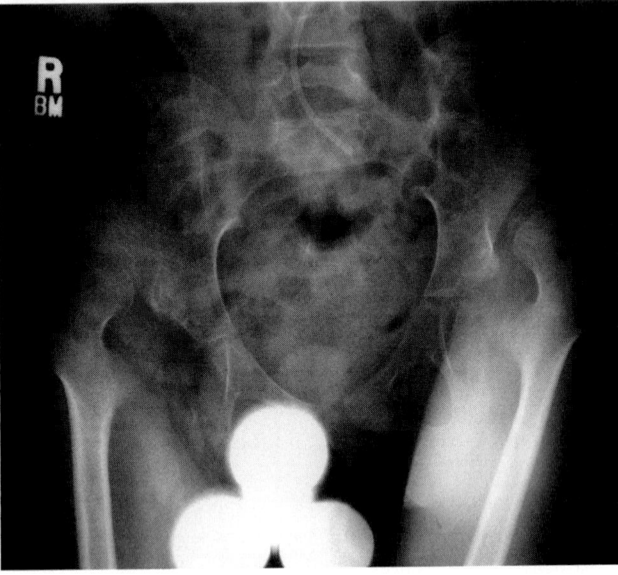

B

Figure 17–14: Hip subluxation–dislocation. **Progressive subluxation leading to dislocation is relatively common in children with spastic quadriplegia and may be seen in those with lesser involvement (diplegia or hemiplegia). Subluxation (A) is incomplete migration of the femoral head from the acetabulum. In a complete dislocation there is no contact between the femoral head and the acetabulum (B). On occasion a "false acetabulum" will develop between the lateral wall of the ilium and the femoral head. From Spiegel DA (2004) Cerebral palsy. In: Pediatric Orthopaedics and Sports Medicine (Dormans JP, ed). Philadelphia: Mosby.**

The preferred approach is to maintain mobile and located hips, and early diagnosis provides the best opportunity to achieve this goal.

- The *pathophysiology* involves the imbalance between strong flexion or adduction and weak extension or abduction; it also involves the development of a fixed adduction contracture. Progressive superior and lateral migration of the femoral head is observed. With long-standing subluxation or dislocation, the femoral head may become deformed, breaking down articular cartilage. Acetabular dysplasia results from asymmetrical pressure from the subluxated femoral head. In contrast to developmental dysplasia of the hip, the area of acetabular deficiency is usually posterior and lateral and may be global.
- Potential problems include pain, seating problems, and difficulties with perineal care. Unilateral dislocation may be associated with pelvic obliquity, asymmetrical sitting pressure, and scoliosis. Although there is some controversy about the likelihood of pain in adulthood, most authors believe that achieving mobile and located hips is an important goal in this population.
- Clinical "at risk" signs include moderate to severe spasticity and a progressive adduction deformity (and usually flexion contracture) with less than 30 degrees passive abduction with the hip in extension. Patients at clinical risk should be followed closely by physical examination, and radiographs should be obtained at periodic intervals.
- The most important radiographic parameter is the *migration percentage* (Figure 17–15), and sequential measurements are used to follow progression of subluxation. A normal migration is less than 30%, and an intermediate risk of progression is seen with a migration of 30 to 60%. Hips with greater than 60% migration will progress to dislocation. Other radiographic findings include coxa valga, a break in Shenton's line, and dysplasia of the acetabulum.
- *Early subluxation* (30–50% migration) is most often treated by an adductor myotomy and iliopsoas lengthening. Soft tissue surgery is most likely to succeed in patients with a clinically at-risk hip and a normal to mildly abnormal migration percentage (approximately 30%). Lengthening of the hamstrings should be considered if there is significant contracture. Nighttime abduction splinting is often recommended, and the role of botox (adductors) as an adjunct to splinting remains to be determined.
- For *moderate subluxation* (>50% migration), proximal femoral varus derotational osteotomy is generally recommended. A pelvic osteotomy may be added if acetabular dysplasia is present (acetabular index > 25 degrees).
- For *dislocation* (>90% migration), both reconstructive and salvage procedures may be considered depending upon the duration of the dislocation, the presence of pain, and the overall medical status of the patient. The approach must be individualized. The status of the articular cartilage is important, and inspection of the femoral head at the time of surgery may be required to finalize the decision.
  - *Reconstructive* surgery typically involves both femoral and pelvic osteotomies, and an open reduction may be required if the migration is greater than 70%. The femoral head may be inspected at the time of open reduction, and a salvage option may be selected if the articular cartilage breaks down significantly.
  - *Salvage* procedures are indicated for chronic, symptomatic dislocations or when inspection of the

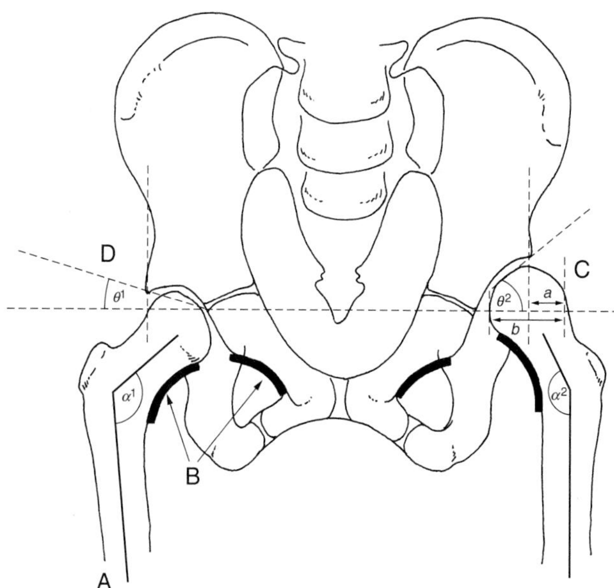

Figure 17–15: Radiographic indices to evaluate hip subluxation. The four major radiographic parameters used to evaluate the spastic hip include the femoral neck–shaft angle (A), Shenton's line (B), Reimer's migration index (C), and the acetabular index (D). In this diagram, the right hip is normal and the left is subluxated. In patients with cerebral palsy, the femoral neck–shaft angle (α^2) may be increased (normal is approximately 135 degrees); however, it is more common to have an "apparent" coxa valga from increased femoral anteversion. Shenton's line is drawn along the medial portion of the femoral neck and should form a smooth arc with a line drawn on the inferior portion of the superior pubic ramus. This arc is typically broken in the presence of subluxation. The migration percentage measures the percentage of the capital femoral epiphysis that lies outside of the lateral margin of the acetabulum and may be used to sequentially follow progressive lateral migration of the femoral head. The migration percentage is distance $a/b \times 100$, and hips with greater than 50 to 60% will nearly always progress to dislocation. The acetabular index (θ) is one way to assess the morphology of the acetabulum. If this measurement is increased above 25 degrees (normal is typically less than 20 degrees), then the acetabulum is dysplastic. From Herring JA, ed (2001) Tachdjian's Pediatric Orthopaedics, 3rd edition, volume 2. Philadelphia: WB Saunders, p 1189.

femoral head reveals evidence of significant damage to the articular cartilage. These include proximal femoral resection, valgus osteotomy, arthrodesis, or prosthetic reconstruction.

Neuromuscular Scoliosis of the Spine

- Scoliosis may be identified in up to 68% of nonambulatory patients with cerebral palsy. Potential problems with progressive or severe deformities include difficulties with the ease of care, inability to adequately maintain sitting balance, pain, and visceral dysfunction (Figure 17–16).[11]

Classification

- According to the Lonstein and Akbarnia classification (Figure 17–17), group I deformities are seen in ambulatory patients and have both a thoracic and a lumbar component. The appearance may be similar to an idiopathic curvature. The pelvis is level. These curves may be well balanced (group IA), or the thoracic curve may be associated with a smaller, fractional curve below which it does not effectively compensate (group IB).
- Group II deformities are seen in nonambulators and involve a thoracolumbar or lumbar curvature that extends into the pelvis. There is significant pelvic obliquity.

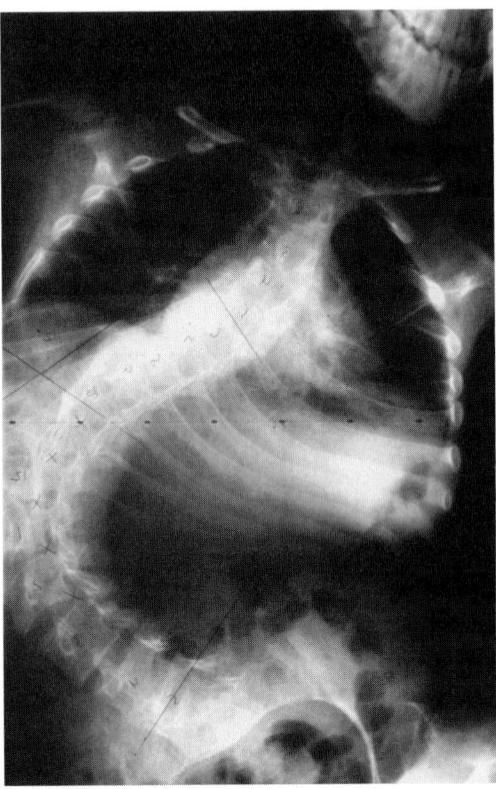

Figure 17–16: Neuromuscular scoliosis. **This nonambulatory patient with spastic quadriplegia developed a severe thoracolumbar curvature with the typical C-shaped appearance. Sitting balance is impaired, and there is associated pelvic obliquity with elevation of the hemipelvis on the concave side of the deformity. From Spiegel DA (2004) Cerebral palsy. In: Pediatric Orthopaedics and Sports Medicine (Dormans JP, ed). Philadelphia: Mosby.**

Treatment Recommendations

- Treatment recommendations depend upon the patient's degree of involvement and the curve variables.
  - Ambulatory patients with hemiplegia or diplegia typically have group I curve patterns, and the management principles are similar to those for idiopathic scoliosis. Bracing with a standard TLSO or a Milwaukee brace is indicated for progressive curvatures of sufficient magnitude in patients with adequate growth remaining.
  - The natural history of scoliosis in the nonambulatory population (significant spasticity or hypotonia and poor trunk control) is different for those with either idiopathic scoliosis or scoliosis associated with ambulatory patients with cerebral palsy. These curves have an earlier onset, are unresponsive to bracing, may progress after skeletal maturity, and are more likely to require surgical intervention. Continued progression is often observed once the curves reach a magnitude greater than 40 degrees.
- Treatment options in the nonambulatory patient must be individualized and depend upon the magnitude of the deformity, the evidence of progression, the functional status of the patient (including cognition), and the desires of the family. Historically, there has been some controversy regarding the indications for such surgery in patients with profound mental retardation.
  - Observation is indicated for smaller curves. For progressive or larger curves, the trend has been to provide support for the trunk to improve sitting balance, facilitate the use of the upper extremities, and, in the case of a brace, possibly delay the need for surgical intervention. Standard bracing programs do not effectively stop curve progression.
  - Positional curve control can be obtained by wheelchair modifications or bracing.
    1. Wheelchair modifications include the various levels of seating support. The minimal level of support includes a firm seat and back. A molded sitting support provides a total contact orthosis to control both the pelvis and the trunk. A variety of commercial seating systems are available.
    2. Whereas the standard thoracolumbosacral orthosis may be poorly tolerated in a significant percentage of patients because of skin or pulmonary problems, the soft spinal orthosis is more comfortable and is usually well tolerated by this patient population. The

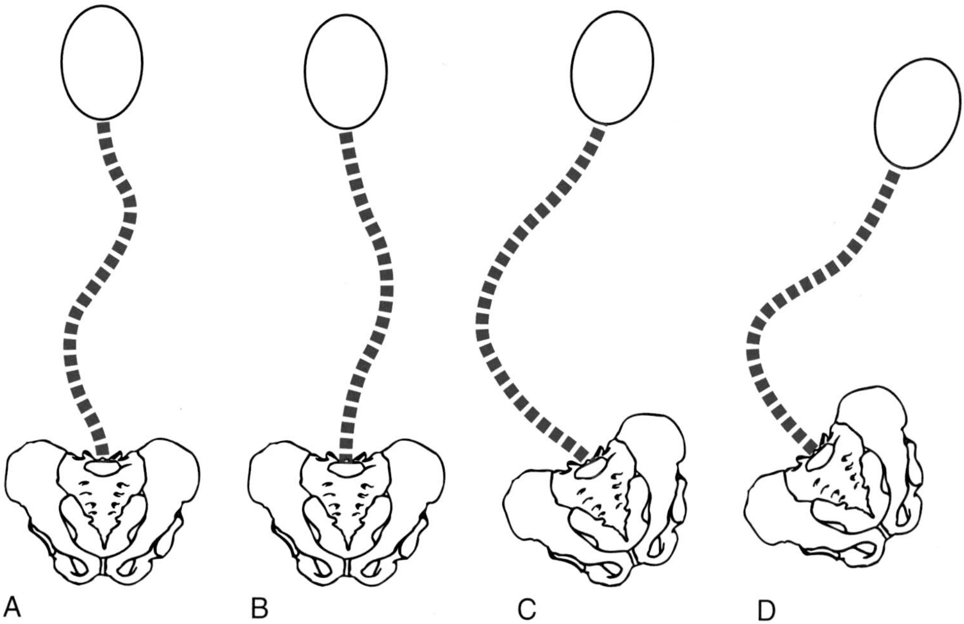

Figure 17–17: Classification of scoliosis in cerebral palsy. Curve patterns in cerebral palsy have been classified into two types. Group I curves are typically seen in ambulatory patients and involve both a thoracic and a lumbar component. These may be balanced, or the thoracic curve may be larger and associated with a fractional, poorly compensated lumbar curve below. Group II curves are seen in the nonambulatory population and include thoracolumbar and lumbar curves associated with pelvic obliquity. From Lonstein JE, Akbarnia B (1983) Operative treatment of spinal deformities in patients with cerebral palsy or mental retardation: An analysis of one hundred and seven cases. J Bone Joint Surg 65A: 43-55.

orthosis serves as a sitting support, which improves sitting balance and may facilitate upper extremity use. Bracing may potentially delay the progression of scoliosis, which in some cases may avoid the need for anterior spinal surgery.

- Proposed benefits of spinal instrumentation and arthrodesis for progressive curves include achieving independent sitting, improving sitting endurance, facilitating upper extremities use, and improving pulmonary status, feeding, and ease of care. Surgery is generally indicated for progressive curvatures beyond 40 degrees or for functional loss (sitting balance and use of upper extremities). Complications are frequent, and a detailed preoperative medical evaluation is essential. Nutritional support may be necessary preoperatively (malnutrition) or postoperatively (ileus and staged anterior and posterior procedures). Mechanisms for delivering nutritional support include both enteral (gastrostomy, jejunal feeding tube, etc.) or parenteral (total parenteral nutrition).

Gait

- A major focus of orthopaedic care in children with cerebral palsy is to improve the quality and energy efficiency of ambulation. Factors that contribute to abnormal ambulation in this population include spasticity, myostatic contractures, bony abnormalities (femoral or tibial torsion and planovalgus feet), muscle imbalance, loss of selective motor control, sensory abnormalities (balance and proprioception), and visual disturbance. Compensatory deviations are also seen and must be differentiated from the primary abnormalities.
- Ambulatory function may be classified as follows: *community ambulator* (walks for extended distances with or without orthotics or an assistive device), *household ambulator* (walks for short distances without support and with or without orthotics or an assistive device), *nonfunctional (therapeutic) ambulator* (walks for limited distances in a therapeutic program), and *nonambulator* (wheelchair bound).[12,13]

Normal Gait in Infants and Toddlers

- Infants usually develop a mature pattern of ambulation by 3 years, and children with cerebral palsy may take 7 years to reach a plateau. Normal toddlers typically have increased flexion at the hip and knee and walk with a wide base to improve balance. The lower extremities are usually in external rotation, and initial contact is typically with a flat foot (rather than a heel strike). The arms are held in abduction (shoulder) and extension (elbow), and reciprocal arm motions usually do not begin until 2 years. When comparing gait parameters of adults with those of toddlers, the adults usually have greater velocity, increased step length, increased time spent in single limb stance, decreased cadence, and a narrow base of support.

Prognosis for Ambulation in Children with Developmental Delay

- Although it is impossible to predict with certainty whether a toddler or child will develop the capacity to ambulate (with or without an assistive device), several authors have outlined criteria that may be predictive.
- According to the Bleck criteria, four primitive reflexes (asymmetrical tonic neck, symmetrical tonic neck, neck righting, and Moro) and three protective reactions (parachute, foot placement, and extensor thrust) are tested in patients older than 1 year. A score of 1 is given for each primitive reflex that is present and for each protective reflex that is absent. The prognosis for ambulation is diminished with the retention of primitive reflexes or with a failure to develop protective reactions. The prognosis is as follows: good (0), guarded (1), and poor (>2).
- Other poor prognostic findings include persistent primitive reflexes beyond 15 months, the inability to achieve head control by 20 months, and the inability to achieve sitting balance by 2 years.

Treatment

- The treatment plan is based upon the bench examination (range of motion, angular and rotational alignment, and degree of spasticity) and the observational gait analysis.

An instrumented motion analysis study may complement the clinical evaluation, especially when multilevel interventions are planned.

Gait Cycle

Prerequisites for a Normal Gait

- Stability during the stance phase
- Clearance during the swing phase
- Appropriate prepositioning of the foot for initial contact
- Adequate step length
- Conservation of energy

Muscle Activity during the Gait Cycle

- Concentric (shortens during contraction)
- Eccentric (lengthens during contraction)
- Isometric (no change in length during contraction)

Phases of the Gait Cycle

- Begins as the heel strikes the ground (Figure 17–18)

Stance Phase (60%)

- Foot is in contact with the floor

Initial Contact and Loading Response

- Ankle plantar flexes passively as the heel strikes the ground
- Hip and knee are flexed
- Muscle action
  - Tibialis anterior decelerates the plantar flexion (eccentric)
  - Hamstrings and hip flexors contract to decelerate the limb (eccentric)

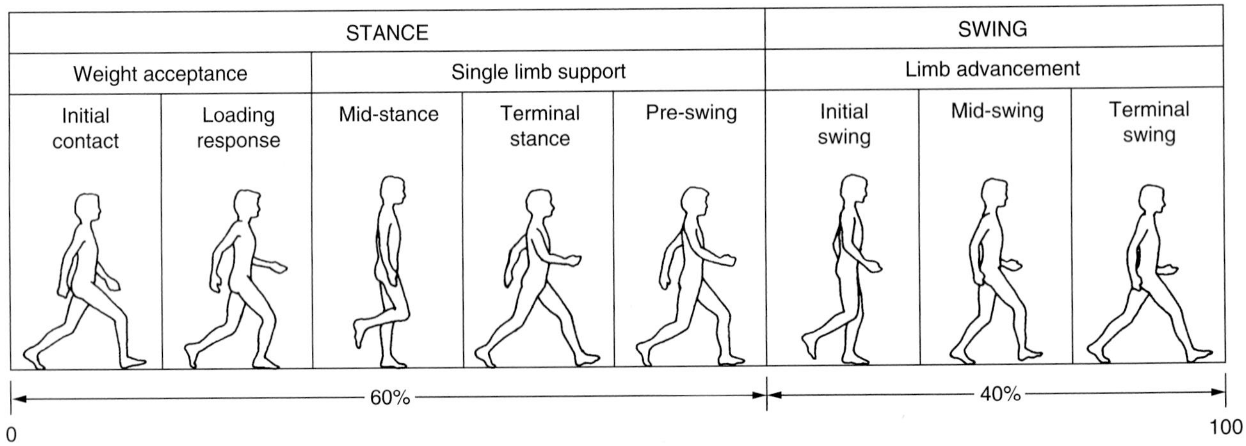

Figure 17–18: The gait cycle includes a stance phase in which the lower extremity is in contact with the ground and a swing phase in which the limb is off the ground. The cycle begins with heel strike. The cycle for the right leg is demonstrated in this figure. From Herring JA, ed (2001) Tachdjian's Pediatric Orthopaedics, 3rd edition, volume 1. Philadelphia: WB Saunders, p 76.

Midstance

- Body advances over the foot
- Foot dorsiflexes as the tibia advances forward
- Extension at the knee and hip

Terminal Stance

- Body continues to advance over the foot
- Muscle action
  - Gastroc–soleus contracts to flex the ankle (concentric), stimulating the heel to rise and preparing for the swing phase

Preswing

- Hip and knee flex passively
- Muscle action
  - Gastroc–soleus contracts to push the limb off the ground

Swing Phase (40%)

- Foot is off the ground, and the goal is to advance the limb and achieve clearance of the foot

Initial Swing

- Hip flexion initiates forward motion of the limb
- Hip and knee are flexed
- Muscle action
  - Tibialis anterior dorsiflexes the foot to help achieve clearance (concentric)

Midswing

- Clearance is achieved
- Hip and knee are still flexed
- Muscle action
  - Tibialis anterior contracts to keep the foot neutral

Terminal Swing

- Deceleration of the limb
- Foot prepares to strike the ground (prepositioning)
- Muscle action
  - Tibialis anterior keeps the foot neutral (eccentric)
  - Quadriceps extend the knee (concentric)
  - Hamstrings decelerate hip flexion and knee extension (eccentric)

Instrumented Motion Analysis

- Instrumented gait analysis is an outstanding research tool, and proposed clinical benefits include helping to refine the operative plan in patients undergoing multiple lower extremity procedures and helping to decide whether tendon transfers are necessary. Prerequisites for a study include the ability to ambulate (with or without an assistive device) and the ability to cooperate (usually children older than 4 years).
- Components of a gait study (in addition to the history, physical examination, and evaluation of a gait video) include the following:
  - *Kinematic data* can be used to reconstruct the relationships among the limb segments during ambulation. Surface markers are placed at various locations on the trunk, pelvis, and lower extremities. Data is collected from a set of cameras (4-12), which identify the location of each surface marker in three dimensions. The data is then processed using computer to reconstruct the relationships among body segments during ambulation (range of motion, velocity, and acceleration of the involved joints).
  - For *kinetic data,* a force plate is employed to collect information that may be used to calculate the magnitude and location of forces around each joint.
  - *Dynamic EMG* is most commonly performed with a surface electrode; however, certain muscle groups (deep and difficult to palpate) such as the tibialis posterior require placement of an electrode within the muscle belly. The technique assesses the activity of each muscle group throughout the gait cycle. Abnormal patterns of activity can be documented, such as when a particular muscle is contracting out of phase or throughout the entire gait cycle. This information helps to plan tendon transfers, such as transfers of the rectus femoris to treat a stiff knee gait or the tibialis posterior to cause a dynamic equinovarus foot deformity.

Common Gait Deviations in Cerebral Palsy

- Gait deviations result from the complex interaction of abnormalities at multiple levels within the extremity, and all pathology must be recognized and treated to obtain the best outcome. A deformity at one level (hip, knee, or foot) may or may not be associated with deformities at other levels, and treating only one level may unmask problems at adjacent levels.[8,12-14]

Hip

- At the hip, a flexion deformity is most common and may be associated with a flexion deformity at the knee. Nonoperative measures include prone positioning and stretching. Surgical treatment involves intramuscular lengthening of the iliopsoas (over the brim).

Knee

- The *crouch gait* pattern increases knee flexion during the stance phase (with or without the swing phase) and may be caused by a hamstring contracture with or without an associated flexion deformity at the hip. Crouching may also compensate for calcaneus, as in the case of an overlengthened tendo Achillis. Patients ambulate with flexion at the hip and knee, and the feet are flat (Figure 17–19). Clinical problems associated with crouching include quadriceps overload, which may gradually elongate the extensor mechanism. Patella alta is commonly observed, which often results in anterior knee pain, patellar sleeve fractures, and late degenerative joint disease. The treatment is to restore adequate muscle length to the hamstrings, iliopsoas, or both and to use the appropriate orthotic support (often a floor reaction AFO).

- The *jump gait* pattern increases knee flexion in the early stance phase with near normal extension during the midstance to late stance phases. The most common cause is a hamstring contracture. Patients are typically flexed at the hip and knee with the foot in equinus. The treatment restores adequate muscle length.
- A *stiff knee gait* results from inadequate knee flexion during the swing phase. The most common cause is inappropriate rectus femoris activity, which delays knee flexion and decreases the range of flexion during the swing phase. This pattern may also be unmasked following hamstring lengthening. The main gait deviation is impaired clearance during the swing phase, and patients may compensate by circumduction, vaulting, and increased pelvic rotation or obliquity. Nonoperative measures include hamstring strengthening, and operative treatment transfers of the rectus femoris to the sartorius, gracilis, or semitendinosus.
- A *recurvatum gait* hyperextends the knee during the midstance to late stance phases, which may be caused by gastroc–soleus contracture or overlengthened hamstrings. Gait deviations include decreased stride length and velocity. Patients may experience posterior knee pain, and degenerative changes may be observed at a long-term follow-up. Treatment lengthens the gastroc–soleus. Occasionally an AFO may be constructed with the plantar flexion stop at several degrees of dorsiflexion to prevent knee hyperextension.

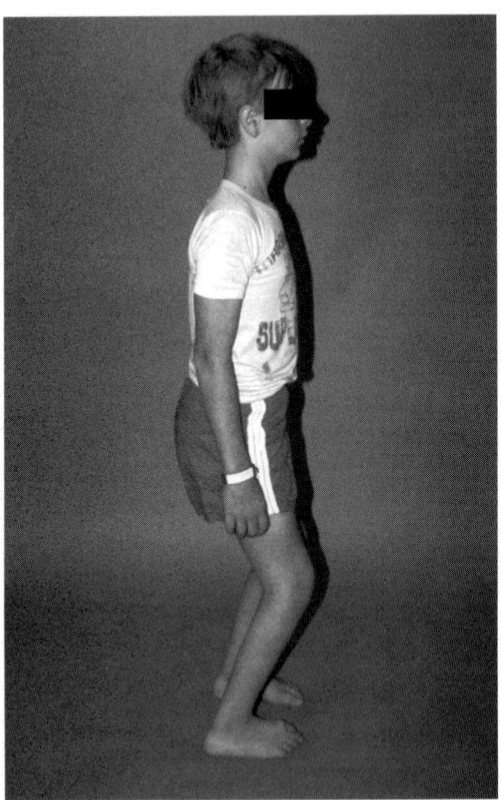

Figure 17–19: This patient is standing in crouch with flexion at both the hip and the knee and excessive dorsiflexion at the ankle. The primary problem in this case might be an overlengthened tendo Achillis with compensatory flexion deformities at both the hip and the knee to maintain balance.

Foot and Ankle

- An *equinus* deformity results from contracture of the gastrocnemius muscle, or both the gastrocnemius and the soleus. The lack of passive ankle dorsiflexion prevents the tibia from advancing over the foot during the stance phase and abolishes the second and third rocker. Equinus may result in knee recurvatum because of the plantar flexion–knee extension couple (posteriorly directed force at the knee). The treatment is lengthening the tendo Achillis (avoid overlengthening) and addressing any proximal contractures within the extremity. Botox injections may provide temporary relief for dynamic deformities, and serial casting may be used to treat myostatic contracture. Not all patients who walk on their toes have an equinus deformity, and examination of the proximal joints is crucial. Flexion contracture at the hip, knee, or both may be compensated for by toe walking (jump gait pattern) in the absence of a gastroc–soleus contracture.
- A *calcaneus* deformity may result from overlengthening of the gastroc–soleus or perhaps gradual elongation caused by coexisting hamstring, hip, or both areas of flexion contractures.

Surgical Treatment of Specific Deformities

- A variety of orthopaedic procedures are employed, often in combination, in the management of deformities of the spine and extremities. The overall philosophy for treatment relates to ambulatory status, which correlates with the degree of neuromuscular involvement. Timing is also important. For lower extremity surgery in ambulatory patients, it is generally held that a plateau in ambulation is reached around 7 years and that efforts to improve a gait surgically should be delayed if possible until this time. The goal is to address as many problems as possible under a single anesthetic, which in a diplegic child might include multiple soft tissue and bony procedures on both lower extremities followed by extensive rehabilitation. In the upper extremity, the patient must be at an age at which cooperation with both the preoperative assessment and the postoperative rehabilitation is possible.

- Preoperative counseling is essential. Expectations should be realistic, and families should be forewarned that some of the deformities may recur with further growth and that subsequent interventions may be required. Families should also be made aware that orthopaedic procedures do not affect other components of the patient's movement disorder, including spasticity, loss of selective motor control, problems with balance, abnormalities in cognition or vision, and underlying weakness.

Procedures

- The muscle–tendon unit is lengthened for myostatic contractures. Lengthening weakens the muscle, and adequate postoperative rehabilitation is mandatory. Overlengthening should be avoided. Techniques include the following:
  - *Myotomy* releases the muscle fibers and is most commonly employed for adduction contracture at the hip or a proximal hamstring release.
  - In an *open tendon lengthening (Z-lengthening),* the tendon is divided and resutured at the appropriate tension.
  - In an *intramuscular lengthening,* the tendinous portion (within the substance of the muscle) is released. Muscles lengthened in this fashion include the gracilis, posterior tibialis, and iliopsoas.
  - *Tendinous recession* is performed at the musculotendinous junction and releases the broad fascial layer that overlies the muscle at this level. Muscles lengthened using this technique include the gastroc–soleus and the semimembranosus.
  - The indications for *tendon release* are limited because of the risk of excessive weakness postoperatively. The technique should be avoided in ambulatory patients but may be considered in nonambulatory patients to improve positioning and ease of care.
- *Tendon transfers* are used to restore muscle balance. The indications for the transfer of an entire tendon are limited because the outcome is generally less predictable in patients with spastic muscle imbalance. There is a higher likelihood of overcorrection, which may result in the opposite deformity. Split tendon transfers are more predictable. Examples include the tibialis posterior or tibialis anterior transfers for dynamic equinovarus of the foot.
- *Osteotomies* are performed to correct rotational or angular deformities.

Lower Extremity

Hip

- An *adduction contracture* (Table 17–1) may internally rotate the extremity and scissor ambulatory patients, or it may result in progressive hip subluxation in nonambulators. Adductor myotomy is performed through a transverse incision centered over the adductor longus. The adductor longus is bluntly dissected and released with care taken to avoid injury to the obturator neurovascular bundle, which lies on the anterior surface of the adductor brevis. A myotomy of the gracilis is then performed, and a partial release of the adductor brevis may be performed if there is residual tightness. In the past, some authors have recommended a neurectomy of the anterior branch of the obturator nerve to prevent recurrence. The current trend is to avoid this procedure because of the risk of an abduction and extension contracture, which may potentially be complicated by an anterior hip dislocation. This contracture may impair the ability to sit. Postoperative care typically involves splinting in abduction to prevent recurrence, in addition to the child's standard physical therapy program.
- *Hamstring contracture* may impair sitting ability in nonambulators, who may vault or slide forward in their wheelchairs. Proximal hamstring release may be performed through a medial approach, essentially an extension of the incision used for an adductor myotomy. The interval is between the anterior border of the gracilis and the adductor magnus. The sciatic nerve lies beside the hamstrings at their origin, and a nerve stimulator may help to avoid injury to this structure.
- *Flexion contracture* often results in a crouched gait, anterior pelvic tilt, and lumbar hyperlordosis. Intramuscular lengthening of the iliopsoas (over the pelvic brim)[15] preserves muscle power and limits the chance of excessive weakness. Excessive weakness may make stair climbing and other activities extremely difficult. An anterior, oblique incision is made just below the anterior superior iliac spine, and the muscle is identified between the sartorius and the femoral sheath. The femoral nerve lies directly on the anterior surface of the iliopsoas, and the tendinous portion of the muscle lies on the posterior surface. The tendinous portion is dissected and released. Postoperative care includes prone positioning for several hours each day and active and passive extension exercises.
- *Progressive subluxation, dislocation,* or both are commonly treated by a proximal femoral osteotomy (usually with an adductor release) with or without an osteotomy of the pelvis[16,17] (Figures 17–20 and 17–21). Patients with dislocation, or more than 70% migration, may require open reduction as well. Open reduction is performed through an anterior approach (also used for the pelvic osteotomy). The goal of proximal femoral derotational

Table 17–1: Common Deformities of the Hip, Knee, and Leg

AMBULATORY STATUS*	HIP	CLINICAL FINDINGS	PROCEDURES	KNEE OR LEG	CLINICAL FINDINGS	PROCEDURES
Ambulatory	Flexion contracture	Crouch Lumbar hyperlordosis	Iliopsoas lengthening (intramuscular)	Flexion contracture	Crouch or jump gait	Hamstring lengthening
	Adduction contracture	Scissoring	Adductor myotomy	Rectus femoris spasticity	Stiff knee gait	Rectus femoris transfer
	Internal femoral torsion	Intoeing or scissoring	Femoral derotational osteotomy	Tibial torsion (internal or external)	Intoeing or outtoeing	Tibial derotational osteotomy
Nonambulatory	Flexion contracture	Lumbar hyperlordosis	Iliopsoas lengthening or release	Extension contracture	Loss of lumbar lordosis Problems with seating balance	Hamstring release (proximal or distal)
	Mild subluxation (migration 30-50%)	Decreased abduction	Adductor or psoas lengthening or release			
	Moderate or severe subluxation (migration > 50%)	Decreased abduction Problems with perineal care Pain	VDRO +/– pelvic osteotomy			
	Dislocation (reconstructive) (migration > 90%)	Chronic pain Problems with perineal care	VDRO +/– pelvic osteotomy +/– open reduction			
	Dislocation (salvage)	Chronic pain Problems with perineal care	Resection Arthroplasty Valgus osteotomy Arthrodesis Prosthesis			

VDRO, varus derotational osteotomy.
* Ambulatory status is important in determining the philosophy of treatment and the most appropriate procedures for problems at the hip, knee, and lower leg. Although muscle releases may be acceptable in nonambulatory patients, lengthening is essential in ambulators to preserve muscle power.

osteotomy is to correct femoral anteversion, and it may be necessary to add varus. The degree of varus should be minimized in ambulatory patients, and derotation alone may be sufficient. Proximal femoral varus will result in abductor insufficiency. If varus is deemed necessary, the neck–shaft angle should be no less than 120 degrees. In nonambulators with subluxation or dislocation, a greater degree of varus is desirable (90-100 degrees). A pelvic osteotomy is indicated in cases with coexisting acetabular dysplasia (acetabular index > 25 degrees). The acetabulum is deficient (rather than maloriented as in developmental hip dysplasia), and a volume-reducing procedure is most popular (differential evolution genetic algorithm, or Dega, and variants) rather than a redirectional osteotomy. The deficiency is most often posterior and lateral but may be global. Other pelvic osteotomies reported in this population include the Chiari osteotomy and the shelf arthroplasty, both of which are more commonly employed for salvage.

– *Femoral osteotomy* is performed through a lateral approach with the patient either prone or supine. A guide pin is inserted parallel to the femoral neck to assess the degree of anteversion and to provide orientation for inserting the chisel (if a blade plate is used). The osteotomy is performed just above the lesser trochanter (derotation will relax the psoas), and the psoas tendon should not be released. Femoral derotation should also improve the mechanical advantage of the abductors. Fixation may be achieved with a blade plate or a hip screw. The distal fragment is laterally rotated to correct the anteversion. In general, the appropriate degree of derotation will provide 30 degrees of medial rotation and 60 degrees of lateral rotation. The guide pin can also be used to gauge the degree of anteversion (the goal is approximately 15 degrees). If varus is added, the shaft should be medialized to maintain the mechanical axis of the limb. Complications include loss of fixation, and a spica cast should be considered in patients with severe spasticity, significant osteopenia, or instability fixation.
– The *pelvic osteotomy* is performed through an anterior approach, and the sciatic notch should be exposed. In the San Diego acetabuloplasty (a similar concept to

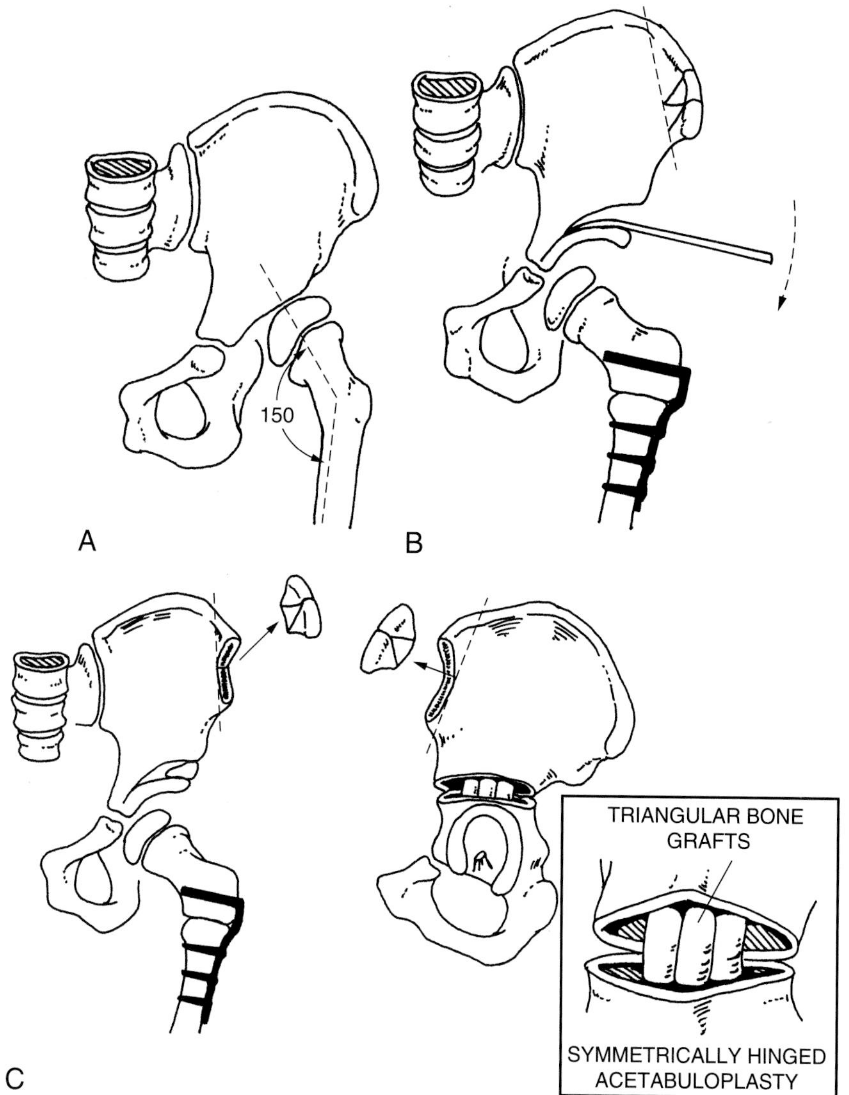

Figure 17–20: Reconstruction for progressive subluxation or early dislocation. In cases with significant subluxation (A), the femoral head is lateralized, and the acetabulum is shallow (acetabular index > 25 degrees). The neck–shaft angle of the proximal femur is increased (150 degrees in this example). The femoral osteotomy (B) corrects rotational malalignment (excessive anteversion) and produces varus (decreases the valgus neck–shaft angle) to better seat the femoral head within the acetabulum. The acetabular osteotomy levers the lateral and posterior acetabular margin downward to reduce volume and provide better coverage for the femoral head. Structural bone grafts are inserted (C) to maintain the degree of correction. From Mubarak SJ, Valencia FG, Wenger DR (1992) One-stage correction of the spastic dislocated hip: Use of pericapsular acetabuloplasty to improve coverage. J Bone Joint Surg 74A: 1349-1352.

DEGA),[16] the osteotomy is made 1 cm from (and parallel to) the acetabular margin. Curved osteotomies are used to deepen the osteotomy in the direction of the triradiate cartilage, and the acetabulum is levered down gently. Structural bone grafts (usually allograft) are then inserted into the gap. The size and shape of grafts may be modified to augment the degree of coverage. Fixation is not required, and patients are placed in a spica cast postoperatively.

- *Chronic subluxation or dislocation* may result in pain from deformation of the femoral head and damage to the articular cartilage. Reconstruction is contraindicated in this setting, and salvage procedures are used to treat chronic pain (Figure 17–22).
  - *Proximal femoral resection* is performed through a lateral approach, and a subtrochanteric osteotomy is performed 3 cm from the lesser trochanter or at the level of the inferior ischial ramus. The proximal femur

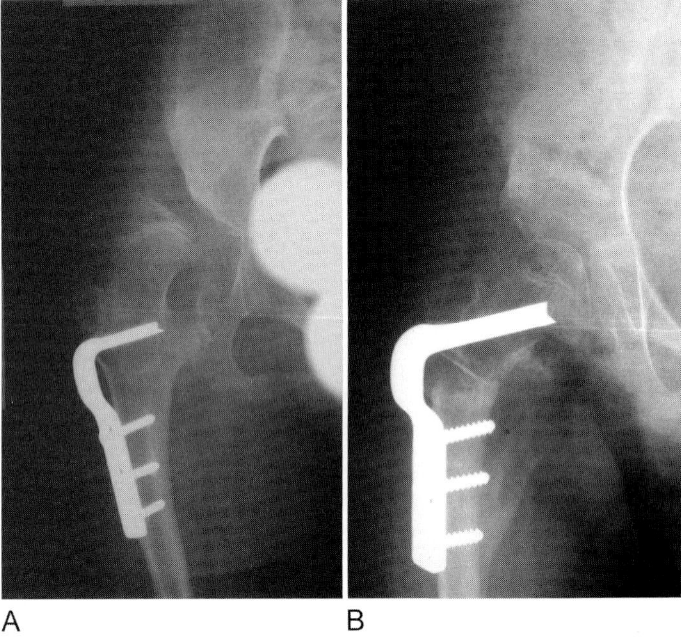

Figure 17–21: Reconstruction for severe subluxation. This 10-year-old female with spastic quadriplegia had previously undergone bilateral femoral osteotomies and soft tissue release but developed recurrence of right hip subluxation (A). She was treated by hardware removal, revision of the femoral varus derotational osteotomy, and a volume-reducing pelvic osteotomy (B).

is extraperiosteally dissected and removed. The hip capsule is repaired over the acetabulum, and the abductors are interposed between the proximal femur and the acetabulum. The quadriceps is sewn over the proximal femur. Postoperative traction is commonly employed for up to 6 weeks, and it may 12 or more months for patients to achieve maximal relief of pain. Both the pain and the spasticity may be greater than before surgery during the initial postoperative period. Complications include heterotopic ossification.

- *Proximal femoral valgus osteotomy* redirects the femoral head from the wall of the ilium and improves abduction (facilitates perineal care). Plate fixation is commonly employed. Problems following the procedure include irritation over the lateral prominence (femoral head) and seating difficulties.
- Arthrodesis has been reported but has a limited role in this population.
- *Prosthetic reconstruction* has been reported infrequently, and the indications remain controversial. Options include total hip arthroplasty and proximal femoral replacement with a humeral prosthesis. The ideal candidate for total hip arthroplasty can walk, stand, or transfer, and the procedure is contraindicated in the setting of significant pelvic obliquity or scoliosis.

Knee

- *Hamstring contracture* (Table 17–1) is extremely common in patients with diplegia and quadriplegia and may be seen in a subset of patients with hemiplegia. Hamstring lengthening is performed distally in ambulatory patients, and most patients can be treated by a medial lengthening, including the semitendinosus (Z-lengthening or intramuscular lengthening), the semimembranosus (recession at musculotendinous junction), and the gracilis (intramuscular lengthening) (Figure 17–23). In deformities of greater severity, a recession of the biceps femoris may also be performed (two transverse cuts in the fascia at the musculotendinous junction). Patients are usually placed in a knee immobilizer for 6 weeks. Complications include genu recurvatum (overlengthening), which is more likely when both the medial and the lateral hamstrings are lengthened. Neurapraxia of the sciatic nerve may rarely complicate acute correction in deformities of greater magnitude (usually those that require lengthening of both the medial and the lateral hamstrings). The pain or dysesthesias may be severe and generally take a significant period to resolve. Increased anterior pelvic tilt (resulting in a crouch) may also complicate hamstring lengthening, especially if the iliopsoas is contracted. Concomitant intramuscular lengthening of the iliopsoas should be performed in the presence of a hip flexion deformity. Hamstring lengthening may also unmask spasticity of the rectus femoris, decreasing knee flexion during the swing phase, which may impair clearance (stiff knee gait).
- *Spasticity of the rectus femoris* may result in a stiff knee gait with impaired clearance (inadequate knee flexion) during the swing phase. Rectus femoris transfer has been shown to increase peak knee flexion and is commonly performed with distal lengthening of the hamstrings.[18] A transverse or oblique incision is made several fingerbreadths from the superior pole of the patella, and the rectus tendon is dissected from the vastus intermedius. Blunt dissection frees

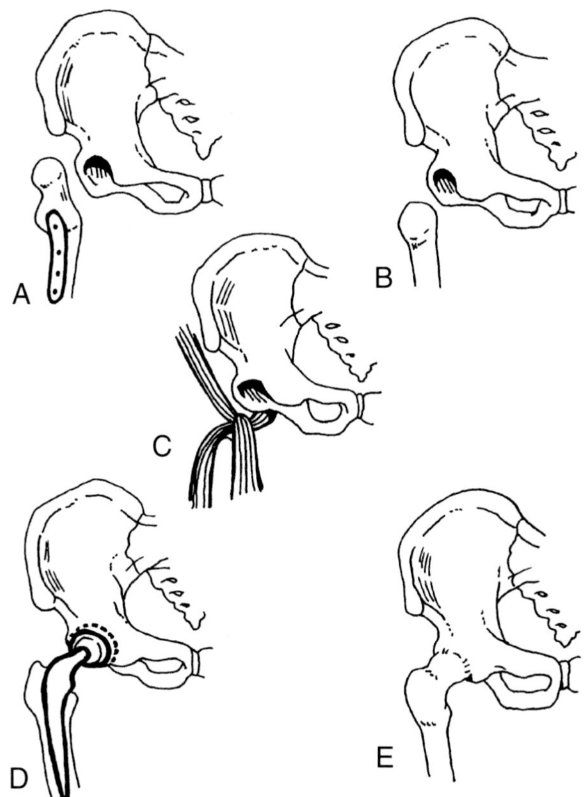

Figure 17–22: Salvage procedures for chronic, symptomatic hip dislocation. Several options are available if the hip dislocation is long standing or if femoral head deformity or degenerative changes in the articular cartilage are present during an attempted open reduction. A, With a valgus osteotomy, the proximal femur is redirected from the acetabulum. This may be combined with interposition of soft tissues. B, A resection arthroplasty removes the proximal end of the femur, most often at the subtrochanteric level. C, Interposition of the hip capsule and abductor muscles is usually performed. D, Total joint arthroplasty replaces the joint with prosthetic components, and some authors have just replaced the proximal femur and left the acetabular side alone. E, Arthrodesis, or fusion, removes the cartilaginous surfaces, realigning the joint in the desired position and securing the joint with hardware to promote permanent healing. Joint replacement and hip fusion are rarely performed. From Dormans JP, Copely LA (1998) Orthopaedic approaches to treatment. In: Caring for Children with Cerebral Palsy: A Teambased Approach (Dormans JP, Pellegrino L, eds). Baltimore: Brookes Publishing, p 155.

the muscle proximally, and the tendon is released distally at the superior pole of the patella. The tendon is transferred to the sartorius, the gracilis, or the semitendonosus.

Foot and Ankle

- Table 17–2 outlines common foot deformities associated with cerebral palsy, clinical findings, and common treatment recommendations.

Equinus Deformities

- Equinus deformities result from contracture of the gastrocnemius or both the gastrocnemius and the soleus. A host of techniques is available for lengthening the tendo Achillis. The decision to use a particular technique depends upon which components of the muscle are contracted and the degree of the contracture. Gastrocnemius recession preserves power for push off (the soleus is left alone) and is less likely to result in overlengthening; however, the rate of recurrence is higher (15-50%). Overcorrection should be avoided because calcaneus deformity is more problematic than residual equinus. This decreases the push off power and results in a crouched gait, especially in the setting of tight hamstrings, hip flexors, or both.

Gastroc–soleus Lengthening

- Refer to Figure 17–24 for the following:
- The *Strayer technique* lengthens the gastrocnemius. The plane between the gastrocnemius tendon and the underlying soleus fascia is developed proximally. The gastrocnemius tendon is released just proximal to where it blends with the soleus fascia to form a conjoined tendon (Achilles tendon). The tendon is then sutured to the underlying soleus fascia at the desired length. Patients are allowed full weight-bearing status in a short leg cast for 6 weeks.
- The Z-lengthening technique addresses both the gastrocnemius and the soleus and is indicated for greater degrees of deformity. This technique has the greatest chance of overlengthening. A short leg cast (a non–weight-bearing cast) is worn for 6 weeks.
- *Sliding lengthening* may be performed using an open or percutaneous technique.
  - Several options are available for percutaneous lengthening. In the White technique, two cuts are made in the tendon. The medial half is sectioned at the insertion into calcaneus, and the lateral half is sectioned more proximally. Forced dorsiflexion is used to achieve correction. In the Hoke technique, three cuts are made in the tendon. A medial cut is made distally and most proximally, and a lateral cut is made centrally. Forced dorsiflexion is used to achieve correction. Aftercare includes a short leg cast (3-6 weeks), and weight-bearing status is permitted.
  - In the open technique, two or three cuts made in tendon under direct visualization, and the foot is dorsiflexed to achieve the desired degree of correction.
  - *Tendinous recession* involves one or more transverse cuts in the aponeurosis (musculotendinous junction). In the Vulpius technique, a Chevron-type cut is made in the aponeurosis of the gastrocnemius and soleus, and the Baker "tongue in groove" technique cuts a central fascial "tongue." This rectangular segment slides distally

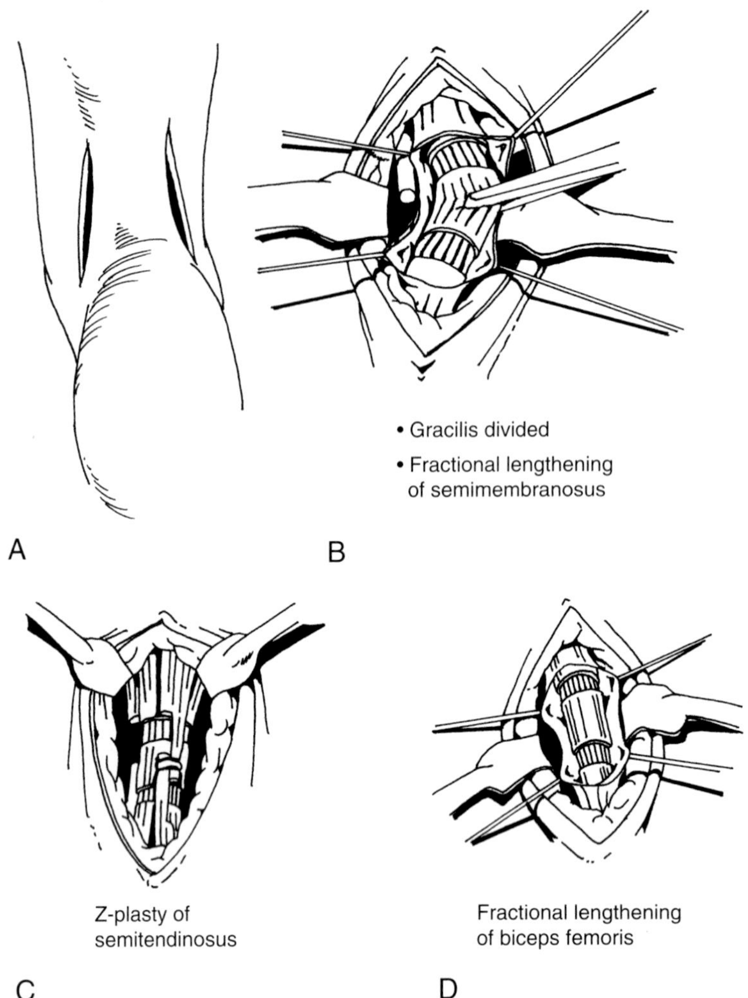

Figure 17–23: Hamstring lengthening. The hamstring muscles include the gracilis, semitendinosus, semimembranosus, and biceps femoris. Surgical lengthening of the medial hamstrings typically involves release or musculotendinous lengthening of the gracilis, Z-lengthening of the semitendinosus, and musculotendinous lengthening of the semimembranosus. With persistent contracture after medial surgery, the biceps femoris may also be lengthened using a musculotendinous technique. Either a long leg cast or a knee immobilizer is usually worn for 5 to 6 weeks after the procedure. From Herring JA, ed (2001) Tachdjian's Pediatric Orthopaedics, 3rd edition, volume 2. Philadelphia: WB Saunders, pp 1171.

and is resutured at the appropriate length. Aftercare involves a short leg cast (3-6 weeks), and weight-bearing status is permitted.

Equinovarus Deformities

- Equinovarus deformities are seen most frequently in the hemiplegic population. Muscle lengthening may be sufficient in milder cases, but a split tendon transfer is usually required to balance the muscular forces. If the deformity is rigid, then an osteotomy of the calcaneus should be added. Either the tibialis anterior or the tibialis posterior may be responsible for the deformity. The confusion test may help to determine which of these is involved. With active flexion of the hip, if the forefoot supinates, the tibialis anterior is likely involved. However, pure dorsiflexion suggests involvement of the tibialis posterior. Instrumented gait analysis provides a more objective way to differentiate between these two muscles, using dynamic EMG.
  - Lengthening of the tibialis posterior muscle is indicated for mild, flexible deformities in younger children. Techniques include distal Z-lengthening and intramuscular lengthening (Frost procedure) near the ankle joint. In the latter, the intramuscular portion of the tendon is isolated and divided. A short leg cast is worn for 6 weeks.
  - Although complete transfer of the tibialis posterior has been associated with a significant prevalence of

Table 17–2: Common Foot Deformities in Cerebral Palsy

DEFORMITY	ETIOLOGY	CLINICAL FINDINGS OR SYMPTOMS	COMMON TREATMENT RECOMMENDATIONS
Equinus	Gastroc–soleus contracture	Limited dorsiflexion Toe walking Component of jump or recurvatum gait pattern Difficulty with clearance during swing phase Difficulty fitting or tolerating an orthosis	Gastroc–soleus lengthening
Equinovarus	Gastroc–soleus contracture Muscle imbalance between inversion and eversion	Hindfoot equinus and varus Internal foot progression Toe walking Difficulty with clearance during swing phase Difficulty fitting or tolerating an orthosis	Gastroc–soleus lengthening Tibialis posterior lengthening Split tendon transfer (tibialis posterior or tibialis anterior) Rancho procedure (split tibialis anterior transfer or intramuscular lengthening of tibialis posterior)
Equinovalgus	Tendo Achillis contracture Peroneal spasticity Weakness of the tibialis posterior Watch for coexisting ankle valgus	Hindfoot equinus and valgus or forefoot abduction Tendo Achillis contracture Callus or breakdown over talar head Medial hindfoot pain Difficulty fitting or tolerating an orthosis	Calcaneal osteotomy (lateral column lengthening) Subtalar arthrodesis Triple arthrodesis (rigid or severe in older patients) Osteotomy or medial malleolar screw epiphysiodesis for coexisting ankle valgus

Equinus and equinovarus deformities are most common and are usually seen in children with spastic hemiplegia. Equinovalgus deformities are seen with some frequency in patients with spastic diplegia. Calcaneus deformities are less common and often occur as a consequence of treatment.

overcorrection into valgus, the *split tibialis posterior transfer* has been successful[19,20] (Figure 17–25). The posterior half of muscle is released distally, and the tendon is split until a point near the ankle. The tendon is then passed posteriorly to the tibia and fibula and secured to the peroneus brevis, usually by weaving. Intramuscular lengthening of the tibialis posterior may be considered at the same time, and gastroc–soleus lengthening is usually performed. A subset of patients will be able to function well without an orthosis.

– The *split tibialis anterior transfer* has also been successful in this population; however, the expected loss of power following transfer exacerbates a foot drop, which will necessitate an AFO. The lateral half of the tibialis anterior is split and transferred to the cuboid. Gastroc–soleus lengthening is usually performed, and the procedure may be combined with intramuscular lengthening of the tibialis posterior (Rancho procedure).

Equinovalgus Deformities

• Equinovalgus deformities are usually associated with gastroc–soleus contracture with or without peroneal spasticity, weakness of the tibialis posterior, or both. These deformities are most common in diplegics and quadriplegics. Patients may experience skin breakdown or pain in the region of the talar head and may have difficulty tolerating their orthoses. More severe deformities may impair ambulation and create difficulties with shoe wear. Hindfoot valgus deformity may occur at the subtalar joint, the ankle joint, or both. Standing anteroposterior radiographs of the ankle should be obtained preoperatively to evaluate the alignment at the ankle joint. Coexisting ankle valgus may be treated by epiphysiodesis or osteotomy. A medial malleolar screw allows gradual correction of ankle valgus and is reversible because the screw may be removed. Patients close to skeletal maturity are usually treated by open epiphysiodesis.

– *Calcaneal osteotomy* (lateral column lengthening) has become a popular technique for managing this deformity[21] (Figure 17–26). An incision is made over the sinus tarsi, and the calcaneus is exposed. The osteotomy is begun 1.5 cm proximal to the calcaneocuboid joint and is directed to exit between the anterior and the middle facets of the subtalar joint. A trapezoidal bone graft (usually an iliac crest allograft) is then inserted into the osteotomy. Lengthening of the gastroc–soleus is usually required. Intramuscular lengthening of the peroneus brevis may also be required, and some surgeons reef the talonavicular joint capsule. One advantage of this technique is that no joints are violated, thereby preserving motion. Complications include graft dislodgement and dorsal subluxation of the calcaneocuboid joint.

– *Subtalar arthrodesis* is another alternative for stabilizing the hindfoot (Figure 17–27). In the Grice extra-articular arthrodesis,[22] an iliac crest or fibular graft is inserted across the subtalar joint with the foot in a reduced position. Problems include nonunion and loss of alignment. The technique described by Dennyson and Fulford employs screw fixation across the talus and calcaneus with cancellous bone grafting. Lengthening

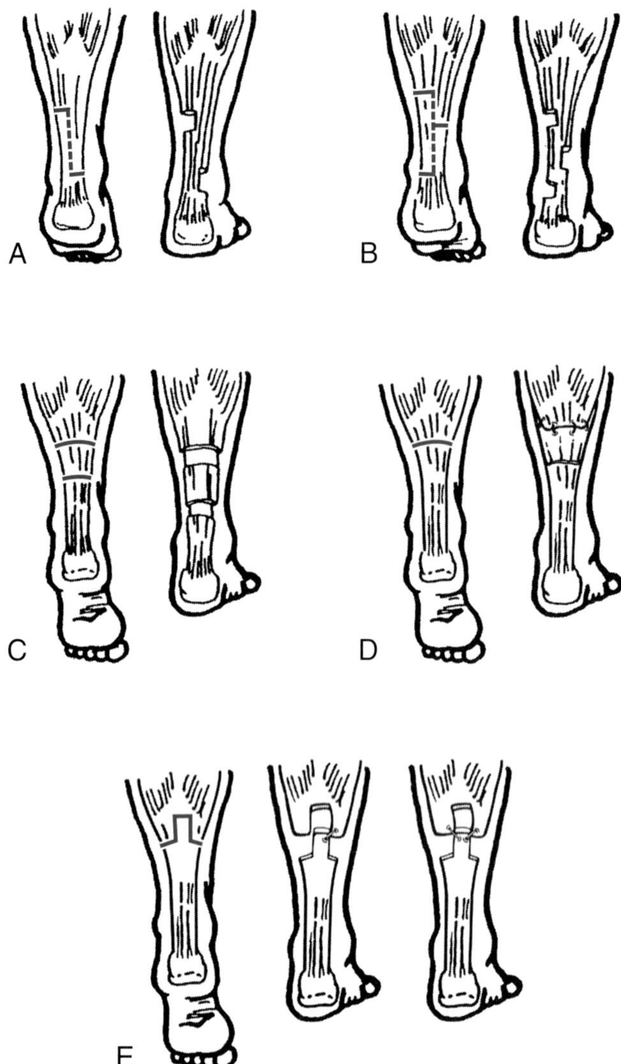

Figure 17–24: Gastroc–soleus lengthening. **Equinus contracture at the ankle may be treated by either an open or percutaneous Z-lengthening or a musculotendinous lengthening of the gastrocnemius with or without the soleus. From Dormans JP, Copely LA (1998) Orthopaedic approaches to treatment. In: Caring for Children with Cerebral Palsy: A Teambased Approach (Dormans JP, Pellegrino L, eds). Baltimore: Brookes Publishing, p 160.**

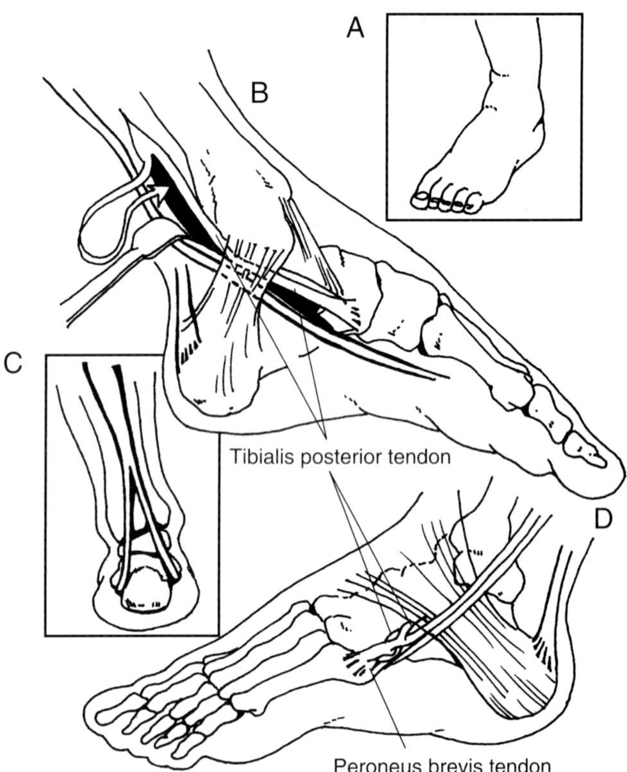

Figure 17–25: Split posterior tibialis tendon transfer. **For a dynamic equinovarus deformity in which the foot is pulled into inversion during the swing phase of gait, a split tibialis posterior tendon transfer achieves better balance by removing some of the deforming force (inversion) and supplementing eversion by rerouting one half of the tendon to the peroneus brevis. From Dutkowski JP (1998) Cerebral palsy. In: Campbell's Operative Orthopaedics, 9th edition (Canale ST, ed), volume 4. St. Louis: Mosby-Year Book, p 3919.**

of the gastrocnemius with or without the soleus is usually required.

- *Subtalar arthrorisis* has been reported but is infrequently performed by orthopaedic surgeons. A staple (or synthetic peg) is placed across the subtalar joint with the foot in the corrected position. Problems include implant migration and synovitis.
- A *triple arthrodesis* is indicated for rigid deformities of greater severity. Because the procedure shortens the foot, it is desirable to wait until early adolescence. A lateral incision is made over the sinus tarsi, and a supplemental medial exposure ensures adequate visualization of the talonavicular joint. The procedure is technically more difficult in the valgus foot, and a graft inserted laterally across the subtalar joint may help to realign the hindfoot in a neutral position (rather than shorten it the medial side).

Hallux Valgus

- Hallux valgus is usually secondary to an equinovalgus foot, often with external tibial torsion. It is important to evaluate and treat the entire extremity. Soft tissue procedures have a higher rate of recurrence in patients with neuromuscular disease. The most reliable procedure is an arthrodesis of the first metatarsophalangeal joint.

Spine

Posterior Spinal Fusion

- Patients are typically instrumented and fused from T2 to the pelvis with segmental spinal instrumentation (fixation at each level). Sublaminar wires or cables are used most frequently, as described by Luque in the late 1970s[25]

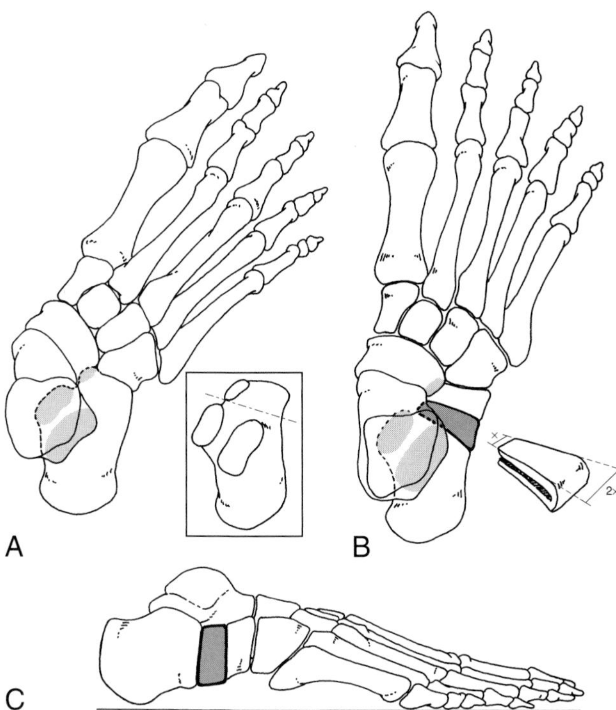

Figure 17–26: Calcaneal osteotomy (lateral column lengthening). **A, One option for managing an equinovalgus deformity of the foot is by lengthening the lateral column of the foot by an osteotomy of the anterior portion of the calcaneus. B and C, A trapezoidal bone graft is inserted into the osteotomy site, which results in a three-dimensional realignment of the bones of the hindfoot. Procedures commonly performed at the same time include gastroc–soleus lengthening and soft tissue reefing to tighten the attenuated structures on the medial side of the foot. From Mosca VS (1995) Calcaneal lengthening for valgus deformity of the hindfoot. J Bone Joint Surg 77A: 500-512.**

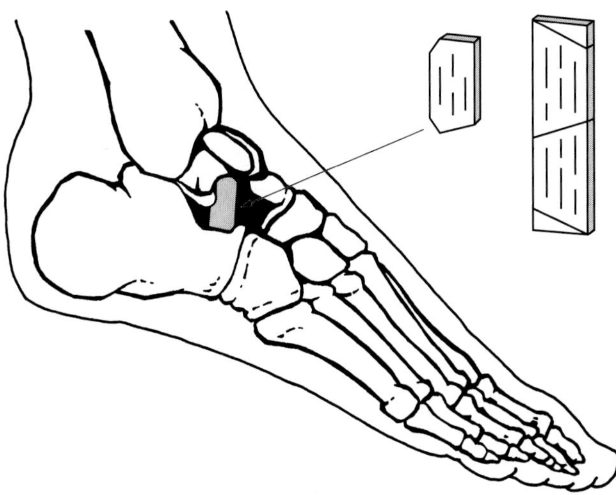

Figure 17–27: Subtalar arthrodesis. **Hindfoot arthrodesis is another technique used to realign the equinovalgus foot. With the Dennyson and Fulford technique, cancellous bone is placed between the talus and the calcaneus, and alignment is secured with a screw. From Grice DS (1952) An extra-articular arthrodesis of the subastragalar joint for correction of paralytic flat feet in children. J Bone Joint Surg 34A: 927-940.**

(Figure 17–28). Supplementary hooks, screws, or both may also be used. For patients with significant pelvic obliquity, fixation to the pelvis is most often achieved with the Galveston technique.[23] Galveston fixation contours the distal portions of each rod to fit within the inner table of the posterior ilium (directed anterior to the sciatic notch toward the acetabulum). The unit rod is a precontoured dual rod construct (made of a single rod) that serves as an alternative to the traditional Luque-Galveston technique[24] (Figure 17–29). Both of these use intrailiac extension of the rods for lumbosacral fixation, although the corrective sequence differs between the two techniques. Alternatives to the intrailiac rod for lumbosacral fixation include intrailiac screws, Dunn-McCarthy fixation, and transiliac screws.[11]

- Bracing is not routinely required postoperatively but should be considered in patients with athetosis, behavioral disorders, or questionable fixation quality.
- Fixation to the pelvis may potentially impair ambulation, and ambulatory patients should be warned preoperatively. In ambulators, consideration can be given to ending the fusion in the lumbar spine, depending on the patient's degree of involvement, the size of the deformity, and any significant pelvic obliquity.
- Complications are frequent in this complex population of patients. Medical complications include urinary tract infection, atelectasis or pneumonia, and ileus. Orthopaedic complications include neurological injury, wound sepsis (deep or superficial), pseudarthrosis, and instrumentation failure. Fracture of one or both rods secondary to fatigue failure from cyclic loading (usually at the thoracolumbar or lumbosacral junction) may occur years after the procedure and suggests the presence of a pseudarthrosis. If the patient is asymptomatic, and correction has not been lost, presumed pseudarthroses may be managed by observation. Those that are symptomatic require revision surgery for grafting and reinstrumentation. Lysis around the intrailiac portions of one or both rods (or screws) is not uncommon and does not necessarily imply pseudarthrosis. Progressive lucency that does not stabilize within the time frame expected for arthrodesis to occur is a more worrisome finding.

Anterior Spinal Release or Fusion

- Anterior spinal release or fusion is indicated in larger, stiffer deformities; deformities with significant pelvic obliquity; or both. Removal of the annulus fibrosus and the disk improves flexibility, and greater correction improves spinal balance and pelvic obliquity. Secondary benefits include an enhanced rate of arthrodesis. Traction

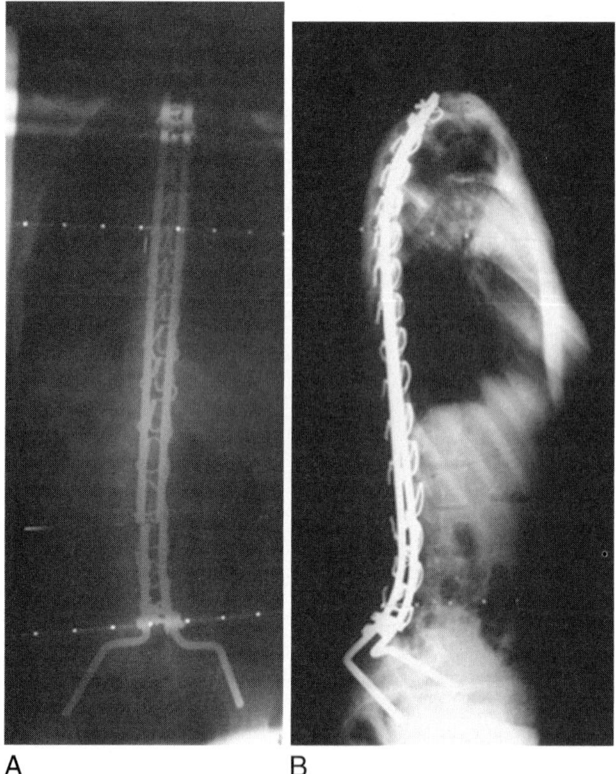

Figure 17–28: Spinal instrumentation for neuromuscular scoliosis. Anteroposterior (A) and lateral (B) radiographs demonstrate the typical spinal construct used to stabilize long neuromuscular curves with pelvic obliquity. Fixation is achieved at each level using sublaminar wires, which are tightened to the spinal rods. The rods extend into the pelvis (iliac wing) on each side to stabilize the lumbosacral junction. Metal cross-links stabilize the construct further by locking the rods to one another. Corrective forces are applied gradually during the sequence of instrumentation. From Spiegel DA (2004) Cerebral palsy. In: Pediatric Orthopaedics and Sports Medicine (Dormans JP, ed). Philadelphia: Mosby.

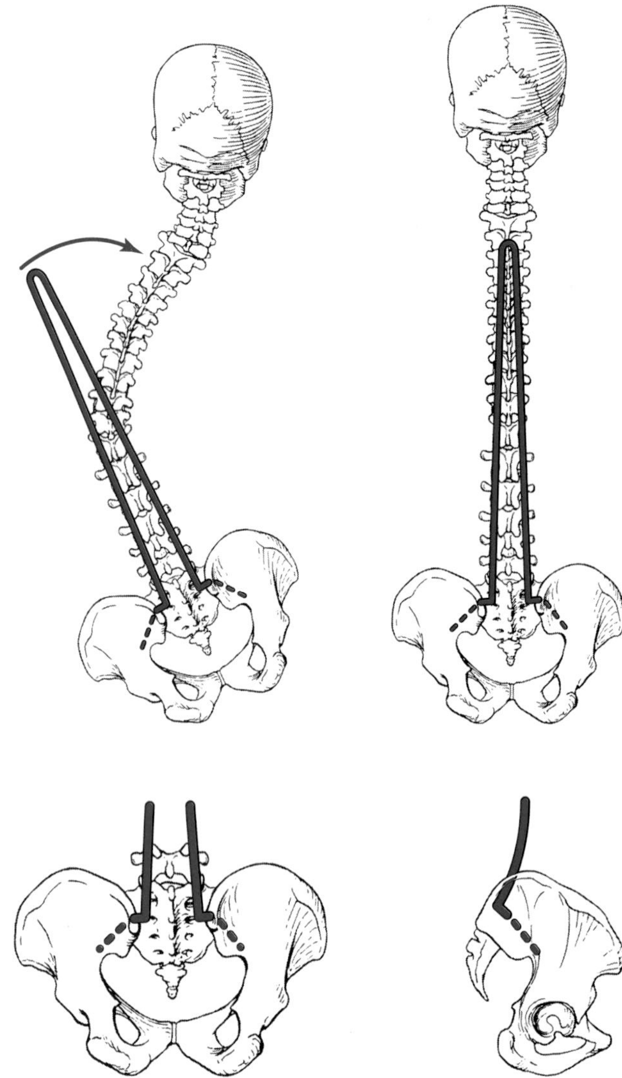

Figure 17–29: The unit rod. The unit rod is a prefabricated spinal rod that incorporates the distal rod bend required for fixation within the inner table of the ilium. The corrective maneuver involves cantilever bending (sublaminar wires are sequentially tightened) once the distal ends of the rod have been secured within the ilium. From Bulman W, Dormans JP, Ecker M, Drummond DS (1996) Posterior spinal fusion for scoliosis in patients with cerebral palsy: A comparison of Luque rod and unit rod instrumentation. J Pediatr Orthop 16: 314-323.

films help to determine which patients may benefit from anterior surgery. Patients with a level pelvis and balanced torso on a traction film can usually be treated with a posterior fusion alone. Supplemental anterior release and fusion are indicated when the curve magnitude is greater than 50 degrees on bending films or with significant trunk imbalance or pelvic obliquity. The higher risk of complications for a combined anterior and posterior spinal fusion must be weighed against the anticipated rewards, and these procedures may be performed on the same day or staged.

Upper Extremity[26]

- Upper extremity problems amenable to surgical intervention are seen most frequently in hemiplegics. Common deformities include internal rotation of the humerus, flexion of the elbow, pronation of the forearm, flexion–ulnar deviation at the wrist or fingers, and adduction of the thumb. All patients have some degree of sensory impairment. Only a limited number of patients with cerebral palsy will benefit from upper extremity surgery, and patient selection is critical to achieving satisfactory results. The goals of surgery are to improve motor function (grasp, release, and pinch), positioning, hygiene, and ease of care. Surgery (muscle lengthening or transfer and joint arthrodesis) helps to correct fixed deformity, to improve joint motion or position, and to treat muscle imbalance. In general, tendon transfers are indicated in patients with higher levels of function, and releases and arthrodesis are more commonly employed in patients with a lower functional level. The ideal candidate for reconstructive surgery has adequate sensory function (stereognosis, proprioception, and light touch), pure spasticity (surgery cannot improve athetosis or dystonia), and the absence of neglect. Volitional use of the extremity is desirable. Selective injections with botox may help in preoperative planning. Realistic goals are essential, and all necessary procedures for reconstructing the extremity should be performed under the same anesthetic if possible.

- An *adduction or internal rotation deformity* of the humerus may respond to soft tissue release.
- *Flexion deformity* is commonly seen at the elbow, and a subset of patients will benefit from lengthening of the biceps (Z-lengthening with release of the lacertus fibrosus) and the brachialis (Chevron fascial release). Occasionally, a release of the origin of the brachioradialis may be required. The extremity is immobilized in extension for several weeks, and splinting is usually recommended to prevent recurrence or gain additional extension.
- *Forearm pronation* deformity can dislocate the radial head. Flexible deformities with a full passive range of motion may respond to release of the pronator teres, and transfer of the pronator teres (to extensor carpi radialis or extensor digitorum communis) can be considered if the muscle is not continuously spastic. If the deformity is severe or rigid, an osteotomy of the radius and a release of the pronator quadratus may be required.
- *Flexion or ulnar deviation at the wrist* may be treated by lengthening the flexor carpi radialis (Z-lengthening), lengthening the flexor carpi ulnaris (intramuscular), and releasing the palmaris longus. The flexor origin may also be released at the medial epicondyle. Options for tendon transfer include the flexor carpi ulnaris to the extensor carpi radialis brevis (Green transfer) or the extensor carpi ulnaris to the extensor carpi radialis brevis. Rigid or severe deformities may be best treated by proximal row carpectomy, arthrodesis, or both. Flexion deformity of the fingers (extrinsic) may be treated by lengthening these muscles by Z-lengthening the tendons, receding the musculotendinous junction, or releasing from their origin proximally.
- *Flexion and adduction of the thumb* (the thumb-in-palm deformity) may be treated by release of the thenar muscle origin with or without releasing the first dorsal interosseous fascia and the first web space. Transfer of the extensor pollicis longus to augment abduction may also be performed. Instability at the first metacarpophalangeal joint may be addressed by capsulodesis, arthrodesis of the sesamoid to the metacarpal head, tenodesis of the extensor pollicis longus to the metacarpophalangeal joint, or arthrodesis of the first metacarpophalangeal joint.
- *Swan neck deformity* of the fingers is treated by soft tissue release and muscle rebalancing.

References

1. Dormans JP, Pellegrino L (1998) Caring for Children with Cerebral Palsy: A Teambased Approach. Baltimore: Brookes Publishing.
   An excellent overview of the all aspects of caring for children with cerebral palsy.

2. Herring JA, ed (2001) Disorders of the brain. In: Tachdjian's Pediatric Orthopaedics, 3rd edition, volume 2. Philadelphia: WB Saunders, pp 1121-1248.
   This outstanding and exhaustive resource describes all aspects of the evaluation and treatment of children with cerebral palsy. The literature review is extensive, and the surgical techniques are well illustrated.

3. Bleck EE (1987) Orthopaedic management in cerebral palsy. Clin Dev Med 99: 100.
   This classic monograph presents a comprehensive overview of orthopaedic problems in cerebral palsy, including causes, orthopaedic and neurological assessment, common problems, and treatment approaches.

4. Staheli LT (1998) Lower limb/torsion. In: Fundamentals of Pediatric Orthopaedics. Philadelphia: Lippincott-Raven Publishers, p 32.

5. Graham K, Aoki K, Autti-Ramo I, Boyd RN, Delgado MR, Gaebler-Spira DJ, Gormley ME, Guyer BM, Heinen F, Holton AF, Matthews D, Molenaers G, Motta F, Garcia Ruiz PJ, Wissel J (2000) Recommendations for the use of botulinum toxin A in the management of cerebral palsy. Gait Posture 11: 67-79.
   This review article (consensus from 15 experts) presents recommendations about the use of intramuscular botulinum toxin A, including patient selection, dosage, administration, and outcome measurement.

6. Steinbok P (2001) Outcomes after selective dorsal rhizotomy for spastic cerebral palsy. Child's Nerv Sys 17: 1-18.
   This is a review of published outcomes based upon categories by the National Center for Medical Rehabilitation Research, including pathophysiology, impairment, functional limitations, disability, and societal limitations. Outcomes were also reviewed in terms of the effect of rhizotomy on orthopaedic surgical procedures and hip subluxation. Sackett's criteria are used to weigh the quality of evidence presented in each article. Rhizotomy decreases spasticity and increases range of motion of the lower limbs. The procedure probably does not influence the need for orthopaedic surgery, and any relationship with progressive hip subluxation remains unclear.

7. Albright AL (1996) Intrathecal baclofen in cerebral palsy movement disorders. J Child Neurol 11 (Suppl 1): S29-S35.

This review article describes the pharmacotherapy, indications or patient selection, technique, results, and side effects or complications of intrathecal baclofen therapy.

8. Winters TF, Gage JR, Hicks R (1987) Gait patterns in spastic hemiplegia in children and young adults. J Bone Joint Surg 69A: 437-441.
   The authors studied 46 patients with spastic hemiplegia by instrumented motion analysis (kinematic sagittal plane data and EMG), and four patterns of gait were identified. The spectrum of deficits ranges from an isolated drop foot (type I) to multilevel soft tissue contractures with or without rotational deformities (type IV).

9. Cooperman DR, Bartucci E, Dietrick E, Millar EA (1987) Hip dislocation in spastic cerebral palsy: Long-term consequences. J Pediatr Orthop 7: 268-276.
   The authors reviewed 38 patients with spastic quadriplegia and hip dislocation (51 hips) at an 18-year follow-up. Of those with unilateral dislocations, 50% developed pain, leading the authors to recommend surgical relocation in this population. Bilateral dislocations were less likely to be painful, and relocation was recommended unless deformity of the femoral head has developed.

10. Bagg MR, Farber J, Miller F (1993) Long-term follow-up of hip subluxation in cerebral palsy patients. J Pediatr Orthop 13: 32-36.
    The authors reviewed 64 subluxated hips at a 19-year follow-up. Risk factors for progression to dislocation include an early age at onset, an increased severity of involvement (cerebral palsy), and a migration greater than 50%. Pain was observed in 8 of 9 dislocated hips (mild to severe), 11 of 24 subluxated hips, and 10 of 31 reduced hips. The severity was greatest in the dislocated hips, and subluxated hips were slightly more painful than reduced hips. Varus derotational osteotomy was effective in preventing dislocation.

11. Lonstein JE, Akbarnia B (1983) Operative treatment of spinal deformities in patients with cerebral palsy or mental retardation: An analysis of one hundred and seven cases. J Bone Joint Surg 65A: 43-55.
    The authors reviewed 109 patients with scoliosis associated with cerebral palsy with or without mental retardation. The authors present a classification method and describe treatment in this difficult patient population.

12. Gage JR, Deluca PA, Renshaw TS (1995) Gait analysis: Principle and applications—Emphasis on its use in cerebral palsy. J Bone Joint Surg 77A: 1607-1623.
    The authors present an analysis of both normal gait and cerebral palsy gait based upon instrumented motion analysis.

13. Davids JR (1997) Normal gait and assessment of gait disorders. In: Lovell & Winters Pediatric Orthopaedics, 4th edition (Morrissey RT, Weinstein SL, eds). Philadelphia: Lippincott-Raven Press, pp 131-156.
    An excellent overview of the gait cycle and common gait deviations.

14. Sutherland DH, Davids JR (1993) Common gait abnormalities of the knee in cerebral palsy. Clin Orthop Rel Res 288: 139-147.
    The authors describe four primary sagittal plane knee abnormalities in ambulatory children with cerebral palsy (crouch, jump, stiff knee, and recurvatum). Common findings on physical examination are described in addition to the causes and the effects on gait.

15. Sutherland DH, Zilberfarb JL, Kaufman KR, Wyatt MP, Chambers HG (1997) Psoas release at the pelvic brim in ambulatory patients with cerebral palsy: Operative technique and functional outcome. J Pediatr Orthop 17: 563-570.
    In this study, 17 patients (29 hips) with flexion deformity at the hip were treated by an intramuscular recession of the psoas tendon at the level of the pelvic brim. The technique is described in detail, and the results of preoperative and postoperative gait analysis are reviewed. Passive hip extension improved 12 degrees, and all patients retained hip flexion strength against some resistance. Both stance phase hip flexion and anterior pelvic tilt improved, and the best results were seen in younger patients.

16. McNerney NP, Mubarak SJ, Wenger DR (2000) One-stage correction of the dysplastic hip in cerebral palsy with the San Diego acetabuloplasty: Results and complications in 104 hips. J Pediatr Orthop 20: 93-103.
    Here, 104 hips underwent a combined procedure including soft tissue release, varus derotational osteotomy, acetabuloplasty (all but 4 hips), and an open reduction (migration > 70%). At a nearly 7-year follow-up, 95% of hips remained located. Of the hips, 5% resubluxated, 8% developed avascular necrosis, and 31% required additional surgical procedures (mostly soft tissue releases) to maintain alignment.

17. Mubarak SJ, Valencia FG, Wenger DR (1992) One-stage correction of the spastic dislocated hip: Use of pericapsular acetabuloplasty to improve coverage. J Bone Joint Surg 74A: 1349-1352.

18. Gage JR, Perry J, Hicks RR, Koop S, Werntz JR (1987) Rectus femoris transfer to improve knee function of children with cerebral palsy. Dev Med Child Neurol 29: 159-165.
    The results of lower extremity soft tissue surgery in patients with spastic diplegia and a stiff knee gait are reviewed both with (37 knees) and without (24 knees) a rectus femoris transfer. Swing phase knee flexion was improved an average of 6.5 degrees more than in the control group, and the arc of knee motion increased 9.5 degrees. Stance phase knee flexion was 8.9 degrees (versus 15 degrees in the control group). The suggested indications for this procedure include continuous activity of the rectus femoris during swing phase and a reduction of greater than 20% in sagittal knee motion.

19. Green NE, Griffin PP, Shiavi R (1983) Split posterior tibial–tendon transfer in spastic cerebral palsy. J Bone Joint Surg 65A: 748-754.
    In this study, 16 equinovarus deformities were treated by split transfer of the tibialis posterior tendon to the peroneus brevis. All but 1 also required lengthening of the tendo Achillis. Patients had inappropriate activity of the tibialis posterior during the swing phase on dynamic EMG. Twelve feet were plantigrade, had no deformity, and did not require

bracing. Fixed hindfoot varus requires a calcaneal osteotomy. Overcorrection was not observed, and there were no cases of postoperative calcaneus deformity.

20. Dutkowski JP (1998) Cerebral palsy. In: Campbell's Operative Orthopaedics, 9th edition (Canale ST, ed), volume 4. St. Louis: Mosby-Year Book, p 3919.

21. Mosca VS (1995) Calcaneal lengthening for valgus deformity of the hindfoot. J Bone Joint Surg 77A: 500-512.
Here, 31 feet with symptomatic hindfoot valgus (8 with cerebral palsy) underwent lateral column lengthening and were followed up at 2.8 years. The osteotomy of the calcaneus extends between the anterior and middle facets, and a trapezoidal bone graft is inserted to both lengthen and adduct the calcaneus. The procedure reliably corrects joint malalignment while preserving motion, thereby avoiding the problems associated with hindfoot arthrodesis. A satisfactory outcome was achieved in all but 2 feet. Most patients will require concomitant tendo Achillis lengthening, and some required additional procedures including medial talonavicular reefing, osteotomy of the middle cuneiform, and lengthening of the peroneus brevis.

22. Grice DS (1952) An extra-articular arthrodesis of the subastragalar joint for correction of paralytic flat feet in children. J Bone Joint Surg 34A: 927-940.

23. Allen BL, Ferguson RL (1982) The Galveston technique for L rod instrumentation of the scoliotic spine. Spine 7: 276-284.
A detailed description of the Galveston technique is presented.

24. Bulman W, Dormans JP, Ecker M, Drummond DS (1996) Posterior spinal fusion for scoliosis in patients with cerebral palsy: A comparison of Luque rod and unit rod instrumentation. J Pediatr Orthop 16: 314-323.
The Luque-Galveston technique (15 patients) was compared with the unit rod technique (15 patients). Instrumentation using the unit rod resulted in a greater average correction of both the coronal curvature (62% versus 49%) and pelvic obliquity (80% versus 50%). Caregiver satisfaction was high in both groups because an improvement in ease of care was seen in 65% (no change in 23%). The complication rate was lower than in earlier studies concerning instrumentation and fusion in this population.

25. Spiegel DA (2004) Cerebral palsy. In: Pediatric Orthopaedics and Sports Medicine (Dormans JP, ed). Philadelphia: Mosby.

26. Waters PM, Van Heest A (1998) Spastic hemiplegia of the upper extremity in children. Hand Clin 14: 119-134.
This review article describes the evaluation and treatment (physical therapy, injections, and surgery) of upper extremity problems in hemiplegia. Surgical procedures for all of the common deformities are presented in detail.

CHAPTER 18

Neuromuscular Disorders of Infancy and Childhood and Arthrogryposis

Harish S. Hosalkar,* Leslie A. Moroz,† Denis S. Drummond,‡ and Richard S. Finkel§

*MD, Resident, Orthopaedic Surgery, University of Pennsylvania, Philadelphia, PA
†BA, Clinical Research Coordinator, Division of Orthopaedic Surgery, The Children's Hospital of Philadelphia, Philadelphia, PA
‡MD, Professor Emeritus, University of Pennsylvania School of Medicine, Philadelphia, PA; Chief Emeritus, Orthopaedic Surgery, The Children's Hospital of Philadelphia, Philadelphia, PA
§MD, Pediatric Neurologist, Director, Neuromuscular Program, Division of Neurology and Neurology Research, The Children's Hospital of Philadelphia, Philadelphia, PA

Pediatric Neuromuscular Disorders

- Infants and children with neuromuscular disorders typically have weakness and hypotonia and less commonly have joint contractures.
- Evaluation of the patient with these issues includes considering disorders of the following:
  - Muscle—Myopathies and dystrophies
  - Neuromuscular junction
  - Peripheral nerve
  - Anterior horn cell
  - Brain and spinal cord
- The most common clinical concerns are delay in motor development, loss of motor skills, poor feeding, insufficient breathing, and musculoskeletal complications.
- Orthopaedic management is an integral component to the care of these patients. Understanding the natural history of each disorder aids the physician in deciding the appropriate type and timing of an intervention.
- Establishing a genetic versus an acquired cause is important for correct prognosis, treatment, and genetic counseling.
- It is helpful to have a timeline for managing pediatric disorders (Table 18–1).

Muscular Dystrophies

Definition

- Muscular dystrophy is a group of primary myopathies genetically determined and characterized by a progressive degeneration of muscle, occasionally present at birth but usually evolving after a latent period of apparently normal development and function. A list of selected inherited diseases of muscle is given in Table 18–2.
- These dystrophic myopathies are conditions with diverse clinical presentations and various degrees of muscle wasting and weakness. They often have characteristic laboratory findings such as elevated serum–muscle enzyme levels, a myopathic pattern on electromyogram (EMG), and characteristic histopathological findings on muscle biopsy.

Table 18–1

Topic and *Intervention* — Time Frame in Years

Birth — 2 — 4 — 6 — 8 — 10 — 12 — 16-20 — 20-30

1. Overview [pre-clinical] [diagnosis][progression of disease..[death..]
Genetic counseling: after the diagnosis has been established and when the parents are emotionally capable of addressing this topic.

2. Gross Motor Skills:
Normal ....
Slowly gaining ....
Plateau phase .... (may be very brief)
Regression in gait ....
Loss of ambulation ....
Regression in upper limb function ....
Maintain mobility:
Bracing ....
Power chair ....
Adaptive equipment:
Hydraulic lift for transfers, toileting ....
Laptop computer ....
School adaptation:
School bus lift and classroom aide ....

3. Musculoskeletal:
Scoliosis ....
Joint Contractures
heel cords ....
tensor fascia lata ....
hamstrings ....
Physiotherapy: ....
Bracing and/or tendon releases (variable) ....
Spinal fusion (variable) ....

4. Pulmonary:
Restrictive lung disease ....
Obstructive sleep apnea ....
Pulmonary function tests (and sleep study?) ....
Annual influenza vaccination ....
Pneumococcal immunization: at time of diagnosis
Non-invasive ventilatory support (variable) ....

5. Cardiomyopathy: ....
Annual ECG ....

6. Obesity: (variable) ....
Nutritional consultation ....

7. Learning Disability: (variable) ....
Psychoeducational evaluation, Individualized Educational Plan (IEP)

8. Depression: (variable) ....
Individualized and family counseling ....
Anti-depressant medication (SSRI) ....

9. Medication:
prednisone, deflazacort (???)...?????.....

Table 18–2: Selected Inherited Diseases of Muscle*

NAME	MODE OF INHERITANCE §	AGE AT PRESENTATION (YEARS)	LONGEVITY (YEARS)
Muscular Dystrophies	**Degenerative Process with Progressive Weakness**		
Duchenne	XR	4	20 on average
Becker	XR	4 to 60	20 to normal
Facioscapulohumeral	AD	3 to 44	Near normal
Limb girdle category	AR>AD	2 to 30	Variable
Emery-Dreifuss	XR>AD	3 to adult	Variable
Congenital	AR	Birth to 2	0 to adult
Congenital Myopathies	**Structurally Abnormal Muscle with Early Onset Weakness and Static or Slowly Improving Strength**		
Myotubular	XR	Birth	Weeks (years)
Centronuclear	AR/AD	Birth to infancy	Normal
Central core	AD	Birth to infancy	Normal
Nemaline	AD/AR	Birth to adult	Variable
Bethlem	AD	Infancy	Normal
Myotonic Disorders	**Mild Weakness, Stiffness, and Difficulty with Muscle Relaxation**		
Myotonic dystrophy	AD	Teens onward	Risk of cardiac arrhythmia in adulthood
Congenital myotonic dystrophy	AD	Birth	25% early mortality
Myotonia congenita	AR>AD	(Childhood) teens onward	Normal

* Adapted from Finkel RS (2001) Muscular dystrophy and myopathy. In: Current Management in Child Neurology (Maria BL, ed). Hamilton, Ontario: BC Decker.
§ Mode of inheritance: *AD*, autosomal dominant; *AR*, autosomal recessive; *XR*, X-linked recessive.
Average at time of diagnosis in years.

- Muscular dystrophies are therefore a heterogeneous group of diseases that present symptoms of muscle weakness and wasting with similar laboratory findings but that differ in the pattern of inheritance, age of onset, distribution of muscle groups involved, and severity and rate of progression.

Historical Aspects

The study of progressive muscle dystrophies began in the midnineteenth century.

Although Meryon was probably the first to make a true observation of muscular dystrophy in 1852, Duchenne published his definitive treatise on "pseudohypertrophic or myelosclerotic muscular paralysis" in 1868. Thomsen described in 1876 a congenital condition associated with delay in relaxation of all skeletal muscles, now known as myotonia congenita or Thomsen's disease. In 1879, Gowers wrote an excellent treatise on pseudohypertrophy in young boys and described his now-famous sign of "climbing up the legs," where the child, to get upright from supine, works his arms up his own legs and body because of severe proximal muscle weakness (Figure 18–1).

The classic description of facioscapulohumeral dystrophy was published by Landouzy and Dejerine in 1884. The categorization of limb girdle muscular dystrophies (LGMD) was introduced by Walton and Nattrass in 1954 but was not characterized effectively until the advent of molecular genetics in the last decade.

Etiology

- Research over the past 20 years has identified the genetic basis of more than 80 neuromuscular disorders.
- Pathophysiology—The identification of the gene or genes responsible for a particular neuromuscular disorder has prompted much investigation into the function and significance of the gene product in the normal muscle cell and into how its absence or alteration leads to cellular dysfunction. Many muscular dystrophies are caused by the absence or reduction of a specific cytoskeletal protein. These proteins are important in the generation of contractile strength or in the preservation of cell integrity with repeated contraction–relaxation. Altered cellular signaling and ion channel dysfunction in the muscle cell membrane are pathophysiological mechanisms in other muscular dystrophies.
- The cause of muscle deterioration in muscular dystrophy is still unknown. It is probably a multifactorial process with a cascade of secondary events that evolve because of a fundamental primary defect in the muscle cell.

Muscle Pathology in the Muscular Dystrophies and Congenital Myopathies

- It is important to note that the routine histopathological examination of muscle does not reliably distinguish

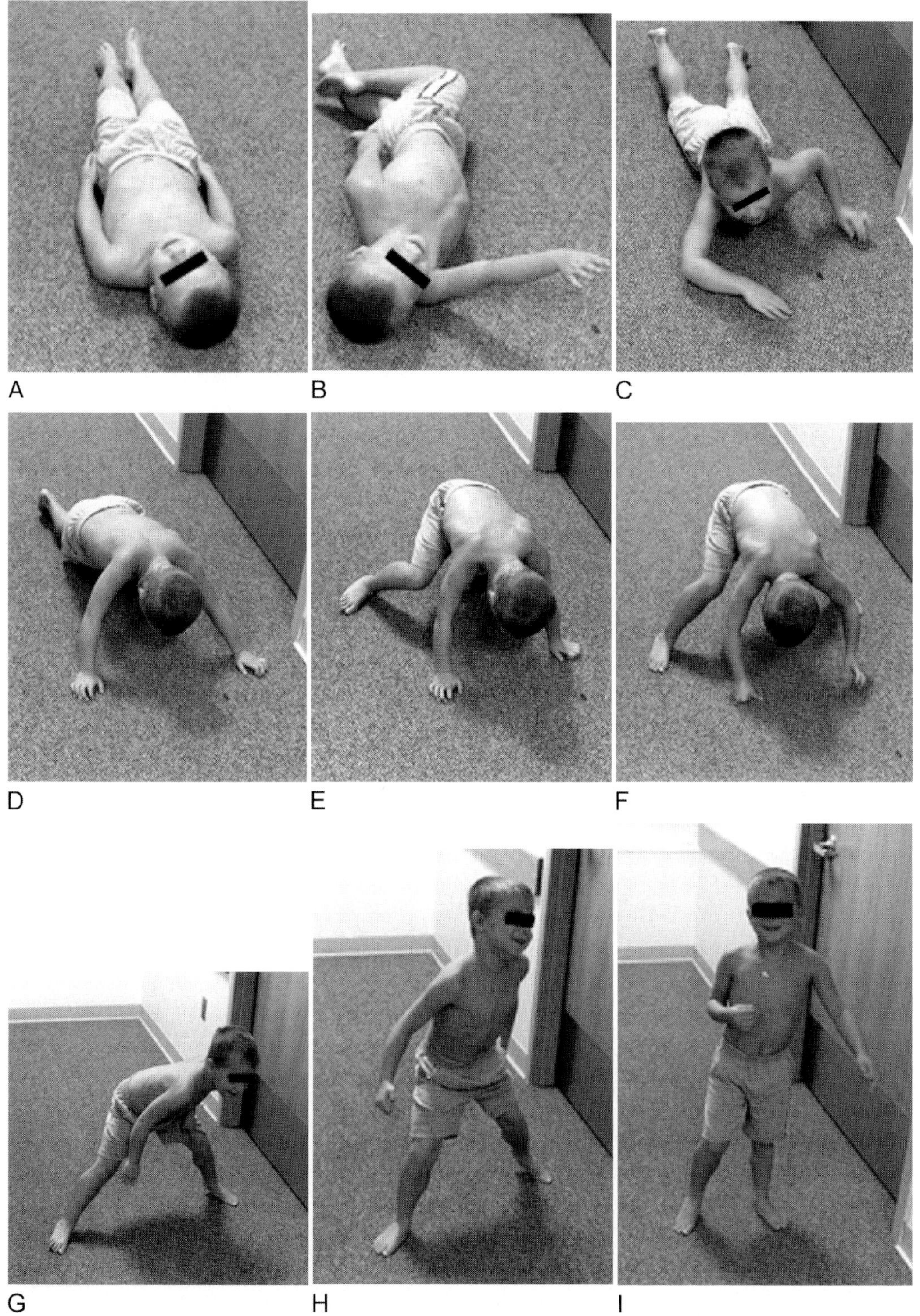

Figure 18–1: The Gowers' maneuver. This demonstrates weakness of the pelvic–femoral musculature. The child lies supine and is asked to stand up without assistance. In the fully positive response, the patient first rolls to the side (A–B) then prone (C) and elevates the trunk (D) and buttocks (E) by pushing up on the outstretched arms (F). The hands then clasp the shins of the extended and widely spaced legs (G), and the trunk is straightened into a vertical stance by walking up the legs with alternative hands (H–I) and thrusting the upper torso and head backward. From Finkel RS, Drummond D (2004) Muscular dystrophy and arthrogryposis. In: Pediatric Orthopaedics and Sports Medicine: The Requisites in Pediatrics (Dormans JP, ed). Philadelphia: Mosby.

among types of muscular dystrophy. The fundamental histopathological changes in the muscles can appear similar in several muscular dystrophies (e.g., Duchenne and limb girdle) or can have minimal structural abnormality (e.g., facioscapulohumeral). The categorization of dystrophies is based on the type of inheritance, pattern of muscle involvement, age of onset, pace of the natural course of the disease, muscle histopathology, and supportive laboratory data.
- The most important pathological features are marked variation in muscle fiber size, increased central nuclei, degenerating and regenerating fibers, and increased endomysial connective tissue, occasionally with adipose and inflammatory foci (Figure 18–2).

Genetics and Molecular Biology

- Genetic research in molecular biology has tremendously enhanced the understanding of the genetic aspects of many of these disorders, and the effect has been revolutionary.
- Since the cloning of the dystrophin gene for Duchenne muscular dystrophy (DMD) and Becker muscular dystrophy in 1985, more than 80 genes for specific muscular dystrophies, myopathies, and ion channel disorders have been identified.
- This has radically changed the clinical approach to evaluating a patient with a suspected muscle disorder because specific molecular genetic testing can in many cases establish a diagnosis without the traditional workup of extensive laboratories, EMG, and muscle biopsy. Specific immunostains that detect a single muscle protein through a fluorescent-tagged monoclonal antibody can provide more specific information about the deficiency of a gene product (e.g., dystrophin absence in DMD). Western blot analysis can further indicate whether the protein in question is absent, reduced in amount, reduced in molecular weight, or reduced in both. Also, the prospect of gene therapy to correct the genetic defect and restore function is on the horizon with the first pilot study in LGMD initiated in 1999. Based on the genetic information, the patient and family can be counseled regarding prognosis, genetic implications, and appropriate treatment options.

Dystrophin

- The dystrophin gene is located in the Xp21 region and spans 2.4 million base pairs. It includes 79 exons (coding regions) that encompass only about 2% of the gene and encode the 427-kDa protein dystrophin. Dystrophin is an intracellular component of the muscle cytoskeleton, linking actin to a complex network of other sarcolemmal proteins that span the muscle cell plasma membrane. It represents 0.01% of skeletal muscle protein.
- The large size of the gene correlates with the high rate of spontaneous mutation (approximately one third of cases). The distribution of dystrophin within skeletal, smooth, and cardiac muscle and within the brain correlates well with the clinical features in DMD and Becker muscular dystrophy.

When to Suspect a Muscle Disease

Hypotonia and Weakness

- At birth—Decreased fetal activity, sluggish newborn reflexes (e.g. Moro reflex), poor head control on traction response (i.e., Moro reflex), slip-through at the shoulder girdle, poor ability to bear weight, sluggish feeding, and increased respiratory effort.
- In infancy or childhood—Occurs especially when progressive. The timing of onset of symptoms and the rate of progression are key factors pointing toward a particular neuromuscular disorder.

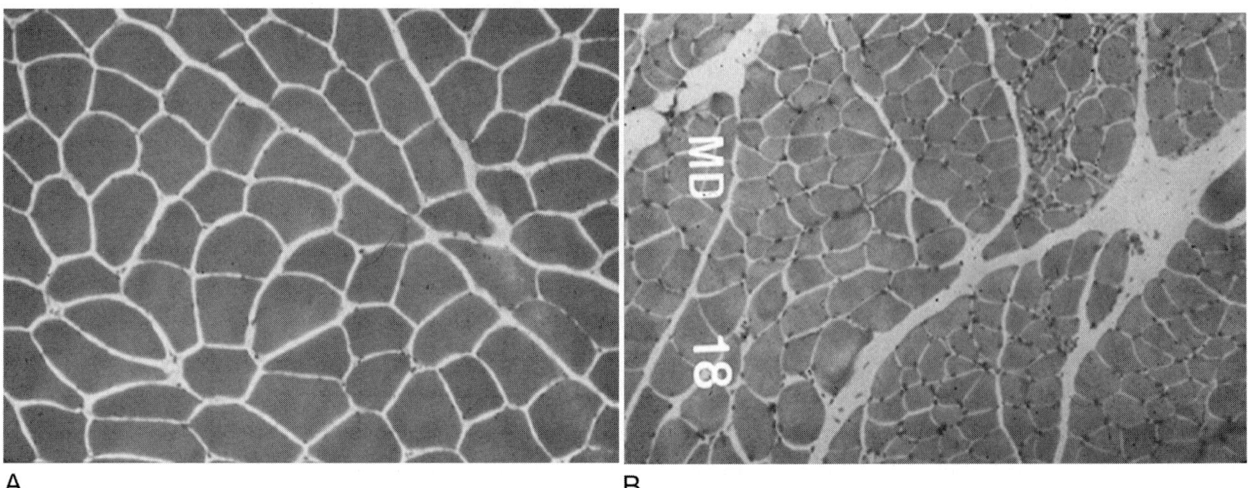

Figure 18–2: When compared with normal muscle (A), histology shows an enlarged central nuclei and variation in the fiber size of dystrophic muscle (B).

- On similar grounds, congenital contractures (e.g., arthrogryposis multiplex congenita) may warrant a neuromuscular evaluation.

Unexplained cardiomyopathy should always prompt a search for an underlying muscular dystrophy or myopathy.

- Family history of a neuromuscular disorder may suggest the need for evaluation of a presymptomatic individual.
- Elevation of serum creatine kinase may be found incidentally and suggests an underlying muscle disease, though modest elevations can also be seen in some neuropathic conditions and in otherwise healthy teenage males.
- The most common symptoms that cause parents to seek consultation are listed in Table 18–3.

Evaluation of a Child with a Suspected Neuromuscular Disorder

- The patient history and clinical examination should be thorough and must include a complete neurological evaluation to enable a differential diagnosis to be made.
- The *history* should focus on important issues such as developmental milestones, age of onset, and details of decline in motor ability (Box 18–1). The biological parents and siblings should also be assessed to diagnose a genetically based disorder.
- The *physical examination* should focus upon the extent and distribution of hypotonia and weakness in the trunk, limb, face, eye, bulbar, and respiratory muscles.
- It is useful to consider neuromuscular disorders in two categories: genetically based and acquired.
  1. *Genetically based* neuromuscular disorders usually present insidiously with fixed weakness and delayed acquisition of motor skills. Table 18–2 summarizes the genetic basis of common conditions. Figure 18–3 illustrates the distribution of weakness in six common muscular dystrophies.
  2. *Acquired* neuromuscular disorders usually have symptoms of rapid or subacute progression of weakness and loss of motor function. Significant muscle pain suggests myositis.
- It is important to search for related diaphragm and chest-wall weakness and cardiomyopathy with pulmonary function testing, chest x-ray film, and EKg or echocardiogram when there is clinical concern or a natural history of risk in these areas.
- The examination of the young infant focuses on functional indicators of weakness such as the extent of head lag on traction from supine to sitting (Figure 18–4), slip-through at the shoulder girdle when held vertically under the arms (Figure 18–5), and capacity to actively bear weight on extended legs. The *scarf sign* also demonstrates shoulder girdle weakness (Figure 18–6).
- For the older infant and young child, the examination considers sitting posture, ability to roll over and sit or pull to a standing position, gait, how the child rises from the supine to a standing position (Gowers' maneuver) or from a chair to a standing position, and ability to climb stairs (Figure 18–7).
- Standard manual muscle testing on the 0 to 5 Medical Research Council scale (Box 18–2) and quantifiable measures of strength using a handheld myometer can be used reliably in a school-aged child of normal intelligence. When used serially, quantified functional measures of endurance (e.g., time to walk or run 30 feet, time to climb four stairs, and Gowers' maneuver) can assess progression of disease and response to treatment.
- The physician should perform the physical examination, noting that some diseases (e.g., DMD and congenital

Table 18–3: Common Presenting Symptoms and Signs of Pediatric Neuromuscular Disorders

GROWTH PHASE	SYMPTOMS AND SIGNS
Infancy	Floppy baby Congenital contractures Poor feeding or failure to thrive Aspiration pneumonia or respiratory insufficiency Slow or delayed development (e.g., not sitting unaided at 9 months or walking independently at 18 months) Poor muscle consistency and tone
Childhood	Tiptoes Has clumsy motor skills Cannot keep up with other children Runs strangely with a waddling gait; falls readily Seems weak when rising from the floor or climbing stairs Fatigues easily Has poor posture—stands with a sway back and pot belly

Box 18–1 Historical Points to Address in Patients with a Suspected Neuromuscular Disorder

- Decreased fetal activity and risk factors of pregnancy or parturition (oligohydramnios, multiple fetus, and breech)
- Age at onset of symptoms or when parents first had concerns
- Distribution of weakness
- Rate of progression versus static process or slow improvement
- Presence of multiple joint contractures
- Early motor milestones
- Loss of skills
- Decline in endurance
- Muscle pain with simple ambulation or with extended exercise
- Related musculoskeletal issues: scoliosis and contractures
- Dysphagia or aspiration and failure to thrive
- Potential cardiac involvement
- Possible ventilatory insufficiency and sleep apnea

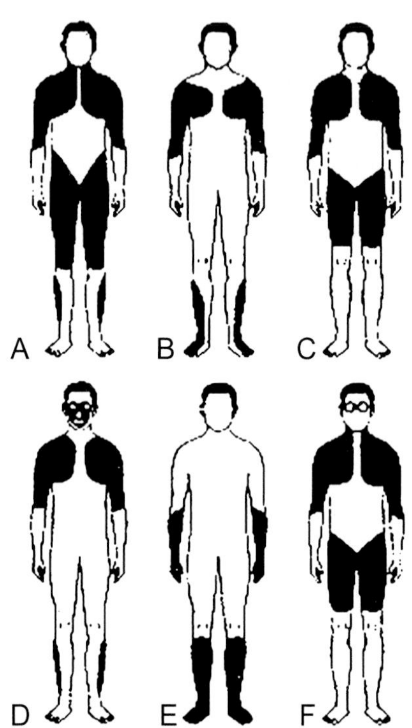

Figure 18–3: Distribution of prominent muscle weakness in different types of dystrophy: Duchenne and Becker (A), Emery-Dreifuss (B), limb girdle (C), facioscapulohumeral (D), distal (E), and oculopharyngeal (F). **Shaded = affected areas. From Emery AE (2002) The muscular dystrophies. Lancet 0359(9307): 687-695.**

myotonic dystrophy) may be accompanied by cognitive delay or mental retardation.

- Muscle tenderness to palpation is a sign of acute inflammation (idiopathic or infectious myositis). In most pediatric neuromuscular disorders, deep tendon reflexes may be normal, reduced, or absent at presentation and usually diminish as the disease progresses.
- The sensory examination will be normal in a myopathy, dystrophy, pure motor neuropathy (spinal muscular atrophy), and neuromuscular junction disorder (myasthenia gravis).[1,2] However, it will be abnormal in hereditary and acquired sensorimotor neuropathies.
- The patient should be evaluated for mental status, seizures, and other central nervous system (CNS) concerns.
- *Contractures* may be evident at birth or may develop in the course of a neuromuscular disorder. Joint contractures are usually caused by weakness, an asymmetry of the muscle power at the joint, and could be contributed by gravitational forces. Thus, finding limitation in joint mobility during examination should always raise the suspicion of underlying weakness and imbalanced strength of the muscles at that joint. Occasionally, contractures may result from a cramped environment *in utero* (e.g., a bifid uterus) such as in arthrogryposis or from an abnormality in collagen type VI. Selected myopathies and dystrophies have distinguishing joint contractures relatively early in the course of weakness and can be an important clue in the diagnosis, as in Emery-Dreifuss muscular dystrophy.
- Features of hypotonia and weakness may also reflect disorders in the CNS and genetic syndromes. In particular, newborns and infants with hypotonia should be scrutinized for any related CNS features, dysmorphic features, or other organ system anomalies that would orient the workup toward a "central" etiology, metabolic disorder, or genetic syndrome rather than a "peripheral" neuromuscular one.[3] Prader-Willi syndrome, for example, is a genetic disorder

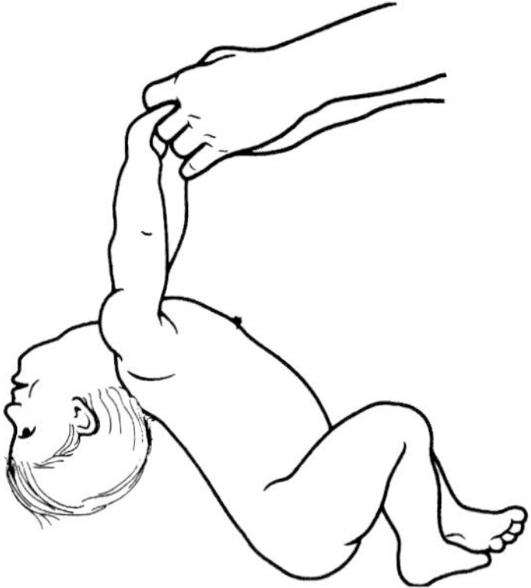

Figure 18–4: Hypotonic posture when held prone. **Reprinted from Bleck EE (2002) Hereditary and developmental neuromuscular disorders. In: Neuromuscular Disorders (Pourmand R, Harati Y, eds). Philadelphia: Lippincott Williams & Wilkins.**

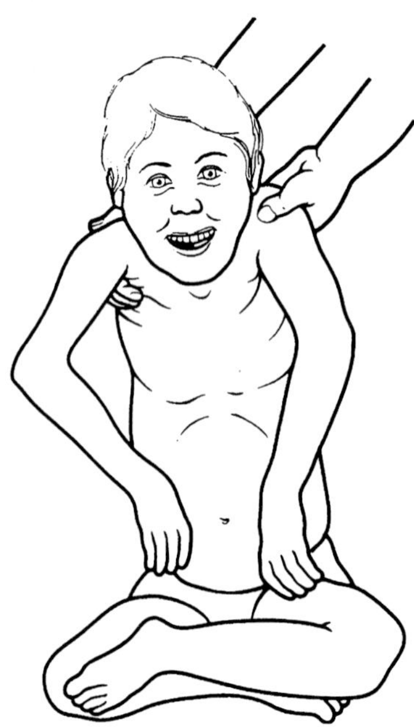

Figure 18–5: Slip-through when held vertically. **Reprinted from Bleck EE (2002) Hereditary and developmental neuromuscular disorders. In: Neuromuscular Disorders (Pourmand R, Harati Y, eds). Philadelphia: Lippincott Williams & Wilkins.**

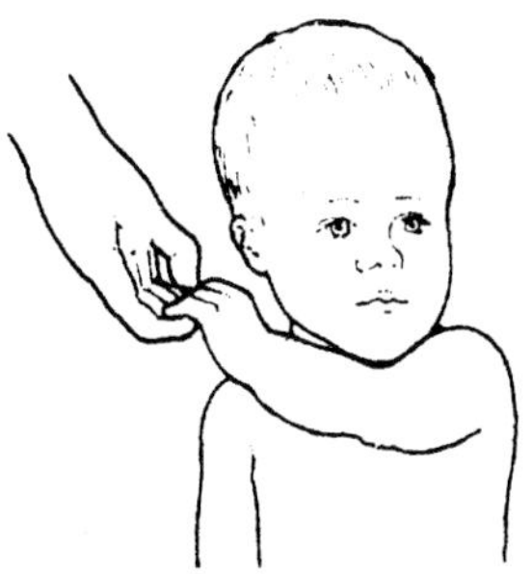
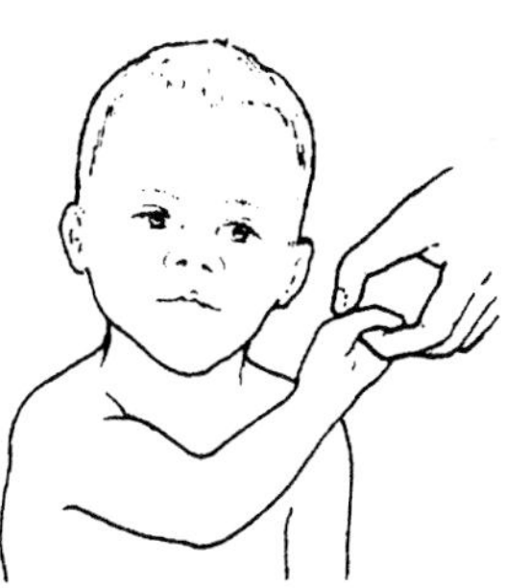

Figure 18–6: Scarf sign. **Reprinted from Bleck EE (2002) Hereditary and developmental neuromuscular disorders. In: Neuromuscular Disorders (Pourmand R, Harati Y, eds). Philadelphia: Lippincott Williams & Wilkins.**

with pronounced hypotonia, weakness, and poor feeding as a neonate that mimics a peripheral neuromuscular disorder. Limb weakness may mimic ataxia, and careful examination is needed to identify this. A focused diagnostic plan can then be pursued that establishes the specific diagnosis in the least invasive, most timely, and most cost-effective manner. The most commonly used diagnostic tests are summarized later in this chapter.

- It is useful to consider neuroanatomical localization, such as anterior horn cell, peripheral nerve, neuromuscular junction, muscle, and connective tissues when constructing a differential diagnosis for a patient with neuromuscular symptoms and signs. Table 18–4 gives examples of diseases for each category.

Laboratory Studies and Diagnostic Testing

- *Serum creatine kinase* is the commonly obtained blood test screening for a disease of muscle and is often elevated 10- to 100-fold in some dystrophies. However, a normal creatine kinase (under about 250 IU) does not exclude a muscle disorder (e.g., some congenital myopathies and facioscapulohumeral dystrophy), nor does it necessarily imply remission of myositis. Recent intramuscular injection, vigorous exercise, or contact sports may cause transiently elevated creatine kinase

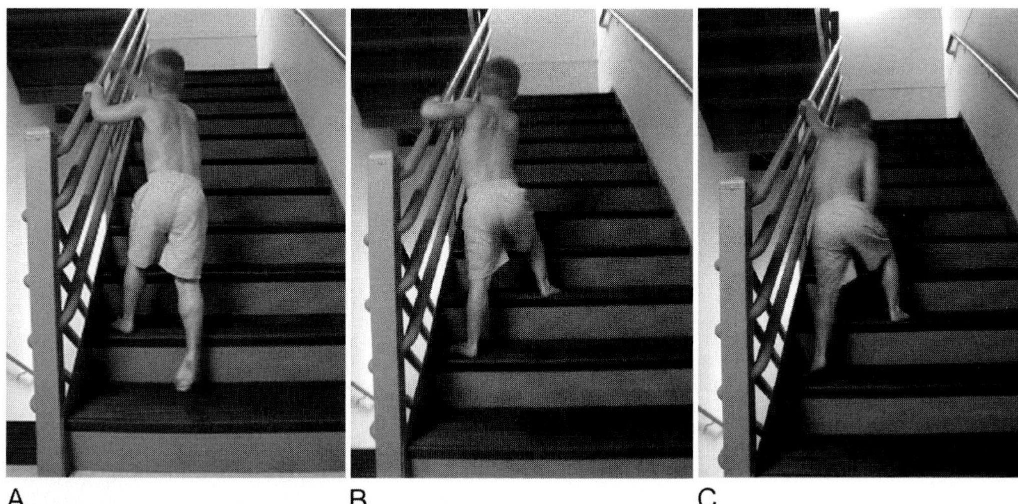

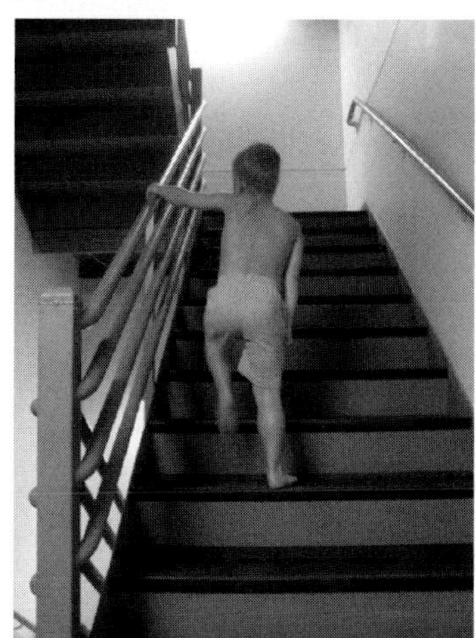

Figure 18–7: A 6-year-old boy with DMD climbing stairs. **Note the need to push off one knee and to pull up using the handrail to ascend one step at a time. From Hosalkar H, Finkel RS, Drummond D (2004) Muscular dystrophy and arthrogryposis. In: Pediatric Orthopaedics and Sports Medicine: The Requisites in Pediatrics (Dormans JP, ed). Philadelphia: Mosby.**

Box 18–2 Medical Research Council Scale of Manual Muscle Testing*

- Grade 0—No evident muscle contraction
- Grade 1—Flicker or trace of muscle contraction
- Grade 2—Active movement with gravity eliminated
- Grade 3—Active movement against gravity
- Grade 4—Active movement against gravity and resistance
  - 4– —Against slight resistance
  - 4—Against moderate resistance
  - 4+ —Against strong resistance
- Grade 5—Normal power

Pending permission from Medical Research Council (UK) (1986) Aids to the Examination of the Peripheral Nervous System, 3rd edition. London: WB Saunders.

levels, which should subside to normal after 2 or 3 days. Persisting elevation of creatine kinase above 1000 IU necessitates further evaluation of an underlying muscular disorder, even in the absence of specific symptoms or signs.

- High levels of serum *aldolase* are often found in muscular dystrophy. The normal serum values are less than about 8. In DMD, values of more than 100 are frequently found. The increase in serum aldolase and creatine kinase is most marked in the early stages of the disease.
- *Blood lactate* and *pyruvate levels* and *carnitine profiles* should be obtained when a mitochondrial disease of the muscle is suspected.
- *Thyroid function studies* are important to consider, but hyperthyroidism is rarely seen in children and congenital hypothyroidism is typically identified in the newborn screen.
- When infectious etiologies are in the differential diagnosis, complete blood count with differential, erythrocyte sedimentation rate, cultures, and in some cases specific antigen studies should be obtained.
- Genetic diagnostic testing for many muscular dystrophies is available from commercial and research laboratories and attempts to identify the specific disease causing a mutation. The National Institutes of Health-sponsored Web site *http://www.geneclinics.org* is an excellent resource for searching for where such testing can be obtained. It also provides current clinical summaries of most genetically based neuromuscular disorders. It is important to work with an expert in neurogenetics to interpret the mutation test results, because benign polymorphisms must be differentiated from disease causing mutations.
- The roles of *EMG and nerve conduction studies* have diminished since the advent of molecular deoxyribonucleic acid (DNA) testing. It remains valuable, however, in differentiating an anterior horn cell, peripheral neuropathy, or neuromuscular junction disorder from a primary disease of muscle and in focusing on a central etiology when both the nerve and muscle parts of the study are normal.
- The role of *muscle biopsy* has also evolved. Evaluation by light microscopy remains important in confirming a suspected dystrophy or myopathy, particularly when clinical features and EMG findings are equivocal. Although specific diagnosis of many dystrophies and myopathies can be established solely by molecular genetic testing, muscle biopsy remains important for evaluating many metabolic disorders and should be performed at a center capable of obtaining and processing the specimen correctly to ensure satisfactory results. In addition, electron microscopy is occasionally useful in defining subcellular aspects of muscle disorders.

Table 18–4: Congenital Anomalies to Search for in Newborns with Arthrogryposis

REGION	ANOMALIES
Head and neck	Craniosynostosis Anomalies of brain cortex Mandibulofacial dysostosis Hypoplasia of the mandible (Pierre Robin sequence) Congenital facial diplegia (Mobius syndrome) Klippel-Feil syndrome
Shoulder girdle	Sprengel's deformity
Spine	Kyphoscoliosis Segmentation disorders Spina bifida Agenesis of sacrum
Cardiovascular system	Congenital heart disease
Genitourinary system	Renal anomalies Ureteral anomalies Cryptorchidism Scrotal defects
Respiratory system	Pneumonia Tracheoesophageal fistula
Abdomen	Inguinal hernia
Extremities	Absence of patellae Syndactylism Constriction bands Synostosis

Technique of Muscle Biopsy

- The ideal muscle for diagnostic biopsy is one clinically affected but not end-stage and has known normative standards. Thus, the vastus lateralis of the quadriceps is often chosen because it is a proximal muscle often affected early in myopathies and dystrophies, easily obtained by open incisional or core needle biopsy, and with well-established age-related standards of normal. The deltoid is the most commonly biopsied muscle of the upper limb. Muscle ultrasound and magnetic resonance imaging (MRI) of the lower limbs are sometimes useful in identifying the optimal muscle to biopsy. Biopsy from the paraspinals during scoliosis repair, the iliopsoas during hip surgery, or the rectus abdominus during gastrostomy tube placement is often unsatisfactory. If an EMG has been performed, the surgeon should select the other side for biopsy to avoid needle artifact.

- The biopsy specimen should be oriented on a tongue blade, placed on damp (not wet) saline-soaked gauze, and transported promptly to the pathology laboratory for processing. A specimen of 400 mg (approximately 0.5 cm^3) is the minimum for a routine biopsy. When metabolic studies are needed, a larger biopsy of 1 g is preferred, and when electron microscopy is requested, a small separate portion of the biopsy should be placed directly into glutaraldehyde (not onto saline-soaked gauze first).
- When general inhalation anesthesia is used for the biopsy procedure, special precautions must be maintained and the anesthesiologist must be alerted to the risk of malignant hyperthermia. Local or spinal anesthesia avoids this potential complication but makes the procedure more challenging for the surgeon because the muscle is not as relaxed and obtaining hemostasis is sometimes less easily secured without the electrocautery. Nonetheless, satisfactory needle core biopsies are often obtained, even in infants, by an experienced surgeon.
- After adequate anesthesia and skin incision, the subcutaneous tissues and fascia are carefully split to expose the muscles. Using double clamps or nonabsorbable sutures approximately 2 cm apart, the muscle is grasped and the sections are made on the outside of the clamps or the sutures. Intramuscular hemorrhage should be carefully prevented. More than one specimen should be usually taken, and it is a good policy to preoperatively discuss the case with the pathologist to review the preservative techniques and the number of specimens, particularly when a metabolic disorder is suspected.

Treatment

- Treatment of the child with a muscular dystrophy is often best coordinated through a neuromuscular clinic with the help of the orthopaedist, neurologist, rehabilitation specialist, cardiologist, pulmonologist, and physical, occupational, and speech therapists. In selected cases a gastroenterologist, nutritionist, geneticist, and social worker are needed as well. The role of the primary care physician is critical in maintaining continuity and in coordinating the evaluation and treatment regimens.
- Once a specific diagnosis has been established, a long-term treatment algorithm can be formulated for that patient based upon the knowledge of the natural history of that condition, noting when particular complications are likely to arise. The treatment goals for patients with a chronic neuromuscular disorder are summarized in Table 18–5.
- Muscular dystrophies have a variety of symptoms that require specific treatments.

Musculoskeletal Treatment

- The treatment of contractures usually begins with passive range of motion stretching or serial casting. Operative procedures may be necessary to obtain optimal alignment and mobility. Proper timing of lower limb tendon releases is critical because selective early surgery may promote and prolong ambulation but surgery late in the ambulatory phase of the disease will often result in good alignment but loss of ambulation.
- Scoliosis is a common manifestation of the muscular dystrophies, particularly DMD and spinal muscular atrophy, and may need stabilization and spinal fusion at the appropriate time during the course of the disease.

Other Systemic Treatment

- Cardiomyopathy and cardiac arrhythmia can occur in several muscle diseases and often warrant screening with an electrocardiogram even for an asymptomatic patient. If abnormal, cardiac consultation should be obtained. Echocardiogram, Holter monitor, and stress testing are done selectively.
- Restrictive lung disease resulting from weakness of the diaphragm and intercostal muscles may be a presenting clinical concern or may arise insidiously in an older child several years after diagnosis. Respiratory complications may arise from a weak cough, preventing effective clearance of secretions and risking aspiration and atelectasis. Older children can be taught "air stacking" breathing techniques that, when used with an abdominal thrust by a caregiver, can significantly increase the cough force. The insufflator–exsufflator provides the child with a weak cough a boost to gain fuller lung expansion during inspiration, a stronger cough, and clearance of secretions.
- Sleep apnea should be addressed in the history. Search for symptoms of noisy breathing or significant pauses in the breathing pattern when asleep, headaches upon awakening, irritability, or excessive daytime somnolence. When present, a sleep study and pulmonary consultation are indicated.
- Noninvasive assisted ventilation (bilevel positive airway pressure) is often used when significant hypoventilation is present. The decision for tracheotomy and full mechanical ventilation requires a detailed long-range review of both the medical and the ethical dimensions of the patient's situation.
- An annual influenza vaccination and the pneumococcal vaccination are recommended for all patients with a chronic neuromuscular disorder and significant respiratory compromise. For infants, respiratory syncytial virus prophylaxis in the winter months is often pursued.
- Adequate nutrition is essential to avoid muscle catabolism during illness and to promote optimal growth. Failure to thrive is a frequent concern in infants with dysphagia.

Table 18–5: Anatomical Approach to the Differential Diagnosis of Genetically Based and Acquired Disorders in Childhood*

ANATOMIC LOCALIZATION	HEREDITARY EXAMPLES		ACQUIRED EXAMPLES
	Hallmark Features	**Typical Presentation**	
Anterior horn cell	*Spinal muscular atrophy* Autosomal recessive Hypotonia and proximal weakness in infants, limb girdle weakness in teens Tongue fasciculations Areflexia Normal intellect and sensation Neurogenic EMG Creatine kinase normal to slightly increased Deletion in survival of motor neurons gene detected in about 98% patients Supportive treatment Genetic counseling	*Type 1*—Werdnig-Hoffmann Disease Diagnosis by 6 months Never achieves sitting unsupported Death usually by 2 years from respiratory insufficiency *Type 2*—Intermediate form Diagnosis 6 months to 2 years Sits but never stands unsupported Variable course, often with long plateau phase Scoliosis *Type 3*—Kugelberg-Welander Disease Diagnosis 2 years to young adult Walks but with proximal weakness Static to slowly progressive course May have long-term survival	*Polio* Disease caused by native virus is rare in immunized populations Rare cases are caused by virulence from revertant mutation of attenuated, oral, live immunization virus Can be caused by other neurotropic viruses (enterovirus or West Nile) Has gastrointestinal symptoms followed by back pain and limb, respiratory, or bulbar weakness Recovery is variable Decline in function (postpolio syndrome) may occur decades later
Peripheral nerve	*Hereditary motor and sensory neuropathy* (e.g., Charcot-Marie-Tooth disease) Usually autosomal dominant; sometimes recessive and X-linked Demyelinating and axonal forms and characteristic nerve conduction findings DNA testing available to confirm the diagnosis in the more common types	Slowly progressive Distal weakness and sensory loss Highly arched feet and hammer toes Foot orthotics and occasional surgery Intrinsic hand wasting and contractures—occupational therapy, adaptive equipment, and occasional tendon transfer surgery	*Acute inflammatory demyelinating polyradiculoneuropathy* (Guillain-Barré Syndrome) Acute weakness, often ascending, may include respiratory failure, facial or bulbar weakness, and ataxia Usually monophasic with good outcome *Chronic inflammatory demyelinating polyneuropathy* More indolent course, often relapsing Treated with immunosuppression
Neuromuscular junction	*Myasthenia Gravis* Usually autoimmune mediated (antiacetylcholine receptor antibodies) means an acquired disorder Congenital syndrome is rare Autosomal more recessive than dominant *Fluctuating weakness and muscle fatigue* First sign may be a medical emergency in respiratory failure	Pure ocular, bulbar, and limb forms versus generalized weakness Characteristic repetitive nerve stimulation decremental response Tensilon (edrophonium) test Immunosuppression therapy Thymectomy for generalized form	*Botulism* Neurotoxin from *Clostridium botulinum* Infantile form is a medical emergency with dysphagia, hypoventilation, generalized hypotonia, and weakness Adult form is from wound infection and may be less severe Characteristic incremental response to repetitive stimulation testing
Muscle *Refer to Table 18–2* A) *Congenital myopathies*	Structural abnormality within the muscle fibers	May be weak at birth or a "floppy baby" Usually static or slow improvement Many genes have been identified that encode for specific muscle cytoskeletal proteins	*Refer to Table 18–3* Infectious, toxic, and idiopathic inflammatory myositis Endocrine-related myopathy
B) *Muscular dystrophies*	Degenerative process of muscle	Occurs from birth to adult years, often with musculoskeletal complications May have significant cardiac and pulmonary compromise Detailed DNA and cellular protein analysis available for most types	

Table 18–5: Anatomical Approach to the Differential Diagnosis of Genetically Based and Acquired Disorders in Childhood*—cont'd

ANATOMIC LOCALIZATION	HEREDITARY EXAMPLES		ACQUIRED EXAMPLES
	Hallmark Features	**Typical Presentation**	
C) Myotonias	Muscle stiffness or slow release of contracted muscle after sustained activity	Usually no or little weakness Congenital form of myotonic dystrophy is more severe	
D) *Mitochondrial and some metabolic muscle diseases*		Mitochondrial cytopathies may have diverse associated features, such as stroke (MELAS), myoclonic epilepsy (MERRF), ophthalmoparesis with retinitis pigmentosa (Kearns-Sayre syndrome), infantile hypotonia, and encephalopathy (Leigh syndrome) Lactic academia is common	
E) *Disorders*	Disorders of glycogen or lipid use	Variable presentation: Hypotonia, weakness, cardiomyopathy, and early demise (Pompe disease, early infantile form, and acid maltase deficiency) Hypotonia and hypoglycemia (glycogenosis, type 3) Muscle cramping, weakness, and myoglobinuria after exercise (McArdle disease, muscle phosphorylase deficiency, carnitine palmityl transferase deficiency type 2, and mitochondrial transport deficiency)	
Collagen and connective tissue	Ligamentous laxity without weakness—benign hyperlaxity, Ehlers-Danlos, and Marfan syndromes Ligamentous laxity with a related myopathy (Ullrich and Bethlem)		
Central nervous system	Congenital brain malformations Destructive processes—postinfectious, hypoxic–ischemic injury, and posthemorrhagic Systemic metabolic disorders		
Genetic syndromes with prominent hypotonia[6]	Trisomy-21 Prader-Willi Smith-Lemli-Opitz		

DNA, deoxyribonucleic acid; *EMG,* electromyogram; *MELAS,* mitochondrial myopathy, encephalopathy, lactic acidosis, and strokelike episodes; *MERRF,* myoclonic epilepsy with ragged red fiber myopathy.

* Examples are presented for conditions of hypotonia with or without weakness.

Short-term supplemental feedings by an indwelling nasogastric tube can be important in an infant with inadequate intake. Gastrostomy tube placement and Nissen type fundoplication is often considered when there is both inadequate intake with dysphagia and gastroesophageal reflux with the risk of aspiration. Such surgery should be contemplated early after such issues arise, because the operative risk once the disease has advanced further may be too high to safely perform the procedure.

Medications

- Corticosteroids have been demonstrated to slow the progression of weakness in DMD and will transiently improve strength in some cases. The optimal dosage of prednisone is 0.75 mg/kg/day, although other regimens have been proposed. There are variable opinions for the optimal time to initiate such treatment and whether to continue once the patient is nonambulant. Annual screening for cataracts and bone density measurements

should be obtained, and the patient should be monitored closely for excessive weight gain, growth retardation, hypertension, glucose intolerance, gastrointestinal bleeding, insomnia, and behavioral changes. The benefit of these drugs for patients with severe Becker muscular dystrophy is probably similar, but in patients with the milder form of Becker muscular dystrophy, the chronic side effects generally outweigh the benefits. The use of corticosteroids in other dystrophies is more empiric and occasionally beneficial.
- Albuterol has demonstrated limited benefit in facioscapulohumeral muscular dystrophy[4] and is being studied in other neuromuscular disorders.
- Creatine increases muscle bulk and strength in exercising athletes but has not been shown to significantly benefit weak neuromuscular patients. Glutamate, selenium, penicillamine with vitamin E, and allopurinol have been used in variably controlled studies of DMD without convincing benefit. The use of such supplements in other muscular dystrophies is empiric.

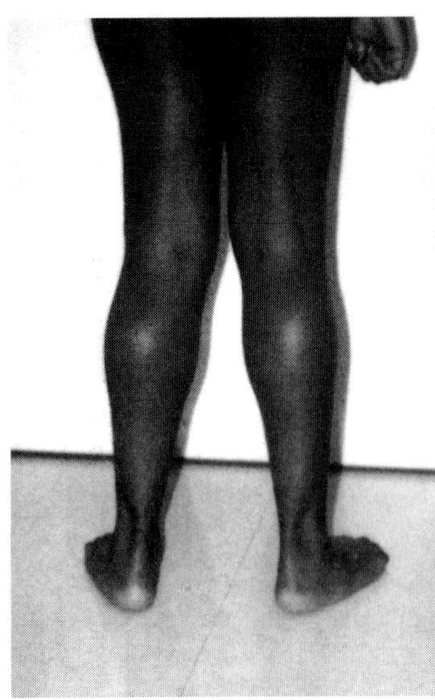

Figure 18–8: Boy with DMD. **Note the marked calf hypertrophy and standing on toes because of Achilles tendon contractures.**

Duchenne Muscular Dystrophy

- DMD is the most common form of muscular dystrophy. It is an X-linked recessive myopathy generally affecting only males. Its incidence ranges from 13 to 33 per 100,000 males, of which one third arise from new mutations.
- The dystrophic process of skeletal muscle associated with DMD is relentlessly progressive, leading to a breakdown of the muscle fibers and replacement of the muscle sarcoplasm with fibrofatty infiltrate. This process causes progressive weakness despite an incongruous increase in the bulk of the muscle mass called *pseudohypertrophy* (Figure 18–8), which is a hallmark for this disease.
- Typically, proximal muscles such as those around the shoulder and hip girdles are involved initially followed by more distally placed muscles. The result is weakness and an inability to resist gravity, leading to frequent falls with difficulty in rising. Again, this is a great hindrance in the use of walking aids.
- *Contractures*—In DMD (and many other neuromuscular disorders) joint contractures typically evolve as weakness progresses beyond grade IV or V of strength (less than active resistance). Contractures are especially common in nonambulatory patients. Typically, patients with DMD develop flexed, abducted, and externally rotated deformities of the hips, which eventually become fixed in position. These patients develop flexion contractures of the knees approaching 90 degrees and stiff equinovarus contractures of both ankles. Often, one type of contracture may influence body positioning and result in the development of other contractures. For example, a patient with flexion deformity of both the hips and the knees, when lying supine in bed, develops tightness in the iliotibial band. The hip abductors shorten, and the patient's hips become fixed in flexion and abduction—the so-called frog-leg position. This may make it difficult for the abducted patient to sit comfortably in a wheelchair because the sides of the chair force adduction.
- *Gait and posture*—With progressive weakness around the hip girdle, walking becomes difficult and could result in frequent falls. The muscles responsible for standing upright, particularly the extensors of the hips and knees, become too weak to sustain an upright stance. Initially, most patients manage an upright stance by a *compensatory posture* marked by hyperlordosis of the spine (Figure 18–9). This extreme lordotic posture shifts the patient's weight distribution so that the weight reaction line runs posterior to the center of rotation for the hips and anterior to the center of rotation for the knees. This compensation is tenuous at best because it is disturbed easily, leading to falls and a feeling of instability. Equinus of the ankles is helpful in maintaining the compensatory posture. Unless there is particularly rapid evolution of Achilles tendon contractures, while the patient is still active and not lordotic, it is *not advisable* in the usual case to surgically correct the equinus because this causes the patient to fall forward, leading to flexion of both the hips and the knees, failure of compensation, and falling. At this stage, a hindfoot release only allows the patient to stand with long leg braces. Accordingly, heel cord lengthening or release is usually postponed until a later stage of the disease if at all.
- *Spinal deformity*—Spinal curvature results from progressive weakening of the paraspinal muscles and is a common component of many neuromuscular conditions. Scoliosis in boys with DMD can usually be observed approximately 2 years after the patient depends on a

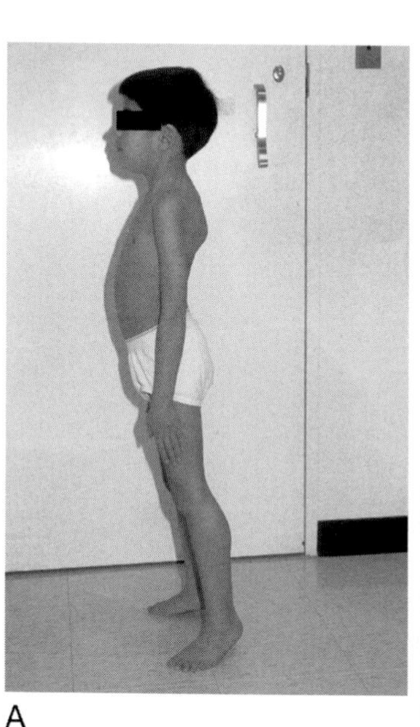

A

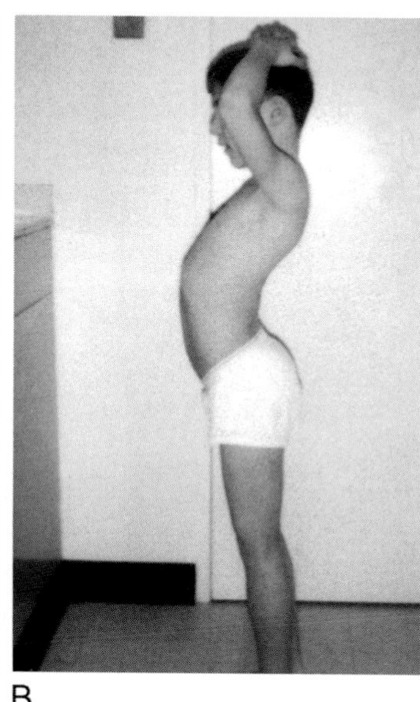

B

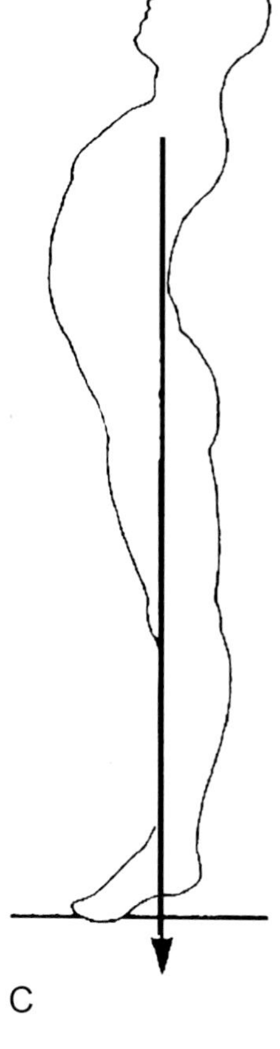

C

Figure 18–9: Compensatory posture in DMD (A and B). Note the relative location of the weight reaction line (C). Reprinted with permission from Siegel IM (1986) Muscle and Its Diseases. Chicago: Year Book Medical.

wheelchair. Initially, the curve is small and may only be appreciated by a radiograph; however, the deformity invariably progresses (Figure 18–10). Because there is some variability in the severity of the disease from patient to patient; and because the severity of the spinal deformity varies with the observed weakness, there is a conflicting prevalence and natural history for scoliosis reported for this population. These differences can be explained by the different follow-up time reported in these studies. However, if observed long enough, virtually all children with DMD will develop a progressive spinal deformity, usually kyphosing scoliosis. The annualized progression averages approximately 10 degrees. Invariably, the rate of progression accelerates with time such that the annualized rate will reach 30 degrees or more. This phenomenon is frequently called *spinal collapse.* Spinal collapse reflects the state of the patient's weakness and the course of the disease. Over time, pulmonary and cardiac status deteriorates and the spinal deformity becomes larger and more rigid (Figure 18–11). Accordingly, surgical correction after the stage of spinal collapse carries a higher risk and greater difficulties than surgery performed before the collapse. In addition, the reported blood loss with surgery after spinal collapse is higher than most other types of neuromuscular scoliosis, although this varies with the stage of the disease at time of surgery.

Management

Limbs

- The main goal of limb surgery is to prolong safe ambulation. The surgeon should try to correct the posture while maintaining all compensatory stabilizing biomechanical factors in individual cases. Maintaining upright weight-bearing status also preserves bone mineralization and allows assistance with transfers even when the patient is nonambulant. However, controversy exists about the value of tendon release and transfer procedures in DMD. This may destroy compensatory posture and adversely effect locomotion after the operation, requiring added bracing and support. Shoulder girdle weakness prohibits the effective use of walking aids, and patients are unable get up from a chair without help. Furthermore, patients are often afraid of falling and may prefer the stability provided by a wheelchair. Weaker patients with a more severe disease course seldom benefit greatly from aggressive surgery.

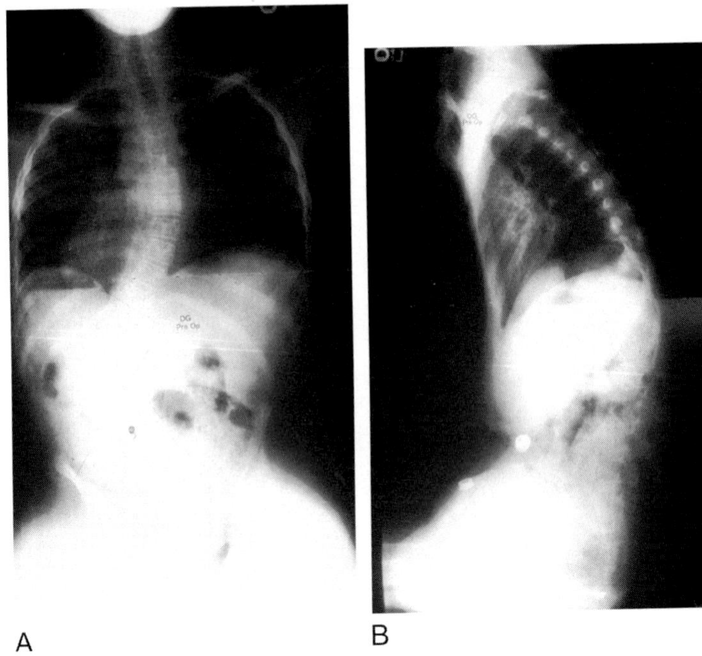

Figure 18–10: Anteroposterior (A) and lateral radiographs (B) demonstrating spinal deformity in DMD.

Hence, limb surgery should be reserved for DMD patients with a less progressive course and for patients with Becker muscular dystrophy who will derive more benefit from surgery.

Foot and Ankle Surgery

- Equinovarus deformity of the foot and ankle could be bothersome in some wheelchair-bound cases: the patients' feet get caught in the wheelchair platforms, they have difficulty with shoe wear, or they find the deformity cosmetically displeasing. Ankle and hindfoot releases can be helpful in these cases.
- Frequently, severe contractures can be partially controlled by the prophylactic nighttime use of modified ankle–foot orthoses. These lightweight plastic braces help the patient to overcome the plantar-directed force of gravity. Although these devises do not eliminate the deformity, they can temporarily limit the progression.
- A simple tenotomy of both Achilles tendons performed early can correct the ankle enough that the foot can be positioned flat or at plantar grade and that shoe wear is facilitated. Later, with disease progression, a more aggressive approach may be needed to correct severe equinovarus contracture with the release of all tight tissues in the posterior and medial aspects of the foot and ankle. In both situations, postoperative bracing is required to prevent recurrent contractures. However, in ambulatory patients with DMD, the equinus position of the ankle is helpful in maintaining balance with compensatory posture. Contracture release in these patients prohibits this compensatory mechanism, and the patients are unable to achieve a balanced stance in the absence of braces that extend from the toes to the upper thighs. This is an important consideration in timing corrective surgery.
- For ambulatory patients, particularly those with Becker muscular dystrophy, the bilateral posteromedial release of the ankles is combined with a transfer of the tibialis posterior tendon from the medial side of the foot and ankle. The tibialis posterior tendon is rerouted through the interosseous membrane that runs between the tibia and the fibula above the ankle and is attached to the midtarsus at the dorsum of the foot. This provides correction, a balanced foot, and some protection against recurrent deformity.

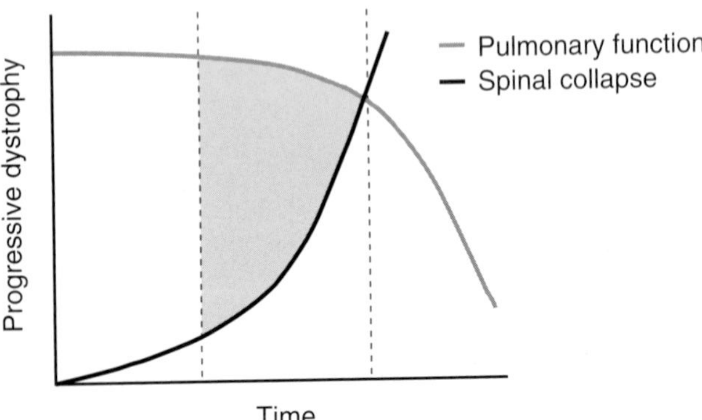

Figure 18–11: Graph of spinal collapse.

Hip and Knee Surgery

- The release of contractures at the hip and knee are less frequently indicated because they occur later in the disease once the goals for the patient have shifted from maintaining upright standing to achieving and maintaining balanced sitting. However, patients who are unable to sit comfortably because of contracted hip abductors may be treated with release of the tensor fascia lata and the anterior fibers of the gluteus medius. Generally, a simple bilateral release may easily address this problem. Percutaneous tendon lengthening procedures are typically well tolerated and effective.

Scoliosis

- The progressive nature of neuromuscular disorders leads to rigid and unbalanced spinal deformities, which eventually interfere with comfortable positioning in a wheelchair, reduce sitting tolerance to a few hours at a time, and cause difficulty in achieving comfortable positioning for sleep. Restrictive lung disease is accentuated on the concave side of the curve because of mechanical restriction in lung expansion. Surgical correction and stabilization with spinal instrumentation and arthrodesis, particularly if done before the curve becomes severe and the disease becomes advanced, is the best way to handle this situation (Figure 18–12).
- The use of a scoliosis brace is never definitive and does not avoid surgery, although it may slow the curve progression and may gain some time to allow somatic growth. Unfortunately, this is not a benefit for conditions such as DMD because the brace only masks the problem while the disease progresses. When bracing is used, the seriousness of the situation becomes apparent later, when the patient has become weaker and the risks involved with surgery are greater. Furthermore, brace wear is often uncomfortable for and poorly tolerated by the child.
- It is essential for the spinal surgery procedure to occur before spinal collapse. Because the natural history for scoliosis with DMD is so predictable, optimal timing for treatment of the deformity can be achieved by obtaining radiographic examinations every 6 months, beginning approximately 2 years after the full-time use of a wheelchair. It is wise to recommend spinal surgery when the curve reaches 30 degrees and certainly before it reaches 50 degrees. Delaying surgery risks spinal collapse, which further complicates DMD with numerous associated health problems.

Preoperative Preparation

The minimum preparation includes the following:

- Cardiac consultation should be used to identify the presence of cardiomyopathy, identify arrhythmia, and assess the risk for cardiac failure. An echocardiogram and an electrocardiogram should be included with this investigation.
- A pulmonary evaluation should determine the pulmonary function, the risk for pulmonary infection, and the potential ventilation needs. This includes a chest radiograph and pulmonary function tests, including lung volumes, maximal inspiratory and expiratory pressures, and blood gases.
- Because of the tendency to bleed more than most other children, testing for an underlying coagulopathy should

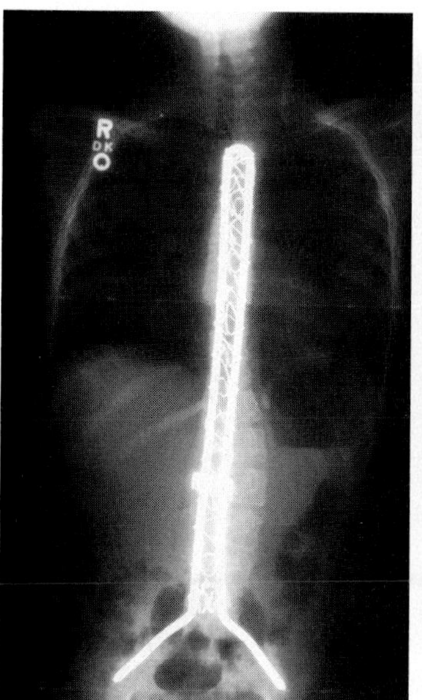

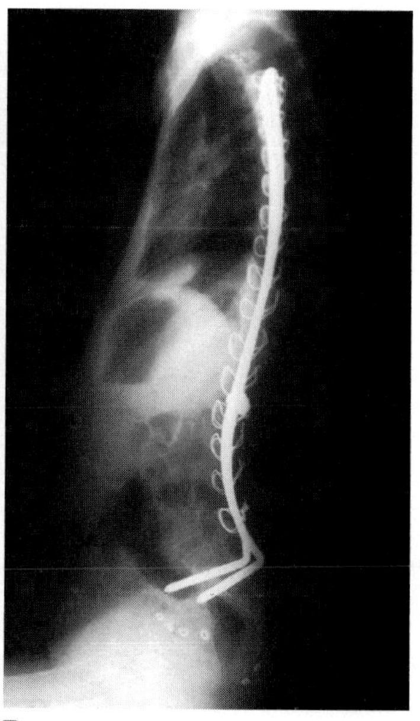

Figure 18–12: Anteroposterior (A) and lateral radiographs (B) showing surgical correction with spinal instrumentation and arthrodesis.

be performed preoperatively and adequate units of blood should be on hand for surgery.

- Experienced anesthesiologists and critical care physicians are required to help manage the patient during and after surgery. These children are at high risk for cardiac and pulmonary complications and should only be managed in tertiary care centers.

Surgical Procedures

- The surgical approach for *spinal correction* is best done through midline posterior exposure. A segmental spinal instrumentation is preferably placed on either side of the midline of the spine. At the same time, a spinal arthrodesis or fusion is done through the facet joints by adding bone graft or a graft substitute. The purchase of the implants through multiple sites of attachment provides load sharing and stability. This should ensure that there will be little loss of correction postoperatively and provides an enhanced chance of obtaining a solid arthrodesis. A brace is not required postoperatively with the biomechanical stability afforded by the segmental spinal instrumentation construct.
- One topic of controversy over this procedure concerns *whether the instrumentation should be extended to the sacrum and pelvis* or stopped at L4. Those that champion stopping short claim similar results in all but a few patients for whom the instrumentation was extended. In addition, shortened instrumentation saves about 1 hour of surgery and therefore decreases associated blood loss. Those who instrument the whole spine claim that it better ensures no further loss of correction of the scoliosis or the pelvic obliquity, thereby reducing the risk of associated unbalanced sitting. These surgeons also note that the patient is generally at their healthiest at the time of the index surgery. Thus, taking the time to instrument the entire spine is necessary to ensure correction that avoids the need for revision surgery—which is not a trivial undertaking. The authors subscribe to the notion that the initial correction should be extended to the sacrum and pelvis (Figures 18–12 and 18–13).
- *Equinus of the ankle* plays an important role in maintaining the compensatory posture, helping to position the weight reaction line anterior to the knees. Disruption of the fragile compensatory posture will cause the patient to fall. Physicians are cautioned to carefully consider all benefits and risks that a given procedure may incorporate. For example, an ill-advised release of the Achilles tendons to correct equinus disturbs this tenuous relationship of position and balance, shifting the weight reaction line posterior to the knees. This causes the knees to flex, and the patient will fall. *The only way that that patient can maintain an upright stance following heel cord release is with a long leg brace, a knee–ankle–foot orthosis.* Thus, if bracing is to be avoided at this time, it is wise to postpone hindfoot release until brace management can be accepted by the patient.

Nonsurgical Management

- *Physical therapy* with passive range of motion is particularly important when there is acute weakness and evolution of contractures. In patients with slowly progressing weakness, the therapist can instruct caregivers in stretching techniques and can guide the family in appropriate activity modification (e.g., swimming, horseback riding, and adapted skiing). Fitting of orthotics or braces and addressing mobility options (e.g., scooter or power chair) are also specialized roles of the physiatrist and physical therapist.

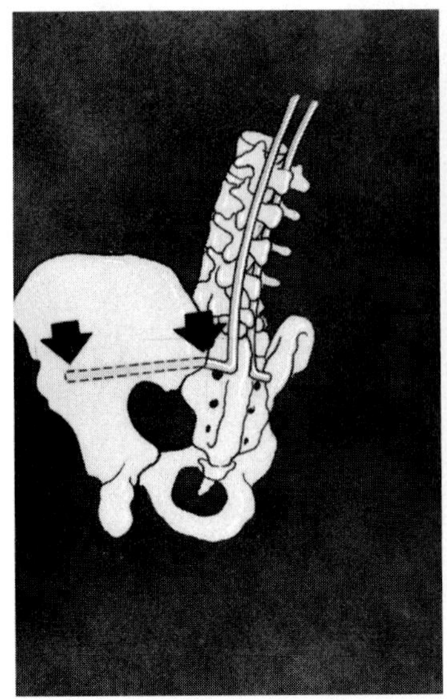

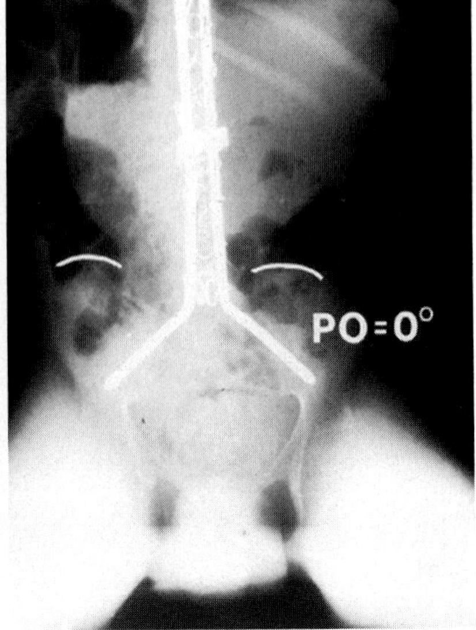

Figure 18–13: Diagrams (A) and radiograph (B) showing the extension of spinal instrumentation to the sacrum and pelvis.

- The *occupational therapist* addresses limitations in fine motor skills and related activities of daily living (dressing, bathing, toileting, food preparation, and eating). Evaluation of home and school settings is often needed to ensure that proper adaptive equipment and safety devices are obtained.
- The *speech therapist* evaluates oral–motor function relating to feeding and speech limitation. In extreme cases, augmentative communications devices can facilitate communication when speech is not possible.
- *Constipation* is a frequent complication when there is abdominal wall weakness and limited fluid intake. This needs to be treated vigorously with adequate fluid intake and the use of fiber added to the diet, fruit juices, senna-based herbal tea or granules, mineral oil preparations, or an occasional suppository.
- The risk of *malignant hyperthermia* in patients with certain muscle diseases undergoing anesthesia needs to be placed prominently in the patient's chart, and the family should be counseled.
- *Psychosocial support* is necessary at home, at school, and in the community. The clinic nurse and social worker are indispensable in inquiring about these issues and in identifying local services. A representative of the Muscular Dystrophy Association (MDA) often attends an MDA-sponsored neuromuscular clinic and offers additional resources, such as regional summer camp programs, funding for diagnostic testing, and some therapeutic support. Several other focused support groups have evolved to provide current information on the diagnosis, treatment options, and research news for their particular topic (e.g., The Parent Project in DMD). A comprehensive listing of these disease-specific support groups can be obtained from the *Exceptional Parent* magazine Web site at *http://www.eparent.com.*
- Box 18–3 illustrates the principal clinical aspects of DMD and related therapeutic interventions for each phase of the disease. This approach can be adapted to other muscular dystrophies and adjusted for the age of onset, rate of progression, and extent of related musculoskeletal, respiratory, and cardiac issues. Characteristic features of other muscular dystrophies including Becker, facioscapulohumeral, LGMD, and congenital muscular dystrophies are listed in Table 18–6.

Future Prospects for Treating Muscular Dystrophies

- New hypotheses about the pathogenesis of a particular disease can be derived from an understanding of the role a particular gene plays in encoding for a specific structural protein or enzyme critical for normal muscle or nerve cell function. Specific adaptive mechanisms within the muscle or nerve cell can then be explored and possibly enhanced with the use of medication. The prospect of gene and stem cell therapies to correct the genetic defect and restore function is on the horizon, with the first pilot human study using a viral vector in LGMD initiated in 1999. Understanding of acquired muscle diseases continues to increase with research. These newer tools allow more accurate diagnosis and assessment of disease activity, thus allowing physicians to counsel the patient and family regarding prognosis, genetic implications, and appropriate treatment options.

Box 18–3 Treatment Goals for Patients with Muscular Dystrophies

- *Maintain strength* through appropriate exercise, weight training, stretching, and possibly the use of medication.
- *Promote safe ambulation* with orthotics, physical therapy, and orthopaedic management of scoliosis and contractures.
- *Maintain mobility* and independence, even when unable to ambulate safely, with the use of a manual or power wheelchair or an electric scooter.
- *Provide adaptive equipment to maintain independence in activities of daily living* at school and at home in recreation and in employment settings.
- *Anticipate and prevent complications* (cardiac, respiratory, nutritional, musculoskeletal, and psychological) with regular physical evaluation, testing, therapy, medication, and surgery.
- *Ensure comfortable and functional sitting.*

Arthrogryposis Multiplex Congenita

Definition

- *Arthrogryposis multiplex congenita* literally means a congenital anomaly in the newborn involving multiple curved joints (Figure 18–14). Although first described by Otto in 1841, Sheldon in 1932 published the first detailed description and called the condition *amyoplasia congenita.*[5]
- It is important to recognize that arthrogryposis is a descriptive term and not an exact diagnosis, because there are at least 150 possible underlying causes.[6]
- Congenital anomalies associated with arthrogryposis are listed in Table 18–7.
- Hall et al. in 1985 considered three main groups:[7]
  1. Classical arthrogryposis multiplex congenita (Figure 18–15) in which the limbs are primarily involved and the muscles are deficient or absent (amyoplasia)
  2. Arthrogryposis with major neurogenic (brain, spinal cord, anterior horn cell, or peripheral nerve) or myopathic (congenital muscular dystrophy, myopathy, or toxic myopathy) dysfunction
  3. Arthrogryposis with other major anomalies and specific syndromes such as diastrophic dysplasia or craniocarpotarsal dystrophy

Table 18–6: Characteristic Features of Other Common Muscular Dystrophies

NAME OF MD	CHARACTERISTIC FEATURES
Becker muscular dystrophy	Sex-linked recessive disease that can pass gene mutation to daughters Later onset and relatively benign course compared with DMD, but wide variation from near-DMD severity to a pure cardiomyopathy or muscle cramping phenotype Muscle biopsy with dystrophin Western blot determination helps to differentiate it from DMD Calf hypertrophy is the most frequent sign Muscle cramps are more common than in other dystrophies Diagnosis rests on clinical presentation, creatine kinase levels, and dystrophin concentration or identifying a dystrophin gene mutation Contractures are rare and do not occur until late Cardiac involvement is variable and can occur in teens even when skeletal muscle strength is relatively strong (does *not* parallel limb weakness) Life expectancy exceeds that of DMD (23-63 years)
Facioscapulohumeral (Landouzy-Dejerine) dystrophy	Mildest form of muscular dystrophies Usually autosomal dominant Onset at any age and expression in either sex Initial involvement of the facial and shoulder girdle muscles (often asymmetric) including the scapular rotators and shoulder abductors Rare occurrence of muscle hypertrophy and joint contractures A normal life span and usually a normal creatine kinase level Identified infantile form is more severe than the adult form and is inherited as an autosomal recessive Earliest presentation is usually facial weakness (difficulty in closing eyelids or pursing the lips), although scapular weakness is the most disabling component of the disorder Scapulothoracic fixation is reasonably effective in stabilizing the winged scapula Scoliosis can occur; when progressive, instrumentation and spinal fusion may be indicated Hyperlordosis may be disabling; if severe and symptomatic, it may necessitate spinal fusion or leave the patient wheelchair bound
Limb girdle dystrophies	15 genetic types identified so far Autosomal recessive more than dominant Males and females equally affected Onset usually in the first decade but occasionally as late as the fourth decade Proximal musculature is more affected than distal, often with a DMD pattern and calf pseudohypertrophy Patients who ambulate until after skeletal maturity may not develop significant scoliosis or contractures Foot drop is rare unlike in the facioscapulohumeral dystrophy Creatine phosphokinase levels are very high Dystrophin deletion testing is negative Muscle biopsy shows dystrophic features Immunostains may show partial secondary reduction in dystrophin Specific testing of other muscle proteins is necessary to establish the diagnosis
Congenital muscular dystrophy	Affects both sexes Creatine phosphokinase is greatly increased No involvement of the dystrophin gene or protein is found Muscle biopsy features a variation of fiber diameter within each fascicle and perimysial and endomysial fibrosis Joint stiffness and contractures may occur Congenital muscular dystrophy can be divided into two types: Type I—Presence or absence of merosin (an extrasarcolemmal protein), with white matter changes on brain MRI scans, where patients show severe weakness and mental retardation Type II—Disorders of glycosylation resulting in severe congenital structural brain malformation (Fukuyama congenital muscular dystrophy, muscle-eye-brain congenital muscular dystrophy, and Walker-Warburg syndrome with lissencephaly) Joint contractures, extensive muscle necrosis, and high creatine phosphokinase levels with retarded motor and intellectual development Usually don't ambulate
Emery-Dreifuss muscular dystrophy	DMD-like presentation in the first decade with early Achilles tendon and elbow flexion contractures as clues Usually X-linked (males) but less commonly autosomal dominant (both sexes) Early cardiac arrhythmia is a major cause of mortality

DMD, Duchenne muscular dystrophy; *MRI,* magnetic resonance imaging.

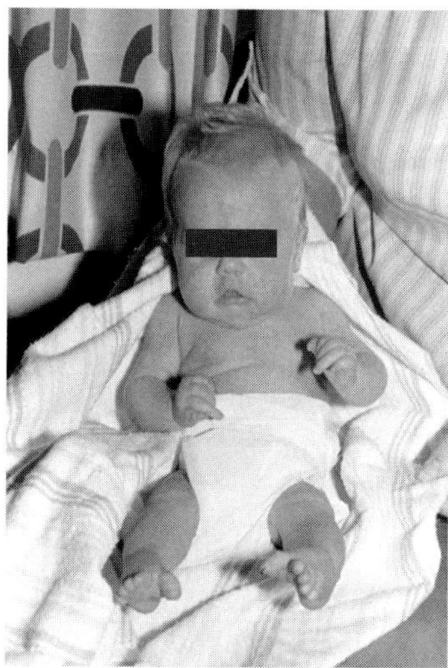

Figure 18–14: Arthrogryposis multiplex congenita. A 32-week premature boy with severe multiple congenital contractures and severe congenital neuropathy. From Finkel RS, Drummond D (2004) Muscular dystrophy and arthrogryposis. In: Pediatric Orthopaedics and Sports Medicine: The Requisites in Pediatrics (Dormans JP, ed). Philadelphia: Mosby.

- Hall noted an incidence of classic arthrogryposis multiplex congenita of 1 in 10,000 live births. In Helsinki, an incidence of 3 in 10,000 live births was reported; there was only 1 case in 56,000 live births in Edinburgh. Based on an apparent increase in the incidence in the 1960s, Wynne-Davies et al. have suggested an infective cause for this rare condition.[8]

Table 18–7: Differential Diagnosis of Congenital Contractures

DISORDERS	DIFFERENTIAL DIAGNOSES
Neurogenic disorders	Spina bifida and spinal disorders Myelodysplasia Sacral and lumbar agenesis Spinal muscular atrophy Fetal neuropathy (toxic and infectious)
Myopathic disorders	(Dystrophia myotonica) Congenital myotonic dystrophy Congenital muscular dystrophy Fetal or congenital myopathy Fetal myasthenia (passive transfer of antibody from mother with myasthenia gravis)
Connective tissue disorders	Marfan syndrome Ehlers-Danlos syndrome
Miscellaneous disorders	Freeman-Sheldon syndrome Turner syndrome Edward syndrome Pterygium syndrome Diastrophic dwarfism

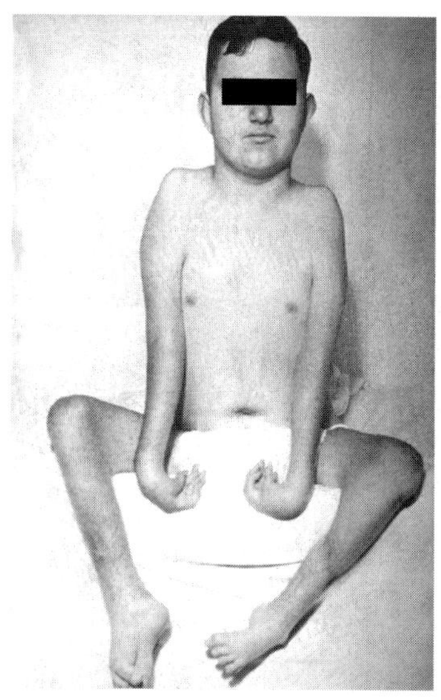

Figure 18–15: Typical contractures in arthrogryposis multiplex congenita.

Clinical Features

- Clinical features include multiple rigid joint deformities with defective muscles but normal sensation. The rigidity of several joints in each case results from both short, tight muscles and capsular contractures. There may be *pterygium* on flexor aspects of contracted joints. There is often absence or fibrosis of muscles or muscle groups.[9,10]
- Normal intellectual development is found in most cases.
- All four limbs are involved in the classical form (amyoplasia congenita), but the condition can also occur only in the upper limbs or only in the lower limbs.[11,12]
- An autosomal dominant variant called *distal arthrogryposis* was described by Hall, in which the hands and feet are severely deformed with only minor contractures proximally and possible development of scoliosis.[6]
- In addition to the multiple joint contractures, the lack of skin creases (cylindrical or tubular limbs) and the deep dimples over the joints are characteristic (Figure 18–16).
- There is dislocation of joints, most commonly the hip (Figure 18–17) but occasionally the knee.
- The trunk is rarely affected.

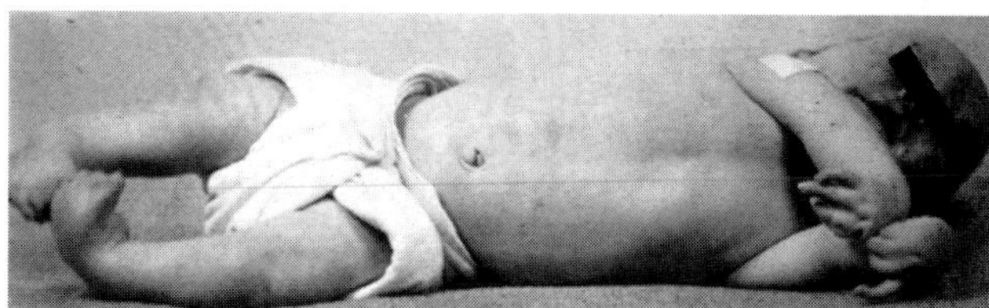

Figure 18–16: Joint contractures, lack of creases in skin, and deep dimples at joints are characteristic of arthrogryposis.

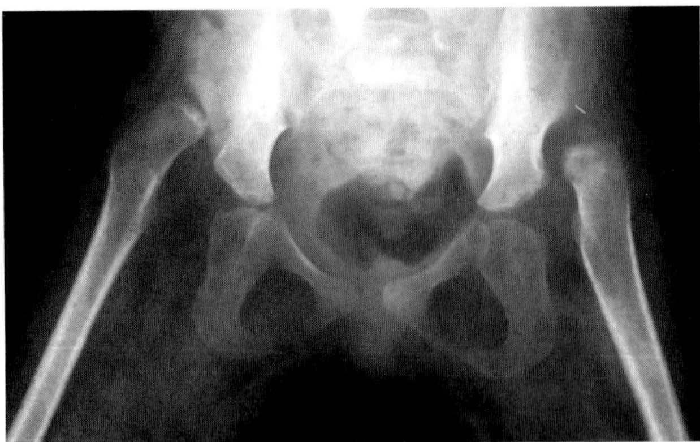

Figure 18–17: Arthrogryposis is often associated with dislocated joints; the hip is most commonly affected.

- Other congenital anomalies such as cryptorchidism, hernias, and gastroschisis may occur.

Etiology

- Arthrogryposis is multifactorial in etiology.[11,13,14]
- Factors liable to produce immobility of the fetus *in utero* may contribute to congenital contractures. Some of these include structural abnormality of the uterus (bifid, large fibroids), oligohydramnios, increased intrauterine pressure, mechanical compression of the fetus, weak fetal movements, breech presentation, and prematurity.
- Inflammatory or infective causes have also been postulated. These include inflammation in joint, muscle, spinal cord, or brain; rubella in early pregnancy; and infection with unknown viruses.
- Whittem proposed on the basis of animal studies that the primary condition is a degeneration of the anterior horn cells occurring in the early months of gestation.
- Wynne-Davies et al. noted an interesting case of a pregnant mother treated with curare for severe tetanus who gave birth to an arthrogrypotic baby. They thus postulated an environmental theory and labeled this *environmental disease of early pregnancy* associated with one or more unfavorable intrauterine factors.[8]

Diagnosis

- Clinical examination remains the best modality for establishing the diagnosis of arthrogryposis. We have found a few factors that are often useful in making a diagnosis. Although not absolute criteria, they are helpful when considered in combination.[13]
- Unlike paralytic disorders, joint deformities of arthrogryposis multiplex congenita are usually stiff or rigid from the beginning with incomplete passive range of motion.
  1. Deformities of arthrogryposis tend to be symmetrical (see Figure 18–15).
  2. The severity of contractures tends to increase toward the periphery of the limb. More proximal joints tend to be less involved, and the trunk is frequently spared. The worse deformities tend to occur in the hands and feet.
- Although arthrogrypotic features are a clinical diagnosis, the clinician must try to establish an etiological diagnosis.
- The orthopaedist, neurologist, geneticist, and pediatrician must participate in diagnosing and managing this condition.
- Radiographs of the extremities with joint involvement are recommended. These may demonstrate congenital bony abnormality and loss of subcutaneous fat and muscle. Radiographs of the whole spine will identify any vertebral anomalies. Computerized tomography or MRI of the brain is useful in establishing or ruling out structural CNS involvement.
- EMG and nerve conduction studies are of limited value and have been used to differentiate the peripheral neuropathic from the myopathic variants.
- A skeletal muscle biopsy is needed when a primary myopathic disorder is suspected unless genetic testing can establish the diagnosis by molecular testing of DNA from peripheral blood.
- Plasma creatine kinase estimation may be done to exclude myopathic disorders. This is best checked on day of life 3 or later once any transient initial increase in creatine kinase from the birth process has subsided.
- If a prenatal ultrasound detects an absence of fetal movement, especially with polyhydramnios, the diagnosis of arthrogryposis can be suspected.
- Histological analysis reveals a small muscle mass with fibrosis and fat between the muscle fibers. Myopathic and neuropathic features may overlap in the same specimen. The periarticular soft tissues are fibrotic.
- Genetic consultation, with chromosome analysis and collagen studies, should be considered when distinct peripheral neuromuscular disorder is not readily apparent.
- The possible differential diagnoses to be considered are listed in Table 18–7.

Prognosis

- The clinician should be able to derive a general prognosis and treatment plan once the diagnosis of arthrogryposis multiplex congenita is established.
- There may be a few functional motor movements near the periphery of the limb. Vigorous occupational therapy and use of hand splints and serial casting can improve the range of motion and functional hand use in many cases of arthrogryposis multiplex congenita when the cause is a non-progressive disorder (e.g., amyoplasia). Surgery, in selected cases, is necessary to obtain more neutral positioning of the wrist and fingers so that the limited degree of strength can be used to optimal biomechanical advantage.
- Recurrence of a corrected deformity is common and is known to occur with growth in a limb in which the periarticular structures are incapable of stretching.

- Arthrogrypotic children have certain positive factors, however, which must be used in their successful management.
  1. Joint instability is not a problem in arthrogryposis unlike is other paralytic conditions.
  2. With a coordinated and team approach to management, there will often be little deterioration from the condition at birth.
  3. There is frequently central sparing and a relatively normal trunk.
  4. A child with normal CNS findings can be expected to have reasonably normal intelligence and, with enough motivation, can contribute to successful management.

Orthopaedic Management of Patients with Arthrogryposis and Multiple Congenital Contractures

It is important to see these patients as early as possible and to start treating the deformities early, because some of them will respond remarkably well to physiotherapy, stretching, and splintage.[9,13,14]

- *Muscle balance* is usually less of a problem than in other paralytic neuromuscular conditions and is easier to achieve. Muscle balance should possibly be established if there are functioning muscles available for transfer.
- *Recurrence of deformity* is the rule because the dense, inelastic soft tissues about the joints do not properly elongate with growth. These structures are considered the key to the successful management of arthrogryposis in a growing child. The surgical implication of this is that the farther the surgery is performed from the joint, the less likely it will have a lasting benefit. In soft tissue release surgeries, therefore, tenotomies are likely to fail if they are not accompanied by capsulotomies. Again, osteotomies to correct deformity or transfer the range of motion to a more useful arc are beneficial but only at or near skeletal maturity; otherwise, the deformity will promptly recur with growth.
- Maximum correction that can safely be achieved is the goal.
- The use of wedging or corrective casts after surgery is of little additional benefit.
- *Range of movement*—Results from passive range of motion stretching varies. Aggressive treatment may appreciably increase the limited range of joint movement or may have little effect. The arc of motion, however, can often be changed into a functionally better position. For example, a fixed flexion deformity of the knee can be changed into an extended position with manipulation even though the range is not increased.
- *Centrifugal involvement*—The severity of the deformity increases toward the periphery of the limb, and the more proximal joints tend to be less involved. Central sparing of the trunk may be noted in most cases. The clinical implication of this is that the useful tendons for transfer are more likely to be found proximally. Also, an uninvolved and flexible trunk may be an asset during training and rehabilitation.
- *Aim of management*—The main aim of management is to achieve maximum functional gain for each patient. Minimum requirements are independent walking, self-care, and ideally the ability to eventually be gainfully employed.[9,13,14]
- *Staging and timing of surgical procedures*—We believe that the maximum benefit from surgical reconstruction of a limb with arthrogryposis is achieved by carefully staging procedures.[9,13,14]
  1. The disabling deformity and contractures should be corrected in the first stage.
  2. The major joints should be then put in a functional arc of motion most adapted to the patient's needs.
  3. In the final stage, tendon transfers are occasionally required to bring motor power to a joint that has been put into its optimum position. The elbow joint is well suited to tendon transfers and has been widely noted to give satisfactory results.

Scoliosis

- In consistency with the principle that the severity of the stiffness and deformity increases toward the periphery of limbs and that the more central or proximal areas are less involved, we believe that central sparing is an important clinical observation.[15]
- A straight, supple, and well-balanced trunk is an important asset in this otherwise crippling disorder, and every effort should be made to maintain this.
- Although relative sparing of the trunk is typical, scoliosis occurs frequently in arthrogryposis because of high incidence of congenital curves. In addition, scoliosis-associated hip contractures and pelvic obliquity occur frequently.
- *Idiopathic scoliosis*—Genetic or idiopathic scoliosis seems to occur as frequently in the arthrogrypotic population as in the general population. The progression and behavior of an idiopathic curve in arthrogryposis is possibly the same as in other children, although it may be more crippling because of the coexisting peripheral deformities.
- *Paralytic scoliosis*—Long paralytic scoliotic curves are sometimes seen in children with the typical neuropathic type of arthrogryposis. Some forms of congenital muscular dystrophy include a "rigid spine" component. The curve is typically seen before the second year and progresses to become long, severe, and eventually rigid. Well-controlled bracing is the treatment of choice in younger children, although surgical management may be necessary in progressive cases.
- *Congenital scoliosis*—These curves are common in arthrogryposis. This is probably consistent with the

other congenital anomalies common in arthrogryposis. Failure of vertebral formation and failure of segmentation have been noted. Klippel-Feil deformity is also found in these patients. These curves must be observed closely, and aggressive treatment such as early surgical fusion may be indicated in the presence of asymmetrical progressive curves.

- *Scoliosis associated with pelvic obliquity*—This is frequently associated with neglected hip deformities that lead to femoropelvic obliquity and is potentially avoidable. Unilateral hip deformity should be particularly watched for and corrected. The trunk can then be kept supple and straight.

Lower Limbs

Foot Involvement

- The most severe deformities in arthrogryposis are known to occur in the foot.
- The rigid foot deformity is usually the clubfoot or equinovarus deformity and, less frequently, a congenital vertical talus deformity.
- The goal of treatment is conversion of the rigid deformed foot into a rigid plantigrade foot.
- Correction of the *hindfoot takes precedence* over that of the forefoot. If heel equinus and varus deformities are corrected, the forefoot deformity usually does not cause a hindrance in walking.
- *Serial stretching (casting)* may sometimes produce a degree of correction. Once it is clear during the course of treatment that conservative treatment will not be successful, surgery should be considered, preferably when the child is ready to walk and ambulate.
- An *extensive posteromedial and posterolateral release* is recommended.[11,13] If the foot fails to correct with even the most extensive soft tissue release or relapses quickly within 2 to 3 years, talectomy may be considered.
- *Talectomy* has been successful in giving good results in these stiff and rigid feet.[16-18] The talus is best approached through a lateral incision as in the case of a triple arthrodesis. We advocate the following principles during surgical correction:
    1. Excision of the talus must be complete because any cartilaginous fragments may grow and cause recurrence of the deformity.
    2. The calcaneus must be positioned below the tibia. Recurrence is common if the posterior release is inadequate or if the tibiocalcaneal reduction is not obtained. We advocate tenotomy of the Achilles tendon in which a segment of the tendon is excised to facilitate the reduction of the calcaneus under the tibia.
    3. During surgery, if total talectomy is found to be inadequate, then the navicular bone may also be excised to correct the deformity.
    4. Talectomy should be followed by immobilization in plaster for at least 10 weeks.
- Recurrence of deformity after talectomy is often difficult to treat. Radical secondary soft tissue release may be required in such cases. Persistent forefoot adduction may require a calcaneocuboid fusion in symptomatic cases. Wedge excision osteotomy in the tarsal region may be useful in the correction of plantaris and cavus deformities. The foot must be sufficiently skeletally mature before osteotomies so that the fusion rate is high.
- The Ilizarov technique and apparatus (Figure 18–18) does offer an opportunity to correct these deformities by gradual distraction and neohistogenesis. Applications of this fixator in the pediatric foot have been fairly successful and satisfactory.[19]
- In older children with neglected or relapsed equinovarus deformity, correction can be best obtained by *triple arthrodesis.* We have found this to be one of the most dependable methods of surgical treatment. Although we have performed this surgery in children as young as 10 years, we prefer to wait until the child is 12 years old. Recurrence is uncommon with this procedure. In rare cases of recurrence of the deformity after triple arthrodesis (at the level of the ankle), a *pantalar arthrodesis* (Figure 18–19) may be offered by an easy conversion of the triple arthrodesis. A *supramalleolar osteotomy* is contraindicated during growth because it invariably fails and is best offered as the last line of defense in the skeletally mature patient.
- Feet deformities with rigid congenital vertical talus may require a thorough posterior release, reduction of the talonavicular dislocation, and lengthening of the tight lateral structures. A satisfactory plantigrade position can

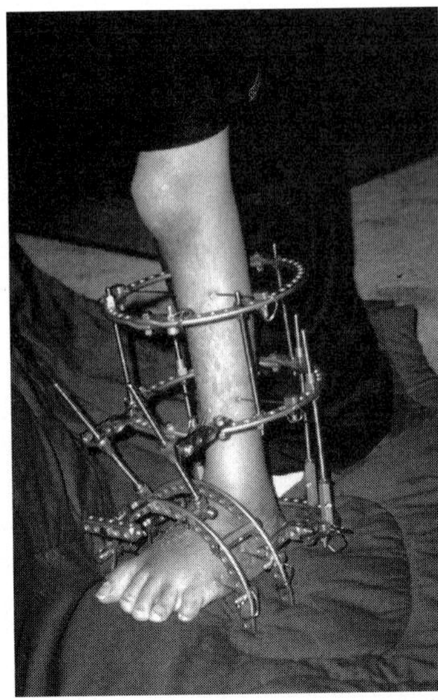

Figure 18–18: Ilizarov fixation device. Photograph courtesy Richard Davidson, MD.

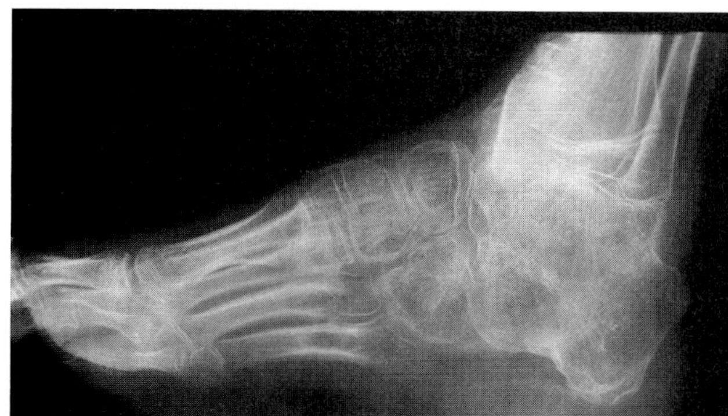

Figure 18–19: Pantalar arthrodesis. Radiograph courtesy Richard Davidson, MD.

be established in most cases, but again stiffness is a common sequela.

Knee Joint

- Both common presentations of the knee deformity, fixed flexion or fixed extension (Figure 18–20), should be initially treated with repeated stretching and splintage.
- The goal is to get the knees straight and to keep them that way with bracing. Extension of the knee is considered the key to later walking. If a flexed knee is neglected, postural hip flexion contractures are likely to ensue. Combined contracture in both hips and knees is not compatible with good gait.
- Nonsurgical management
  - Manipulation and plaster casting in the younger child has been successful in a large population of our patients. It is important to note that although the arc of motion is changed to a more extended position, the range is not increased. Even if complete extension may not be obtained, the knee joints are usually stable and mild flexion deformities are compatible with a good gait pattern.
- Surgical management

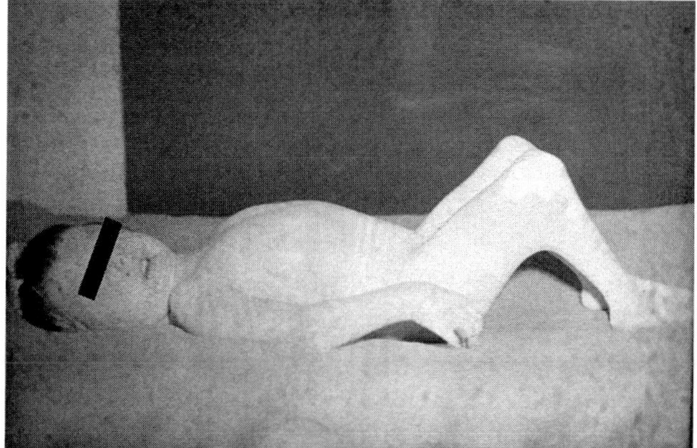

Figure 18–20: Fixed flexion of the knees in a boy with arthrogryposis multiplex congenita.

  - Deformities not responding to soft tissue stretching may need surgical intervention.
  - It is advisable to plan the timing of knee surgery in keeping with the treatment plan for the foot. For example, if the foot requires immobilization with the knee flexed, then the knee flexion correction should be staged subsequent to the foot management. On the other hand, if the knee is in fixed extension, it is better to correct the knee extension before operation on the foot so that the foot can be immobilized with a flexed knee.
  - The main principle in knee surgery in arthrogryposis is to transfer the fixed arc of knee movement into the most useful range because a significant gain in the range is often not achievable.
- Surgeries for release of fixed flexion often involve extensive soft tissue release of all posterior structures except the neurovascular bundle at the back of the knee. Medial and lateral incisions may be used instead of a midline longitudinal incision to minimize problems with wound healing. Serial plasters with gradual stretching in the postoperative period are extremely helpful in achieving further knee extension. Long-term splintage is then required to maintain the knee position.[20]
  - In older children that risk vascular compromise with extensive soft tissue release and stretching, bony shortening (of the lower femur) may be performed to achieve adequate knee extension. On the other hand, osteotomies for the correction of deformities in arthrogryposis should be delayed until near skeletal maturity to avoid progressive or recurrent deformity.
  - Fixed hyperextension of the knee may respond reasonably well to serial stretching and casting. In severe cases that fail to respond to stretching, an extensive muscular release with quadricepsplasty may be necessary to correct the knee position. Splintage and knee support are likely to be required on a long-term basis.[14]
  - The Ilizarov fixator again provides a useful alternative to surgical release or in cases of failed surgery, especially in the older patient.[19]

Hip Joint

- A common finding at birth in arthrogrypotic patients is stiffness of the hips in flexion, abduction, and external rotation.
- The two most common involvements of the hips are fixed contractures and hip dislocation (Figure 18–17).
- Fixed contractures in arthrogryposis of the hips tend to be in the frog position with severe abduction and external rotation components. These are sometimes more problematic than hip dislocations. They hinder walking or ambulating and can be difficult to treat.
  - *Management*—It is important to correct the knee deformity before attempting any surgical intervention

and correction at the hip. With knee correction at an early stage, the results of hip deformity correction are encouraging. In some cases surgical release may be required and should be carefully weighed with the presentation of the whole lower limb and not just the hip joint. For example, in a patient with contractures of the hip and knee, failure to correct the flexed knee will lead to failure of hip surgery.

– Surgical treatment

1. *Growing child*—Full correction is not easily obtainable with soft tissue release procedures. There are often adhesions around the femoral neck, and total capsulectomy carries with it the risk of avascular necrosis. Also, subtrochanteric osteotomy in the growing child usually fails. Recurrence is usually unavoidable with skeletal growth.
2. *Skeletally mature child*—If the child is able to ambulate with compensatory lordosis, it is best to wait until skeletal maturity and then hope for lasting correction with subtrochanteric osteotomy.

- Arthrogryposis may lead to unilateral or bilateral dislocation of hips. Dislocations are usually stable and, if the pelvis is well balanced, are consistent with a good gait. Treatment of hip dislocation is often not easy because closed reduction invariably fails, and stiffness and persistent flexion deformity usually follow open reduction. Diagnosis can be difficult clinically because the marked stiffness may be a limiting factor for demonstrating the hip instability clinically.
- If the hips are dislocated, in most cases they are not reducible on abduction. They should not be splinted if irreducible. Splinting in such cases may lead to avascular necrosis.
- *Bilateral dislocations* tend to be high and stable, are usually symmetrical, and tend to have a fairly balanced pelvis. This is often consistent with a good gait, and it may be advisable to leave them alone because it is often not possible to get a satisfactory result on both sides and attempts to do so may lead to more stiffness with a high chance of repeated dislocation.
- In cases of *unilateral dislocation,* there is a risk of progressive pelvic obliquity and secondary scoliosis. We therefore believe it is often worth reducing the dislocated hip, especially in the infant and the younger child. Open reduction should be done as soon as the child is healthy enough and knee flexion contractures have been controlled. Excessive delays make the procedure more technically demanding and the reduction more difficult to achieve.

Upper Limbs

Unlike management of lower limbs in which independent walking is the main goal, management of upper extremities in arthrogryposis requires considerable caution because prognosis for successful treatment depends more on the extent of the deformity and on the patient's intelligence. The minimum requirements for the patient are the ability to feed and attend to personal hygiene.[11,13]

Timing

- Again, in contrast to the lower limbs in which surgery cannot be postponed because of a risk of delayed walking, operations on upper limbs can be postponed for several years. Interestingly, arthrogrypotic children develop a remarkable ability to move well with their upper limbs despite the complexities of these deformities, developing a surprising amount of dexterity. Therefore surgical intervention should be weighed carefully in these cases (Figure 18–21).

Planning

- *Both limbs should be considered as a unit.*
  – The general principle that the arc of joint motion can be changed but not increased should be remembered. A reasonable expectation at the end of treatment is that the patient should ideally be able to move one hand to his mouth and the other to his anus, but still be capable of opposing both hands. This is important to consider because children with severe hand deformities and weakness depend on the integrated use of both hands (bimanual opposition) to perform any task that normal people do with one hand. In addition, the patient must be able to push himself out of a chair.
- *Shoulder and elbow joints should be considered as a unit.*
  – The rotation of the shoulder is an important factor on which the axis of the elbow joint motion largely depends. Therefore, if elbow surgery is contemplated to enable the hand to reach the mouth, a severely fixed and internally rotated shoulder should be simultaneously corrected.
- *Procedures performed in one joint may affect another.*
  – We have noticed that Steindler's flexorplasty performed to achieve motor power for the elbow increases flexion contractures of the wrist and fingers (Figure 18–22).
  – Carpectomy performed for wrist deformity may improve flexion contractures of the fingers by causing relative lengthening of the long flexors.

Physiotherapy

- Physiotherapy, with stretching and splintage, makes a major contribution to obtaining motion in the stiff joints. Detailed assessment by a physical therapist and an occupational therapist is necessary before embarking upon any surgical intervention, and surgery should possibly be deferred until 4 years.

Shoulder Joint

- The typical deformity is adduction and internal rotation. Although shoulder weakness is common, these children can develop remarkable trick movements; therefore surgical intervention may rarely be indicated.

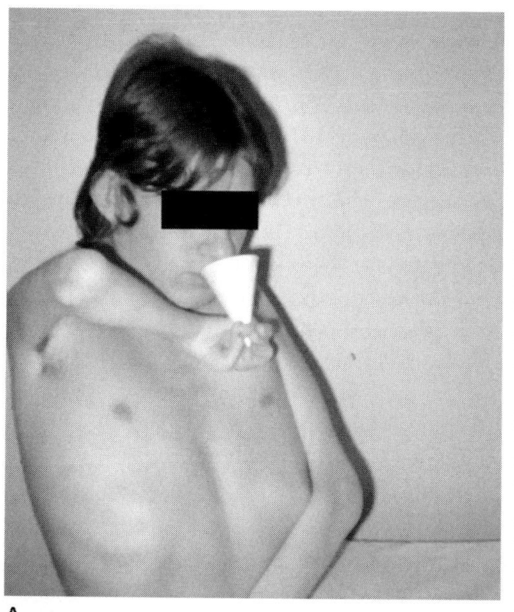

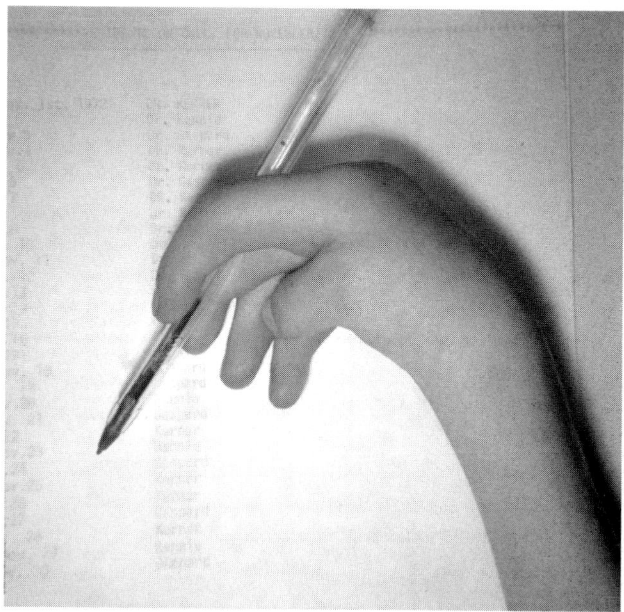

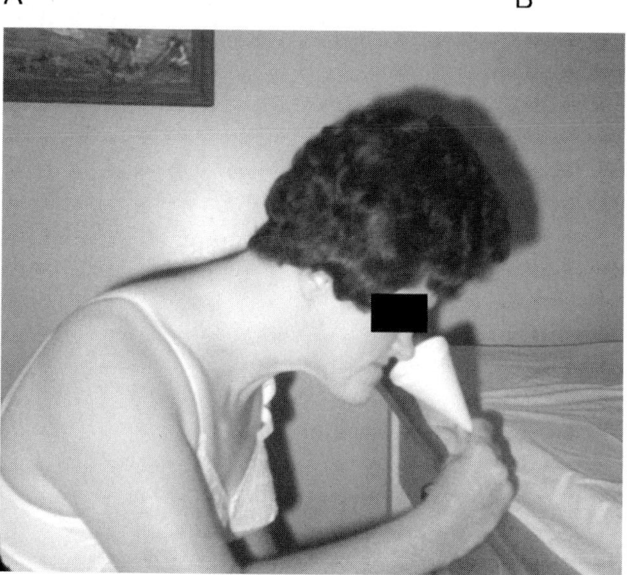

Figure 18–21: Upper limb functionality in two different patients with arthrogryposis multiplex congenita (A–C).

- Adduction itself is not troublesome because usually there is enough passive abduction for self-care and surgery is rarely required. Fixed internal rotation at the shoulder can in some cases jeopardize the axis of elbow motion. In severe cases, a simple external rotation osteotomy may be performed in the upper humerus to bring the forearm and hand into a more functional position[21].

Elbow Joint

- The two noted common involvements of the elbow are fixed extension contracture and fixed flexion contracture. Both these conditions respond well to stretching and physical therapy and can be controlled well in infancy.
- Once the child is ambulating, activities such as crutch walking, toileting, and pushing from a chair or a seated position essentially need active elbow extension. Therefore it is important not to inadvertently damage the active extension mechanism while intending to improve active flexion.
- Passive flexion can be surgically achieved by a posterior soft tissue release of the elbow, lengthening of the triceps, and a posterior capsular and collateral ligament release. This can restore a useful arc of motion, and further procedures may not be even necessary in most cases.
- In candidates for which a value of increased active flexion can be established, active power could be provided in multiple ways:

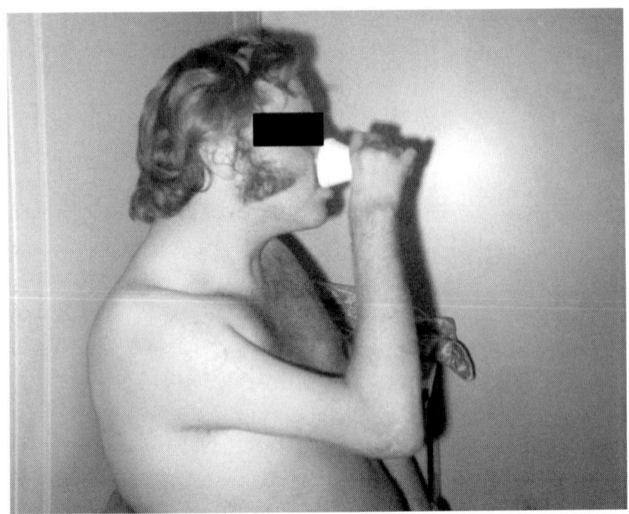

Figure 18–22: Upper limb functionality after Steindler's flexorplasty.

1. A Steindler's flexorplasty procedure advancing the flexor origin up the humerus with possible reinforcement with extensor origin advancement may be performed. This can essentially be performed only if the flexor and extensor group of muscles are sufficiently strong (Figure 18–22).
2. Transfer of the triceps tendon to the radius may be performed and can become a strong and active flexor. However, there is loss of active extension, which could lead to severe functional impairment in most cases.
3. Pectoralis major muscle transfer has also been proposed for achieving active elbow flexion, although it may not be possible in some cases because of the technical difficulties (absent biceps tendon) or an extensive and unacceptable scar.

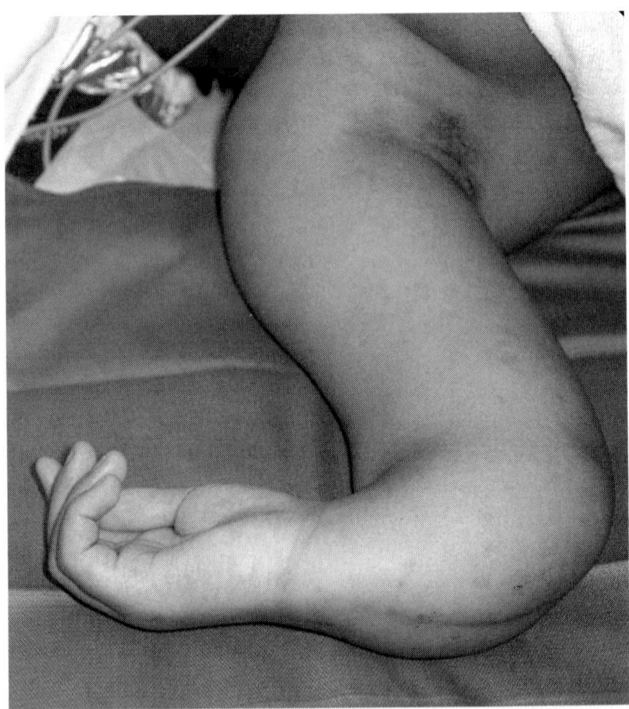

A

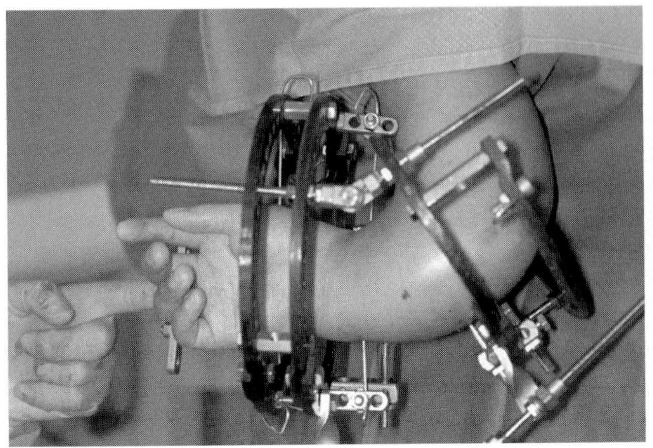

B

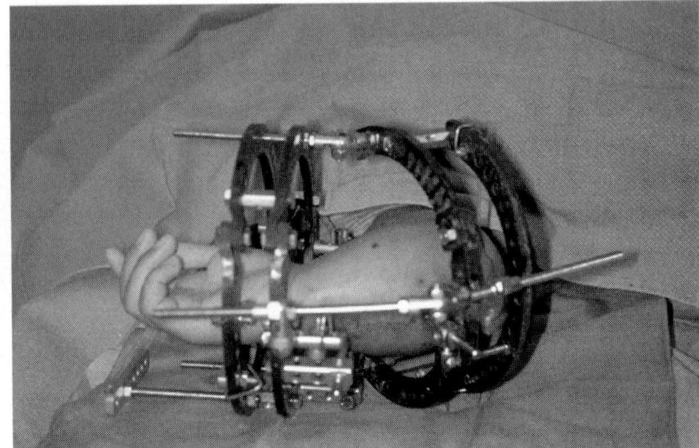

C

Figure 18–23: (A) Shows the patient prior to surgery. (B–C) An Ilizarov fixation device used to correct forearm contractures. Photographs courtesy Richard Davidson, MD.

- Elbow and forearm soft tissue contractures can be successfully corrected using the Ilizarov fixator in many cases (Figure 18–23).

Wrist and Hand

- The wrist is often involved in a flexion contracture, and the fingers may be curved and stiff. Thumb adduction (thumb-in-palm) deformity is also common.
- Manipulation, stretching, and splintage (especially early)[22] can be important in establishing mobility and range. Interestingly, the flexed position of the wrist is functional and may not need intervention. Surgical corrections involving partial or complete carpectomy have been described and often show high incidence of recurrence of deformity with growth.
- Finger stiffness is extremely difficult to correct in these cases, and surgery is rarely indicated. Most patients adapt extremely well to the finger stiffness and are impressive in their functioning abilities. Release of thumb adductors and web space enlargement are useful in correcting the thumb deformity.
- Wrist arthrodesis for functional or cosmetic gain may be considered at or near skeletal maturity.

Summary

Early recognition and counseling of parents is extremely important in this condition, which could be extremely distressing both to the parents and the patients. There is a tendency for the deformity to recur throughout growth; therefore long-term stretching, splintage, and orthoses are often necessary. The classical form of the condition is nonprogressive with intact sensations; therefore patients benefit significantly from proper choice of surgery and can remain active and functional in adult life.

References

1. Finkel RS (2001) Muscular dystrophy and myopathy. In: Current Management in Child Neurology (Maria BL, ed). Hamilton, Ontario: BC Decker.
2. Shapiro F, Specht L (1993) The diagnosis and orthopaedic treatment of childhood spinal muscular atrophy, peripheral neuropathy, Friedreich ataxia, and arthrogryposis. J Bone Joint Surg Am 75(11): 1699-1714.
3. Darras BT (1997) Neuromuscular disorders in the newborn. Clin Perinatol 24(4): 827-844.
4. Emery AE (2002) The muscular dystrophies. Lancet 359(9307): 687-695.
5. Herring J, ed (2001) Tachdjian's Pediatric Orthopedics. Philadelphia: WB Saunders.
6. Hall JG, Reed SD, Greene G (1982) The distal arthrogryposes: Delineation of new entities—Review and nosologic discussion. Am J Med Genet 11(2): 185-239.
7. Hall JG (1985) Genetic aspects of arthrogryposis. Clin Orthop (194): 44-53.
8. Wynne-Davies R, Williams PF, O'Connor JC (1981) The 1960s epidemic of arthrogryposis multiplex congenita: A survey from the United Kingdom, Australia, and the United States of America. J Bone Joint Surg Br 63B(1): 76-82.
9. Tachdjian MO, ed (1990) Pediatric Orthopedics. Philadelphia: WB Saunders.
10. Dee R (1988) Miscellaneous neuromuscular disorders of orthopaedic interest. In: Principles of Orthopaedic Practice (Dee R, Mango E, Hurst LC, eds). New York: McGraw-Hill pp 455-476.
11. Williams PF (1985) Management of upper limb problems in arthrogryposis. Clin Orthop (194): 60-67.
12. Drummond DS, Cruess RL (1978) The management of the foot and ankle in arthrogryposis multiplex congenita. J Bone Joint Surg Br 60(1): 96-99.
13. Drummond DS, Siller TM, Cruess RL (1974) Management of arthrogryposis multiplex congenita. Instruct Course Lect 23: 79-95.
14. Fixsen J (2002) Arthrogryposis multiplex congenita. In: Children's Orthopaedics and Fractures (Benson MK, JF, Macnicol MF, Parsch K, eds). Philadelphia: Churchill Livingstone pp 293-298.
15. Drummond DS, Mackenzie DA (1978) Scoliosis in arthrogryposis multiplex congenita. Spine 3(2): 146-151.
16. Green AD, Fixsen JA, Lloyd-Roberts GC (1984) Talectomy for arthrogryposis multiplex congenita. J Bone Joint Surg Br 66(5): 697-699.
17. Hsu LC, Jaffray D, Leong JC (1984) Talectomy for club foot in arthrogryposis. J Bone Joint Surg Br 66(5): 694-696.
18. D'Souza H, Aroojis A, Chawara GS (1998) Talectomy in arthrogryposis: Analysis of results. J Pediatr Orthop 18(6): 760-764.
19. Brunner R, Hefti F, Tgetgel JD (1997) Arthrogrypotic joint contracture at the knee and the foot: Correction with a circular frame. J Pediatr Orthop B 6(3): 192-197.
20. Murray C, Fixsen JA (1997) Management of knee deformity in classical arthrogryposis multiplex congenita (amyoplasia congenita). J Pediatr Orthop B 6(3): 186-191.
21. Lloyd-Roberts GC, Harris NH, Chrispin AR (1978) Anteversion of the acetabulum in congenital dislocation of the hip: A preliminary report. Orthop Clin North Am 9(1): 89-95.
22. Jones KL (1997) Smith's Recognizable Patterns of Human Malformation (Jones KL, ed). Philadelphia: WB Saunders.

Bibliography

Neuromuscular Texts

Dubowitz V (1989) Color Atlas of Muscle Disorders in Childhood. Chicago: Year Book Medical Publishers.

A superb out-of-print atlas with pictures and brief descriptions of the main neuromuscular disorders of childhood. Find it in your medical library.

Dubowitz V (1995) Muscle Disorders in Childhood, 2nd edition. Philadelphia: WB Saunders.
A more detailed description of pediatric neuromuscular disorders, including many of the newer genetic discoveries.

Schapira AHV and Griggs RC, eds (1999) Muscle diseases. In: Blue Books of Practical Neurology, volume 24. Boston: Butterworth-Heinemann.
An excellent more recent text on both genetically based and acquired muscle diseases in children and adults.

Engel A, Franzini-Armstrong C, eds (2004) Myology, 3rd edition. New York: McGraw-Hill.
A detailed two-volume reference text.

Professional Resources

Dubowitz V, ed. Neuromuscular Disorders (journal published eight times per year). Amsterdam: Elsevier Science Pergamon Press.
Clinical trial information: http://clinicalstudies.info.nih.gov/ and http://www.centerwatch.com.
The Web links provide monthly updates on an extensive list of gene locations for nuclear and mitochondrial mutations for inherited myopathies, dystrophies, neuropathies, ion channel disorders, ataxias, and congenital myasthenic syndromes.

Patient Resources

General

Muscular Dystrophy Association (USA)—800-572-1717, http://www.mdausa.org.

Muscular Dystrophy Association (Canada)—800-567-2873, http://www.mdac.ca.

Adaptive recreational organizations: Adventures in Movement for the Handicapped (aimkids@siscom.net) and American Alliance for Health, Physical Education, Recreation and Dance—(http://www.aahperd.org).

Specific, Disease-Focused Resources

DMD-Becker muscular dystrophy: The Parent Project—800-714-5437, http://www.parentdmd.org.

Inflammatory myopathy: Myositis Association of America—http://www.myositis.org.

Spinal muscular atrophy: Families of Spinal Muscular Atrophy—http://www.fsma.org.

Arthrogryposis multiplex congenita: AVENUES support group—http://www.sonnet.com/avenues.

Hereditary sensory and motor neuropathy: Charcot-Marie-Tooth Association—http://www.charcot-marie-tooth.org.

Acute inflammatory demyelinating polyneuropathy: Guillain-Barré Syndrome Foundation International—http://www.guillain-barre.com.

Mitochondrial disorders: United Mitochondrial Disease Foundation—http://www.umdf.org.

Myasthenia gravis: Myasthenia Gravis Association of America—http://www.myasthenia.org.

Orthopaedic topics—http://www.orthoseek.com.

CHAPTER 19

Neuromuscular Disorders

Myelomeningocele

Benjamin D. Roye

MD, MPH, Attending Surgeon, Division of Pediatric Orthopaedics, Department of Orthopaedic Surgery, Beth Israel Medical Center, New York, NY

Introduction

- Neuromuscular diseases have two broad categories: hereditary and acquired (Box 19–1).
  - Acquired neuromuscular disease, such as cerebral palsy, spina bifida, and polio, may occur as early as the first month of gestation.
  - Hereditary diseases include muscular dystrophies (e.g., Duchenne's and Beckers), spinal muscular atrophy, congenital myopathies, and Friedrich's ataxia.
- After cerebral palsy, spina bifida is the most common neuromuscular disease with an incidence of approximately 2 per 10,000 live births in the United States.[1]
- Spina bifida has a wide range of disease severity, from the subclinical spina bifida occulta to a complete thoracic level paralysis from rachischisis.
- Orthopaedic problems are common and include spinal deformity (scoliosis and kyphosis), hip dislocation, equinovarus and calcaneovalgus foot deformities, fractures, and lower extremity contractures.
- Patients with neuromuscular disease are complicated with multiple nonorthopaedic problems including the following:
  - Bowel or bladder incontinence
  - Pressure sores
  - Hydrocephalus
  - Tethered cord
  - Arnold-Chiari malformation
  - Latex allergy—This is an *immunoglobulin E-mediated reaction*. Prophylactic latex precautions from birth have greatly reduced the incidence of this problem.[2]
- The multiple problems experienced by these patients demand treatment with a multidisciplinary team. The best format for this seems to be through a single multidisciplinary clinic: "one-stop shopping." Involved health care providers should include the following:
  - Neurosurgery—Neurosurgeons close the defect, ventriculoperitoneal shunts, and tethered cord.
  - Orthopaedic surgery—Surgeons treat bone and joint deformities with orthoses and surgery.
  - Urology—These providers manage urinary continence problems caused by a neurogenic bladder, a common problem in this muscle group.
    1. Clean, intermittent catheterization has been shown to be safe and effective for these children.[3]
    2. Pharmacological treatment with oral anticholinergic agents has a role, but many children do not tolerate the side effects.
    3. Rarely, bladder augmentation may be considered.
    4. Vigilant care of urinary issues can prevent infections and permanent damage to the renal parenchyma.[4]
  - Nursing—Nurses are critical in providing patient–parent education, especially in the realm of pressure sore prevention and care, and in coordinating bowel and catheterization regimens for incontinence.
  - Physical and occupational therapy—Therapists have been shown to accelerate the development of gross and fine motor skills when working to maximize function and independence. Early intervention programs have been demonstrated to significantly decrease the

Box 19–1 Neuromuscular Disorders

Hereditary

Muscular dystrophies
- Duchenne
- Becker

Charcot-Marie-Tooth disease
Friedrich ataxia
Spinal muscular atrophy

Acquired

Cerebral palsy
Poliomyelitis
Arthrogryposis—Can be inherited (10%)
Neural tube defects
- Spina bifida
- Anencephaly

number of surgeries, improve locomotion, and increase the probability of normal schooling.[5]

  - Orthotists—Children with neuromuscular disease require many types of orthoses to maintain joints in normal positions and to facilitate different activities of daily living, especially walking.
- Neurological level—The *most proximal level that functions in a clinically significant manner* is defined as the neurological level (Box 19–2). For a muscle group to be considered clinically functional, it must be able to at least resist gravity.
  - The neurological level can deteriorate with time, which should raise suspicions. This may indicate a worsening hydrocephalus, an ascending syrinx, or a symptomatic tethered cord. Any rapid deterioration necessitates an aggressive workup that may include a computerized tomography (CT) scan of the head and magnetic resonance imaging (MRI) of the head, spine, or both in addition to a shunt evaluation (Box 19–3).

Embryology, Etiology, and Prevention

- Development of the spinal cord (Figure 19–1)
  - The neural plate is derived from the ectoderm in the trilaminate embryo.
  - Between gestational days 24 and 26, the plate tubularizes to form the neural tube.

Box 19–2 What's in a Level?

The neurological motor level of a child with myelomeningocele is defined by the most distal nerve root functioning in a clinically significant manner and able to resist at least gravity.

Box 19–3 Evaluating Deterioration

Neurological deterioration should be rapidly and aggressively worked up to rule out a reversible or treatable condition. Common causes of deterioration include ventriculoperitoneal shunt problems and a syrinx.

  - The neural tube goes on to differentiate into the spinal cord, the peripheral nerves, and the pia, arachnoid, and dura mater that line the central nervous system.
- Diagnosis of neural tube defects can usually be made prenatally.
  - Elevated levels of maternal α–feto protein between weeks 15 and 18 of pregnancy can indicate a neural tube defect. False-positive results can occur with twin pregnancies and other obstetric complications.
  - Elevated serum α-fetoprotein should be followed with amniocentesis or ultrasound to confirm the diagnosis. Ultrasound can demonstrate evidence for a neural tube defect as early as week 10 of gestation.
- There are two competing etiological theories of spina bifida: Von Recklinghausen proposed a primary failure of neural tube closure, and Morgagni espoused a secondary rupture of closed neural tube.
  - In either case, the problem probably occurs in the fourth week of gestation before the mother knows she is pregnant.
  - Longitudinal ultrasonographic studies suggest a progressive deformity throughout gestation, including Arnold-Chiari malformation, ventriculomegaly, and clubfeet.
- Familial factors also play a role in the etiology of spina bifida.
  - The sibling of a child with a neural tube defect has a 2 to 4% risk of neural tube defect.[6] If there are two or more siblings with neural tube defect, the risk increases to 10 to 25%.[7]
- Environmental factors have been implicated in causing neural tube defects.
  - The use of valproic acid (an antiseizure medication) during pregnancy[8] and inadequate maternal folate levels[9,10] have been associated with an increase in the rate of spina bifida.
- Prevention programs have increased awareness of the need for maternal folic acid supplementation (Box 19–4).
  - When initiated at least 1 month before pregnancy, supplementation has been shown to reduce the risk of neural tube defects by 50%.[11]
  - Grain-product enrichment with folic acid initiated in 1996 resulted in a 19 to 25% reduction in live births with spina bifida over 5 years.[12,13]

NEURULATION

1a SHAPING:

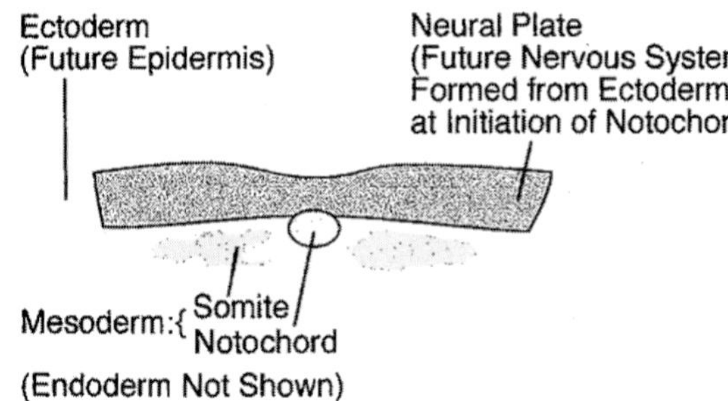

1b FOLDING:

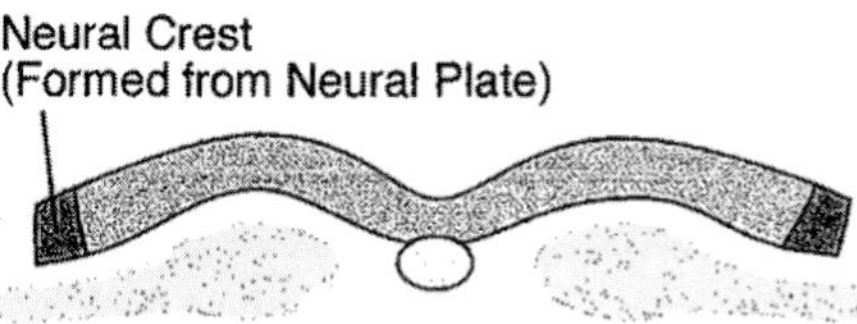

2 ELEVATION:

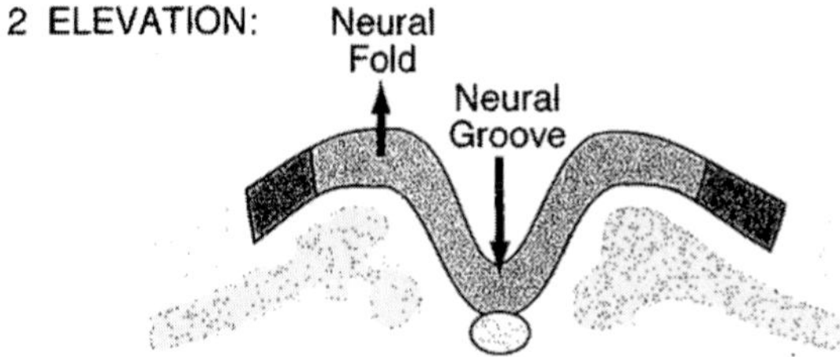

3 CONVERGENCE:

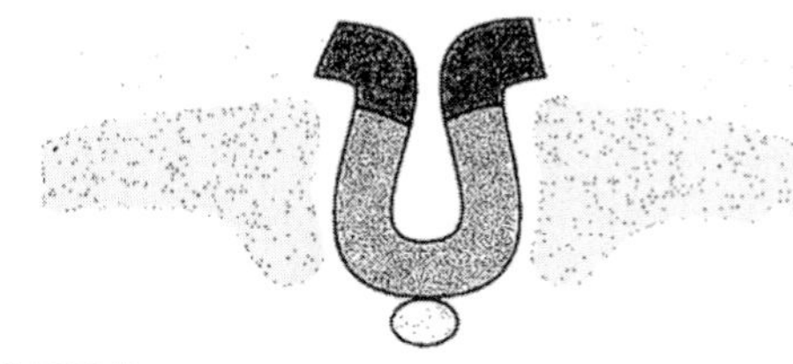

4a CLOSURE:

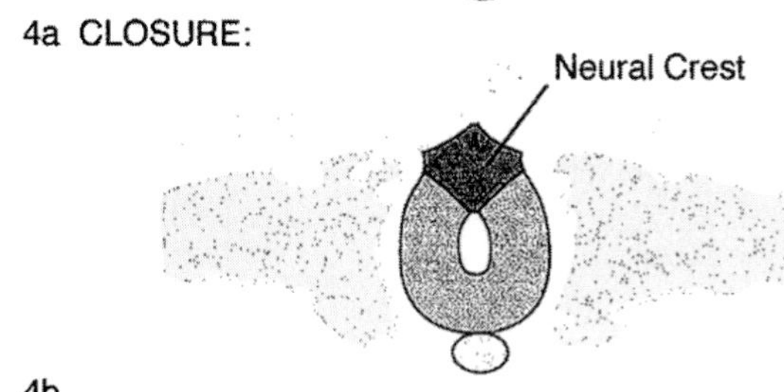

4b

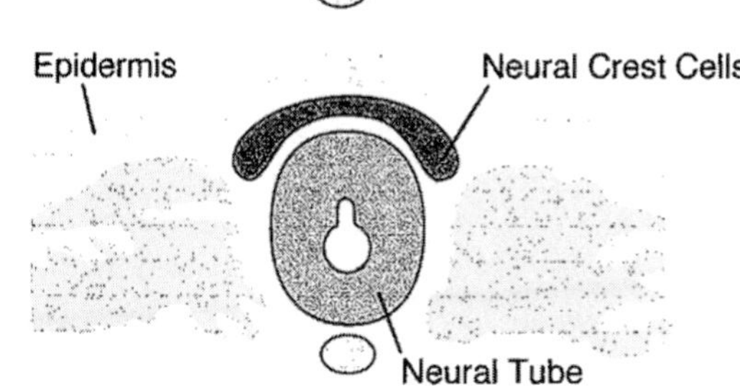

Figure 19–1: Schematic of neural tube formation during the first four weeks of gestation.

Box 19–4 An Ounce of Prevention

Defects in folic acid metabolism have been strongly correlated with neural tube defects, and folic acid supplementation is associated with declining rates of neural tube defects. Women considering having children should be strongly encouraged to take folic acid before becoming pregnant.

Range of Defects and Associated Anomalies

- Neural tube defects cover a range of deformities, from the typically benign spina bifida occulta to the devastating rachischisis. We list the most common types of neural tube defects affecting the spinal cord and some of the associated anomalies.
- Spina bifida occulta occurs when the posterior elements of the vertebrae are bifid but the meninges and cord remained within spinal canal (Figure 19–2). This typically asymptomatic condition may be present in up to 15% of the population.
  - There is a rare association with tethered cord syndrome and diastematomyelia, so any neurological symptoms should spark a workup that includes an MRI of the spine.
- *Spina bifida cystica* is a general term referring to a herniation of the meninges, with or without neural elements, through a posterior defect in the spinal column.

Subtypes

Meningocele

- Meningocele is herniation of meningeal cyst through a defect in posterior vertebral elements with the neural elements remaining within the spinal canal. These children are typically neurologically intact.

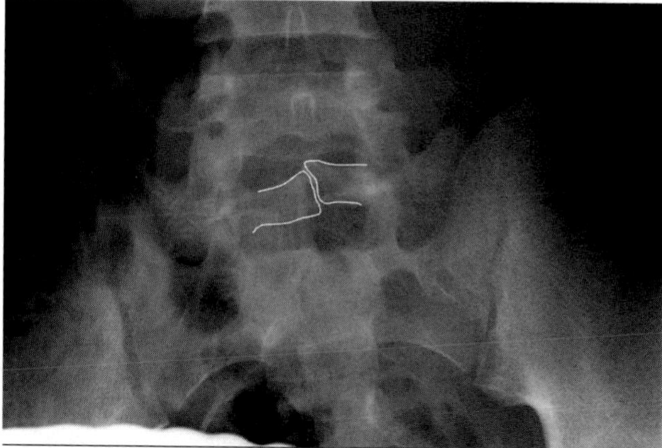

Figure 19–2: Radiograph of a young woman with spina bifida occulta at S1.

Myelomeningocele

- Myelomeningocele is herniation of the meninges with the spinal cord and/or the spinal nerve roots through a defect in posterior vertebral elements. This condition represents approximately 90% of spina bifida cystica (Figure 19–3).
  - Neurological defects are the rule in this group, and the neurological level is strictly defined as the lowest (caudal most) level with *clinically significant function*. A functional muscle must be able to resist at least gravity.
  - Cognitive impairment is also common in this group, although some children are high functioning with relatively minor learning disabilities.
  - Common associated anomalies include hydrocephalus, Arnold-Chiari lesions, and tethered cords.

Myelocele

- Also known as rachischisis or myeloschisis, myelocele is the rarest and most devastating form of spina bifida cystica. The neural plate fails to tabularize, leaving neural plate tissue exposed with no overlying tissue cover.

Lipomeningocele

- A skin-covered defect with a subcutaneous lipoma is connected to an intraspinal lipoma through a fibrofatty stalk. Motor–sensory defects are common, as are issues with urinary continence.

Associated Anomalies

Hydrocephalus

- A dilation of the cerebral ventricles from accumulation of cerebrospinal fluid (CSF) (Figure 19–4).
  - This condition is seen in 80% of cases of spina bifida cystica[14] and results from a derangement in the flow of CSF.
  - In spina bifida cystica, the derangement may be secondary to an Arnold-Chiari malformation (described later in this chapter).

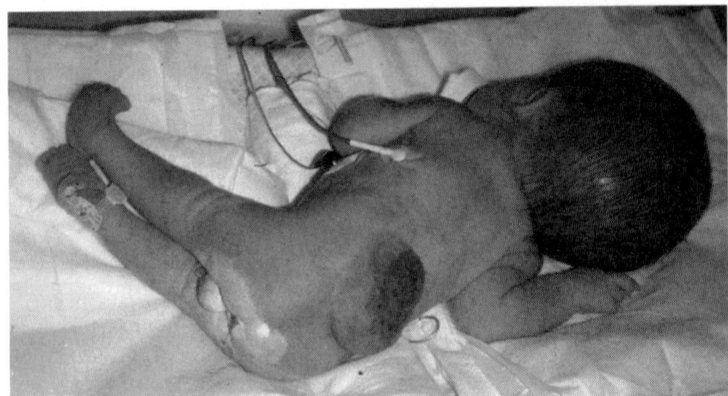

Figure 19–3: Unrepaired myelomeningocele. Photograph of a newborn with an unrepaired myelomeningocele. Note the clubfeet and the extensile posturing of the knees.

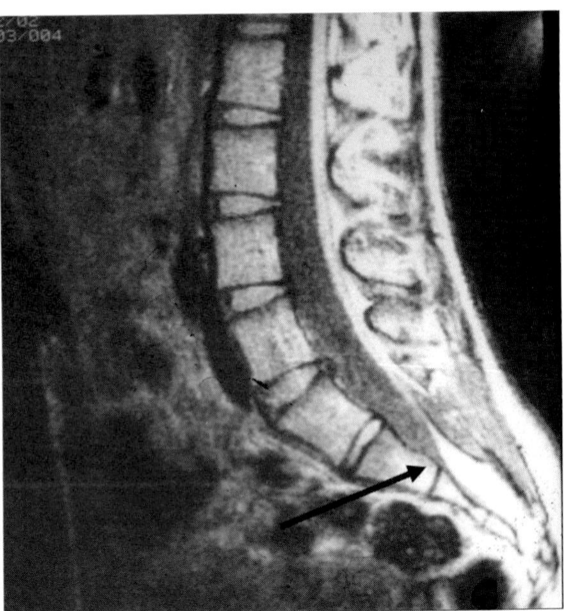

Figure 19–4: Tethered cord. Normally the spinal cord terminates at the L1 or L2 level in the conus. In this MRI, the conus can be seen in the midsacral region, a clear indication of tethering. Although most children with myelomeningocele may show MRI evidence of a tether, unless they demonstrate neurological deterioration, surgical release is usually not indicated. Note that this child also has a fatty lesion near the end of the cord, a lipomeningocele.

  - Treatment consists of placement of a ventriculoperitoneal shunt soon after diagnosis.

Hydromyelia

- Also known as a syrinx, hydromyelia is an accumulation of CSF within the spinal cord (Figure 19–5).
  - Although occasionally asymptomatic, these lesions can cause neurological deterioration.
  - When they are symptomatic they require neurosurgical decompression.

Arnold-Chiari Malformation

- An Arnold-Chiari malformation is a herniation of the cerebellum through the foramen magnum. There are two types.
  - Type I—Herniation of cerebellar tonsils only. Flow of CSF is typically unimpeded in this less severe variant (Figure 19–6).
  - Type II—Herniation of cerebellar vermis through the foramen magnum. This type is highly associated with spina bifida cystica, and it impairs the drainage of CSF from the ventricles leading to hydrocephalus. This more severe herniation may be caused by the loss of CSF through a neural tube defect *in utero*. Herniations have been shown to reduce spontaneously after fetal repair of myelomeningocele.[15]

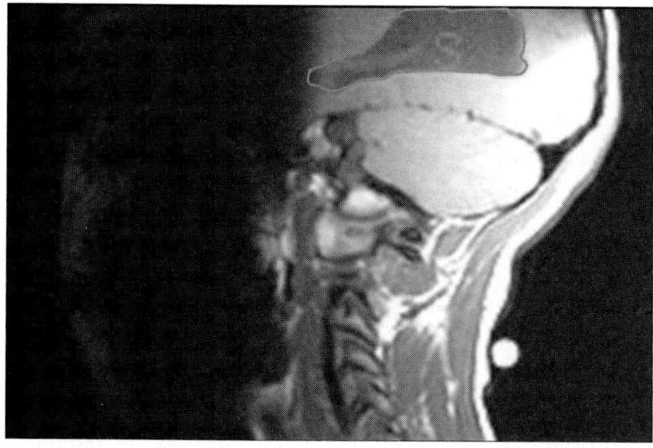

Figure 19–5: Hydrocephalus, or abnormally large cerebral ventricles, are typically caused by abnormalities in CSF flow and are commonly seen in children with myelomeningocele. In this MRI, the dilated fourth ventricle can be seen as the large, dark structure in the brain.

Tethered Cord

- This fibrous band connecting the conus medullaris (the caudal terminus of the spinal cord) to the bony sacrum prevents the normal cranial migration of the conus with growth (Figure 19–7).
- MRI evidence suggests that tethering is present in nearly 100% of myelomeningocele cases. However, neurosurgical release indicated *only* with neurological deterioration (Box 19–5).

Diastematomyelia

- This split in the spina cord is associated with a bony or cartilaginous septum (Figure 19–8).
- Treatment requires neurosurgical resection of the septum.

Nonneurological Issues

- Aside from the often-severe neurological deficits, children with spina bifida can have a variety of other problems that must be considered when coordinating their care.

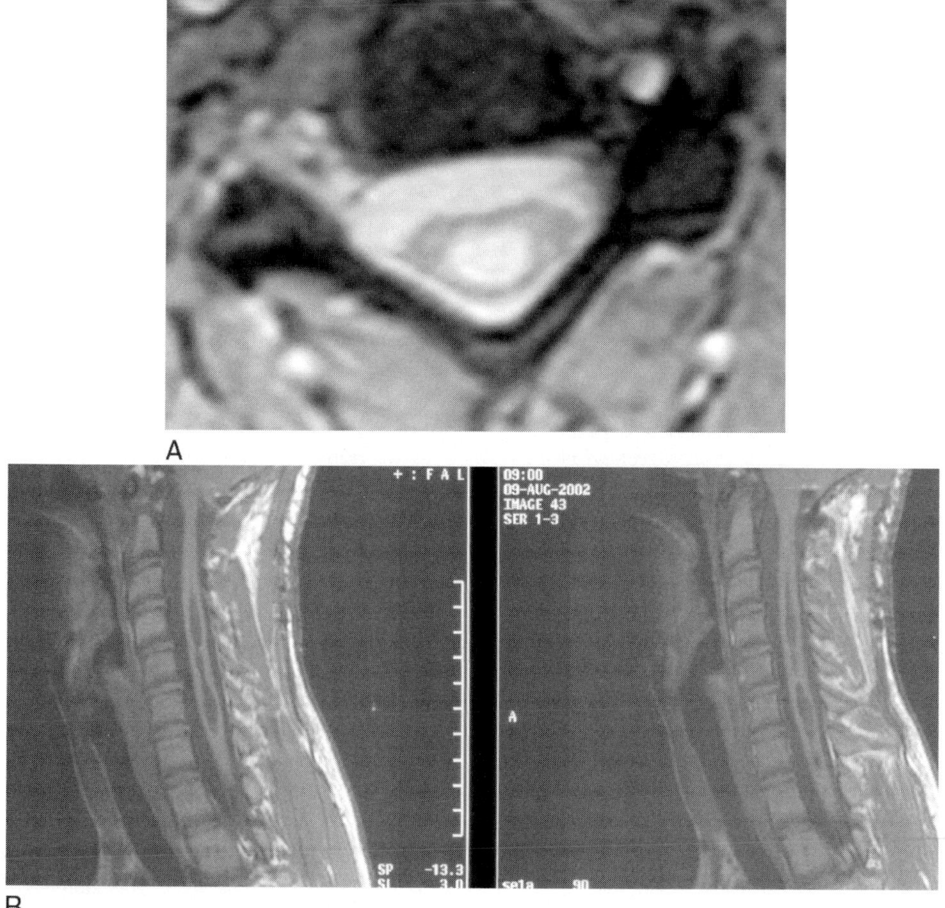

Figure 19–6: Syrinx, or hydromyelia, is an abnormal collection of CSF within the spinal cord. Pressure from this fluid can damage the spinal cord and deteriorate neurological function. In this MRI, the bright signal in the middle of the gray spinal cord on cross-sectional (A) and sagittal (B) cuts represents the syrinx.

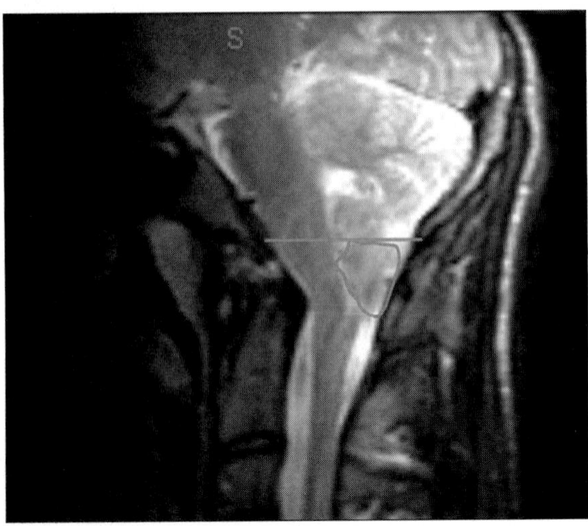

Figure 19–7: Arnold-Chiari I malformation. In this lesion, the cerebellar tonsils *(outlined)* can be seen herniating below the level of the foramen magnum *(straight line)*. In the type II lesions, the cerebellar vermis herniates as well, which can result in the disruption of CSF flow and hydrocephalus.

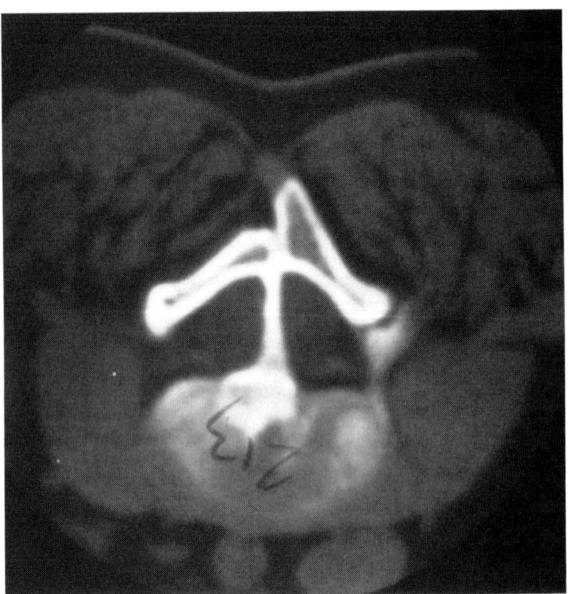

Figure 19–8: This axial CT scan demonstrates a bony septum through the middle of the spinal canal, a condition known as diastematomyelia.

- Latex allergies, mediated by IgE, were extraordinarily common in children **with** spina bifida cystica,[16] probably because of repeated exposures in the first year.[17] The recent initiation of universal latex precautions from birth in this population has dramatically reduced the incidence of latex hypersensitivity (Box 19–6).[2]
- Malignant hyperthermia, a severe and often fatal reaction to anesthesia, has been reported to be more likely in this population.[18] When it occurs, this problem is treated with emergent administration of intravenous dantrolene, which should be readily available in the operating room.
- Skin breakdown and pressure sores are major problems for these children. Approximately 60% of these children develop pressure sores somewhere over their backs or legs. Their sensory deficits place them at increased risk for this problem. They are unable to feel the ischemic pain from unchecked pressure over a bony prominence that leads to skin breakdown.
  - Treatment requires local wound care and often elimination of the bony prominence.
  - The prominence can be treated by either resection or realignment.
  - We recommend realignment over resection when possible (Box 19–7).
  - Resection of a bony prominence without treating the underlying problem leads to recurrence of the pressure point.
- Infection in either pressure sores or operative wounds can be difficult to eradicate and requires a multidisciplinary approach.
  - Nursing care provides education for primary prevention, but when problems do occur, they provide day-to-day wound care. Lately there has been increasing use of continuous low-pressure suction dressings to accelerate healing.
  - The skills of a plastic surgeon may be required for wound debridement and closure.
  - Orthopaedic surgeons perform realignment procedures or bony resections to relieve pressure from a bony prominence. As mentioned, realignment is preferred over resection because recurrence is less likely.
  - For wounds in the pelvic region, general surgeons may be enlisted to create a bowel diversion to redirect stool from the wound.

Initial Evaluation and Treatment

- Spina bifida cystica is frequently diagnosed *in utero*.
  - In the second trimester, 80 to 90% of neural tube defects can be detected by an increased maternal serum

Box 19–5 Spinal Cord Tethering

Nearly all children with myelomeningocele have evidence of spinal cord tethering on MRI, but release is reserved for those with neurological deterioration. Radiographic evidence of tethering is not, by itself, indication for surgical release.

Box 19–6 Avoid Latex

Once nearly universal, the incidence of IgE-mediated latex allergies has plummeted with the institution of universal latex precautions at birth in children with myelomeningocele.

Box 19–7 To Resect or Not To Resect?

Anytime bony resection is considered to treat a nonhealing pressure ulcer, consider the possibility of a realignment procedure. Realignment can often provide longer-lasting and more predictable results.

Box 19–8 Fetal Surgery

Recent evidence suggests that fetal surgery to close neural tube defects reduces the incidence of hydrocephalus and improves the ultimate neurological level. However, more studies and longer follow-up are needed before this could be recommended as the standard-of-care treatment.

α-fetoprotein.[19] False-positive results do occur (e.g., with multiple gestations), and the screening must be combined with a more detailed study.
  - Amniocentesis between the weeks 15 and 16 of gestation can provide more detailed information with fetal α-fetoprotein levels.
  - Ultrasound can provide anatomical evidence of spina bifida at weeks 10 to 14 of gestation (Figure 19–9)[20] and in some cases even earlier.[21]
- *In utero* surgery is being performed at several centers across the country.[22]
  - Treating spina bifida before the child is even born may improve the ultimate neurological level. Amniotic fluid is caustic to the exposed neural elements, and reducing the time the nerves are exposed to the amniotic fluid may limit the damage.
  - Early studies suggest there is a decrease in the incidence of Arnold-Chiari malformations,[15] hydrocephalus, and the need for shunting (Box 19–8).[23]
  - Despite its potential promise, *in utero* surgery is risky for mother and child alike, and standard treatment still consists of urgent closure of the defect after birth.
- A ventriculoperitoneal shunt is placed to treat hydrocephalus when present.
- The initial orthopaedic examination typically occurs after neurosurgical closure of the defect (Box 19–9). In an infant, the key parts of the examination are to document spontaneous movement, muscle tone, and reflexes.
  - Accurately determining the neurological level is difficult until the child is older and able to follow commands.[24]
  - The neurological examination needs to be constantly monitored because the motor and sensory levels are not static and may deteriorate. The importance of constantly monitoring the neurological level cannot be overstated.

Upper Extremity Problems

Problems in the upper extremities are ubiquitous in this population, although they do not typically require orthopaedic intervention.[25]

- Arms, although not usually directly affected by the spinal lesion, can have problems with strength and coordination.

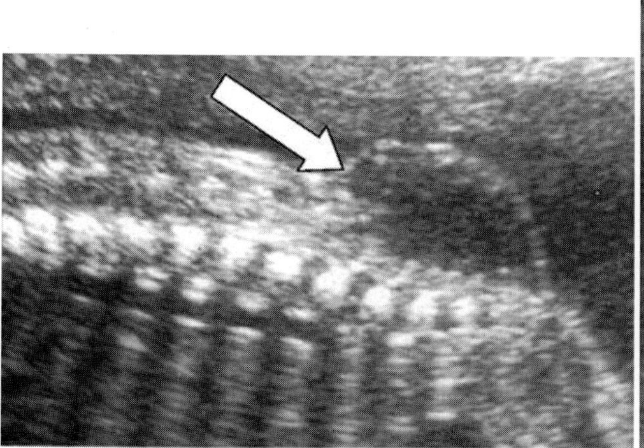
A

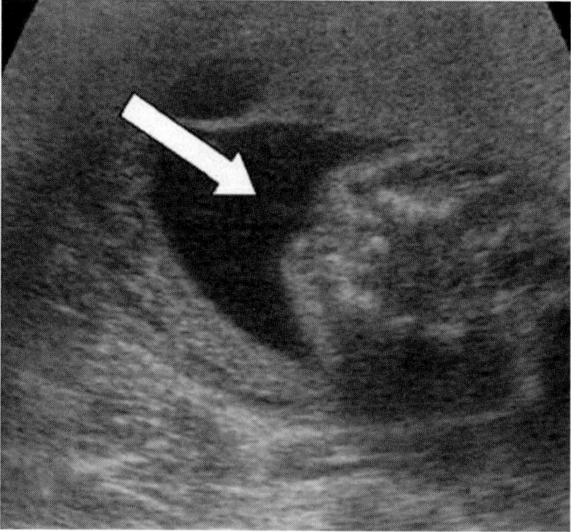
B

Figure 19–9: Fetal ultrasound with myelomeningocele.[20] Late first-trimester ultrasound can detect neural tube defects with great accuracy, especially when used with screening maternal α-fetoprotein levels. These ultrasounds demonstrate a lumbar level myelomeningocele in both the sagittal (A) and the axial (B) planes. From Aubry MC, Aubry JP, Dommergues M (2003) Sonographic prenatal diagnosis of central nervous system abnormalities. Childs Nerv Syst 19(7-8): 391-402.

Box 19–9 Initial Treatment

The initial orthopaedic examination should be performed after the neurosurgeons close the defect.

The motor and sensory levels are difficult to pinpoint until the child is older and develops some language abilities.

The neurological level needs to be constantly monitored it may not remain constant and any rapid deterioration necessitates an immediate workup to rule out a reversible cause such as a shunt problem or a syrinx.

- These difficulties are often secondary to brain damage resulting from hydrocephalus.[26]
- An ascending syrinx is another possible cause of upper extremity dysfunction.

- The occupational therapist plays a central role in dealing with upper extremity problems.[27]
- Deteriorating problems in the upper extremity should prompt an aggressive workup. There are several treatable causes of worsening function, including shunt blockage and a syrinx.

Lower Extremity Deformity

Lower extremity problems are a major source of disability for children with spina bifida cystica and frequently require orthopaedic intervention. The following sections describe the major problems seen from the hips to the toes.

Hip Deformity

- Deformity in the hip can range from contractures to subluxation to frank dislocation (Figure 19–10).
- The risk of developing a deformity relates to neurological level, but it is not specifically related to volitional muscle imbalance caused by the lesion.[24] Imbalance caused by spasticity seems a more likely culprit.
  - For example, despite the great muscle imbalance across a hip with an L4 level lesion (hip flexors function well but extensors and abductors are weak) there is a relatively low rate of dislocation. However, despite the complete paralysis across the hip seen in high lumbar and thoracic level lesions, there is a higher rate of hip subluxation and dislocation.[28]
  - Therefore prophylactic surgery to correct volitional muscle imbalance is not recommended.
- Specific treatment of a hip deformity depends on the neurological level, the specific deformity, and the individual child's function (Box 19–10).
- For children with high-level lesions (at or above L2), walking is sometimes possible early in life with extensive bracing and therapy.
  - There is little, if any, meaningful strength across the hip in this group, and deformity is usually secondary to positioning and spasm.

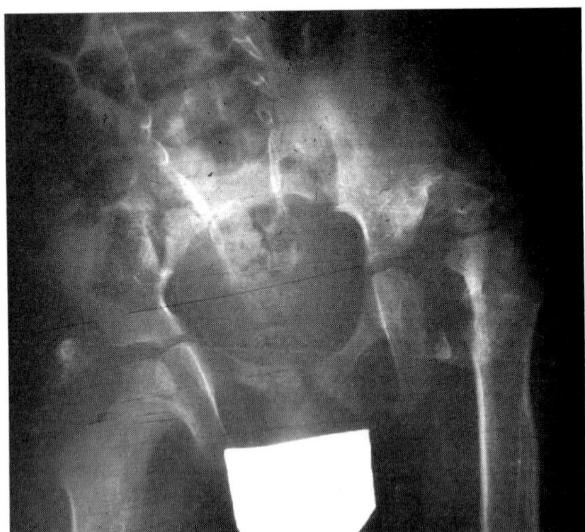

Figure 19–10: Hip dislocation. This radiograph demonstrates a high left hip dislocation with the formation of a pseudoacetabulum on the iliac wing. These unilateral dislocations lead to pelvic obliquity that can create seating problems and pressure sores.

  - Hip instability, even when unilateral, is not a source of disability in this group and generally does not require treatment.[29]
- However, preventing or treating the flexion deformities common in this group are critical to providing these children a chance to ambulate.
  - Although they typically don't walk beyond the age of 10, walking should be encouraged because of the physiological (increased bone density) and psychosocial benefits.[30]
  - Contractures can lead to hip subluxation and dislocation and problems with fitting orthoses.
  - Physical therapy and splinting play an important role in preventing and treating mild hip flexion contractures.
  - The extensive orthoses these patients need to walk require the hips to be extended although not necessarily located.
  - Soft tissue releases may be indicated for flexion contractures greater than 20 degrees to maintain

Box 19–10 Principles of Treating Hip Dysplasia

- Maintain hip flexibility to allow bracing and positioning.
- Soft tissue releases (iliopsoas and adductors) are commonly needed.
- For thoracic or upper lumbar lesions, reserve osteotomies for children with pressure sores or severe flexion contractures.
- For L3-L4 lesions, literature is controversial.
- In ambulatory patients, a level pelvis is important.
- Treat hip subluxation in children with functional quadriceps and stable neurological level.
- Aggressively treat hip pathology in lesions at or below L5.

bracing and ambulation. An anterior hip release usually involves the iliopsoas, sartorius, rectus femoris, tensor fascia lata, and hip capsule.
  - Ultimately, a flexible hip is more important than a reduced hip, and multiple surgeries are generally not indicated because they can lead to stiffness and difficulty with bracing and positioning.
  - Osteotomies, although rarely indicated, can be useful in treating severe flexion deformities (greater than 60 degrees) or treating pressure sores resulting from the hip deformity.
- Flexion, abduction, and external rotation contractures are common in children with total paralysis across the hips and in the legs because of the posture they assume as infants (Figure 19–11). Awareness of this problem and the use of prophylactic splinting and physical therapy can often prevent this deformity from becoming a major problem.
  - Soft tissue releases are useful for contractures that persist despite conservative measures. Releasing the tensor fascia lata usually improves the abduction contracture. Treatment of flexion contractures was described previously.
  - Subtrochanteric osteotomies may be required for persistent external rotation contractures.
- Isolated abduction contractures, when unilateral, can lead to spinal obliquity and scoliosis. Treatment consists of splinting and physical therapy followed by tensor fascia lata release if necessary.

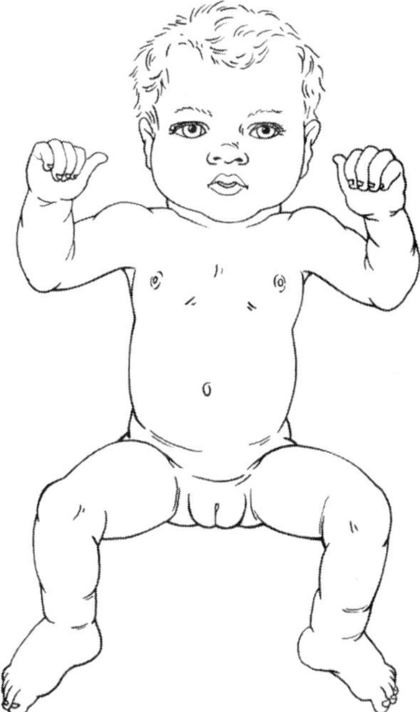

Figure 19–11: Infant posturing with high-level paraplegia. This drawing demonstrates the typical posturing of an infant with a thoracic level myelomeningocele. The contractures they tend to develop, hip flexion and external rotation, mimic this posture.

- Adduction contractures can lead to pelvic obliquity and problems with ambulating, positioning, pressure sores, and peroneal hygiene. When nonoperative measures fail, an open adductor release is indicated. The adductors longus and brevis and the gracilis are released through a transverse incision over the adductor longus.
- Most children with midlumbar lesions (L3-L4) are ambulatory with varying bracing requirements. However, the wide range of function in this group makes recommending broad treatment strategies difficult and controversial.
  - Some patients in this group are born with a teratological hip dislocation, but most develop problems related to an imbalance between the abductors and the adductors or to spasticity.
  - Regardless of the cause, hip subluxation or dislocation complicates 50 to 70% of these cases and is a source of controversy. Studies have alternately shown hip dysplasia to have a negative effect on ambulation[31] and to have no effect on ambulation.[32]
- Many recommend reserving surgical treatment for ambulatory children with a unilateral hip dislocation, strong quadriceps, and a stable neurological level.
  - Unilateral dislocations are of greater concern because they interfere with ambulation by creating pelvic obliquity and leg length discrepancy.
  - Unilateral hip instability is also associated with scoliosis, but interestingly there is no correlation between the side of instability and the direction of the curve.[33]
  - Bilateral dislocations have been shown not to have a negative effect on function,[34] so they do not typically warrant treatment unless they are associated with a significant fixed flexion contracture.
  - Treatment of hip dysplasia in the first year is particularly challenging, with a 50% failure rate.[35,36]
- Multiple procedures have been described with the goal of producing a balanced, stable hip.
- Surgical treatment begins with an open hip reduction including an anterior release and bony correction of any acetabular and femoral dysplasia as necessary.
- Muscle transfers have been recommended to dynamically balance the hip to prevent recurrence.
  - Myotomies may improve balance, but they reduce stability.
  - The once popular transfer of the iliopsoas to the greater trochanter has fallen out of favor. This is because of the problem with hip extension contractures that develop because the psoas is transferred out of phase.[37]
  - Transfer of the external oblique to the greater trochanter increases the extensor moment on the hip and has been shown to improve gait pattern

and reduce or eliminate requirements for bracing. Combining this procedure with a transfer of the adductors and tensor fascia lata posteriorly to the gluteus maximus may further improve results.[38]
  - Outcomes may be improved if surgery is delayed until the child has learned to walk.[37]
- Children with low neurological levels (L5 or below) are typically high functioning and have a low incidence of significant hip pathology. Hip dysplasia should be treated aggressively in this population, as it would be in an otherwise normal child, to best preserve their function.

Knee Deformity

- Knee flexion contractures are probably the most common knee deformity and are a particular problem in patients with a thoracic or high lumbar level.
  - Small contractures (less than 10 degrees) can be treated with serial casting.
  - Large contractures (greater than 30 degrees) require a posterior release.
  - Problems with wound closure and tightness of neurovascular structures may preclude a complete acute correction, and the soft tissue release may need to be followed by serial casting to obtain complete correction.
  - Treatment may not be required in nonambulatory children unless the deformity interferes with positioning, transfers, or hygiene.
- Knee extension contractures are seen in individuals with both high neurological and mid-neurological levels.
  - In infancy, serial casting is usually adequate to obtain 90 degrees of flexion.[39]
  - Older children who walk may function adequately with a knee extension contracture, but serial casting can sometimes improve function in those whose ambulation is impaired.
  - When casting fails to adequately improve flexion, a soft tissue lengthening of the extensor mechanism is the next step. Several procedures have been described, including a Z-plasty of the extensor mechanism and a V-Y lengthening of the quadriceps.[40] An anterior capsulotomy may also be required to obtain maximal correction. Patients without meaningful leg power may benefit from a simple patellar tendon release to facilitate seating.[41]
- Valgus deformity at the knee is rare and does not typically require orthopaedic intervention. Contracture of the iliotibial band has been described to cause distal femoral valgus that may progress despite release.
- Clinically significant knee arthropathy has also been described in ambulatory young adults with spina bifida.
  - Abnormal walking mechanics may lead to a degenerative arthropathy.[42] This problem should be discussed with younger patients and their families because regular use of forearm crutches can reduce the impact on the knees and prevent this problem.[43]
  - Charcot arthropathy is described in the next section.

Foot and Ankle Deformity

- Similar to the hip, the development of foot and ankle deformities bears little relation to spontaneous motor activity.[44]
  - Approximately 75% of patients with spina bifida cystica develop a significant deformity that requires treatment, including many patients with high and midlevel lesions that have no meaningful power across their ankles.[44]
  - Reflex spasticity plays an etiological role in some, although upward of 75% of deformities occur in the absence of spasticity.
  - Deformities present at birth may be secondary to intrauterine positioning.
  - The overall goals of treating foot and ankle problems are to create a braceable plantigrade foot to facilitate ambulation and positioning and to prevent skin problems.

Clubfoot Deformity

- The clubfoot, or equinovarus, deformity affects 30 to 50% of children with spina bifida cystica.
- In this deformity, the hindfoot is usually rigidly fixed in equinus and varus, often with midfoot cavus and forefoot adductus and supination (Figure 19–12).
- Clubfeet not only can impair walking ability but also can create seating problems when the feet cannot sit properly on footrests. Left unchecked, this deformity can lead to the formation of pressure sores, especially on the dorsolateral foot.
- Often present at birth, these deformities are rigid and resistant to nonoperative measures. Casting may still be used to prevent progression and buy time until surgery can be performed.
- The aggressive approach to surgical treatment of clubfoot in children with spina bifida cystica sets it apart from the idiopathic clubfoot. A complete pantalar release is performed with tenotomies or excision of all contracted tendons to eliminate the deforming forces.
  - Tendon lengthening is not recommended because of the high incidence of recurrent deformity.
  - Tendon transfers usually fail because the transferred tendon is often out of phase. Because it loses a strength grade, it often cannot provide adequate support.
  - Even though they are not contracted, the anterior tibialis and peroneal tendons should be released in the child with an L5 motor level to prevent a calcaneus deformity (Box 19–10).[37]

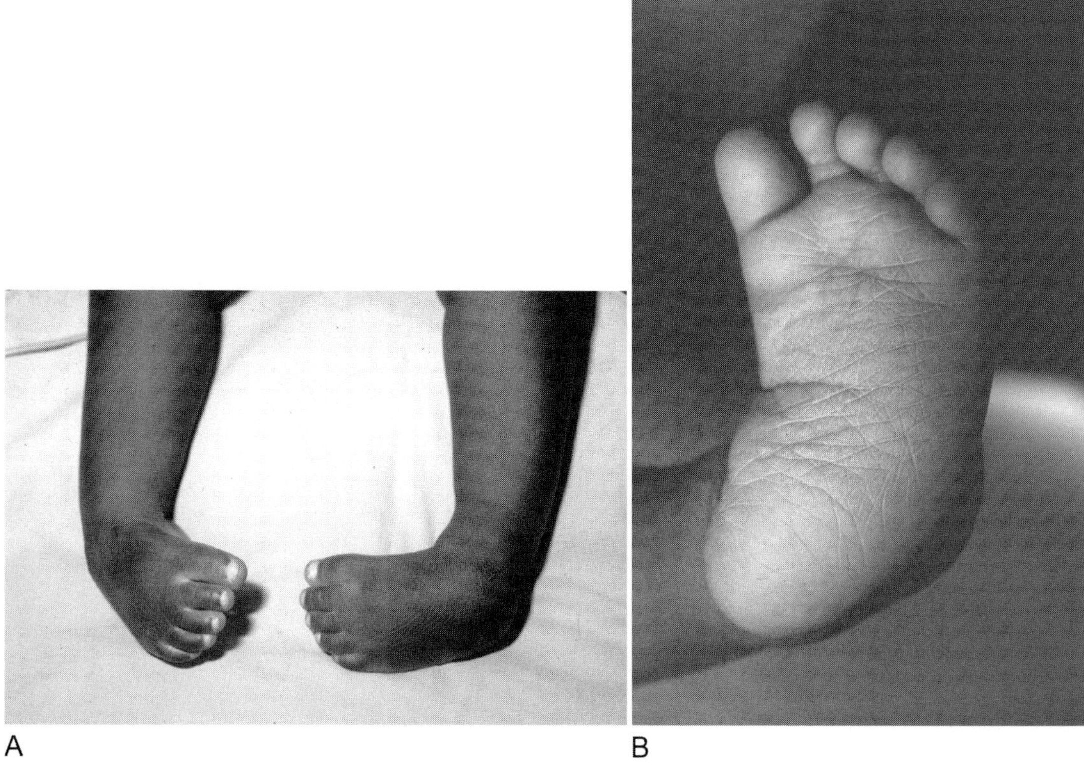

Figure 19–12: **Clubfoot.** Note the equinus and varus (A) of the ankle (hindfoot) and the adducted forefoot with a deep medial skin crease (B). When viewed from the medial side, the deep creases in both the midfoot and the hindfoot are evident (C).

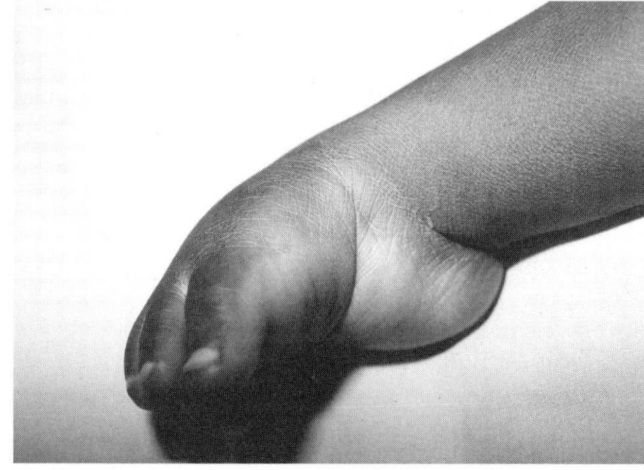

- Skin and incisional problems are common partly because of the severe nature of the deformity.
  - Tension across the skin or closure must be avoided. Skin slough results in scar formation and scar contracture that can lead to recurrence.
  - Some recommend carrying the medial arm of the incision over the dorsum of the foot to reduce tension on a medial skin bridge.[37]
  - Tissue expanders and rotational pedicle flaps have also been described to address this problem.
- Despite postoperative splinting, recurrence is still common.
  - Recurrent deformity may be treated by talectomy and splinting.

Calcaneus and Calcaneovalgus Deformities

- Calcaneus and calcaneovalgus deformities are seen in about 30% of this population (Figure 19–13). They typically lead to the same functional and skin problems as the clubfoot.
  - This deformity often results from a tibialis anterior muscle that is spastic or pulling against a weak or paralyzed gastrocnemius; thus this deformity is most frequently seen in children with L5- or S1-level paralysis.
  - In some cases, calcaneovalgus is caused by a vertical talus where the midfoot and forefoot are dorsiflexed

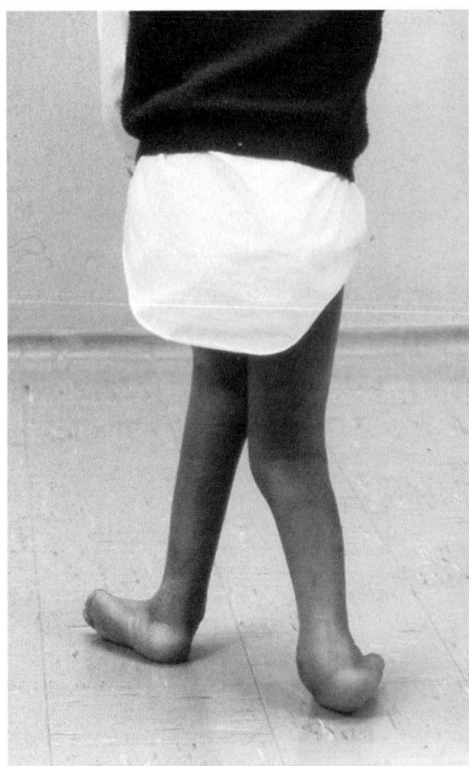

Figure 19–13: This child demonstrates a calcaneovalgus deformity in both feet, which limits his ambulatory ability.

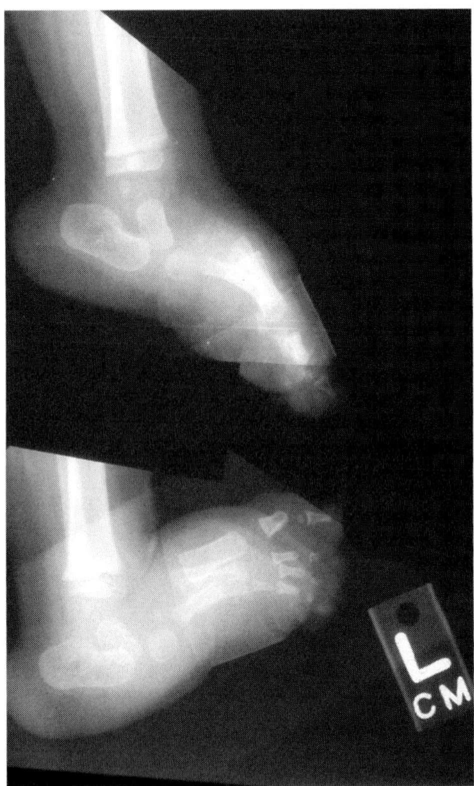

Figure 19–14: The vertical or oblique talus can be confused with the clubfoot. The diagnostic *sine qua non* is the persistence of a plantar flexed talus relative to the calcaneus when the foot is brought into dorsiflexion, as seen in these x-ray films.

on a rigid, plantar flexed talus (Figure 19–14). Occasionally, this entity can be confused with a clubfoot if the forefoot is in equinus, but careful examination will reveal fixed calcaneus of the hindfoot.

- Flexible deformities may respond to stretching or casting, although holding these feet in a brace after correction can be challenging.
- Anterior soft tissue release, including the peroneals, tibialis anterior, extensor hallucis longus, and extensor digitorum longus, can greatly facilitate bracing.[45] Tibialis anterior tendon transfer has been described,[46,47] but the transferred muscle is out of phase and has not been found to change bracing needs.[48]
- Achilles tenodesis has been described with good results for calcaneus with minimal valgus deformity,[49] although stretching of the Achilles can occur over time.

Planovalgus Deformity

- Valgus without calcaneus can also occur in the subtalar joint, ankle, or both. It is commonly associated with a flat foot, the so-called planovalgus deformity (Figure 19–15).
- A valgus deformity presents a problem, especially in the ambulatory child or when the deformity places the medial foot at risk for pressure sores.
- Treatment depends on the rigidity and the specific location of the deformity.
  - Flexible deformities can be treated with casting and bracing, although this rarely provides adequate long-term results.
  - To correct subtalar valgus, a wide subtalar release and (usually) an extra-articular subtalar arthrodesis are required.[50,51] Tibiotalar fusions are to be avoided because of the unacceptable complication rate.
  - Distal tibial valgus can be corrected with either a closing wedge supramalleolar osteotomy in skeletally mature patients or a hemiepiphysiodesis in skeletally immature children.
  - When externally rotated, the ankle joint may require a supramalleolar derotational osteotomy.

Cavus Deformities

- Cavus deformities typically occur in children with sacral level lesions. This deformity is usually caused by unopposed pull of the tibialis anterior muscle and toe flexors, so clawing of the toes is a commonly associated deformity (Figure 19–16).
  - Flexible deformities can sometimes be contained in an ankle–foot orthosis (AFO). Brace compliance can be a problem because sacral level paraplegics are highly functional and will shed their braces, so a plantar release may be required.

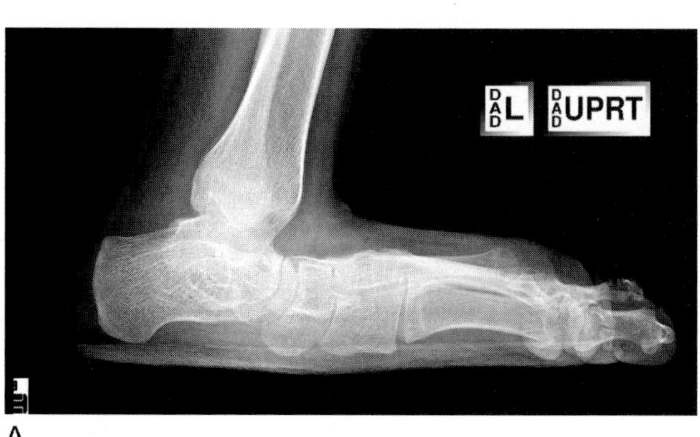

A

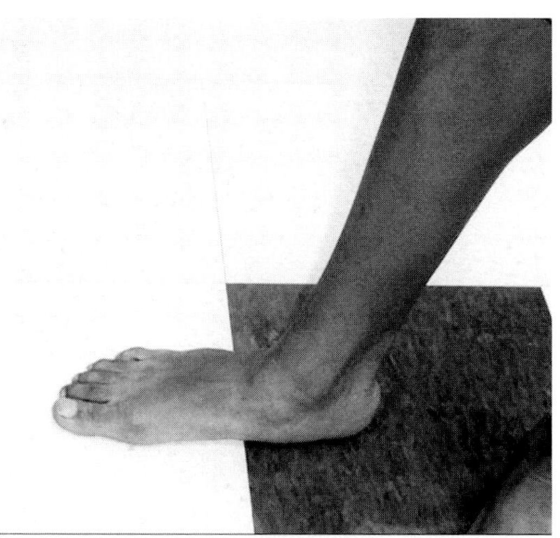
B

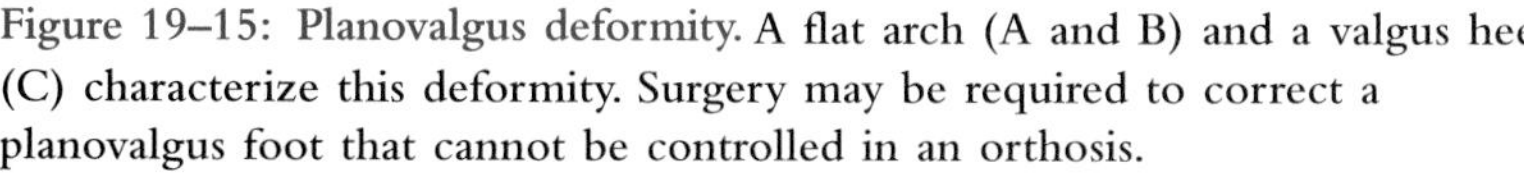
Figure 19–15: Planovalgus deformity. A flat arch (A and B) and a valgus heel (C) characterize this deformity. Surgery may be required to correct a planovalgus foot that cannot be controlled in an orthosis.

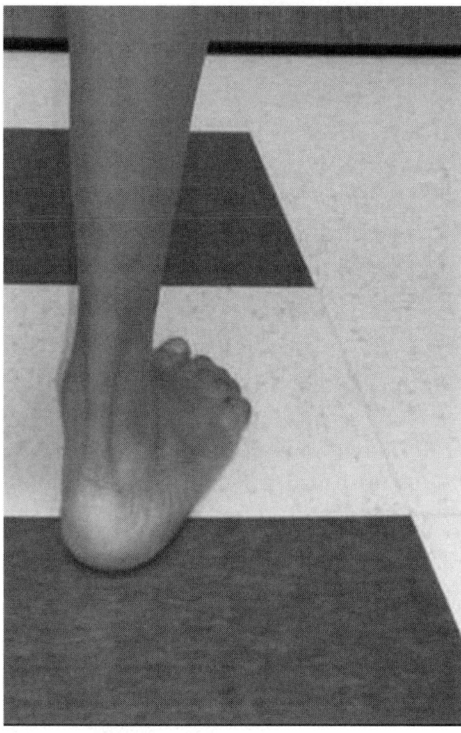
C

- Claw toes can usually be treated simply with flexor tenotomies.
- Rigid deformities in older children may require a closing wedge first metatarsal osteotomy or, when the calcaneus is dorsiflexed, a calcaneal osteotomy. A tibialis anterior lengthening should also be performed. An out-of-phase transfer to the calcaneus will not be successful.[37]
- For a cavovarus deformity, a tibialis anterior transfer to the middle of the foot with or without a posteromedial release can be helpful.
- Other described transfers include the extensor longus tendons to the metatarsal heads to correct cavus and a peroneal brevis transfer for a cavovalgus deformity.

Charcot Arthropathy

- Charcot arthropathy is a relatively uncommon complication in this population with an incidence of about 1%. It seems to occur in ambulatory children with a motor level at or below L4 and a sensory level slightly higher.[52]
- A red, swollen foot may precede radiographic changes by several weeks or even months. Aggressively treating

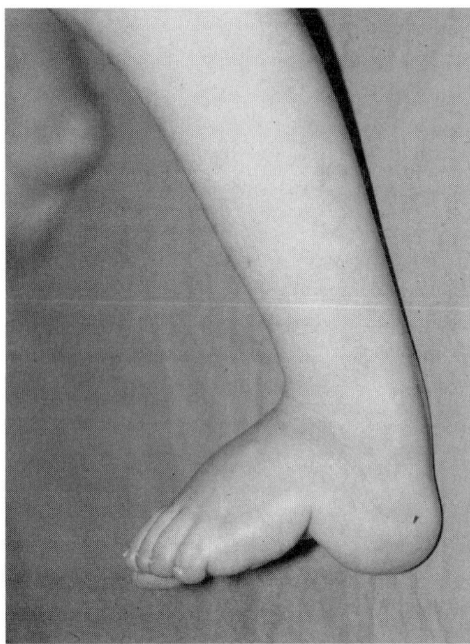

Figure 19–16: This severe cavus deformity occurred in a young girl with a sacral level myelomeningocele. Note the midfoot crease evident even on the lateral side of the foot.

suspected Charcot arthropathy at this stage with immobilization and non–weight-bearing status offers the best chance of a successful outcome.[37]

- Once typical radiographic changes of joint fragmentation become evident, outcomes become less satisfying (Figure 19–17).
  - Months of immobilization may be necessary until all skin changes resolve and there is radiographic evidence of healing.
  - Once healed, continued protection with an orthosis is recommended to protect against further injury.
- Although the ankle is the most commonly affected joint, Charcot arthropathy has been described in the knee and hip in children with myelomeningocele.

Pathological Fractures

- Disuse osteopenia and even osteoporosis occur in children with myelomeningocele as they lose the ability to ambulate. The combination of sensory loss with bone loss greatly increases the risk for a pathological fracture.
- The overall incidence of pathological fracture in this population is around 20%, with a much higher incidence in thoracic level paraplegics (69%).[53]
- These fractures do not occur in ambulatory patients with low-level sacral lesions and can be delayed or prevented by encouraging other patients to bear weight.
- These fractures are often not recognized at the time of injury because they are painless.
- Their symptoms are similar to those of an infection with a swollen, red limb, often associated with fever (Box 19–11). Knowledge of these fractures is essential to prevent a delay in diagnosis with an unnecessary workup for infection.
- Supracondylar femur fractures are the most common type and can look like a septic knee (Figure 19–18).
- Treatment consists of brief immobilization with a cast or fracture brace because these fractures usually heal quickly with exuberant callus.
- Rarely, pathological fractures in this population may be secondary to metabolic problems such as renal osteodystrophy or vitamin C deficiency.[30]

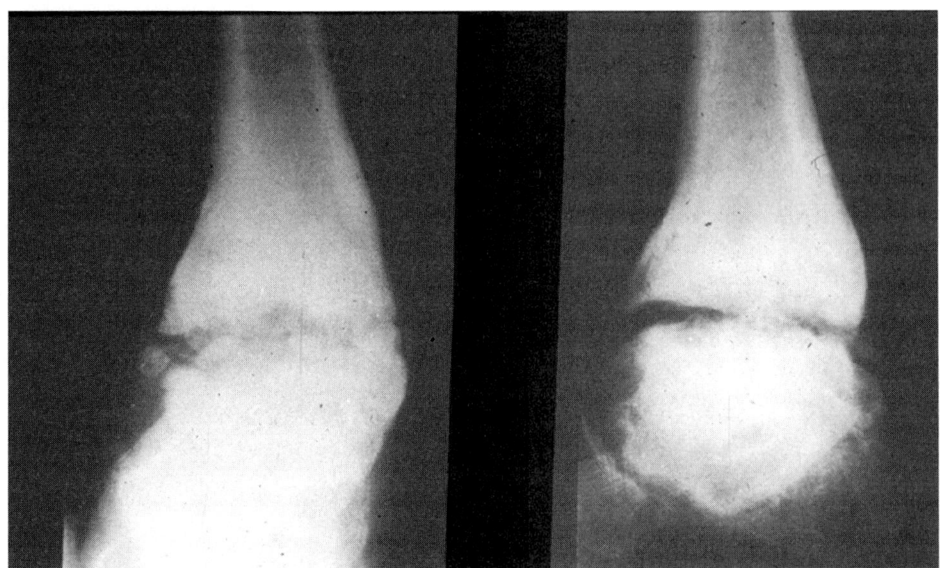

Figure 19–17: Charcot arthropathy. These anteroposterior and lateral radiographs show complete destruction and fragmentation of the ankle joint.

Box 19–11 Septic Joint?

A red swollen knee, even with fever, is most likely a pathological fracture. Make sure to carefully examine and take x-ray film of children with these symptoms to avoid delaying the diagnosis of fracture.

Spinal Deformity

Scoliosis and kyphosis complicate approximately 50%[33,54] of all cases of spina bifida cystica. In addition to the common paralytic curves, upward of 15% may be congenital curves.[55]

Scoliosis

- Scoliosis in this population has been defined as curves with a Cobb angle greater than 20 degrees (Figure 19–19). Most curves develop early in life, but about 40% of curves develop after 9 years and may first appear in patients 15 years old (Box 19–12).[33]
- Children with a thoracic neurological level or a thoracic level for their last intact laminar arch have a 90% incidence of scoliosis.[33] Those with a level below L4 have an incidence closer to 10%.
- Community ambulators have half the incidence of scoliosis as noncommunity ambulators.[33]

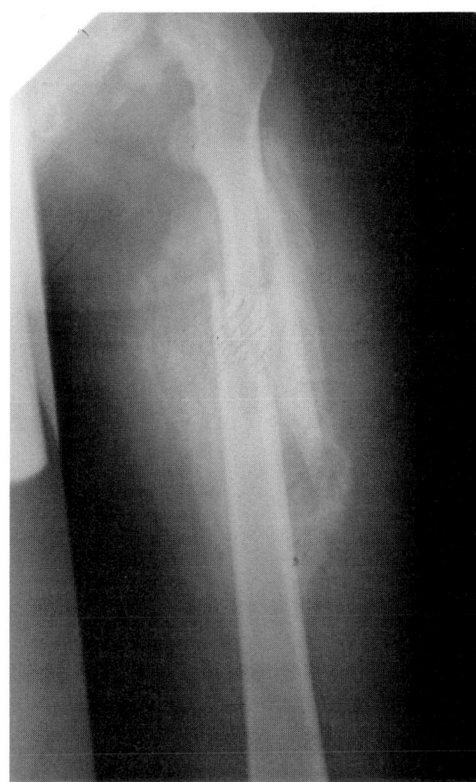

Figure 19–18: Pathological supracondylar femur fracture. The anteroposterior radiograph of a left femur demonstrates a several-weeks-old femur fracture with exuberant callous formation.

Box 19–12 Spinal Deformity—Not Just for the Young

Although scoliotic and kyphotic deformities are common early in life, many curves develop after the age of 9 and may present as late as 15 years.

Most curves are progressive and not responsive to brace treatment. Although surgery is often recommended, complication rates are high and reoperation is not unusual.

- Rapidly progressive curves or curves associated with deteriorating neurological level should be imaged with MRI to rule out a possible syrinx.[56] Neurosurgical decompression of a syrinx has been documented to stabilize or even improve the scoliosis.[57]
- Even mild scoliosis can affect balance and impair walking and sitting ability. As the curve progresses, pelvic obliquity may develop followed by pressure sores. Large curves can cause pain, make positioning in a chair nearly impossible, and even affect cardiopulmonary function.[58,59]
- Curves greater than 20 degrees documented to progress are generally considered candidates for posterior fusion and instrumentation because they progress. Although a Swedish study found there could be a role for brace therapy in this population,[60] most Americans favor operative treatment.[61]
- The overall complication rate of surgery is nearly 50%, and each patient requires, on average, 1.5 procedures.[62]

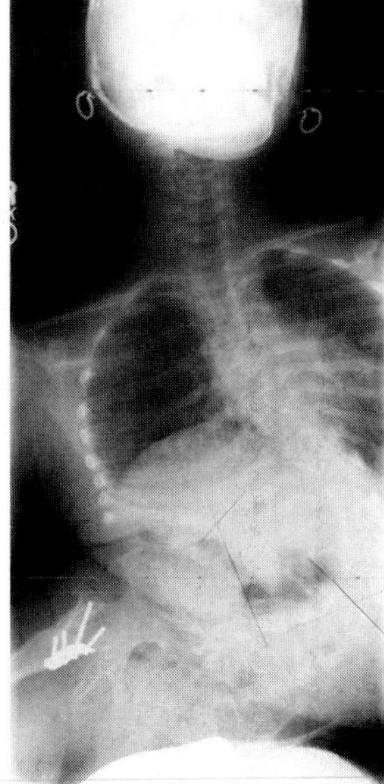

Figure 19–19: This seated anteroposterior radiograph demonstrates a severe 110-degree scoliosis in a girl with myelomeningocele. Note the severe pelvic obliquity and the hardware in the right hip from prior surgery for a hip dislocation.

  - Hardware problems are seen in 15%[62,63] to 30%[64,65] of cases, and deep infections affect 8%[62,66] to 33%.[67]
  - Ventriculoperitoneal shunt failure, a potentially fatal complication, can also be seen after spine surgery.[66]
- Getting the wound to heal after correcting a severe deformity is a particularly vexing problem (Figure 19–20). Plastic surgeons are sometimes used to raise local flaps to facilitate low-tension closures.

Kyphosis

- Kyphosis, particularly common (>30%) in thoracic level paraplegics, can also be of congenital or paralytic origin.
- Short, acute S-shaped curves progress (Figure 19–21) more rapidly (8 degrees/year) than long, gentle C-shaped curves (3 degrees/year).
- Kyphosis causes multiple problems including loss of truncal height, difficulty sitting and looking forward, and skin ulceration over the gibbus. Increased abdominal pressure can cause respiratory compromise from loss of diaphragmatic breathing, and loss of access to the anterior abdominal wall can lead to problems caring for or creating urinary diversions or stomas.[68]
- These curves are progressive and not responsive to bracing. Bracing itself can cause skin and respiratory problems.
- Therefore, despite the high complication rate, surgery is the treatment of choice.
  - Infection, problems with skin healing, hardware failure, recurrence, and death have all been well described in this group.[69,70]
  - The goals of kyphosis surgery include improving truncal balance and seating, freeing the upper extremities for useful tasks, and improving skin problems.

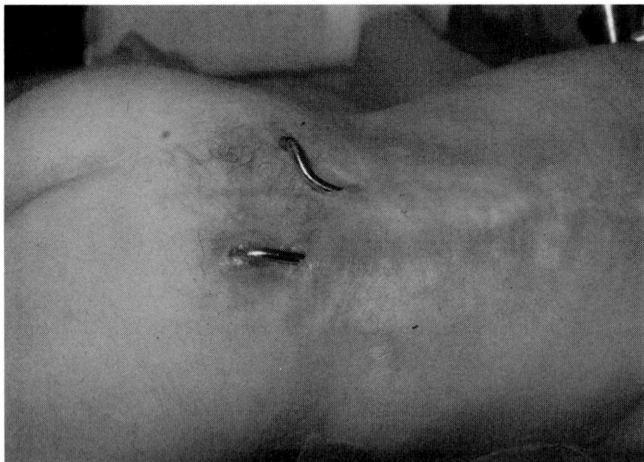

Figure 19–20: Wound breakdown. **This unfortunate girl had a spine fusion for severe scoliosis and had skin breakdown over her hardware. Obtaining adequate skin coverage in children with myelomeningocele for surgical procedures can be a major challenge, especially in the spine.**

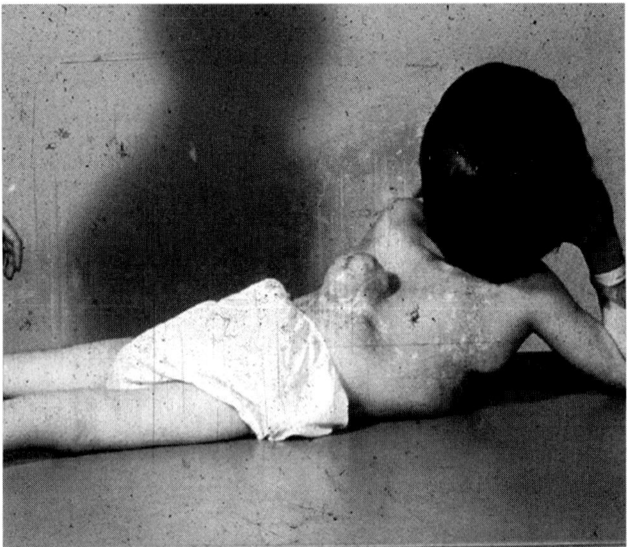

Figure 19–21: **This photograph shows a young boy with a severe, short kyphosis that has become a gibbus deformity measuring 180 degrees on x-ray film. Surgical treatment to relieve skin breakdown and the obvious positioning difficulties usually involves resection vertebrae in the apex of the deformity.**

  - The skeletally immature child poses a challenging problem. Spinal fusion may not be advisable because without spinal growth there will be inadequate room for the abdominal and thoracic organs resulting in pulmonary insufficiency.
    1. Instrumentation without fusion can buy time until the child is large enough for a definitive fusion.
    2. In very small children, apical wiring of posterior elements may be adequate. An extraperiosteal Luque wiring technique is required in most children older than 1 or 2 years.
    3. In older children and adolescents, fusion (to the pelvis) is usually possible at the time of the index procedure.
  - Spinal shortening may be required in severe deformities because the abdominal great vessels tether the kyphosis anteriorly. To shorten the spine in skeletally immature patients, partial excision of the periapical vertebrae with creation of a posterior tension band creates both immediate correction and the potential for gradual, long-term correction when the anterior column grows against the surgically tethered posterior elements. In severe, rigid curves, excision of the gibbus has been described with positive results.
  - Skin closure may be difficult, and plastic surgeons are often employed to raise local flaps to facilitate wound closure.

Ambulation and Use of Orthoses

A working knowledge of the gait cycle is necessary to understand how the many orthoses used in children with myelomeningocele work to facilitate ambulation (Box 19–13).

Gait Cycle

- The two main phases of the gait cycle, stance and swing, can each be broken into several parts.

Stance Phase

- *Stance phase* occurs anytime a foot is in contact with the ground. By convention the gait cycle begins in stance phase.
  - Stance begins with *heel strike,* with the knee extended and the hip slightly flexed, as the ankle dorsiflexors contract concentrically to keep the forefoot off the ground.
  - The limb begins to accept the weight of the body during *loading response* as the hip begins to extend and the ankle slowly plantar flexes against the eccentrically firing dorsiflexors.
  - *Midstance* occurs when the center of gravity is directly over the ankle and the foot is flat on the ground.
  - This is immediately followed by *terminal stance,* with dorsiflexion of the ankle against an eccentrically firing gastroc–soleus complex when the body's center of gravity moves forward.
  - The stance phase terminates with *toe off* when the now tensioned gastroc–soleus complex actively plantar flexes the ankle propelling the body forward.

Swing Phase

- *Swing phase* describes gait with the foot off of the ground.
  - *Initial swing* requires hip flexion, knee flexion, and ankle dorsiflexion to keep the forefoot clear of the ground.
  - In *midswing* and *terminal swing,* the knee and hip begin to extend, moving the foot forward and down while the ankle dorsiflexors fire to keep the forefoot clear of the ground. When heel strike occurs, swing phase ends and another cycle begins.

Orthoses

- The "simple" act of walking requires coordination of several major muscle groups across three joints, and a disturbance in any area will affect the gait pattern.

Box 19–13 Proper Use of Orthoses

Orthoses improve function by holding joints in a position advantageous for proper function. They can improve gait and function when used properly, even allowing ambulation in children with thoracic level paraplegia.

Orthoses cannot correct deformity; rather, they are designed to maintain a position passively achievable.

- Orthotics cannot correct a rigid deformity but rather are used to stabilize joints and replace muscles that are not functioning normally to improve, if not normalize, gait.
- Knowledge of the basic types of orthoses is important for all individuals involved in the care of children with myelomeningocele.
- As the size and complexity of the brace increases, so do the weight and the energy required to walk. In addition, bigger, bulkier braces, especially in older children, may adversely affect compliance.
- The AFO is one of the most commonly used braces in orthopaedics (Figure 19–22).
  - The basic *AFO* holds the foot in a neutral position at the cost of ankle and subtalar motion. However, for the child with a weak tibialis anterior muscle (innervated by L4-L5) who cannot clear the floor during swing phase, this brace can greatly improve gait.[71]
  - The *floor reaction AFO* is open posteriorly and closed anteriorly over the proximal tibia. This anterior pad creates a posteriorly directed force to the knee during stance, helping to compensate for a weak gastrocnemius and improving a crouch gait.
  - A variety of custom AFOs can be used to hold flexible or surgically corrected foot deformities in an advantageous position. These braces can be constructed to control dorsiflexion and plantar flexion, heel varus and valgus, and forefoot supination and pronation.

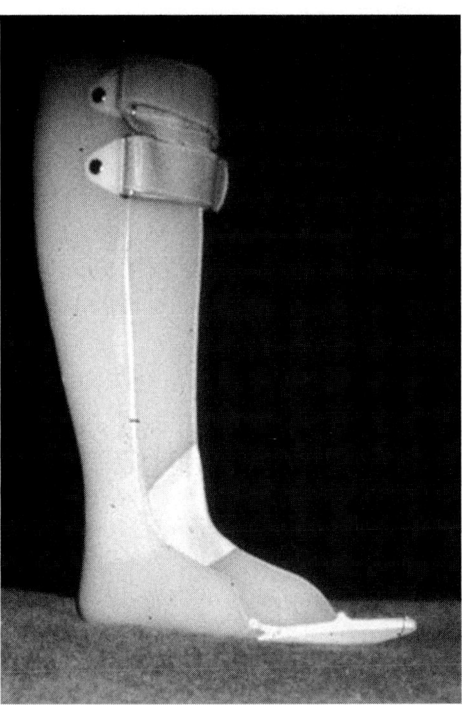

Figure 19–22: This solid AFO helps to control ankle equinus and, with the raised sides, can help to control ankle varus and valgus. Some models have hinged ankles, and most have straps crossing ankle and foot to hold the foot down.

- Children with weak quadriceps muscles (L3-L4) usually require help with knee stabilization and may benefit from a *knee–ankle–foot orthosis* (KAFO) (Figure 19–23). The quadriceps are important in gait both to extend the knee during the swing phase and to hold the knee straight during the stance phase. The KAFO can prevent unwanted knee flexion during stance with properly placed anterior pads and drop locks on the knee hinge.[71]
- The next stage of bracing, the *hip–knee–ankle–foot orthosis* (HKAFO), can help to position the legs of children with low or midlumbar motor levels and severe torsional problems (Figure 19–24). Some patients with profound quadriceps weakness may also benefit from the HKAFO.
- Weakness about the hip and a propensity toward hip flexion contractures in children with upper lumbar motor levels often makes the HKAFO less functional. In these cases, the *reciprocating gait orthosis* (RGO) is a better choice.
  - If L1 motor function is intact, the psoas major can flex the hip.
  - The RGO coordinates the motion of both legs so that when one hip is actively flexed the other passively extends.
- Thoracic level paraplegics have no volitional control of any muscles of ambulation and require the cumbersome *thoracic–hip–knee–ankle–foot orthosis* if they are to walk.
  - This brace supports the entire lower body and can be used as a stander or for walking if combined with Lofstrand crutches or a walker.

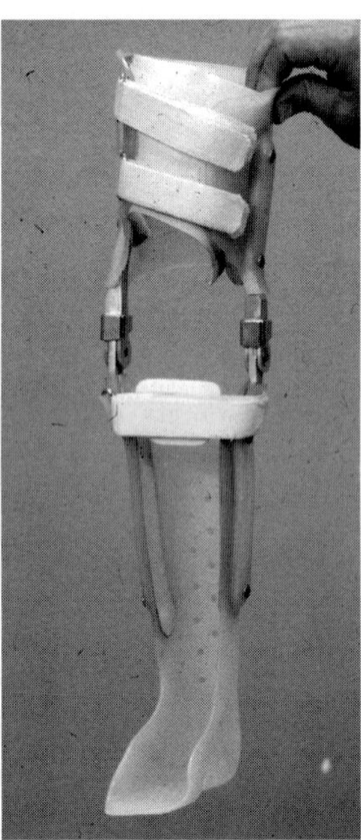

Figure 19–23: This KAFO helps to control both the knee and the ankle joints. The knee hinges can be locked or unlocked depending on the level of voluntary control of the knee.

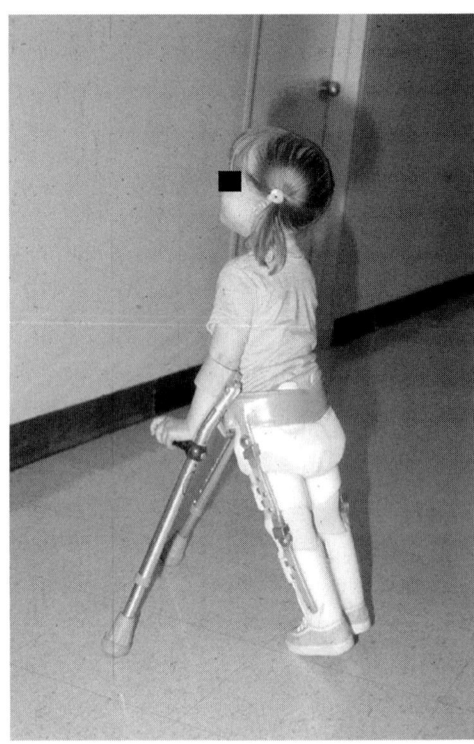

Figure 19–24: HKAFO. This brace helps to control the entire lower extremity and can facilitate ambulation in children with high lumbar lesions.

  - Another option for these children is the swivel walker, which converts the side-to-side motion of the thorax into forward motion with a swiveling base.[71]

Summary

- Myelomeningocele represents a fairly wide range of disease severity from the highly functional, ambulatory child with a sacral level lesion to the totally debilitated child with a thoracic level lesion.
- Treatment begins at, if not before, birth and requires constant vigilance from a multidisciplinary team that includes the orthopaedist among its many members.
- Treatment of deformity in this population needs to be individualized to the patient. The patient's functional, intellectual, and emotional development must all be factored into the equation with the deformity when deciding on appropriate treatment.
- Surgery has a high complication rate in this population, but unfortunately nonoperative measures are not effective for many of their problems.

References

1. National Center for Health Statistics (2000) Trends in spina bifida and anencephalus in the United States, 1991-2000. In: NCHS Health E-Stats. Hyattsville, MD: U.S. Department of Health and Human Services, Centers for Disease Control.

2. Nieto A, Mazon A, Pamies R, Lanuza A, Munoz A, Estornell F, Garcia-Ibarra F (2002) Efficacy of latex avoidance for primary prevention of latex sensitization in children with spina bifida. J Pediatr 140(3): 370-372.

   A good review article documenting the decrease in latex allergies in children with myelomeningocele when latex precautions are initiated at birth (or before).

3. Madersbacher H (2002) Neurogenic bladder dysfunction in patients with myelomeningocele. Curr Opin Urol 12(6): 469-472.

4. McCoy R (ed) (2002) Urological management of spina bifida (including management of urinary tract infections). Aust Fam Physician 31(1): 84-87.

5. Rudeberg A, Donati, F Kaiser G (1995) Psychosocial aspects in the treatment of children with myelomeningocele: An assessment after a decade. Eur J Pediatr 154(9 Suppl 4): S85-S89.

6. Seller MJ, Nevin NC (1984) Periconceptional vitamin supplementation and the prevention of neural tube defects in south-east England and Northern Ireland. J Med Genet 21(5): 325-330.

   One of the first studies to document the importance of periconceptional folic acid supplementation in reducing the incidence of neural tube defects.

7. Carter CO, Evans K (1973) Children of adult survivors with spina bifida cystica. Lancet 2(7835): 924-926.

8. Weinbaum PJ, Cassidy SB, Vintzileos AM, Campbell WA, Ciarleglio L, Nochimson DJ (1986) Prenatal detection of a neural tube defect after fetal exposure to valproic acid. Obstet Gynecol 67(3 Suppl): 31S-33S.

9. Laurence KM, Carter CO, David PA (1968) Major central nervous system malformations in South Wales: II—Pregnancy factors, seasonal variation, and social class effects. Br J Prev Soc Med 22(4): 212-222.

10. Pendleton HJ (1969) Acute folic acid deficiency of pregnancy associated with oral ulceration and anencephaly. Proc R Soc Med 62(8): 834.

    First article associating neural tube defects with folic acid metabolism.

11. American Academy of Pediatrics Committee on Genetics (1999) Folic acid for the prevention of neural tube defects. Pediatrics 104(2 Pt 1): 325-327.

    Position statement by the American Academy of Pediatrics recommending the routine use of folic acid in women considering child birth and the Food and Drug Administration's fortification of grain products with folic acid.

12. Honein MA, Paulozzi LJ, Mathews TJ, Erickson JD, Wong LY (2001) Impact of folic acid fortification of the U.S. food supply on the occurrence of neural tube defects. Jama 285(23): 2981-2986.

    Major study relating the drop in the rate of neural tube defects to the initiation of folic acid fortification of bread in the United States.

13. Erickson JD (2002) Folic acid and prevention of spina bifida and anencephaly: 10 years after the U.S. Public Health Service recommendation (Introduction). Morbid Mortal Week Rep 51(RR-13): 1-3.

14. Rintoul NE, Sutton LN, Hubbard AM, Cohen B, Melchionni J, Pasquariello PS, Adzick NS (2002) A new look at myelomeningoceles: functional level, vertebral level, shunting, and the implications for fetal intervention. Pediatrics 109(3): 409-413.

15. Tulipan N, Hernanz-Schulman M, Lowe LH, Bruner JP (1999) Intrauterine myelomeningocele repair reverses preexisting hindbrain herniation. Pediatr Neurosurg 31(3): 137-142.

    Important article documenting the success of intrauterine repair of myelomeningocele in reducing Chiari malformations. This and other articles have shown a reduction in the incidence of hydrocephalus requiring shunting.

16. Alenius H, Palosuo T, Kelly K, Kurup V, Reunala T, Makinen-Kiljunen S, Turjanmaa K, Fink J (1993) IgE reactivity to 14-kD and 27-kD natural rubber proteins in latex-allergic children with spina bifida and other congenital anomalies. Int Arch Allergy Immunol 102(1): 61-66.

17. Degenhardt P, Golla S, Wahn F, Niggemann B (2001) Latex allergy in pediatric surgery is dependent on repeated operations in the first year of life. J Pediatr Orthop 1(4): 401-403.

18. Anderson TE, Drummond DS, Breed AL, Taylor CA (1981) Malignant hyperthermia in myelomeningocele: A previously unreported association. J Pediatr Orthop 1(4): 401–403.

19. Yates JR, Ferguson-Smith MA, Shenkin A, Guzman-Rodriguez R, White M, Clark BJ (1987) Is disordered folate metabolism the basis for the genetic predisposition to neural tube defects? Clin Genet 31(5): 279-287.

    This is the first article to suggest that a role for a defect in folate metabolism, and not just dietary intake, may contribute to neural tube defects.

20. Aubry MC, Aubry JP, Dommergues M (2003) Sonographic prenatal diagnosis of central nervous system abnormalities. Childs Nerv Syst 19(7-8): 391-402.

21. Blaas HG, Eik-Nes SH, Isaksen CV (2000) The detection of spina bifida before 10 gestational weeks using two- and three-dimensional ultrasound. Ultrasound Obstet Gynecol 16(1): 25-29.

22. Adzick NS, Sutton LN, Crombleholme TM, Flake AW (1998) Successful fetal surgery for spina bifida. Lancet 352(9141): 1675-1676.

23. Bruner JP, Tulipan N, Paschall RL, Boehm FH, Walsh WF, Silva SR, Hernanz-Schulman M, Lowe LH, Reed GW (1999) Fetal surgery for myelomeningocele and the incidence of shunt-dependent hydrocephalus. JAMA 282(19): 1819-1825.

24. Broughton N (1998) The hip. In: Menelaus' Orthopaedic Management of Spina Bifida Cystica (Broughton N, Menelaus M, eds). Philadelphia: WB Saunders, 135-144.

    Menelaus's classic textbook on spina bifida is a must read for anyone taking care of children with this disorder. Several chapters are cited in this bibliography, but the hip chapter is particularly helpful in organizing a controversial and confusing subject.

25. Turner A (1985) Hand function in children with myelomeningocele. J Bone Joint Surg Br 67(2): 268-272.

26. Mazur JM, Menelaus MB, Hudson I, Stillwell A (1986) Hand function in patients with spina bifida cystica. J Pediatr Orthop 6(4): 442-447.
   A case series of 143 patients in whom extensive testing of upper extremity function that revealed better function in lumbar and sacral level lesions than in thoracic level lesions. This study also found a strong negative correlation between hydrocephalus and upper hand function.

27. Abery CA, Galvin JL (1998) Physiotherapy and occupational therapy. In: Menelaus' Orthopaedic Management of Spina Bifida Cystica (Broughton N, Menelaus M, eds). Philadelphia: WB Saunders, pp 77-93.

28. Broughton NS, Menelaus MB, Cole WG, Shurtleff DB (1993) The natural history of hip deformity in myelomeningocele. J Bone Joint Surg Br 75(5): 760-763.
   A review of more than 1000 children with myelomeningocele found that, contrary to common belief, there was no associating between hip contractures–instability and muscle imbalance.

29. Fraser RK, Bourke HM, Broughton NS, Menelaus MB (1995) Unilateral dislocation of the hip in spina bifida: A long-term follow-up. J Bone Joint Surg Br 77(4): 615-619.

30. Mazur JM, Shurtleff D, Menelaus M, Colliver J (1989) Orthopaedic management of high-level spina bifida: Early walking compared with early use of a wheelchair. J Bone Joint Surg Am 71(1): 56-61.

31. Lee EH, Carroll NC (1985) Hip stability and ambulatory status in myelomeningocele. J Pediatr Orthop 5(5): 522-527.
   Review of 32 ambulatory children with myelomeningocele who underwent a hip stabilization procedure for subluxated or dislocated hips. The authors recommend this treatment plan because at a 4-year follow-up 83% of the hips were still stable and 78% of the children were community ambulators.

32. Bazih J, Gross RH (1981) Hip surgery in the lumbar level myelomeningocele patient. J Pediatr Orthop 1(4): 405-411.
   Review of 74 ambulatory patients with myelomeningocele that found that reduction of a dislocated hip did not improve function, contrary to the findings in Lee and Carroll's paper.[31]

33. Trivedi J, Thomson JD, Slakey JB, Banta JV, Jones PW (2002) Clinical and radiographic predictors of scoliosis in patients with myelomeningocele. J Bone Joint Surg Am 84A(8): 1389-1394.
   This retrospective study of 141 children found that about 50% of cases of myelomeningocele develop scoliosis. Contrary to conventional wisdom, they found that more than 40% of curves developed after 9 years and that they continued to develop until the age of 15. They recommended redefining scoliosis in this group as curves greater than 20 degrees because smaller curves tended to spontaneously regress.

34. Heeg M, Broughton NS, Menelaus MB (1998) Bilateral dislocation of the hip in spina bifida: A long-term follow-up study. J Pediatr Orthop 18(4): 434-436.
   In this minimum 10-year follow-up review, the authors found that hips with good range of motion and a level pelvis were more important for ambulation than a reduced bilateral hip dislocation.

35. Breed AL, Healy PM (1982) The midlumbar myelomeningocele hip: Mechanism of dislocation and treatment. J Pediatr Orthop 2(1): 15-24.

36. Tosi LL, Buck BD, Nason SS, McKay DW (1996) Dislocation of hip in myelomeningocele: The McKay hip stabilization. J Bone Joint Surg Am 78(5): 664-673.

37. Lindseth RE (2001) Myelomeningocele. In: Lovell and Winter's Pediatric Orthopaedics (Morrissy RT, Weinstein SL, eds). Philadelphia: Lippincott Williams & Wilkins, pp 601-632.

38. Phillips DP, Lindseth RE (1992) Ambulation after transfer of adductors, external oblique, and tensor fascia lata in myelomeningocele. J Pediatr Orthop 12(6): 712-717.
   This retrospective review on 47 patients undergoing muscle transfers about the hip found gait improvement in 37 of 41 patients available at a 4-1/2-year follow-up with reduced requirements for bracing and ambulatory aids.

39. Menelaus M (1998) The knee. In: Menelaus' Orthopaedic Management of Spina Bifida Cystica (Broughton N, Menelaus M, eds). Philadelphia: WB Saunders, pp 129-134.

40. Dias LS (1982) Surgical management of knee contractures in myelomeningocele. J Pediatr Orthop 2(2): 127-131.
   The authors report their surgical results on 38 knee contractures and recommend radical flexor releases for flexion deformities and a V-Y quadriceps plasty for extension deformities. Prolonged splinting postoperatively is emphasized to prevent recurrence, especially for flexion deformities.

41. Sandhu PS, Broughton NS, Menelaus MB (1995) Tenotomy of the ligamentum patellae in spina bifida: management of limited flexion range at the knee. J Bone Joint Surg Br 77(5): 832-833.

42. Williams JJ, Graham GP, Dunne KB, Menelaus MB (1993) Late knee problems in myelomeningocele. J Pediatr Orthop 13(6): 701-703.

43. Greene WB (1999) Treatment of hip and knee problems in myelomeningocele. Instr Course Lect 48: 563-574.

44. Broughton NS, Graham G, Menelaus MB (1994) The high incidence of foot deformity in patients with high-level spina bifida. J Bone Joint Surg Br 76(4): 548-550.
   This consecutive series of 124 children found a nearly 90% incidence of foot deformity in spina bifida, of which nearly 80% underwent operative correction. Interestingly, spasticity was not present in most of the feet and was uncommon in equinus feet (17%).

45. Rodrigues RC, Dias LS (1992) Calcaneus deformity in spina bifida: Results of anterolateral release. J Pediatr Orthop 12(4): 461-464.

46. Fraser RK, Hoffman EB (1991) Calcaneus deformity in the ambulant patient with myelomeningocele. J Bone Joint Surg Br 73(6): 994-997.

47. Bliss DG, Menelaus MB (1986) The results of transfer of the tibialis anterior to the heel in patients who have a myelomeningocele. J Bone Joint Surg Am 68(8): 1258-1264.
    The authors report long-term results on 25 patients with tibialis anterior transfer for calcaneus deformity and found less than 10% of the transferred muscles were functioning in a plantigrade foot. The best outcomes were found in children older than 5 years undergoing surgery without spasticity.

48. Janda JP, Skinner SR, Barto PS (1984) Posterior transfer of tibialis anterior in low-level myelodysplasia. Dev Med Child Neurol 26(1): 100-103.

49. Stevens PM, Toomey E (1988) Fibular–Achilles tenodesis for paralytic ankle valgus. J Pediatr Orthop 8(2): 169-175.

50. Aronson DD, Middleton DL (1991) Extra-articular subtalar arthrodesis with cancellous bone graft and internal fixation for children with myelomeningocele. Dev Med Child Neurol 33(3): 232-240.

51. Lee Y, Grogan T, Mosely C (1990) Extra-articular arthrodesis in myelodysplasia. Orthop Trans 14: 590.

52. Nagarkatti DG, Banta JV, Thomson JD (2000) Charcot arthropathy in spina bifida. J Pediatr Orthop 20(1): 82-87.
    This multicenter study undertook to document the prevalence of Charcot arthropathy in spina bifida patients. They found this complication in only about 1% of cases.

53. Barnett J, Menelaus M (1998) Pressure sores and pathological fractures. In: Menelaus' Orthopaedic Management of Spina Bifida Cystica (Broughton N, Menelaus M, eds). Philadelphia: WB Saunders, pp 51-65.

54. Bowman RM, McLone DG, Grant JA, Tomita T, Ito JA (2001) Spina bifida outcome: A 25-year prospective. Pediatr Neurosurg 34(3): 114-120.
    This article documents one institution's experience with spina bifida into adulthood. At a 25-year follow-up, these patients had undergone many surgeries and had a mortality rate of nearly 25%. The authors stress the importance of creating a network of care for these complicated patients as they enter adulthood.

55. Samuelsson L, Eklof O (1988) Scoliosis in myelomeningocele. Acta Orthop Scand 59(2): 122-127.

56. Samuelsson L, Bergstrom K, Thuomas KA, Hemmingsson A, Wallensten R (1987) MR imaging of syringohydromyelia and Chiari malformations in myelomeningocele patients with scoliosis. AJNR Am J Neuroradiol 8(3): 539-546.

57. Hall PV, Campbell RL, Kalsbeck JE (1975) Meningomyelocele and progressive hydromyelia: Progressive paresis in myelodysplasia. J Neurosurg 43(4): 457-463.

58. Carstens C, Paul K, Niethard FU, Pfeil J (1991) Effect of scoliosis surgery on pulmonary function in patients with myelomeningocele. J Pediatr Orthop 11(4): 459-464.
    This retrospective review demonstrated improvements in pulmonary function in 8 of 13 patients despite the requirement for anterior thoracic surgery in many of them.

59. Banta JV, Park SM (1983) Improvement in pulmonary function in patients having combined anterior and posterior spine fusion for myelomeningocele scoliosis. Spine 8(7): 765-770.

60. Muller EB, Nordwall A (1994) Brace treatment of scoliosis in children with myelomeningocele. Spine 19(2): 151-155.
    In this study out of Sweden, the authors conclude that brace treatment is a viable option in this population because 13 of 21 patients completed an average of 2.5 years of brace treatment without further progression of their curve.

61. Torode I, Dickens D (1998) The spine. In: Menelaus' Orthopaedic Management of Spina Bifida Cystica (Broughton N, Menelaus M, eds). Philadelphia: WB Saunders, pp 145-167.

62. Banit DM, Iwinski HJ Jr, Talwalkar V, Johnson M (2001) Posterior spinal fusion in paralytic scoliosis and myelomeningocele. J Pediatr Orthop 21(1): 117-125.
    This review of the authors' experience with 50 posterior spinal fusions for scoliosis using mostly segmental instrumentation had a complication rate of nearly 50% with an average of 1.5 procedures per patient. The deep infection rate was 8%, and the pseudarthrosis rate was 16%. Although these reports are improved from nonsegmental techniques, the authors still recommend anterior and posterior fusion to reduce the pseudarthrosis rate.

63. Stella G, Ascani E, Cervellati S, Bettini N, Scarsi M, Vicini M, Magillo P, Carbone M (1998) Surgical treatment of scoliosis associated with myelomeningocele. Eur J Pediatr Surg 8(Suppl 1): 22-25.

64. Parsch D, Geiger F, Brocai DR, Lang RD, Carstens C (2001) Surgical management of paralytic scoliosis in myelomeningocele. J Pediatr Orthop B 10(1): 10-17.

65. Geiger F, Parsch D, Carstens C (1999) Complications of scoliosis surgery in children with myelomeningocele. Eur Spine J 8(1): 22-26.

66. Mazur J, Menelaus MB, Dickens DR, Doig WG (1986) Efficacy of surgical management for scoliosis in myelomeningocele: Correction of deformity and alteration of functional status. J Pediatr Orthop 6(5): 568-575.
    The authors report the results of 49 spinal fusions for scoliosis in patients with myelomeningocele. They found that sitting balance was improved in approximately 70% of cases involving posterior fusion but in only 28% of isolated anterior cases. Ambulation was adversely affected in most cases involving anterior fusion and in 27% of cases involving isolated posterior fusion.

67. Osebold WR, Mayfield JK, Winter RB, Moe JH (1982) Surgical treatment of paralytic scoliosis associated with myelomeningocele. J Bone Joint Surg Am 64(6): 841-856.

68. Eckstein HB, Vora RM (1972) Spinal osteotomy for severe kyphosis in children with myelomeningocele. J Bone Joint Surg Br 54(2): 328-333.

69. Houfani B, Meyer P, Merckx J, Roure P, Padovani JP, Fontaine G, Carli P (2001) Postoperative sudden death in two adolescents with myelomeningocele and unrecognized arrhythmogenic right ventricular dysplasia. Anesthesiology 95(1): 257-259.

70. Winston K, Hall J, Johnson D, Micheli L (1977) Acute elevation of intracranial pressure following transection of nonfunctional spinal cord. Clin Orthop 128: 41-44.

71. Phillips D (1998) Orthotics. In: Menelaus' Orthopaedic Management of Spina Bifida Cystica (Broughton N, Menelaus M, eds). Philadelphia: WB Saunders, pp 67-76.

Index

Page numbers followed by "b" indicate boxes; "f," figures; "t," tables.

A

Abdominal injury trauma, 41
Abdominal reflexes, 31
Abuse, child, 111b
Accessory navicular, 216–217
Acetabular fractures, 87, 88f, 133–134, 135f
Achondroplasia, 281, 354
  clinical features, 354–355
  medical problems, 356
  orthopaedic considerations, 356–357
  radiographic findings, 355–356
Acquired coxa vara, 261
  clinical presentation, 262
  epidemiology, 262
  etiology, 262
  natural history, 262
  radiographic findings, 262
  treatment, 262
Acromioclavicular joint, injuries around, 80, 81f
Acromioclavicular separation, 146
Acute osteochondral fractures, 144
Adduction contracture, 423, 425f
Adolescent Blount disease, 203
Adolescent idiopathic scoliosis, 272–273
  bracing, 273, 274f
  observation, 273
  surgery, 273–276, 277f
  treatment options, 273
    observation and bracing, 273
    surgery, 273–276, 279f
Aggrecan, 9
Aggressive fibromatosis, 330–332
Aitken classification, 258, 259f, 259t
Albright's syndrome, 312
Alkaline phosphatase, 8
Allen's test, 166b
Amputations in upper extremity disorders, 171–173
Aneurysmal bone cyst, 316–318
Angiomatosis, 328
Ankle
  cerebral palsy and, 425, 432, 440, 445–448
  deformity and neuromuscular disorders, 492
  muscular dystrophies and surgery on, 468
  musculoskeletal examination, 27, 28f
  orthoses, 432
  sports medicine, 152–154
Ankylosing spondylitis, juvenile, 412
Anterior cruciate ligament
  injuries, 100–101
  tears, 150–151
Anterior spinal release or fusion, 449–450
Apical ectodermal ridge, 4
Apical vertebra, 270
Apoptosis, 8–9
Appendicular skeleton, 3
Arnold-Chiari malformation, 486–487
Arteriovenous malformations, 327
Arthritis
    chronic arthritis
Arthritis (*Continued*)
  classifications, 407–408
  connective tissue diseases with associated
    chronic arthritis, 413–414
  juvenile psoriatic arthritis, 411
  juvenile rheumatoid arthritis, 409–411
  poststreptococcal reactive arthritis, 412
  reactive arthritis, 412
  septic arthritis, 176, 408–409
  transient synovitis *versus* septic arthritis, 408–409
  viral arthritis, 413
Arthrogryposis multiplex congenita, 471–473
  clinical features, 473–474
  definition, 471–473
  diagnosis, 474
  elbow joint, 479–481
  etiology, 474
  foot involvement, 476–477
  hand, 481
  hip joint, 477–478
  knee joint, 477
  lower limbs, 476–478
  management of, 475
  physiotherapy, 478
  prognosis, 474–475
  scoliosis, 475–476
  shoulder joint, 478–479, 480f
  upper limbs, 478–481
  wrist, 481
Arthropathy associated with inflammatory bowel
    disease, 412
Articular cartilage components, 404b
Articular joint development, 4
Asymmetrical tonic neck reflex, 30–31f
Atlantoaxial instability, 121–124
Atlantoaxial rotary instability, 122
Atlas fractures, 119–120
Avascular necrosis, 112f, 237
Avulsion fractures, 132–133
Axial skeleton, 3

B

Babinski reflex, 31f
Back pain, 285–286, 287b
Baclofen and cerebral palsy, 428
Barlow test, 228f
Benzodiazepines and cerebral palsy, 428
Blount disease, 201–202, 203f
Bone cysts
  aneurysmal, 316–318
  simple, 314–316
  unicameral, 314–316
Bones
  carpal bone fractures, 54–55
  formation or ossification, 4
  fracture scans, 42
  growth and development, 6
    cell proliferation, 6
    chondrocyte hypertrophy, 6–7
Bones (*Continued*)
    collagens in the growth plate, 7
    growth plate chondrocytes, life cycle of, 6
    growth plate regulation, 6
    growth plate zones, 6
    growth slowdown lines, 7f
    long bones, growth of, 6
    parameters influencing rate of growth, 6
    parathyroid hormone-related peptide, 6
    physeal closure, 7
    physiological epiphysiodesis, 7
    skeletal maturity, 7
    unanswered questions about growth, 6
    vascular invasion, 6
  long bones, anatomy of, 5
  metabolic disorders of. *See* Bones, metabolic
    disorders of
  technetium-99m bone scan, 249–250
Bones, metabolic disorders of, 386
  calcium homeostasis, 386
  hyperparathyroidism, 388–400
  hypervitaminosis A, 400
  hypervitaminosis D, 400–401
  hypoparathyroidism, 400
  hypophosphatasia, 392
    clinical features, 392–393
    radiographic findings, 392–393
    treatment, 393
  idiopathic juvenile osteoporosis, 397
  mineral metabolism, 386–388
  osteogenesis imperfecta, 393–394
    clinical features, 394, 395f
    diagnosis, 394–395
    radiographic findings, 394, 395f
    Shapiro classification, 394b
    Sillence classification, 394b
    treatment, 395–397
  osteopetrosis, 398, 399f
  osteoporosis, 397
  parathyroid disorders, 398–400
  parathyroid hormone, 387
  phosphorus homeostasis, 386
  renal osteodystrophy, 390
    clinical findings, 390–391
    radiographic features, 391
    treatment, 391–392
  rickets, 388, 389b
    clinical features, 389
    diagnosis, 390
    laboratory findings, 389
    radiographic findings, 389–390,
      391f
    treatment, 391–392
    vitamin D-resistant rickets, 389
  scurvy, 401
  serum calcium, 387–398
  vitamin D, 387
Bone tumors
  bone origin, tumors of, 294–311

Bone tumors (*Continued*)
- common locations of pediatric bone tumors, 292t
- musculoskeletal infections, 346, 347f
- upper extremity disorders, 180

Borrelia burgdorferi, 344
Botulinum toxin A and cerebral palsy, 428–430
Boutonniere deformity, 169
Brachial plexus palsy, 190–191
- diagnosis, 192
- management, 192–193
- microsurgery, 193
- natural history, 193
- shoulder weakness and deformity, 193–194

Burns of the upper extremities, 173–174
Burr-down technique, 296–297
Burst fractures, 124–125, 126f

C
Cadence, 13
Caffey disease, 44
Calcaneovalgus deformities, 493–494
Calcaneovalgus foot, 213
Calcaneus, fractures of, 110
Calcaneus deformities, 493–494
Calcium homeostasis, 386
Camptodactyly, 187
Capillary malformations, 327
Capitellum and trochlea, articular fractures of, 76
Carpal bone fractures, 54–55
Cartilaginous origin, tumors of, 302–307
Cavus deformities, 494–495, 496f
Central deficiencies and upper extremity disorders, 183–184, 185f
Cerebral palsy, 188–190, 279
- adduction contracture, 423, 425f
- ankle, 425, 440, 445–448
- ankle-foot orthoses, 432
- anterior spinal release or fusion, 449–450
- assistive devices, 431, 432f
- asymmetrical tonic neck reflex, 421
- ataxic, 420
- baclofen, 428
- balance and coordination, 422
- basal ganglia, 422
- benzodiazepines, 428
- botulinum toxin A, 428–430
- cerebellar dysfunction, 422
- classification, 419–420
- clinical evaluation, 421–425
- coexisting medical problems, 419
- common gait deviations in cerebral palsy, 439–440
- dantrolene sodium, 428
- definition, 418, 419b
- diagnosis, 418
- dorsal rhizotomy, 430
- dyskinetic, 420
- epidemiology, 418
- equinovalgus deformities, 447–448, 449f
- equinovarus deformities, 446–447, 448f
- equinus deformities, 425, 428f, 445
- etiology, 418
- extensor thrust, 422
- femoral rotational examination, 423, 425f
- flexion contracture, 423–424, 426f
- foot, 425, 429f, 440, 445–448
- foot placement reaction, 422
- gait, 437–440
- Gallant reflex, 421

Cerebral palsy (*Continued*)
- gastroc-soleus lengthening, 445, 448f
- geographical classification, 420–421, 432–437
- grasp reflex, 421
- hallux valgus, 448
- head and trunk righting, 421
- hip and, 423, 439, 441–444, 445f
- history, 421
- iliopsoas, 423
- infantile reflexes, 421
- instrumented motion analysis, 439
- intramuscular injections, 428–431
- intrathecal baclofen, 430–431
- knee, 423–425, 439–442, 444–445, 446f
- Landau reaction, 421
- lateral prop reaction, 422
- lower extremity, 441–448
- management of spasticity, 426
- Moro reflex, 421
- musculoskeletal assessment, 422–423
- neurological examination, 421
- neuromuscular hip dysplasia, 434–436
- neuromuscular scoliosis of the spine, 436–437
- normal gait in infants and toddlers, 437–438
- oral medications, 426–428
- orthoses, 431–432, 433f, 434f
- parachute response, 422
- patterns of injury to the central nervous system, 419
- phenol, 430
- physical and occupational therapy, 431–432
- physiological classification, 420
- posterior spinal fusion, 448–449, 450f
- postural reactions, 421
- prognosis for ambulation in children with developmental delay, 438
- protective reactions, 422
- pyramidal dysfunction, 422
- range of motion, 423
- rectus femoris contracture, 424, 426f
- risk factors, 418–419
- rotational examination, 424–425, 427f
- segmental rolling, 421
- sensory function, 423
- spasticity, treatment of, 426–432
- spinal orthoses, 432
- spine, 448–450
- Staheli test, 423, 424f
- surgical treatment, 440–451
- symmetrical tonic neck reflex, 421
- Thomas test, 423, 424f
- tibia, 423–425
- tizanidine, 428
- tone reduction, 426
- tonic labyrinthine reflex, 421
- upper extremity, 423, 450–451
- upper extremity orthoses, 432, 434f

Cervical spine, 116, 117b
- deformities, 286–288
- injuries, 119–123
- musculoskeletal examination of, 18f

Charcot arthropathy, 498–499
Child abuse, 111b
Childhood polymyositis, 414
Chondroblastoma, 304–305
Chondrodysplasia punctata, 375
- clinical features, 375
- medical problems, 376
- orthopaedic considerations, 376

Chondrodysplasia punctata (*Continued*)
- radiographic findings, 375–376

Chondroectodermal dysplasia, 360
- clinical features, 360
- medical problems, 360
- orthopaedic considerations, 361
- radiographic findings, 360, 361b

Chondrogenesis, 8
Chondromyxoid fibroma, 305
Chronic arthritis
- classifications, 407–408
- connective tissue diseases with associated chronic arthritis, 413–414

Circulation and upper extremity disorders, 160
Clavicle shaft fractures, 80
Cleft hand, characteristics of, 184t
Cleidocranial dysplasia, 379
- clinical features, 379–380
- orthopaedic considerations, 380
- radiographic findings, 380

Clinodactyly, 187
Clubfoot, 208–211, 495–496
Cobb angle, 269
Compartment syndrome, 45, 170
Compression fractures in spine trauma, 123–124
Congenital, 1
Congenital anomalies and upper extremity disorders, 181–188
Congenital coxa vara, 257
- Aitken classification, 258, 259f, 259t
- classification, 258–259
- clinical presentation, 259–260
- etiology, 259
- Gillespie classification, 258–259, 260f
- radiographic findings, 260, 261f
- treatment, 260–261, 262f

Congenital kyphosis, 283
Congenital pseudarthrosis of the tibia, 204–205
Congenital scoliosis, 281–283
Congenital vertical talus, 213, 214f
Connective tissue diseases with associated chronic arthritis, 413–414
Contractures and musculoskeletal examinations, 17
Coronal limb abnormalities, 199–206
Coxa vara, 255
- acquired coxa vara, 261
  - clinical presentation, 262
  - epidemiology, 262
  - etiology, 262
  - natural history, 262
  - radiographic findings, 262
  - treatment, 262
- congenital coxa vara, 257
  - Aitken classification, 258, 259f, 259t
  - classification, 258–259
  - clinical presentation, 259–260
  - etiology, 259
  - Gillespie classification, 258–259, 260f
  - radiographic findings, 260, 261f
  - treatment, 260–261, 262f
- developmental coxa vara, 255
  - clinical presentation, 255
  - epidemiology, 255
  - etiology, 255
  - natural history, 256
  - radiographic findings, 255–256, 257f
  - treatment, 256–257, 260f
- femoral anteversion, 263

Cozen fractures, 102–103b

Curly toe, 220
Cysts
  bone cysts
    aneurysmal, 316–318.
    simple, 314–316
    unicameral, 314–316
  epidermal inclusion cysts, 179
  upper extremity disorders, 177, 179

D
Dantrolene sodium and cerebral palsy, 428
Deep tendon reflexes, 28
Deep vein thrombosis, 45
Deformation, 1
Deformity, 1, 17
Delbert classification, 86b
Developmental, 1
Developmental coxa vara, 255
  clinical presentation, 255
  epidemiology, 255
  etiology, 255
  natural history, 256
  radiographic findings, 255–256, 257f
  treatment, 256–257, 258f
Developmental dysplasia and dislocation of the hip, 225
  avascular necrosis, 237
  Barlow test, 228f
  clinical presentation, 227–230
  etiology, 226–227
  hip development in developmental dysplasia of the hip, 226
  incidence, 226–227
  infants, 228–229, 230f, 232–234
  Klisic test, 230f
  magnetic resonance imaging, 231
  natural history, 232–233
  neonate, 227–228
  newborns, 233–236
  normal hip development, 225–226
  older than 2 years, 235–236
  Ortolani maneuver, 228f
  pathophysiology, 225–227
  radiography, 230–231, 232f
  residual acetabular dysplasia, 236–237
  risk factors, 226–227
  screening criteria, 231–232
  sequelae and complications, 236–237
  6 months to 2 years, 234–235
  treatment, 233–236
  ultrasound, 230
  walking child, 229–230
Developmental reflexes, 28
Development and growth. *See* Growth and development
Diastematomyelia, 487, 488f
Diastrophic dysplasia, 361–362
  clinical features, 362
  medical problems, 363
  orthopaedic considerations, 363
  radiographic findings, 362–363
Discoid lateral meniscus, 148–150
Disruption, 1
Distal radius and ulna fractures, 55–57f, 58f
Distal radius and ulna injuries, 57–59f
Distal tibial transition fractures, 107f, 108f
Dorsal rhizotomy, 430
Down's (trisomy 21) syndrome, 287–288
Duchenne muscular dystrophy, 280, 466–467
Dyschondrosteosis (Leri-Weill syndrome), 378
  clinical features, 378
  diagnosis, 379
  orthopaedic considerations, 379
  radiographic findings, 378–379
Dysplasia, 1
  developmental dysplasia and dislocation of the hip. *See* Developmental dysplasia and dislocation of the hip
  neuromuscular hip dysplasia, 434–436
  osteofibrous dysplasia, 312–314
  residual acetabular dysplasia, 236–237
  skeletal. *See* Skeletal dysplasias
Dysplasia epiphysealis hemimelica, 304
Dystrophin, 458

E
Elbow
  arthrogryposis multiplex congenita, 479–481
  dislocations, 74f–75
  fractures, *See* Elbow fractures
  musculoskeletal examinations, 21, 23f
  thrower's elbow, 140
Elbow fractures, 68–69
  capitellum and trochlea, articular fractures of, 76
  elbow dislocations, 74f–75
  lateral condyle fractures, 71f–73
  lateral epicondyle fractures, 76
  medial condyle fractures, 76
  medial epicondyle fractures, 73f–74
  nursemaid's elbow, 75, 76f
  rare elbow injuries, 76, 77f
  supracondylar fractures, 68–71f
  T-condylar distal humerus fractures, 76, 77f
Eilis-van Creveld syndrome, 360–361
Embryology, 2–3
  neuromuscular disorders, 484, 485f
  spinal disorders, 265–266
  upper extremity disorders, 181
Enchondroma, 180, 305–307
Eosinophilic granuloma, 346
Epidermal inclusion cysts, 179
Epstein-Barr virus, 413
Equinovalgus deformities, 447–448, 449f
Equinovarus deformities, 446–447, 448f
Equinus deformities, 425, 428f, 445
Ewing sarcoma, 293b, 320–323
Exostosis, 180, 302–304
Extensor tendon injuries, 168

F
Fat embolism, 46
Felon, 175
Femoral anteversion, 263
Femoral epiphysis, slipped capital. *See* Slipped capital femoral epiphysis
Femoral rotational examinations, 423, 425f
Femur growth and development, 11
Femur injuries, 90t, 90f–93f, 94f
  evaluation, 92
  5–10 years, 93f
  management, 92f
  older than 11 years, 93, 94f
  treatment, 92–93t
  younger than 5 years with an isolated injury, 92–93
Fibroma, 308–311
Fibromatosis, 330
Fibromatosis, aggressive, 330–332
Fibrous cortical defect, 308–311
Fibrous dysplasia, 311–312
Fibrous origin, tumors of, 179, 308–314
Fibrous tissue origin, tumors of, 330–332
Fibula, 11
Fibula hemimelia, 205
Fifth metatarsal fractures, 154–155, 156f
Finger deformities, mallet, 49–50f, 51f, 168–169
Fingertip amputations, 50–51
Fingertip injuries, 170–171, 172f
Flatfoot (planovalgus), 211
Flexible planovalgus foot, 211–213
Flexion-distraction injuries, 124, 125f
Flexor tendon injuries, 167–168
Flexor tenosynovitis, 175–176
Floating knee, 112f
Foot, 110–111
  ankle-foot orthoses, 432
  arthrogryposis multiplex congenita and, 476–477
  calcaneovalgus foot, 213
  calcaneus, fractures of, 110
  cerebral palsy and, 425, 429f, 432, 440, 445–448
  deformities, 206–218, 495
  growth, 12
  ingrown toenail, 220
  lesser toe deformities, 220
  metatarsals, fractures of, 111
  midfoot, fractures of, 110–111
  midfoot sprains, 154–155
  muscular dystrophies and surgery, 468
  musculoskeletal examinations, 27, 28f
  musculoskeletal infections, 345, 346b, 346f
  neuromuscular disorders, 493
  phalanges, fractures of, 111
  talus, fractures of, 110
Foot cavus, 217–218
Foot pain, 218–220
Forearm
  fractures. *See* Wrist and forearm fractures
  musculoskeletal examinations, 21–22, 23f, 24f
Foreign bodies and upper extremity disorders, 177
Fractures, 36–38f, 39, 42f, 44
  acetabular fractures, 87, 88f, 133–134, 135f
  acute osteochondral fractures, 144
  altered fracture patterns, 36
  arthrogram, 42
  atlas fractures, 119–120
  avulsion fractures, 132–133
  bone scans, 42
  calcaneus, 110
  carpal bone fractures, 54–55
  classification, 38, 39f, 42
  clavicle shaft fractures, 80
  in compression, 36, 37f, 123–124
  computerized tomography, 42
  Cozen fractures, 102–103b
  definition, 42
  distal radius and ulna fractures, 55–57f, 58f
  distal tibial transition fractures, 107f, 108f
  elbow. *See* Elbow fractures
  fifth metatarsal fractures, 154–155, 156f
  foot injuries, 110–111
    calcaneus, fractures of, 110
    metatarsals, fractures of, 111
    midfoot, fractures of, 110–111
    phalanges, fractures of, 49f, 111
    talus, fractures of, 110
  forearm. *See* Wrist and forearm fractures
  growth plate injury, 42–43f

Fractures (*Continued*)
hand injuries
carpal bone fractures, 54–55
metacarpal fractures, 52–54f
phalangeal fractures, 49f
humeral shaft fractures, 76–77, 78f
imaging of pediatric fractures, 42f–43f
knee, 94–107f, 108f
Cozen fractures, 102–103b
distal tibial transition fractures, 107f, 108f
isolated tibia shaft fractures, 104–106f
patella, fractures of, 99–100f, 101f, 102f, 148
proximal tibia metaphyseal fractures, 102–103, 104f
proximal tibia physeal fractures, 103–104f
tibial and fibular shaft fractures, 104, 105f
tibial spine, fractures of, 94–98
classification, 94–95f
complications, 98
evaluation, 95
management, 95–98
tibial tubercle avulsion, fractures of, 98t, 98f–99f
imaging, 98
management, 99f
physical examination, 98
lateral condyle fractures, 71–73
lateral epicondyle fractures, 76
magnetic resonance imaging for acute fractures, 42
medial condyle fractures, 76
medial epicondyle fractures, 73f–74
metaphyseal distal radius and ulnar fractures, 59f–60f
metatarsals, fractures of, 111
Monteggia fractures, 64f–65f
odontoid fractures, 120, 121f
open fractures, classification of, 42
open fractures and lower extremity trauma, 112
osteochondral fractures, acute, 144
overgrowth after fracture, 39
patella, fractures of, 99–100f, 101f, 102f, 148
pathological fractures, 496, 497b, 497f
pelvic fractures, 87–89f, 131, 132f, 146–147
Peterson classification, 38, 39f
phalanges, fractures of, 49f, 111
physeal fractures, 37–38
physeal growth disturbances, 39
plain films, 42
proximal humerus fractures, 77–78, 79f
proximal tibia metaphyseal fractures, 102–103, 104f
proximal tibia physeal fractures, 103–104f
proximal ulna fractures, 66
radius, 55–57f, 58f
diaphyseal fractures, 61–62f, 63f
proximal radius fractures, 65–66f
remodeling, 37, 38f
Salter-Harris classification, 38, 39f
soft tissue factors, 37
spine trauma, 123–124
stable pelvic ring fractures, 131
stress fractures, 109f–110b, 144–145
supracondylar fractures, 68–71f
T-condylar distal humerus fractures, 76, 77f
in tension or torsion, 36, 37f
tibial spine fractures, 94–98
classification, 94–95f
complications, 98
evaluation, 95
management, 95–98
sports medicine, 151–152

Fractures (*Continued*)
tibial transition fractures, 107f, 108f
tibial tubercle avulsion, fractures of, 98t, 98f–99f
imaging, 98
management, 99f
physical examination, 98
tibial tubercle fractures, 152
tillaux fractures, 154
toddler's fractures, lower extremity trauma, 107–109f
transitional fracture patterns, 36–37, 38f
triplane fractures, 154, 155f
ulna, 55–57f, 58f, 61–63f, 66
wrist. *See* Wrist and forearm fractures
Freiberg infraction, 218–219
Friedreich ataxia, 281

G

Gait and gait analysis, 31–32
cerebral palsy, 437
common gait deviations in cerebral palsy, 439–440
gait, 437–440
normal gait in infants and toddlers, 437–440
gait cycle, 13, 31–32, 502
maturation of gait, 13
musculoskeletal examination, 31–32
cadence, 31
gait cycle, 31–32
motion analysis laboratory, 33f–34b
normal gait, prerequisites for, 32
step length, 31
step period, 31
stride length, 31
stride period, 31
neuromuscular disorders, 502
Galeazzi fractures, 60–61f
Gastroc-soleus lengthening, 445, 448f
Gaucher's disease, 346–347
Genitourinary injury, 41
Genu valgum, 204
Gillespie classification, 258–259, 260f
Glasgow coma scale, 41t
Glenohumeral joint subluxation and dislocation, 78–80
Glomus tumors, 178, 179f
Growth and development, 1, 2b, 2f
aggrecan, 9
alignment, 11
alkaline phosphatase, 8
ambulation, beginning, 13
apical ectodermal ridge, 4
apoptosis, 8–9
appendicular skeleton, 3
articular joint development, 4
axial skeleton, 3
basic growth considerations, 9–10
bones, 6
cell proliferation, 6
chondrocyte hypertrophy, 6–7
collagens in the growth plate, 7
formation or ossification, 4
growth plate chondrocytes, life cycle of, 6
growth plate regulation, 6
growth plate zones, 6
growth slowdown lines, 7f
long bones, growth of, 6
parameters influencing rate of growth, 6
parathyroid hormone-related peptide, 6

Growth and development (*Continued*)
physeal closure, 7
physiological epiphysiodesis, 7
skeletal maturity, 7
unanswered questions about growth, 6
vascular invasion, 6
cadence, 13
chondrogenesis, 8
concepts, 2
congenital, 1
control of development, 3
deformation, 1
deformity, 1
developmental, 1
developmental red flags, 12
disruption, 1
dysplasia, 1
embryology, 2–3
femur, 11
fibula, 11
foot growth, 12
gait, maturation of, 13
gait cycle, 13
growth plate, origin of, 4
growth plate chondrocytes, 8
hip growth, 10–11
Hueter-Volkmann's law, 3b
integrins, 9
limb rotational alignment, 4
lower limb growth, 11
malformation, 1
matrix metalloproteases, 8
matrix vesicles, 8
mechanical influences on growth, 3b
motor milestones, 12b
neurodevelopmental "norms," 12–13
normal values for rotational alignment in children, 11
origin of the profession, 2b
packaging problems, 1
postnatal foot growth, 12
predicting growth remaining to equalize limb lengths, 11
problems in growth, 2
production problems, 1
secondary centers of ossification, 4
skeletal system, 4
apophysis, 5
bipolar physes, 5
cartilage formation zone, 5
cartilage transformation zone, 5
growth zone, 5
Lappet formation, 5
long bones, anatomy of, 5
perichondral fibrous ring of LaCroix, 5
periosteum, 6
physis, 5
skeletal functions, 4
skeleton, 4
spherical physes, 5–6
zone of Ranvier, 5
spine growth, 10
stance phase, 13
step length, 13
straight-line graph method, 11
stride length, 13
swing phase, 13
tibia, 11
tibiofemoral angle changes with growth, 11

Growth and development (*Continued*)
upper extremity growth, 12
vascular endothelial growth factor, 9
velocity, 3f, 13
Westh and Menelaus method, 11
Wolffs law, 3b
Growth plate, origin of, 4
Growth plate chondrocytes, 8
Gymnast's wrist, 140–141

H
Hallux valgus, 448
Hand disorders and injuries, 47–49f
arthrogryposis multiplex congenita, 481
carpal bone fractures, 54–55
dislocations, 55
fingertip amputations, 50–51
fingertip injuries, 170–171, 172f
mallet finger deformities, 49–50f, 51f, 168–169
metacarpal fractures, 52–54f
musculoskeletal examination, 21–22, 23f, 24f
nail bed injuries, 51–52f
phalangeal fractures, 49f
thumb hypoplasia, 188, 189f, 189t
Hand tumors, malignant, 180–181
Head injury, 40, 41t
Hemangiomas, 178, 324–326
Hepatitis B, 415
Hip
arthrogryposis multiplex congenita, 477–478
disorders of. *See* Hip disorders
examinations and cerebral palsy, 423
growth, 10–11
injuries of. *See* Hip injuries
muscular dystrophies and surgery, 469
rotation, 197, 198f
Hip disorders, 224, 253
cerebral palsy, 439, 441–444, 445f
coxa vara. *See* Coxa vara
developmental dysplasia and dislocation of the hip, 225
avascular necrosis, 237
Barlow test, 228f
clinical presentation, 227–230
etiology, 226–227
hip development in developmental dysplasia of the hip, 226
incidence, 226–227
infant, 228–229, 230f
infants younger than 6 months, 233–236
Klisic test, 230f
magnetic resonance imaging, 231
natural history, 232–233
neonate, 227–228
newborns, 233–236
normal hip development, 225–226
older than 2 years, 235–236
Ortolani maneuver, 228f
pathophysiology, 225–227
radiography, 230–231, 232f
residual acetabular dysplasia, 236–239
risk factors, 226–227
screening criteria, 231–232
sequelae and complications, 236–237
6 months to 2 years, 234–235
treatment, 233–236
ultrasound, 230
walking child, 229–230
history, 224
Hip disorders, (*Continued*)
idiopathic chondrolysis of the hip, 253
clinical presentation, 253
differential diagnosis, 254
epidemiology, 253
etiology, 253
natural history, 254
radiographic findings, 253–254
treatment, 254
inspection, 224
Legg-Calve-Perthes disease. *See* Legg-Calve-Perthes disease
manipulation, 224–225
musculoskeletal examination, 22–24f, 25f
neuromuscular disorders, 490–492
neuromuscular hip dysplasia, 434–436
observation, 224
palpation, 224–225
physical examination, 224
slipped capital femoral epiphysis. *See* Slipped capital femoral epiphysis
Trendelenburg sign, 225f
Hip injuries, 85–90
acetabulum, fractures of, 87f, 88f
Delbert classification, 86b
pelvis, fractures of, 87–89f
soft tissue injuries of, 89f–90
Hueter-Volkmann's law, 3b
Humeral shaft fractures, 76–77, 78f
Humerus
proximal humerus fractures, 77–78, 79f
and shoulder region, fractures of, 76–82
T-condylar distal humerus fractures, 76, 77f
Hydrocephalus, 486, 487f
Hydromyelia, 486, 487f
Hyperparathyroidism, 398–400
Hypervitaminosis A, 400
Hypervitaminosis D, 400
Hypochondroplasia, 357
clinical features, 357–358
diagnosis, 358
orthopaedic considerations, 358
radiographic findings, 358
Hypoparathyroidism, 400
Hypophosphatasia, 392
clinical features, 392–393
radiographic findings, 392–393
treatment, 393

I
Idiopathic chondrolysis of the hip, 253
clinical presentation, 253
differential diagnosis, 254
epidemiology, 253
etiology, 253
natural history, 254
radiographic findings, 253–254
treatment, 254
Idiopathic genu valgum, 204
Idiopathic juvenile osteoporosis, 397
Idiopathic scoliosis, adolescent, 272–273
bracing, 273, 274f
observation, 273
surgery, 273–276, 277f
treatment options, 273–276, 277f
Idiopathic scoliosis, infantile, 276–278
Idiopathic scoliosis, juvenile, 276
Iliopsoas, 423–424, 426f
Infantile cortical hyperostosis, 44f
Infantile idiopathic scoliosis, 276–278
Infection
musculoskeletal. *See* Musculoskeletal infections
neonatal infections, 345
upper extremity disorders, 174–176
Inflammatory bowel disease, arthropathy associated with, 412
Ingrown toenail, 220
Integrins, 9
Intestinal injury, 41
Intrathecal baclofen and cerebral palsy, 430–431
Isolated tibia shaft fractures, 104–106f

J
Jansen metaphyseal chondrodysplasia, 378
Joint anatomy, 403
Joint development, 403–405
Joint pathoanatomy, 405
Juvenile ankylosing spondylitis, 412
Juvenile bunion, 219–220
Juvenile dermatomyositis, 414
Juvenile idiopathic scoliosis, 276
Juvenile psoriatic arthritis, 411
Juvenile rheumatoid arthritis, 409–411

K
Kanavel's signs of flexor tenosynovitis, 175b
Kingella Kingae, 343
Klippel-Feil syndrome, 286–287
Klisic test, 230f
Knee
arthrogryposis multiplex congenita, 477
cerebral palsy, 423–425, 439–440, 444–445, 446f
deformity and neuromuscular disorders, 492
floating knee, 112f
injuries, *See* Knee injuries
muscular dystrophies and surgery, 469
musculoskeletal examination, 24–27b, 27f
Knee injuries
anterior cruciate ligament injuries, 100–101
Cozen fractures, 102–103b
distal tibial transition fractures, 107f, 108f
fractures, 94–107f, 108f
Cozen fractures, 102–103b
distal tibial transition fractures, 107f, 108f
isolated tibia shaft fractures, 104–106f
patella, fractures of, 99–100f, 101f, 102f, 148
proximal tibia metaphyseal fractures, 102–103, 104f
proximal tibia physeal fractures, 103–104f
tibial and fibular shaft fractures, 104, 105f
tibial spine, fractures of, 94–98
classification, 94–95f
complications, 98
evaluation, 95
management, 95–98
tibial tubercle avulsion, fractures of, 98t, 98f–99f
imaging, 98
management, 99f
physical examination, 98
isolated tibia shaft fractures, 104–106f
lateral collateral injuries, 102
ligament injuries, 100–102
medial collateral injuries, 101
meniscal injuries, 102
patella, fractures of, 99–100f, 101f, 102f, 148
patellofemoral injuries, 102
posterior cruciate ligament injuries, 101
proximal tibia metaphyseal fractures, 102–103, 104f

Knee injuries (*Continued*)
proximal tibia physeal fractures, 103–104f
tibial and fibular shaft fractures, 104, 105f
tibial spine, fractures of, 94–98
classification, 94–95f
complications, 98
evaluation, 95
management, 95–98
tibial tubercle avulsion, fractures of, 98t, 98f–99f
imaging, 98
management, 99f
physical examination, 98
Kniest dysplasia, 363–364
clinical features, 364
medical problems, 365
orthopaedic considerations, 365
radiographic findings, 364–365
Köhler disease, 218
Kyphosis, 498

L
Landau reaction, 421
Langerhans cell histiocytosis, 318–319, 321f
Laparotomy, 41
Larsen syndrome, 380–381
clinical features, 381
orthopaedic considerations, 381–382
radiographic findings, 381
Lateral collateral injuries, 102
Lateral condyle fractures, 71–73
Lateral epicondyle fractures, 76
Legg-Calve-Perthes disease, 237
classification systems, 239–241
clinical presentation, 238
diagnosis, 241–242
epidemiology, 238
etiology, 237
natural history, 242
nonoperative treatment, 243
operative treatment, 243–245
pathogenesis of deformity, 237
patterns of deformity, 237–238
physical examination, 238
prognosis, 242
prognostic factors, 241
radiographic findings, 238–242
radiographic results, classification of, 241, 242t
radiographic stages, 238–239, 240t
treatment, 242–245
Leg length inequality and angular deformity, 112
Leri-Weill syndrome, 378
clinical features, 378
diagnosis, 379
orthopaedic considerations, 379
radiographic findings, 378–379
Lesser toe deformities, 220
Leukemia, 323, 346
Ligament injuries
knee injuries, 100–102
sports medicine, 148–151
Limb rotational alignment, 4
Lipoma and upper extremity disorders, 179–180
Lipomeningocele, 486
Liver laceration, 41
Lower extremities
ankle. *See* Ankle
arthrogryposis multiplex congenita, 476–478
cerebral palsy, 441–448
disorders. *See* Lower extremity disorders
Lower extremities (*Continued*)
foot. *See* Foot
knee. *See* Knee
leg length inequality and angular deformity, 112
neuromuscular disorders, 490–496
sports-specific injuries, 146–148
trauma. *See* Lower extremity trauma
Lower extremity disorders, 197
accessory navicular, 216–217
adolescent Blount disease, 203
Blount disease, 201–202, 203f
calcaneovalgus foot, 213
clubfoot, 208–211
congenital pseudarthrosis of the tibia, 204–205
congenital vertical talus, 213, 214f
coronal limb abnormalities, 199–206
curly toe, 220
fibula hemimelia, 205
flatfoot, 211
flexible planovalgus foot, 211–213
foot cavus, 217–218
foot deformities, 206–218
foot pain, 218–220
Freiberg infraction, 218–219
genu valgum, 204
hip rotation, 197, 198f
idiopathic genu valgum, 204
ingrown toenail, 220
juvenile bunion, 219–220
Kohler disease, 218
lesser toe deformities, 220
macrodactyly, 220
metabolic disease, 201, 202f
metatarsus adductus, 198, 206–207
multiple hereditary exostoses, 204
physical examination of limb rotation, 198–199, 200f
polydactyly, 220
rotational abnormalities, 197–199
Sever's disease, 119
skeletal dysplasias, 201
skewfoot, 207–208
syndactyly, 220
tarsal coalition, 215, 216f
tibial bowing, 204
tibial rotation, 197–198
toe walking, 205–206
trauma, 199–201
Lower extremity trauma, 85, 199–201
avascular necrosis, 112f
child abuse, 111b
complications, 112
femur injuries. *See* Femur injuries
floating knee, 112f
foot injuries. *See* Foot
hip injuries. *See* Hip injuries
knee injuries. *See* Knee injuries
leg length inequality and angular deformity, 112
multiple trauma, 111–112
open fractures, 112
stress fractures, 109f–110b
toddler's fractures, 107–109f
Luque-Galveston technique, 278
Lyme disease, 413
Lymphatic malformations, 327

M
Macrodactyly, 187–188, 220
Maffucci's syndrome, 328
Malformation, 1
Mallet finger, 49–50f, 51f, 168–169
Marfan's syndrome, 281
Matrix metalloproteases, 8
Matrix vesicles, 8
McKusick metaphyseal chondrodysplasia, 377–378
Medial collateral injuries, 101
Medial condyle fractures, 76
Medial epicondyle fractures, 73f–74
Meningocele, 485
Meniscal injuries
knee injuries, 102
sports medicine, 148–151
Metabolic disease of the lower limbs, 201, 202f
Metabolic disorders, bones. *See* Bones, metabolic disorders of
Metacarpal fractures, 52–54f
Metaphyseal chondrodysplasia, 377
Jansen metaphyseal chondrodysplasia, 378
McKusick metaphyseal chondrodysplasia, 377–378
Schmid metaphyseal chondrodysplasia, 377
Metaphyseal distal radius and ulnar fractures, 59f–60f
Metaphyseal fibrous defect, 308–311
Metatarsals, fractures of, 111
Metatarsus adductus, 198, 206–207
Metatropic dysplasia, 358
clinical features, 359
medical problems, 359–360
orthopaedic considerations, 360
radiographic findings, 359
Midfoot, fractures of, 110–111
Midfoot sprains, 154–155
Mineral metabolism, 386–388
Monteggia fractures, 64f–65f
Motor function and upper extremity disorders, 161, 162t
Motor milestones, 12b
Mucopolysaccharidoses, 371–372
clinical features, 372
orthopaedic considerations, 373
radiographic findings, 372–373
Multiple enchondromatosis, 307, 309f
Multiple epiphyseal dysplasia, 373–374
clinical features, 374
orthopaedic considerations, 375
radiographic findings, 374
Multiple epiphyseal exostoses
clinical features, 383f
orthopaedic considerations, 383–384
radiographic findings, 383, 384f
Multiple hereditary exostoses, 204, 382
Muscular dystrophies
anatomical approach to the differential diagnosis, 464t–465t
ankle surgery, 468
definition, 454–456
diagnostic testing, 462–463
Duchenne muscular dystrophy, 280, 466–469
dystrophin, 458
etiology, 456
evaluation, 459–461
foot surgery, 468
genetics, 458
hip surgery, 469
historical aspects, 456, 457f
hypotonia, 458–459
inherited diseases of muscle, 456t
knee surgery, 469
laboratory studies, 461–462

Muscular dystrophies (*Continued*)
limbs, 467–468
malignant hyperthermia, 471
medications, 465–466
molecular biology, 458
muscle biopsy, technique of, 462–463
muscle pathology, 456–458
nonsurgical management, 470–471
occupational therapy, 471
physical therapy, 470
preoperative preparation, 469–470
psychosocial support, 471
scoliosis, 469
speech therapy, 471
surgical procedures, 470
treatment, 463–471
weakness, 458–459
Muscular origin, tumors of, 332–334
Musculoskeletal examination, 15
abdominal reflexes, 31
ankle, 27, 28f
asymmetrical tonic neck reflex, 30–31f
Babinski reflex, 31f
cadence, 31
cerebral palsy, 422–423
cervical spine, 18f
child's perinatal questionnaire, 16b
contractures, 17
deep tendon reflexes, 28
deformity, 17
developmental reflexes, 28
direction of joint motion, 18b
elbow, 21, 23f
foot, 27, 28f
forearm, 21–22, 23f, 24f
gait and gait analysis, 31–32
cadence, 31
gait cycle, 31–32
motion analysis laboratory, 33f–34b
normal gait, prerequisites for, 32
step length, 31
step period, 31
stride length, 31
stride period, 31
gait cycle, 31–32
hand, 21–22, 23f, 24f
hip, 22–24f, 25f, 26f
knee, 24–27b, 27f
mother's prenatal questionnaire, 16b
motion analysis laboratory, 33f–34b
motor developmental milestones, 16b
motor innervation, 29b
muscle-tendon units crossing two joints, 17b
neurological examination, 27–28b, 29t
abdominal reflexes, 31
asymmetrical tonic neck reflex, 30–31f
Babinski reflex, 31f
deep tendon reflexes, 28
developmental reflexes, 28
motor innervation, 29b
palmar grasp reflex, 28–29f
parachute reaction, 29–30f
pathological knee diagnosis based on tenderness, 27b
sensation, 31
startle reflex, 29
stepping reflex, 29, 30f
symmetrical tonic neck reflex, 30f
normal gait, prerequisites for, 32
Musculoskeletal examination (*Continued*)
normal knee alignment by age, 17b
orthopaedic history, 15–16
palmar grasp reflex, 28–29f
parachute reaction, 29–30f
pathological knee diagnosis based on tenderness, 27b
physical examination, 16–27
range of motion, 17–18b
sensation, 31
shoulder, 19–21f, 22f
spasticity, 17b
startle reflex, 29
step length, 31
step period, 31
stepping reflex, 29, 30f
stride length, 31
stride period, 31
symmetrical tonic neck reflex, 30f
thigh, 24–27b, 27f
thoracolumbar spine, 18–19, 20f, 21f
wrist, 21–22, 23f, 24f
Musculoskeletal infections, 337
anatomy, 337–338
antibiotics, 347–348
bone tumors, malignant, 346, 347f
Borrelia burgdorferi, 344
causative organisms, 342–344
classification methods, 342
diagnosis, 346–347
eosinophilic granuloma, 346
epidemiology, 350
follow-up, 349–350
foot, 345, 346b, 346f
Gaucher's disease, 346–347
historical features in the evaluation of pediatric musculoskeletal infection, 338b
Kingella Kingae, 343
laboratory tests, 340–342
leukemia, 346
mycobacterium tuberculosis, 344
myelodysplasia with fracture, 347
neisseria gonorrhoeae, 343
Neisseria meningitidis, 343
neonatal infections, 345
pelvis, 345
physical examination, 338, 339b
radiological examination, 338–340, 341t
sickle cell disease, 347
spine, 344
Staphylococcus aureus, 342
streptococcus pneumoniae, 343
streptococcus pyogenes, 342
surgical decision making, 348–349
treatment, 347–348, 350
unusual manifestations of subacute and chronic infections, 350
Musculoskeletal tumors, 290
aggressive fibromatosis, 330–332
Albright's syndrome, 312
aneurysmal bone cyst, 316–318
angiomatosis, 328
arteriovenous malformations, 327
biopsy, 293–294
bone origin, tumors of, 294–308
capillary malformations, 327–328
cartilaginous origin, tumors of, 302–308
chondroblastoma, 304–305
chondromyxoid fibroma, 305
Musculoskeletal tumors (*Continued*)
classification, 291b, 294
clinical presentations of pediatric musculoskeletal tumors, 291b
common locations of pediatric bone tumors, 292t
computed tomography, 293
dysplasia epiphysealis hemimelica, 304
enchondroma, 305–307
evaluation, 290–294
Ewing sarcoma, 293b, 320–323
exostosis, 302–304
fibroma, 308–311
fibromatosis, 330
fibrous cortical defect, 308–311
fibrous dysplasia, 311–312
fibrous origin, tumors of, 308–314
fibrous tissue origin, tumors of, 330–332
hemangiomas, 324–326
history, 290, 291b
Langerhans cell histiocytosis, 318–319, 321f
leukemia, musculoskeletal manifestations of, 323
lymphatic malformations, 327
Maffucci's syndrome, 328
magnetic resonance imaging, 293
metaphyseal fibrous defect, 308–311
multiple enchondromatosis, 307, 309f
muscular origin, tumors of, 332–334
nerve origin, tumors of, 328–330
neurofibroma, 328, 330f
neurolemmoma, 328
nonossifying fibroma, 308–311
osteoblastoma, 297–298
osteochondroma, 302–304
osteofibrous dysplasia, 312–314
osteoid osteoma, 294–297
burr-down technique, 296–297
clinical findings, 295
radiographic and histological features, 295, 296f
treatment, 295–297
osteosarcoma, 293b, 298–302
classic high-grade osteosarcoma, 298–300, 301f
conventional osteosarcoma, 298–300, 301f
high-grade surface osteosarcoma, 302
parosteal osteosarcoma, 300–302
periosteal osteosarcoma, 302
surface or juxtacortical osteosarcoma, 300–302
peak ages of common pediatric musculoskeletal tumors, 291t
periosteal chondroma, 308
peripheral nerve sheath tumors, malignant, 392–330, 331f
peripheral neuroectodermal tumor, 319–323
physical examination, 291
radiograph examination, plain, 291–293
radionuclide scans, 293
rhabdomyosarcoma, 332–334
soft tissue tumors, 323–334
surgical stages, 294t
synovial cell sarcoma, 334
treatment, 294, 295f, 295t
unicameral bone cyst, 314–316
vascular malformations, 325t, 326–328
vascular tumors, 324–328
venous malformations, 327
Mycobacterium tuberculosis, 344
Myelocele, 486
Myelodysplasia, 279, 349
Myelomeningocele, 486

N
Nail bed injuries, 51–52f
Nail injuries, 170–171, 172f
Necrosis, avascular, 112f, 237
Neisseria gonorrhoeae, 343
Neisseria meningitidis, 343
Neonatal infections, 345
Nerve injury, 166–167
Nerve origin, tumors of, 327–330
Neurodevelopmental "norms," 12–13
Neurofibroma, 328
Neurofibromatosis, 281, 282f
Neurolemmoma, 328
Neurological examinations, 27–28b, 29t, 423
Neuromuscular disorders, 454, 483–484, 500
  ambulation, 499–500
  ankle deformity, 492
  Arnold-Chiari malformation, 486–487
  arthrogryposis multiplex congenita. *See* Arthrogryposis multiplex congenita
  associated anomalies, 485–487
  calcaneovalgus deformities, 493–494
  calcaneus deformities, 493–494
  cavus deformities, 494–495, 496f
  cerebral palsy. *See* Cerebral palsy
  Charcot arthropathy, 495–496
  clubfoot deformity, 492–493
  diastematomyelia, 487, 488f
  embryology, 484, 485f
  etiology, 484
  foot deformity, 492
  gait cycle, 499
  hip deformity, 490–492
  hydrocephalus, 486, 487f
  hydromyelia, 486, 487f
  initial evaluation and treatment, 488–489, 490b
  knee deformity, 492
  kyphosis, 498
  latex allergies, 487–488, 489b
  lipomeningocele, 486
  lower extremity deformity, 490–496
  meningocele, 485
  muscular dystrophies. *See* Muscular dystrophies
  myelocele, 486
  myelomeningocele, 486
  nonneurological issues, 487–488
  orthoses, use of, 499–500
  pathological fractures, 496, 497b, 497f
  planovalgus deformity, 494, 495f
  prevention, 484, 485b
  range of defects, 485–487
  scoliosis, 497–498
  spinal deformity, 497–498
  tethered cord, 486–487, 488b, 488f
  upper extremity disorders, 188–194, 492–493
Neuromuscular hip dysplasia, 434–436
Neuromuscular scoliosis, 278–281, 282f, 436–437
Nodular tenosynovitis, 179
Nonossifying fibroma, 308–311
Nursemaid's elbow, 75, 76f

O
Occiput-C1 dislocations, 119
Odontoid fractures, 120, 121f
Open fractures and lower extremity trauma, 112
Origin of the profession, 2b
Ortolani maneuver, 228f
Osgood-Schlatter disease, 141, 142f
Osteoblastoma, 297–298
Osteochondral fractures, acute, 144
Osteochondritis dissecans, 143–144
Osteochondrodysplasias. *See* Skeletal dysplasias
Osteochondroma (exostosis), 180, 302–304
Osteofibrous dysplasia, 312–314
Osteogenesis imperfecta, 281, 393–394
  clinical features, 394, 395f
  diagnosis, 394–395
  radiographic findings, 394, 395f
  Shapiro classification, 394b
  Sillence classification, 394b
  treatment, 395–397
Osteoid osteoma, 294–297
  burr-down technique, 296–297
  clinical findings, 295
  radiographic and histological features, 295, 296f
  treatment, 295–297
Osteomyelitis, 45
Osteopetrosis, 398, 399f
Osteoporosis, juvenile idiopathic, 397
Osteosarcoma, 293b, 298–302
  classic high-grade osteosarcoma, 298–300, 301f
  conventional osteosarcoma, 298–300, 301f
  high-grade surface osteosarcoma, 302
  parosteal osteosarcoma, 300–302
  periosteal osteosarcoma, 302
  surface or juxtacortical osteosarcoma, 300–302

P
Packaging problems, 1
Palmar grasp reflex, 28–29f
Parachute reaction, 29–30f
Parathyroid disorders, 398–400
Parathyroid hormone, 387
Paronychia, 174–175
Parvovirus, 413
Patella, fractures of, 99–100f, 101f, 102f, 148
Patellar dislocation, 147–148
Patellofemoral injuries, 102
Pathological fractures, 496, 497b, 497f
PauciJRA, 411
Pelvic fractures, 87–89f, 131, 132f, 146–147
Pelvis and musculoskeletal infections, 345
Pelvis trauma, 116, 127
  acetabular fractures, 133–134, 135f
  anatomy, 127–128
  associated injuries, 129–130
  avulsion fractures, 132–133
  classification, 130–131
  imaging, 128–129
  physical examination, 128
  stable pelvic ring fractures, 131
  Torode and Zieg classification pediatric pelvic fractures, 130t
  unstable pelvic fractures, 131, 132f
Periosteal chondroma, 308
Peripheral nerve sheath tumors, malignant, 392–330, 331f
Peripheral neuroectodermal tumor, 319–323
Peterson classification, 38, 39f
Phalanges, fractures of, 49f, 111
Phenol and cerebral palsy, 430
Phosphorus homeostasis, 386
Physeal distal radius and ulna injuries, 57–59f
Planovalgus, 211
Planovalgus deformity, 494, 495f
Plastic deformation of the radius, ulna, or both, 63
Polydactyly, 186–187, 220
PolyJRA, 410–411
Polymyositis, childhood, 414
Posterior cruciate ligament injuries, 101
Posterior spinal fusion, 448–449, 450f
Poststreptococcal reactive arthritis, 412
Production problems, 1
Proximal humerus fractures, 77–78, 79f
Proximal radius fractures, 65–66f
Proximal tibia metaphyseal fractures, 102–103, 104f
Proximal tibia physeal fractures, 103–104f
Proximal ulna fractures, 66
Pseudoachondroplasia, 370
  clinical features, 370
  orthopaedic considerations, 370–371
  radiographic findings, 370, 371f
Pseudoaneurysms and upper extremity disorders, 178, 179f
Pseudosubluxation, 288
Psoriatic arthritis, juvenile, 411
Pyogenic granulomas and upper extremity disorders, 178, 179f

R
Radius
  deficiency, 181–183
  diaphyseal fractures, 61–62f, 63f
  fractures, 55–57f, 58f
    diaphyseal fractures, 61–62f, 63f
    proximal radius fractures, 65–66f
  injuries, 57–59f
  plastic deformation of the radius, 63
  proximal radius fractures, 65–66f
Range of motion in musculoskeletal examinations, 17–18b
Reactive arthritis, 412
Rectus femoris contracture, 424, 426f
Reiter syndrome, 412
Renal osteodystrophy, 390
  clinical findings, 390–391
  radiographic features, 391
  treatment, 391–392
Residual acetabular dysplasia, 236–237
Rhabdomyosarcoma, 332–334
Rheumatic fever, 412
Rheumatoid arthritis, juvenile, 409–411
Rickets, 388, 389b
  clinical features, 389
  diagnosis, 390
  laboratory findings, 389
  radiographic findings, 389–390, 391f
  treatment, 391–392
  vitamin D-resistant rickets, 389
Rotational abnormalities, 197–199
Rotational examination in cerebral palsy, 424–425, 427f
Rubella, 413

S
Salter-Harris classification, 38, 39f
Salter-Harris fracture types, 47, 48f
Sarcoidosis, 414
Scheuermann's kyphosis, 283–284
Schmid metaphyseal chondrodysplasia, 377
Scoliosis, 469, 470f
  adolescent idiopathic scoliosis, 272–273
    bracing, 273, 274f
    observation, 273
    surgery, 273–276, 277f
    treatment options, 273–276, 277f
  arthrogryposis multiplex congenita, 475

Scoliosis (*Continued*)
congenital scoliosis, 281–283
infantile idiopathic scoliosis, 276–278
juvenile idiopathic scoliosis, 276
neuromuscular disorders, 497–498
neuromuscular scoliosis, 278–281, 282f, 436–437
Scurvy, 400–401
SEA syndrome, 411
Seddon's classification of nerve injury, 190t
Sensation, 30
Sensibility and upper extremity disorders, 160
Septic arthritis, 176, 408–409
Serum calcium, 387–388
Sever disease, 142–143, 219
Shoulder
arthrogryposis multiplex congenita, 478–479, 480f
dislocation, 145–146
fractures of, 76–82
musculoskeletal examinations, 19–21f, 22f
thrower's shoulder, 139–141
Sickle cell disease, 347
Simple bone cysts, 314–316
Sinding-Larsen-Johansson syndrome, 141–142
Skeletal dysplasias, 353–354
achondroplasia, 354
clinical features, 354–355
medical problems, 356
orthopaedic considerations, 356–357
radiographic findings, 355–356
chondrodysplasia punctata, 375
clinical features, 375
medical problems, 376
orthopaedic considerations, 376
radiographic findings, 375–376
chondroectodermal dysplasia, 360
clinical features, 360
medical problems, 360
orthopaedic considerations, 361
radiographic findings, 360, 361b
classification of skeletal dysplasias, 354b, 355b
cleidocranial dysplasia, 379
clinical features, 379–380
orthopaedic considerations, 380
radiographic findings, 380
diastrophic dysplasia, 361–362
clinical features, 362
medical problems, 363
orthopaedic considerations, 363
radiographic findings, 362–363
dyschondrosteosis, 378
clinical features, 378
diagnosis, 379
orthopaedic considerations, 379
radiographic findings, 378–379
Ellis-van Creveld syndrome, 360–361
hypochondroplasia, 357
clinical features, 357–358
diagnosis, 358
orthopaedic considerations, 358
radiographic findings, 358
Kniest dysplasia, 363–364
clinical features, 364
medical problems, 365
orthopaedic considerations, 365
radiographic findings, 364–365
Larsen syndrome, 380–381
clinical features, 381
orthopaedic considerations, 381–382
radiographic findings, 381

Skeletal dyplasias (*Continued*)
lower limb disorders, 201
metaphyseal chondrodysplasia, 377
Jansen metaphyseal chondrodysplasia, 378
McKusick metaphyseal chondrodysplasia, 377–378
Schmid metaphyseal chondrodysplasia, 377
metatropic dysplasia, 358
clinical features, 359
medical problems, 359–360
orthopaedic considerations, 360
radiographic findings, 359
mucopolysaccharidoses, 371–372
clinical features, 372
orthopaedic considerations, 373
radiographic findings, 372–373
multiple epiphyseal dysplasia, 373–374
clinical features, 374
orthopaedic considerations, 375
radiographic findings, 374
multiple epiphyseal exostoses
clinical features, 383f
orthopaedic considerations, 383–384
radiographic findings, 383, 384f
multiple hereditary exostoses, 382
pseudoachondroplasia, 370
clinical features, 370
orthopaedic considerations, 370–371
radiographic findings, 370, 371f
spinal abnormalities, 356t
spondyloepiphyseal dysplasia congenita, 365
clinical features, 365, 366f
medical problems, 365
orthopaedic considerations, 367, 369f
radiographic findings, 365, 366f–368f
spondyloepiphyseal dysplasia tarda, 367
clinical features, 367
orthopaedic considerations, 370
radiographic findings, 369–370
Skeletal system
apophysis, 5
bipolar physes, 5
cartilage formation zone, 5
cartilage transformation zone, 5
growth zone, 5
Lappet formation, 5
long bones, anatomy of, 5
perichondral fibrous ring of LaCroix, 5
periosteum, 6
physis, 5
skeletal functions, 4
skeleton, 4
spherical physes, 5–6
zone of Ranvier, 5
Skewfoot, 207–208
Skin, 161–164
Slipped capital femoral epiphysis, 245
classification, 245–246
clinical presentation, 247–248
complications, 252
computerized tomography, 249–250
degree of slippage, treatment to reduce, 250
epidemiology, 247
etiology, 246–247
further slippage, treatment to prevent, 250–252
magnetic resonance imaging, 250
natural history, 250
prophylactic pinning of the contralateral hip, 252
radiographs, 248–249

Slipped capital femoral epiphysis (*Continued*)
salvage procedures, 252
technetium-99m bone scan, 249–250
treatment, 250–252
ultrasonography, 250
Soft tissue
sports medicine injuries, 138–139
tumors, 177–180, 324–334
upper extremity disorders, 160, 161–164
Spasticity and musculoskeletal examinations, 17b
Spina bifida, 279–280
Spinal disorders, 265
achondroplasia, 281
adolescent idiopathic scoliosis, 272–273
bracing, 273–274f
observation, 273
surgery, 273–276, 277f
treatment options, 273–276, 277f
anatomy, 265
apical vertebra, 270
back pain, 285–286, 287b
bony structures, 266
cerebral palsy, 279
cervical spinal deformities, 286–288
Cobb angle, 269
congenital kyphosis, 283
congenital scoliosis, 281–283
Down's syndrome, 287–288
Duchenne muscular dystrophy, 280
embryology, 265–266
Friedreich ataxia, 281
history, 266–267
infantile idiopathic scoliosis, 276–278
juvenile idiopathic scoliosis, 276
Klippel-Feil syndrome, 286–287
laboratory studies, 272
Luque-Galveston technique, 278
Marfan's syndrome, 281
myelodysplasia, 279
neurofibromatosis, 281, 282f
neurological examination, 268b
neurological levels, 268b
neuromuscular disorders, 497–498
neuromuscular scoliosis, 278–281, 282f
osteogenesis imperfecta, 281
physical examination, 266–267, 268b, 270t
pseudosubluxation, 288
radiological examination, 267–272
Scheuermann's kyphosis, 283–284
spina bifida, 279
spinal dysraphism, 279
spinal maturation, 266
spinal muscular atrophy, 280
spondylolisthesis, 284–285
spondylolysis, 284–285
stable vertebra, 270
torticollis, 287
transitional vertebra, 269
Spinal orthoses, 432
Spine
cerebral palsy, 448–450
cervical spine, 116, 117b
deformities, 286–288
injuries, 119–123
musculoskeletal examinations, 18f
disorders. *See* Spinal disorders
growth, 10
musculoskeletal infections, 344
posterior spinal fusion, 448–449, 450f

Spine (*Continued*)
thoracolumbar spine, 116–117
injuries, 123–127
musculoskeletal examinations, 18–19, 20f, 21f
trauma. *See* Spine trauma
Spine trauma, 116
atlantoaxial instability, 121–122
atlantoaxial rotary instability, 122
atlas fractures, 119–120
burst fractures, 124–125, 126f
cervical spine, 116, 117b
cervical spine injuries, 119–123
compression fractures, 123–124
flexion-distraction injuries, 124, 125f
mechanisms of pediatric spine injury, 117–118
Occiput-C1 dislocations, 119
odontoid fractures, 120, 121f
physical examination, 118
radiologic examination, 118–119, 120b
spinal cord injury without radiographic abnormality, 125–127
spondylolisthesis, 120–121, 122f
subaxial cervical spine injuries, 122–123
thoracolumbar spine, 116–117
thoracolumbar spine injuries, 123–125
unique characteristics of the pediatric cervical spine, 119b
Splenic laceration, 41
Spondyloarthropathies, 411–413
Spondyloepiphyseal dysplasia congenita, 365
clinical features, 365, 366f
medical problems, 365
orthopaedic considerations, 367, 369f
radiographic findings, 365, 366f–368f
Spondyloepiphyseal dysplasia tarda, 367
clinical features, 367
orthopaedic considerations, 370
radiographic findings, 369–370
Spondylolisthesis, 120–121, 122f, 284–285
Spondylolysis, 284–285
Sports medicine, 138, 156
acromioclavicular separation, 146
acute osteochondral fractures, 144
ankle injuries of the young athlete, 152–154
anterior cruciate ligament tear, 150–151
chronic injuries, 139–145
discoid lateral meniscus, 148–150
fifth metatarsal fractures, 154–155, 156f
gymnast's wrist, 140–141
ligament injuries, 148–151
lower extremity, sports-specific injuries, 146–148
meniscal injuries, 148–151
midfoot sprains, 154–155
Osgood-Schlatter disease, 141, 142f
osteochondritis dissecans, 143–144
overuse injuries, 139–145
patellar dislocation, 147–148
patellar fractures, 148
pelvic avulsion fractures, 146–147
Sever disease, 142–143
shoulder dislocation, 145–146
Sinding-Larsen-Johansson syndrome, 141–142
soft tissue injuries, 138–139
sprain, 138
strain, 138–139
stress fractures, 144–145
thrower's elbow, 140
thrower's shoulder, 139–140
tibial spine fractures, 151–152
Sports medicine (*Continued*)
tibial tubercle fractures, 152
tillaux fractures, 154
triplane fractures, 154, 155f
upper extremity injuries, acute, 145–146
Sprains, 138
Stable pelvic ring fractures, 131
Stable vertebra, 270
Staheli test, 425, 426f
Stance phase, 13
Staphylococcus aureus, 342
Startle reflex, 29
Step length, 13, 31
Stepping reflex, 29, 30f
Strains, 138–139
Streptococcus pneumoniae, 343
Streptococcus pyogenes, 342
Stress fractures, 109f–110b, 144–145
Stride length, 13, 31
Subaxial cervical spine injuries, 122–123
Supracondylar fractures, 68–71f
Swan neck deformity, 169
Swing phase, 13
Symmetrical tonic neck reflex, 30f
Syndactyly, 185–186, 220
Synostosis, 188
Synovial cell sarcoma, 334
Synovial disorders, 403, 415–416
anatomy, 403–405
arthropathy associated with inflammatory bowel disease, 412
articular cartilage components, 404b
childhood polymyositis, 414
classifications of chronic arthritis, 407–408
clinical features, 405–406
connective tissue diseases with associated chronic arthritis, 413–414
diagnosis, 408
diagnostic imaging, 407
Epstein-Barr virus, 413
evaluation, approach to, 406
hepatitis B, 413
joint anatomy, 403
joint development, 403–405
joint pathoanatomy, 405
juvenile ankylosing spondylitis, 412
juvenile dermatomyositis, 414
juvenile psoriatic arthritis, 411
juvenile rheumatoid arthritis, 409–411
laboratory evaluations, 406–407
Lyme disease, 413
medical treatments, 414
overall function, 415
parvovirus, 413
pauciJRA, 411
physical examinations, 406
physical therapy, 414–415
polyJRA, 410–411
poststreptococcal reactive arthritis, 412
prevention of worsening deformity, 415
radiographic examination, 407
reactive arthritis, 412
Reiter syndrome, 412
rheumatic fever, 412
rubella, 413
sarcoidosis, 414
SEA syndrome, 411
spondyloarthropathies, 411–413
surgical treatment, 415
Synovial disorders (*Continued*)
systemic lupus erythematosus, 413
systemic onset JRA, 409–410
transient synovitis *versus* septic arthritis, 408–409
treatment, 416–415
varicella, 413
vasculitis-associated arthritis, 414
viral arthritis, 413
Systemic lupus erythematosus, 413
Systemic onset JRA, 409–410

T

Talus, fractures of, 110
Tarsal coalition, 215, 216f
T-condylar distal humerus fractures, 76, 77f
Tendon injuries
extensor tendon injuries, 168
flexor tendon injuries, 167–168
upper extremity disorders, 167–170
Tethered cord, 487
Thighs and musculoskeletal examinations, 24–27b, 27f
Thomas test, 423, 424f
Thoracic injury, 40–41
Thoracolumbar spine, 116–117
injuries, 123–125
musculoskeletal examinations, 18–19, 20f, 21f
Thrower's elbow, 140
Thrower's shoulder, 139–140
Thumb hypoplasia, 188, 189f, 189t
Tibia
cerebral palsy, 423–425
congenital pseudarthrosis of the tibia, 204–205
growth and development, 11
isolated tibia shaft fractures, 104–106f
proximal tibia metaphyseal fractures, 102–103, 104f
proximal tibia physeal fractures, 103–104f
Tibial bowing, 204
Tibial rotation, 197–198
Tibial spine fractures, 94–98
classification, 94–95f
complications, 98
evaluation, 95
management, 95–98
sports medicine, 151–152
Tibial transition fractures, 107f, 108f
Tibial tubercle avulsion, fractures of, 98t, 98f–99f
imaging, 98
management, 99f
physical examination, 98
Tibial tubercle fractures, 152
Tillaux fractures, 154
Tizanidine and cerebral palsy, 428
Toddler's fractures, lower extremity trauma, 107–109f
Toe walking, 205–206
Torode and Zieg classification pediatric pelvic fractures, 130b
Torticollis, 287
Transient synovitis *versus* septic arthritis, 408–409
Transitional vertebra, 269
Transverse deficiencies, 184–186
Trauma, 36
abdominal injury, 41
activities not recommended by the American Academy of Pediatrics, 40
behavioral risk factors, 39
Caffey disease, 44f
compartment syndrome, 45

Trauma (*Continued*)
complications, 45
deep vein thrombosis, 45
environmental risk factors, 39–40
epidemiology, 39–40, 43
examination of polytrauma patient, 40
fat embolism, 45
fractures, *See* Fractures
genitourinary injury, 41
Glasgow coma scale, 41t
growth disturbance, 45
head injury, 40, 41t
imaging for abuse, 44
individual risk factors, 39
infantile cortical hyperostosis, 44f
intestinal injury, 41
laparotomy, 41
liver laceration, 41
lower extremities. *See* Lower extremity trauma
morbidity, determinants of, 40
nonaccidental injury, 43–45
osteomyelitis, 45
overgrowth after fracture, 39
pelvis. *See* Pelvis trauma
Peterson classification, 38, 39f
physeal growth disturbances, 39f
physical examination, 44
physiological factors, 40
polytrauma management, 40–42
prevention, 45–46
residual disability, 45
Salter-Harris classification, 38, 39f
spine. *See* Spine trauma
splenic laceration, 41
stiffness, 45f
surgery, 42
thoracic injury, 40–41
Trendelenburg sign, 225f
Triplane fractures, 154, 155f
Trisomy 21 syndrome, 287–288
Trochlea and capitellum, articular fractures of, 76
Tumors
fibrous origin, tumors of, 179, 308–314
fibrous tissue origin, tumors of, 330–332
glomus tumors, 178, 179f
hand tumors, malignant, 180–181
muscular origin, tumors of, 332–334
musculoskeletal. *See* Musculoskeletal tumors
soft tissue tumors, 177–180, 323–334
upper extremity disorders, 176–181
vascular tumors, 177–179, 324–328

U

Ulna
deficiency, 183, 184t
fractures, 55–57f, 58f, 61–63f, 66
injuries, 57–59f
plastic deformation of the radius, ulna, or both, 63
proximal ulna fractures, 66
Unicameral bone cysts (simple bone cysts), 314–316
Unstable pelvic fractures, 131, 132f
Upper extremity disorders, 194
Allen's test, 166b
amputations, 171–173
arthrogryposis multiplex congenita, 478–481
Upper extremity disorders (*Continued*)
bone tumors, benign, 180
boutonniere deformity, 169
brachial plexus palsy, 190–191
diagnosis, 192
management, 192–193
microsurgery, 193
natural history, 193
shoulder weakness and deformity, 193–194
burns, 173–174
camptodactyly, 187
central deficiencies, 183–184, 185f
cerebral palsy, 188–190, 423, 450–451
circulation, 160
cleft hand, characteristics of, 184t
clinodactyly, 187
compartment syndrome, 170
congenital anomalies, 181–188
cysts, 177
distant flaps, 164, 165f
embryology, 181
enchondroma, 180
epidermal inclusion cysts, 179
extensor tendon injuries, 168
felon, 175
fibrous tumors, 179
fingertip injuries, 170–171, 172f
flexor tendon injuries, 167–168
flexor tenosynovitis, 175–176
foreign bodies, 177
free flaps, 164, 165f
general history, 159
glomus tumors, 178, 179f
hand tumors, malignant, 180–181
hemangiomas, 178
history, 159, 177
imaging, 177
infection, 174–176
injury, 159–174
Kanavel's signs of flexor tenosynovitis, 175b
limb anomalies, classification of, 181, 182b
lipoma, 179–180
local flaps, 163
macrodactyly, 187–188
mallet finger, 168–169
motor function, 161, 162t
nail injuries, 170–171, 172f
nerve injury, 166–167
neuromuscular disorders, 188–194, 492–493
nodular tenosynovitis, 179
osteochondroma, 180
paronychia, 174–175
physical examination, 159–160, 177
polydactyly, 186–187
primary wound closure, 163
pseudoaneurysms, 178, 179f
pyogenic granulomas, 178, 179f
radial deficiency, 181–183
regional flaps, 164
Seddon's classification of nerve injury, 190t
sensibility, 160
septic arthritis, 176
skeleton, 160
skin, 161–164
skin grafts, 163–164
Upper extremity disorders (*Continued*)
soft tissue, 160
soft tissue injury, 161–164
soft tissue tumors, benign, 177–180
swan neck deformity, 169
syndactyly, 185–186
synostosis, 188
tendon injury, 167–170
thumb hypoplasia, 188, 189f, 189t
transverse deficiencies, 184–185
tumors, 176–181
ulnar deficiency, 183, 184t
vascular injury, 164–166
vascular malformations, 178
vascular tumors, 177–179
Upper extremity growth, 12
Upper extremity injuries, 47, 48f, 82
acromioclavicular joint, injuries around, 80, 81f
clavicle shaft fractures, 80
elbow fractures. *See* Elbow fractures
forearm fractures. *See* Wrist and forearm fractures
glenohumeral joint subluxation and dislocation, 78–80
hand disorders and injuries. *See* Hand disorders and injuries
humeral shaft fractures, 76–77, 78f
humerus and shoulder region, fractures of, 76–82
proximal humerus fractures, 77–78, 79f
sports medicine, 145–146
wrist fractures. *See* Wrist and forearm fractures
Upper extremity orthoses, 432, 434f

V

Varicella, 413
Vascular endothelial growth factor, 9
Vascular injury and upper extremity disorders, 164–166
Vascular malformations, 178, 325t, 326–328
Vascular tumors, 177–179, 324–328
Vasculitis-associated arthritis, 414
Velocity, 13
Venous malformations, 327
Viral arthritis, 413
Vitamin D, 387
Vitamin D-resistant rickets, 389

W

Wolffs' law, 3b
Wrist
arthrogryposis multiplex congenita, 481
fractures. *See* Wrist and forearm fractures
gymnast's wrist, 140–141
musculoskeletal examination, 21–22, 23f, 24f
Wrist and forearm fractures, 55–66f
distal radius and ulna fractures, 55–57f, 58f
Galeazzi fractures, 60–61f
metaphyseal distal radius and ulnar fractures, 59f–60f
Monteggia fractures, 64f–65f
physeal distal radius and ulna injuries, 57–59f
plastic deformation of the radius, ulna, or both, 63
proximal radius fractures, 65–66f
proximal ulna fractures, 66
radius and ulna diaphyseal fractures, 61–62f, 63f
shafts of the radius and ulna, injuries to, 61–65